Peripheral Endovascular Interventions

Second Edition

Springer

New York
Berlin
Heidelberg
Barcelona
Hong Kong
London
Milan
Paris
Singapore
Tokyo

Rodney A. White, MD
Chief, Division of Vascular Surgery,
Harbor–UCLA Medical Center, Torrance, California.
Professor of Surgery, UCLA School of Medicine,
Los Angeles, California

Thomas J. Fogarty, MD
Professor of Surgery,
Stanford University Medical Center,
Stanford, California

Editors

Peripheral Endovascular Interventions

Second Edition

With 293 Illustrations, 51 in Full Color

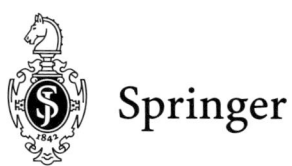

Rodney A. White, MD
Chief, Division of Vascular Surgery
Harbor–UCLA Medical Center
Torrance, CA 90509, USA
and
Professor of Surgery
UCLA School of Medicine
Los Angeles, CA, 90095, USA

Thomas J. Fogarty, MD
Professor of Surgery
Stanford University Medical Center
Stanford, CA 90509, USA

Library of Congress Cataloging-in-Publication Data
Peripheral endovascular interventions / [edited by] Rodney A. White, Thomas J. Fogarty.
    p. cm.
  Includes bibliographical references and index.
  ISBN 0-387-98444-5 (hbk.: alk. paper)
  1. Peripheral vascular diseases—Endoscopic surgery.
2. Blood-vessels—Endoscopic surgery. 3. Intravenous catheterization.
4. Arterial catheterization.
I. White, Rodney A. II. Fogarty, Thomas J.
RD598.5 .P4742 1998
617.4′13059—ddc21   98-44697

Printed on acid-free paper.

First edition © 1996 by Mosby.

© 1999 Springer-Verlag New York, Inc.
All rights reserved. This work may not be translated or copied in whole or in part without the written permission of the publisher (Springer-Verlag New York, Inc., 175 Fifth Avenue, New York, NY 10010, USA), except for brief excerpts in connection with reviews or scholarly analysis. Use in connection with any form of information storage and retrieval, electronic adaptation, computer software, or by similar or dissimilar methodology now known or hereafter developed is forbidden.
The use of general descriptive names, trade names, trademarks, etc., in this publication, even if the former are not especially identified, is not to be taken as a sign that such names, as understood by the Trade Marks and Merchandise Marks Act, may accordingly be used freely by anyone.
While the advice and information in this book are believed to be true and accurate at the date of going to press, neither the authors nor the editors nor the publisher can accept any legal responsibility for any errors or omissions that may be made. The publisher makes no warranty, express or implied, with respect to the material contained herein.

Production coordinated by Chernow Editorial Services, Inc., and managed by Timothy Taylor; manufacturing supervised by Thomas King.
Typeset by Best-set Typesetter Ltd., Hong Kong.
Printed and bound by Maple-Vail Book Manufacturing Group, York, PA.
Printed in the United States of America.

9 8 7 6 5 4 3 2 1

ISBN 0-387-98444-5 Springer-Verlag New York Berlin Heidelberg SPIN 10662927

Preface to the Second Edition

The first edition of *Peripheral Endovascular Interventions* was developed to furnish a comprehensive review of the subject for individuals from different disciplines. It offered a thorough overview of accepted techniques and methods, as well as information needed to adapt endovascular technologies to clinical practice. Additional sections briefly discussed new concepts so that the reader was kept informed of future developments.

Since the publication of the first edition in 1996, the field has rapidly evolved and several new technical advances have occurred. The utility and utilization of imaging techniques, particularly ultrasound and spiral Computed Tomography, and several new devices, including endovascular prostheses, have matured. Therefore, several new chapters have been added to provide detailed discussions of these advances and provide a overview of their potential for clinical application. An additional group of new chapters addresses specific topics, including disobliteration techniques, inferior vena caval filters, brachocephalic angioplasty, tibioperioneal angioplasty, and endoscopic first rib resection. Other developing areas discussed in detail include laparoscopic aortic procedure, endoluminal radiation therapy, and carotid angioplasty and stenting. Approximately 40% of the material in this edition is new, and the entire text updated to reflect the current status of peripheral endovascular treatments.

As with the first edition, our intention is not to recommend or promote the use of endovascular methods before they are proven by appropriate clinical studies, but rather to provide a detailed assessment of potential advantages. To accomplish this goal, we have made timely production and publication of this book a priority.

Rodney A. White, MD
Thomas J. Fogarty, MD

Preface to the First Edition

Catheter-based diagnosis and treatment of vascular diseases has evolved over the last several decades, with a recent increase occurring in the utility of the therapeutic methods. This development has been stimulated by several factors including miniaturization of interventional devices and imaging technologies, and an emphasis on the utilization of minimally invasive, cost-effective treatments that reduce the economic impact of health care delivery. As part of this evolution, the development and adaption of new interventional techniques and devices has produced a continual need for updating and training physicians in several subspecialties regarding the use of these methodologies. This requires not only adapting the technologies to current clinical practice but also establishing educational training curriculum in subspecialty fellowship programs.

Because endovascular technologies are of multispecialty interest, a review of the entire scope of fundamental information regarding each aspect of the field is required to furnish a comprehensive review that will provide specific utility for individuals from different disciplines. For this reason, we have undertaken the development of this text to satisfy two goals. The first is to provide a broad overview of the entire range of topics for clinicians with little or no background relative to the subject matter. Secondly, those with some familiarity will find definitive informational material to allow adaptation of endovascular technologies to their current clinical practice.

To adequately understand and safely use catheter-based interventional therapies, knowledge of a number of topics beyond the clinical indications and techniques for applying endovascular methods is required. A thorough understanding of the pathophysiology of vascular disease, safety issues regarding interventional devices and imaging methods, and a comprehension of fundamental biomaterials concepts is needed. These topics are addressed in detail and represent relatively mature aspects of this field that are otherwise characterized by continual change in devices and techniques as the field expands.

Additional sections of the book attempt to introduce and briefly discuss new concepts that may be of utility in the future, such as endoluminal prostheses, catheter-based drug delivery systems, and percutaneous vascular sealing devices. The obvious liability in including these topics in the text is that some may not be adopted or practical for broad clinical application. In this regard, it is not our intent to recommend or promote the use of investigational endovascular methods before they are proven by appropriate clinical studies, but rather to provide a detailed assessment of potential advances. To accomplish this goal, we have made timely production and publication of this book a priority so that information presented is as current as possible.

Rodney A. White, M.D.
Thomas J. Fogarty, M.D.

Contents

Preface to the Second Edition v
Preface to the First Edition vii
Contributors xiii

PART I INTRODUCTION

1 Evolution of Endovascular Therapy:
   Diagnostics and Therapeutics 3
   Thomas J. Fogarty and Amitava Biswas

2 Pathophysiology of Vascular Disease 11
   Christopher K. Zarins and Seymour Glagov

PART II COMPONENTS OF AN ENDOVASCULAR PRACTICE

3 Training and Credentialing in Endovascular Surgery 33
   G. Patrick Clagett and Kenneth E. McIntyre Jr.

4 Assessment of Vascular Patients
   and Indications for Therapy 41
   Christian de Virgilio

5 Establishing an Endovascular Service 53
   Rodney A. White and Thomas J. Fogarty

6 Anesthesia for Endovascular Procedures 59
   Daniel F. Grum

7 Intraprocedural Monitoring 93
   Lawrence N. Sampson, Juan Ayerdi, and Sushil K. Gupta

8 Postintervention Surveillance of
   Endovascular Procedures 103
   John P. Henretta and Kim J. Hodgson

9   Safety Considerations for Endovascular Surgery 119
    George E. Kopchok

PART III FACILITIES AND EQUIPMENT FOR ENDOVASCULAR INTERVENTION

10 Endovascular Suite Design 133
    Edward B. Diethrich

11 Image Production and Visualization Systems: Angiography, US, CT, and MRI 143
    Suzanne M. Slonim and Lewis Wexler

12 Preoperative and Postoperative Spiral CT Evaluation of Patients Undergoing Placement of Endovascular Stent-Grafts 161
    Irwin Walot

13 Angioscopy: Instrumentation, Techniques, and Applications 177
    Arnold Miller and Juha P. Salenius

14 Intravascular Ultrasound Imaging 195
    Martin R. Back, George E. Kopchok, and Rodney A. White

PART IV ENDOVASCULAR INSTRUMENTATION AND DEVICES

15 Biomaterials: Considerations for Endovascular Devices 219
    Martin R. Back and Rodney A. White

16 Catheter Skills 247
    Edward V. Kinney, Thomas J. Fogarty, and Christine E. Newman

17 Devices and Techniques for Vascular Access: Utility and Limitations of Current Methods 259
    Rodney A. White and Thomas J. Fogarty

18 Balloon Angioplasty 269
    John V. White, Ibrahim G. Eid, Amit Kharod, and Sherry Scovell

19 Catheter Thromboembolectomy 289
    Thomas J. Fogarty, Amitava Biswas, and Christine E. Newman

20 Disobliteration Techniques 309
    Gwan H. Ho and Frans L. Moll

Contents

21 Intravascular Stents 321
    Vimal Murthy, Himanshu Shah, and Michael C. Dalsing

22 Laser Angioplasty 353
    Warren S. Grundfest

23 Intraluminal Grafts: Historical Perspectives 361
    Marco Scoccianti and Rodney A. White

24 Endovascular Treatment of Traumatic Arteriovenous
    Fistulas and Pseudoaneurysms and of Arterial
    Occlusive Disease 371
    Carlos E. Donayre

25 Endovascular Repair of Thoracic Aortic Aneurysms 383
    Bradley B. Hill, Christopher K. Zarins,
    and Thomas J. Fogarty

26 Techniques, Case Selection, and Pitfalls Associated with
    Endovascular Aneurysm Repair 391
    Robert C. Allen and Thomas J. Fogarty

27 Inferior Vena Caval Filters: Impact of
    Endovascular Technology 403
    Mary C. Proctor and Lazar J. Greenfield

PART V SPECIALIZED ENDOVASCULAR TECHNIQUES

28 PTA and Stenting of Subclavian and
    Innominate Arteries 413
    Amir Motarjeme

29 Role of Angioplasty in Limb Salvage 423
    D.E. Schwarten

30 Carotid Angioplasty and Stenting 429
    Edward B. Diethrich

31 Complications and Troubleshooting 445
    Frank J. Criado, Omran Abul-Khoudoud,
    and Eric Wellons

32 Thrombolysis: Peripheral Arterial Applications 455
    Carlos E. Donayre and Kenneth Ouriel

33 Combined Surgical and Endovascular Approaches 481
    James May and Geoffrey H. White

34 Laparoscopic Aortic Surgery 497
    Carlos R. Gracia and Yves-Marie Dion

35 Endovenous Surgery 515
    John J. Bergan and Patricia E. Thorpe

| 36 | Thoracic Outlet Syndrome: Endoscopic Transaxillary First Rib Resection and Thoracodorsal Sympathectomy for Causalgia | 531 |

Bernardo D. Martinez

| 37 | Prevention of Lesion Recurrence in Endovascular Devices | 539 |

Ted R. Kohler and Alexander W. Clowes

| 38 | Endoluminal Radiation Therapy | 555 |

Rudolf P. Tutein Nolthenius and Frans L. Moll

| 39 | Local Drug Delivery: New Approaches in Endovascular Therapies | 565 |

Aaron V. Kaplan

| 40 | Management of the Percutaneous Access Site | 577 |

James W. Vetter

| 41 | Endovascular Chemotherapy Delivery | 591 |

Dat Nguyen and Stanley R. Klein

Index 621

Contributors

Omran Abul-Khoudoud, MD
Division of Vascular Surgery, The Union Memorial Hospital, Baltimore, MD 21218, USA

Robert C. Allen, MD
Chief, Division of Vascular and Endovascular Surgery, Sanger Clinic, Carolinas Medical Center-Carolinas Heart Institute, Charlotte, NC 28203, USA

Juan Ayerdi, MD
Department of Vascular Surgery, Guthrie Clinic and Robert Packard Hospital, Sayre, PA 18840, USA

Martin R. Back, MD
Section of Vascular Surgery, Department of Surgery, University of South Florida College of Medicine, Tampa, FL 33606, USA

John J. Bergan, MD
Professor of Surgery, Loma Linda University Medical Center, University of California, San Diego, CA, USA

Amitava Biswas, MD
Division of Vascular Surgery, Stanford University Medical Center, Stanford, CA 94305-5450, USA

G. Patrick Clagett, MD
Professor and Chairman, Division of Vascular Surgery, University of Texas Southwestern Medical Center, Dallas, TX 75235-9157, USA

Alexander W. Clowes, MD
Professor of Surgery, University of Washington, Seattle VA Medical Center, Seattle, WA 98108, USA

Frank J. Criado, MD
Chief, Division of Vascular Surgery, Director, Endovascular Program, The Union Memorial Hospital, Baltimore, MD 21218, USA

Michael C. Dalsing, MD
Indiana University School of Medicine, Department of Surgery, Wishard Memorial Hospital, Indianapolis, IN 46202, USA

Christian de Virgilio, MD
Division of Vascular Surgery, Harbor-UCLA Medical Center, Torrance, CA 90509, USA

Edward B. Diethrich, MD
Arizona Heart Institute, Phoenix, AZ 85064, USA

Yves-Marie Dion, MD
Associate Professor of Surgery, Centre Hospitalier Universitaire de Québec, Université Laval Québec, Québec, Montreal, Canada

Carlos E. Donayre, MD
Division of Vascular Surgery, Department of Surgery, Harbor-UCLA Medical Center, Torrance, CA 90509, USA

Ibrahim G. Eid, MD
Department of Surgery, Division of Vascular Surgery, Temple University Hospital, Philadelphia, PA 19140, USA

Thomas J. Fogarty, MD
Professor of Surgery, Stanford University Medical Center, Stanford, CA, 90509, USA

Seymor Glagov, MD
Professor, Department of Pathology, University of Chicago, Chicago, IL 60637, USA

Carlos R. Gracia, MD
Director, California Laparoscopic Institute, San Ramon, CA 94583, USA

Lazar J. Greenfield, MD
Department of Surgery, University of Michigan Hospitals, Ann Arbor, MI 48109-0436, USA

Daniel F. Grum, MD
Chief, Department of Anesthesiology, Memphis Regional Medical Center, Associate Professor of Anesthesiology, University of Tennessee Health Sciences Center, Memphis, TN 38163, USA

Warren S. Grundfest, MD
Director, Division of Laser Research and Technology Development, Department of Surgery, Cedars Sinai Medical Center, Los Angeles, CA 90048, USA

Sushil K. Gupta, MD
Department of Vascular Surgery, Guthrie Clinic and Robert Packard Hospital, Sayre, PA 18840, USA

John P. Henretta, MD
Section of Peripheral Vascular Surgery, Department of Surgery, Southern Illinois University School of Medicine, Springfield, IL 62794-1312, USA

Bradley B. Hill, MD
Division of Vascular Surgery, Stanford University, Stanford, CA 94305-5642, USA

Gwan H. Ho, MD
Department of Vascular Surgery, St. Antonius Hospital, 3435 CM Nieuwegein, The Netherlands

Kim J. Hodgson, MD
Section of Peripheral Vascular Surgery, Department of Surgery, Southern Illinois University School of Medicine, Springfield, IL 62794-1312, USA

Aaron V. Kaplan, MD
Cardiac Catheterization Laboratory, VA Medical Center, Palo Alto, CA 94304, USA

Amit Kharod, MD
Department of Surgery, Division of Vascular Surgery, Temple University Hospital, Philadelphia, PA 19140, USA

Edward V. Kinney, MD
Division of Surgery, Baptist East Hospital, Surgical Care Associates, Louisville, KY 40207, USA

Stanley R. Klein, MD
Division of Vascular Surgery, Department of Surgery, Harbor-UCLA Medical Center, Torrance, CA 90509, USA

Ted R. Kohler, MD
Puget Sound Health Care System, Department of Veterans Affairs, Seattle, WA 98108, USA

George E. Kopchok, MD
Division of Vascular Surgery, Harbor-UCLA Medical Center, Torrance, CA 90509, USA

Bernardo D. Martinez, MD
Division of Vascular Surgery, St. Vincent Mercy Medical Center, Toledo, OH 43608, USA

James May, MD
Department of Surgery, Royal Prince Alfred Hospital, University of Sydney, Sydney, NSW 2006, Australia

Kenneth E. McIntyre Jr., MD
Department of Surgery, St. Paul Medical Center, Dallas, TX 75235, USA

Arnold Miller, MD
Assistant Clinical Professor of Surgery, Harvard University Medical School, Metrowest Medical Center, Department of Surgery, Natek, MA 01760, USA

Frans L. Moll, MD
Department of Vascular Surgery, St. Antonius Hospital, 3435 CM Nieuwegein, The Netherlands

Amir Motarjeme, MD
Midwest Vascular Institute, Downers Grove, IL 60515, USA

Vimal Murthy, MD
Department of Surgery, Indiana University School of Medicine, Wishard Memorial Hospital, Indianapolis, IN 46202, USA

Christine E. Newman, MD
Support Services Manager, Division of Vascular Surgery, Stanford University Medical Center, Fogarty Business and Engineering Offices, Stanford, CA 94305-5450, USA

Dat Nguyen, MD
Department of Surgery, Harbor-UCLA Medical Center, Torrance, CA 90509, USA

Rudolf P. Tutein Nolthenius, MD
Department of Vascular Surgery, St. Antonius Hospital, 3435 CM Nieuwegein, The Netherlands

Kenneth Ouriel, MD
Chief, Division of Vascular Surgery, Cleveland Clinic Foundation, Cleveland, OH 44195, USA

Mary C. Proctor, MD
Department of Surgery, University of Michigan Hospitals, Ann Arbor, MI 48109-0436, USA

Juha P. Salenius, MD
Department of Surgery, Metrowest Medical Center, Natek, MA 01769, USA

Lawrence M. Sampson, MD
Department of Vascular Surgery, Guthrie Clinic and Robert Packard Hospital, Sayre, PA 18840, USA

Contributors

D.E. Schwarten, MD
Director of Vascular Services, Northside Cardiology, St. Vincent Hospital, Indianapolis, IN 46260, USA

Marco Scoccianti, MD
Staff Vascular Surgeon, Division of Vascular Surgery and Laboratory of Vascular Pathology, IDI-IRCC, 00100 Rome, Italy

Sherry Scovell, MD
Department of Surgery, Division of Vascular Surgery, Temple University Hospital, Philadelphia, PA 19140, USA

Himanshu Shah, MD
Department of Radiology, Indiana University School of Medicine, Wishard Memorial Hospital, Indianapolis, IN 46202, USA

Suzanne M. Slonin, MD
Department of Radiology, Division of Cardiovascular and Interventional Radiology, Stanford University Medical Center, Stanford, CA 90509, USA

Patricia E. Thorpe, MD
Chief, Division of Interventional Radiology, Associate Professor of Radiology and Surgery, Creighton University, St. Joseph's Hospital, Omaha, NE 68131, USA

James W. Vetter, MD
Cardiovascular Medicine, Redwood City, CA 94062, USA

Irwin Walot, MD
Department of Radiology, Harbor-UCLA Medical Center, Torrance, CA 90509, USA

Eric Wellons, MD
Division of Vascular Surgery, Director, Endovascular Program, The Union Memorial Hospital, Baltimore, MD 21218, USA

Lewis Wexler, MD
Department of Radiology, Stanford University Medical Center, Stanford, CA 90509, USA

Geoffrey H. White, MD
Royal Prince Alfred Hospital, Department of Surgery, University of Sydney, Sydney, NSW 2006, Australia

John V. White, MD
Department of Surgery, Division of Vascular Surgery, Temple University Hospital, Philadelphia, PA 19140, USA

Rodney A. White, MD
Chief, Division of Vascular Surgery, Harbor–UCLA Medical Center, Torrance, CA 90509, USA, and Professor of Surgery, UCLA School of Medicine, Los Angeles, CA 90095, USA

Christopher K. Zarins, MD
Professor of Surgery, Division of Vascular Surgery, Stanford University Medical Center, Stanford, CA 94305-5450, USA

Part I
Introduction

1
Evolution of Endovascular Therapy: Diagnostics and Therapeutics

Thomas J. Fogarty and Amitava Biswas

Interest in the workings of the circulation goes back to the ancient Greeks: Hippocrates and Galen both wrote about their findings in the heart and blood vessels. The pulmonary circulation was first described by an Arab physician, Ibn Al-Nafiis, in 1230, and no less a figure than Leonardo da Vinci had a keen interest in the hydrodynamic properties of blood. However, it was Harvey's description of the circulation in 1628 that truly marked the beginnings of our modern understanding of the vasculature. Since then, great strides have been made in our understanding of vascular disease, leading to the development of endovascular methods for both diagnosis and treatment.[1]

Although endovascular therapy, the manipulation of pathology by an intraluminal approach, is a relatively recent concept, it has a rich history. The history of endovascular therapy can be divided into two 30-year periods. The first 30 years, from about 1929 to 1959, was an era of diagnostics, during which a number of cardiac and vascular diagnostic procedures were rapidly developed (Table 1-1). The second 30 years, from 1960 to the present, can be considered the era of therapeutics, which saw the development of interventional modalities such as embolectomy, angioplasty, and atherectomy (Table 1-2). Although many investigators were involved in the conception, design, and implementation of various diagnostic and therapeutic innovations, a number of individuals and events stand out as pivotal in significantly advancing the field as a whole and in bringing endovascular therapy to the point at which it is today. It is interesting to note the multidisciplinary nature of the advances that have been made in this evolution; the joint participation of cardiologists, surgeons, and radiologists has been critical to the evolution of the current technology of endovascular therapy. From a developmental standpoint, this is a field to which no one discipline can lay sole claim.

First 30 Years: Era of Diagnostics (1929–1959)

Roentgen's discovery of x-ray images of bones in 1895 set off a flurry of medical activity, with physicians seeking ever more ways to use the new technology. Angiograms of cadavers were taken as early as 1896, and experiments to elucidate the vasculature of live animals were attempted shortly thereafter. In both these cases, as well as in early attempts to visualize the extremities of living patients, the limiting factor proved to be the lack of a suitably nontoxic contrast agent. In 1927 the Portuguese neurologist Egas Moniz finally succeeded in using a 22% sodium iodide solution to visualize the cerebral circulation.[2]

Arteriography—Dos Santos

Moniz's colleague and countryman, the surgeon Renaldo Dos Santos (Figure 1-1), felt that Moniz's technique would be well applied to the extremities. With his associates, Augusto Lamas

TABLE 1–1. Partial List of Significant Developments in Endovascular Diagnostics

Developer	Year	Instrument	Use
Dos Santos	1929	Needle	Visualization
Forssmann	1929	Coax catheter	Physiologic
Cournand	1941	Coax catheter	Clinical diagnosis
Seldinger	1953	Guide	Percutaneous access
Sones	1959	Coax catheter	Coronary visualization

TABLE 1–2. Partial List of Noteworthy Contributions to Endovascular Therapeutics

Developer	Year	Instrument	Use
Fogarty	1963	Coax balloon	Removal
Dotter	1964	Coax catheter	Dilate
Grüntzig	1974	Coax balloon	Dilate
Palmaz	1984	Stent	Stent
Simpson	1985	Coax cutter	Removal
Parodi	1990	Stent/graft	Graft

and Jose Pereira Caldas, Dos Santos seized on Moniz's breakthrough to develop arteriography and aortography.[3] Using these new techniques, they were able to not only demonstrate arterial conditions such as atherosclerosis, aneurysms, and ischemic paralysis but also to look at vessel changes in osteomyelitis and tumors. Dos Santos and his group were able to see atheromatous plaques, obstructions, irregular contours of vessels, and collaterals. In their 1931 book, they published 100 peripheral arteriograms and 300 lumbar aortograms, encompassing pathologic findings in various inflammatory conditions and tumors.[1] This work paved the way for the future development of vascular visualization.

Cardiac Catheterization—Forssmann and Cournand

At the same time that Dos Santos was beginning his pioneering work in the peripheral vasculature, Werner Forssmann, a surgical intern in Berlin just out of medical school (Figure 1–2), was about to conduct another landmark experiment. Until this time, physicians had been very wary of trying to access the heart directly. However, Forssmann felt that it should be possible to insert a catheter into the right side of the heart through a venous channel and thereby monitor cardiac pressures, obtain blood for analysis, and administer therapeutic agents. His superiors flatly refused to allow him

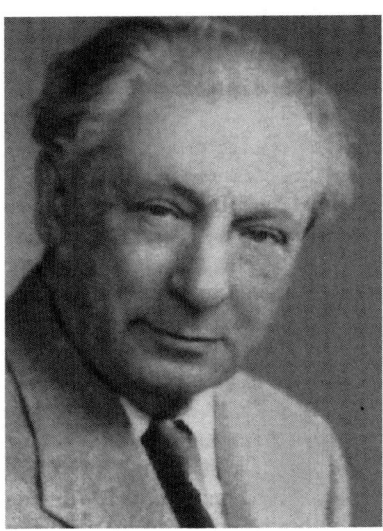

FIGURE 1–1. Renaldo Dos Santos, MD, pioneer surgeon and original developer of diagnostic arterial visualization techniques and technologies.

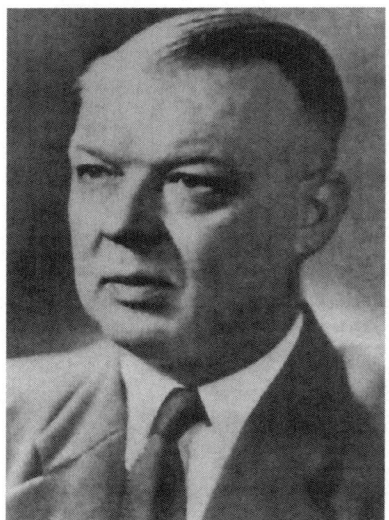

FIGURE 1–2. Werner Forssmann, MD, physician credited with developing endovascular diagnostics by courageously demonstrating the potential for cardiac assessment using catheter technology.

to attempt this experiment in any patient, including himself. However, he persisted, and in 1929, working behind a screen where no one could see him, he inserted a ureteral catheter into his own basilar vein. After fighting off another physician who wanted to remove the catheter, Forssmann proceeded to advance the catheter into his right ventricle by watching the reflection of his fluoroscopic image in a mirror. This experiment constituted the first use of a cardiac catheter in a living human, and it marked a turning point in the development of endovascular diagnosis.

It was to be another decade before the potential of Forssmann's experiment would be realized. It was not until 1941, when Andre Cournand began his landmark work in cardiopulmonary physiology,[4] that the power of cardiac catheterization became apparent. Cournand was able to refine the design of the catheter, adding curved ends to lessen trauma and incorporating double lumens to measure two cavities at once. However, his major contribution was not the instruments he used but what he did with them. He and his colleagues were able to take pressure readings in the right heart, determine blood volumes using dye techniques, catheterize the pulmonary artery, and determine changes in cardiac output in response to physical activity.[5] All of these procedures could now be accomplished without significant harm to the patient, demonstrating the practical utility of a catheter-based technology. For his efforts, Cournand was awarded the 1956 Nobel Prize in Physiology or Medicine, which he shared with Dickinson Richards and, at Cournand's insistence, Werner Forssmann.

Vascular Access—Seldinger

Vascular access remained a problem at this time. To get an artery for catheter placement or contrast injection, one had to either make a surgical cutdown of the area or insert the catheter percutaneously through a large-bore needle. Both methods left something to be desired. A cutdown was time consuming. Catheterizing through a needle required a hole larger than the catheter, which carried the risk of perivascular bleeding. The problem was solved in 1953 by a Swedish radiologist, Sven Ivar Seldinger. His breakthrough was to insert a flexible guidewire through a relatively small-bore needle and then remove the needle, leaving the wire in place. Subsequently, a larger catheter could be inserted over the guidewire.[6] The Seldinger technique allowed the passage of a catheter through a hole smaller than itself. This method, which continues to be used today for venous and arterial cannulation, was a significant developmental advance in endovascular therapy.

Coronary Angiography—Sones

The next major step in vascular visualization was accomplished by a cardiologist, F. Mason Sones. In 1958, Sones and his colleagues were already performing left heart catheterization through a femoral or brachial access site. Sones was interested in visualizing the coronary arteries, but he found that placement of contrast medium at the ascending aorta—or even into the sinus of Valsalva near the orifice of the coronary arteries—was unsatisfactory. Then one day as he was preparing a left ventriculogram, he paused for a cigarette and history was made.[7] The catheter tip slipped into the right coronary artery, gave an excellent picture of the vessel and its branches, and sent the patient into asystole. In the absence of a defibrillator, the patient's forceful cough came in time to avoid disaster. However, the development of direct-current countershock made the procedure more feasible. Sones designed a tapered woven catheter that allowed him direct access to the coronary arteries, and in 1962 he published a landmark collection of coronary arterial images taken in 1020 patients.[8]

Other Diagnostic Modalities

Since the early days of vascular imaging, many new and exciting techniques have emerged, and the field continues to grow. Intravascular ultrasound—the invasive use of ultrasound to generate high-resolution images of vessels, ducts, or organs—began in the 1950s with research directed toward measuring and recording cardiac motion. The application of ultrasound technology to the peripheral vasculature occurred shortly thereafter. To date, intravascular ultrasound has been used in conjunction with atherectomy and with both balloon and laser angioplasty. At present, research is continuing to find ways to use ultrasound to take advantage of the density differentials in calcified plaques to provide better guidance for therapeutic procedures.

Perhaps the most exciting development in vascular imaging is angioscopy—the direct visualization of the blood vessels. The first application of endoscopy in the vasculature was in the heart. However, as less invasive cardiac diagnostic techniques became more reliable, the impetus for the further development of cardioscopic technology decreased. For the last 30 years, angioscopy has been focused on the peripheral vessels, including both arteries and veins. It has been repeatedly demonstrated that angioscopy is an ideal method to directly evaluate the results of numerous vascular procedures—allowing the immediate correction of any procedural errors. Endarterectomy, arterial reconstruction, angioplasty, embolectomy, and atherectomy have all been effectively evaluated by angioscopy. It has proven to be one of the most promising new endovascular technologies.

Other diagnostic modalities that have been developed in recent years include radionuclide scanning and the vascular application of computed tomography (CT) and magnetic resonance imaging (MRI). Research continues in this field, and it is probable that we can look forward to even more new and exciting diagnostic options.

Second 30 Years: Era of Therapeutics (1960–1990)

It must of course be remembered that diagnosis is only half the story of the development of endovascular procedures. Ultimately, the goal is not only to describe the vascular pathology but to manipulate it in the interest of the patient. Manipulation can be done in a number of ways. The pathology can be removed, pulverized, shaved, or disrupted; alternatively, a device can be put in place to mitigate the consequences of pathology. In the three decades since Sones' work, we have seen a flowering of endovascular therapeutic techniques designed to remedy vascular disease. Just as in the development of diagnostic methods, many people were involved in creating and perfecting the therapeutic methods we have today. However, a few events and personalities stand out as pivotal.

Embolectomy—Fogarty

The earliest disease entity to be approached intraluminally was embolic occlusion. Ischemic injury from such events resulted in severe morbidity, and until the early 1960s there was no resort for the problem other than a major operation requiring large and multiple incisions. These patients all had severe associated cardiac risk; therefore prolonged anesthesia carried a high operative risk. There was no standard technique or instrumentation to manage this difficult patient group. Then in 1961 the balloon embolectomy catheter was introduced, and its results were reported by Thomas Fogarty and colleagues in 1963.[9] The instrument was composed of a hollow pliable catheter body with a soft elastomeric balloon situated at the tip. In use, the catheter tip with the deflated latex balloon was passed through and beyond the area of occlusion. Once past the embolus, the balloon was inflated and the catheter withdrawn toward the arteriotomy, the inflated balloon pulling the embolic material as it was retracted. The catheter was passed both antegrade and retrograde from a small femoral cutdown. This approach marked the first conversion of a previously complicated and potentially dangerous open procedure into a safe, relatively easy endovascular procedure, using a much smaller incision and performed under local anesthesia. This was to be the beginning of endovascular therapy and of less invasive interventions.

Balloon Angioplasty—Dotter/Grüntzig

The next major milestone in the evolution of endovascular therapy was the application of catheter-based techniques to the problem of atherosclerotic stenosis. Charles Dotter (Figure 1–3) was professor and chairman of radiology at the University of Oregon, where Fogarty was a first-year surgical resident. Dotter knew of Fogarty's work, but in 1964 his interest was in treating chronic occlusions percutaneously. That year, he passed an 8F Teflon catheter over a guidewire into an elderly woman with ischemic gangrene who had refused amputation. After the first catheter was in place, he passed a 12F Teflon catheter over it to further dilate the stenotic segment.[10]

In Europe, this catheter-based angioplasty was refined by several clinicians using modified catheters, but Dotter and Fogarty made the next advance. In 1965, Dotter used a balloon catheter made by Fogarty with two balloons wrapped over one another to give extra thickness. Once the tip was in the vicinity of the iliac stenosis, expansion of the balloon caused an increase in the lumen diameter. The balloon was deflated and removed through a very small incision. Fourteen years later, this first balloon angioplasty was still patent.[11]

In 1974, Andreas Grüntzig made a fundamental improvement in the balloon angioplasty catheter by changing the balloon material from the latex of the embolectomy balloon to polyvinyl chloride.[12] This was a less elastomeric material than the latex balloon and allowed more force to act on the plaque rather than to distend away from the atheroma (as was intended in the design of the embolectomy balloon). Grüntzig began his angioplasty work in the peripheral circulation,[12] but his main interest was the heart. He is best remembered for the introduction of coronary angioplasty, which quickly became (and remains) one of the most common endovascular procedures. In 1982, John Simpson developed the movable guidewire concept, which further advanced the ease and versatility of coronary angioplasty.[13]

In the 1980s, some investigators began trying to use laser energy to disrupt atheromatous plaque. These laser methods began with much interest and fanfare. However, the high cost of setting up a workable system coupled with the persistent problem of vessel perforation and the difficulty of the procedure itself all combined to make laser angioplasty less practical than originally hoped. It is possible that better integration of visualization modalities and computer-directed laser systems could make laser angioplasty worthwhile in the future.

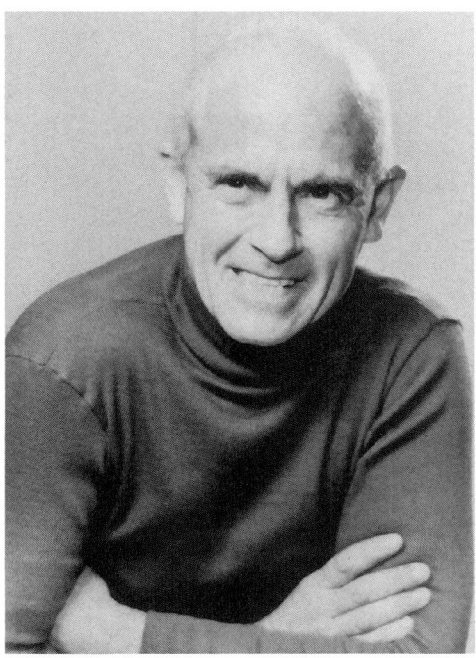

FIGURE 1–3. Charles Dotter, MD, "father of interventional radiology," who developed endovascular techniques and demonstrated the utility of catheter-mediated therapies in the radiology setting at the University of Oregon Medical School and Health Sciences Center.

Atherectomy—Simpson

About the same time that lasers were being developed, John Simpson (Figure 1–4) developed the idea of mechanically removing atheroma from diseased vessels. In 1988 he coined the term *atherectomy*, referring to a catheter-based technique to physically remove obstructing atheroma from the vessel lumen. It was felt that this approach would have a number of advantages over balloon angioplasty. In particular, it was intended to reduce restenosis rates because the atherectomy device would selectively cut and remove the atheromatous material from the vessel wall and

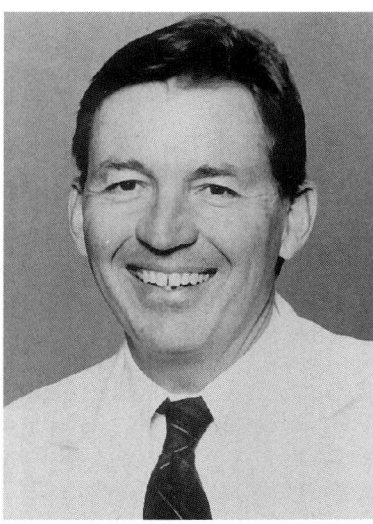

FIGURE 1–4. John B. Simpson, MD, cardiologist and innovator of catheter-mediated techniques for treating coronary artery atherosclerosis.

leave behind a smooth luminal surface. To achieve this aim, Simpson developed the directional atherectomy catheter, which consists of a cylindrical metal housing containing a drumlike cutting element located at the end of a dual-lumen catheter. The cylinder has a cutting window on one side and an inflatable balloon on the opposite side. Inflating the balloon brings the plaque into the cutting window, where it is shaved off with the cutting element and stored in a collecting chamber at the distal end of the catheter for subsequent removal. This device remains the most widely used atherectomy device today, and it has been associated with fairly low long-term restenosis rates—particularly with eccentric lesions. It is interesting to note that Simpson and Fogarty collaborated on the initial design and clinical application of directional atherectomy.[14] This collaboration occurred at Sequoia Hospital, a small community hospital 6 miles north of Stanford, California, where both Simpson and Fogarty had previously worked.

Several other approaches to atherectomy have been developed, including the transluminal extraction catheter (TEC), which contains an open-ended cutter at the distal end of a catheter assembly. This device cuts atheroma located in front of it rather than to the side, as does the Simpson AtheroCath. Thus, it is not "directional." An attached vacuum provides continuous suction to prevent embolization of plaque particles. This design also allows a better approach to total occlusions. Other mechanical plaque disruption catheters that are often called atherectomy devices may be better referred to as atheroablation devices because they do not actually remove atheroma. Instead, they use a high-speed rotational catheter with a spinning tip to pulverize the plaque into particles presumably too small to cause microembolization. Unfortunately, microembolization remains a problem with both of these types of devices, and efforts continue to reduce and eliminate this serious problem.

Stents and Stent-Grafts

Embolectomy and atherectomy were developed to remove the source of arterial occlusion. Angioplasty and atheroablation were intended to disrupt pathology. Another aspect of endovascular therapy was the insertion of a device to circumvent the effects of pathology. The first devices introduced endovascularly were venous filters in the inferior vena cava to prevent pulmonary embolism. In 1958,[15] M.S. De Weese and colleagues passed a grid of silk sutures across the vena cava to trap large embolic material that came up from the pelvis and extremities. Mobin-Uddin, Greenfield, and Roehm applied less invasive endovascular technology to venous implants for venous thromboembolic disease. The idea of introducing a synthetic device endovascularly to manage vascular disease was quickly seized on for use in the arterial system. In fact, Dotter had suggested the idea of a mechanical arterial scaffold in 1964, but it was not until Julio Palmaz's experience with a balloon-expandable wire stent that the technique became a clinical practicality.

Julio Palmaz introduced his first stent in 1985[16] and then developed a refined version in 1986.[17] Palmaz's original stent was a continuous steel wire with silver-soldered cross points; his later one was made of stainless steel tubing with eight rows of slots. When the stent was expanded, the slots opened to form diamond-shaped spaces. This design allowed more resistance to radial collapse than meshlike stents such as the Medinvent, but it was not flexible. Palmaz's stent had application in areas where radial strength was critical and the distances were relatively short, such as the coronary arteries. The stent was delivered to the stenotic site via a catheter and then expanded to its open configuration by balloon inflation. For the first time, a stent was shown to be relatively nonthrombogenic (a significant problem with previous stents). Although clinicians are still concerned about the problem of long term stenosis, stent technology has rapidly evolved to a state where it has been shown to be highly efficatious in large bore vessels. Consequently, it's utility is now recognized by surgeons who have currently accepted it as a viable method to treat stenotic lesions.

The most recent implantable device to enter the endovascular field is the endograft. Introduced by J.C. Parodi (Figure 1–5) in 1991, it marks the first significant minimally invasive approach for the treatment of aneurysms. First termed as its name implies, the stent-graft, is a combination of a vascular stent, which provides support, with an enveloping graft material that lines the spaces in the stent. The idea is to introduce the device endovascularly to the affected site and secure it in place by friction or hooks in such a manner that the endograft bridges the aneurysm. Thus, blood flow is diverted through the endograft and never gets to the actual aneurysm. This mechanism is intended to prevent rupture.

Endograft technology is important because it has the potential to replace traditional open aneurysm repair which is a major procedure associated with significant morbidity and mortality. The technology has also been successfully applied to thoracic aortic aneurysms. To date, however, the procedure is still in the investigational stages, and long-term results are currently being obtained.

Conclusion

Endovascular therapy is a multidisciplinary field, involving contributions from surgeons, cardiologists, radiologists, physicists, and engineers. It is also a growing field destined to have a fascinating future because it addresses many issues that are of prime importance in medicine and society today. The problems and pathologies that endovascular therapy seeks to remedy are some of today's most common chronic medical problems in the world's developed countries and are a significant cause of morbidity and mortality. Furthermore, the methods used and under development are geared toward replacing the complicated open procedures of the past with simpler, quicker, minimally invasive procedures of the future. Medically, these procedures decrease the risk to the patient and allow a quicker return to normal daily functions. In this era of cost containment and fiscal responsibility, endovascular therapies can decrease operating-room time, hospitalization time, and overall time to recovery. In a very real sense, the proven endovascular techniques have actually delivered "more for less." Today, work continues to further refine

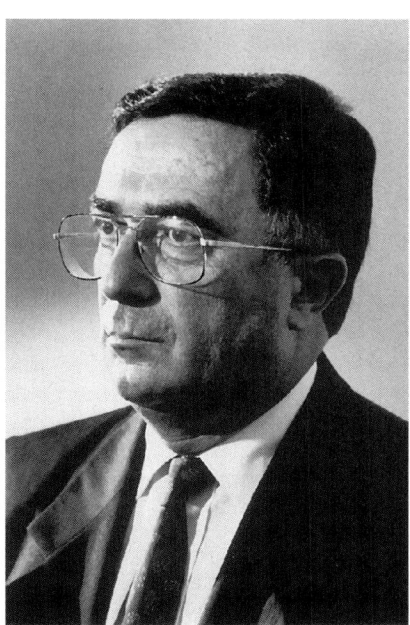

FIGURE 1–5. Juan C. Parodi, MD, vascular surgeon and designer who advanced the clinical techniques and applications for the transluminally placed endovascular endograft.

existing technologies and to develop additional innovations to serve this purpose.

References

1. Doby T: *Development of angiography and cardiac catheterization*, Littleton, Mass, 1976, Publishing Sciences Group.
2. Moniz E: Arterial encephalography: its importance in the location of cerebral tumors, *Revue Neurologique* 48:72, 1927. Reprinted in Viega-Pires J, Grainger R, editors: *Pioneers in angiography: the Portuguese school of angiography*, Boston, 1987, MTP Press.
3. Dos Santos R: Arteriography of the limbs, with the collaboration of Augusto Lamas and J Pereira Caldas, *Medicina Contempanea* 1929. Reprinted in Viega-Pires J, Grainger R, editors: *Pioneers in angiography: the Portuguese school of angiography*. Boston, 1987, MTP Press.
4. Cournand A, Ranges H: Catheterization of the right auricle in man, *Proc Soc Exp Biol Med* 46:462, 1941.
5. Cournand A: Cardiac catheterization: development of the technique, its contributions to experimental medicine and its initial applications in man, *Acta Med Scand* 579(suppl):7, 1975.
6. Seldinger S: Catheter replacement of the needle in percutaneous arteriography, a new technique, *Acta Radiol* 39:368–376, 1953.
7. Loop F: F Mason Sones, Jr, M.D. (1918–1985), *Ann Thor Surg* 43:237–238, 1987.
8. Sones F, Shirey E: Cine coronary arteriography, *Mod Con Cardiovas Dis* 31:735, 1962.
9. Fogarty T, Cranley J, Krause R, et al: A method for extraction of arterial emboli and thrombi, *Surg Gynecol Obstet* 116:241–244, 1963.
10. Dotter C, Judkins M: Transluminal treatment of arteriosclerotic obstruction: description of a new technic and a preliminary report of its application, *Circulation* 30:654–670, 1964.
11. Dotter C: Transluminal angioplasty: a long view, *Radiology* 135:561–564, 1980.
12. Grüntzig A, Hopf H: Perkutane rekanalisation chroischer arterieller verschlusse mit neuen dilatationskatheter: modification der Dotterteknik, *Dtsch Med Wochenschr* 99:2502–2551, 1974.
13. Simpson J, Baim D, Robert E et al: A new catheter system for coronary angioplasty, *Am J Cardiol* 49:1216–1222, 1982.
14. Simpson J, Selmon M, Robertson G et al: Transluminal atherectomy for occlusive peripheral vascular disease, *Am J Cardiol* 61:96G–101G, 1988.
15. DeWeese M, Hunter D: A vena cava filter for the prevention of pulmonary emboli, *Bulletin de la Societe Internationale de Chirurgie* 1:1–9, 1958.
16. Palmaz J, Sibbitt R, Reuter S et al: Expandable intraluminal graft: preliminary study, *Radiology* 156:72–77, 1985.
17. Palmaz J, Sibbitt R, Tio F et al: Expandable intraluminal vascular graft: a feasibility study, *Surgery* 99:199–205, 1986.

2
Pathophysiology of Vascular Disease

Christopher K. Zarins and Seymour Glagov

Vascular disease is the major cause of morbidity and mortality in Western civilization. Its manifestations include heart attacks, strokes, lower extremity occlusive disease, and aneurysmal disease, and its predominant underlying cause is atherosclerosis. Although atherosclerosis is a generalized disorder of the arterial tree associated with well-known risk factors—including hyperlipidemia, hypertension, cigarette smoking, and diabetes mellitus—its clinical expression tends to be focal. Not all individuals with extensive risk factors develop atherosclerotic plaques, and many patients with extensive atherosclerotic plaques have no recognized risk factors. Moreover, morbidity and mortality usually result from localized plaque deposition at certain vulnerable sites in the arterial tree rather than from diffuse disease. For example, the carotid arteries, coronary arteries, and lower extremity arteries are particularly susceptible to plaque formation, whereas the upper extremity arteries are rarely involved. Some arteries with small plaques may become occluded, whereas other arteries with large and extensive plaques may retain a normal lumen caliber. Still others may become aneurysmally enlarged.

The responses of arterial smooth muscle and endothelial cells to physiologic and pathologic stimuli promote the initiation and progression of atherosclerotic plaque. Because there is a close integration between the mechanical and metabolic functions of arteries, an alteration of one type of stimulus affects other aspects of the pathogenetic process. A large body of descriptive clinical and experimental data on the general appearance of human atherosclerotic lesions exists, but the precise initiating and perpetuating pathogenic mechanisms remain obscure. The factors determining lesion composition, rate of enlargement, organization, and disruption still require elucidation. This chapter reviews the pathophysiology of atherosclerosis as it affects the artery wall and considers the factors that affect plaque localization and the mechanisms that are likely to lead to stenoses and aneurysms.

Atherosclerotic Process

Atherosclerosis is not necessarily a continuous process leading inexorably to artery stenosis or other clinically significant complications. Plaque formation involves an interaction among systemic risk factors and local conditions in the lumen and artery wall in the context of a living tissue capable of healing and remodeling. The evolution of atherosclerotic lesions is a combination of initiating and sustaining processes, adaptive responses, and involutional changes. Despite the available experimental data concerning plaque progression and regression, the natural history of atherosclerotic lesions in humans is poorly understood.

Plaque Initiation

Plaque initiation refers to the earliest detectable biochemical and cellular events leading to or preceding the formation of atherosclerotic lesions. Possible mechanisms of plaque initiation have been the subject of extensive study. Principal research foci have included altered endothelial function or turnover resulting in increased permeability, oxidative alteration of insudated lipids by endothelium, and the subsequent ingress of macrophages.[1] Other possible factors include various stimuli to smooth muscle proliferation, such as circulating mitogens[2]; limitations of transmural transfer or egress related to the composition and organization of subendothelial tissues and media[3]; and high levels of specific lipoprotein cholesterol fractions.[4] Each of these factors is associated with early lesion development in experimental models, and each may also be related to one or more epidemiologically identified risk factors. Although none has been directly implicated yet in the mural disturbance that leads to plaque formation, some or several of these stimulating mechanisms may well prove to be significant.

Endothelial injury and the response to this injury have been proposed as critical and essential first steps in plaque pathogenesis.[5] According to this response-to-injury hypothesis,[6] the endothelial lining of arteries can be damaged or denuded by several factors, including mechanical forces such as shear stress and hypertension, chemical agents such as homocysteine or excessive lipids, immunologic reactions, or hormonal dysfunction. Responses to such injuries include platelet deposition, release of platelet-derived growth factor, leukocyte adhesion and diapedesis, cellular proliferation, and lipid deposition.[7-9] According to this theory, local, repeated endothelial injury or denudation would determine the location of plaque formation.

There is, however, growing recognition that there is no direct evidence for the response-to-injury hypothesis. There is no in vivo evidence of spontaneous endothelial injury or disruption, with or without platelet adherence, in areas at risk for future lesion development.[10,11] In animal models, experimentally induced endothelial cell denudation is transient and is restored by rapid regeneration. In addition, there is no direct evidence that experimentally induced endothelial injury or denudation results in eventual sustained lesion formation,[12] even in the presence of hyperlipidemia. On the contrary, strong experimental evidence suggests that the formation of intimal plaques requires the presence of a continuous endothelial covering.[10,12-14] Moreover, the role of platelets in atherogenesis remains unclear, and platelet-derived growth factor can be isolated from tissue other than platelets.[15]

More recent research has investigated other possible initiating processes. Altered endothelial function may be linked to an inflammatory response to injury, characterized by leukocyte adhesion, diapedesis and cell proliferation, smooth muscle cell migration, and macrophage foam cell formation. This response is accompanied by lipid accumulation—including cholesterol, cholesterol esters, and triglycerides—in both cell types. The pathobiology of this lipid accumulation process may be attributable to increased lipoprotein infiltration, coupled with dysregulation of the cholesterol ester cycle and cholesterol efflux processes. Lipid accumulation may be enhanced by a process in which T cells, macrophages, and smooth muscle cells release specific biologic response modifiers that participate in the dysregulation of lipid metabolism.[16,17]

Very old people who have no clinically manifest atherosclerotic disease during life often have substantial and advanced atherosclerotic plaques at autopsy. It is obvious that these people's longevity and good health did not stem from the prevention of plaque initiation or formation; rather, their lack of atherosclerotic disease symptoms must be attributable to the stable nature of the plaque, control of its progression, adequate artery adaptation, and prevention of lesion complications.

Plaque Progression

Plaque progression refers to the continuing increase in intimal plaque volume, which may cause narrowing of the lumen and obstruction of blood flow. Plaque progression may be rapid or slow, continuous or episodic. Rates of plaque accretion may vary with its stage of development, its composition, and its cell population. Some of these variables may be modulated by clinical risk factors; others may be related to changes in circulation and wall composition that are associated with lesion growth. At the tissue level, plaque progression involves cellular migration, proliferation, and differentiation; intracellular and extracellular lipid accumulation; extracellular matrix accumulation; and degeneration and cell necrosis. Evolution and differentiation of plaque organization and stratification are also characteristics of progression.

Artery Wall Responses

Artery wall responses to intimal plaque accumulation serve to maintain an adequate lumen channel. The formation of a fibrous cap, the sequestration of necrotic and degenerative debris, the persistence of a regular and round lumen cross section, and the adaptive enlargement of the artery are all aspects of an overall adaptive and healing process (Figure 2–1). If plaque enlargement is accompanied by these responses, plaque progression is well tolerated. Lumen diameter and blood flow can be maintained even with advanced and extensive lesions.

The primary artery wall response to atherosclerotic plaque deposition is arterial enlargement. It is not uncommon to have a twofold enlargement of atherosclerotic arteries, with little or no alteration in lumen cross-sectional area. The compensatory enlargement of the affected artery segment tends to limit the stenosing effect of the enlarging intimal plaque (Figure 2–2). Such enlargement of atherosclerotic arteries has been demonstrated in experimental atherosclerosis[18–20]; in human coronary,[21,22] carotid,[23] and superficial femoral arteries[24]; and in the abdominal aorta. The mechanism by which this enlargement occurs is unclear. Possible explanations include adaptive responses to altered blood flow on the segment of artery wall that is free of plaque formation or direct effects of the plaque on the subjacent artery wall. Focal intimal plaque deposition decreases lumen diameter. The resulting increased local blood flow velocity and wall shear stress induces dilatation of the artery to restore baseline levels of shear stress. In addition, atrophy of the media underlying the plaque could cause outward local bulging of the artery to maintain an adequate lumen caliber

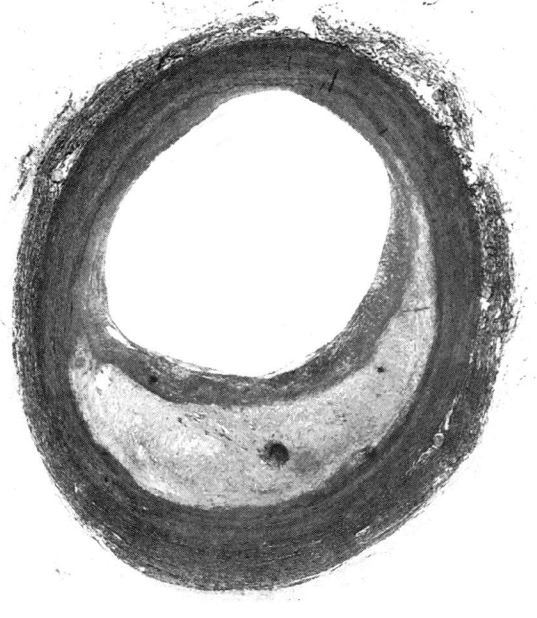

FIGURE 2–1. Cross section of a well-adapted atherosclerotic artery. Artery enlargement in response to increasing intimal plaque tends to preserve a normal lumen caliber. Lumen contour remains round and the eccentric lipid-rich necrotic core of the plaque is walled off from the lumen by a fibrous cap containing elastic lamellae that resembles the media.

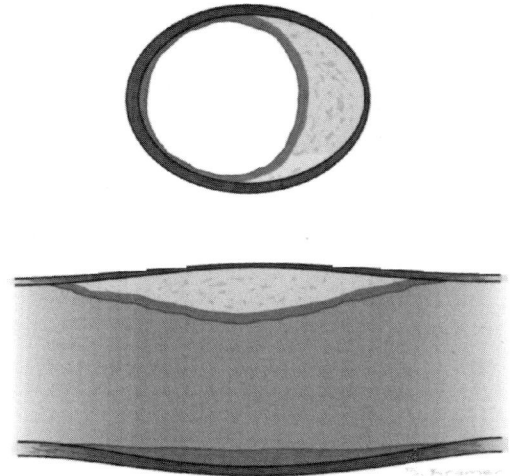

FIGURE 2–2. Arterial wall compensatory changes in response to increasing atherosclerotic plaque. The fibrous cap sequesters the plaque contents from the lumen, and artery enlargement prevents lumen stenosis.

(Figure 2–3). Thus an increase in intimal plaque volume appears to engender an increase in artery size.

In arteries such as the human left main coronary artery, compensatory enlargement keeps pace with increases in intimal plaque. Such enlargement can maintain a normal or near-normal lumen caliber and is effective in preventing lumen stenosis until the cross-sectional area of the plaque occupies approximately 40% of the area encompassed by the internal elastic lamina (Figure 2–4). Further plaque enlargement or complication appears to exceed the ability of the artery to enlarge. The result is lumen stenosis.[21] Thus atherosclerosis is fundamentally a dilating rather than a constricting disorder of arteries.

Understanding the processes that regulate plaque development, differentiation, and healing is the key to determining why one plaque progression results in unfavorable complications—such as stenosis, ulceration, or thrombosis—and another does not. Rates of cell proliferation, lipid deposition, fibrous cap formation, necrosis and healing, calcification, and inflammation may vary over time. They may also differ with location at the same point in time. Such differences probably account for the wide spectrum of morphologic changes seen in plaques in a given patient at any one time.

Plaque Regression

Plaque regression refers to a discernible decrease in intimal plaque volume. This decrease may be precipitated by a number of factors, including resorption of lipids or extracellular matrix, cell death, or migration of cells out of the plaque.

Animal Studies

In atherosclerotic animal models, significant reduction in lesion volume resulted when experimentally elevated serum lipid levels were markedly reduced by diet alteration or lipid-lowering drugs.[25-27] Although lesions experimentally induced by an atherogenic diet

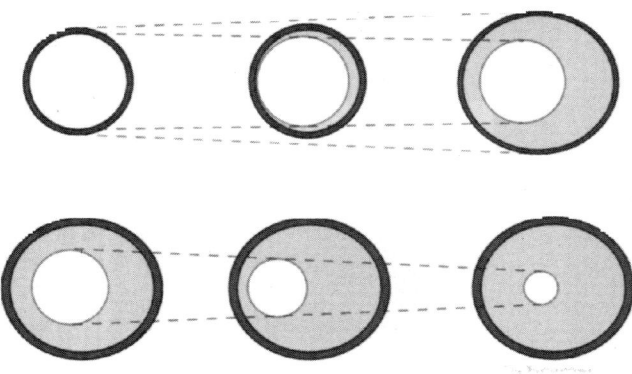

FIGURE 2–3. Arterial enlargement can prevent lumen stenosis when intimal plaque occupies more than 40% of the area encompassed by the internal elastic lamina. Further plaque enlargement and circumferential plaque formation usually result in lumen stenosis. (Adapted from Glagov S, Weisenberg E, Zarins CK et al: Compensatory enlargement of human atherosclerotic coronary arteries, *N Engl J Med* 316:1371–1375, 1987.)

2. Pathophysiology of Vascular Disease

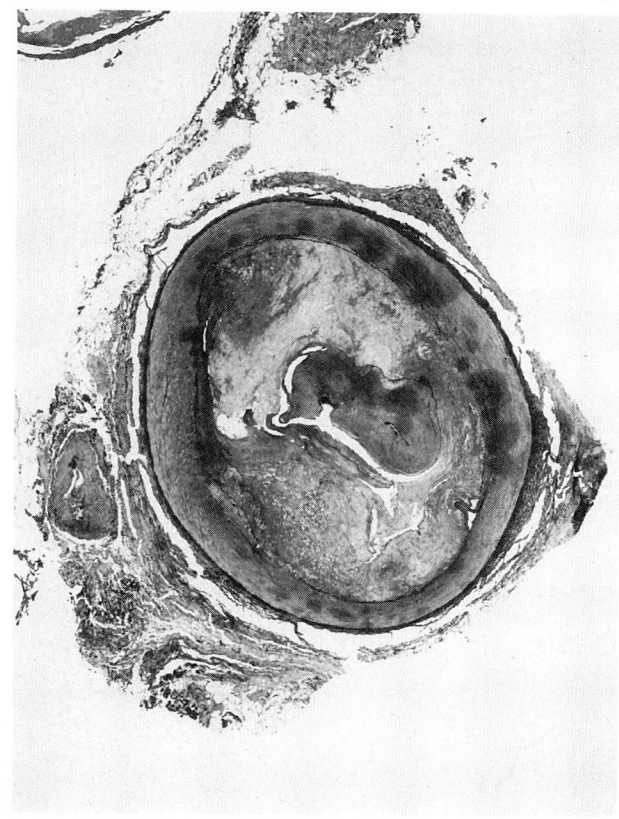

FIGURE 2–4. Cross section of occluded atherosclerotic artery. Intimal plaque deposition exceeding the arterial compensatory mechanisms resulted in lumen stenosis. Thrombosis of the stenotic vessel resulted in occlusion of the lumen.

respond readily, the response is not uniform. For example, coronary and aortic lesions in monkeys tend to regress, but carotid lesions appear to be resistant.[28] In swine, severe, long-standing lesions are much more resistant to regression than early foam cell lesions.[29] In most animal studies, induction and regression periods occur over a matter of months, It is unclear whether human lesions, which may have accumulated over decades, would also decrease significantly.

Human Studies

In human trials, apparent regression of atherosclerotic lesions in coronary[30–32] and peripheral arteries has been documented by serial contrast arteriography. In each of these trials, results are based on luminal changes observable by angiography rather than on direct evidence of plaque regression. The fact that each trial has demonstrated simultaneous progression *and* regression of different lesions during the course of treatment indicates the complexity of the process.

Although plaque regression is usually considered to be simply resorption of plaque material, it may proceed by various mechanisms. Changes in plaque metabolism may result in dissolution of the fibrous cap, ulceration and erosion, and embolization of the necrotic core (Figure 2–5). Also, *apparent regression* may take place when the rate of artery wall enlargement exceeds the rate of plaque deposition. As indicated previously, most human studies performed to date have used angiography, which provides information only on lumen diameter and contour—not on the volume and composition of the atherosclerotic lesion itself. Despite continued plaque progression, arteriography will show no change if intimal plaque deposition and artery wall enlargement keep pace. If arterial enlargement exceeds plaque deposition, the angiographic evidence will indicate

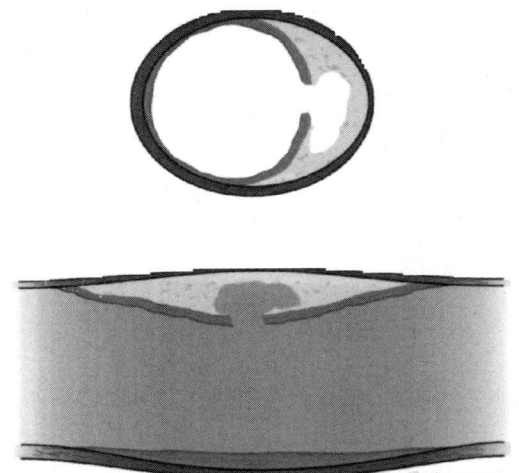

FIGURE 2–5. Erosion of the protective fibrous cap exposes the necrotic lipid core of the plaque. This erosion can result in embolization of plaque contents or accumulated platelets and thrombi. It may also promote plaque fissuring, dissection hemorrhage, and thrombosis.

regression, even if plaque deposition continues.[33] These phenomena occur at the outset of plaque formation in some vessels and, in some locations, are quite prominent. Direct assessment of the plaque and artery wall, as well as of lumen caliber, will be necessary to achieve certainty about reduction in lesion volume or regression of atherosclerosis in humans.

Although the desirability of plaque regression may seem like an a priori assumption, regression regimens could alter plaque composition and organization in unfavorable ways, especially in plaques with soft, semifluid, or pultaceous contents. These alterations could lead to plaque ulceration or disruption, release of plaque debris, and thrombosis or embolism. In certain circumstances, the plaque may provide mechanical support to the artery wall (particularly in cases of well-organized sclerotic plaques). This support may be especially significant when there has been medial atrophy underneath the plaque. Under these circumstances, plaque dissolution could leave a weakened artery wall and the potential for aneurysm formation. Experimental studies have shown that aneurysms form in monkeys undergoing cholesterol-lowering regression regimens.[34–35] Further studies of the direct effects of regression regimens on plaques and the artery wall are needed, and the specific effects of regression on well-established atherosclerotic plaques must be defined. As alternative therapeutic goals, arrest or control of progression, plaque stabilization, and enhancement of artery wall adaptation might be considered.

Plaque Complication

Clinical sequela of atherosclerotic lesions are usually caused by plaque complications. Complications such as plaque disruption or ulceration may result in the exposure of plaque components to the circulation, resulting in occlusive or embolizing thrombi (Figure 2–6). The susceptibility of plaques to disruption, fracture, or fissuring probably depends on plaque structure, composition, and consistency. Plaques may be relatively soft and pliable, friable or cohesive, densely sclerotic, or calcific and brittle. Some plaques have well-formed fibrous caps, similar in architecture and thickness to a normal artery wall, that effectively sequester the plaque and its contents from the lumen. In others, the necrotic interior is separated from the lumen by endothelium alone or

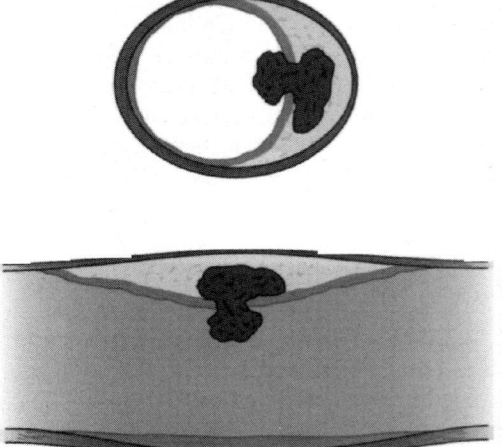

FIGURE 2–6. Fibrous cap erosion and plaque fissuring exposes a thrombogenic surface to the lumen, promoting local thrombosis.

by only a narrow zone of connective tissue.[36] Activation of macrophages and mediators of inflammation with release of cytokines and proteolytic enzymes can result in fibrous cap erosion and alteration of the plaque and artery wall structure and composition; and it may induce local thrombogenic conditions. Local mechanical stresses resulting from sudden changes in pressure, flow, or pulse rate—or those arising from torsion and bending in relation to organ movements—may then precipitate disruption of friable or brittle plaques with embolization or thrombosis.

Hemodynamic Influences in Atherosclerosis

Hemodynamic influences are important determinants of structure and function of both normal and atherosclerotic arteries. Variations in lumen diameters and in vessel curvatures and branchings produce local disturbances in the primary flow field as blood courses through the arterial tree. These disturbances result in regions of varied shear stress and boundary conditions with areas of flow separation, secondary flow patterns, and disordered flow. The complexity of flow conditions at specific sites is exacerbated by the pulsatile nature of blood flow. Branch points are particularly vulnerable to plaque formation and are characterized by wide variations in hemodynamic conditions. Thus it is not surprising that a wide variety of hemodynamic variables have been implicated in plaque pathogenesis. These include high and low wall shear stress, flow separation and stasis, oscillation of flow, turbulence, and hypertension.[37]

Wall Shear Stress

Wall shear stress (π_w) in arteries is the tangential drag force produced by blood moving across the endothelial surface. It is described by the Hagen-Poiseuille formula:

$$\pi_w = \frac{4\mu Q}{\pi r^3}$$

where μ = viscosity of blood, Q = blood flow, and r = radius. Wall shear stress is a function of the velocity gradient of blood near the endothelial surface. Its magnitude is directly proportional to blood flow and blood viscosity and inversely proportional to the cube of the vessel radius. Thus a small change in vessel radius will have a large effect on wall shear stress. Shear stress has an immediate and direct effect on endothelial cells, which respond to increases in shear stress by releasing nitric oxide, producing relaxation of artery wall smooth muscle cells and vasodilation (Figure 2–7).

It was originally thought that high shear stress potentiated plaque formation by producing endothelial injury and disruption, thereby exposing the underlying artery wall to circulating platelets and lipids.[4-5] It is now recognized that endothelial cells can withstand very high

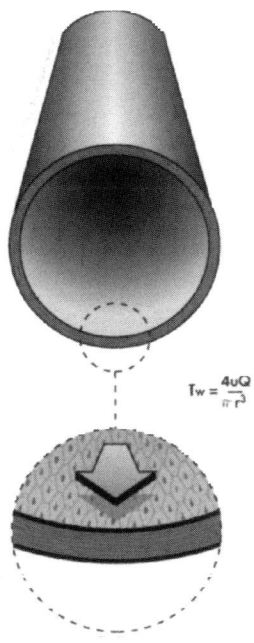

FIGURE 2–7. Wall shear stress is the drag force on the endothelial surface and is directly proportional to blood flow and inversely proportional to the cube of the vessel radius. Endothelial cells respond to increased shear by releasing endothelial-derived relaxing factor (EDRF). Small increases in lumen radius will have a large effect on reducing wall shear stress.

levels of shear and that the reported high shear-induced in vivo endothelial abnormalities were experimental artifacts.[38] Plaques form in areas of low wall shear stress rather than in those of high shear stress. In fact, areas of high shear appear to be relatively spared of plaque formation.[39] This phenomenon may serve to limit the rate of plaque deposition in developing stenoses, which produce local elevations in wall shear stress.

In experimental atherosclerosis, the earliest lesions develop at the upstream rims of aortic ostia, which are regions of low shear stress. Similar plaque localization has been noted in humans. It has been suggested that low wall shear stress rates may retard the mass transport of atherogenic substances away from the vessel wall, resulting in increased accumulation of lipids.[40] Low shear stress may also interfere with turnover of substances at the endothelial surface that are essential for both artery wall nutrition and maintaining optimal endothelial metabolic function.[41]

Flow Field Changes

Alterations in the vessel geometry result in local flow field changes. Such changes occur at branch points and curvatures and are most prominent in the carotid bifurcation because of the presence of the carotid sinus.[42] The carotid sinus is a widened area of the proximal internal carotid artery ad has twice the cross-sectional area of the distal internal carotid artery. The internal carotid has a low resistance outflow with high diastolic flow, whereas the external carotid has a relatively high resistance outflow bed. The geometric characteristics of the carotid bifurcation and differences in outflow resistance result in a unique flow field at the bifurcation. These characteristics of the carotid sinus create a large area of *flow separation and stasis* along its outer wall (Figure 2-8). As flow from the common carotid artery enters the bifurcation, flow streamlines are compressed toward the flow divider and inner wall of the internal carotid artery, an area of rapid laminar flow and high shear stress. Plaque formation does not occur in this area. Rather, the earliest intimal plaques develop along the outer wall of

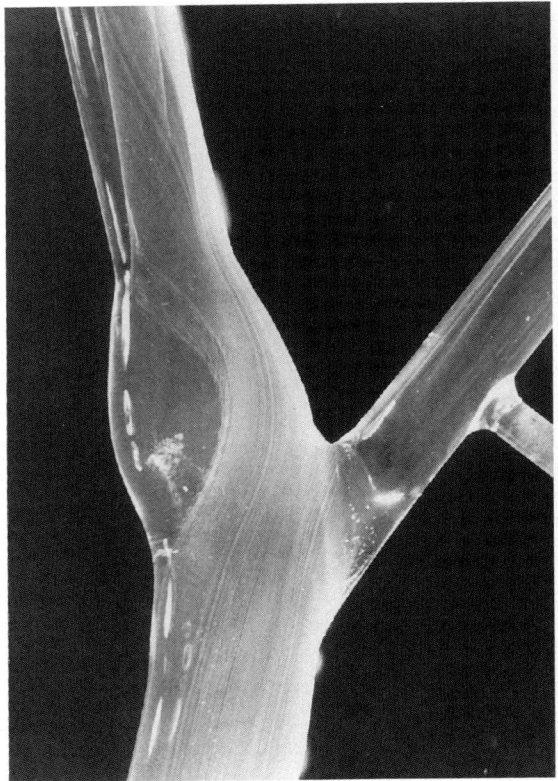

FIGURE 2-8. Glass model carotid bifurcation with hydrogen bubble flow visualization, demonstrating large area of flow separation along the outer wall of the internal carotid sinus. This is an area of low flow velocity, low wall shear stress, and increased particle residence time and is the region of the carotid bifurcation most susceptible to plaque deposition.

the sinus, a region of low flow velocity and shear stress in which a large area of flow separation develops. Late, complicated, stenotic, and ulcerated lesions also tend to develop in this region.[43] In flow-separation areas, there is a reversal of axial flow and slow fluid movement upstream. This area is also a zone of complex secondary flow patterns, including counterrotating helical trajectories. Flow reattaches distally in the sinus. The distal internal carotid, which has relatively rapid axial flow throughout its cross section, is almost always free of plaque (Figure 2-9).

2. Pathophysiology of Vascular Disease

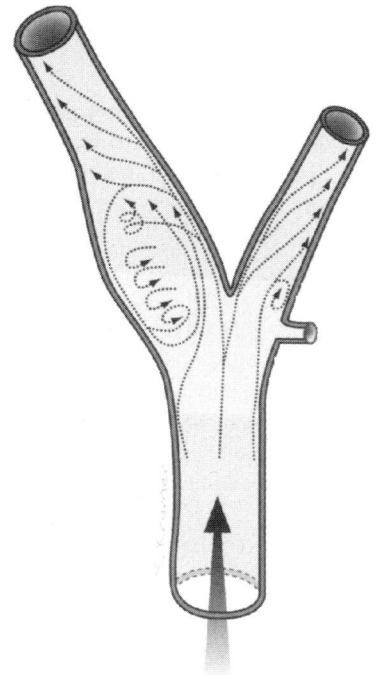

FIGURE 2–9. Carotid bifurcation flow field. Flow streamlines are skewed toward the inner wall of the carotid bifurcation, where flow is laminar and velocity and shear stress are high. The outer wall of the carotid sinus is characterized by a region of low and oscillating shear stress with vortex formation, retrograde flow, and irregular flow patterns. This is the region susceptible to plaque formation.

Particle Residence Time

Particles are present in the outer region of the carotid sinus, in the area of flow separation and low flow velocity, for a significantly longer period of time than along the inner wall. This is referred to as *increased particle residence time* and is associated with elevated plaque formation. Atherogenic particles would therefore have a greater opportunity to interact with the vessel wall. Time-dependent lipid-particle–vessel-wall interactions would thus be facilitated in this region, making plaque formation more likely. Increased particle residence time would also increase the probability of the deposition or vessel-wall adhesion of blood-borne cellular elements that may play a role in atherogenesis.[44] Flow separation has been shown to favor deposition of platelets in vitro,[45] which may stimulate cell proliferation and induce intimal thickening and plaque formation. Radiographic and ultrasound studies in patients have confirmed the presence of flow separation and stasis in this outer wall region of the carotid bifurcation (see Figure 2–9).[46]

Oscillation of Flow

Under conditions of pulsatile flow, dynamic features of the flow field become prominent. The differences between steady flow and pulsatile flow are most prominent along the outer wall of the carotid sinus. Along the inner wall of the carotid sinus, pulsatile flow conditions are similar to those seen under steady flow conditions.[47] Flow remains laminar, with high flow velocity and shear stress. Although there are fluctuations in the magnitude of velocity and shear, there is no change in velocity or shear stress directional vectors.

In contrast, along the outer wall where plaque forms, pulsatile flow produces an *oscillating shear* stress pattern. During early systole, the region of flow separation disappears and there is forward flow throughout the cross-sectional area of the sinus. However, during late systole, the region of separation and flow reversal becomes prominent along the outer wall. There is also a reversal in the shear stress directional vector.[47] During diastole, pulsatile flow conditions are similar to those seen under steady flow conditions. These alternating positive and negative shear stress vectors (oscillations) along the outer wall of the carotid sinus have been shown to correlate strongly with early plaque deposition.[48]

Thus variations in shear stress direction associated with pulsatile flow may lead to increased endothelial permeability, whereas even relatively high shear stresses that remain unidirectional may not be injurious.[49] The oscillating shear stress pattern may cause an increased ingress of plasma constituents through the endothelial monolayer because of its effects on the stability of intercellular junction. Because endothelial cells normally align in the direction of flow[50] in an overlapping arrangement, changing shear stress may cause cyclic shifts in the relationship between shear stress direction and the orientation of intercellular overlapping borders. This hypothesis is supported by studies showing increased permeability of cultured, confluent endothelial cells that have been subjected to changes in shear stress.[51] Also, increased Evans blue dye staining has been observed in relation to differences in endothelial organization[52] that may be attributable to changing flow patterns. Oscillation of shear stress direction is a systolic event. Therefore the number of such oscillations is directly related to the number of systoles, or *heart rate*, which has been implicated as an independent risk factor in coronary atherosclerosis.

Turbulence

Turbulence results from the random movement of elements in a flow field. Turbulence in blood flow is dependent on blood flow velocity, artery diameter, and blood viscosity. Causes of focal turbulence include extreme or abrupt changes in geometry resulting from intraluminal projections, severe stenoses, or other obstacles in the flow stream.[53] Although turbulent flow has often been implicated as a factor in plaque pathogenesis,[54,55] neither experimental atherosclerosis studies nor in vitro observations in the model carotid bifurcation support this suggestion.

Various flow field disturbances, such as flow separation, recirculation, and vortex formation, occur in the arterial tree under both normal and abnormal conditions. However, turbulence only develops in the presence of abnormal geometry such as stenoses or shunts. Also, various studies have shown that regions immediately distal to severe stenoses, which are characterized by significant turbulence,[56,57] are free of atherosclerotic lesion.[58-60]

In the region where plaques form in the human carotid bifurcation, there is a zone of complex secondary and tertiary flow patterns, including counterrotating helical trajectories; but, there is no turbulence.[61] This lack of turbulence holds true under a wide range of Reynolds' numbers and flow conditions, including both steady and pulsatile flow. Furthermore, in vivo noninvasive studies of carotid arteries in normal human subjects using pulsed Doppler ultrasound have not observed turbulence.[62] In areas of early plaque formation in the normal carotid bifurcation, turbulence may develop late as a result of severe carotid stenosis. Thus turbulence may be a result, rather than a cause, of atherosclerotic plaques.

Hypertension

Postmortem studies have revealed that hypertension is associated with an increase in both the extent and severity of atherosclerosis.[63] Numerous epidemiologic studies have implicated hypertension in the development of serious complications of atherosclerosis in humans, such as myocardial infarction and stroke.[64-66] Nevertheless, recent clinical data revealed no significant difference in the development of myocardial infarction or stroke between patients with and without control of mild to moderate hypertension. These data suggest that a combination of factors interacting with hypertension may be important.[67]

The effects of other local hemodynamic variables may influence the effects of hypertension in different portions of the arterial tree. For example, hypertension is known to be a more important factor in cerebrovascular disease and stroke than in coronary artery or peripheral occlusive disease.[65] Severe atherosclerosis can occur in clinically normotensive individuals, and vessels distal to stenoses can be spared, even in the presence of elevated blood pressure. So hypertension may potentiate or enhance atherogenesis but in itself may not be a necessary atherogenic factor.

Experimental studies of hypertension as an important etiologic factor in plaque pathogenesis have produced ambivalent results.[60,68-70] Inhibition of plaque deposition, despite the presence of hypertension and marked hyperlipidemia, was associated with a decreased pulse pressure,[38,60] decreased wall motion,[71] and decreased arterial wall metabolism.[72] Hypertension enhanced experimental plaque formation and plaque progression but inhibited plaque regression,[73,74] despite reduction of hypercholesterolemia. These observations suggest that factors other than blood pres-

2. Pathophysiology of Vascular Disease

sure per se may be of primary importance in atherogenesis.

Plaque Localization

Several major arterial sites are especially prone to plaque formation and the development of advanced atherosclerotic lesions, whereas others are relatively resistant. The coronary arteries, carotid bifurcation, infrarenal abdominal aorta, and iliofemoral vessels are particularly susceptible, whereas the thoracic aorta, common and distal internal carotid, mesenteric, renal, intercostal, mammary, and upper extremity arteries tend to be spared.[75] As discussed previously, the selective localization of plaques that evolve into clinical symptoms has been attributed to differences in local hemodynamic patterns. Although plaques may develop in straight vessels, they are usually located at bifurcations or bends, where hemodynamic variations are especially likely.

Susceptible Regions of the Arterial Vasculature

Carotid Artery Bifurcation

The carotid bifurcation is especially susceptible to plaque formation, with focal plaque deposition occurring principally at the origin of the internal carotid artery (Figure 2–10). In contrast, plaque does not tend to occur in the proximal common and distal internal carotid arteries. The distribution of lesions at this site is probably associated with the hemodynamic conditions created by the special geometry of the carotid bifurcation, as described previously.

As plaques enlarge at the outer wall of the carotid bifurcation, they modify the geometric configuration of the lumen. These modifications favor subsequent plaque formation on the side and inner walls. In its most advanced and stenotic form, atherosclerotic disease at the carotid bifurcation involves the entire circumference of the sinus, including the region of the flow divider. Nevertheless, plaques in this area remain largest and most complicated at the outer and side walls of the carotid bifurcation. Characteristic hemodynamic conditions at this site, including the turbulence underlying the characteristic bruit, may also compromise the integrity of existing carotid plaques and contribute to their tendency to fissure, ulcerate, and embolize.

Coronary Arteries

The coronary arteries are particularly prone to the development of atherosclerosis.[76] Predisposing factors include the geometric configuration of the vessels and their branches, the mechanical torsion and flexions of the vessels

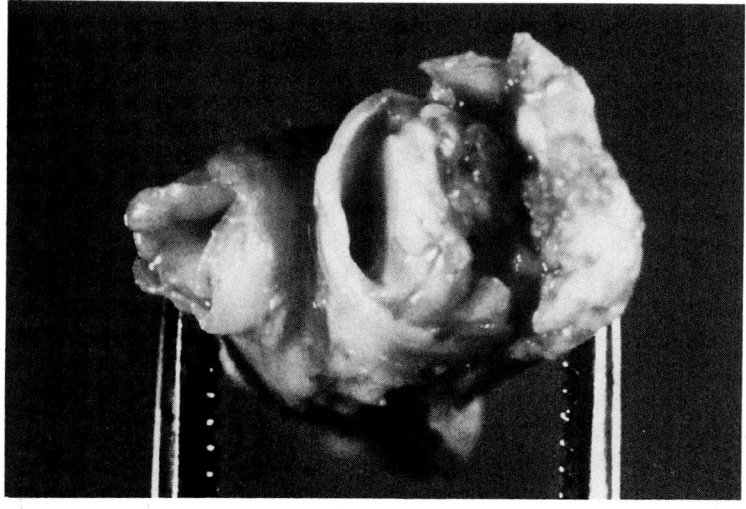

FIGURE 2–10. Atherosclerotic plaque removed from carotid bifurcation, viewed on end demonstrating internal and external branches. Plaque is most prominent along outer wall of carotid sinus. Inner wall of internal carotid has minimal intimal thickening.

associated with cardiac motion, and the special reactivity of the smooth muscle in these arteries to vasoactive substances and nervous impulses. In addition, the selective localization of plaque in the left coronary artery opposite the flow divider at the bifurcation of the left circumflex indicates the presence of hemodynamic relationships similar to those prevailing at the carotid bifurcation.[76] This is a region characterized by low flow velocity and low and oscillating wall shear stress opposite the flow divider.[77] If oscillation of shear stress direction, which occurs mainly during systole, is a major factor in plaque localization, the coronary arteries may have a higher vulnerability than other systemic arteries. The coronary arteries experience two systolic episodes and one diastolic episode of flow acceleration and deceleration during each cardiac cycle. Coronary arterial flow decreases initially in systole, increases briefly when peak systolic aortic pressure exceeds intracoronary pressure, and decreases again during the remainder of systole.[78] Flow reversal during systole has been demonstrated with tachycardia and in concentric left ventricular hypertrophy.

Because phasic fluctuation in coronary flow is predominantly a systolic occurrence, both the frequency and magnitude of oscillations in shear stress direction should be directly dependent on heart rate. Thus the preferential localization of plaques in the coronary arteries may be related to the fact that the coronary arteries experience at least twice as many oscillations of flow velocity over time as other major arteries. A modest change in heart rate has a remarkable cumulative effect on flow conditions in the coronary arteries.

In experimental studies, sinoatrial node ablation in cynomolgus monkeys resulted in a 20% reduction in mean heart rate. After 6 months on an atherogenic diet, animals with a low heart rate had a 50% reduction in coronary artery atherosclerotic plaque.[79] Heart rate has also been directly implicated as an independent risk factor in human coronary atherosclerosis. A number of major prospective clinical studies have found that high heart rates in men at rest are predictive of future coronary heart disease[80,81]; conversely, low heart rates appear to protect against coronary atherosclerosis.[82] Although increased resting heart rate seems to correlate significantly with an atherogenic lipid profile in sedentary men,[83] both theoretic and experimental evidence suggests that hemodynamic factors associated with cyclic myocardial contraction selectively predispose the coronary arteries to atherosclerosis.

Abdominal Aorta

Although atherosclerotic plaques are regularly found in the adult human thoracic aorta, they are often less abundant, complicated, or calcific than those found in the abdominal aorta. Clinically significant aortic plaque is generally most likely to be found in the abdominal region of the aorta, below the level of the renal arteries. Plaque complications in this region include obstruction, ulceration, thrombus formation, and (potentially) aneurysmal degeneration. The differences in atherogenic susceptibility between the thoracic and abdominal aortas may be related to differences in flow conditions, in mural architecture, or in vasa vasorum distribution and aortic wall nutrition. Suprarenal flow volume is largely independent of skeletal muscular activity. In contrast, infrarenal flow volume is largely dependent on the muscular activity of the lower extremities. Therefore reduced physical activity results in an overall reduction in flow volume and velocity in the infrarenal segment. The long-term effect of reduced flow velocity may be accentuated by the tendency of the aorta to enlarge with age. In addition, the media of the thoracic aorta is well furnished with vasa vasorum, but that of the abdominal aorta is relatively avascular. These differences in medial nutrition may enhance the atherogenic susceptibility of the abdominal aortic segment.

Superficial Femoral Artery

There is no widely accepted explanation for the discrepancy between the incidence of atherosclerotic plaque in the upper and lower extremity arteries. Recognized differences in the two areas include hydrostatic pressure and variations in volume flow depending on the level of physical activity. As in the abdominal aorta, the relative inactivity of a sedentary life style, associated with low flow rates and diminished shear stress, may tend to increase rates of plaque deposition in these arteries.[84]

Cigarette smoking and diabetes mellitus are the risk factors most closely associated with atherosclerotic disease of the lower extremities, but their specific mechanisms of action are unknown. Arterial medial density in the lower extremities may be increased because of the chronically heightened smooth muscle tone induced by nicotine use. Such a change could interfere with the transluminal transfer of materials entering the intima, facilitating accumulation of atherogenic materials. Occlusive plaque of the superficial femoral artery tends to be predominantly located at the adductor canal. Possible explanations for this location include repeated mechanical trauma, limitations on vessel compliance, or restrictions on compensatory enlargement because of the closely applied adductor magnus tendon.[24]

Aneurysm Formation

Aneurysmal enlargement is the most dramatic degenerative change affecting the human aorta. Most patients with aortic aneurysms have evidence of significant atherosclerosis in the coronary arteries, carotid bifurcation, and/or the lower extremity arteries. Although a causative relationship has not been proven, increasing knowledge of the atherosclerotic process and its effect on the artery wall supports a close pathogenetic relationship between atherosclerosis and aneurysm formation.[85]

Arterial Enlargement

As previously noted, arterial enlargement occurs in response to atherosclerosis and tends to compensate for the increase in intimal plaque area. The rate of enlargement in response to atherosclerotic plaque may vary in different segments of the coronary tree under varying conditions. In the human aorta, enlargement is seen both with increasing age and with increasing atherosclerotic plaque. However, whereas the primary determinant of thoracic aortic size is age, the primary determinant of abdominal aortic size is the amount of intimal plaque. This may explain the particular susceptibility of the abdominal aorta to aneurysmal development.

Medial Thinning

In atherosclerosis, the media frequently becomes thin and disappears under large plaques (Figure 2–11). It is not clear whether this thinning is related to the mechanism of atherosclerotic enlargement or to the erosive effects of plaque components on the artery wall. Cavitary excavations of the media, frequently noted in lipid-rich areas of the plaque, may be associated with regions of macrophage invasion and inflammation. Under atherosclerotic conditions, collagen and fibrous tissue collect in the adventitia and calcification occurs within the plaque and media. The presence of these materials in the aortic wall may compensate for loss of the media and may even provide structural support. Aortic enlargement can occur in atherosclerosis only if the aortic wall matrix fibers of collagen and elastin are degraded and/or resynthesized in new proportions. Simple passive distention will not permit the aorta to enlarge in excess of its diastolic dimensions without rupture. Thus proteolytic enzymes must be activated for adaptive atherosclerotic arterial enlargement to take place. During active, rapid enlargement, which characterizes aneurysmal development, proteolytic activities would probably be much larger and perhaps less controlled. Indeed, increased collagenase, elastase, and metalloproteinases have been demonstrated in aortic aneurysms, with maximal concentrations noted in those that are rapidly enlarging or ruptured.[86–88] In experimental studies, enzymatic destruction of the medial matrix architecture results in dilatation and rupture of the aorta.[89] Experimental mechanical injury that destroys the medial lamellar architecture can result in aneurysm formation.[90] These observations underscore the importance of the media in maintaining the integrity of the aorta.

Human atherosclerotic aneurysms, particularly those of the abdominal aorta, are charac-

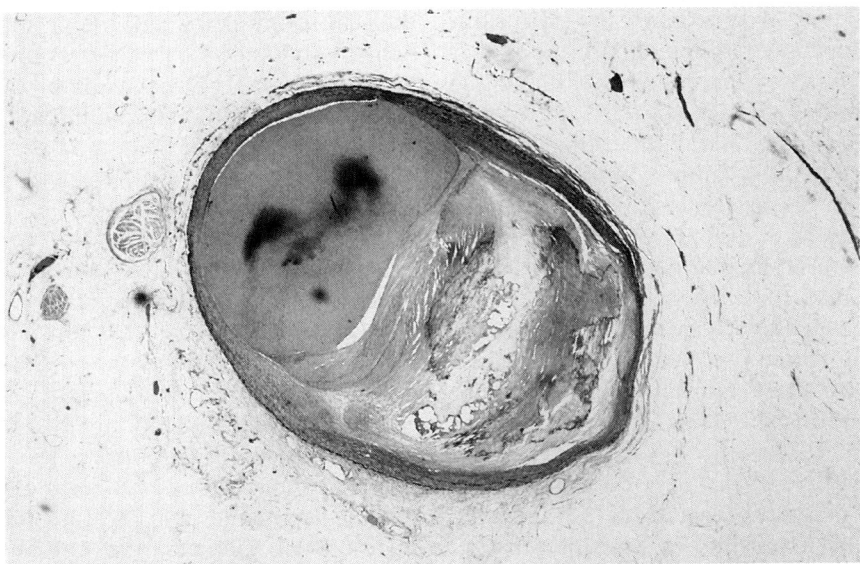

FIGURE 2–11. Prominent thinning of the media underneath atherosclerotic plaque. Note loss of medial lamellar architecture. This may predispose to subsequent aneurysmal degeneration if the plaque ulcerates or regresses.

terized by extensive atrophy of the media. The normal lamellar architecture is almost totally effaced, and the aortic wall is replaced by a narrow fibrous band. There are also atrophic changes in the overlying atherosclerotic lesions; plaques may be thinned and left with little residual lipid. Fibrosis and calcification may predominate. Human abdominal aortic aneurysms are rarely found without evidence of atherosclerosis. Atherosclerotic plaques are usually prominent in the neck of the aneurysm and the iliac vessels, and they frequently occur posteriorly along the lumbar ostia.

Mechanism of Aneurysm Formation in Atherosclerosis

Observations of human atherosclerotic arteries suggest a possible mechanism for aneurysm formation. Intimal plaque deposition is accompanied by a compensatory arterial enlargement and by atrophy of the aortic media underlying the plaque. Stable, fibrotic, or calcified atherosclerotic plaques, well nourished by vasa vasorum, may provide structural support to the aortic wall, particularly in association with adventitial fibrogenesis, which is characteristic of atherosclerosis. Late in the atherosclerotic process when the aorta is enlarged, plaque may undergo senescence. This process may be accompanied by reduction in plaque volume and alteration in composition, in ulceration, or in regression resulting in lumen enlargement. Tensile support may thus become insufficient, and progressive aneurysmal enlargement may follow (Figure 2–12).

In some atherosclerotic plaques, metabolic alteration in plaque lipid composition may stimulate macrophage activity and inflammation and promote proteolytic activity. The balance between plaque formation, artery wall adaptation, and matrix protein synthesis and degradation probably plays a major role in aneurysmal pathogenesis. Aneurysms appear to occur at a relatively late phase of plaque evolution, when atrophy of the plaque and media are predominant, rather than at an earlier phase of atherosclerosis, when cell proliferation, fibrogenesis, and sequestered lipid accumulation are predominant.

2. Pathophysiology of Vascular Disease

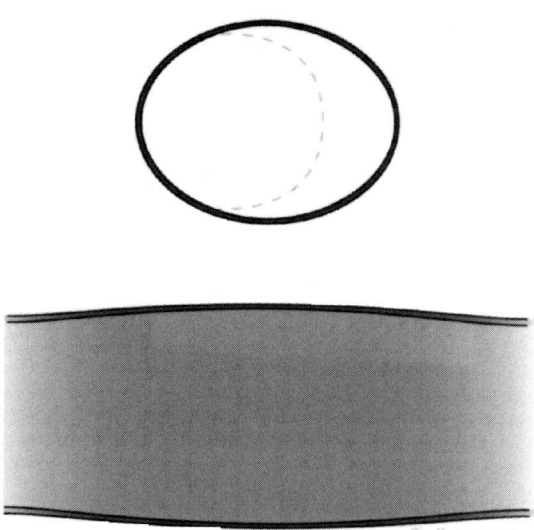

FIGURE 2–12. Possible mechanism of atherosclerotic aneurysmal degeneration. Enlargement of the atherosclerotic aorta may be associated with significant medial thinning and loss of elastic architecture beneath atherosclerotic plaques. Under these circumstances, the plaque may provide structural support to the aortic wall. Plaque dissolution resorption and regression would act to enlarge the lumen. The plaque resorptive process may be promoted by macrophage release of proteolytic enzymes, which may weaken the susceptible aortic wall. The enlarged atherosclerotic aorta and thinned aortic wall would result in increased mural tension with progressive aneurysmal dilation.

Experimental Observations

In animal models, diet-induced atherosclerosis produces arteries with lipid-laden intimal plaques and artery wall responses—such as compensatory arterial enlargement and medial degeneration—similar to those found in human atherosclerosis. Arterial enlargement in coronary, carotid, and superficial femoral arteries of primates limits lumen stenosis in a manner similar to that seen in human arteries.[18–20] Particularly in primate species (which are more susceptible to aneurysm formation in atherosclerosis), plaque formation and artery enlargement are also associated with destruction of medial architecture.[90] Experimental destruction of aortic medial architecture, both by mechanical methods alone and by mechanical injury combined with hyperlipidemia, has also been shown to produce aneurysms.[91]

Our own experience with more than 500 nonhuman primates that were fed high-cholesterol, high-fat diets to induce experimental atherosclerosis has demonstrated that aneurysms form only in animals maintained on atherogenic diets for prolonged periods of time. The cynomolgus monkey, in which diet-induced atherosclerosis produces destruction of the media, is much more prone to the development of aneurysms than the rhesus monkey, in which atherosclerotic destruction of the media rarely occurs. In cynomolgus monkeys, aneurysms developed in 13% of animals maintained on atherogenic regimens for more than 12 months. Histologic studies of these primate aneurysms showed evidence of aortic wall thinning with destruction of the medial lamellar architecture and of plaque atrophy.[92]

Of particular note in these primate experiments is the relationship between plaque regression and aneurysm formation. In a controlled trial of cholesterol lowering, significant aneurysmal enlargement of the abdominal aorta was noted only in those monkeys undergoing atherosclerotic regression. Aneurysmal enlargement was associated with significant reduction in plaque volume and medial thickness in the abdominal aorta.[93] These data are consistent with the hypothesis that the atherosclerotic process plays a significant role in the pathogenesis of aneurysms and that plaque regression and medial thinning may be important factors in this process.

Others have reported aneurysm formation with experimental diet-induced atherosclerosis in several species of monkeys and canines.[90,94] In these studies, aneurysms have been observed only after extended exposure to atherogenic regimens—suggesting that aneurysm formation occurs at a later stage in the atherosclerotic process. This is consistent with the observation that patients undergoing operation for abdominal aortic aneurysms tend to be approximately 10 years older than those undergoing operation for occlusive disease.[95]

Conclusion

Atherosclerosis is a degenerative process of the arterial tree that has various local effects on the artery wall. Specific hemodynamic forces are important in plaque localization. Intimal plaque deposition is counterbalanced by compensatory artery wall responses, such as fibrous cap formation and artery enlargement. The fibrous cap sequesters the plaque from the arterial lumen, and compensatory arterial enlargement serves to preserve a normal lumen caliber. Erosion of the fibrous cap may lead to ulceration, thrombosis, and embolization. Regression of plaque contents may be associated with release of proteolytic enzymes. Erosion of the artery wall may result in progressive aneurysmal enlargement. Stenoses may develop as a result of inadequate compensatory enlargement or excessive plaque deposition. Occlusion is usually caused by superimposed thrombosis. The simultaneous occurrence of differing rates of plaque deposition and differing types of artery wall responses engender the variety and heterogeneity of the clinical manifestations of atherosclerosis. Further understanding of the cellular and molecular mechanisms underlying the atherosclerotic process will improve our ability to control the disease.

References

1. Ross R: The pathogenesis of atherosclerosis—an update, *N Engl J Med* 314:488, 1986.
2. Benditt EP, Barrett T, McDougall JK: Viruses in the etiology of atherosclerosis, *Proc Natl Acad Sci USA* 80:6388, 1983.
3. Caro CG: Transport of material between blood and wall in arteries. *Ciba Found Symp* 12:127, 1973.
4. Ross R, Harker L: Hyperlipidemia and atherosclerosis, *Science* 193:1094, 1976.
5. Ross R: The pathogenesis of atherosclerosis: an update, *N Engl J Med* 314:488–500, 1986.
6. Ross R, Glomset J: The pathogenesis of atherosclerosis, *N Engl J Med* 295:369, 1976.
7. Ross R: Atherosclerosis: a problem of the biology of arterial wall cells and their interactions with blood components, *Arteriosclerosis* 1:293, 1981.
8. Ip JH, Fuster V, Badimon L et al: Syndromes of accelerated atherosclerosis: role of vascular injury and smooth muscle proliferation, *J Am Coll Cardiol* 15:1667–1687, 1990.
9. Schwartz S, Heimark R, Majesky M: Developmental mechanisms underlying pathology of arteries, *Physiol Rev* 70:1177–1209, 1990.
10. Zarins CK, Taylor KE, Bomberger RA et al: Endothelial integrity at aortic ostial flow dividers, *SEM* 3:249–254, 1980.
11. Taylor KE, Glagov S, Zarins CK: Preservation and structural adaptation of endothelium over experimental foam cell lesions, *Arteriosclerosis* 9:881–894, 1989.
12. Reidy MA: Biology of disease: a reassessment of endothelial injury and arterial lesion formation, *Lab Invest* 53:513, 1985.
13. Falcone DJ, Hajjar DP, Minick CR: Lipoprotein and albumin accumulation in re-endothelialized and de-endothelialized aorta, *Am J Pathol* 114:112, 1984.
14. Dzau VJ, Gibbons GH, Cooke JP et al: Vascular biology and medicine in the 1990s: scope, concepts, potentials, and perspectives, *Circulation* 87:705, 1993.
15. Di Corleto PE, Bowen-Pope DF: Cultured endothelial cells produce a platelet-derived growth-like factor protein, *Proc Natl Acad Sci USA* 80:1919, 1983.
16. Hajjar DP, Pomerantz KB: Signal transduction in atherosclerosis: integration of cytokines and the eicosanoid network, *FASEB J* 6:2933, 1992.
17. Pomerantz K, Hajjar D: Eicosanoids in regulation of arterial smooth muscle cell phenotype, proliferative capacity, and cholesterol metabolism, *Arteriosclerosis* 9:413, 1989.
18. Bond MG, Adams MR, Bullock BC: Complicating factors in evaluating coronary artery atherosclerosis, *Artery* 9:21, 1981.
19. Beere PA, Glagov S, Zarins CK: Experimental atherosclerosis at the carotid bifurcation of the cynomolgus monkey, *Atheroscler Thromb* 12:1245, 1992.
20. Armstrong ML, Heistad DD, Marcus MI et al: Structural and hemodynamic responses of peripheral arteries of macaque monkeys to atherogenic diet, *Arteriosclerosis* 5:336, 1985.
21. Glagov S, Weisenberg E, Zarins CK et al: Compensatory enlargement of human atherosclerotic coronary arteries, *N Engl J Med* 316:1371, 1987.
22. Zarins CK, Weisenberg E, Kolettis G et al: Differential enlargement of artery segments in response to enlarging atherosclerotic plaques, *J Vasc Surg* 7:386, 1988.

23. Masawa N, Glagov S, Bassiouny H et al: Intimal thickness normalizes mural tensile stress in regions of increased intimal area and artery size, *Arteriosclerosis* 8:621a, 1988.
24. Blair JM, Glagov S, Zarins CK: Mechanism of superficial femoral artery adductor canal stenosis, *Surg Forum* 41:359, 1990.
25. Malinow MR: Experimental models of atherosclerosis regression, *Atherosclerosis* 48(2):105, 1983.
26. Wissler RW, Vesselinovitch D: Combined effects of cholestyramine and probucol on regression of atherosclerosis in rhesus monkey aortas, *Appl Pathol* 1(2):89, 1983.
27. Stary HC: Regression of atherosclerosis in primates, *Virchows Arch [A]* 383:117, 1979.
28. Clarkson TB, Bond MG, Bullock BC et al: A study of atherosclerosis regression in Macaca mulatta. V. Changes in abdominal aorta and carotid and coronary arteries from animals with atherosclerosis induced for 38 months and then regressed for 24 or 48 months at plasma cholesterol concentrations of 300 or 200 mg/dl, *Exp Mol Pathol* 41(I):96, 1984.
29. Daoud AS, Jarmolych J, Augustyn JM et al: Sequential morphologic studies of regression of advanced atherosclerosis, *Arch Pathol Lab Med* 105(5):233, 1981.
30. Blankenhorn DH, Nessim SA, Johnson BL et al: Beneficial effects of combined colestipolniacin therapy on coronary atherosclerosis and coronary venous bypass grafts, *JAMA* 257:3233, 1987.
31. Brown G, Albert JJ, Fisher LD et al: Regression of coronary artery disease as a result of intensive lipid-lowering therapy in men with high levels of apolipoprotein B, *N Engl J Med* 323:1290, 1990.
32. Buchwald H, Varco RL, Matts PJ et al: Effect of partial ileal bypass surgery on mortality and morbidity from coronary heart disease in patients with hypercholesterolemia: report of the Program on the Surgical Control of the Hyperlipidemias (POSCH), *N Engl J Med* 323:946, 1990.
33. Zarins CK, Zatina MA, Glagov S: Correlation of postmortem angiography with pathologic anatomy: quantitation of atherosclerotic lesions. In Bond MG et al, editors: *Clinical diagnosis of atherosclerosis: quantitative methods of evaluation*, New York, 1983, Springer-Verlag.
34. Zarins CK, Glagov S, Wissler RW et al: Aneurysm formation in experimental atherosclerosis. Relationship to plaque evolution, *J Vasc Surg* 12(3):246, 1990.
35. Zarins CK, Xu C-P, Glagov S: Aneurysmal enlargement of the aorta during regression of experimental atherosclerosis, *J Vasc Surg* 15:90, 1992.
36. Glagov S, Zarins CK, Giddens DP et al: Atherosclerosis: what is the nature of the plaque? In Strandness DE Jr et al, editors: *Vascular diseases: current research and clinical applications*, Orlando, Fla, 1987, Grune & Stratton.
37. Glagov S, Zarins CK, Giddens DP et al: Hemodynamics and atherosclerosis, *Arch Pathol Lab Med* 112:1018–1031, 1988.
38. Zarins CK, Bomberger RA, Glagov S: Local effects of stenosis: increased flow velocity inhibits atherogenesis, *Circulation* 64(suppl II):II-221–II-227, 1981.
39. Bassiouny HS, Lieber BB, Giddens DP et al: Quantitative inverse correlation of wall shear stress with experimental intimal thickening, *Surg Forum* 39:328–330, 1988.
40. Caro CG, Fitz-Gerald JM, Schroter RC: Atheroma and arterial wall shear: observation, correlation and proposal of a shear dependent mass transfer mechanism for atherogenesis, *Proc R Soc Lond B Biol Sci* 117:109–159, 1971.
41. Robertson AJ Jr: Oxygen requirements of the human arterial intima in atherogenesis, *Prog Biochem Pharmacol* 4:305–316, 1968.
42. Giddens DP, Zarins CK, Glagov S: Response of arteries to near-wall fluid dynamic behavior, *Appl Mech Rev* 43(5):S96–S102, 1990.
43. Zarins CK, Giddens DP, Bharadvaj BK et al: Carotid bifurcation atherosclerosis: quantitative correlation of plaque localization with flow velocity profiles and wall shear stress, *Circ Res* 53:502–514, 1983.
44. Gerrity RG, Goss JA, Soby L: Control of monocyte recruitment by chemotactic factor(s) in lesion-prone areas of swine aorta, *Arteriosclerosis* 5:55–66, 1985.
45. Parmentier EM, Morton WA, Petschek HE: Platelet aggregate formation in a region of separated blood flow, *Phys Fluids* 20:2012–2021, 1981.
46. Fox JA, Hugh AE: Static zones in the internal carotid artery: correlation with boundary layer separation and stasis in model flows, *Br J Radiol* 43:370–376, 1976.
47. Ku DN, Giddens DP: Pulsatile flow in a model carotid bifurcation, *Arteriosclerosis* 3:31–39, 1983.
48. Ku DN, Giddens DP, Zarins CK et al: Pulsatile flow and atherosclerosis in the human carotid bifurcation: positive correlation between plaque

location and low and oscillating shear stress, *Arteriosclerosis* 5:293–302, 1985.
49. Fry DL: Hemodynamic forces in atherogenesis. In Scheinberg P, editor: *Cerebrovascular disease*, New York, 1976, Raven Press.
50. Nerem RM, Levesque MJ, Cornhill JF: Vascular endothelial morphology as an indicator of the pattern of blood flow, *J Biomech Eng* 103:171–176, 1981.
51. Dewey CF, Bussolari SR, Gimbrone MA et al: The dynamic response of vascular endothelial cells to fluid shear stress, *J Biomech Eng* 103:177–185, 1981.
52. Fry DL: Responses of the arterial wall to certain physical factors, *Ciba Found Symp* 12:93–125, 1973.
53. Giddens DP, Khalifa AMA: Turbulence measurements with pulsed Doppler ultrasound employing a frequency tracking method, *Ultrasound Med Biol* 8:427–437, 1982.
54. Davies PF, Remuzzi A, Gordon EJ et al: Turbulent fluid shear stress induces vascular endothelial cell turnover in vitro, *Proc Natl Acad Sci USA* 83:2114–2117, 1986.
55. Gutstein WH, Farrell GA, Armellini C: Blood flow disturbance and endothelial cell injury in pre-atherosclerotic swine, *Lab Invest* 29:134–149, 1973.
56. Lieber BB: Ordered and random structures in pulsatile flow through constricted tubes, thesis, Atlanta, Ga, 1985, Georgia Institute of Technology.
57. Khalifa AMA, Giddens DP: Characterization and evolution of post-stenotic flow disturbances, *J Biomech* 14:279–296, 1981.
58. Ku DN, Zarins CK, Giddens DP et al: Reduced atherogenesis distal to stenosis despite turbulence and hypertension (abstr), *Circulation* 74 (suppl 2):II-334, 1986.
59. Coutard M, Osborne-Pellegrin MJ: Decreased dietary lipid deposition in spontaneous lesions distal to a stenosis in the rat caudal artery, *Artery* 12:82–98, 1983.
60. Bomberger RA, Zarins CK, Taylor KE et al: Effect of hypotension on atherogenesis and aortic wall composition, *J Surg Res* 28:402–409, 1980.
61. Bharadvaj BK, Mabon RF, Giddens DP: Steady flow in a model of the human carotid bifurcation: part II. laser doppler anemometer measurements, *J Biomech Eng* 15:363–378, 1982.
62. Ku DN, Giddens DP, Phillips DJ et al: Hemodynamics of the normal human carotid bifurcation: in vitro and in vivo studies, *Ultrasound Med Biol* 11:13–26, 1985.
63. Glagov S, Rowley DA, Kohut R: Atherosclerosis of human aorta and its coronary and renal arteries, *Arch Pathol Lab Med* 72:558–571, 1961.
64. Chabanian AV: The influence of hypertension and other hemodynamic factors in atherogenesis, *Cardiovasc Dis* 26:177–196, 1983.
65. Kannel WB, Schwartz MJ, McNamara PM: Blood pressure and risk of coronary heart disease: the Framingham study, *Dis Chest* 56:43–52, 1969.
66. Robertson WB, Strong JP: Atherosclerosis in persons with hypertension and diabetes mellitus, *Lab Invest* 18:538, 1969.
67. Medical Research Council Working party: MCR trial of treatment of mild hypertension: principal results, *Br Med J* 291:97–104, 1985.
68. Breterton KN, Day AJ, Skinner SL: Hypertension-accelerated atherogenesis in cholesterol-fed rabbits, *Atherosclerosis* 27:79–87, 1977.
69. Bomberger RA, Zarins CK, Glagov S: Subcritical arterial stenosis enhances distal atherosclerosis. Resident Research Award, *J Surg Res* 30:205–212, 1981.
70. Hollander W, Madoff I, Paddock J et al: Aggravation of atherosclerosis by hypertension in a subhuman primate model with coarctation of the aorta, *Circ Res* 38(suppl 2):63, 1976.
71. Lyon RT, Runyan-Hass A, Davis HR et al: Protection from atherosclerotic lesion formation by reduction of artery wall motion, *J Vasc Surg* 5(3):413–420, 1987.
72. Cozzi PJ, Lyon RT, Davis HR et al: Aortic wall metabolism in relation to susceptibility and resistance to experimental atherosclerosis, *J Vasc Surg* 7(5):706–714, 1988.
73. Zarins CK, Bomberger RA, Taylor KE et al: Artery stenosis inhibits regression of diet-induced atherosclerosis, *Surgery* 88:86–92, 1980.
74. Xu C-P, Glagov S, Zatina MA et al: Hypertension sustains plaque progression despite reduction of hypercholesterolemia, *Hypertension* 18(2):123–129, 1991.
75. McGill HC Jr: Atherosclerosis: problems in pathogenesis. In Paoletti R, Gotto AM, editors: *Atherosclerosis reviews*, New York, 1977, Raven Press.
76. Montenegro MR, Eggen DA: Topography of atherosclerosis in the coronary arteries, *Lab Invest* 18:586–593, 1968.
77. Tang TD, Giddens DP, Zarins CK et al: Velocity profile and wall shear measurements in a model

human coronary artery, *Adv Bio Eng ASME* 17:261–263, 1990.
78. Granata L, Olsson RA, Huvos A et al: Coronary inflow and oxygen usage following cardiac sympathetic nerve stimulator in unanesthetized dogs, *Circ Res* 16:114, 1965.
79. Beere PA, Glagov S, Zarins CK: Retarding effect of lowered heart rate on coronary atherosclerosis, *Science* 226:180–182, 1984.
80. Schroll M, Hagerup LM: Risk factors of myocardial infarction and death in men aged 50 at entry, *Dan Med Bull* 24:252, 1977.
81. Dyer AR, Persky V, Stamler J et al: Heart rate as a prognostic factor for coronary heart disease and mortality: findings in three Chicago epidemiologic studies, *Am J Epidemiol* 112:736, 1980.
82. Williams PT, Wood PD, Haskell WL et al: The effects of running mileage and duration on plasma lipoprotein levels, *JAMA* 247:2674, 1982.
83. Williams PT, Haskell WL, Vranizan KM et al: Associations of resting heart rate with concentrations of lipoprotein subfractions in sedentary men, *Circulation* 71:441, 1985.
84. Ku DN, Glagov S, Moore JE Jr et al: Flow patterns in the abdominal aorta under simulated post-prandial and exercise conditions: an experimental study, *J Vasc Surg* 9:309–316, 1989.
85. Zarins CK, Glagov S: Aneurysms and obstructive plaques: differing local responses to atherosclerosis. In Bergan JJ, Yao J, editors: *Aneurysms: diagnosis and treatment*, ed 1, New York, 1982, Grune & Stratton.
86. Busuttil RW, Abou-Zamzam AM, Machleder HI: Collagenase activity of the human aorta: a comparison of patients with and without abdominal aortic aneurysm, *Arch Surg* 116:1373–1378, 1980.
87. Menashi S, Campa JS, Greenhalgh RM et al: Collagen in abdominal aortic aneurysm: typing, content, and degradation, *J Vasc Surg* 6:578–582, 1987.
88. Brophy CM, Marks WH, Reilly JM et al: Decreased tissue inhibitor of metalloproteinases (TIMP) in abdominal aortic aneurysm tissue: a preliminary report, *J Surg Res* 50:653–657, 1991.
89. Dobrin PB, Baker WH, Gley WC: Elastolytic and collagenolytic studies of arteries: implications for the mechanical properties of aneurysms, *Arch Surg* 119:405–409, 1984.
90. DePalma RG, Koletsky S, Bellon EM et al: Failure of regression of atherosclerosis in dogs with moderated cholesterolemia, *Atherosclerosis* 27:297–310, 1977.
91. Zatina MA, Zarins CK, Gewertz BL et al: Role of medial lamellar architecture in the pathogenesis of aortic aneurysms, *J Vasc Surg* 1:442–448, 1984.
92. Zarins CK, Glagov S, Vesselinovitch D et al: Aneurysm formation in experimental atherosclerosis: relationship to plaque evolution, *J Vasc Surg* 12:246–256, 1990.
93. Zarins CK, Xu C, Glagov S: Aneurysmal enlargement of the aorta during regression of experimental atherosclerosis, *J Vasc Surg* 15:90–101, 1992.
94. Strickland HL, Bond MG: Aneurysms in large colony of squirrel monkeys (Saimiri sciureus), *Lab Anim Sci* 33:589–592, 1983.
95. Clark ET, Gewertz BL, Bassiouny HS et al: Current results of elective aortic reconstruction for aneurysmal and occlusive disease, *J Vasc Surg* 31:438–441, 1990.

Part II
Components of an Endovascular Practice

3
Training and Credentialing in Endovascular Surgery

G. Patrick Clagett and Kenneth E. McIntyre Jr.

The explosive interest in minimally invasive endoluminal repair of occlusive lesions and aortic aneurysms and the extension of this technology to the repair of traumatic lesions, arteriovenous malformations, and fistulas is having a major impact on the direction of training in vascular surgery. Although the durability and long-term success of endoluminal procedures are only beginning to be known (especially in comparison to conventional, open vascular surgical procedures), it is likely that vascular repairs performed transluminally will comprise a significant portion of vascular surgical practice in the future. A large body of preliminary work suggests that this approach offers a potentially better method to treat a significant proportion of vascular surgical cases because of reduced morbidity and mortality and enthusiastic patient acceptance.[1] It has been estimated that within the next decade one-third to one-half of vascular prosthetic reconstructions currently carried out by open surgical approaches could be replaced by endovascular prostheses inserted percutaneously or by open means from a remote access site.[1] The inference is clear: If these devices prove successful over time, a significant amount of conventional vascular surgery will become obsolete.

Current Training and Credentialing

There are no current requirements for formal training in endovascular surgery as part of the conventional 1-year training experience in general vascular surgery. The most recent Accreditation Council for Graduate Medical Education (ACGME) requirements spelled out in the Graduate Medical Education Directory (green book) states "that the residents have an ***acquaintance*** with the methods and techniques of angiography and ***competence in the interpretation*** of angiographic findings." [emphasis added][2] In contrast, the ACGME special requirements for residency training in vascular and interventional radiology include graduation from an approved residency in diagnostic radiology and a minimum of 1 year of additional training. During this year experience with 500 cases including those involving arteriography, venography, angioplasty, and related percutaneous revascularization procedures, embolotherapy, and percutaneous placement of endovascular prostheses, stents, and inferior vena cava filters must be documented.[2]

It is clear that vascular surgery training programs must incorporate endovascular surgery and related technologies into their curricula. A simple "acquaintance" with diagnostic angiography and an ability to interpret angiograms will no longer be adequate to meet the needs of vascular surgical trainees. Many vascular surgery fellowships are changing to incorporate endovascular training because program directors recognize the pressing need to make the necessary modifications to be compatible with the changing landscape in vascular surgery. In a survey conducted by the Association of Program Directors in Vascular Surgery, 80% of program directors thought that formal, "hands-on" endovascular surgery training was an essential or important component for vascular surgical trainees. Another 16% thought that endovascular surgical training was helpful but not essential, and only a few, 6%, replied that it was not important or relevant.[3]

Despite the wide recognition of the need for endovascular training, the experience offered by most training programs is variable and, in many cases, incomplete. According to the best currently available data, fewer than one-half of all programs offer some formal training in percutaneous arterial puncture and catheter/guidewire techniques for arteriography and device placement.[3] Alarmingly, only one-fifth of vascular surgery training programs provide an experience that would meet the minimal standards for credentialing as outlined by the Society of Vascular Surgery/International Society for Cardiovascular Surgery, North American Chapter's Ad Hoc Committee on Endovascular Surgery Credentialing and Training for Vascular Surgeons in 1993.[4] This group has recently updated their recommendations. At least 100 catheterizations and 50 interventions that may include percutaneous or intraoperative approaches are required for individual credentialing for endovascular surgery privileges. The credentialee must demonstrate that he or she performed at least one-half of these procedures as the primary interventionalist.[5] These credentialing standards, as well as those recommended by other specialty organizations, are shown in Table 3–1.

Increasing pressure to alter training programs to incorporate this technology is coming from the trainees themselves. Although not formally surveyed, one frequently hears this concern among former, present, and future trainees. Former trainees who have not had endovascular surgery experience lack a competitive advantage when entering the practice arena. Current trainees are keenly aware of this situation and in many instances seek informal arrangements to gain training by "hanging out" with interventional radiologists and cardiologists at their institutions. These solutions, although creative, are fraught with the dangers inherent in any nonformalized training experience. When interviewed, future trainees frequently inquire about the ability to receive a formal endovascular experience as part of the fellowship.

Criteria for Training Programs

Acceptance of the premise that endovascular surgery training is an important component of vascular surgical education generates a series of difficult questions: (1) What should be taught? (2) How much should be taught? (3) Who should teach it? Clear answers to these and related questions are difficult because of the rapidly changing and evolving nature of endovascular technology and the multidisciplinary interest in patients with conditions amenable to this approach.

What Should Be Taught?

The elements of what should be taught have been thoughtfully summarized elsewhere.[4,5]

TABLE 3–1. Number of Procedures Required for Credentialing

Procedure	SCVIR	SCAI	ACC[a]	AHA[a]	SVS/ISCVS[a]
Catheterizations	200	100/50[b]	100	100	100/50[b]
Interventions	25	50/25[b]	50	50/25[b]	50/25[b]
Live demonstration	Yes	Yes	Yes	Yes	Yes

From White RA, Hodgson KJ, Ahn SS et al: Endovascular interventions training and credentialing for vascular surgeons, J Vasc Surg 1999; 29(1):177–186.
SCVIR, Society of Cardiovascular and Interventional Radiology; SCAI, Society for Cardiac Angiography and Interventions; ACC, American College of Cardiology; AHA, American Heart Association; SVS/ISCVS, Society for Vascular Surgery/International Society for Cardiovascular Surgery.
[a] Includes knowledge of thrombolytic therapy.
[b] As primary interventionalist.

Because the vascular surgical trainee has completed a residency in general surgery, is currently undergoing intensive training in the medical and surgical management of vascular disease, and may have different goals for application of endovascular techniques, the training experience is vastly different from that of interventional radiology. In most instances the goal of the vascular surgeon is to use these techniques as *adjunctive* measures to *complement*, not replace, surgical therapy.

Percutaneous arterial puncture for introduction of guidewires, catheters, and devices should represent no impediment to vascular surgical trainees. The Seldinger technique for percutaneous cannulation of vessels is commonly employed by both radiologists and cardiologists, who perform most of their procedures through the femoral or axillary arteries. General surgery residents have experience with percutaneous placement of femoral or radial arterial catheters for monitoring blood pressure. Furthermore, residents frequently use this method for introducing other devices, such as large venous (subclavian, internal jugular, femoral) catheters for trauma resuscitation, hemodialysis access, hyperalimentation, chemotherapy, central venous and pulmonary artery pressure monitoring, and vena caval filters. Most vascular surgical fellows have significant experience with percutaneous vascular access for catheter introduction and are qualified to perform percutaneous femoral and axillary arterial punctures for endovascular access. A trainee with little or no experience may develop this skill by performing 10 to 15 percutaneous insertions under the guidance of an individual skilled in these techniques.

Radiologic imaging techniques are an important component of endovascular surgical therapy. Most surgeons are familiar with using C-arm fluoroscopic units for placing central venous access catheters and vena caval filters. Although mobile imaging units are generally available in operating rooms, the quality of the images produced by most of these machines is inferior compared to those produced by the fixed, high-resolution, image-enhanced systems that are currently used in most interventional radiology and cardiology suites. Despite this shortcoming, the newest generation of digital C-arm fluoroscopy units have overcome many previous limitations. With these high quality mobile units that incorporate freeze-frame and road mapping technology, successful and reproducible results with endovascular procedures are consistently obtainable.[6] Although this equipment is not available in all operating rooms at present, it is likely that this situation will change with the increasing use of endovascular devices that require open, surgical access from a peripheral site. It is highly desirable that trainees learn how to use sophisticated imaging systems and be completely trained in radiation safety guidelines. This should not be a major obstacle to obtaining endovascular training and could be easily incorporated into the curriculum by developing a liaison with interventional radiologists or cardiologists, who are in charge of this equipment in most institutions.

Most vascular surgical training programs place appropriate emphasis on the importance of correct interpretation of angiograms, and trainees in vascular surgery should be fully competent in this area. Although few training programs incorporate percutaneous diagnostic angiography in their formal training, all trainees should be able to perform angiography competently in the operating room in order to evaluate reconstructive procedures. The Ad Hoc Committee on Endovascular Surgery Credentialing and Training for Vascular Surgeons has recommended that at least 100 catheterizations be documented to meet the requirements for credentialing.[5] This experience can be partially obtained in the operating room during open vascular surgical procedures, but the need to learn percutaneous arterial cannulation cannot be overly emphasized.

Complete knowledge of the pharmacology and toxicity of angiographic contrast agents is important. Vascular surgical trainees should already be familiar with these issues because of experience managing patients who have had adverse reactions to such agents. Knowledge of radiation safety and x-ray exposure are also important to incorporate into formal training. These guidelines are readily obtainable because individual institutional policies are in place to comply with state licensing requirements for controlling and monitoring radiation safety.

Training in guidewire placement has an essential role in endovascular interventions because guidewires constitute the main method to safely introduce, position, and manipulate endovascular devices. Safe positioning of guidewires requires finely developed technical skills and expertise in imaging. Most trainees have developed some of these skills through their familiarity with placing venous catheters and related devices. However, a higher level of competence is required to perform guidewire cannulation of selected branch vessels and to pass wires across tightly stenotic or occluded lesions without causing perforation or dissection. These skills can be incorporated into a formal training program with appropriate supervision in the operating room or the angiography suite. In addition, models have been developed to simulate diseased arteries, allowing the trainee to learn guidewire manipulation in a stress-free environment. Because vascular surgical trainees have extensive knowledge of the physical characteristics of atherosclerotic and occlusive lesions encountered during their operative experience and so presumably are technically proficient, guidewire skills can be rapidly acquired. Knowledge regarding the various types of guidewires and information about their physical properties is easily obtained through individual instruction, didactic lectures, hands-on symposia, and available literature.

Training with specific devices and procedures varies with each institution's experience in evolving technologies, patient populations, and the preferences and expertise of the instructors. Of the currently available devices and techniques, balloon angioplasty with or without stent placement is considered the standard for comparing other devices. As shown in Table 3-1, other specialties have defined their credentialing criteria as they relate to interventions that may include balloon dilation, stent placement, or both. Many surgeons have become highly skilled in the use of balloon dilation with or without stent placement in conjunction with open surgical procedures. The Society for Vascular Surgery/International Society for Cardiovascular Surgery (SVS/ISCVS) Ad Hoc Committee on Credentialing and Training for Vascular Surgeons has recommended that 50 balloon dilations be documented as a minimum standard for credentialing in endovascular surgery.[5] Many other devices have been or will be developed, but balloon dilation remains the most widely accepted procedure and should continue to be the prototype for training. *Intraoperative* balloon dilation performed on appropriate lesions and for the proper indications probably represents the easiest method by which vascular surgeons can teach vascular surgical trainees in most institutions. Finally, the trainee must have reasonable experience with the use of stents in both the arterial and venous positions. The use of stents to treat arterial occlusive disease has grown so rapidly they are often applied in areas without proven scientific benefit. Experience with the use of stents can also be obtained in the operating room setting. The early-generation mobile imaging systems make accurate intraoperative stent deployment challenging. In addition, a new group of "stent-related" complications have been described (both during and following the procedure), and the trainee must be able to recognize and treat them.[7,8]

How Much Should Be Taught?

The next issue is **how much to teach**. This question is clearly the most sensitive because it raises the specter of "turf wars" with interventional radiologists, cardiologists, and vascular medicine specialists. The goal of training should not be to transform vascular surgeons into interventional radiologists or attempt to replace radiologists. Most vascular surgeons involved in placing endoluminal prostheses readily admit that close collaboration with interventional radiologist colleagues is necessary for the successful deployment of these devices. Adjunctive balloon angioplasty, stent placement, and other creative catheter or guidewire manipulations are often necessary to achieve satisfactory positioning, smooth luminal contours, and tightly sealed junctions with the native vessel. These skills are clearly beyond the entry level of many surgeons interested in this discipline. However, intimate knowledge of the potential variation in atherosclerotic and degenerative lesions, the vascular exposure required for placement of endoluminal prostheses, and the ability to deal with immediate and long-term complications resulting in conversion to an open surgical procedure remain important knowledge and skills possessed only by competent vascular surgeons.[5] Furthermore, these procedures are currently performed under general anesthesia with full invasive monitoring. Many of these procedures have proven to be long, are complicated, and are associated with major blood loss.

These considerations, along with the potential for immediate life- and limb-threatening complications, continue to mandate principal involvement by a competent vascular surgical team. Endoluminal placement of vascular prostheses, by necessity, involves a close, collaborative relationship between vascular surgeons and interventional radiologists. Therefore the goal of training for vascular surgeons should be to become fully competent to participate successfully in this collaboration. To this end, the skills detailed above are an absolute necessity. A secondary goal would be to give the trainee competence to successfully carry out combined procedures, such as intraoperative balloon angioplasty with stent placement complemented by infrainguinal bypass. If vascular surgeons trained in endovascular techniques restrict their activities to these areas, there should be no turf issues with other specialists.

Who Should Teach?

The final issue relates to who should teach endovascular techniques to vascular surgical trainees. In the context of a training program, the individual who teaches endovascular techniques should be an experienced vascular surgeon or interventionalist—optimally both. Ideally, vascular surgeons teach the trainees. According to a recent poll from the Association of Program Directors in Vascular Surgery, this clearly was the case in 80% of the programs where endovascular techniques were formally taught.[3] However, in many instances, teachers of vascular surgery do not possess the requisite skills to be competent instructors. In these situations a formal rotation during fellowship on the interventional and diagnostic angiography service is the most desirable alternative. The amount of "hands-on" experience would likely be variable, but the trainee would at least obtain knowledge of the fundamentals to carry to the operating room.

Invitations to interventional radiologists to come to the operating room and participate in combined procedures is a good way to encourage their involvement in an environment controlled by a vascular surgeon. This experience in cross-fertilization obviates the crude approach of "See one, do one, teach one!" To further encourage involvement with interventional radiologists, a reciprocal offer could be made whereby the interventional radiology trainee could rotate on the vascular surgery service or noninvasive vascular laboratory to gain more in-depth knowledge of vascular disease.

Another method of obtaining this training is to have the vascular surgery trainee rotate on a cardiac catheterization service. Although this solution is less than ideal because the interventions are different for the coronary circulation, the trainee would at least gain experience in the Seldinger technique of femoral artery puncture, radiation safety procedures, and some catheter and guidewire skills. The length of rotations on the interventional radiology and cardiology services would have to be defined according to the experience available at individual institutions, but 6 to 8 weeks seems to be the interval being applied in most situations.

Sadly, local politics and turf issues preclude successful implementation of endovascular surgery training in many institutions. This was clearly the case for a significant proportion of respondents (25%) in the survey conducted by the Association of Program Directors in Vascular Surgery.[3] These program directors simply stated that interventional radiologists and cardiologists were unwilling to train a vascular surgical trainee at their institution. Another reason for not offering endovascular surgery training during fellowship was the perceived lack of cases encountered during a given fellowship at some institutions. This, along with the unwillingness of other specialists to train vascular surgeons, creates a significant problem in many training programs. It is hoped that with time this unfortunate attitude will change. In the meantime other creative solutions are needed.

A potential solution to this problem is to encourage extramural rotations at suitable facilities. Again, the Association of Program Directors in Vascular Surgery has conducted an informal poll to assess the availability of such training situations. The amount, quality, and appropriateness of such training are unknown and remain to be verified. It clearly represents a less than ideal method of obtaining this training, but some possibilities exist for interested program directors. In conjunction with this and other methods of training, there are multiple "hands-on" courses offered by reputable individuals and institutions around the United States, and they are proliferating with increasing frequency. These courses should not constitute the main venue for training, however, as they are by necessity short (2 to 5 days in length) and do not provide the amount of experience necessary to receive credentialing. Unfortunately, these methods offer a short-term remedy to a chronic problem that must be addressed if the vascular surgical trainee is to graduate with the knowledge and appropriate skills required to perform endovascular surgery.

Moore et al. described a futuristic approach to training "the vascular disease specialist."[9] By combining the knowledge and skills of vascular surgery, interventional radiology, and vascular medicine, a new department with a modern training program and novel curriculum would be established. The department would be comprised of four divisions: vascular medicine, vascular surgery, vascular intervention, and vascular imaging.[9] The ultimate goal of such a training program is to have a single category of trainee who would be exposed to all aspects of the diagnosis and treatment of vascular diseases.

Conclusion

Endovascular surgery training should be available to all vascular surgery trainees. According to the Association of Program Directors in Vascular Surgery survey, most programs are currently offering, or plan to offer, endovascular surgery training in the near future. One certainly hears a desire for this training voiced by vascular surgery fellowship applicants and disappointment among former vascular surgery trainees that this program was not more readily available in the past. Despite the enthusiasm for this technology, formal training for vascular fellows is widely variable and should become more standardized. The minimum case load for credentialing standards as published by the SVS/ISCVS Ad Hoc Committee on Endovascular Surgery Credentialing and Training for Vascular Surgeons should be a target for training experience. It is important for program directors and trainees to document and record this experience for future credentialing and, possibly, accreditation purposes.

The mode and manner of obtaining this training as part of the vascular fellowship experience is probably less important than the quality of the training. Continuous experience throughout a 1-year fellowship or an intramural or extramural separate rotation would be equally appropriate. Individuals teaching vascular surgery trainees include vascular surgeons, interventional radiologists, interventional cardiologists, and vascular medicine specialists. The teachers depend on local circumstances and expertise. All are acceptable so long as appropriate indications are followed and outcomes are carefully monitored.

The education of vascular surgeons who successfully complete training but have had no exposure to endovascular cases during their fellowship remains a significant problem. It is hoped that as more vascular surgery training programs develop liaisons with interventional radiologists teaching programs in endovascular surgery will become more widespread and training will become available to former fellows. The availability of postgraduate training programs will undoubtedly parallel the growth, development, and commercial success of endoluminal prostheses for the treatment of aortic aneurysms. As this technology advances, one will most likely see a proliferation of courses devoted to this discipline. The situation is analogous to that engendered by the development of laparoscopic cholecystectomy and

4
Assessment of Vascular Patients and Indications for Therapy

Christian de Virgilio

Evaluation of the vascular patient requires a systematic approach that begins with the history and physical examination, generally followed by noninvasive studies to obtain a more quantitative estimation of the degree of vascular compromise. The decision to perform more invasive studies or to proceed to endovascular therapy must be individualized but is dependent in large part on the findings of the history, physical examination, and noninvasive studies. The following sections outline the principles of vascular patient assessment and the indications for endovascular therapy.

History and Physical Examination of the Ischemic Lower Extremity

A thorough history and physical examination are essential components of the assessment of vascular patients. Risk factors for atherosclerosis, such as smoking, diabetes, hyperlipidemia, and familial predisposition, must be identified. Evidence of coronary or cerebrovascular involvement should be sought. In most instances the status of the lower extremity vascular bed can be accurately defined by a carefully obtained history. The site of pathology can be further localized by a diligent physical examination. It is imperative that the examiner determine early whether the patient's complaints represent acute or chronic arterial insufficiency, as this information greatly affects the timing of the intervention.

Chronic Arterial Insufficiency

Patients with chronic arterial insufficiency most often complain of pain in the extremity. The location, character, and duration of the pain provide vital information and help distinguish arterial disease from other causes of extremity pain. The pain of arterial insufficiency takes on one of two forms: intermittent claudication or ischemic rest pain.

Claudication is described as a cramping or aching pain brought on by exercise that is relieved by rest. Thigh and buttock claudication usually signify aortoiliac disease. Associated impotence increases the likelihood of bilateral iliac disease. Isolated calf claudication suggests disease in the superficial femoral artery (SFA), although aortoiliac disease occasionally is the cause. The physical examination helps make the distinction. Patients with aortoiliac disease have diminished femoral pulses and bruits, whereas those with isolated SFA disease have normal femoral pulses and diminished popliteal pulses.

When assessing a patient for possible arterial insufficiency, it is important to remember that other disease processes can mimic claudication. Osteoarthritis of the hip or knee joint can cause similar symptoms, but the pain is not reproducible at a predictable walking distance and not immediately relieved by rest. Osteophytic narrowing of the lumbar canal leading to neurospinal compression can be confused with aortoiliac disease, but the weakness is relieved by leaning over and worsened by increasing lumbar lordosis.

Ischemic rest pain is considered a sign of more advanced arterial insufficiency. It usually occurs at night, involves the foot, and is relieved by placing the foot in a dependent position. It is sometimes confused with the burning discomfort of diabetic neuropathy, though the latter is not relieved by dependency.

Other signs of severe arterial ischemia should be sought. Calf muscle atrophy, loss of hair, atrophy of the skin, skin appendages, and subcutaneous tissue are indicative of advanced ischemia. The skin takes on a shiny, scaly appearance. The finding of severe pallor on leg elevation followed by a deep rubor on dependency (Buerger's sign) further supports severe ischemia.[1]

Acute Arterial Insufficiency

The presentation of acute arterial insufficiency is frequently dramatic. Sudden onset of severe extremity pain, pallor, and pulselessness may progress to paresthesia and paralysis (the five Ps). All five Ps are not necessarily present, however, so they cannot be used to grade the severity of the ischemia.

Three categories of severity of acute lower extremity ischemia have been adopted by the Society for Vascular Surgery/International Society for Cardiovascular Surgery (SVS/ISCVS) committee on reporting standards: viable, threatened, and irreversible.[2] A *viable* extremity (category I) has no continuing ischemic pain, no neurologic deficit, and adequate skin capillary return; and there are clearly audible Doppler signals in a pedal artery.[2] A *threatened* extremity (category II) has more severe ischemia, but it is still reversible if prompt revascularization is achieved. Arterial Doppler signals are not clearly audible in the foot, though venous signals are present. Category II is further divided into marginally threatened (IIa) and immediately threatened (IIb) ischemia. With *marginally* threatened ischemia, patients may complain of numbness and minimal sensory loss in the toes, without continuous pain.[2] *Immediately* threatened limbs have continuous ischemic pain with detectable loss of sensation above the toes, a continuing lack of all sensation in the toes, any motor loss, or a combination of these factors.[2] Patients with *irreversible* ischemia have profound sensory loss and muscle paralysis extending above the foot. Arterial and venous Doppler signals are absent, as is capillary refill. Muscle rigor or skin marbling may be present. Irreversible ischemia requires major amputation or results in permanent neuromuscular damage regardless of therapy.[2]

It is important to differentiate between embolic and thrombotic causes of acute ischemia, as the etiology of the ischemia may have therapeutic implications. *Embolic* arterial occlusion should be suspected in patients who have no antecedent history of chronic arterial insufficiency. Pulse examination in the uninvolved extremities is often normal. A history of recent myocardial infarction or atrial fibrillation point to a cardiac source of the embolus. Bilateral toe gangrene in the face of good pedal pulses (blue toe syndrome) suggests an aortic source of the embolus: from an aortic aneurysm or an atherosclerotic plaque. *Thrombotic* arterial occlusion occurs most often in the setting of underlying progressive atherosclerosis. Volume depletion or a sudden drop in cardiac output may be contributing factors. The patient often reports a long-standing history of claudication or ischemic rest pain. Physical examination, in addition to the findings of an acutely ischemic extremity, may reveal evidence of diffuse atherosclerosis with diminished pulses and bruits in the uninvolved extremities.

Noninvasive Studies

Following the history and physical examination, noninvasive studies are undertaken to provide a more objective and quantitative assessment of the degree of ischemia. The decision of which noninvasive tests to perform is dictated in part by the acuity and severity of the ischemia. The minimum assessment includes interrogation of the distal artery with

Continuous-Wave Doppler

A great deal of information can be gleaned from the audible signal of a continuous-wave nondirectional, handheld Doppler test. Normal arterial signals are biphasic or triphasic.[3] The first sound corresponds to high-velocity forward flow during systole. The second sound results from reversed flow during early diastole. Flow reversal occurs in high-resistance vascular beds (e.g., normal extremity arteries). Some vessels rely on continuous forward flow during diastole (e.g., internal carotid and renal arteries); and, as such, their resistance is low. The second sound is absent in these arteries. The third sound represents forward flow during late diastole.

In the presence of extremity ischemia peripheral resistance falls, and the second sound disappears. As ischemia worsens, the signal becomes monophasic or absent. According to the SIS/ISCVS criteria for acute ischemia, absent arterial signals correlate with threatened or irreversible ischemia and should prompt an attempt to elicit adjacent venous signals. Inaudible venous signals generally signify irreversible ischemia.

Ankle-Brachial Index and Segmental Pressures

The ankle-brachial index (ABI) is obtained by measuring the highest pressure at the ankle using continuous-wave Doppler and dividing the result by the highest arm pressure. The normal ABI averages 1.1 as the pressure in the ankle is 12 to 24 mm greater than that in the arm in the supine position.[3] If the index is diminished, segmental pressures are measured to further localize the site of obstruction. Segmental pressures are performed by sequentially placing a pneumatic cuff around the upper thigh, above the knee, around the calf, and at the ankle and measuring the pressure at each position. A pressure drop of more than 15 mm Hg from one site to the next suggests that a hemodynamically significant stenosis is present in the artery with the lower pressure.[3]

The ABI determines whether hemodynamically significant arterial disease is present. A normal ABI indicates that significant disease is unlikely. If the ABI is normal and the clinical index of suspicion remains high, the ABI should be repeated following exercise. The increased flow generated by exercise may accentuate the pressure drop across a fixed stenosis. ABI readings of more than 1.2 are also considered abnormal. Medial calcification, as seen in diabetics, results in noncompressible vessels and is one cause of spuriously elevated ankle pressures.

The degree of ABI diminution is related to the severity of the ischemia. The ankle pressure is reduced by at least 10 mm Hg by a single 50% or greater *stenosis* and by 53 mm Hg and 61 mm Hg in the presence of an SFA and iliac *occlusion*, respectively.[3] Pressure drops of more than 50 mm Hg suggest multilevel obstruction. In general, in patients with claudication the ABI is of 0.59 ± 0.15, in patients with rest pain 0.26 ± 0.13, and in patients with gangrene 0.05 ± 0.08.[4] By using the ABI and segmental pressures in combination with the history and physical examination one can determine the level of disease and estimate whether the lesion represents a stenosis or an occlusion. For example, a patient with unilateral thigh claudication, a diminished femoral pulse with a bruit, an ankle pressure of 100 mm Hg, and an arm pressure of 120 mm Hg (ABI 0.83) can be predicted to have an isolated iliac *stenosis*. Conversely, a patient with calf claudication and foot rest pain, absent femoral, popliteal, and pedal pulses, an ankle pressure of 30 mm Hg, and an arm pressure of 120 mm Hg (ABI 0.25) likely has both iliac and SFA *occlusions*.

Digital pressures are a valuable adjunct to the segmental pressure measurements. Digital pressures may enable the examiner to localize arterial disease to the pedal or digital arteries. When evaluating lower extremity ischemia, the digital pressure is particularly useful in diabetics, as medial calcification rarely involves the digital arteries. The normal toe pressure is 24 to 41 mm Hg less than the brachial pressure, and the corresponding normal toe-brachial index is

0.89 ± 0.16.[4] Toe pressures below 30 mm Hg correlate with nonhealing of toe ulcers or amputation sites.[4]

Pulse Volume Recording

The pulse volume recording (PVR) relies on air plethysmography to produce waveforms that correlate with pulsatile arterial flow. The PVR, which can be calibrated to provide a semi-quantitative estimate of the degree of obstruction, is particularly useful in two settings: (1) The toe PVR is helpful for determining the need for revascularization in the diabetic patient with a foot ulcer or gangrene who has a spuriously elevated ABI. The absence of pulsatile arterial flow on a PVR in such a patient indicates severe arterial obstruction. (2) The PVR is a valuable intraoperative tool. Performed immediately before and after an intervention (i.e., bypass, angioplasty) it can detect improvement or deterioration of the pulsatile arterial flow.

Transcutaneous Oximetry

Transcutaneous measurement of the oxygen pressure ($tcPO_2$) is another helpful tool when evaluating severe limb ischemia. The $tcPO_2$ has been used to predict the healing of ischemic ulcers, determine the level of amputation, and predict the success of revascularization postoperatively.[5,6] Like the PVR, $tcPO_2$ is valuable in the diabetic patient with a foot ulcer or gangrene and falsely elevated ankle pressures. One study found that ischemic ulcers were unlikely to heal when $tcPO_2$ measurements in the foot were less than 30 mm Hg.[7] The ulcers healed when the $tcPO_2$ was at least 38 mm Hg.

Duplex Ultrasonography

Duplex ultrasonography combines a real-time, high-resolution image of the vessel wall and lumen with Doppler signal analysis. The ultrasound image localizes the plaque and characterizes its morphology. It may also demonstrate abnormalities such as aneurysm formation, intraluminal thrombus, intraplaque hemorrhage, and dissection (Figures 4–1, 4–2).

Analysis of the Doppler signal includes three components: spectral analysis, velocity waveforms, and color-flow imaging. *Spectral analysis* detects stenoses by identifying abnormalities in blood flow patterns. Stenoses from atherosclerotic plaques interrupt laminar flow and produce more random movements of blood cells.[8] These more random movements create spectra with a wide range of frequencies and amplitudes. Spectral broadening is the term used to describe the resultant wide frequency band. Specific criteria have been established for calculating the percent diameter reduction for carotid and lower extremity lesions based on spectral analysis of pulsed Doppler signals. For carotid stenosis, the criteria are based on the peak systolic frequency, end-diastolic frequency, and degree of spectral broadening.[8] For

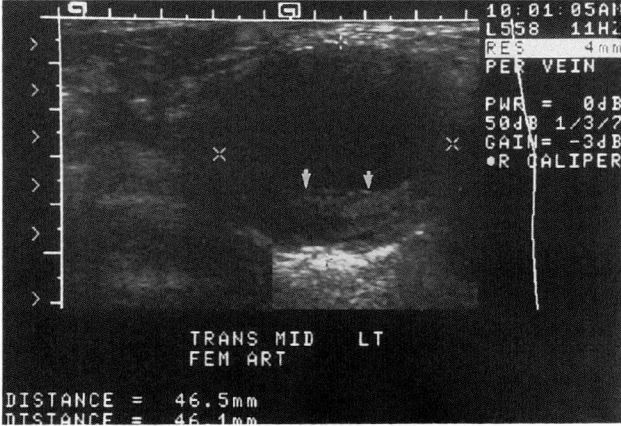

FIGURE 4–1. Ultrasonography of left groin reveals a 4.6 × 4.6 cm common femoral artery aneurysm (*cursors*). Thrombus is visible posteriorly (*arrows*).

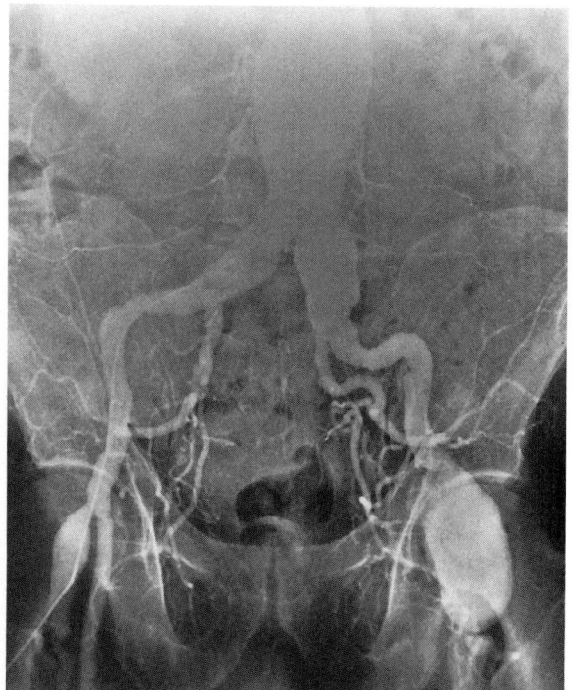

FIGURE 4–2. Aortogram of same patient as in Figure 4–1 demonstrates aneurysmosis. In addition to the left common femoral artery aneurysm, aortic, bilateral common iliac, and right superficial femoral artery aneurysms are present. The classic slow blood flow velocity makes angiographic assessment difficult.

lower extremity stenosis, the velocity waveforms are adjuncts utilized in the analysis. The normal extremity artery has a triphasic waveform that corresponds to the audible Doppler signals previously described. In the presence of an arterial stenosis, peripheral resistance distally decreases, eliminating the flow reversal phase. With severe stenosis, the waveform *distal* to the stenosis becomes monophasic, with a low, rounded peak. The waveform *within* the stenosis, on the other hand, demonstrates a markedly increased peak systolic velocity. *Color-flow* imaging provides flow information of the entire image in real time. The specific information produced by the color includes the direction of flow and an estimate of the mean frequency. Color-flow imaging does not allow as precise calculation of the degree of stenosis as does spectral analysis.[8] The technique is particularly useful when scanning a long length of artery. Color changes that correspond to an increased frequency can be rapidly identified. The examiner can then focus the spectral analysis to that area. Color-flow imaging is also helpful when interrogating deeply located vessels, as the color makes it easy to distinguish vessels from adjacent structures.

In addition to the evaluation of carotid and extremity arteries, duplex ultrasonography is well established for use in the diagnosis of deep venous thrombosis. It is also utilized in the evaluation of renal and mesenteric artery stenosis. More recently, color duplex ultrasonography has been used intraoperatively to assess the adequacy of repair following carotid endarterectomy and of renal and mesenteric revascularization.[9,10] Intraoperative color duplex scanning is especially valuable following transaortic renal endarterectomy, as the distal endpoint is not visualized (Figures 4–3, 4–4). Hemodynamically significant intimal flaps are

FIGURE 4–3. Intraoperative duplex scan shows a 50% diameter stenosis at the origin of the right renal artery (*cursors*).

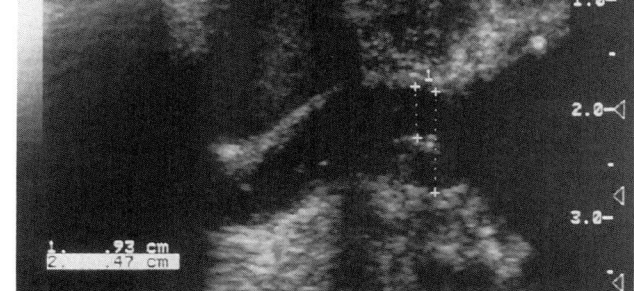

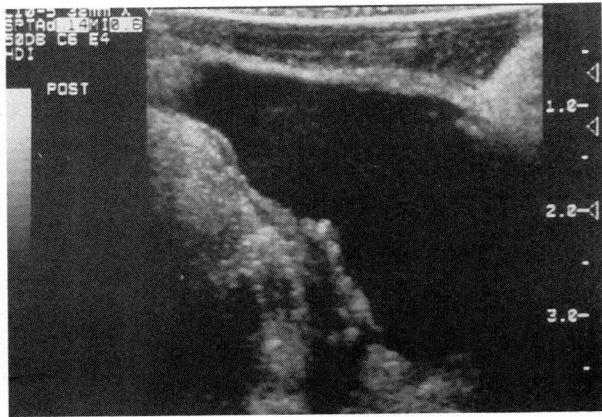

FIGURE 4–4. Intraoperative duplex scan of the renal artery in the same patient as in Figure 4–3 following transaortic renal endarterectomy shows a wide open renal orifice without an intimal flap.

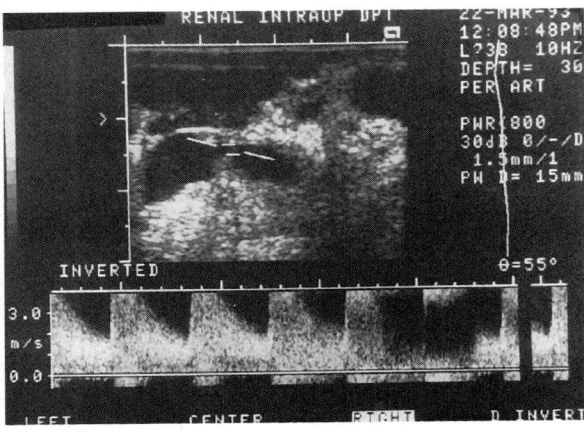

FIGURE 4–5. Intraoperative duplex scan of the renal artery in a different patient following transaortic endarterectomy demonstrates an intimal flap. Markedly elevated velocity (>3.0 m/s) and spectral broadening indicate that the lesion is hemodynamically significant.

readily identified and corrected intraoperatively (Figures 4–5, 4–6).

Computed Tomography

Standard computed tomography (CT) plays a larger role in the assessment of aortic aneurysm than atherosclerotic occlusive disease. The CT scan gives information on aneurysm size, involvement of the renal and iliac arteries, and other unexpected findings, such as horseshoe kidney, retroaortic left renal vein, inferior vena cava duplication, and malignancy (Figures 4–7, 4–8). Detection of a horseshoe kidney on CT should prompt arteriography to define the frequently anomalous renal arteries.[11] (Figure 4–9).

When assessing a patient for possible endoluminal aortic aneurysm repair, CT scanning

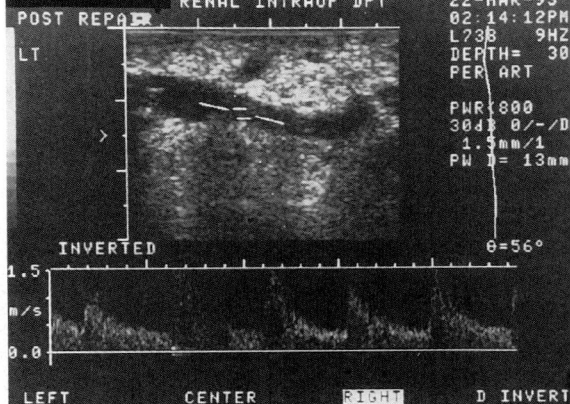

FIGURE 4–6. Intraoperative duplex scan of the same patient as in Figure 4–5 after the intimal flap was repaired. Velocity in the renal artery now approximates aortic velocity.

FIGURE 4–7. Computed tomography demonstrates an aortic aneurysm with a retroaortic left renal vein (*arrows*).

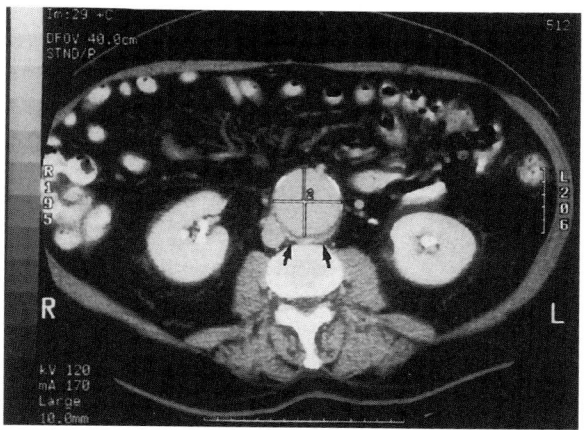

FIGURE 4–8. Computed tomography shows the intraabdominal portion of a thoracoabdominal aneurysm. A horseshoe kidney (*arrows*) is draped anteriorly across the aneurysm. (From de Virgilio C, Gloviczki P, Cherry K et al: Renal artery anomalies in patients with horseshoe or ectopic kidneys: the challenge of aortic reconstruction, *Cardiovasc Surg*, 4:413–420, 1995.)

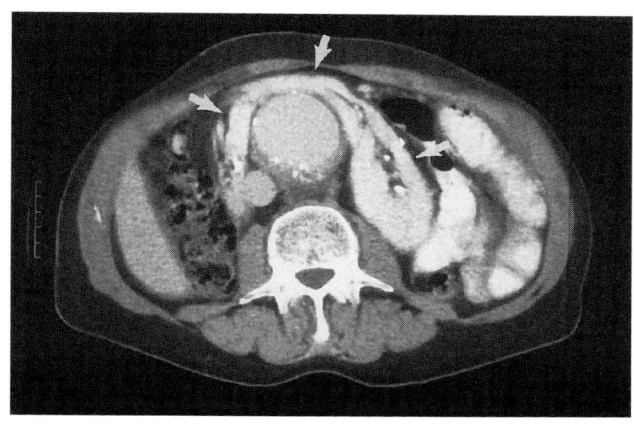

FIGURE 4–9. Aortogram of a different patient with an infrarenal aortic aneurysm demonstrates three renal arteries (*arrows, arrowhead*) supplying the horseshoe kidney. (From de Virgilio C, Gloviczki P, Cherry K et al: Renal artery anomalies in patients with horseshoe and ectopic kidneys: the challenge of aortic reconstruction, *Cardiovasc Surg*, 4:413–420, 1995.)

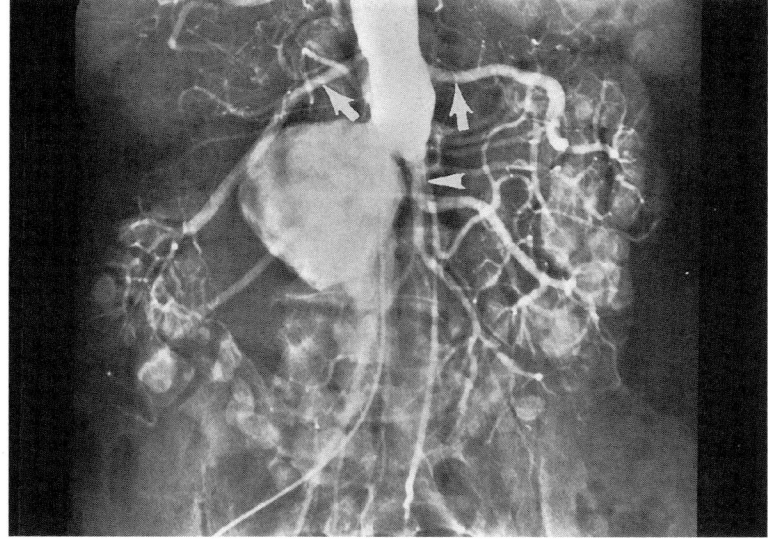

has some limitations. Because the cuts are 5 to 10mm thick, CT is less able than angiography to properly identify the neck of the aneurysm.[12] It is also less able to measure the length and diameter of the proximal aneurysm neck, particularly if the aorta is angulated or tortuous.[12] The precise origins of the renal arteries also can be difficult to localize with CT, and accessory renal arteries are readily missed (Figure 4–10).

Ultrafast CT is an imaging modality that acquires a multilevel sequence of scans within a fraction of a second.[13,14] The entire aorta can be scanned in seconds, thereby minimizing motion artifacts due to patient movement, respiration, and cardiac cycle. The injection of contrast bolus is optimized to improve vascular enhancement via the rapid acquisition technique. Ultrafast CT is ideal for detecting thoracic aneurysms or thoracic aortic dissection. It has also been used to detect intracardiac tumors, assess coronary artery bypass patency, and quantify the degree of native coronary artery calcification.

Spiral CT angiography (CTA) creates three-dimensional images of the aorta and its branches. The advantage of this technique lies in its ability to perform rapid-sequence acquisition and a cross-sectional reconstruction in any plane. Data collected from a single contrast injection can create images in many three-dimensional views. Vessel images are displayed without superimposed overlying structures. Contrast is injected through an antecubital vein, thereby avoiding the risks of arterial puncture associated with standard angiography. Spiral CTA is useful for assessing the abdominal aorta and its branches. It may play a role in evaluating aortic aneurysm and dissection. In aortic aneurysmal disease it can measure the aortic diameter and residual aortic lumen, locate main and accessory renal arteries, and visualize associated stenoses or atheromatous plaques.[15] It has recently been used for assessing the suitability of endovascular repair of aortic aneurysms (discussed in detail in Chapters 23–26). In aortic dissection, spiral CTA can demonstrate the true and false lumens and the perfusion source of the visceral vessels.

Magnetic Resonance Angiography

Magnetic resonance angiography (MRA) is used to evaluate the aorta and the carotid, renal, and lower extremity arteries. MRA forms

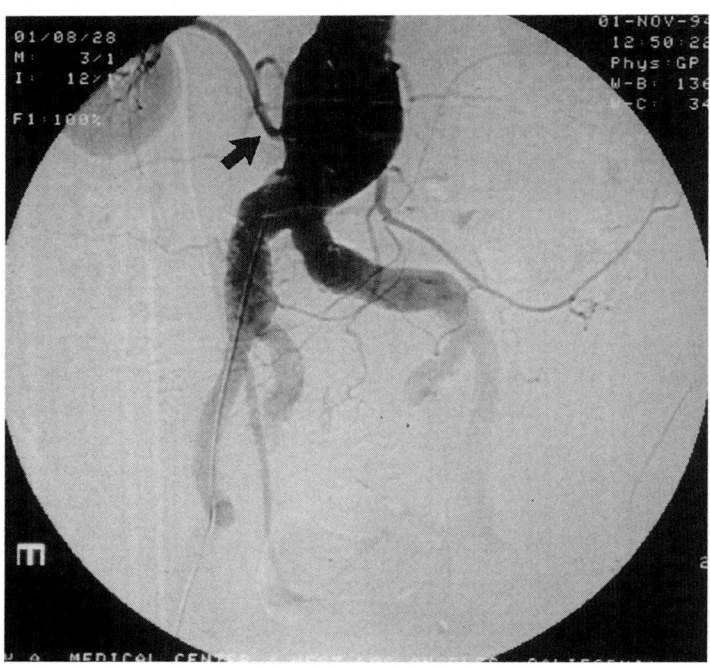

FIGURE 4–10. Aortogram demonstrates an aortic aneurysm with a large anomalous right renal artery (*arrow*) arising from the body of the aneurysm. The anomalous renal artery was not detected on computed tomography.

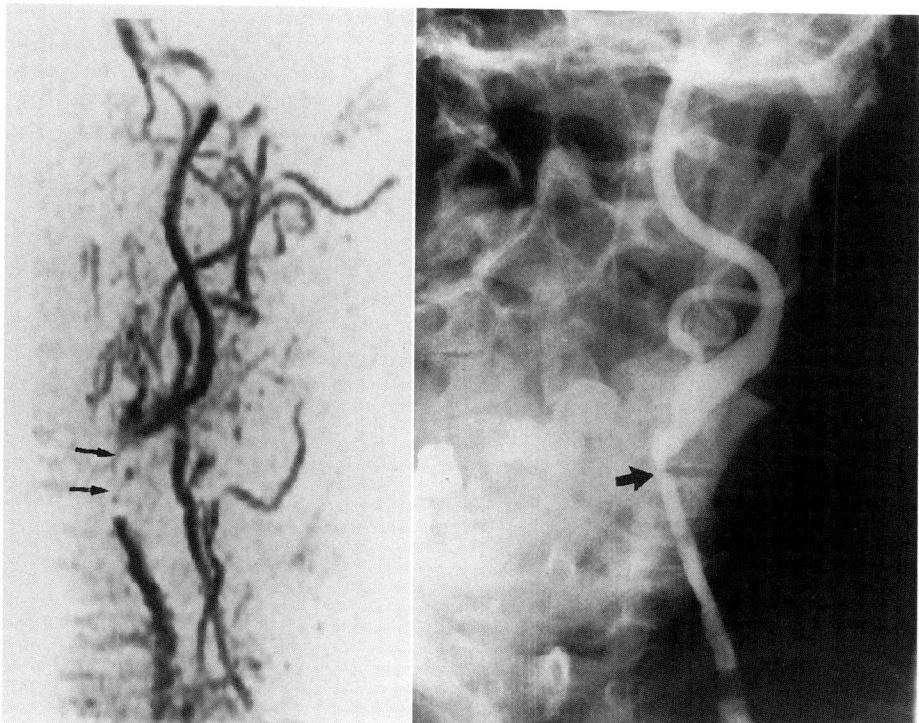

FIGURE 4–11. **A**, Magnetic resonance angiography of the carotid bifurcation demonstrates a signal void in the distal common carotid artery (*arrows*) with distal reconstitution consistent with an occlusion versus a high grade stenosis. **B**, Arteriography revealed a high grade common carotid stenosis (*arrows*).

an image of blood flow based on physical differences between moving and stationary protons. The signal intensity is a reflection of the velocity and flow patterns of moving protons within the bloodstream. An occluded vessel is represented on MRA as an area of signal void. A major advantage of MRA is that it does not require the use of catheters or intravenous contrast. MRA also has several disadvantages. It tends to overestimate the degree of stenosis. A high grade stenosis may create a long signal void on MRA and appear occluded (Figures 4–11, 4–12). Thus MRA has some limitations in the assessment of high grade carotid stenoses, where the distinction between an occluded vessel and a tight stenosis is crucial. MRA may also fail to detect stenoses less than 50%, and it has limited ability to visualize accessory renal arteries or branch renal artery stenosis.

Magnetic resonance angiography has proven useful in several clinical settings. In patients with impaired renal function or contrast allergy, it avoids the use of intravenous contrast. It has been used to detect main renal artery stenosis. In one study, MRA was 100% sensitive and 94% specific for detecting the presence of main renal artery stenoses of more than 50% when compared to standard angiography.[16] However, it has not yet been adopted as the screening test of choice for renovascular hypertension. MRA is also helpful in patients with lower extremity ischemia. Cambria and colleagues observed 98% agreement between MRA and standard angiography in 24 patients with lower extremity occlusive disease; in 6 patients bypass grafts were successfully performed based solely on MRA.[17] In another study, Owens and coworkers detected suitable distal target vessels on MRA in 17% of patients that were not seen on

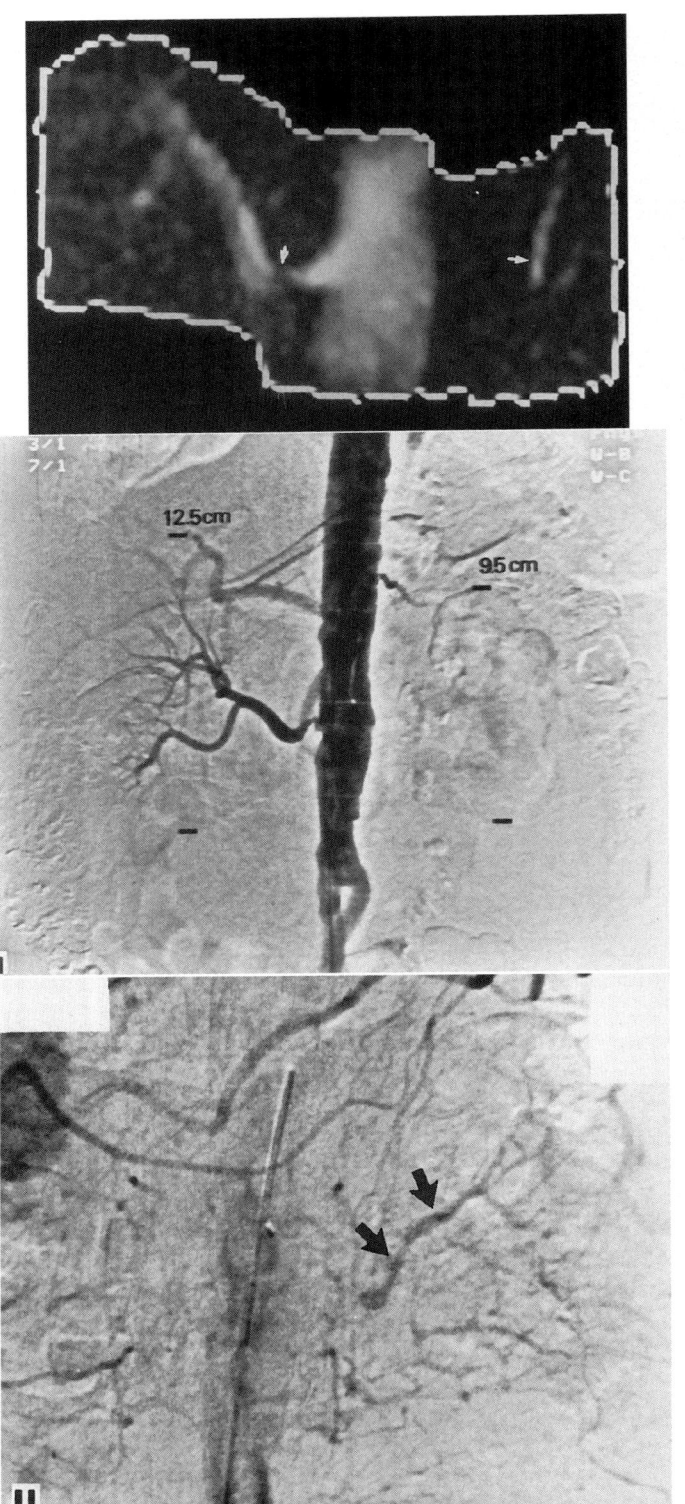

FIGURE 4–12. **A**, Magnetic resonance angiography of the renal arteries demonstrates a long signal void of the left renal artery with a distal renal artery branch reconstitution (*arrow*). A short signal void is seen on the right renal artery (*arrow*). **B**, Arteriography confirmed a left renal artery occlusion and a high grade stenosis of the right renal artery. Measurements indicate the length of the renal parenchyma. **C**, Delayed arteriographic views confirmed distal reconstitution of a left renal artery (*arrows*), which was suitable for bypass.

standard angiography.[18] More recently, Carpenter and associates performed 78 peripheral vascular procedures based on MRA alone; only two minor discrepancies were noted between the preoperative MRA and the intraoperative completion arteriogram.[19]

Patient Selection

Patient selection for endovascular intervention must be individualized. To make a proper decision, multiple factors must be taken into consideration. First, the indication for intervention must be clear to both the patient and the physician. Is the problem acutely limb threatening, chronically life style limiting, or asymptomatic? In general, the indications for intervention in patients with lower extremity atherosclerotic disease include severe life style limiting claudication, ischemic rest pain, nonhealing ulcer, gangrene, and asymptomatic graft stenosis detected on routine postoperative surveillance.

Once the indication is identified, the interventionalist must be aware of the natural history of the problem in order to make an informed decision. One area of great controversy is the role of invasive therapy, if any, in patients with lower extremity claudication *without* limb threat. Various factors have been identified in claudicants that predict disease progression and the eventual need for intervention. Such factors include a history of smoking more than 40 pack-years, a history of diabetes, an initial ankle pressure less than 70 mm Hg, an initial ABI less than 0.5, toe pressure less than 40 mm Hg, and a significant drop in ABI during follow-up.[20] In one series, no patient with an initial ABI of 0.7 or more required amputation over a 6.5-year follow-up.[21]

Life expectancy of the patient and associated co-morbid conditions also comprise essential information. Lower extremity atherosclerosis is a marker for diffuse atherosclerosis. In one study the 5-year mortality in patients with an initial ABI of less than 0.5 was 50%.[22] Most of the deaths were due to myocardial infarction or stroke. Therefore, particular attention should be paid to eliciting signs of concomitant symptomatic coronary and carotid disease. Many patients with claudication cannot perform exercise cardiac testing. Other means of noninvasive cardiac testing should be considered, such as dipyridamole thallium imaging.

Finally, prior to embarking on endovascular intervention the physician must determine how amenable the lesion is to this treatment and the probable long-term outcome. Short-segment stenoses of the common iliac artery are particularly amenable to balloon angioplasty. Such a lesion could be predicted on physical examination by the presence of a diminished femoral pulse with a bruit, although such patients likely suffer only from intermittent claudication, still a controversial indication for treatment. It is important in such a situation that the patient be well informed about the potential risks and benefits.

When planning intervention in patients with ischemic rest pain, a nonhealing ulcer, or gangrene, it must be remembered that they typically have multilevel disease. Thus adequate revascularization may require multiple angioplasties or a combination of angioplasty and surgical bypass. Long segments of diffuse disease and long occlusions are less amenable to angioplasty.

References

1. Rutherford R: Evaluation and selection of patients for vascular surgery. In Rutherford R, editor: *Vascular surgery*, Philadelphia, 1989, Saunders.
2. Rutherford R, Baker JD, Ernst C et al: Recommended standards for reports dealing with lower extremity ischemia: revised version, *J Vasc Surg* 26:517–538, 1997.
3. Sumner D: Objective diagnostic techniques: the role of the vascular laboratory. In Rutherford R, editor: *Vascular surgery*, Philadelphia, 1989, Saunders.
4. Kinney EV, Bandyk DF, Towne JB: The vascular laboratory in clinical care: part I, *Surg Rounds* September: 765–777, 1991.
5. Osmundson PJ, Rooke TW, Hallett JW: Effect of arterial revascularization on transcutaneous oxygen tension of the ischemic extremity, *Mayo Clin Proc* 63:897–902, 1988.
6. White RA, Nolan L, Harley D et al: Noninvasive evaluation of peripheral vascular disease using

transcutaneous oxygen tension, *Am J Surg* 144:68, 1982.
7. Cina C, Kastamouris A, Megerman J et al: Utility of transcutaneous oxygen tension measurements in peripheral arterial occlusive disease, *J Vasc Surg* 1:362–369, 1984.
8. Zierler RE: Physiologic basis of hemodynamic measurement. In White R, Hollier L, editors: *Vascular surgery: basic science and clinical correlations*, Philadelphia, 1994, Lippincott.
9. Dougherty MJ, Hallett JW Jr, Naessens JM et al: Optimizing technical success of renal revascularization: the impact of intraoperative color-flow duplex ultrasonography, *J Vasc Surg* 17:849–857, 1993.
10. Bandyk DF, Mills JL, Gahtan V et al: Intraoperative duplex scanning of arterial reconstructions: fate of repaired and unrepaired defects, *J Vasc Surg* 20:426–433, 1994.
11. De Virgilio C, Gloviczki P, Cherry K et al: Renal artery anomalies in patients with horseshoe and ectopic kidneys: the challenge of aortic reconstruction, *Cardiovasc Surg* 4:413–420, 1995.
12. Donayre C, Ivancev K, White R: Patient selection and preoperative assessment. In Chuter T, Donayre C, White R, editors: *Endoluminal vascular prostheses*, Boston, 1995, Little Brown.
13. Bleiweis MS, Greorgiou D, Milliken JC et al: Ultrafast computed tomography of the heart and great vessels. In Cavaye DM, White RA, editors: *A text and atlas of arterial imaging*, London, Chapman & Hall.
14. Thompson BH, Stanford W: Electron beam computed tomographic imaging of aortic aneurysms and dissections, *J Invas Cardiol* 6:213–227, 1994.
15. Rubin GD, Walker PJ, Dake MD et al: Three-dimensional spiral computed tomographic angiography: an alternative imaging modality for the abdominal aorta and its branches, *J Vasc Surg* 18:656–665, 1993.
16. Farrugia E, King BF, Larson TS: Magnetic resonance angiography and detection of renal artery stenosis in a patient with impaired renal function, *Mayo Clin Proc* 68:157–160, 1993.
17. Cambria R, Yucel E, Brewster D et al: The potential of lower extremity revascularization without contrast arteriography: experience with magnetic resonance angiography, *J Vasc Surg* 17:1050–1057, 1993.
18. Owens R, Carpenter J, Baum R et al: Magnetic resonance imaging of angiographically occult runoff vessels in peripheral occlusive disease, *N Engl J Med* 326:1577–1581, 1992.
19. Carpenter JP, Baum RA, Holland GA et al: Peripheral vascular surgery with magnetic resonance angiography as the sole preoperative imaging modality, *J Vasc Surg* 20:861–871, 1994.
20. Walsh DB, Cronenwett JL: Natural history of atherosclerosis in the lower extremity, carotid, and coronary circulations. In White RA, Hollier LH, editors: *Vascular surgery: basic science and clinical correlations*, Philadelphia, 1994, Lippincott, 1994.
21. Jelnes R, Gaardsting O, Jensen KH et al: Fate in intermittent claudication: outcome and risk factors, *BMJ* 293:1137, 1986.
22. O'Riordan DS, O'Donnell JA: Realistic expectations for the patient with intermittent claudication, *Br J Surg* 78:861, 1991.

5
Establishing an Endovascular Service

Rodney A. White and Thomas J. Fogarty

The components of an idealized endovascular service are described in many areas throughout this text. Although institutions desire to form endovascular services with significant forethought and planning, in most cases they evolve based on the expertise of individual clinicians who have an interest in adapting newer treatment methods to specific illnesses that occur in the particular patient population. In many cases, this may have occurred as interventional radiologists applied their diagnostic imaging and catheter-based skills to the percutaneous treatment of vascular lesions. In addition, peripheral endovascular methods have been applied by surgeons who have maintained their diagnostic radiographic skills and began to use endovascular methods as techniques evolved. Cardiologists also treat peripheral vascular lesions. They use the peripheral vessels to improve access for cardiac interventions or as a part of a combined peripheral and coronary intervention.

Each subspecialty has specialized skills that influence the efficacy and safe utility of endovascular methods, with the idealized endovascular specialist being an individual who has extensive knowledge of both catheter-based interventional methods and surgical techniques. The future vascular specialist may be trained in all of these areas. Many institutions are assessing the need for endovascular training and are evaluating the optimal way to accomplish this goal. In the interim, practicing physicians in various subspecialties will be modifying their practice to accommodate the use of endovascular surgical methods. This entails establishing methods to provide training and facilities for application of the methods in an environment that maximizes involvement of appropriate subspecialties. The role of individuals will vary from institution to institution, depending on the particular expertise of those involved and the institutional capabilities to accommodate to the new methods.

The key to establishing an endovascular service in a particular institution relies on assessing multiple variables, including the needs of the patient population being served, the expertise of individual vascular subspecialists within the institution, and the adequacy of facilities and equipment to accommodate the procedures. The ideal way to establish an endovascular service is to establish an agreement among the involved subspecialties (i.e., vascular surgeons, interventional radiologists, and cardiologists) to determine the optimal location to perform the procedures. Because each interventional group has its own procedure suite, the choice of facility obviously depends on the adequacy of each facility, the complexity and potential risk of procedures, the expertise of the physicians, and the determination of the interventional specialist who will head the endovascular team. The cost of upgrading and redesigning existing suites or the creation of a new facility will in large part determine the location.

Endovascular Physicians

Although the organization of the endovascular team will be determined by the expertise and interest of various subspecialties and the qualities of interventional facilities, two types of clinical skills are required. Interventional catheter-based manipulation and imaging skills are needed for both diagnostic and therapeutic interventions, and surgical skills are required to help determine the indications for endovascular therapy compared with conventional surgical treatment. Surgical expertise is also needed to treat possible complications of endovascular mishaps that may require either emergent or elective surgical correction. A combination of interventional catheter skills and diagnostic skills might be provided by an appropriately trained cardiovascular or vascular surgeon, although currently the usual scenario in most settings is that the endovascular team consists of both interventional radiologist(s) and/or cardiologist(s) and vascular surgeon(s). Although some institutions have been unable to address the development of a service because of either facility constraints or political controversies among the subspecialties, many hospitals are developing congenial arrangements that fulfill the needs of all involved parties.

Several guidelines have been proposed addressing the credentialing and training for various subspecialists to perform endovascular interventions; there are many points of agreement regarding the essentials for safe application of the technologies.[1-6] Although there are points of disagreement in these documents, ongoing conversations among the involved interventional groups are resolving the remaining issues and delineating mechanisms for addressing controversial areas for establishing an endovascular service in various types of institutional environments. The essentials of establishing an effective environment are those that stimulate the training, credentialing, and practice for the idealized vascular specialist of the future and those that provide facilities that accommodate the needs of the endovascular team.

Endovascular Facilities

Facilities and equipment for endovascular suites are addressed in more detail in other chapters. The important aspects of these topics that are relevant to establishing an endovascular service relate to identifying the facilities that have adequate imaging and interventional capabilities to perform the therapeutic procedures. The initial facility may be a prototype interventional suite that is used during the organizational phase of developing the endovascular service. This facility might later be upgraded, or a new facility may be established as a second stage once the direction and make-up of the endovascular team has been constituted.

If the endovascular efforts are to be focused on conventional catheter-based methods such as balloon angioplasty, conventional radiographic and cardiology catheterization suites are both adequate to perform these interventions. If more sophisticated procedures requiring either the intraluminal introduction of larger devices through surgical incisions or the insertion of implantable prostheses such as intraluminal grafts are to be performed, then facilities that are built to accommodate sterile procedures and conversion to emergency surgical interventions are required.[7] Currently, most interventional suites do not have this capability. Conversion of an operating room by acquiring appropriate imaging equipment satisfies the need for sterility and enables conversion to an open surgical procedure when required. The other alternative is to modify existing interventional rooms to meet these needs. Obviously, specialized facilities built within or adjacent to the operating room best accommodate this need, although very few institutions presently have this potential. Figure 5–1 illustrates a special procedure suite that combines the imaging requirements of a high-quality mobile cinefluoroscopy unit, carbon fiber table, and sterile room environment with full anesthesia capabilities.

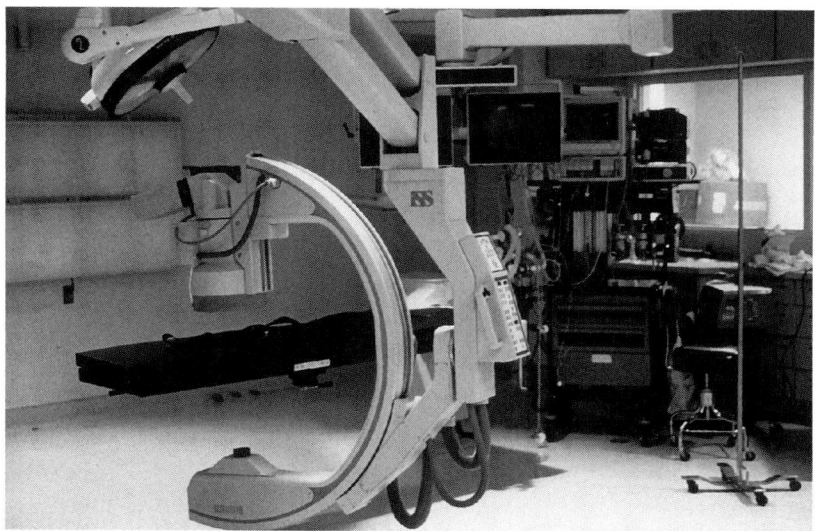

FIGURE 5–1. Endovascular interventional procedure suite that combines high-quality mobile cinefluoroscopy with a sterile environment and full anesthesia service.

Selection and Quality Assurance of Endovascular Procedure

In the current environment, the endovascular specialist needs skills that are a combination of those acquired in several subspecialty training environments. The most effective approach is to base the endovascular service on the combined clinical diagnostic and therapeutic skills of all involved subspecialties and to determine the appropriateness for interventions based on decisions made during a regularly scheduled endovascular conference. This format should be used to assess and plan diagnostic strategies for patients, interpret the outcomes of diagnostic studies, and use this information to determine the most appropriate form of therapy. The sessions are also extremely important for demonstrating the results of chosen modalities, reporting long-term follow-up, and determining outcome assessment parameters. The conference can be used to identify limitations and indications of established and developing therapies and to identify issues that are appropriate for future quality assurance evaluations. In this manner, all appropriate parties are involved in determining the efficacy of therapy and for reviewing cases that may require interventions if complications occur during the treatment.

Endovascular Suite Operational Considerations

Several considerations are integral to developing appropriate operational plans for an endovascular suite. These include the issues listed in Box 5–1. Although many of these are addressed in various sections of this text, several are pertinent to establishing an endovascular service and are reviewed in this discussion.

Scope of Service

The scope of services in the endovascular suite will be determined by the type of available equipment and facilities and the expertise of the interventional physicians. In many institutions, the use of procedures such as balloon dilation, thrombectomy, and administration of thrombolytic agents is currently performed to varying degrees in both interventional radiology and cardiology suites and in operating

> **Box 5–1. Endovascular Suite Operational Plans**
>
> - Scope of services
> - Patient scheduling and hours of operation
> - Preprocedure patient selection and preparation
> - Patient monitoring during procedures
> - Postprocedure recovery mechanisms
> - Equipment and supplies (inventory control)
> - Staff
>   - Nurses
>   - X-ray technicians
>   - Anesthetists
>   - Interventional physicians
> - Staff inservice
>   - Procedure protocols
>   - Emergency procedures
> - Patient follow-up monitoring and quality assessment

Patient Scheduling and Hours of Service

Patient scheduling and available hours for endovascular services will be determined by the facilities being used in a particular institution and the scope of available procedures. For institutions equipped with facilities that can accommodate the variety of options that have been described, including those requiring a sterile environment and vascular surgical involvement, no further consideration is required. On the other hand, major considerations are involved when the scope of procedures to be performed are being increased and require either major renovations or establishing new collaborative arrangements between subspecialty services. In this situation, the availability of support staff and facility scheduling options may be factors limiting the hours of availability.

Patient Selection, Procedural Considerations, and Recovery Mechanisms

Patients amenable to endovascular therapy present by one of two mechanisms. Outpatients who have been selected using conventional criteria can be admitted the day of the procedure. Other candidates for endovascular treatment are identified from the inpatient services.

Preinterventional screening includes the diagnostic evaluation, physical examinations, and imaging evaluations described in other areas in this text. Additional preinterventional evaluation including blood chemistries, hematology, and coagulation factors are essential in either outpatient or inpatient settings.

During the procedures, monitoring is determined by the level of anesthesia required to perform the procedure. Conscious sedation protocols can be used for many percutaneous interventions, although anesthesia standby or administration of regional or general anesthesia is required for some of the more advanced endovascular interventions such as the insertion of endoluminal prostheses. In more advanced cases, where a sterile field is

rooms. Application of other endovascular techniques such as vena cava filter placements, atherectomy procedures, and stent deployment are reserved to areas with high-quality imaging systems (i.e., cinefluoroscopy, intravascular ultrasound, and/or angioscopy) used by skilled interventionists interested in offering a broad spectrum of services.

Future endovascular practices will require an amalgamation of conventional facilities and physician skills. Evolving complex procedures using implantable devices such as endoluminal prostheses require not only high-resolution imaging but also a sterile environment and physicians with sophisticated catheter skills, vascular surgical judgment, and operative expertise. Each institution must address the considerations regarding the scope of services to not only establish an endovascular service but also incorporate evolving methods in an effective and safe manner.

required and the patients are prepped for potential emergent surgical interventions, the role of anesthesia for preoperative, intraoperative, and postoperative care and monitoring is mandatory.

After performance of the endovascular procedure, recovery may be accomplished in an outpatient recovery area if the patients are to be discharged home after recovery. Alternatively, the patients are returned to a conventional postoperative recovery area before returning to their hospital beds.

Equipment and Supplies

Equipment and supplies for an endovascular suite should be identified by a separate hospital code for purchasing and inventory analysis. By this mechanism one can assess the cost efficacy of procedures and assure availability of supplies that are needed for interventions. Many endovascular devices such as balloon catheters and guidewires have special indications that are not easily accomplished using another device. For this reason, it is usually wise to order supplies in pairs and to have an inventory mechanism that accurately tracks and replaces consumables.

Other issues regarding the purchasing, maintenance, and safety issues of endovascular devices are discussed extensively in other chapters in this text. A complete appraisal of the needs of a particular institution are obviously determined by local institutional resources and needs.

Endovascular Procedure Room Staffing

Staff requirements for an endovascular suite will depend on the evolution of new services, particularly those that may require an environment that assimilates sterile procedures, such as an operating room. In this case, nursing and anesthesia staff have an integral role in assuring appropriate preparation and setup of instruments, for preparing the interventional environment, and for preoperative and postoperative care and monitoring the patient. For conventional endovascular therapies such as balloon angioplasty that are performed using local anesthesia, no personnel or monitoring beyond that which is usually available is required. For more complex procedures, the additional personnel requirements should be anticipated.

All individuals involved in endovascular procedures should be fully informed regarding endovascular concepts with regular inservice conferences that update new techniques and methods. Broad-based comprehensive educational activities are required to ensure ongoing quality function of the service.

Patient Follow-up, Monitoring, and Quality Assessment

Postprocedural assessment of interventions is needed on a routine basis and should be assessed and recorded using recommended standards.[8] Quality assessment of performance should be reviewed weekly at the interventional conference, with complications referred for quality assurance review by the department supervising endovascular procedures.

References

1. String ST, Brener BJ, Ehrenfeld WK et al: Interventional procedures for the treatment of vascular disease: recommendations regarding quality assurance, development, credentialing criterion, and education, *J Vasc Surg* 9:736–739, 1989.
2. White RA, Hodgson KJ, Ahn SS et al: Endovascular interventions training and credentialing for vascular surgeons, *J Vasc Surg* (in press).
3. Spies JB, Bakal CW, Burke DR et al: Guidelines for percutaneous transluminal angioplasty, *Radiology* 177:619–626, 1990.
4. Spittell JA, Creager MA, Dorros G et al: Recommendations for peripheral transluminal angioplasty: training and facilities, *J Am Coll Cardiol* 21:546–548, 1993.
5. Wexler L, Dorros G, Levin DC et al: Guidelines for performance of peripheral percutaneous transluminal angioplasty, *Cathet Cardiovasc Diagn* 2:128–129, 1990.
6. Levin DC, Becker GJ, Dorros G et al: Training standards for physicians performing peripheral angioplasty and other percutaneous peripheral vascular interventions, *Circulation* 86:1348–1350, 1992.

7. Veith FJ, Abbott WM, Yao JST et al: Guidelines for development and use of transluminally placed endovascular prosthetic grafts in the arterial system, *J Vasc Surg* 21:670–685, 1995.

8. Ahn S, Rutherford R, Becker G et al: Reporting standards for lower extremity arterial endovascular procedures, *J Vasc Surg* 17:1103–1107, 1993.

6
Anesthesia for Endovascular Procedures

Daniel F. Grum

The field of cardiovascular anesthesiology is well established, with dedicated specialists, extra-year fellowship programs to provide subspecialty training, its own national specialty society, and a variety of specialty textbooks for reference. The practice of cardiovascular anesthesiology has centered around intraoperative general anesthetic management and intensive care of the vascular patient. The emerging multidisciplinary field of endovascular therapy brings different requirements to this practice. Anesthesiologists now must recognize the distinct logistic and clinical requirements that distinguish the inpatient cardiovascular surgical patient from the endovascular outpatient, since many of the latter will be able to undergo procedures requiring only pain management with monitored anesthesia care. Analgesic management differs from anesthesia, which modifies or suspends a variety of normal physiologic functions and carries risks and complications, necessitating additional effort and expense to avoid these unwanted effects. Recent advances in management of analgesia and sedation have made preservation of normal physiologic function in the operating room possible through the control of pain. This management will find appropriate application during endovascular procedures. The distinction will take advantage of the anesthesiologist's consultative pain management skills and may eventually limit administration of anesthesia to operative surgical procedures.

This chapter includes a review of the pharmacology of both new and accepted drugs in cardiovascular anesthesia. Operative cardiovascular anesthesia is reviewed from the point of local sedation, regional, and general anesthesia. The principles by which each may be satisfactorily accomplished are discussed. Risk management, preoperative preparation of the patient, and contemporary concepts of continuous quality improvement are critically assessed. The implications of these factors as they relate to the organization and management of an endovascular service are also briefly presented.

Pharmacology of Endovascular Analgesia and Anesthesia

Drugs administered to the endovascular patient to provide analgesia, sedation, or anesthesia often have profound effects on the cardiovascular system directly and through interaction with chronically and acutely administered cardiovascular agents. Therapeutic strategy must be individualized with consideration for these effects.

Analgesic and Anesthetic Agents and Adjuvants

Premedicants

Although an anticholinergic agent is not usually given as a premedicant to cardiovascular patients, specific indications such as the need to decrease bronchial secretions during awake fiberoptic intubation do arise. The unpredictable increase in heart rate, especially with administration of atropine, is the major adverse side effect. Because of the potential for hallucinations and delerium, there is little reason to recommend scopolamine alone as a sedative. However, its combination with morphine is still a widely used premedicant for vascular patients. Glycopyrrolate, a quaternary ammonium compound that has little penetration of the blood-brain barrier, will not affect the level of consciousness, raises heart rate much less than does atropine or scopolamine, and is an adequate antisialagogue. Anticholinergics reduce lower esophageal sphincter tone and may therefore increase the possibility for gastric reflux. They do not affect either gastric volume or pH. The H_2 receptor antagonists, cimetidine, ranitidine, and famotidine, all decrease gastric volume and increase pH. The risk of aspiration is best reduced when one of them is used before anesthetic induction in combination with metoclopramide, which promotes gastric emptying. This produces results superior to using oral sodium citrate (Bicitra) with or without intravenous (IV) metoclopramide. Although cimetidine decreases activity of P-450 mixed function oxidases and decreases hepatic blood flow, any effect on drug metabolism is seldom clinically important.

Tranquilizers

Diazepam is used less frequently than in prior decades because of its prolonged action, pain upon IV injection, its painful and unpredictable absorption, and slow onset of action from intramuscular sites. A potential advantage of diazepam is a nitroglycerin-like effect on patients with coronary artery disease.[1] Lorazepam has a long terminal elimination half-life, and its long duration of action can be a disadvantage. Midazolam has the shortest elimination half-life, its anxiolytic effects dissipating in about 60 minutes. Its pharmacokinetics are unaffected by age, but as with other benzodiazepines the dose should be reduced in the elderly because of apparent age-related effects on pharmacodynamics. It is particularly suitable for short procedures but must be supplemented by a narcotic to attenuate hemodynamic alterations to stress. Attention to timing of administration is important. Small IV sedative doses of either midazolam (0.05 mg/kg) or diazepam (10 to 12 mg total) have insignificant hemodynamic effects, but both produce significant decreases of mean arterial pressure (MAP) and systemic vascular resistance (SVR) when given to patients receiving fentanyl.[2] Flumazenil, a benzodiazepine antagonist, has been used (0.24 ± 0.10 mg) to reverse diazepam sedation (mean 11.4 ± 4.4 mg) in cardiac catheterization patients without significant alteration in hemodynamic or ventilatory parameters.[3] Rapid distribution coupled with a high rate of extraction by the liver contribute to a relatively short duration of action. Hence, one must be aware of the possible need for repeat dosage. The butyrophenone droperidol has anxiolytic and antiemetic properties and stimulates hypoxic ventilatory drive.[4] However, it may potentiate the ventilatory depressant effect of other sedatives and narcotics, and a significant percentage of patients may experience dysphoria. Nonanesthesiologists frequently order the antihistamines promethazine (Phenergan) or hydroxyzine (Vistaril) as a premedicant. Antihistamines potentiate the action of other drugs with sedative properties, have relatively long durations of action, cause greater irritation at the injection site than alternative agents mentioned above, have inferior anxiolytic, amnestic, and sedative properties compared with midazolam,[5] and do not prevent nausea and vomiting. Therefore there is little to recommend their use.

Analgesics

Hemodynamic effects of typical premedicant doses of morphine are usually minimal in the supine patient. Onset after IV administration is in 5 to 10 minutes, peak action occurs in 15 to 30 minutes, and duration persists for 4 to 6 hours. Because morphine causes vasodilation of both resistance and capacitance vessels, even modest doses can produce orthostatic hypotension.[6] This is worsened by acute and chronic hypovolemia. Hypotension can also be produced by histamine release. Its central depressant effect is readily potentiated by other sedatives. It is inadequate as an anesthetic in relatively healthy patients and promotes increased blood loss and increased fluid requirements.

Fentanyl (Sublimaze), a potent synthetic opioid, has a rapid onset and short duration of action and causes little depression of myocardial contractility or change in SVR or pulmonary vascular resistance (PVR). It is commonly used with sedatives as an adjunct to regional anesthesia or local infiltration to facilitate minor procedures. Its ventilatory depression is synergistic with benzodiazepines; care should be exercised when using this combination. High-dose fentanyl with modest doses of a hypnotic agent is widely used to provide anesthesia for major cardiovascular surgery because it does not depress left ventricular function while preventing cardiovascular and electrocardiographic alterations during induction and intubation. Along with its analogs, fentanyl is best administered by continuous IV infusion for anesthesia. Although high plasma and central nervous system concentrations are rapidly achieved after a single large bolus, their rapid decline may cause insufficient narcosis at the time of maximal stimulation. Continuous infusion of fentanyl has been demonstrated to block the hemodynamic and hormonal responses to intraoperative nociceptive stimuli,[7,8] although this effect is inconsistent and is favorably influenced by the presence of chronic β-adrenergic blockade.[9] Although most hypotension after fentanyl administration is probably related to associated bradycardia, care must be exerted in patients with increased sympathetic tone, since induction with fentanyl can unmask hypovolemia and cause a significant decrease in blood pressure.[10,11] This may be due to inhibition of central sympathetic outflow that is unrelated to analgesia or other sensory depressant effects.[12] Because high-dose fentanyl causes prolonged ventilatory depression and need for postoperative ventilatory support, it may not be suitable for minor procedures of short duration.

Sufentanil is 8 to 10 times more potent than fentanyl in humans. As with other opioids, pharmacokinetics and pharmacodynamics vary with age. Equipotent doses of IV sufentanil and fentanyl have the same time to onset of action.[13] Care must be taken when using sufentanil with sedative agents because of the potential for profound ventilatory depression. When used to provide general anesthesia, sufentanil is at least as effective as fentanyl in providing hemodynamic stability during induction[14] and noxious intraoperative stimuli,[7] in spite of its ability to reduce SVR.[15] Similar to fentanyl, this stability is variable and influenced by patient demographics and the presence of chronically administered vasoactive drugs.

Alfentanil is 5 to 10 times less potent than fentanyl when given by IV bolus. Onset of action is rapid, with peak effect occurring in 1.0 to 1.5 minutes, and duration is short. It is therefore a valuable analgesic for supplemental use with sedation. When combined with propofol, it can be used to provide total IV anesthesia of short duration with rapid emergence in suitable cases. Although it may not provide a similar degree of hemodynamic stability in cardiac surgery compared with sufentanil or fentanyl,[14,16] investigations reviewing more than 2000 patients suggest that choice of anesthetic technique does not influence outcome.[17,18] Cardiovascular stability when using sufentanil may be improved by avoiding the heavy use of adjuvant sedative-hypnotic agents.

Meperidine, in contrast to other opioids, in anesthetic doses causes significant hypotension, tachycardia, and myocardial depression and therefore is not used for this purpose. This can also occur when used as an analgesic in doses of 2.0 to 2.5 mg/kg.[19,20]

Agonist-antagonist opioids such as nalbuphine and butorphanol are appealing analgesics for general use because of their low risk of inducing ventilatory depression. However, there is a ceiling effect regarding analgesic potency. Supplementation of inhalation anesthesia produces a reduction of anesthetic concentration of only 8% to 11%, compared with the 63% or 65% reductions made possible by using morphine[21] or fentanyl, respectively.[22] Butorphanol, unlike fentanyl and its congeners or nalbuphine, can increase systemic and pulmonary artery pressures, pulmonary capillary wedge pressure (PCWP), PVR, and cardiac work.[23] Therefore it should be used cautiously if at all in patients with cardiomyopathy or other conditions in which pulmonary artery pressures are elevated. Attenuation of cardiovascular and hormonal responses to surgical stimuli is lacking with nalbuphine.[24] This factor and a very high rate of negative subjective assessments by patients[25] is found with other drugs in this class and limits their use in cardiovascular and endovascular anesthesia.[26]

That opiates can increase muscle tone and cause severe rigidity has been known for decades, although the mechanism is not clearly understood. Muscle rigidity is not due to a direct action on muscle fibers, since it can be decreased or prevented by predosing with a neuromuscular blocker. It may be related to the production of the catatonic state that all opiates can produce, although a more complex role of the central nervous system is undoubtedly involved. The increase in muscle tone rapidly progresses to stiffness occurring particularly in the thoracic and abdominal muscles. Glottic closure is an inconsistent finding, but an association with the decrease in pulmonary compliance and functional residual capacity may result in the patient being unable to breathe spontaneously or to have ventilation assisted by bag and mask. Rigidity is associated with increases in pulmonary artery, central venous, and intracranial pressures. Although not well studied, the incidence appears to increase with rapid injection, large doses, and increasing age of the patient. Administration of succinylcholine will rapidly terminate the episode and facilitate assisted ventilation but result in a patient who will be paralyzed for several minutes. Attempts to block or attenuate rigidity using subanesthetic pretreatment with benzodiazepines have been inconsistent in their results.

The endeavor to develop an opiate that causes better hemodynamic stability, that is more potent, and that is faster in onset and shorter in duration than existing agents continues. Remifentanil, an opioid undergoing testing in humans, produces rapid onset of profound analgesia. It has a unique ester linkage that enables it to undergo rapid metabolism (ester hydrolysis) by circulating and nonspecific tissue esterases into inactive compounds.[27] It has a small volume of distribution and an extremely short half-life. The time to recovery after discontinuation of a remifentanil infusion does not appear to be influenced by the duration of administration, total dose, or patient age, weight, or gender.[28] Potential advantages are several: (1) rapid IV titration of the drug to desired effect, (2) lack of accumulation, (3) reduced to absent incidence of postinfusion narcotic side effects, and (4) a route of metabolism unaffected by renal or hepatic disease, with positive implications for use in medically compromised patients. There is obvious application for this type of agent in maintenence of safe, short-lasting pain relief for procedures not requiring a general anesthetic, in cases where rapid emergence from anesthesia is desirable, and in provision of rapidly titratable postoperative pain management. Further studies will be necessary to delineate the clinical utility of this most promising drug.

General Anesthetic Induction Agents

Commonly used anesthetic induction agents such as thiopental and etomidate decrease myocardial oxygen consumption but at the expense of decreasing left ventricular loading conditions and/or contractility.[29,30] Furthermore, the hemodynamic response to airway manipulation and intubation is not limited by these agents, necessitating the use of one of the narcotics described previously. Thiopental can be used safely for induction in normal patients and in those with compensated heart disease. Caution must be exercised in those with either left or right ventricular failure, cardiac tamponade, or hypovolemia. A similar caveat may be offered for propofol, although the rapid emergence from sedation resulting from its large volume of distribution and rapid metabolism is an advantage in appropriate clinical situations. Induction with diazepam, whether by bolus injection or slow infusion, is characterized by short-term amnesia, hemodynamic stability, lack of depression of myocardial contractility, and decreased myocardial oxygen consumption in patients with either coronary artery or valvular heart disease. Undesirable features include pain on injection, a significant incidence of thrombophlebitis, long duration of action, and a tendency to accumulate in the elderly. Diazepam has the potential for cardiovascular depression when used with a narcotic, possibly because diazepam ablates normal sympathetic tone.[31] It therefore should be used cautiously in patients with hypovolemia and cardiac tamponade. The rapid onset, short duration of action, and rapid plasma clearance require that a continuous infusion of midazolam be minimized when used to supplement narcotic anesthesia. Flumazenil can effectively reverse sedation produced when midazolam is used either as a component of total IV anesthesia or in the intensive care unit. However, flumazenil must be used carefully in this situation, since it can produce central nervous system effects (e.g., nausea and vomiting, agitation, seizures) in patients either receiving large doses of benzodiazepines or suffering from an overdose.

Characteristics of etomidate, although offering no advantages over other induction agents in healthy patients, may be preferred in situations requiring rapid anesthetic induction in patients with hypovolemia, cardiac tamponade, or low cardiac output. Many studies document the hemodynamic stability after etomidate induction in both normal patients and those with cardiac disease. Although similar to the use of ketamine in this respect, etomidate does not increase heart rate and PVR, which may limit the use of the former agent. Etomidate also produces the least change in myocardial oxygen balance of available IV induction agents.[32] Although there is considerable detailed information about the effects of IV induction doses of these agents, knowledge of the effects of prolonged, steady-state infusion on hemodynamics, and drug interactions with other anesthetic and cardiovascular agents is still lacking.

Volatile Anesthetic Agents

Extensive descriptions of the cardiovascular effects of inhalation anesthetics are found in general anesthesiology and cardiovascular specialty textbooks and need not be repeated here. The effects of volatile agents and their comparative pharmacology are described at equipotent minimal alveolar concentrations (MACs). MAC is the inspired alveolar concentration analog to an ED_{50} of a nongaseous drug. Halothane causes a dose-dependent decrease in cardiac output, accompanied by hypotension, although the overall effect on SVR is small. Halothane has a proarrhythmic effect in combination with β-adrenergic drugs in doses that would not have any effect on cardiac rhythm in the awake patient. Enflurane, like all inhalation anesthetics, produces dose-dependent ventilatory depression and hypercarbia in the spontaneously ventilating patient and blunts hypoxemic and hypercarbic ventilatory drive to a greater extent than does halothane. Although light and moderate levels of anesthesia produce decreases in blood pressure similar to that found with either halothane or isoflurane, deep levels of enflurane anesthesia can produce profound hypotension resulting from decreases in both cardiac output and SVR. The dose-dependent decrease in SVR is the most important factor in the hypotension produced by isoflurane. Cardiac output is usually well maintained, even during moderately deep anesthesia. Isoflurane among contemporary volatile agents is considered to be the most potent coronary artery vasodilator. Dilation of resistance vessels may compromise oxygen supply distal to a coronary stenosis by decreasing poststenotic perfusion pressure.[33] Although about 20% of patients with coronary artery disease have "steal prone" coronary anatomy, isoflurane-induced vasodilation seldom has clinical significance. Isoflurane may be the preferred volatile agent for procedures involving the carotid or middle cerebral arteries because of its ability to lower critical regional cerebral blood flow.[34]

Volatile agents are seldom used alone to provide anesthesia for cardiovascular patients but rather are most commonly used to augment anesthetic depth to attenuate hypertension and tachycardia that may occur from surgical stress. Although both halothane and isoflurane are effective in controlling surgically induced hypertension, the differences in their direct effects on cardiovascular mechanics mentioned previously are important. The decrease in blood pressure by halothane is achieved by a decrease in cardiac output, whereas SVR may remain high.[35,36] Ventricular filling pressures can remain elevated, a situation that may not be tolerated by a compromised myocardium. Conversely, isoflurane primarily decreases SVR, thereby promoting increased stroke volume with a decrease in PCWP.[29] The latter reduces wall tension with a favorable effect on subendocardial perfusion. Thus even though both halothane and isoflurane have negative inotropic effects, the greater decrease in vascular resistance caused by the latter allows left ventricular function to improve when it is used to control intraoperative hypertension.

Although nitrous oxide continues to be a safe and commonly used agent, its use in cardiovascular patients is controversial. In the 1980s, animal studies suggested that addition of nitrous oxide may induce myocardial ischemia, results that were not confirmed clinically in humans.[37] However, nitrous oxide has been found to constrict epicardial vessels in dogs[38] and to significantly depress the cardiac index in patients with end-diastolic pressures more than 15 mm Hg.[39] Desflurane is a new volatile anesthetic that has recently been introduced into clinical practice in the United States. Its low blood gas solubility (similar to that of nitrous oxide) facilitates rapid induction and adjustments in the depth of anesthesia and permits quicker emergence. Although originally thought to have cardiovascular properties similar to that of its isomer isoflurane in healthy patients, recent studies show that this is true only under steady-state-equivalent MAC conditions. A rapid increase in desflurane concentration to 1.5 MAC after anesthetic induction causes transient increases in sympathetic activity, plasma epinephrine concentration, and vasopressin secretion, thus promoting increases in heart rate (more than 30 beats per minute) and arterial blood pressure (more than 30 mm Hg).[40] This occurs at an increased inspired concentration that does not provide an excessive depth of anesthesia or constitute an overdose. Although a similar observation had been earlier made in patients with coronary artery disease, 9% of whom experienced electrocardiographic signs of ischemia,[41] this dosing technique had been accepted practice when using volatile agents in healthy patients. The duration of anesthesia preceding the increase in administered concentration does not influence this cardiovascular response, although subsequent step increases in concentration produce an attenuated hormonal and hemodynamic alteration.[42] A similar pattern of hemodynamic change has subsequently been observed using isoflurane, but with the dose-response shifted markedly to the right (at 3.5 MAC).[43] The changes produced by desflurane, and to a lesser degree by isoflurane, are potentially hazardous to select patients and illustrate the risks of anesthesia, even when well researched and accepted agents are used.

Neuromuscular Blocking Agents

The commonly used nondepolarizing muscle relaxants seldom have a deleterious effect on hemodynamics in healthy patients. Pancuronium can increase heart rate and thereby cause myocardial ischemia during high-dose fentanyl anesthesia in patients with coronary artery disease, an effect attenuated by administration of a benzodiazepine.[44] Doxacurium, pipecuronium, vecuronium, rocuronium, and atracurium have minimal hemodynamic effects. With these agents, histamine release (and potential hypotension) and vagal blockade are prominent only at doses 2 and 3 times the ED_{95} or with rapid injection. It is important to note that the patient's underlying cardiovascular physiology, chronic cardiovascular medications, and any acutely administered anesthetic agents all precondition the response to the muscle relaxant used. Thus vecuronium and fentanyl can result in a severe decrease in heart rate.[45] Similarly, a patient with poor ventricular function, taking a chronic β-adrenergic blocker for angina pectoris, and who is sedated may not have a tachycardic response to pancuronium.

It is also important to remember that muscle relaxants do not have sedative or amnestic properties and therefore require concomitant administration of a hypnotic when used in the intensive care unit. Use of intermittent boluses of a long-acting agent in amounts ranging from one-fifth to one-third of the original dose, titrated to a measured or monitored effect, can maintain an adequate level of paralysis either during surgery or in the intensive care unit. Total dose and cost can be lessened by continuous IV administration via a controlled infusion device, titrated to effect using a blockade monitor to assess response to a "train-of-four." The kidney is the primary route of elimination for the longer-acting agents such as pancuronium, metocurine, doxacurium, and pipecuronium, none of which undergo significant metabolism. Vecuronium and rocuronium also undergo significant clearance by the liver, which results in intermediate duration of action. Dosages of the latter agents must be modified accordingly in the presence of either renal or hepatic disease. Alternatively, an agent not dependent on the diseased organ system can be used. Such an alternative would be atracurium, which is deactivated by Hoffman elimination (spontaneous chemodegradation at physiologic temperature and pH) and by metabolism by nonspecific plasma esterases into inactive compounds. The resultant lack of dependence on an organ system for elimination makes it unique among the nondepolarizing agents.

The depolarizing agent succinylcholine is seldom used other than to facilitate endotracheal intubation. The advantage of a short recovery time after prolonged continuous infusion carries the risk of phase two block (i.e., it resembles a prolonged nondepolarizing agent blockade). Mivacurium is a new nondepolarizing neuromuscular blocking agent that is metabolized by human plasma cholinesterase and undergoes ester hydrolysis in the liver. Time to recovery compares favorably with that for vecuronium and atracurium.[46] As with those agents, it is a suitable choice to maintain paralysis by a continuous infusion.

Local Anesthetics

Local anesthetics are classified into two groups that differ in chemical structure, site of action, metabolism, and allergic potential. The amides (lidocaine, mepivicaine, bupivacaine, etidocaine) are relatively stable in solution, are generally metabolized in the liver, and exhibit little potential to produce an allergic reaction. The esters (procaine, 2-chloroprocaine, tetracaine, cocaine) are relatively unstable in solution, undergo ester hydrolysis for deactivation, and can cause allergic reactions primarily through sensitivity to para-aminobenzoic acid, a primary metabolite. The success of regional anesthesia can be influenced by technical skill, site of administration, addition of a vasoconstrictor, use of local anesthetic mixtures, carbonation, and physiologic variables such as renal failure. Time to onset, density, and duration of the block vary directly with dosage. The greatest separation between sensory and motor blockade is exhibited by bupivacaine.

All local anesthetics have systemic effects. Systemic toxicity primarily involves the cardiovascular and central nervous systems. Lidocaine and other older anesthetics produce preconvulsant manifestations such as lightheadedness and dizziness, numbness, tingling lips, ringing ears, or drowsiness. Severe toxicity manifests as confusion, slurring of speech, twitching, muscle tremors, and frank convulsions. High blood levels can result in cardiac arrest. All local anesthetics have direct effects on vascular smooth muscle and exert a dose-dependent negative inotropic effect that varies directly with nerve conduction blocking potential.[47] Therefore cardiac depression is greatest with tetracaine, bupivacaine, and etidocaine. The central nervous system prodrome may be absent with bupivacaine or etidocaine overdose, with full cardiac arrest presenting first. Bupivacaine may produce severe cardiac arrhythmias, and resuscitation may be extremely difficult because of the high degree of binding to cardiac muscle. The effect on the peripheral vascular system is usually biphasic,[48] with low and high concentrations producing vasoconstriction and vasodilation respectively. Conversely, cocaine, which may be used topically to facilitate nasotracheal intubation, generally causes vasoconstriction. Obviously, careful attention to technique, including aspiration to check for an intravascular location of the needle, is mandatory for safety. I have observed bradycardia, prolonged PR-interval, and hypotension relatively refractory to treatment for several hours in a patient who received as little as 2 ml of 0.5% bupivacaine from an improperly administered intraoperative intercostal block for postoperative pain relief. Since hypoxemia, hypercarbia, and acidosis potentiate the myocardial depressant action of local anesthetics, treatment consists of oxygen, ventilatory support and control of the airway, and fluid administration, with inotropic support and anticonvulsant therapy as indicated.

Drug Interactions

Life expectancy has increased dramatically in the United States in recent years. The fastest-growing segment of the population is the percentage in its eighth decade of life. Increased sophistication in the care of the elderly has eliminated advanced age and illness as major restrictions to surgical intervention. Patients presenting for endovascular surgery characteristically are relatively old, have coexisting cardiovascular and pulmonary disease, and frequently are taking several chronic medications that have implications for anesthetic management. This section discusses the potential anesthetic interactions of the most frequently used cardiovascular medications.

Nitroglycerin and Sodium Nitroprusside

The dilating effect of nitroglycerin (NTG) occurs predominantly in the venous circulation. Dilation of arteriolar resistance vessels occurs only at relatively high doses that are easily obtained by IV use although not by chronic oral therapy.[49] Because chronic antianginal therapy with NTG usually does not affect SVR, MAP, or diastolic blood pressure, there is minimal interaction with drugs used for general anesthesia. In contrast, IV administration is often synergistic with the vasodilating properties of volatile anesthetics. Additionally, the negative inotropic effect of these agents can severely compromise cardiac output in a vasodilated patient. NTG may prolong the neuromuscular blockade produced by pancuronium.[50]

Sodium nitroprusside (SNP) is frequently used as an alternative to NTG for treatment of perioperative hypertension. Unlike NTG, low doses of SNP primarily decrease arterial blood pressure and can in high doses cause redistribution of coronary blood flow away from ischemic myocardium.[51] It may be wise to avoid its use with isoflurane, which can also cause an intracoronary steal, although there are no controlled studies to suggest a detrimental effect of this combination. When used to control proximal arterial hypertension during crossclamping of the thoracic aorta, SNP has been shown to increase cerebral spinal fluid pressure (probably from an increase in cerebral blood flow and cerebral blood volume) and to decrease spinal cord and renal blood flow in dogs[52] but not to change spinal cord perfusion pressure in humans before crossclamping.[53] SNP should be used cautiously to lower intraoperative hypertension to preoperative values in procedures in which there is a documented risk of ischemia to the brain or to the spinal cord.

Both NTG and SNP can produce arterial hypoxemia by inhibiting hypoxemic pulmonary vasoconstriction. Methemoglobinemia, although rare, has been reported after excessive IV infusion of SNP. Treatment is with 100% oxygen and methylene blue, 2 g/kg. SNP inhibits platelet function to a greater degree than does NTG. NTG infusion rates above 3 µg/kg/min may cause heparin resistance through a qualitative antithrombin III abnormality.[54]

β-Adrenergic Antagonists

The debate about whether to discontinue β-adrenergic antagonists before surgery and anesthesia has long since been resolved in favor of administration of the patient's usual dose up to surgery, restarting the drug as soon as possible postoperatively. However, their negative inotropic effect is additive with that of increasing concentrations of the volatile anesthetic agents. Propranolol causes additive slowing of heart rate and atrioventricular (AV) node conduction with halothane, enflurane, and isoflurane.[55-57] Circulatory depression in the presence of propranolol is greatest with enflurane. Bronchospasm is the primary noncardiac adverse effect of β-adrenergic blocking agents. In awake patients, bronchospasm causes an increase in the work of breathing, maldistribution of ventilation, and a ventilation-perfusion mismatch resulting in hypoxemia. These effects can be ameliorated by inhalation anesthesia, but the initial severe increase in airway pressures during positive pressure ventilation decreases venous return to the heart, which may cause a subsequent fall in cardiac output and systemic blood pressure. Although the cardioselective β-blockers are less likely to produce this effect, all drugs of this class should be used with caution if at all in patients requiring aminophylline or $β_2$-agonists to maintain adequate bronchiolar mechanics.[58,59]

Calcium Entry Blockers

A diverse class of structurally and pharmacologically dissimilar drugs, calcium entry blockers have a broad spectrum of implications for anesthesia. Verapamil, when used perioperatively with high-dose narcotic anesthesia in patients with a normal heart, causes a decrease in SVR without any change in cardiac output or AV conduction time.[60] However, it decreases heart rate and peak left ventricular pressure in animals when used with volatile agents[61] and can cause AV dissociation in patients anesthetized with enflurane. In both animal and human studies, enflurane is less well tolerated than isoflurane or halothane in combination with verapamil. When administered IV to patients on chronic β-adrenergic blocker therapy and anesthetized with halothane, verapamil decreases MAP, myocardial contractility, and cardiac index.[62] Studies and case reports suggest that it may seriously reduce skeletal muscle contractility when given to patients with neuromuscular disease[63] or in those given even modest doses of neuromuscular blocking agents.[64,65] Verapamil has been recommended as adjunctive therapy for malignant hyperpyrexia, but some studies question its efficacy and demonstrate additive myocardial depression,[66] hyperkalemia, and cardiovascular collapse[67] when used with dantrolene, the major therapy for this condition. In spite of these potential drug interactions, the current recommendation is to continue verapamil perioperatively because of the even greater risk of rebound hypertension and myocardial ischemia.

Adverse effects of diltiazem are rare, and it may exert a stabilizing action against the arrhythmogenic effect of halothane.[68] Nifedipine has a high incidence of minor side effects such as headache, dizziness, nausea, and vomiting, which may increase risk in the perianesthetic period. Both nifedipine and nicardipine reduce SVR with little effect on cardiac output or heart rate in patients under narcotic anesthesia. Although it appears to have an additive depressant effect on myocardial contractility in combination with volatile anesthetic agents, cardiac output remains unchanged, probably because of a decrease in SVR.[69,70] Chronic administration should not be interrupted.

Diuretics

Although the most common recommendation is to withhold diuretic therapy on the day of operation unless necessary for immediate treatment of volume overload, the risks and benefits of continuation of diuretic therapy into the perioperative period are not well studied. The major anesthetic concern is their effect on fluid and electrolyte balance. Anesthetic induction may precipitate severe hypotension and tachycardia in patients with unrecognized hypovolemia. Hypokalemia is associated with an increased incidence of arrhythmias, and acute potassium replacement may be dangerous in and of itself. Diuretic therapy can potentiate the action of neuromuscular blocking agents.[71]

Common Antihypertensive Agents

Perioperative continuation of vasodilators such as minoxidil and hydralazine is recommended to prevent withdrawal symptoms. Serious interactions with anesthetics have not been reported. α-Adrenergic blocking agents such as prazosin and phenoxybenzamine may inhibit the normal response to indirect-acting vasopressors when used to treat hypotension. The afterload reduction caused by these drugs may augment the hypotensive effect of anesthetic agents that decrease preload. Therapy with clonidine and other $α_2$-agonists should be continued up to operation to prevent rebound hypertension. However, the response to IV ephedrine in both awake and anesthetized patients is enhanced by oral premedication with clonidine. Intraoperative requirements for IV sedatives and opiates and maintenance dosages of volatile anesthetics are diminished. However, time to recovery from anesthesia is considerably prolonged. The depletion of central norepinephrine stores caused by guanethidine may produce the functional equivalent of denervation hypersensitivity, resulting in exaggerated and reduced hemodynamic responses to direct- and indirect-acting sympathomimetics, respectively. Reserpine causes a response to vasopressors similar to that of guanethidine and may potentiate the action of sedatives and volatile anesthetics. The increase in venous capacitance and decrease in arteriolar resistance caused by angiotensin-converting enzyme inhibitors can lead to a significant reduction in blood pressure during induction of general anesthesia. The implications of α-adrenergic blocking agents such as prazosin, terazosin, and phenoxybenzamine relate to their effect on the peripheral circulation. Drugs that reduce preload may cause an unexpected hypotensive response, and the effects of modest blood loss during surgery can be exaggerated. The response to catecholamines may be attenuated. The reflex response to hydralazine therapy can produce a modest hyperdynamic circulation (with increases in heart rate and stroke volume) and may precipitate angina pectoris in patients with coronary artery disease. Minoxidil, now also used to promote hair growth in balding people, can cause tachycardia and pulmonary hypertension.

Antiarrhythmic Agents

Except in unusual circumstances, antiarrhythmic drugs should be continued up to the time of operation and restarted as soon as possible afterward. Volatile anesthetics, ketamine, and droperidol may reduce, whereas succinylcholine, diazepam, and neostigmine can increase, the incidence of digoxin-induced ventricular arrhythmias during anesthesia. Of greater concern during anesthesia is the avoidance of hypokalemia, acid-base disturbances, interaction with other cardiovascular agents such as quinidine, and other situations that can lead to an increased serum digitalis level. The adverse effects of most antiarrhythmics that are of concern to the anesthesiologist, in addition to their propensity to cause arrhythmias themselves, mostly involve the potential for hypotension (Class IA agents); central nervous system manifestations such as ataxia, tremor, and disorientation (Class IB agents); and bradycardia or ventricular tachycardia (Class IC agents). The ability of quinidine therapy to dramatically increase the plasma digitalis concentration and thereby produce digitalis toxicity is always a concern.

The high potential for perianesthetic complications in patients taking amiodarone warrant discussion of the risk-to-benefit ratio between the cardiologist and anesthesiologist. The risk of subjecting the patient to a life-threatening arrhythmia while prolonging the date of the operation during discontinuation of the drug must be weighed against the risk of hypotension (that is relatively resistant to vasopressor therapy) and mortality under anesthesia.[72] Bretylium causes the equivalent of a denervated state by blocking catecholamine release, thereby causing an exaggerated and diminished response to direct- and indirect-acting sympathomimetic drugs, respectively. Few data are available on the use and side effects of adenosine intraoperatively.

Anesthesia for Endovascular Procedures

Development of endovascular anesthesia is in its infancy. Hence, implications must be drawn from the body of existing knowledge regarding anesthesia for vascular surgical procedures and known cardiovascular and neurologic effects of anesthetics. Advances in anesthetic and cardiac pharmacology have facilitated better control of intraoperative cardiovascular and respiratory function, which in turn has improved the outcome of vascular surgery patients. However, the choice of an anesthetic technique should depend on more than its effect on cardiac, pulmonary, and cerebral physiology or on convenience to patient or surgeon. Surgery, and possibly many endovascular interventions, produce a neuroendocrine stress response and alterations in other organ functions. Several consequences of this response are especially important to endovascular surgery patients, since they often are already at increased risk for cardiac dysfunction and adverse metabolic effects such as hypercoagulability. The choice of anesthetic may have important implications regarding amelioration of these negative effects and thus on postoperative patient outcome.

Physiologic Response to Surgery and Anesthesia

The increased secretion of catabolically acting, and inhibition of anabolically acting, hormones precipitated by surgery causes a hypermetabolic state. Postoperatively, glucose, amino acids, and fat from tissue stores are released. Surgical stress also induces changes in the coagulation and fibrinolytic systems,[73] which often result in a hypercoagulable state. This is not compounded by general anesthesia with volatile agents, whose metabolic effects are minimal and of short duration. Similarly, neither etomidate nor high dose opioids, which inhibit the catabolic hormonal response to surgery, have any effect on the postoperative response. As early as 1908, Crile proposed that neuroblockade would block adverse effects of nociception and might improve operative outcome. It indeed appears that blockade of the surgical stress response by local anesthetic inhibition of the nociceptive pathway from the surgical field to the central nervous system has a beneficial effect on postoperative catabolism. Important factors include the operative site (less effective stress inhibition with abdominal or thoracic than with lower extremity procedures), duration of the neural blockade, and timing (more effective when blockade is instituted before surgery than postoperatively).[73] Although neither epidural nor spinal anesthesia have any important effect on coagulation or fibrinolysis, thromboembolic events also are reduced and graft patency is improved,[74,75] probably secondary to the improved blood flow resulting from peripheral vasodilation. Most studies on neural blockade have been done using high concentrations of local anesthetics, so no conclusions can be offered regarding the inhibitory effects of lower, analgesic doses.

Risk of postoperative cardiovascular complications appears to be related to the hemodynamic changes, such as intraoperative hypertension and hypotension and increased myocardial oxygen demand, induced by the surgical stimulus.[77] Regional anesthesia, by reducing or preventing reflex responses leading to alterations in blood pressure and increased demands on the heart, might have a beneficial effect on postoperative outcome. However, outcome data are conflicting.[77-80] Research suggests that preservation rather than ablation of autonomic nervous system function is important in cardiac well-being. Not only is autonomic impairment associated with increased risk of adverse cardiac events in the awake patient with angina pectoris or myocardial infarction, but it seems to be related to the extent of hemodynamic instability after induction of anesthesia.[81] Such autonomic imbalance (low-frequency sympathetic predominance) that accompanies myocardial infarction might be responsible for the increased morbidity and mortality that occurs after surgery in patients with recent infarction. The gradual improvement in infarction-related autonomic dysfunction over 3 to 12 months could be one explanation why cardiac risk is greatly diminished when elective surgery is delayed until 6 months after infarction.[82] Finally, preservation of reflex regulation of coronary vascular resistance[83] and of cardiac-vagal cardiac reflexes[84] plays an important role in the termination of ischemic events. Reflexes that reduce heart rate, decrease myocardial oxygen demand, and appear to counteract or lessen the likelihood of sympathetic hyperactivity appear to be important in reducing the severity of ischemia. Digitalis, which augments cardiopulmonary reflex activity, functions similarly. Therefore other cardiac and anesthetic agents that preserve beneficial aspects of autonomic function could be expected to be safer than those that inhibit them. To this effect it might be significant to note that induction with etomidate preserves the normal reflex sympathoexcitation associated with hypotension, whereas thiopental and propofol abolish it. A fentanyl anesthetic, in combination with a benzodiazepine, reduces arterial baroreflex function less than does anesthesia with a volatile agent. The long-recognized decrease in heart rate that accompanies high-dose narcotic administration is obviously an advantage in patients with ischemic heart disease. Premedication with clonidine produces hemodynamic stability, decreases both IV and volatile anesthetic requirements during induction and maintenance,[85,86] and significantly decreases oxygen uptake throughout anesthesia while reducing heart rate and MAP into the postoperative period.[87,88] Both short-acting (e.g., atracurium, vecuronium, rocuronium) and long-acting (e.g., doxacurium and pipecuronium) neuromuscular blocking agents have little effect on heart rate, mean arterial blood pressure, and cardiac index, in contrast to pancuronium, which has pronounced vagolytic and sympathomimetic effects that may predispose patients to myocardial ischemia.[89] The clinical implications of these findings are unclear, since most studies have been conducted on patients treated with β-adrenergic blockers, calcium channel blockers, or both. Also, the magnitude of the stress response caused by endovascular surgery is largely unknown. However, the construction of an anesthetic regimen that preserves favorable autonomic reflexes and that could possibly reduce cardiac morbidity and mortality in patients with high cardiac risk has merit.

Approach to Anesthesia for Endovascular Procedures

The objectives of the anesthesiologist are to provide a pain-free environment, facilitate surgery, and decrease morbidity and mortality. To do so, the anesthesiologist must have a thorough understanding of the surgical and anesthetic risks involved, basic physiology, the pharmacology of the drugs at his or her disposal, and the reliability of various monitoring modalities. Due consideration must also be given to the choice of whether to provide regional, general, or local anesthesia with sedation, the physiologic consequences of these alternatives, and the desires of the patient. Cost effectiveness of anesthetic techniques is becoming an ever-increasing factor and should be determined using statistical process control (see p. 85).

Carotid and Intracranial Procedures

Many endovascular procedures are often performed under a regional anesthetic technique or using a local anesthetic field block with sedation. Among them are procedures involving treatment of an intracranial aneurysm or arteriovenous malformation and of vertebral and carotid artery lesions such as an intracavernous aneurysm or traumatic arteriovenous fistula. Choosing a local anesthetic for these cases evokes the same controversy existing over the potential advantages of regional versus general anesthesia for carotid endarterectomy. Advocates of regional techniques cite the ability to continuously monitor the central nervous system, a lower incidence of perioperative myocardial infarction, increased perioperative hemodynamic stability, reduced stress response, and cost savings secondary to decreased intensive care. Demonstrable improvement in outcome from a regional technique remains equivocal. Studies in which mostly regional techniques are evaluated without a control group have yielded impressive results. However, when regional and general techniques are compared in the same practice, results are inconclusive. Studies comparing the incidence of perioperative blood pressure instability similarly are inconclusive, except that postoperative blood pressure appears to be more stable when a regional technique is used. When techniques are subjected to financial analysis, patients having regional anesthesia incur a cost saving, primarily from a decreased postoperative use of the intensive care unit.

Endovascular surgery patients often require intensive perioperative monitoring because these patients can have systemic manifestations of atherosclerotic vascular and coronary artery disease. They are at risk for cardiac and cerebral ischemia, which can be diagnosed with appropriate monitoring and treated accordingly. Because the major source of morbidity and mortality in these patients is cardiac in origin, appropriate electrocardiogram (ECG) monitoring remains mandatory. Leads II and V5 should be used because of their combined high sensitivity for detecting ischemic changes. Arterial cannulation for beat-to-beat monitoring of systemic blood pressure is indicated for patients undergoing complicated carotid procedures. Blood pressure should be checked in both arms to check for a possible wide discrepancy, a somewhat common finding in patients with carotid and peripheral vascular disease. Cannulation should be accomplished in the arm with the higher blood pressure to prevent errors in hemodynamic management that are based on an erroneously low reading. Monitoring for cerebral ischemia is controversial. This has been especially true regarding open carotid procedures, since the majority of neurologic deficits after carotid endarterectomy have been thromboembolic rather than secondary to ischemia caused by carotid crossclamping.[90] A positive influence of monitoring the electroencephalogram (EEG) on clinical outcome remains to be proven.[91] Studies measuring the utility of a pulmonary artery catheter and transesophageal echocardiography (TEE) regarding outcome also have produced contradictory results. Whether their use, singly or together, will be of benefit in endovascular procedures is best left to statistical process analysis (see p. 85). Routine monitoring for all cases should include oximetry, capnography, measurement of systemic blood pressure in some manner, and body temperature.

If local anesthetic infiltration with sedation is chosen to facilitate an endovascular procedure, careful attention must still be paid to preoperative preparation. The patient should arrive at the operative facility in time for adequate management of aspiration prophylaxis and preoperative sedation. The former begins with appropriate NPO status. Although controversial, it is still prudent to recommend that patients remain NPO for at least the traditional 8 hours before the procedure, regardless of whether a field block, regional anesthetic, or general anesthetic is planned. It is important to reinterview patients on the day of surgery regarding their NPO status, since this admonition is sometimes disregarded. Some patients indulge in a late heavy meal just before midnight, which increases risk of aspiration. Therefore a recommedation not to ingest solid food after 9 PM is preferable to the standard NPO past midnight. Antiaspiration prophylaxis continues with administration of an appropriate H_2 receptor antagonist. Because oral dosage (ranitidine 150mg) requires 1.5 to 3.0 hours to attain peak effect, if the patient presents for same day surgery, he or she should arrive several hours before the procedure. Although IV ranitidine (50mg) peaks faster, it is not more efficacious than when given orally and is considerably more expensive. Oral sodium citrate can be used as a supplement on arrival to the operating suite. It is advisable to undertake the above steps in all patients who might require emergency anesthetic intervention, even though the original intent is to perform the endovascular procedure using local anesthetic infiltration and sedation.

Preoperative sedation must be timed appropriately to allay fear, permit a smooth transition to the procedure room, and effect a short recovery. Because any sedative can cause drowsiness, the patient must be observed and be provided a safe location in which to await the procedure. A benzodiazepine will accomplish the goals of sedation and anxiolysis with fewer side effects better than will alternatives.[92] Pain on intramuscular injection is avoided and the risk of overdosage minimized when they are given orally. Diazepam, 10 to 15 mg, given 90 minutes before the procedure is a good choice and will produce minimal synergistic sedation with perioperative narcotics. Alternatively, midazolam, 15 mg, may be used, but at a risk of incurring a slower recovery.

Monitored sedation during the procedure often is the safest and most efficient method of managing a patient for an endovascular procedure. Nonetheless, it must be undertaken with intravascular access and full patient monitoring in place before beginning the procedure. Vital signs should be continually observed at not greater than 5-minute intervals and more often as required. Patient cooperation is best maintained intraoperatively through a combination of constant communication and IV administration of a sedative and narcotic. IV midazolam has a faster onset and offset than does diazepam, although it does not have the latter's ability to produce retrograde amnesia. It may be given in incremental doses of 0.5 to 1.0 mg and supplemented with a short-acting narcotic such as fentanyl, 1 to 2 µg/kg, or alfentanil, 10 to 20 µg/kg. The latter has the advantage of having a faster onset and offset. An appropriately trained and credentialed individual should be assigned sole responsibility for administering sedation and monitoring the patient. This should not be an added responsibility for a circulating nurse, who will frequently have his or her attention diverted from the patient to meet the needs of the endovascular proceduralist. Often patients will benefit from the administration of a short-acting hypnotic such as sodium thiopental or propofol at the beginning of the vascular access cutdown or during a critical part of the procedure. These agents should only be administered by an anesthesiologist or delegated nurse anesthetist because of the associated risk of compromising the integrity of the patient's airway and ventilatory status.

Techniques of regional anesthesia for neck and intracranial endovascular procedures include deep cervical plexus block, superficial cervical plexus block, and local infiltration. Contraindications to regional block include patient refusal, patient anticoagulation, clotting abnormalities, and infection at the site of the proposed block. As with local field block, it is prudent to begin an IV infusion, attach the patient to basic monitors, and acquire baseline values before administering the block or any adjuvant sedation. Premedication should provide anxiolysis sufficient to ensure patient cooperation during placement of the needle but not to sedate the patient to a degree where assessment of neurologic function becomes difficult either before or after the procedure. Either diazepam, 10 mg, given orally or midazolam titrated to effect by IV administration currently most closely approaches these requirements. An H_2 receptor antagonist should be given as described previously. Although the deep plexus originates from the first through fourth cervical (C_1 to C_4) nerve roots, the block is directed toward C_2 to C_4, since the first root carries no sensory fibers. The roots course through the intervertebral foramina, running behind the vertebral artery and out to the transverse processes, where they split into the ascending and descending branches, which form the deep and superficial cervical plexus. This anatomy explains why the risks related to deep plexus block, although rare in experienced hands, can be severe. The vertebral artery can be pierced in the attempt to locate the transverse processes, which serve as landmarks for needle position. The main hazard is intravascular injection of local anesthetic, which can cause seizure activity even if small amounts are injected. Although seizures are typically of very short duration, the associated cardiovascular instability and potential for hypoxemia are poorly tolerated in this patient population. That one should always aspirate to detect blood or cerebral spinal fluid before injecting a local anesthetic cannot be emphasized enough. If the needle should pass intrathecally through the intravertebral foramen, there is a small risk of producing spinal anesthesia, which would necessitate cardiopulmonary support until resolved. A successful deep plexus block can produce ipsilateral phrenic nerve paralysis, which is usually of little clinical consequence, even in patients with chronic obstructive lung disease. The major drawback to a regional technique is the potential for a procedural complication involving one or more of the following: loss of consciousness, cardiovascular collapse, inability of the patient to protect the airway, ventilatory arrest, or seizure activity. Emergency intervention including assisted ventilation, endotracheal intubation, and cardiopulmonary resuscitation may be required, necessitating compromise of a sterile surgical field in the neck or temporary cessation of the endovascular procedure at a critical, inopportune time, Furthermore, pharmacologic therapy for seizure activity or for a mild ischemic cerebral event may itself compromise the patient's state of consciousness and ability to maintain ventilation.

A supplemental bolus of alfentanil may be used before placing the block. The rapid plasma-effect site equilibration of alfentanil results in a peak effect in 1 to 2 minutes and in a smaller dose requirement. Although the patient should be profoundly analgesic while the block is being placed, the reduced dose requirement compared with sufentanil and fentanyl results in a rapid offset.[93] A regional technique often requires the intraoperative use of sedatives to quell anxiety for all but the least apprehensive patient. Unfortunately, heavy use of a benzodiazepine may actually cause a state in which cooperation is decreased and in any case may compromise the ability to continuously assess cerebral function. Reversal of benzodiazepine sedation and overdose by flumazenil is dramatic. However, elimination of flumazenil is more rapid than that of midazolam, and resedation is possible. A modest dose of a benzodiazepine (midazolam 1 to 2 mg) with low-dose ketamine (0.1 mg/kg) may produce a comfortably sedate patient who is easily arousable for neurologic assessment while avoiding the complications caused by large doses of ketamine or midazolam alone. Heavy use of ketamine can cause untoward side effects such as loss of airway protection, a hyperdynamic circulation, increased intracerebral pressure, lack of cooperation, and emergence phenomena. Alternatively, propofol infusion allows more precise control of sedation than is possible with midazolam. Its rapid onset of action permits rapid upward titration in anticipation of a surgical stimulation, and a similarly rapid offset facilitates rapid recovery. Since propofol is a potent ventilatory depressant, it should be administered only by an anesthesiologist or other personnel trained in acute airway management.

If a general anesthetic is chosen for an intracranial or carotid endovascular procedure, the anesthesiologist must balance benefits to the central nervous system against what may be best for the patient with suspected coronary artery disease. A further goal is to have the patient awake and responsive as soon after completion of the procedure as possible. The role a specific anesthetic technique plays in overall outcome is controversial. Current data suggest that when the incidence of tachycardia, hypertension, and dysrhythmias is factored out, there appears to be no significant difference in severe outcome between the use of halothane, fentanyl, isoflurane, and enflurane.[94] Most evidence points to the ability of the anesthesiologist, not any specific technique, as the main determinant of outcome. Although myriad anesthetic regimens are possible, there are salient features of management of the cardiac patient that hold true for all techniques. Induction should be more deliberate than in those patients who can tolerate a wider range of hemodynamic changes, using careful titration of hypnotics and narcotics, cardiovascular drugs, and fluids. Most often an IV narcotic technique, supplemented by a volatile inhalation agent and an IV sedative, is used. A neuromuscular blocking agent is chosen either to counteract the hemodynamic effects of the above (e.g., the vagolytic effects of pancuronium to counteract the slow heart rate produced by fentanyl) or for its lack of appreciable effect on the cardiovascular system.

More specifically, etomidate induction has less effect on hemodynamics than does thiopental and lowers the cerebral metabolic rate for oxygen consumption. The hemodynamic response to laryngoscopy and endotracheal intubation can be attenuated by administration of a small dose of narcotic before anesthetic induction. If one chooses to maintain anesthesia with a volatile agent, isoflurane may be the best choice because it supports the lowest critical blood flow without producing cerebral ischemia.[95,96] Isoflurane can produce an isoelectric electroencephalogram in lower concentrations than other agents and appears to produce a metabolic profile similar to that when barbiturates are used to induce cerebral isoelectricity.[97] However, isoflurane has been reported to cause an intracoronary steal that may be detrimental in some patients with coronary artery disease.[98] Patients in whom volatile anesthetic agents are not well tolerated may be anesthetized using a total IV anesthetic technique. Propofol in combination with a short-acting narcotic offers several advantages. Unlike thiopental, concentrations of propofol that cause cerebral isoelectricity are well below those that cause a decrease in myocardial contractility. However, when used with a narcotic, a propofol dose ranging from one that produces light sedation (25–50 µg/kg/min) to deep sedation (50–75 µg/kg/min) will often suffice, especially when a neuromuscular blocking agent is added, because of the minimal surgical stimulation caused by endovascular procedures. The high clearance of propofol and the rapid emergence from sedation that follows its discontinuance permit neurologic evaluation rapidly after termination of anesthesia. Recovery from the volatile agent desflurane is even faster but is accompanied in a high percentage of patients by nausea and vomiting[99] and by the risk of a sudden increase in sympathetic activity and catecholamine concentration if the concentration is suddenly increased (see previous discussion).

The choice of narcotic supplement is determined by the expected duration of the endovascular procedure. In spite of the rapid terminal half-life of alfentanil, the time required for a 50% decrease in effect site concentration after an infusion dosed to maintain a constant opioid concentration is actually slower than that for sufentanil if the duration of the infusion is less than 8 hours. Sufentanil is highly fat-soluble; this sequestration in fat not only produces a long terminal half-life but also increases the ability of its high clearance to produce a rapidly decreasing plasma drug concentration after discontinuation of an infusion.[100] Therefore sufentanil may be a better choice than alfentanil for a procedure lasting less than 8 hours. Conversely, alfentanil may be the opiate of choice if rapid emergence is desired in a procedure lasting longer than 8 hours. The choice of neuromuscular blocker may also be determined by the duration of the case. Pancuronium may be used to facilitate endotracheal intubation, its vagolytic effect being offset by the vagomimetic action of a narcotic infusion. For shorter cases or in patients in whom greater cardiovascular stability is required, a newer agent or succinylcholine may be employed. Pipecuronium and doxacurium (long-acting agents) and rocuronium, vecuronium, and atracurium (short-acting agents) are best administered by continuous infusion and titrated to effect using a neuromuscular blockade monitor to facilitate rapid offset of paralysis.

Complications may be more difficult to detect under general anesthesia. Somatosensory evoked potentials can detect ischemia in both cortical and subcortical structures but can be influenced by general anesthesia. Monitoring with the compressed spectral array or with the density spectral array observes the cortical surface and may miss focal subcortical ischemia. The EEG in general is affected by sensory stimulation, body temperature, acid-base balance, serum glucose level, and premedicant and anesthetic drugs. In the event of focal cerebral ischemia, thiopental may provide some cerebral protection, although it appears to be of little use in global ischemia.[101,102] Further protection may be offered using calcium channel antagonists. Nimodipine administered before and after ischemic events improves neurologic outcome[103] and reduces mortality.[104] Since elevated blood glucose at the time of an ischemic cerebral event has been correlated with worsened outcome,[105] fluid maintenance by IV infusion with a crystalloid solution without glucose may be indicated.

Anesthesia in the Cardiac Catheterization Suite

Because many children have cardiac lesions that are amenable to correction in the catheterization suite, the anesthesiologist in attendance must be well acquainted with the pathophysiology of congenital heart disease and with pediatric anesthetic management. Thorough preoperative assessment is mandatory, since as many as 25% of patients with congenital heart disease have associated abnormalities involving other organ systems.[106] Airway anomalies are of particular significance. Hypoxemia, hypercarbia, and acid-base changes with resultant catecholamine release occurring because of airway compromise with sedation or during anesthetic induction can alter PVR, which in turn can affect intracardiac shunt direction. Sufficient data should be available regarding the child's cardiopulmonary reserve to assist in planning anesthetic management.

Safe management depends on optimal communication between the cardiologist, surgeon, and anesthesiologist for preoperative preparation. There has been much debate regarding the timing of withholding food and liquid in the pediatric population. Neonates and infants usually can be given clear liquids until 2 to 3 hours before the procedure, whereas in older children solid foods are withheld after midnight and clear liquids administered 3 to 4 hours before the procedure commences. Premedication will vary with the child's age and overall physical status. Neonates and infants often require no premedication; minimal sedation will usually suffice in children 9 to 12 months old. Premedication is best given orally to prevent crying and oxygen desaturation. Midazolam (0.5 mg/kg) alone or pentobarbital (2–4 mg/kg) with meperidine (2–3 mg/kg) will provide effective sedation and facilitate mask induction of anesthesia. Often nothing more than a compassionate conversation will suffice in children of grade school age and older. When IV sedation is planned, intramuscular premedication (ketamine 4–8 mg/kg and atropine 10 µg/kg, or a ketamine-midazolam-atropine combination) often is preferable, since it more reliably allows for a cooperative child during placement of an IV catheter.

The decision regarding anesthetic management of the pediatric patient will depend on the nature of the lesion and of the interventional procedure, the patient's physical condition, and the preference of the anesthesiologist. Sedation may be accomplished using one of a variety of hypnotic drugs. We favor IV ketamine (0.5–1.0 mg/kg loading dose, 10–20 µg/kg/min maintenance). Alternatively, IV midazolam (25–100 µg/kg loading dose, 0.25–1.0 µg/kg/min maintenance) or propofol (250–750 µg/kg loading, 10–50 µg/kg/min maintenance) may be administered. One must remember that either a supplemental narcotic bolus or infusion may produce severe ventilatory depression. Attention must be paid to monitoring the adequacy of ventilation and oxygenation, as well as basic cardiovascular parameters. The ECG, pulse oximetry, capnography, and body temperature are mandatory. The decision to use invasive procedures such as arterial, central venous, or pulmonary artery cannulation or echocardiography should be individualized after discussion among cardiologist, surgeon, and anesthesiologist.

Severely compromised children may not tolerate sedation without becoming hypoxemic and will require general anesthesia. General anesthesia facilitates control of ventilation and oxygenation and possible prevention of the increase in PVR that accompanies the effects of hypoventilation. Inhalation anesthesia with isoflurane and a narcotic supplement is usually acceptable. However, patients with decreased myocardial contractility or poor ventricular pump function may not tolerate the myocardial depression caused by any inhalation agent. Induction and maintenance with ketamine or with a narcotic by continuous infusion are acceptable alternatives.

Adult interventional cardiac catheterization procedures provide an equally daunting challenge. In the past, the anesthesiologist usually was summoned only to help during emergency resuscitation of patients experiencing complications during a procedure or to assume a role as early as possible in the management of the patient requiring emergency surgical intervention. However, procedures are now being done that often require the presence of an anesthesiologist from beginning to finish, such as percutaneous transluminal coronary angioplasty (PTCA) or stent insertion in high-risk patients, percutaneous balloon valvuloplasty (PBV), and catheter ablation of reintrant tachyarrhythmias.

Controversy still exists regarding the role of the anesthesiologist. PTCA, intracoronary stent placement, directional atherectomy, and laser ablation can be accomplished in most patients without assistance from the anesthesiology department. Such procedures are even performed in hospitals without surgical backup. Yet many centers keep an operating room and anesthesiology team on standby in case of an extreme emergency. When anesthesia is required, it is usually either for emergency PTCA or for a related complication. General anesthesia with enflurane has been demonstrated to be safe in the former situation for patients undergoing PTCA for acute myocardial infarction.[107] An added benefit of general anesthesia might be lower plasma catecholamine levels and promotion of hemodynamic stability.[108] However, it must be recognized that hypotension under general anesthesia can worsen myocardial ischemia. A narcotic-based technique probably will provide the most stable setting in the ischemic patient, since it will not depress myocardial contractility. Since all volatile halogenated anesthetics have the ability to vasodilate coronary arteries at high administered concentrations, high doses probably should be avoided during ischemia to avoid the risk of intracoronary steal. In emergency situations with profound cardiovascular collapse, only amnestic drugs should be used until the patient is safely placed on cardiopulmonary bypass. In cases where emergency surgery is required, IV access, any arterial or pulmonary artery cannulation, and especially the brachial or femoral sheath used for access during PTCA should be left in place for use in the operating room. Monitoring consideration for general anesthesia follows the guidelines mentioned previously.

Intravenous sedation will usually facilitate most PBV procedures. When general anesthesia is required, the anesthesiologist must plan pharmacologic management in accordance with the hemodynamic pathophysiology of the lesion and anticipate the needed alterations in hemodynamic management once the valvular stenosis has been relieved. Management is essentially similar to that provided for open surgical correction of either pulmonary, mitral, or aortic valvular stenosis. Sedation is all that is usually required for radiofrequency ablation procedures. Direct current (DC) procedures produce nerve and muscle simulation, which can cause patient movement and displacement of the catheter at the time the current is administered, or complications such as diaphragmatic or esophageal rupture.[109] General anesthesia with muscle relaxation is indicated to prevent these complications. Endotracheal intubation should be accomplished to protect against aspiration should intragastric pressures rise secondary to DC stimulation. A continuous IV anesthetic technique using propofol, supplemented by a narcotic, is usually sufficient and does not affect intracardiac conduction. Use of an intermediate-acting neuromuscular blocker (vecuronium, rocuronium, or atracurium) will provide profound muscle relaxation, allow for multiple ablation attempts as required, and allow quick recovery from paralysis.

Abdominal and Lower Extremity Procedures

Many of these procedures can be accomplished using local infiltration at the vascular cutdown site. Sedation then must be adequate to produce a cooperative patient who will not move during the critical moments of the operation. During lengthy correction of vascular stenoses of the lower extremity, this is often wishful thinking. Patients become restless when required to remain in one position for several hours, and oversedation in the attempt to produce a cooperative patient often produces the opposite result. Therefore, in many centers, patients undergo a regional or general anesthetic.

Selection of a general anesthetic technique involves considerations similar to those detailed previously. As with carotid surgery, the major morbidity and mortality for abdominal and lower extremity vascular procedures is cardiac in origin. However, many of the traditional perioperative cardiac risk factors are lacking, or at least diminished, during an endovascular procedure. Fluid shifts associated with open surgical procedures may be reduced, hemodynamic consequences of clamping and unclamping the aorta absent, pulmonary compromise lessened, requirements and complications of blood transfusion minimized, and the general stress response attenuated. As a result, the extensive monitoring usually employed during anesthesia for open surgical procedures can often be minimized. Since the large swings in afterload that commonly occur with aortic crossclamping will be absent, invasive monitoring can often be limited to central venous cannulation to monitor fluid balance, if there is no evidence of left ventricular failure. This also provides easy central venous administration of volume and cardiovascular drugs as necessary. The necessity for arterial cannulation can be individualized. Standard monitoring of dual lead ECG, pulse oximetry, capnography, and body temperature is assumed.

The choice of anesthetic technique involves the same considerations detailed above. However, operations involving the lower extremity, in contrast to carotid and intracranial procedures, allow for the option of maintaining the patient's ventilation by mask rather than with an endotracheal tube. This technique may be selected in patients not requiring intubation for airway protection or controlled ventilation because of poor pulmonary status. The stress of endotracheal intubation is avoided, as are the agents needed to facilitate this maneuver. Assisted ventilation is most easily accomplished when a volatile agent is used as the primary anesthetic, although the small degree of stimulation caused by many endovascular procedures may also permit a narcotic-sedative technique that permits spontaneous ventilation. The primary danger is that the patient may "lighten" and move at an inopportune moment.

Regional analgesia or anesthesia may have potential benefits, both in decreasing the stress response to surgery and in improving myocardial performance. Epidural anesthesia can be associated with attenuation of the hypercoagulable state after major vascular surgery, resulting in a lower incidence of thrombotic events.[100] However, since endovascular patients may be receiving anticoagulants, a major potential risk is development of an epidural hematoma. In patients receiving nonsteroidal antiinflammatory drugs (NSAIDs), the associated risk is controversial and largely undetermined. Although Horlocker et al. showed that epidural and spinal anesthesia can be safely performed, there is a higher incidence of traumatic placement (blood aspiration through the needle or catheter).[111] Traumatic needle placement may be significant, since a study demonstrated that 62% of spinal hematomas occurred when placement was described as such.[112] One should be aware that the platelet defect of most NSAIDs reverses in 3 to 5 days, but that of aspirin persists for 1 week and may not be accurately detectable by use of the bleeding time.[113] Risk is increased if patients are simultaneously receiving perioperative anticoagulants.[114] The decision to use a regional anesthetic should be individualized in these patients.

The risk of spinal hematoma from central neural blockade is still considered prohibitive in patients with a known coagulopathy who have received thrombolytic therapy within 24 hours and probably in fully anticoagulated patients. Patients receiving one or two doses of warfarin usually will not have an elevated prothrombin time and may have a regional anesthetic. Similarly, regional blockade may be administered to patients receiving subcutaneous low-dose heparin if the dose is not administered within 4 to 6 hours of the anesthetic procedure. Epidural and spinal anesthesia have been used safely in patients before systemic anticoagulation, provided heparin is not given for at least 1 hour after needle placement.[110,115] When the epidural catheter is no longer needed for anesthesia or postoperative analgesia, it ideally should not be removed until 4 to 6 hours after the last heparin dose and heparin not restarted for at least 1 hour afterward. Current monitoring of coagulation should be undertaken to avoid excess anticoagulation. Patients should be clinically monitored for at least 1 day to assess for signs and symptoms of a peridural hematoma.

If regional anesthesia is chosen, premedication should be minimal to ensure that the patient is awake enough to cooperate during positioning to facilitate the technique. Subsequent supplementation with an IV hypnotic can be accomplished as needed during or after the procedure. A lumbar epidural site is preferred, and an anesthetic concentration sufficient to effect motor function is administered to produce a target operative site that is free from movement if the procedure is anticipated to be lengthy or the patient apt to be restless. A continuous technique allows titration to the desired effect and emergence from any motor blockade soon after the procedure is completed. Sedation is titrated to the desired effect. Alternatively, an analgesic mixture of a local anesthetic with or without a narcotic (bupivacaine 0.25% alone or bupivacaine 0.125% with fentanyl 5µg/ml) at 10ml/hr after an initial bolus injection and with supplemental sedation should produce sufficient analgesia in the cooperative patient. Use of the catheter can continue in the recovery room to provide analgesia with a local anesthetic, supplemented with a narcotic, in a concentration that allows motor function. The resultant postoperative hemodynamic stability also argues for consideration of a regional technique.

The same caveats that pertain to central neural blockade in any patient with cardiovascular disease are relevant for the endovascular patient. Onset of the block can be unexpectedly precipitous and have severe hemodynamic consequences. Therefore careful fluid loading and judicious dosing of the local anesthetic must be employed. An initial local anesthetic volume of 10 ml or less should be used, with additional doses titrated to effect. It is important not to rush during initiation of a regional technique lest the potential benefit of the technique be eliminated by a preventable cardiovascular complication. There are no significant hemodynamic advantages among the available local anesthetics, and the choice of agent can be determined by the following: (1) required analgesic depth, (2) desired degree of motor blockade, and (3) duration of action. Subdural erosion of the catheter is a rare but potentially serious complication. When analgesic epidural doses are employed, onset of spinal blockade will slowly progress over approximately 20 to 60 minutes. This gradual onset of spinal blockade results in a progressive loss of motor function of the lower extremities. Subdural erosion with injection of a local anesthetic in a concentration high enough to produce motor blockade can produce spinal blockade in several minutes. Frequent monitoring of lower limb motility is useful, with immediate discontinuation of the epidural infusion should unplanned impairment of muscle strength develop. Epidural anesthesia has also been used to supplement general anesthesia for major vascular surgery in an effort to decrease the stress response. Use of a combined technique is probably unnecessary for endovascular procedures.

Spinal anesthesia has been a durable anesthetic technique for decades. The risks associated with airway management are diminished, and it is likely that many of the same benefits accrue regarding ablation of the stress response as with epidural anesthesia. However, the predictably rapid sympathectomy and resultant precipitous fall in systemic blood pressure contraindicate the technique in most seriously ill cardiovascular patients. Dural puncture headache remains a source of patient dissatisfaction, in spite of a greatly lowered incidence when using a thin-gauge, pencil-point needle. Purported advantages of spinal anesthesia are speed and reliability. However, failure rates approximate those for the epidural technique, and speed of onset is of dubious value because of the associated hypotension. There should be adequate time to establish epidural analgesia or anesthesia for almost all endovascular procedures. In patients for whom there is insufficient time to use an epidural technique, spinal anesthesia can be considered. However, the time constraints of emergency circumstances may also preclude giving an adequate volume preload, thus increasing the risk of hypotension. Nonetheless, spinal anesthesia remains a viable alternative in selected patients.

Postoperative Pain Management

Acute postoperative pain is a natural consequence of tissue injury and is the result of extrinsic and intrinsic (including expectations) physiologic factors. There is disagreement over the severity and significance of postoperative pain and hence over the choice of measures taken to relieve it. However, pain is as severe as the patient states it is. Recognition of individual patient differences and preferences, rather than adherence to a preconceived regimen, is the key to satisfactory pain management. Techniques such as epidural analgesia (with local anesthetics, narcotics, or both), patient-controlled analgesia (PCA), and transcutaneous electrical nerve stimulation (TENS) were developed in response to deficiencies with intramuscular narcotics "as needed" after major surgery and have all been shown to have merit. Ketorolac, currently the only NSAID approved for pain relief by parenteral administration, has advantages over traditional narcotics. It does not produce sedation or ventilatory depression. Its analgesic capability may be all that is required after endovascular procedures in which postoperative pain is of modest intensity.

6. Anesthesia for Endovascular Procedures

Postoperative surgical pain inadequately treated may enhance the stress response and cause complications. Another negative aspect of pain after major surgery is its impact on pulmonary mechanics, ventilation and oxygenation, and delaying weaning from mechanical ventilation. In one study, adverse pulmonary and endocrine responses in a small group of high-risk surgery patients were shown to be less when postoperative epidural analgesia was used compared with parenteral narcotics. Patients with epidural analgesia spent fewer days in the intensive care unit and hospital postoperatively, although this did not reach statistical significance. Hospital costs were significantly less.[116] Although not ideal, epidural analgesia may be the most effective modality for reducing the stress response to lower abdominal and lower extremity surgery in part because it can be initiated before surgical stress. However, demonstrations of improvement in outcome, duration of hospitalization, and cost are mostly conspicuous by their absence.[117] Furthermore, there should be insignificant pulmonary compromise from either a local anesthetic with sedation or a general anesthetic in the vast majority of patients for endovascular procedures. This should not be surprising for this patient population where the vascular cutdown may be the only significant nidus of pain. With the growing emphasis on cost effectiveness of all therapy, in what way do the techniques of pain relief fit? Further research is required to address the cost of improvement in patient outcome and satisfaction from new technologies.[118]

Endovascular Anesthesia Service

Organization

The organization of the anesthesiology service will depend, in general, upon the following characteristics: (1) presence/absence of a resident-teaching service, (2) whether certified registered nurse anesthetists (CRNAs) are used, (3) magnitude of the patient population, and (4) financial considerations.

Both the academic and nonacademic service should have a dedicated staff with its own section chief. The chief ideally will possess management, organizational, and leadership skills and not be appointed merely as a reward for clinical expertise, research, or friendship. Staffing should be adequate to provide 24-hour coverage for emergency situations without overtaxing personnel. The usual scholarly environment should characterize the academic department. Clinical service to patients, teaching, education, and research should all be provided. In both academic and nonacademic environments, the entire anesthesiology staff should be encouraged to attend teaching rounds and clinical conferences with surgical and medical colleagues. Faculty from all three departments should participate in a combined quality assurance meeting.

The anesthesiology service chief should participate in the design and equipment selection of the endovascular suite. Each non-operating-room site will have its own unique limitations and requirements. Considerations of importance to the anesthesiologist are listed in Box 6–1. Anesthesia and monitoring equipment for endovascular procedures in which the anesthesiology service participates must be of the same sophistication and quality as that in the cardiovascular operating room. This must include the ability to directly measure arterial, central venous, and pulmonary artery pressures, to evaluate cardiac output, to monitor transcutaneous oxygen saturation and end-tidal carbon dioxide tension, and to measure arterial and mixed venous blood gases. If the endovascular procedure is done outside of the operating room (such as in the cardiac catheterization suite), provision for prompt transfer to the surgical suite should be available in cases where complications mandate surgical intervention. Admission into an intensive care facility should be available, since endovascular procedures will typically be performed on patients at high risk for cardiovascular complications. Respiratory therapy and intensive care ventilators should be immediately available. Anesthesiologists can provide valuable service in this area even if they are not directly responsible for the primary management of intensive care patients. Their knowledge of anesthetic agents, muscle relaxants, vasoactive drugs, airway manage-

> **Box 6–1. Logistic Considerations for Anesthesia**
>
> Physical layout
>   Interview/holding area
>   Induction room
>   Access to room
>   Lighting
> Equipment/location
>   Suction
>   Oxygen/nitrous oxide sources
>   Monitors
>   Anesthesia machine
>   Medication storage
>   Emergency cart
>   Defibrillator
>   Emergency medications
>   Backup equipment
>   Oxygen tanks
>   Suction
>
> Patient considerations
>   Access to patient by anesthesiologist
>   Patient positioning
>   Safety precautions
>   Radiation/noise
>   Temperature
>   Transportation
>   Routing
>   Portable monitors
>   Portable oxygen
>   Emergency access to operating room
>   Access to intensive care unit
> Personnel
>   Training
>   Safety precautions
>   Backup support

ment, and the effects of surgery and anesthesia on pulmonary function qualifies them as pharmacologic and physiologic consultants in the intensive care unit (ICU).

The anesthesiology service chief, in conjunction with the chair of the department, should have an advisory role in the development of protocols, not only for the operating room suite, but for the use of sedative and analgesic drugs and for monitoring guidelines in areas where direct participation by anesthesiology staff is not required. This participation is specified by the Joint Commission on Accreditation of Healthcare Organizations (JCAHO) regulations in its 1994 manual and applies to any setting in which a patient receives, for any purpose, by any route, and anesthetic or sedation (with or without analgesia) for which there is a reasonable expectation that in the manner used the sedation or analgesia will result in the loss of protective reflexes in a significant number of patients.[119] Although areas in which the nonanesthesiologist physician delegates the administration of sedatives and the task of patient monitoring have traditionally been left untouched by such regulations, current trends in health care are changing this attitude. The absence of oversight that can allow a physician to get in over his or her head is slowly being changed by state regulations, by consumer standards that demand tighter control over outcomes, and by a 1994 JCAHO initiative to begin accrediting health care networks.[120] Mandated regulations will involve training, education, and provision for adequate space, equipment, and monitoring before, during, and after procedures.

Does safety monitoring make a difference? Although evaluation of intraoperative data suggests that there has been a decline in the number and severity of intraanesthetic deaths,[121,122] there is no conclusive proof that monitoring practices such as pulse oximetry and capnography improve patient outcome.[123,124] However, the goal of safety monitoring is to provide the earliest possible warning of danger. Since the most serious incidents involving anesthesia and sedation continue to relate to ventilation and oxygenation, it is understandable that the American Society of Anesthesiology (ASA) has made oximetry a standard of care and virtually mandates capnography.[125] Uniform quality of anesthesia service throughout a hospital or clinic does not necessarily mean identical care. However, anesthesia and sedation are the same wherever they are given, and patients deserve a high standard of care and safety regardless of location. Since there is presently no national consensus regarding monitoring standards outside of the operating room, the individual institution will have to develop a comprehensive quality plan for the safe provision of analgesia and anesthesia throughout the facility.

Controversy exists regarding whether CRNAs should administer anesthesia or sedation to high-risk patients undergoing cardiovascular procedures. Current ASA Guidelines for Delegation of Technical Anesthesia Functions to Non-physician Personnel acknowledge that "while optimal anesthesia care involves a one-to-one relationship between anesthesiologist and patient, manpower shortages may necessitate the utilization of non-physician personnel to perform technical functions ... under the personal direction of an anesthesiologist or other qualified physician."[126] In many practices, a CRNA who has met the technical and intellectual requirements established by the hospital administers monitored anesthesia care to appropriately selected patients, with a staff anesthesiologist supervising and being immediately available to intervene during emergencies. Since most patients undergoing endovascular procedures will have a relatively high number of medical problems, and since there is currently no lack of competent anesthesiologists who have elected to obtain additional emphasis on cardiovascular practice, the question of a shortage of all physician anesthesia personnel is now debatable. Changes in the delivery of medical care and in reimbursement for services are rendering obsolete the argument that CRNAs are more cost effective as well. Lack of consensus in the medical community may mean that the marketplace will ultimately determine the answer to the question regarding use of CRNAs.

The size of the practice is a major determinant in the availability of anesthesia coverage. A correlation exists between the size of the hospital and the availability of "in-house" 24-hour coverage by an anesthesiologist.[127] Other factors include the ratio of anesthesiologists to resident staff or CRNAs, the ratio of providers to operating rooms, surgical scheduling, the likelihood of a non-operating-room procedure requiring emergency transfer to the operating room, and the extent of departmental involvement in the ICU. There has been debate over the maximum number of continuous workhours spent by a given practitioner, and New York has enacted laws limiting the hours that residents and emergency physicians may work consecutively.[128] Although objective data on this subject is inconclusive,[129,130] the greater the scale of involvement by anesthesiologists, the greater the need for additional personnel to provide safe service.

Managed care has put downward pressure on reimbursement of individual specialists. Equitable revenue-sharing arrangement in the future is a management issue that will increasingly play an important role and cannot be ignored. Unfortunately, many health maintenance organization (HMO) contracts require a hospital to be a full-service institution. Small departments that overextend themselves in an attempt to preserve income lose economy of scale and exert negative pressure on the quality of care. Departments with staffing adequate to provide the service being mandated by the marketplace and by regulating agencies must be compensated fairly in return.

Managing Anesthetic Risk

Administration of anesthesia to patients with cardiovascular disease is a safe procedure. This statement is confirmed by clinical experience nationwide and in editorial commentary.[131,132] The basic risks inherent to the administration of anesthesia, such as drug interactions, complications of vascular access, pulmonary aspiration, hemodynamic aberrations, dental trauma, hypothermia, and awareness, are not unique to the patient with cardiovascular disease. Incidence may be increased because such patients typically take a large number of drugs chronically, require more invasive vascular access and monitoring devices, and have a more unstable cardiovascular system. Several variables have been extensively studied as preoperative predictors of cardiac risk for anesthesia.[133,134] Investigations of the effect of advanced age, hypertension, diabetes mellitus, angina pectoris, and old myocardial infarction, factors common in patients with vascular disease, on anesthetic risk have yielded eqivocal results. Others, such as arrhythmias, congestive heart failure, and recent (within 6 months) myocardial infarction (MI) have been largely unquestioned predictors of cardiac morbidity.[135]

Traditional anesthetic risk assessment has been narrow in focus in that it has centered on preoperative preparation and intraoperative management. However, morbidity from increased risk is but one form of patient outcome. There is risk, financial as well as medical, from incorporating expensive technology into clinical practice merely to provide more information that links one form of outcome (morbidity) with what is accepted clinical practice. Society is demanding that the net benefit (e.g., risk of the procedure, risk of acting on false-positive or false-negative results, cost, and patient benefits including clinical outcome) be examined. For example, presence of a reversible defect during dipyridamole thallium scintigraphy (DTS), a very expensive procedure, was demonstrated to be an important predictor of cardiac ischemic events after peripheral vascular surgery[136] and to aid in stratifying risk when used in conjunction with patient clinical characteristics.[137] Attempts to duplicate these results with DTS have yielded variable results regarding risk[138] and negative utility regarding risk stratification.[139] DTS has a relative lack of specificity and low predictive value because of a high incidence of false-positive results. The latter may cause referral for unnecessary invasive testing and surgery, thus augmenting patient risk without any currently demonstrated improvement in outcome. Thus a procedure lauded at anesthesiology meetings in the late 1980s as perhaps being the definitive test for cardiac risk is now often questioned as yet another sophisticated and expensive diagnostic technique of indeterminant value for use in a large group of at-risk patients.

Furthermore, even the opinion regarding the predictive value of recent MI has been challenged.[140,141] Use of invasive monitoring to facilitate tight control of intraoperative blood pressure and heart rate followed by monitoring and aggressive treatment in the ICU for 1 to 2 days postoperatively dramatically decreased reinfarction rates compared with those previously published.[142-145] Although the monetary cost of this aggressive management is high, it must be viewed in the context of the cost to treat the high incidence of perioperative MI in vascular patients and the dollar cost to society of the high mortality rate in this subset. Standardized clinical trials are unlikely to provide a solution to this dilemma of cost-to-benefit analysis. The studies of Wells and Kaplan[141] and Rao et al.[140] suggest that a multidisciplinary perioperative approach to minimizing cardiac risk should be undertaken. Therefore the solution to the question of risk management may depend on using the industrial management technique of statistical process control (SPC) in which all input variables (i.e., patient clinical profile; various preoperative tests; invasive or surgical procedure performed; other perioperative interventions by cardiologist, anesthesiologist, or surgeon; drug therapy) are measured against output (e.g., clinical result, duration of stay, complication rate, cost) in a large ongoing database (see the discussion on p. 86).

Further evidence supporting a perioperative approach to risk management is offered in a study by Mangano et al. in which the only factor correlating with an increase in all adverse cardiac outcomes was postoperative ischemia.[146] Multivariate analysis showed a lack of correlation with other prior or concurrent clinical factors or perioperative events, such as cardiac risk index, history of MI or congestive heart failure, or preoperative or intraoperative ischemia. The authors suggest greater emphasis on patient care in the postoperative period with specific attention to prevention of ischemia.

The implications of ischemia in the outpatient setting is similarly detailed.[147] The importance of postoperative ischemia has been demonstrated for the specific subset of vascular surgery patients.[148] Predictors of postoperative ischemia in one study were shown to be: (1) electrocardiographic evidence of left ventricular hypertrophy, (2) hypertension history, (3) diabetes mellitus, (4) definite coronary artery disease, and (5) digoxin use.[149] Another study from the same hospital population demonstrated that, even in patients at high risk of cardiac complications, noncardiac causes of in-hospital mortality are more common after noncardiac surgery, further redrawing attention to factors such as hypertension, impaired renal function, and limitation of activity.[150] Thus it appears that we may have gone full circle in the assessment of risk factors but still do not know which tests or therapy to order when.

Whether these findings are applicable to patients nationwide is debatable, since it is possible that the risk profile of a black male patient in Memphis, Tennessee, differs from that of a white female patient in Los Angeles. Results mentioned above illustrate the need for an individualized control process in each practice setting. Independent multivariate cause-and-effect studies will most likely be required to delineate both the risks for subsets of patients in different practice settings throughout the nation and what tests and therapy should be ordered to identify and minimize them.

Patient Evaluation and Consultation

Except for emergencies, the patient interview and discussion of anesthetic management ideally will occur at least several days before any elective procedure. This is best accomplished in an outpatient preoperative clinic, where the appropriate history and physical examination, laboratory assessment, and preanesthesia interview can be coordinated in one patient visit. The logistic advantages of this system are well documented and have been shown to convey time and economic benefits to the surgeon and anesthesiologist, as well as the patient.[151] The presumed complexity of surgery is most often the primary or sole determinant used by third-party payors to select which procedures are appropriate for outpatient or same-day surgery admission. As procedures become less invasive, the risk of anesthesia will often supersede that of the surgery. Early evaluation by the anesthesiologist allows time for further medical workup when indicated and for discussion between the anesthesiologist, internist, and surgeon regarding any special perioperative management. The anesthesiologist must be aware of any potential circumstances that could necessitate changing the anesthetic management from one involving monitored sedation with or without local anesthesia to one requiring an emergency general anesthetic.

The preanesthetic evaluation includes a detailed review of personal and familial medical and surgical histories, allergies and adverse drug reactions, current illness, and medication use and abuse. The physical examination must be documented. The extent of laboratory assessment will depend on the medical condition of the patient, the planned procedure, and to some extent the likelihood of any emergency surgery that may be required. Although these patients will present with the same medical profile as those who in prior years would undergo major cardiac and vascular surgery, the lesser degree of invasiveness and potentially lower anesthetic risk may require a less extensive patient workup. This will need to be determined by a detailed analysis of cause-and-effect data regarding input (i.e., preoperative workup) and output (i.e., clinical results, morbidity, mortality) of each clinical practice. Blood for type and screen or crossmatch should be drawn as warranted.

The pertinent risks, benefits, and expectations of the anesthetic plan must be fully discussed and documented. The intent is to inform, not frighten or coerce, the patient. If a detailed discussion is warranted, anxiety can be assuaged by assistance from a well-trained and informed nurse and by the consultant who will perform the endovascular procedure. Documentation must include a description of the planned anesthetic management, patient acknowledgment of the potential risks and expected benefits, and a statement that patient questions were invited and answered and that the patient wishes to proceed with the anesthetic.

Changing consumer attitudes regarding quality of care make it desirable to have a consistent and objective measure of patient satisfaction. A standardized questionnaire, filled out when the patient is discharged and in the absence of the anesthesiologist, will provide a reliable undirected opinion. Continuous analysis of questionnaire results (outcome) can be used to direct continuous improvement of the service provided and to supply information for

---

Box 6–2. Endovascular Anesthesia Survey

Please circle YES or NO to each question.
- Did an anesthesiologist provide service during your procedure?   YES   NO
- Were the risks and benefits of anesthesia clearly explained?   YES   NO
- Did you have a spinal, epidural, or nerve block?   YES   NO
- Were you satisfied with the effect of the block?   YES   NO
- Did you receive intravenous sedation with the nerve block?   YES   NO
- Were you satisfied with the result of the sedation?   YES   NO
- Did you have a local anesthetic with sedation?   YES   NO
- Were you satisfied with this technique for pain relief?   YES   NO
- Did you have a general anesthetic?   YES   NO
- Were you satisfied with your general anesthetic?   YES   NO
- How would you rate the anesthesia team member who took care of you?
   a. Professional   YES   NO
   b. Pleasant   YES   NO
   c. Considerate   YES   NO
   d. Indifferent   YES   NO
   e. Inconsiderate/rude   YES   NO

Comments:

Name (optional):   Date of delivery (optional):

---

departmental quality assurance initiatives (Box 6–2).

Total Quality Management

Discussions of traditional intradepartmental guidelines regarding policies and procedures, risk management and quality of care, and granting of credentials can be found in standard anesthesiology textbooks and derive in part from statements by the JCAHO and from the Standards, Guidelines, and Statements of the ASA. Institutional compliance with JCAHO standards is virtually mandatory, since the majority of states require JCAHO accreditation to qualify for licensure. JCAHO requires and pays particular attention to preoperative and postoperative assessment and the quality assurance (QA) mechanisms of individual departments and of the organization. The QA mechanism must record the occurrence of deviation from clinical indicators of quality that are based on important aspects of care. The circumstances of any deviation must be investigated, causation for the deviation from acceptable standard established, communication with the care provider undertaken, and a plan for corrective action established. JCAHO indicators and measurements are based on retrospective analysis of adverse events that are presumed to be related to quality care. However, there are no guidelines for the measurement of variations in clinical care that account for the occurrence of adverse outcomes. Therefore it is a system that merely counts incidents but that fails to measure cause and effect and thereby facilitate quality improvement.

The ASA has recently endorsed an approach that makes no a priori judgments about relevance of clinical indicators. Rather, it is an occurrence-driven QA process in which a department committee determines the relevance of a clinical incident to anesthetic management.[152] The process classifies the type of management error, determines the nature of its cause (e.g., none, mechanical, human) and origin (e.g., inadequate knowledge, inadequate data, disregarding of data), grades the severity of the outcome according to preset criteria, and reports corrective action back to the practitioner. A computerized database of adverse clinical incidents is developed that facilitates tracking of individual performance, as well as comparison with other practitioners and with department norms. However, it is still an occurrence-driven process subject to the limitations of retrospective peer review,[153] does not generate an ongoing stream of cause-and-effect data, and fails to facilitate specific quality improvement measures for department-wide policies.

The United States is in the midst of a health care reformation that has led to experimentation with concepts designed to monitor, manage, and compare performance of health care providers employing techniques borrowed from industrial management. Physicians have heard of the terms *total quality management* (TQM) and *continuous quality improvement* (CQI), but most have little understanding of their underlying principles. These concepts derive from activity-based vendor supply and integrated accounting systems. They provide a framework for continuous improvement and innovation and address outcome in terms of consumer (patient, third party payor, industry), rather than provider (physician), expectations.

The collective term for this process is statistical process control (SPC). Derived from Japanese industrial management principles, it has three important tenets for medical CQI: (1) outcome (quality) must be measured if control and improvement are to occur, (2) information to make statistically valid improvements in quality can be derived through analysis of variation found in outcome, and (3) use of control charts and skeleton diagrams can help to define sources of variation to facilitate the process.

The endovascular practice is a good choice to demonstrate the utility of industrial management and quality techniques because the information collected by each member of the team is of vital importance to all the other members. However, the interpretation and significance of data are likely to be different among the anesthesiologist, cardiologist, surgeon, and nurse; and data collection and transcription are likely to differ significantly as well. This variation can delay and complicate the flow of patient care. Use of a single control chart that delineates all aspects of patient care, and on which all vital patient parameters and therapeutic modalities are listed, can help the team draw statistically valid conclusions (SPCs) from the same ongoing flow of patient data, eliminate duplication of recorded data, and save valuable time and expense.

The SPCs can also form the basis of TQM and QA through the use of cause-and-effect diagrams and control charts. The former is a management tool that tracks all events of a manufacturing process and relates them to various outcome measurements.[154] This TQM technique requires creation of a flowchart/skeleton diagram (clinical pathway) that describes how the process of clinical care provided by the department for a clinical subset of patients should be organized. This is similar in structure to the algorithms that have appeared as teaching aids in medical textbooks. Input such as care provider, laboratory tests and results, and modalities of technical and pharmacologic anesthetic treatment serve as input parameters into the patient database. Clinical results, cost, and solicited feedback on consumer satisfaction serve as outcome (quality) measures in the database. Use of this database can enable the department to observe changes in outcome based on changes in input parameters.

The departmental database should be part of (or fully integrate with) the endovascular patient and hospital databases. This facilitates collection of a large amount of ongoing patient information from which valid conclusions regarding clinical effectiveness of interdepartmental resource utilization, cost effectiveness, and patient satisfaction can be obtained. SPC techniques can thus be used to replace traditional peer review and to identify areas in which individual and total processes of patient care can be improved. It may ultimately help physicians play the central role in facilitating changes in the delivery of health care that are consumer oriented and keep reform out of the control of outside agencies.

References

1. Cote P, Guerret P, Bourassa MG: Systemic and coronary hemodynamic effects of diazepam in patients with normal and diseased coronary arteries, *Circulation* 50:1210, 1974.
2. Tomichek RC, Rosow CE, Schneider RC et al: Cardiovascular effects of diazepam-fentanyl anesthesia in patients with coronary artery disease, *Anesth Analg* 61:217, 1982.
3. Geller E, Halpern P, Chernilar J et al: Cardiorespiratory effects of antagonism of diazepam sedation with flumazenil in patients with cardiac disease, *Anesth Analg* 72:207, 1991.
4. Ward DS: Stimulation of hypoxic ventilatory drive by droperidol, *Anesth Analg* 63:106, 1984.
5. Fragan RJ, Funk DI, Avram MF et al: Midazolam vs hydroxyzine as intramuscular premedicant, *Can Anaesth Soc J* 30:136, 1983.
6. Drew JH, Dripps RD, Conroe JH Jr: Clinical studies on morphine. II. The effect of morphine upon the circulation of man and upon the circulatory and respiratory responses to tilting, *Anesthesiology* 7:44, 1966.
7. Hynynen M, Takkunen O, Salmenpera M et al: Continuous infusion of fentanyl or alfentanil for coronary artery surgery. Plasma opiate concentrations, hemodynamics and postoperative course, *Br J Anaesth* 58:1252, 1986.
8. Hynynen M, Lehtinen A-M, Salmenpera M et al: Continuous infusion of fentanyl or alfentanil for coronary artery surgery. Effects on plasma cortisol concentration, beta-endorphin immunoreactivity and arginine vasopressin, *Br J Anaesth* 58:1260, 1986.
9. de Lange S, Boscoe MJ, Stanely TH et al: Comparison of sufentanil-O_2 and fentanyl-O_2 for coronary artery surgery, *Anesthesiology* 56:112, 1982.
10. Tomicheck RC, Rosow CE, Philbin DM et al: Diazepam/fentanyl interaction, hemodynamic and hormonal effects in coronary artery surgery, *Anesth Analg* 62:881, 1983.
11. Reeves JG, Kissin I, Fournier SE et al: Added negative inotrophic effect of a combination of diazepam and fentanyl, *Anesth Analg* 63:97, 1984.
12. Flacke JW, Davie LJ, Flacke WE et al: Effects of fentanyl and diazepam in dogs deprived of autonomic tone, *Anesth Analg* 64:1053, 1985.
13. Scott JC, Cooke JE, Stanski Dr: Electroencephalographic quantitation of opioid effect: comparative pharmacodynamics of fentanyl and sufentanil, *Anesthesiology* 74:34, 1991.
14. Miller DR, Wellwood M, Teasdale SJ et al: Effects of anesthetic induction on myocardial function and metabolism: a comparison of fentanyl, sufentanil and alfentanil, *Can J Anaesth* 35:219, 1988.
15. Howie MB, McSweeney TD, Lingam RP et al: A comparison of fentanyl-O_2 and sufentanil-O_2 for cardiac surgery, *Anesth Analg* 64:877, 1985.
16. Rucquoi M, Camu F: Cardiovascular responses to large doses of alfentanil and fentanyl, *Br J Anaesth* 55:233S, 1983.
17. Tumen KJ, McCarthy RJ, Spiess BD et al: Does choice of anesthetic agent significantly affect outcome after coronary artery surgery? *Anesthesiology* 70:189, 1989.
18. Slogoff S, Keats AS: Randomized trial of primary anesthetic agents on outcome of coronary artery bypass operations, *Anesthesiology* 70:179, 1989.
19. King BD, Elder JD, Dripps RD: The effect of intravenous administration of meperidine upon the circulation of man and upon the circulatory response to tilt, *Surg Gyn Obstet* 94:591, 1952.
20. Stanley Th, Liu WS: Cardiovascular effects of meperidine-N20 anesthesia before and after pancuronium, *Anesth Analg* 56:669, 1977.
21. Murphy MR, Hug CC: The enflurane-sparing effect of morphine, butorphanol, and nalbuphine, *Anesthesiology* 57:489, 1982.
22. Murphy MR, Hug CC: The anesthetic potency of fentanyl in terms of its reduction of enflurane MAC, *Anesthesiology* 57:485, 1982.
23. Popio KA, Jackson DH, Ross AM et al: Hemodynamic and respiratory effects of morphine and butorphanol, *Clin Pharmacol Ther* 23:281, 1978.
24. Weiss BM, Schmid ER, Gattiker RI: Comparison of nalbuphine and fentanyl anesthesia for coronary artery bypass surgery. Hemodynamics, hormonal response and postoperative respiratory depression, *Anesth Analg* 73:521, 1991.
25. Lake CL, Duckworth EN, DiFazio CA et al: Cardiovascular effects of nalbuphine in patients with coronary or valvular heart disease, *Anesthesiology* 57:498, 1982.
26. Okutani R, Kono K, Kinoshita O et al: Variations in hemodynamic and stress hormonal responses in open heart surgery with buphrenorphine/diazepam anesthesia, *J Cardiothorac Anesth* 3:401, 1989.
27. Glass SA, Hardman D, Kamiyama Y et al: Preliminary pharmacokinetics and pharmacodynamics of an ultra-short-acting opioid:

Remifentanil (G187084B), *Anesth Analg* 77:1031, 1993.
28. Westmoreland CL, Hoke JF, Sebel PS et al: Pharmacokinetics of remifentanil (G187084B) and its major metabolite (G190291) in patients undergoing elective surgery, *Anesthesiology* 79:893, 1993.
29. Sear JW: Intravenous anesthetics. In Anaesthesia for the compromised heart, *Bailleres Clin Anaesthesiol* 3:217, 1989.
30. Chraemmer-Jorgensen B, Hoillemd-Carlsen PP et al: Left ventricular performance monitored by radionuclide cardiography during induction, *Anesthesiology* 62:278, 1985.
31. Flacke JW, Davis JD, Flacke WE et al: Effects of fentanyl and diazepam in dogs deprived of autonomic tone, *Anesth Analg* 64:1053, 1985.
32. Kettler D, Sonntag H, Wolfram-Donath U et al: Haemodynamics, myocardial function, oxygen requirement, and oxygen supply of the human heart after administration of etomidate. In Doenick A, editor: *Anaesthesiology and resuscitation*, Berlin, 1977, Springer-Verlag.
33. Reiz S, Balfours E, Sorensen MB et al: Isoflurane—a powerful coronary vasodilator in patients with coronary artery disease, *Anesthesiology* 59:91, 1983.
34. Messick JM, Casement B, Sharbrough FW et al: Correlation of regional cerebral blood flow with EEG changes during isoflurane anesthesia for carotid endarterectomy, *Anesthesiology* 66:344, 1987.
35. Bastard OG, Carter JG, Moyers JR et al: Circulatory effects of isoflurane in patients with ischemic heart disease. A comparison with halothane, *Anesth Analg* 63:635, 1984.
36. Hesse W, Arnold B, Schulte-Sassee U et al: Comparison of isoflurane and halothane when used to control hypertension in patients undergoing coronary bypass surgery, *Anesth Analg* 62:15, 1983.
37. Cahalan MK, Prakash O, Rulf ENR et al: Addition of nitrous oxide to fentanyl anesthesia does not induce myocardial ischemia in patients with ischemic heart disease, *Anesthesiology* 67:925, 1987.
38. Wilkowski DA, Sill JC, Bonta W et al: Nitrous oxide constricts epicardial coronary arteries without effect on coronary arterioles, *Anesthesiology* 66:659, 1987.
39. Balasarawathi K, Kumar P, Rao TL et al: Left ventricular end diastolic pressure as an index for nitrous oxide use during coronary artery surgery, *Anesthesiology* 55:708, 1981.
40. Ebert TJ, Muzi M: Sympathetic hyperactivity during desflurane anesthesia in healthy volunteers, *Anesthesiology* 79:444, 1993.
41. Helman JD, Leung JM, Bellows WH et al: A comparison of desflurane and sufentanil in patients undergoing coronary artery surgery, *Anesthesiology* 77:47, 1992.
42. Weiskopf RB, Eger EI, Noorani M et al: Repetitive rapid increases in desflurane concentration blunt transient cardiovascular stimulation in man, *Anesthesiology* 81:843, 1994.
43. Yli-Hankala A, Randell T, Seppala T et al: Increases in hemodynamic variables and catecholamine levels after a rapid increase in isoflurane concentration, *Anesthesiology* 78:266, 1993.
44. Haggmark S, Hohner P, Ostman M et al: Comparison of hemodynamic, electrocardiographic, mechanical, and metabolic indicators of intraoperative myocardial ischemia in vascular surgical patients with coronary artery disease, *Anesthesiology* 70:19, 1989.
45. Savarese JJ, Lowenstein E: The name of the game: no anesthesia by cook book, *Anesthesiology* 62:70, 1985.
46. Ali HH, Savarese JJ, Embree PB et al: Clinical pharmacology of mivacurium chloride infusion (BW B1090U0): Comparison with vecuronium and atracurium, *Br J Anaesth* 61:541, 1988.
47. Block A, Covino BG: Some effects of local anesthetic agents on cardiac conduction and contractility, *Reg Anesth* 6:55, 1982.
48. Johns RA, DeFazio CA, Longnecker DE: Lidocaine constricts or dilates rat arterioles in a dose-dependent manner, *Anesthesiology* 62:141, 1985.
49. Bassenge E, Holtz J, Kinadeter H et al: Threshold dosages of nitroglycerin for coronary artery dilation, afterload reduction and venous pooling in conscious dogs. In Lichtlen PR, Engel HJ, Schey I et al, editors: *Nitrates III*, Berlin, 1981, Springer-Verlag.
50. Glisson SN, Sanchez MM, El-Etr AA et al: Nitroglycerin and neuromuscular blockage produced by gallamine, succinylcholine, d-tubocurarine and pancuronium, *Anesth Analg* 59:117, 1980.
51. Mann T, Cohn PF, Holmen BL et al: Effects of nitroprusside on regional myocardial blood flow in coronary artery disease, *Circulation* 57:732, 1978.
52. Gelman S, Reves JG, Fowler et al: Regional blood flow during thoracic aortic crossclamping

and sodium nitroprusside infusion in dogs (abstract), *Anesth Analg* 62:245, 1983.
53. Grum DF, Svensson LG: Changes in cerebrospinal fluid pressure and spinal cord perfusion pressure prior to cross-clamping of the thoracic aorta in humans, *J Cardiothorac Vasc Anesth* 5:331, 1991.
54. Becker RC, Corrao JM, Bovill EG et al: Intravenous nitroglycerin-induced heparin resistance: a qualitative antithrombin III abnormality, *Am Heart J* 119:1254, 1990.
55. Henriksson Ba, Biber B, Haggendal J et al: Cardiovascular effects of enflurane and asphyxia during long-term beta-adrenoceptor blockade, *Acta Anaesthesiol Scand* 29:363, 1985.
56. Horan BF, Prys-Roberts C, Roberts JG et al: Haemodynamic responses to isoflurane anaesthesia and hypovolemia in the dog and their modification by propranolol, *Br J Anaesth* 49:179, 1979.
57. Roberts JE, Foex P, Clark TNS et al: Hemodynamic interactions of high dose propranolol treatment and anaesthesia in the dog. 1. Halothane dose response studies, *Br J Anaesth* 48:315, 1976.
58. Gerber JG, Nies AS: Beta-adrenergic blocking drugs, *Ann Rev Med* 36:145, 1985.
59. Greefhorst APM, Van Herwaarden CLA: Comparative study of the ventilatory effects of three beta$_1$-selective blocking agents in asthmatic patients, *J Clin Pharmacol* 20:417, 1981.
60. Kates RA, Kaplan JA: Cardiovascular responses to verapamil during coronary artery bypass graft surgery, *Anesth Analg* 62:21, 1983.
61. Marijic J, Zelijko J, Bosnjakj et al: Effects and interaction of verapamil and volatile anesthetics on the isolated perfused guinea pig heart, *Anesthesiology* 69:914, 1988.
62. Schulte-Sasse V, Hess W, Markschies-Hornung A et al: Combined effects of halothane anesthesia and verapamil on systemic hemodynamics and LV myocardial contractility in patients with ischemic heart disease, *Anesth Analg* 63:791, 1984.
63. Zalman F, Perloff JK, Durant NN et al: Acute respiratory failure following verapamil in Duchenne's muscular dystrophy, *Am Heart J* 105:510, 1983.
64. Kraynack BL, Lawson NW, Ginautas et al: Effects of verapamil on indirect muscle twitch response, *Anesth Analg* 62:827, 1983.
65. Jones RM, Cashman JN, Casson WR et al: Verapamil potentiation of neuromuscular blockade: failure of reversal with neostigmine, but prompt reversal with edrophonium, *Anesth Analg* 64:1021, 1985.
66. Roewer LS, Rumberger E, Bode H et al: Electrophysiological and mechanical interactions of verapamil and dantrolene on isolated heart muscle, *Anesthesiology* 63:A274, 1985.
67. Salzman LS, Kates RAS, Corke BC et al: Hyperkalemia and cardiovascular collapse after verapamil and dantrolene administration in swine, *Anesth Analg* 63:473, 1984.
68. Iwatsuki N, Katoh M, Ono K et al: Antiarrhythmic effect of diltiazem during halothane anesthesia in dogs and in humans, *Anesth Analg* 64:964, 1985.
69. Spiss CK, Zadrocilck E, Weinmayr-Goettel M et al: Nifedipine induced hypotension in man: hemodynamic response during isoflurane and halothane anesthesia, *Anesthesiology* 63:A93, 1985.
70. Schulte-Sasse V, Hess W, Markschies-Hornung A et al: Cardiovascular interactions of halothane anesthesia and nifedipine in patients subjected to elective coronary artery bypass surgery, *Thoracic Cardiovasc Surg* 31:261, 1983.
71. Miller RD: Enhancements of d-tubocurarine neuromuscular blockade in man, *Anesthesiology* 45:422, 1967.
72. Liberman BA, Teasdale SJ: Anaesthesia and amiodarone, *Can Anaesth Soc J* 32:629, 1985.
73. Kehlet H: Modification of responses to surgery by neural blockade: clinical implications. In Cousins MJ, Bridenbaugh PO, editors: *Neural blockade in clinical anesthesia and management of pain*, Philadelphia, 1987, JB Lippincott.
74. Jorgensen LN, Rasmussen LS, Nielsen PT et al: Antithrombotic efficacy of continuous extradural analgesia after knee replacement, *Br J Anaesth* 66:8, 1991.
75. Kehlet H: Influence of regional anaesthesia on postoperative morbidity, *Ann Chir Gynaecol* 73:171, 1984.
76. Reiz S: Myocardial ischaemia associated with general anesthesia, *Br J Anaesth* 61:68, 1988.
77. Gelman S, Laws HL, Potzick J et al: Thoracic epidural vs balanced anesthesia in morbid obesity: an intraoperative and postoperative hemodynamic study, *Anesth Analg* 59:902, 1980.
78. Reinhart K, Foehring U, Kersting T et al: Effects of thoracic epidural anesthesia on systemic hemodynamic function and systemic oxygen supply-demand relationship, *Anesth Analg* 69:360, 1989.

79. Rawal N, Sjostrand U, Christoffersson E et al: Comparison of intramuscular and epidural morphine for postoperative in the grossly obese, *Anesth Analg* 63:583, 1984.
80. Scott NB, Kehlet H: Regional anaesthesia and surgical morbidity, *Br J Surg* 75:299, 1988.
81. Burgos LG, Ebert TJ, Asiddao CB et al: Increased intraoperative cardiovascular morbidity in diabetics with autonomic neuropathy, *Anesthesiology* 70:591, 1989.
82. Schwartz PJ, Zaza A, Pala M et al: Baroreflex sensitivity and its evolution during the first year after myocardial infarction, *J Am Coll Cardiol* 12:629, 1988.
83. Trimarco B, Chierchia S, Lembo G et al: Prolonged duration of myocardial ischemia in patient with coronary heart disease and impaired cardiopulmonary baroreceptor sensitivity, *Circulation* 81:1792, 1990.
84. Deferrari GM, Vanou E, Stramba-Badiale M et al: Vagal reflexes and survival during acute myocardial ischemia in conscious dogs with healed myocardial infarction, *Am J Physiol* 261:73, 1991.
85. Maze M, Tranquilli W: Alpha-1 adrenoceptor agonists: defining the role in clinical anesthesia, *Anesthesiology* 74:581, 1991.
86. Segal IS, Jarvis DJ, Duncan SR et al: Clinical efficacy of oral-transdermal clonidine combinations during the perioperative period, *Anesthesiology* 74:220, 1991.
87. Quintin L, Viale JP, Annat G et al: Oxygen uptake after major abdominal surgery: effect of clonidine, *Anesthesiology* 74:236, 1991.
88. Quintin L, Roudot F, Roux C et al: Effect of clonidine on the circulation and vasoactive hormones after aortic surgery, *Br J Anaesth* 66:108, 1991.
89. Ferres C, Carson I, Lyons S et al: Haemodynamic effects of vecuronium, pancuronium and atracurium in patients with coronary artery disease, *Br J Anaesth* 59:305, 1987.
90. Blume WT, Ferguson GG, McNeil DK: Significance of EEG changes at carotid endarterectomy, *Stroke* 17:891, 1986.
91. Roizen MF: Anesthetic goals for operations to relieve or prevent cerebrovascular insufficiency. In Roizen MF, editor: *Anesthesia for vascular surgery*, New York, 1990, Churchill Livingstone.
92. Raeder JC, Breivik H: Premedication with midazolam in outpatient general anesthesia: a comparison of morphine, scopolamine, and placebo, *Acta Anaesthesiol Scand* 31:509, 1987.
93. Shafer SL, Varvel JR, Aziz N et al: The pharmacokinetics of fentanyl administered by computer controlled infusion pump, *Anesthesiology* 73:1091, 1990.
94. Forrest JB, Rehder K, Cahalan MK et al: Multicenter study of general anesthesia III. Predictors of severe perioperative adverse outcomes, *Anesthesiology* 76:3, 1992.
95. Casement B, Messick J, Milde L et al: "Critical" CBF during isoflurane anesthesia in man (abstract), *Anesthesiology* 63:A406, 1985.
96. Michenfelder JD, Sundt TM, Fode N et al: Isoflurane when compared to enflurane and halothane decreases the frequency of cerebral ischemia during carotid endarterectomy, *Anesthesiology* 67:336, 1987.
97. Newberg LA, Milde JH, Michenfelder JD: The cerebral metabolic effects of isoflurane at and above concentrations that suppress cortical electric activity, *Anesthesiology* 59:23, 1983.
98. Reiz S, Ostman M: Regional coronary hemodynamics during isoflurane nitrous oxide in patients with ischemic heart disease, *Anesth Analg* 64:570, 1985.
99. Wrigley SR, Fairfield JE, Jones RM et al: Induction and recovery characteristics of desflurane in day case patients: a comparison with propofol, *Anaesthesia* 46:615, 1991.
100. Shafer SL: *Intravenous anesthesia: new drugs and techniques*, 44th annual refresher course lectures and clinical update programs. American Society of Anesthesiologists Annual Meeting, Washington, DC, Oct 1993.
101. Smith AL, Hoff JT, Nielsen SL et al: Barbiturate protection in acute focal cerebral ischemia, *Stroke* 5:127, 1974.
102. Ward JD, Becker DP, Miller DJ et al: Failure of prophylactic barbiturate coma in the treatment of severe head trauma, *J Neurosurg* 62:383, 1985.
103. Steen PA, Gisvold SE, Milde JH et al: Nimodipine improves outcome when given after complete cerebral ischemia in primates, *Anesthesiology* 62:406, 1985.
104. Gelmers H, Gorter K, De Weerdt C et al: A controlled trial of nimodipine in acute ischemic stroke, *N Engl J Med* 319:203, 1988.
105. Pulsinelli WA, Levy DE, Sigbee B et al: Increased damage after ischemic stroke in patients with hyperglycemia with or without established diabetes mellitus, *Am J Med* 74:540, 1983.
106. Rashkind WJ: Historical aspects of surgery for congenital heart disease, *J Thorac Cardiovasc Surg* 84:619, 1982.

107. de Bruijn NP, Hlatky MA, Jacobs JR et al: General anesthesia during percutaneous transluminal coronary angioplasty: results of a randomized controlled clinical trial, *Anesth Analg* 68:201, 1989.
108. Kates RA, Stack RS, Hill RF et al: General anesthesia for patients undergoing percutaneous transluminal coronary angioplasty during acute myocardial infarction, *Anesth Analg* 65:815, 1986.
109. Sebag C, Lavergne T, Millat B et al: Rupture of the stomach and esophagus after attempted transcatheter ablation of an accessory pathway by direct current shock, *Am J Cardiol* 63:890, 1989.
110. Tuman KJ, McCarthy RJ, March RJ et al: Effects of epidural anesthesia and analgesia on coagulation and outcome after major vascular surgery, *Anesth Analg* 73:696, 1991.
111. Horlocker TT, Wedel DJ, Offord KP: Does preoperative antiplatelet therapy increase the risk of hemorrhagic complications associated with regional anesthesia? *Anesth Analg* 70:631, 1990.
112. Owens EL, Kasten GW, Hessel EA: Spinal hematoma after lumbar puncture and heparinization, *Anesth Analg* 65:1201, 1986.
113. Ferris VA, Swanson E: Aspirin usage and perioperative blood loss in patients undergoing unexpected operations, *Surg Gynecol Obstet* 156:439, 1983.
114. Ruff RL, Dougherty JH: Complications of lumbar punctures following anticoagulation, *Stroke* 12:879, 1981.
115. Rao TLK, El-Etr AA: Anticoagulation following placement of epidural and subarachnoid catheters: an evaluation of neurologic sequelae, *Anesthesiology* 55:618, 1981.
116. Yeager MP, Glass DD, Neff RK et al: Epidural anesthesia and analgesia in high-risk surgical patients, *Anesthesiology* 68:729, 1987.
117. Ballantyne JC, Carr DB, Chalmers TC et al: Postoperative patient-controlled analgesia: meta-analysis of initial randomized controlled trials, *J Clin Anesth* 5:182, 1993.
118. Youngstrom P: Financial aspects of patient controlled analgesia—stimulus for development in a changing environment. Proceedings from the Patient Controlled Analgesia Symposium, the University of Wales College of Medicine, Naples, Fla, 1993.
119. *1994 Accreditation manual for hospitals*. Surgical and Anesthesia Services. Joint Commission on Accreditation of Healthcare Organizations. Oakbrook Terrace, Ill, 1993, The Commission.
120. Borzo G: New anesthesia rules, *Am Med News* 38:13, 1994.
121. Tinker JH, Dull DL, Caplan RA: Role of monitoring devices in prevention of anesthetic mishaps: a closed claims analysis, *Anesthesiology* 71:541, 1989.
122. Eichorn JH: Prevention of intraoperative anesthesia accidents and related severe injury through safety monitoring, *Anesthesiology* 70:572, 1989.
123. Duncan PG, Cohen MM: Pulse oximetry and capnography in anesthetic practice: an epidemiologic appraisal, *Can J Anaesth* 38:619, 1991.
124. Mooer TJ, Johannessen NW, Espersen K et al: Randomized evaluation of pulse oximetry in 20,802 patients: II. Perioperative events and postoperative complications, *Anesthesiology* 78:445, 1993.
125. American Society of Anesthesiologists: *Standard for basic intra-operative monitoring* (October 1986 and last amended October 1992), Park Ridge, Ill, 1992, The Society.
126. American Society of Anesthesiologists: *Guidelines for delegation of technical anesthesia functions to non-physician personnel*, Park Ridge, Ill, 1994, The Society.
127. Gibbs CP, Krischer J, Peckam BM et al: Obstetric anesthesia: a national survey, *Anesthesiology* 65:298, 1986.
128. State of New York: *Official compilation of codes, rules, and regulations of the State of New York*, Chapter 5 (Health), Subchapter A, Part 405.4, 1989.
129. Deaconson TF, O'Hair DP, Levy MF et al: Sleep deprivation and resident performance, *JAMA* 260:1721, 1988.
130. Storer JS, Floyd HH, Gill WL et al: Effects of sleep deprivation on cognitive ability and skills of pediatric residents, *Acad Med* 64:29, 1989.
131. Roizen MF: Can the anesthesiologist reduce myocardial morbidity after vascular surgery? *J Cardiothorac Vasc Anesth* 5:424, 1991.
132. Killip T: Anesthesia in major noncardiac surgery, *JAMA* 268:252–253, 1992.
133. Goldman L, Caldera DL, Nussbaum SR et al: Multifactorial index of cardiac risk in noncardiac surgical procedures, *N Engl J Med* 297:845–850, 1977.
134. Detsky AS, Abrams HB, Forbath N et al: Cardiac assessment for patients undergoing noncardiac surgery. A multifactorial clinical risk index, *Arch Intern Med* 146:2131, 1986.

135. Mangano DT: Preoperative assessment of cardiac risk. In Kaplan JA, editor: *Cardiac anesthesia*, ed 3, Philadelphia, 1993, WB Saunders.
136. Boucher CA, Brewster DC, Darling RC et al: Determination of cardiac risk by dipyridamole-thallium imaging before peripheral vascular surgery, *N Engl J Med* 312, 389, 1985.
137. Eagle KA, Coley CM, Newell JB et al: Combining clinical and thallium data optimizes preoperative assessment of cardiac risk before major vascular surgery, *Ann Intern Med* 110:859, 1989.
138. Mangano DT, London MJ, Tubau JF et al: Dipyridamole-thallium-201 scintigraphy as a preoperative screening test: a reexamination of its predictive potential, *Circulation* 84:493, 1991.
139. Marwick TH, Underwood DA: Dipyridamole thallium imaging may not be a reliable screening test for coronary artery disease in patients undergoing vascular surgery, *Clin Cardiol* 13:14, 1990.
140. Rao TK, Jacobs KH, El-Etr AA: Reinfarction following anesthesia in patients with myocardial infarction, *Anesthesiology* 59:499, 1983.
141. Wells P, Kaplan JA: Optimal management of patients with ischemic heart disease for non-cardiac surgery by complementary anesthesiologist and cardiologist interaction, *Am Heart J* 102:1029, 1981.
142. Tarhan S, Moffit E, Taylor WF et al: Myocardial infarction after general anesthesia, *JAMA* 220:1451, 1972.
143. Steen PA, Tinker JH, Tarhan S: Myocardial reinfarction after anesthesia and surgery, *JAMA* 239:2566, 1978.
144. Eerola M, Arola R, Kaukinen S et al: Risk factors in surgical patients with verified preoperative myocardial infarction, *Acta Anaesthesiol Scand* 24:219, 1980.
145. Hertzer NR: Fatal myocardial infarction following lower extermity revascularization. Two hundred seventy-three patients followed six to eleven postoperative years, *Ann Surg* 193:4, 1981.
146. Mangano DT, Browner WS, Hollenberg M et al: Association of postoperative myocardial ischemia with cardiac morbidity and mortality in men undergoing non-cardiac surgery, *N Engl J Med* 323:1791, 1990.
147. Mulcahy D, Fox K: Therapeutic implications of ischemia in the ambulatory setting, *Prog Cardiovasc Dis* 34:413, 1992.
148. Raby KE, Barry J, Creager MA et al: Detection and significance of intraoperative and postoperative myocardial ischemia in peripheral vascular surgery, *JAMA* 268:222, 1992.
149. Hollenberg MH, Mangano DT, Browner WS et al: Predictors of postoperative myocardial ischemia in patients undergoing noncardiac surgery, *JAMA* 268:205, 1992.
150. Browner WS, Li J, Mangano DT: In-hospital and long-term mortality in male veterans following noncardiac surgery, *JAMA* 268:228, 1992.
151. Pasternak LR: Outpatient anesthesia. In Rogers MC, Tinker JH, Covino BG et al, editors: *Principles and practice of anesthesiology*, vol 2, St. Louis, 1993, Mosby.
152. Vacanti CJ, Vitez TS: How quality assurance and the peer review process can help your department. In *Peer review in anesthesiology, 1993*. Park Ridge, Ill, 1993, American Society of Anesthesiologists.
153. Kaplan RA, Posner KL, Cheney FW: Effect of outcome on physician judgments of appropriateness of care, *JAMA* 265:1957, 1991.
154. Cause and effect diagram (CE diagram). In Ishikawa IA: *Guide to quality control*, revised English edition, ed 2, Tokyo, 1986, Asian Productivity Organization.

7
Intraprocedural Monitoring

Lawrence N. Sampson, Juan Ayerdi, and Sushil K. Gupta

The goals of intraprocedural monitoring during endovascular interventions include maintenance of patient safety and assurance of short-term and long-term success. Endovascular procedures by definition are carried out without direct operative exposure, and a form of monitoring, usually angiography, is a fundamental part of the procedure. The ideal monitoring technique is inexpensive, low risk, not cumbersome, and able to visualize ongoing progress to decrease morbidity and predict short-term and long-term failure. Postoperative surveillance has become standard practice in vascular surgery; intraoperative assessment is a basic part of the program to improve procedural outcomes.

The stakes in terms of success of endovascular procedures are high. Frequently the impetus for performance of the "less invasive" procedure is that the patient has significant medical co-morbidity, making traditional open procedures risky. Emergent conversion to open procedures or for salvage of an early postprocedural complication carries all the risks of an emergency procedure in a high risk patient. Although endovascular procedures are considered "low risk" and mortality is low, failures are not innocuous in terms of clinical outcome. Table 7–1 lists periprocedural complications from percutaneous transluminal angioplasty. In one report failure of iliac percutaneous transluminal angioplasty (PTA) led to a worsening clinical status in 10.3% of cases, with resultant amputation in 4.3%. Failure of femoropopliteal PTA led to worsening clinical status in 8.5%, with amputation necessary in 15.8%.[1] With carotid angioplasty and stent placement, failure may result in stroke with no tenable open salvage procedure. For endovascular stent-grafting of aneurysms, endoleaks may represent failure of intraoperative monitoring. Although such leaks may not necessitate open intervention, they clearly increase the need for surveillance.[2]

In this chapter we discuss the criteria for success, technology for anatomic and physiologic monitoring, and issues related to specific interventions.

Criteria of Success for Endovascular Interventions

The postprocedural results of endovascular interventions must ultimately be judged on the basis of clinical, hemodynamic, anatomic, and imaging criteria. Such standards have been developed for occlusive disease, aneurysmal disease, and lower extremity arterial endovascular procedures.[3–7] For occlusive disease, clinical success is defined as improvement by at least one category of limb ischemia (Table 7–2).[4,5] Patients with tissue loss must reach at least a level of claudication to be considered improved. Hemodynamic success equates with an improvement of the ankle-brachial index (ABI) of more than 0.15 or an improvement in the ABI of more than 0.10 if there is accompanying clinical improvement. The ABI cannot be used as a gauge of hemodynamic success in

TABLE 7–1. Complications from Arteriography

Mechanical complications
  Bleeding
  Hematoma
  False aneurysm
  Arteriovenous fistula
  Arterial wall laceration
  Intimal wall dissection
  Thrombosis
  Embolism
Contrast-related complications
  Allergic reactions
  Nephrotoxicity
  Fluid overload

patients with noncompressible vessels. In this setting, improvement in hemodynamic category level using pulse volume recording (PVR) or Doppler waveform recordings may be used. Using imaging techniques, anatomic success is defined as a residual luminal stenosis of less than 30% of normal diameter.[7]

Intraprocedural measures of success include anatomic and hemodynamic measures. Techniques for assessing anatomic measures of success include angiography, intravascular ultrasonography, and duplex scanning. Techniques for monitoring hemodynamic success include pull-back pressures, volume and flow measurements, transcranial duplex ultrasonography, PVR, sensory evoked potentials, percutaneous oxygen monitoring, and piezoelectric pulse monitoring. Some of these procedures are a fundamental part of the endovascular armamentarium at the present time, whereas the role of others has yet to be defined.

Anatomic Monitoring

Angiography

Intraoperative arteriography has long been considered the gold standard for intraoperative monitoring of peripheral revascularization procedures and is advocated as routine during infrainguinal bypass procedures.[8] Angiography, of course, is an integral part of most endovascular procedures, such as balloon angioplasty, atherectomy, laser angioplasty, intravascular stenting, and thrombolytic therapy. Angiography is done before, during, and after these endovascular interventions (Figures 7–1, 7–2).

There is a small but definable risk with angiography (Table 7–1). AbuRhama and associates[9] reported in a series of 707 arteriograms an overall complication rate of 14.3%, of which 7.1% were major complications; the mortality

TABLE 7–2. Clinical Categories of Chronic Limb Ischemia

Category		Clinical description	Objective criteria
Grade 0	0	Asymptomatic; no hemodynamic significant occlusive disease	Normal treadmill/stress test
Grade I	1	Mild claudication	Completes treadmill exercise[a]; AP after exercise <50 mm Hg but >25 mm Hg less than BP
	2	Moderate claudication	Between categories 1 and 3
	3	Severe claudication	Cannot complete treadmill exercise and AP after exercise <50 mm Hg
Grade II	4	Ischemic rest pain	Resting AP < 40 mm Hg, flat or barely pulsatile ankle or metatarsal PVR; TP > 30 mm Hg
Grade III	5	Minor tissue loss—nonhealing ulcer, focal gangrene with diffuse pedal ischemia	Resting AP < 60 mm Hg, ankle or metatarsal PVR flat or barely pulsatile; TP < 40 mm Hg
	6	Major tissue loss—extending above TM level, functional foot no longer salvageable	Same as category 5

From Rutherford RB, Flanigan DP, Gupta SK et al: Suggested standards for reports dealing with lower extremity ischemia, *J Vasc Surg* 4:80–94, 1986.
AP, ankle pressure; BP, brachial pressure; PVR, pulse volume recordings; TP, toe pressure; TM, transmetatarsal.
[a] Five minutes at 2 mph on a 12% incline.

FIGURE 7–1. A 48-year-old man with a 1-week history of right calf claudication and numbness was found on examination to have a cool, mottled right foot with no popliteal or pedal pulses. **A**, Angiogram reveals thrombosis of the popliteal artery. Note the corresponding pulse monitoring tracing using a piezoelectric monitor. **B**, Angiogram after thrombolysis with corresponding tracing.

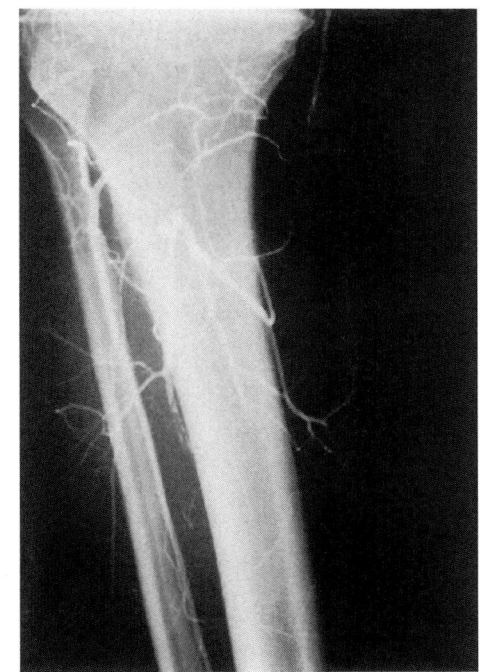

rate was 0.7%. These complications can be devastating to patients who are often already in a high risk category. Furthermore, this technique offers no hemodynamic assessment of the procedure's success. Although completion angiography has a sensitivity of 90%, specificity of 98%, and accuracy of 97%,[7] the hemodynamic consequences of equivocal lesions can be of uncertain significance.

It is in this situation where adjunctive means of intraprocedural monitoring can be of benefit in further delineating whether and when further manipulations using endovascular or operative approaches are needed. Equivocal lesions can be evaluated using these other adjunctive means, thereby avoiding the subjectivity of having only angiographic assessment, additional patient discomfort, and the dangers of repeated injections of contrast and radiation exposure in an attempt to delineate the lesion more clearly. Thus, the use of angiography can be made more judicious and directed. Other

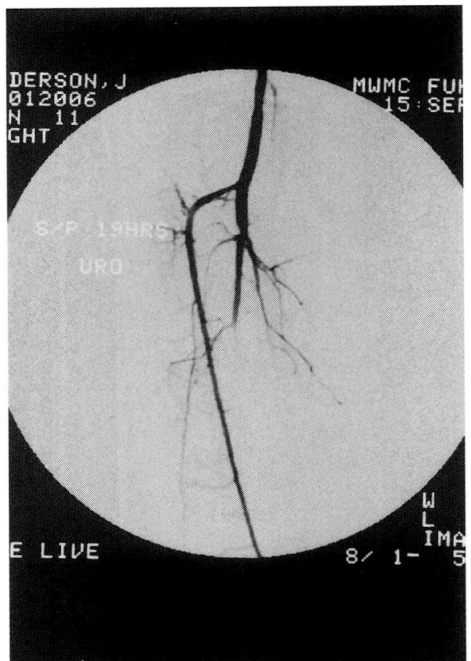

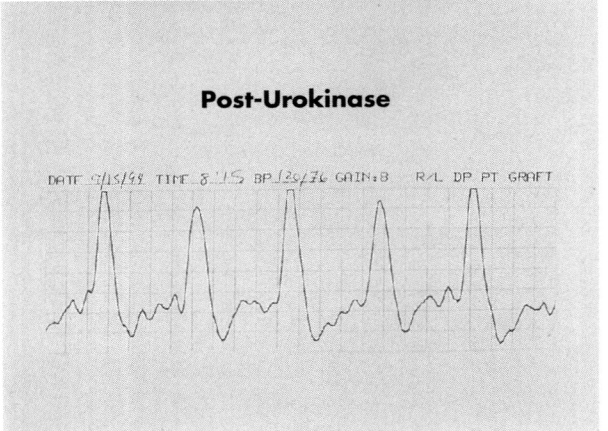

FIGURE 7–1. *Continued.*

intraoperative monitoring techniques may also call attention to the occurrence of complications such as embolization, perforation, or thrombosis.

Intravascular Ultrasonography

Whereas angiography offers a global assessment of a given segment of the arterial tree (i.e., a roadmap), intravascular ultrasonography (IVUS) offers a detailed view of local wall pathology, and the relationship of stents or other devices to the vessel wall. As technology improves, IVUS will ultimately be able to provide real-time imaging of balloon angioplasty, stent deployment, and stent-graft deployment, providing needed information about the relationship of balloons, stents, and grafts to the vessel wall and other anatomically important landmarks such as the renal artery. IVUS is a more sensitive predictor of angioplasty outcome than angiography and more accurately determines stent expansion, leading to improved patency.[10,11] Limitations of this technique are its inability to evaluate blood flow, determine length of stenosis, depict collat-

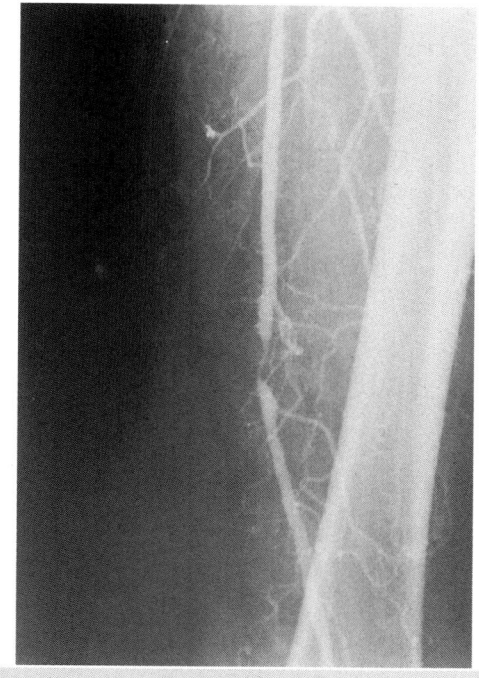

FIGURE 7–2. A 67-year-old woman with a 3-month history of progressively worsening claudication of the right calf. **A**, Angiogram reveals focal stenosis of a superficial femoral artery. Note the corresponding pulse monitoring tracing using a piezoelectric monitor before PTA. **B**, Angiogram after successful PTA and the corresponding tracing.

eral blood vessels, and traverse vessels of small caliber.[12] It may also require a large amount of fluid for irrigation and may increase the likelihood of complications because of additional manipulations.

Duplex Ultrasonography

Although in some centers duplex ultrasonography has supplanted arteriography for intraoperative assessment during carotid, renal, and lower extremity reconstructions, its role in endovascular procedures is less clear. For open procedures the application of duplex is straightforward: The probe is placed directly on the vessel or bypass graft in the region of interest. Duplex ultrasonography offers some significant benefits: Continuity between intraoperative and postoperative surveillance, lack of radiation and contrast materials, and established criteria of clinical significance. However, it seems unlikely that a cumbersome technique would supplant arteriography or IVUS, which are a fundamental part of most endovascular procedures. Because most endovascular procedures are carried out at a distance from the

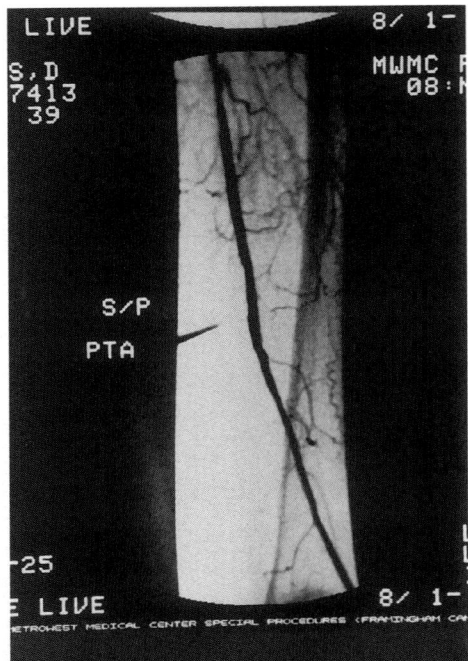

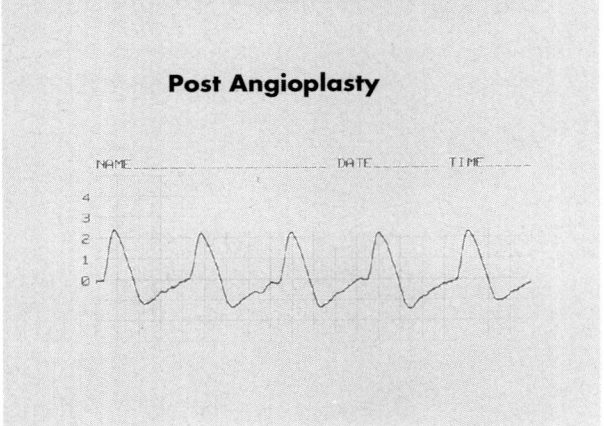

Figure 7–2. *Continued.*

pathology, the application of the probe would involve a separate field. Duplex ultrasonography requires a trained operator and does not provide information regarding the distal runoff.

Hemodynamic Monitoring

Pull-Back Pressures

The role of pull-back pressures in the diagnosis of occlusive disease is well established.[13] Pull-back pressures define hemodynamically significant lesions, and their association with clinical outcomes has been established. They are a basic part of angioplasty procedures.[14]

Transcranial Doppler Ultrasonography

The use of intraoperative transcranial Doppler ultrasonography (TCD) monitoring allows hemodynamic evaluation of blood flow velocity in the middle cerebral artery and detection of microemboli. TCD examination effectively assesses the collateral circulation and permits prompt detection of ischemic changes secondary to embolism or spasm. The number of microemboli during carotid endarterectomy dissection may correlate with perioperative neurologic complications;[15] this has not been documented for carotid angioplasty or stenting.[16] TCD analysis has suggested that embolism is more frequent with percutaneous transluminal angioplasty than with primary stent placement.[17]

Pulse Volume Recording

Pulse volume recording has been advocated as a means of intraoperative monitoring during peripheral revascularization.[18,19] This procedure is not invasive and requires no special skill or training. Other advantages include the fact that it can be used even in the presence of calcified vessels, it is easily repeatable, and it is not dependent on systemic-physiologic factors.[18] It has been long known that during revascularization procedures PVR provides an immediate, consistent physiologic assessment of the success of the intervention.[19]

Volume and Flow Measurements

Another method for routinely monitoring the physiologic consequences of revascularization is measurement of blood flow using electromagnetic flowmetry,[20] laser Doppler flowmetry, transit time flowmetry, and Doppler flowmetry.[21] For distinguishing between these possibilities, the flow response to vasodilation is important.[20] Failure to respond to papaverine strongly suggests obstruction. Only a variable correlation has been found between flow and the angiographic assessment of runoff. Flow measurements should not be taken as an accurate prognostic test of patency.[22] Flow rates have not been predictive of technical complications or graft outcome.[23]

Percutaneous Oxygen Monitoring

Local cutaneous circulation, as a reflection of tissue blood supply, has been used as another means of noninvasive monitoring in the setting of carotid and lower extremity occlusive disease.[24,25] It has been advocated as a means of immediately evaluating the severity of peripheral vascular disease and assessing the adequacy of its treatment. A consistent relation exists between PaO_2 and transcutaneous oxygen tension ($PtcO_2$). $PtcO_2$ has been found to increase immediately after restoration of blood flow and reach a maximum within 25 minutes.[26] Transcutaneous carbon dioxide tension ($PtcCO_2$) monitoring has also been used in conjunction with $PtcO_2$.[27] Whereas successful revascularization is accompanied by a rapid, marked increase in $PtcO_2$, a slow, low increase suggests a complication or poor runoff, indicating the need for additional intraprocedural examinations such as angiography.[26]

Continuous Piezoelectric Pulse Sensor

A novel technique used to monitor limb perfusion during surgical revascularization is the piezoelectric pulse sensor (Pulse Check; Cardiovascular Concepts, Portola Valley, CA). Readily adapted to endovascular procedures, this device consists of ultrathin 28 μm thick polyvinylidine fluoride film applied to a tissue with 0.9 kg tension. It converts tissue displacement by arterial pulsation to electrical signals via a transducer (Figure 7–3). These signals are then displayed as visual waveforms that provide continuous real-time assessment of distal perfusion. The need for arteriography in the intraprocedural setting can be reduced or eliminated by the use of this sensor.[27,28] Being able to see a quantifiable change in the amplitude of the distal pulse can help the surgeon properly assess the hemodynamic significance of residual lesions after an intervention (Figures 7–1, 7–2).[29]

Manual palpation and handheld Doppler evaluations of pulses are subjective, intermittent, and often not available because of the presence of digital segmental disease. A high level of correlation has been found between the pulse sensor and flowmetry and between the sensor and intraluminal pressure measurements.[30] Often patients with peripheral vascular disease have gangrenous extremities that

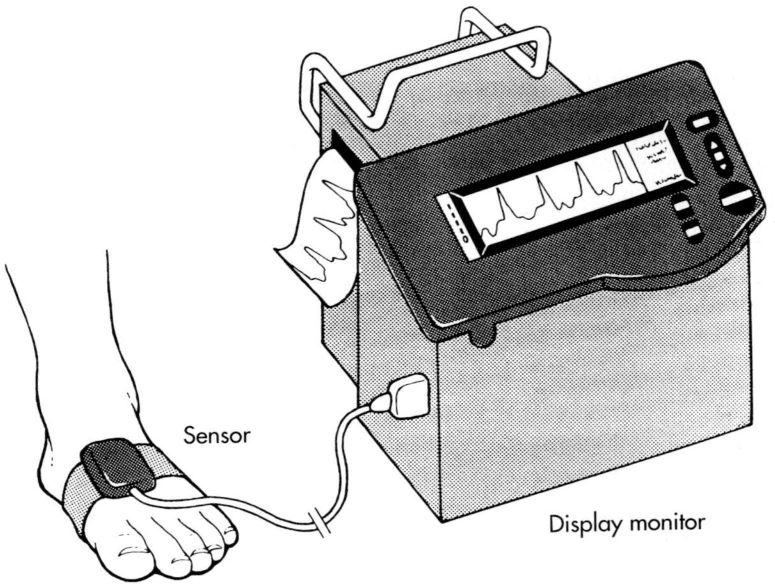

FIGURE 7–3. Pulse monitoring device.

require dressings, which make repeated examination of the foot cumbersome. The utility of this sensor device lies in its ability to be applied to the foot covered or wrapped by dressings while continuing to give an ongoing assessment of perfusion during the revascularization procedure. The pulse check monitor system may have value in operating rooms, recovery rooms, intensive care units, and radiology suites.[31] The device also removes the variability of time-consuming and subjective methods of assessing limb perfusion, such as continuous-wave Doppler sonography, skin temperature, capillary refill, and pulse palpation.[32] The piezoelectric sensor has been used during surgical revascularization procedures on 30 limbs of 22 patients. The procedures have included thromboembolectomy, bypass, and aortic surgery. Experience with this device after femoropopliteal and femoral-distal bypasses has shown good correlation between the change in the amplitude of the pulse signal with the change in ABI.[33]

Hashemi and associates[31] found a linear correlation between the change in amplitude and shape of the waveform and incremental changes in perfusion pressure. The piezoelectric pulse sensor fuunctions well in the dorsalis pedis artery position with good sensitivity. However, this sensitivity is lost at the posterior tibial artery position because of anatomic limitations that do not allow secure placement of the sensor on the skin.

Conclusion

Endovascular interventions represent viable alternatives to surgical revascularization. Ensuring the adequacy of the results continues to be as important as it is during surgical procedures. This concern with outcome may be even more prevalent because endovascular procedures are often undertaken in high risk patients who tolerate emergency reinterventions poorly. A variety of modalities have been used to monitor the success of revascularization using hemodynamic and anatomic criteria. Although limitations are encountered with each of the modalities, the piezoelectric pulse sensor holds promise as an ideal intraprocedural monitoring device.

References

1. Johston KW, Sniderman KW: Complications of percutaneous transluminal angioplasty of peripheral arterial occlusive disease. In

Bernhard VM, Towne JB, editors: *Complications in vascular surgery*, St Louis, 1991, Quality Medical Publishing.
2. Matsumura JS, Moore WS: Clinical consequences of periprosthetic leak after endovascular repair of abdominal aortic aneurysm, *J Vasc Surg* 27:606–613, 1998.
3. Rutherford RB, Flanigan DP, Gupta SK et al: Suggested standards for reports dealing with lower extremity ischemia, *J Vasc Surg* 4:80–94, 1986.
4. Rutherford RB, Baker JD, Ernst CB et al: Recommended standards for reports dealing with lower extremity ischemia: revised version, *J Vasc Surg* 26:517–538, 1997
5. Johnston KW, Rutherford RB, Tilson MD et al: Suggested standards for reporting arterial aneurysms, *J Vasc Surg* 13:452–458, 1991.
6. Ahn SS, Rutherford RB, Johnston KW et al: Reporting standard for infrarenal endovascular abdominal aortic aneurysm repair, *J Vasc Surg* 25:405–410, 1997.
7. Ahn SS, Rutherford RB, Becker GJ et al: Reporting standards for lower extremity arterial endovascular procedures: Society for Vascular Surgery/International Society for Cardiovascular Surgery, *J Vasc Surg* 17:1103–1107, 1993.
8. Mills JL, Fujitani RM, Taylor SM: Contribution of routine intraoperative completion arteriography to early infrainguinal bypass patency, *Am J Surg* 164:506–511, 1992.
9. AbuRahma AF, Robinson PA, Boland JP et al: Complications of arteriography in a recent series of 707 cases, factors affecting outcome, *Ann Vasc Surg* 7:122–129, 1993.
10. Reid DB, Diethrich EB, Marx P, Wrasper R: Intravascular ultrasound assessment in carotid interventions, *J Endovasc Surg* 3:203–210, 1996.
11. Arko F, Mettauer M, McCollough R et al: Use of intravascular ultrasound improves long-term clinical outcome in the endovascular management of atherosclerotic aortoiliac occlusive disease, *J Vasc Surg* 27:614–623, 1998.
12. Heil JM, Rinecker H, Huber A: Possibilities of interventional ultrasound (IVUS) in intraoperative diagnostic and quality control in peripheral vascular surgery, *Thorac Cardiovasc Surg* 39(suppl):252–254, 1991.
13. Archie JP: Physiologic studies to document severity of aortoiliac occlusive disease. In Ernest CB, Stanley JC, editors: *Current therapy in vascular surgery*, ed 3, Mosby, 1995, St Louis.
14. Rholl KS: Percutaneous aortoiliac intervention in vascular disease. In Baum S, Pentecost MJ, editors: *Abram's Angiography*, Boston, 1997, Little Brown, p 230.
15. Ackerstaff RG, Jansen C, Moll FL et al: The significance of microemboli detection by means of transcranial Doppler ultrasonography monitoring in carotid endarterectomy, *J Vasc Surg* 21:963–969, 1995.
16. Crawley F, Clifton A, Buckenham T et al: Comparison of hemodynamic cerebral ischemia and microemboli signals detected during carotid endarterectomy and carotid angioplasty, *Stroke* 28:2460–2464, 1997.
17. Benichou H, Bergeron P: Carotid angioplasty and stenting, will periprocedural Doppler monitoring be important? *J Endovasc Surg* 3:217–223, 1996.
18. O'Hara PJ, Brewster DC, Darling RC et al: The value of intraoperative monitoring using the pulse volume recording during peripheral vascular reconstructive operations, *Surg Gynecol Obstet* 15:275–281, 1981.
19. O'Donnell TF, Cossman D, Callow AD: Noninvasive monitoring, a prospective study comparing Doppler systolic occlusion pressure and segmental plethysmography, *Am J Surg* 135:539–546, 1978.
20. Sounnenfeld T: Electromagnetic flowmetry for intraoperative monitoring, *Vasa* 11:178–182, 1982.
21. Lundell A, Bergqvist D: Intraoperative flow measurements in vascular reconstruction, *Am Chir Gynaecol* 81:187–191, 1992.
22. Bernhard VM: Intraoperative monitoring of femorotibial bypass grafts, *Surg Clin North Am* 54:77–84, 1974.
23. Barnes RW: Intraoperative monitoring in vascular surgery, *Ultrasound Med Biol* 12:919–926, 1986.
24. Slavin KV, Dujovny M, Ausman JI et al: Clinical experience with transcranial cerebral oximetry, *Surg Neurol* 42:531–540, 1994.
25. Samson RH, Gupta SK, Goldstein R et al: Evaluation of peripheral arterial disease using a transcutaneous oxygen tension sensor. In: Huch R, Huch A, editors: *Continuous transcutaneous blood gas monitoring*. Basel, 1983, Marcel Dekker, pp 689–695.
26. Quian S, Iwai T, Sato S et al: Evaluation of the measurements of the intraoperative transcutaneous partial pressure oxygen ($PtcO_2$) as a prognostic indicator in vascular reconstruction, *Surg Today* 22:523–529, 1992.

27. Kram HB, Shoemaker WC: Use of transcutaneous O_2 monitoring in the intraoperative management of severe peripheral vascular disease, *Crit Care Med* 11:482–483, 1983.
28. Fogarty TJ et al: Monitoring distal extremity perfusion with the pulse amplitude monitor during cardiovascular reconstruction, *Cardiovasc Surg* 20:303–305, 1992.
29. Fogarty TJ, Hermann GD: New techniques for cloth extraction and managing acute thromboembolic limb ischemia. In Veith FJ, editor: *Current critical problems in vascular surgery*, vol 3, St Louis, 1991, Quality Medical Publishing.
30. Gupta SK, Dietzek AM Veith FJ et al: Use of piezoelectric sensor for monitoring vascular grafts, *Am J Surg* 160:182–186, 1990.
31. Hashemi HA, Katz ML, Carter AP et al: The piezoelectric pulse sensor device, a prospective evaluation, *Ann Vasc Surg* 8:367–371, 1994.
32. Cavaye DM, Tabbara MR, Kopchok GE et al: Continuous piezoelectric pulse sensor monitoring of peripheral vascular reconstructions, *Vasc Surg* 20:718–722, 1992.
33. Girishkumar H, Landa R, Gupta S et al: Continuous, non-invasive perioperative monitoring of lower extremity pulses following vascular procedures [abstract]. Presented at the XXI World Congress of The International Society for Cardiovascular Surgery, Sept. 12–15, Lisbon.

Color Plate

PLATE 1 Persistent arteriovenous fistula noted after in situ bypass. The high diastolic flow is the key to this diagnosis.

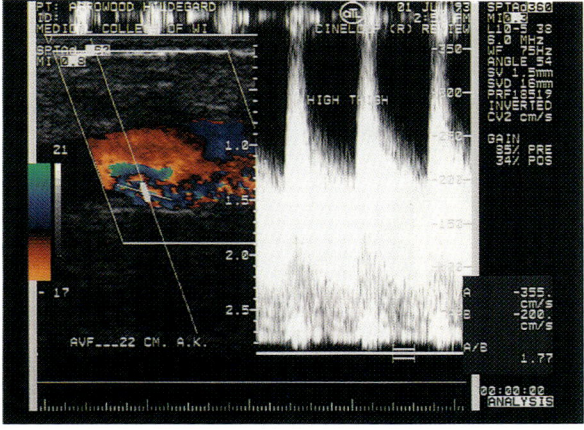

PLATE 2 Proximal anastomotic stenosis. There is high peak systolic flow velocity (>450 cm/sec) with spectral broadening.

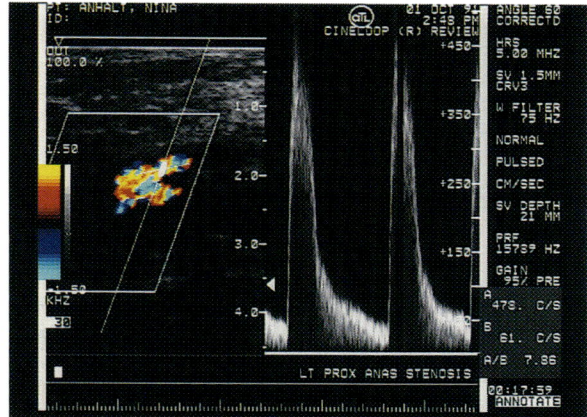

PLATE 3 Waterhammer type of signal that denotes a failing vein graft. Systolic velocity is 20 cm/sec.

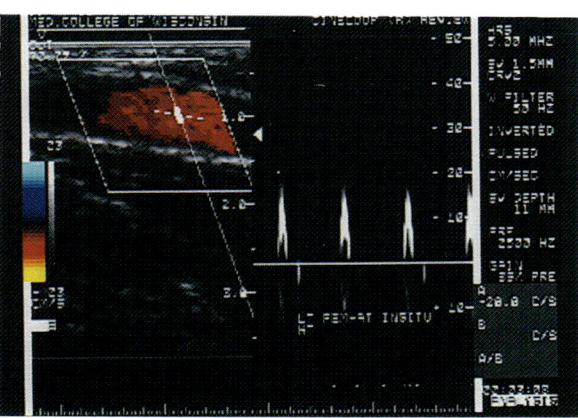

Color Plate

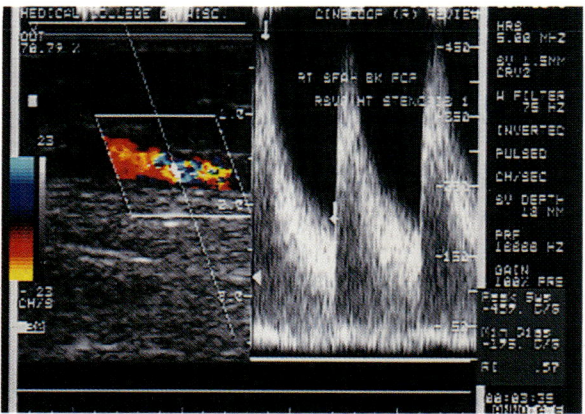

PLATE 4 Greater than 75% stenosis noted in in situ femoral distal graft. Peak systolic velocity is greater than 450cm/sec with marked spectral broadening.

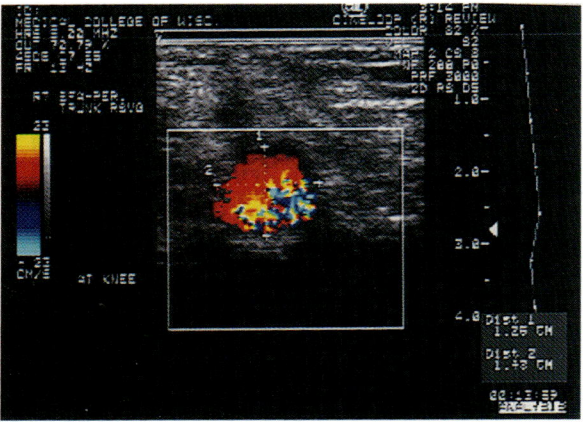

PLATE 5 Aneurysmal degeneration of a vein graft measuring 1.25 × 1.43 cm.

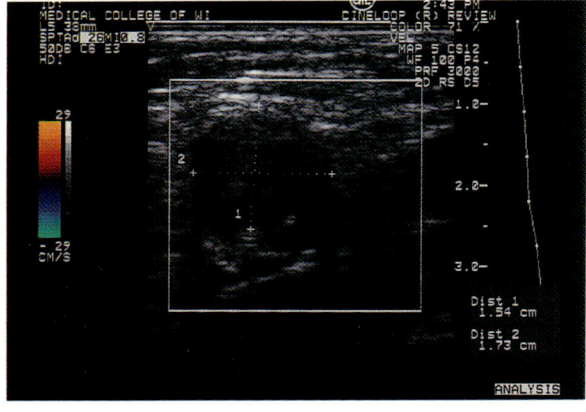

PLATE 6 Thrombus occludes 75% of diameter of graft of polytetrafluoroethylene in situ anastomosis.

8
Postintervention Surveillance of Endovascular Procedures

John P. Henretta and Kim J. Hodgson

As endovascular therapies gain increased acceptance for the treatment of vascular disease, postintervention surveillance becomes more critical. The underlying rationale for routine, systematic follow-up is multifactorial. The primary reason is to improve the results of treatment by detecting failures or recurrences early enough in their course that their correction is as minimally involved as possible. It has been well demonstrated, for example, that correction of a threatened saphenous vein bypass improves its patency when compared to simple observation.[1-3] This finding is thought to be applicable to endovascular therapies as well: Treatment of a recurrent stenosis with a second endovascular procedure, perhaps with supplemental stenting, is more likely to be initially technically successful and durable than an attempt to recannulate an occlusion that results from ignoring the recurrence. Furthermore, treatment of an occlusion may require thrombolysis, which has its own inherent risks. The advantages of close postintervention surveillance become even more obvious when dealing with an artery feeding an end-organ (e.g., the renal artery), in which case progression to occlusion may cause irretrievable organ injury.

Surveillance of interventions is also valuable as a means to evaluate new or evolving forms of therapy. As surgical reconstructions (the "gold standard") are being challenged by corresponding endovascular techniques, the need for a comparison of the two modalities to establish efficacy is readily apparent. Such comparison requires scheduled, objective evaluation over long periods. Unfortunately, there are no long-term results of prospective randomized series of endovascular revascularizations, making it difficult to ascertain the appropriate role for endovascular intervention in a number of anatomic areas and clinical circumstances. For example, although the use of stents has resulted in an initial technical success rate approaching 100% for the endovascular treatment of renal artery stenoses,[4,5] long-term data are lacking. Moreover, a recent report indicates a concerning 2.5-fold risk of significant restenosis in stented renal arteries compared to those not treated with stents.[6]

Finally, as health care delivery systems are restructured and third party payers award contracts to physicians or physician groups, cost containment and patient outcome data will undoubtedly play a role in these decisions. Therefore, a widely accepted, uniform method of follow-up is mandatory if bona fide comparisons are to be made. Reporting standards applicable to the determination of initial and long-term success must be developed. Furthermore, they must be based on evaluative means and criteria that are widely available and accepted, reasonably economical, and clinically relevant. Only then can widespread adoption of these criteria be anticipated and meaningful data produced.

Endovascular Reporting Standards for Occlusive Disease

In 1991 Rutherford and Becker[7] proposed reporting standards for evaluating the results of surgical and percutaneous therapy for peripheral arterial occlusive disease, observing that the nonstandardized reporting common at the time could translate into 5-year iliac angioplasty patency rates ranging from 52% to 89% for the same group of patients. They attempted to classify vascular disease and stratify its significance before and after treatment. Evaluation parameters and definitions of successful treatment outcomes were proposed, as were reportable associated complications. This topic was revisited by an ad hoc subcommittee of the Society for Vascular Surgery (SVS) and the International Society for Cardiovascular Surgery (ISCVS) in 1993,[8] in which more specific definitions of success for endovascular procedures were proposed. A three-parameter evaluation matrix was developed based on anatomic, hemodynamic, and clinical criteria assessed at the time of intervention, at patient discharge, and at all follow-up evaluations. To be classified as a successful intervention it is stipulated that all three parameters must demonstrate significant improvement, defined below, at all time intervals.

Anatomic evaluation pertains to the extent of recanalization achieved at the site of intervention as assessed by an imaging modality. At the time of the intervention the threshold for success is less than a 30% residual stenosis, and the modality typically used to assess the result is arteriography, though intravascular ultrasonography (IVUS) could provide a similar assessment. Follow-up evaluations usually rely on duplex ultrasound examinations, for which no 30% stenosis criterion exists, which presumably is why the threshold for anatomic success during the follow-up phase is defined as less than a 50% re-stenosis, whether assessed by duplex ultrasonography or a subsequent angiographic or IVUS evaluation. The anatomic evaluation is the only parameter that looks expressly at the treated region and assesses the degree of recanalization achieved and maintained.

The second requirement for success pertains to the extent of alleviation a patient experiences in the clinical symptoms and relies heavily on the clinical categories outlined by Rutherford et al. in 1986.[9] To qualify as a clinical success patients must improve by at least one clinical category after the intervention. There are inconsistencies, however, with regard to patients with claudication, as under the Rutherford et al. classification scheme a one-category improvement would render them asymptomatic, yet elsewhere in this publication it is stated that it takes only a 50% or more improvement in walking distance for the intervention to be defined as successful. Other problems when applying these standards are readily apparent when one considers that under these guidelines it is impossible to have an "early" (defined as "in-hospital") success in patients with ischemic ulceration unless such patients are kept in the hospital until all of their ulcers heal. Similarly, asymptomatic patients who undergo an endovascular intervention for graft preservation can never be considered to have undergone a successful procedure because they cannot improve by one clinical category, being asymptomatic to begin with.

Finally, the third parameter of evaluation involves hemodynamic success, which is defined as an improvement of the ankle-brachial index (ABI) of at least 0.15. However, if the patient meets the thresholds for success in both the anatomic and clinical categories, an ABI increase of only 0.10 can be used to indicate a hemodynamic success. This criterion is yet another illogical recommendation in these proposed standards because if success in all three parameters is required to declare an interventional success, the threshold for hemodynamic success is functionally 0.10. Furthermore, in the commonly encountered patient with incompressible vessels, the relatively qualitative modalities of pulse-volume recording and Doppler waveform recording are used to determine hemodynamic success. Additionally, in patients with superficial femoral artery occlusions it is suggested that the thigh-brachial index be used for pre- and postintervention evaluation.

Dilemma of Defining Success

Despite the best intentions of the SVS/ISCVS committee, their proposed reporting standards have come under much criticism, and several authors have proposed substantial modifications.[10–12] Even one of the authors of the SVS/ISCVS document has gone on to state that their recommendations were never intended to require success in all three parameters for the procedure to be considered successful overall, "only that each [of the parameters] be reported using uniform criteria."[13] Although revised reporting standards are reportedly in development,[13] there is presently no consistency in the definitions used in the literature, which continues to make the evaluation of different treatment modalities and outcomes problematic. Contributing to the confusion is the fact that reporting standards may need to be different for comparing two endovascular modalities ("apples to apples") than they would be when comparing an endovascular to a surgical revascularization ("apples to oranges"), as distinctly different issues, discussed below, are on the table.

Evaluating the initial and long-term results of endovascular interventions for occlusive disease can be viewed in two distinctly different ways. The first pertains to the technical success of the procedure itself, as measured by the reestablishment of an appropriately sized flow channel through a specific location in a vessel undergoing treatment. This measure of success is appropriate when comparing the results of two endovascular procedures, such as angioplasty alone compared to angioplasty with supplemental stenting. By assessing the initial and long-term results of such interventions it may be possible to determine the most effective modality for recanalizing a particular type of occlusive lesion in a specific anatomic area. This type of analysis can also be used to assess the technical competence of a particular endovascular therapist using the available endovascular tools to recanalize vessels.

The second method of analyzing the results of peripheral interventional procedures for occlusive disease looks at the overall benefits of the procedure to the patient, typically in terms of improvement in clinical and hemodynamic indices. This method represents a more global evaluation of the intervention in that it assesses both the success of reestablishing a suitable flow channel and the overall success of the procedure in augmenting limb blood flow. Therefore this type of analysis addresses the question of whether an endovascular intervention was the most suitable form of revascularization for the patient as much as it attests to the adequacy of the recanalization achieved. However, because it is possible and common for an intervention to recanalize a vessel successfully without an improvement in these other parameters, this method of analysis should not be used to pass judgment on the efficacy of a particular method of intervention or on the skills of the interventionalist. Rather, such analysis is most appropriate to answer the question of the applicability of an interventional procedure to a given clinical situation when compared to surgical revascularization, as the latter typically bypasses all significant occlusive lesions and the former addresses only a limited area of disease.

Surveillance Protocols for Endovascular Treatment of Occlusive Disease

All patients considered for endovascular treatment of arterial occlusive disease should undergo preprocedural evaluation by way of all three parameters: clinical, hemodynamic, and anatomic. Although ankle pressure determinations alone may suffice for the hemodynamic component, the common coexistence of significant superficial femoral disease mandates the measurement of segmental limb pressures, or at least thigh and ankle pressures, to facilitate documenting hemodynamic success in this group of patients. Similarly, if the ankle vessels are incompressible, Doppler waveform or pulse-volume recordings can be performed. Patients with near-normal resting indices undergoing treatment for claudication should undergo an exercise evaluation to document their maximal walking distance and their ankle pressure response to exercise for subsequent postintervention comparison. This protocol also allows categorization of the clinical parameters using the chronic limb ischemia scale recommended by the SVS/ISCVS Ad Hoc Committee on Reporting Standards.[9] These criteria should also be utilized to grade severe degrees of limb ischemia, giving a complete and quantifiable characterization of the clinical consequences of the patient's occlusive lesions.

Anatomic categorization of the lesion undergoing treatment is typically performed by way of angiography at the time of the intervention. Preprocedural duplex ultrasonographic evaluation, however, may allow a more directed, focused angiographic evaluation. Furthermore, duplex scanning may provide more accurate information about the hemodynamic significance of a lesion, as even multiple-plane angiography is misleading in some instances. IVUS is an additional tool that can evaluate the anatomic characteristics of a vessel before and after intervention. These other options notwithstanding, arteriography is considered the standard preprocedure and initial postprocedure anatomic test to determine successful intervention.

The term "initial technical success" means different things to different people, but it is generally taken to mean a postintervention residual stenosis of less than 30%. Although this definition may be suitable for lesions not amenable to the measurement of hemodynamic parameters (e.g., renal or carotid arteries), when on-table hemodynamic measurements can be made most investigators believe they should be included in the definition of initial technical success. For the anatomic evaluation, biplanar angiography remains the most common modality, but IVUS measurements are also suitable. Duplex ultrasonography is not sufficient, as initial technical success requires a less than 30% residual stenosis, for which there are presently no substantiated duplex criteria. Hemodynamic documentation of a successful intervention can be obtained by a variety of means. The most accurate is simultaneous determination of pressure in a central artery (e.g., the aorta) and an arterial segment just downstream of the treated lesion. Another approach is to perform "pull-through" pressure measurements, whereby a pressure-transduced catheter is retracted from the upstream side to the downstream side of a lesion while pressure measurements are being recorded. With both of these methods, a pressure differential of more than 5 mm Hg is generally taken to indicate a failed intervention or one in need of more work. Unfortunately, the latter approach requires loss of a guidewire crossing of the lesion, which may be problematic if further intervention is required. Pull-through pressures can also be obtained with the guidewire remaining across the dilated lesion if the catheter is of sufficient size that the guidewire does not obturate it so much as to influence the recorded pressure. Pull-through pressures cannot be assumed to be accurate when the catheter across the lesion originates from the upstream side, as the very presence of the catheter across the lesion may obturate it sufficiently to reduce the pressure on the downstream side of the lesion. If pressures are measured in this way and no gradient is detected, it can be presumed that no pressure gradient exists. A final method of hemodynamic evaluation at the time of the procedure is the use of pharmacologic vasodilatation to "stress" the results of the intervention. Typically, 100 to 200 µg nitroglycerin or 10 to 20 mg papaverine is injected intraarterially into the distribution of the vessel that was dilated. A decline in subsequent pressure measurements of more than 20 mm Hg downstream of the lesion indicates a hemodynamically significant residual stenosis.

Following successful intervention, reevaluation intervals are somewhat arbitrary but often include evaluation of all three parameters at the time of discharge and at 1, 3, and 6 months, with follow-up every 6 months after that. Clinical categorization at the time of discharge may be irrelevant, as ulcers would not have had sufficient time to heal and puncture-associated discomfort may preclude an earnest attempt to ambulate. The need for anatomic evaluation (duplex scan) at discharge is somewhat controversial because early changes in the endothelium (e.g., edema or hemorrhage) may falsely elevate the velocity across a treated segment of vessel.[14–16] Nonetheless, others have suggested a correlation of early duplex abnormalities and late failure.[17,18] Predischarge thigh and ankle pressure determination, however, should be performed for subsequent comparison.

It is recommended that all three assessments be performed at subsequent follow-up intervals. From the clinical standpoint, objective documentation of absolute walking distance through exercise treadmill testing is preferred but is often omitted owing to cost, patient acceptance, or the patient's inability to perform the test. A change in the resting ABI of more than 0.15 is thought to be significant, whether it is an increase over the pretreatment level indicating a successful intervention or a decrease, indicative of a failed intervention or recurrent stenosis. Anatomic follow-up is generally performed with duplex ultrasonography, for which the accuracy and efficacy have been well documented.[19,20] Criteria for positivity on duplex scanning include complete absence of flow, indicating complete occlusion of the vessel, or doubling of the velocity in a region of the vessel compared to that in the segment immediately proximal, indicating a more than 50% stenosis in the high-velocity region (Figure 8–1, see color plate).

Guidelines for the postintervention surveillance of renal or other visceral artery occlusive lesions are less well defined. Because renal lesions are typically asymptomatic, the only "clinical" parameter that can be assessed is the patient's blood pressure control, which unfortunately is typically multifactorial in nature. Furthermore, hemodynamic parameters are also impossible to assess noninvasively. Therefore the mainstay of surveillance of renal artery endovascular interventions is duplex scanning (Figure 8–2, see color plate), which we usually perform at discharge and at 1 month and every 6 months thereafter. Although specific criteria vary among vascular laboratories, the accuracy of duplex ultrasonography for detecting renal artery stenoses is well established.[21,22] Duplex scan findings indicating a recurrent stenosis, especially in the face of worsened hypertension, warrants angiographic confirmation and possible reintervention (Figure 8–3, see color plate).

At present, carotid angioplasty is an experimental procedure that may or may not become the standard of care in the future. Specific surveillance criteria have not yet been established, but it is reasonable to infer that duplex ultrasonographic scanning will constitute the mainstay of this endeavor using already well-established diagnostic criteria. Obviously, the development of clinical symptoms, though not necessarily indicative of restenosis, implies failure of the intervention to accomplish its goal and may warrant further evaluation with angiography.

Endovascular Reporting Standards for Aneurysmal Disease

The new, rapidly evolving field of endoluminal grafting has brought with it an entirely new set of definitions, some of which are more concretely defined than others. It is intuitive that endografting procedures performed for occlusive disease should be subject to the same criteria of success that have been established for standard angioplasty and stent procedures, as both are performed in an effort to alleviate symptoms caused by vascular obstructions. Endoluminal grafting of aneurysmal disease, however, has entirely different determinants of success, as the goal of these procedures is to exclude a segment of a vessel from continuity with the bloodstream. Therefore blood flow within the aneurysm sac following endograft placement may represent failure to isolate the aneurysm from systemic arterial pressure, leaving the patient unprotected from the risk of rupture. Although this situation may represent a "leak" through the graft or one of its arterial junctions, the blood remains contained within the aneurysm sac; therefore the situation does not have the severe ramifications of a leaking aneurysm. Consequently, the term *endoleak* has been coined to refer to this situation; and two distinctly different types of endoleak, believed to have significantly

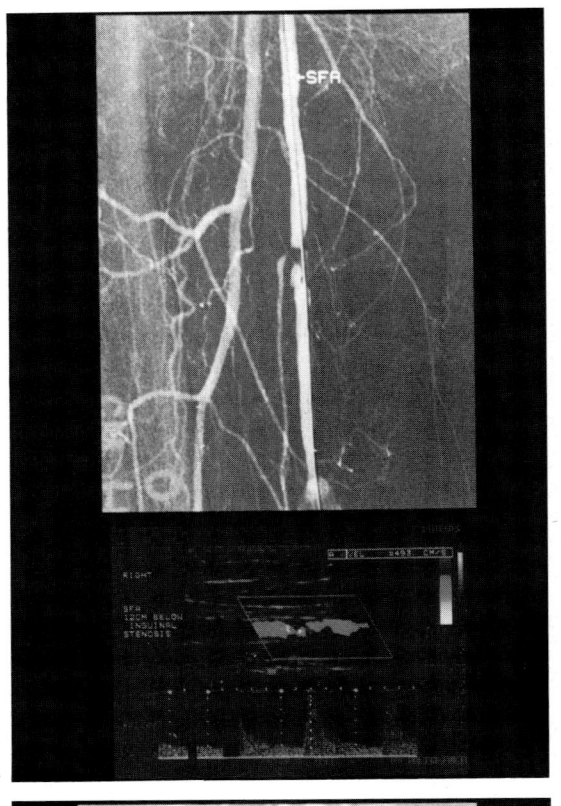
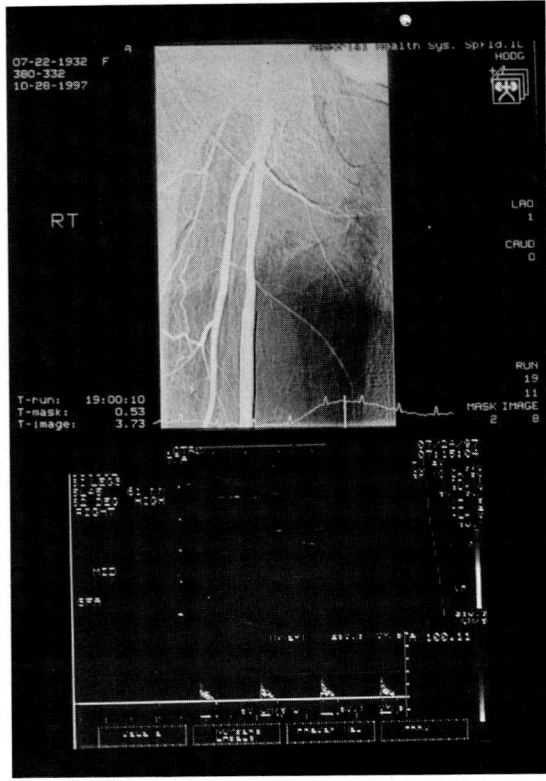
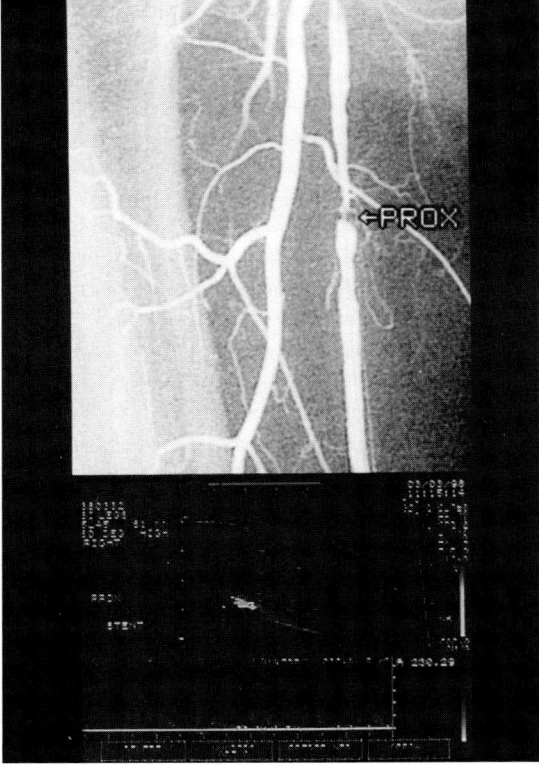
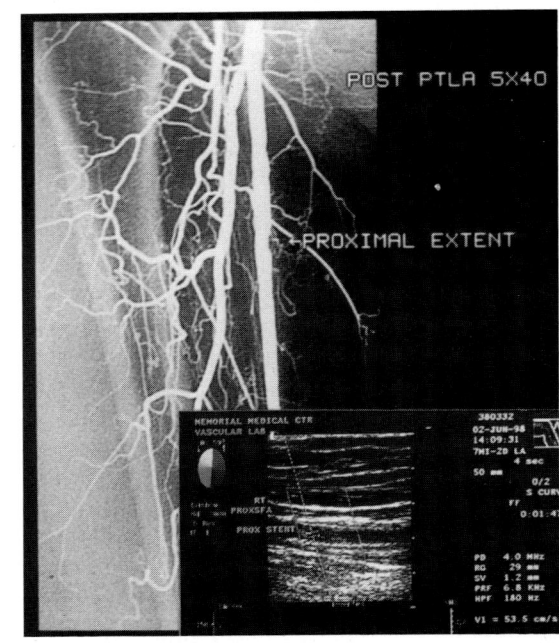

different clinical consequences, have been described.[23]

A graft-related endoleak refers to blood flow within the aneurysm sac originating from the graft itself, one of its modular junctions, or one of the junctions of the graft and the native arterial system. In this situation the aneurysm continues to be subjected to systemic arterial pressure and remains at risk for rupture. In contrast, a non-graft-related endoleak represents flow within the aneurysm sack that originates from a collateral vessel, such as a lumbar artery or the inferior mesenteric artery. Typically this flow enters the aneurysm sac from one vessel and exits via another owing to a pressure gradient between the two. This type of endoleak is believed to involve lower pressures and therefore to be associated with less risk of aneurysm rupture. Furthermore, non-graft-related endoleaks appear to have higher rates of spontaneous thrombosis than graft-related endoleaks. Consequently, it is important to be able not only to detect endoleaks but to differentiate between the two types.

Reporting standards for endoluminal repair of infrarenal abdominal aortic aneurysms have been recently published.[23] Although a detailed review is beyond the scope of this chapter, the essence of the criteria is documentation of aneurysm exclusion without the presence of complications, such as compromise of critical branch vessels. Late follow-up evaluations must note no development of graft thrombosis, infection, or migration or the enlargement of the aneurysm sac, which is generally taken to indicate failure to exclude the aneurysm. Successful aneurysm exclusion cannot always be determined at the time of graft implantation owing to the inherent porosity of the graft fabric or suture holes in the fabric associated with the attachment of the supporting stent structure. Consequently, the attainment of "initial" technical success is generally determined at 48 hours, at which time many but not all of the initial benign endoleaks have sealed. Although these reporting standards stipulate a 48-hour cutoff for endoleak resolution for the procedure to be deemed successful, this distinction is arbitrary and has no basis in science. Of greater value is the sequential reevaluation of early endoleaks to document the time at which they resolve. If they persist beyond 3 months, most would urge more aggressive evaluation and treatment, if indicated.

Surveillance Protocols for Endo-Grafted Abdominal Aortic Aneurysms

At present, the mainstay of surveillance of endografted aneurysms is spiral computed tomography (CT) with intravascular contrast, although color-flow duplex Doppler scanning may be a less-invasive suitable alternative (Figure 8–4, see color plate). CT scanning permits the aneurysm sac to be examined for the presence of contrast agent, which would indicate an endoleak.[23–27] At times the pattern of contrast distribution within the aneurysm sac indicates the source of the leak and guides further evaluation and treatment, particularly if it indicates a graft-related endoleak for which treatment is mandatory. Because the consequences of an untreated graft-related endoleak

---

FIGURE 8–1. **A**, Angiogram and corresponding color-flow duplex scan of a high grade stenosis of the superficial femoral artery (*SFA*) proximal to the origin of an SFA–popliteal bypass graft detected on routine graft surveillance. Peak systolic velocity within the stenosis measured 493 cm/s. **B**, After PTA and Wallstent treatment of the SFA stenosis with a successful anatomic result shown by angiography and color-flow duplex scanning, which revealed a peak systolic velocity of 100 cm/s in the stented region. **C**, Stenosis of the SFA just proximal to the previously treated region detected at 8 months by a color-flow duplex scan, revealing peak systolic velocities of 230 cm/s. **D**, Early identification of the graft-threatening SFA stenosis allowed treatment with balloon angioplasty, with an excellent angiographic result. It maintained patency of the bypass graft without recurrent stenosis, seen by color-flow duplex scanning at 3 months. (See color plate).

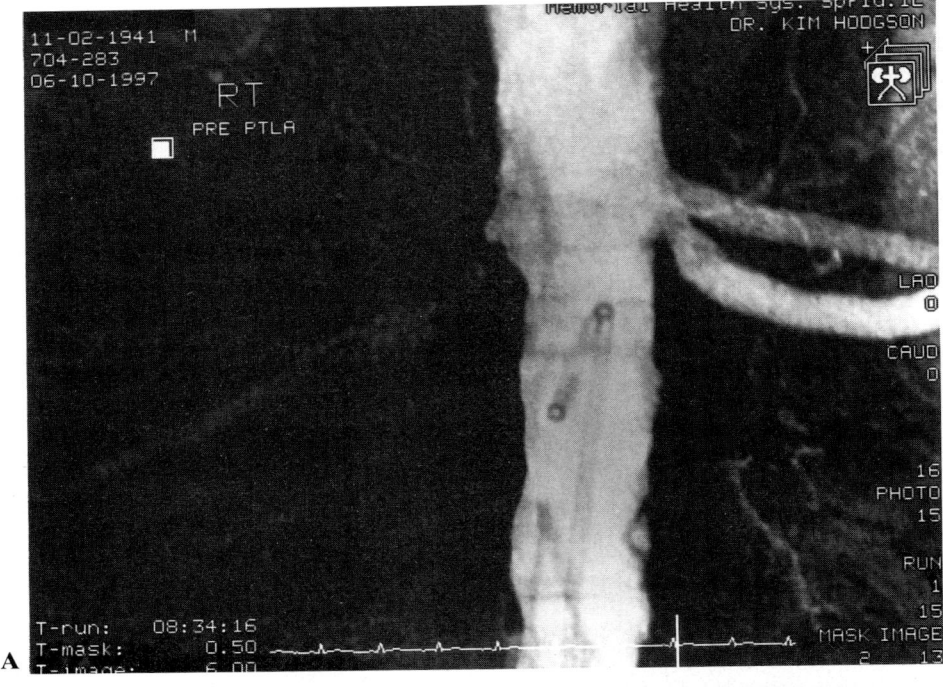

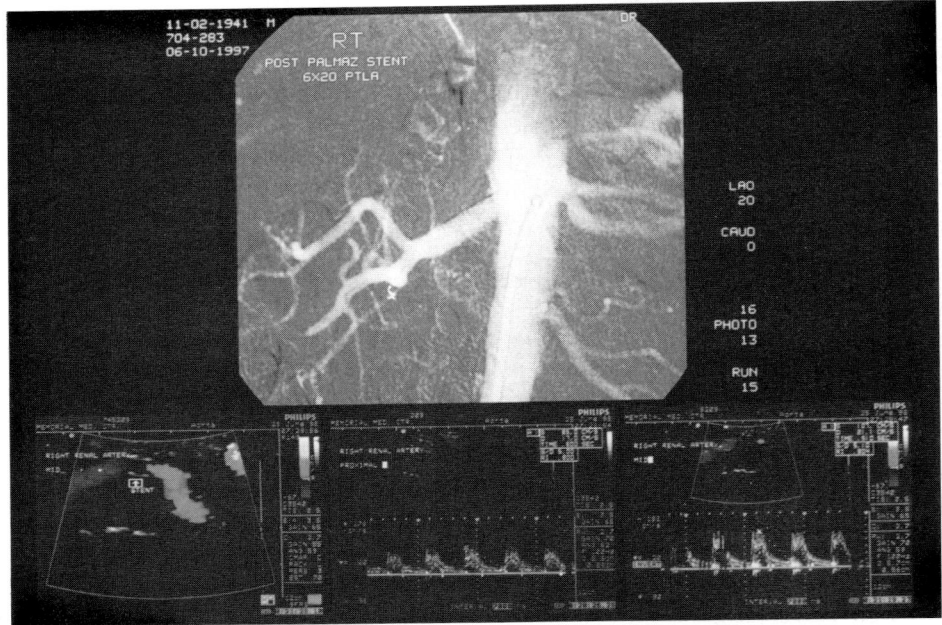

FIGURE 8–2. **A**, Preintervention angiogram of a high-grade right renal artery stenosis showing faint filling of the right renal artery. There was no apparent flow-channel connection to the aorta. **B**, After angioplasty and Palmaz stenting with an excellent angiographic result. Subsequent color-flow duplex scanning at 1 year demonstrates continued anatomic success with no elevation of flow velocitiy in the renal artery. (See color plate).

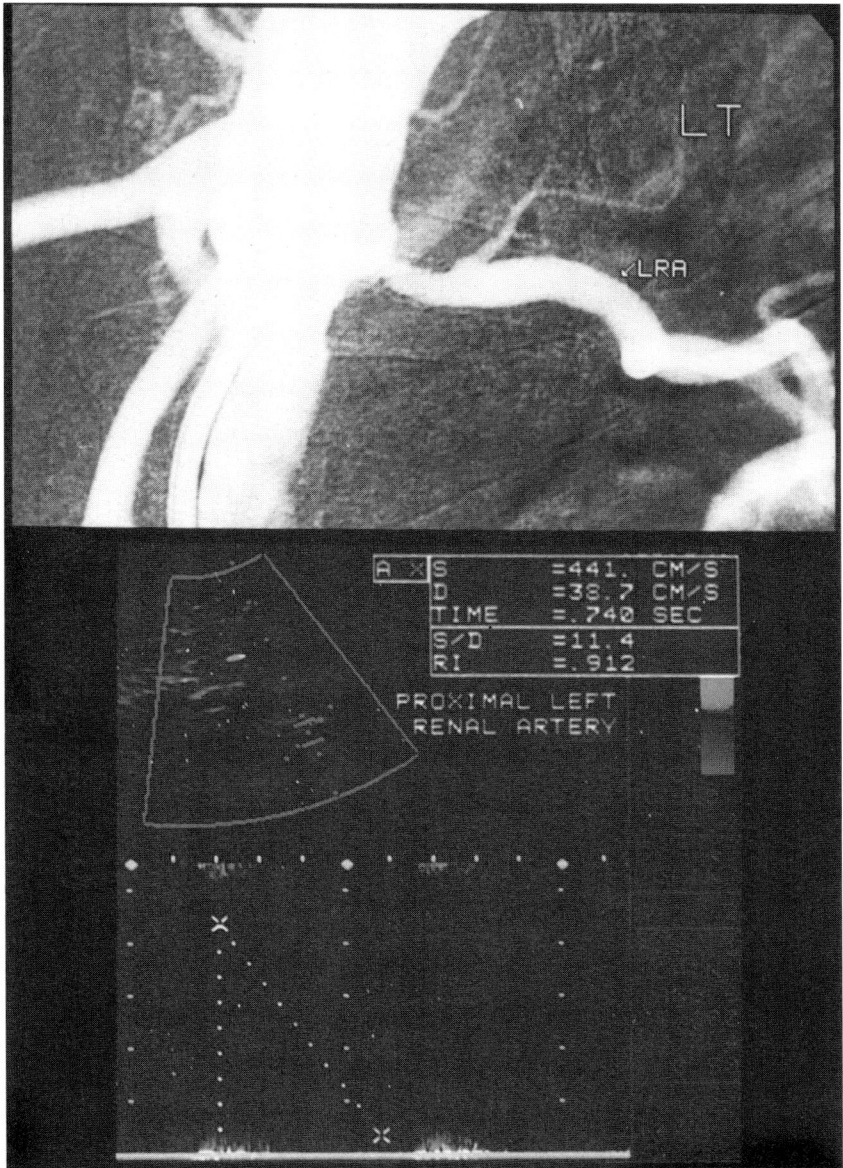

FIGURE 8–3. **A**, Surveillance color-duplex scanning of a dilated and stented left renal artery (*LRA*) revealed peak systolic velocities of 441 cm/s. Neointimal hyperplasia is apparent within the stent. **B**, Although complete recanalization of the left renal artery could not be achieved, leaving a 20% residual stenosis, the subsequent velocity dropped to 113 cm/s. (See color plate).

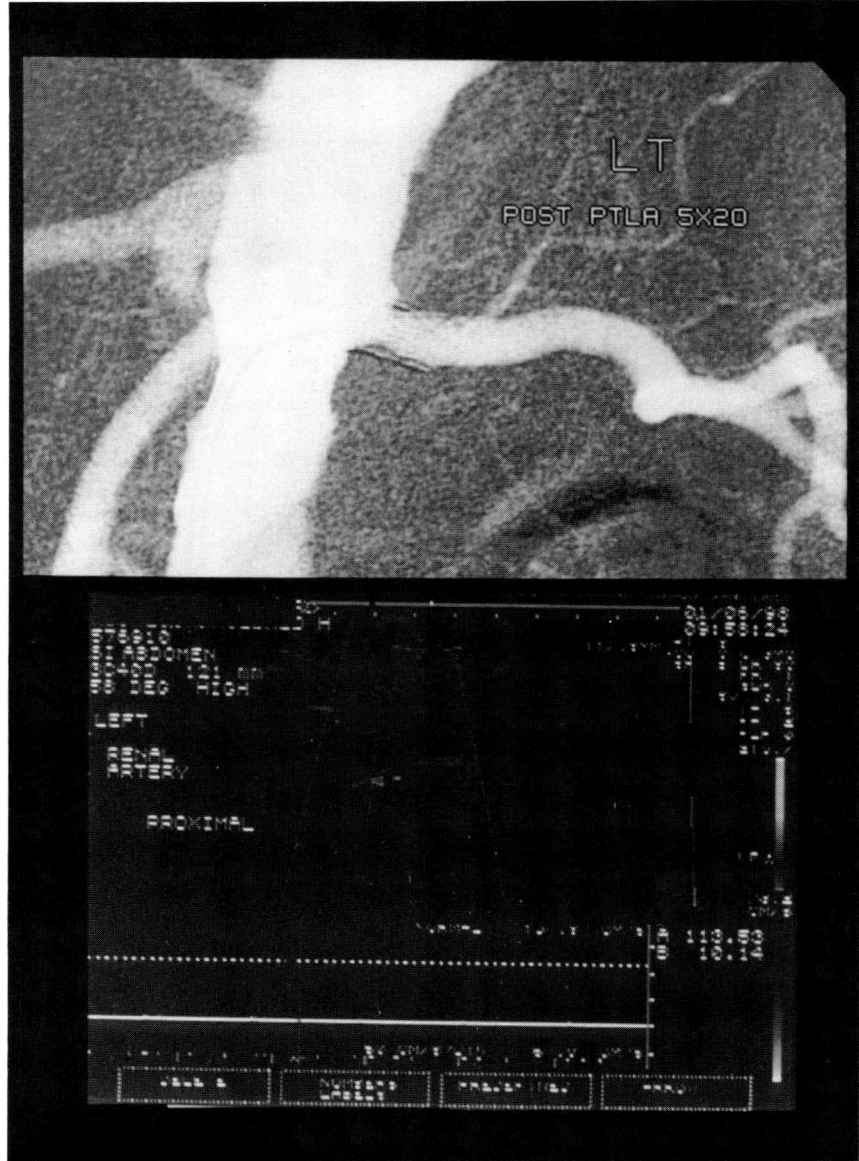

FIGURE 8–3. *Continued.*

8. Postintervention Surveillance of Endovascular Procedures

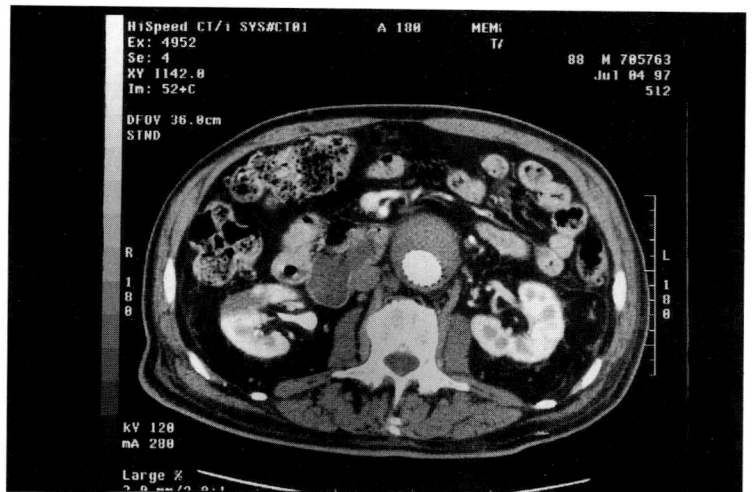

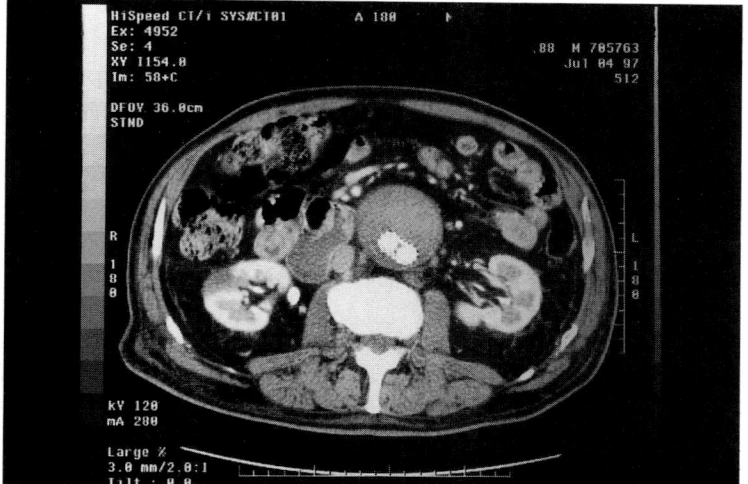

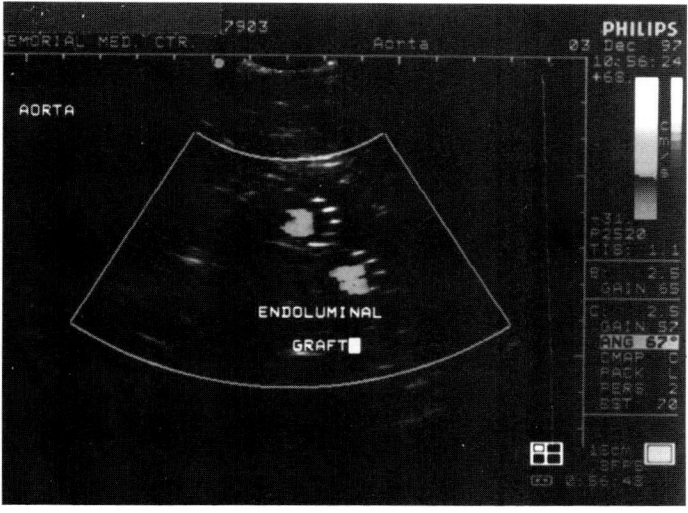

FIGURE 8–4. **A**, Spiral CT scan through the aortic component of an endograft with no evidence of contrast outside the graft. **B**, Spiral CT scan through the iliac components of an endograft with no evidence of contrast outside the graft. **C**, Color-flow duplex Doppler evaluation of the bifurcated region of an endograft demonstrating continued patency without apparent flow signals outside the endograft. (See color plate).

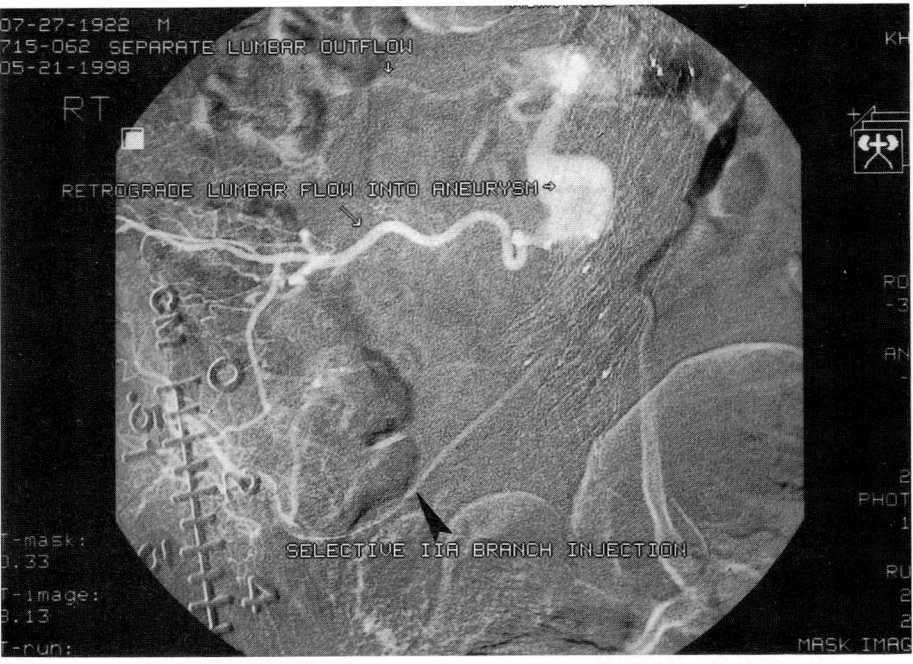

FIGURE 8–5. Selective contrast injection into a branch of the right internal iliac artery demonstrating collateral filling of a lumbar artery, which subsequently fills the aneurysm sac before exiting through another lumbar artery.

can be so dire, a CT scan indicating that the endoleak is non-graft-related is generally not considered sufficient documentation of this etiology without confirmatory testing. We advocate angiographic evaluation of all graft–graft and graft–vessel junctions to ensure that they appear sound. Furthermore, selective contrast injection into the internal iliac and superior mesenteric arteries may demonstrate the collateral pathway feeding the endoleak, ensuring the correct classification and in some instances permitting therapeutic embolization (Figure 8–5). Three-dimensional reconstruction of the CT scan often helps elucidate the nature and origin of endoleaks (Figure 8–6, see color plate). Although a variety of therapeutic options are available for addressing both types of endoleak, a detailed discussion of endoleak management is beyond the scope of this chapter.

Color flow duplex scanning offers a noninvasive means of interrogating aortic endografts for the presence of endoleaks (Figure 8–7, see color plate).[26] Patency of the graft and the major adjacent branches (e.g., renal and internal iliac arteries) can also be determined, as can the overall diameter of the aneurysm sac. The use of power Doppler sonography may further increase the sensitivity of the test, but the negative predictive value of all types of duplex scanning is suboptimal because of the low flow associated with many endoleaks. Large leaks,

FIGURE 8–6. **A**, Surveillance CT scan reveals contrast outside the endograft, indicative of an endoleak. **B**, Three-dimensional CT reconstruction indicates that the source of the endoleak is the endograft–iliac artery junction (*arrow*). **C**, Subsequent angiographic confirmation of the source of the endoleak allowed coil embolization. **D**, Following coil embolization of the outflow lumbar artery and the endoleak track, no further flow is noted within the aneurysmal sac. (See color plate).

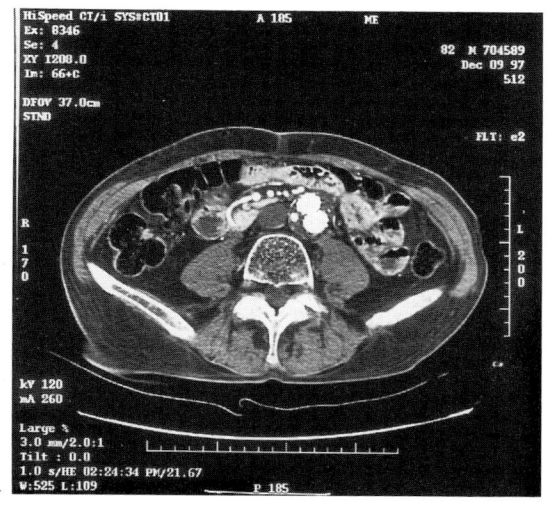
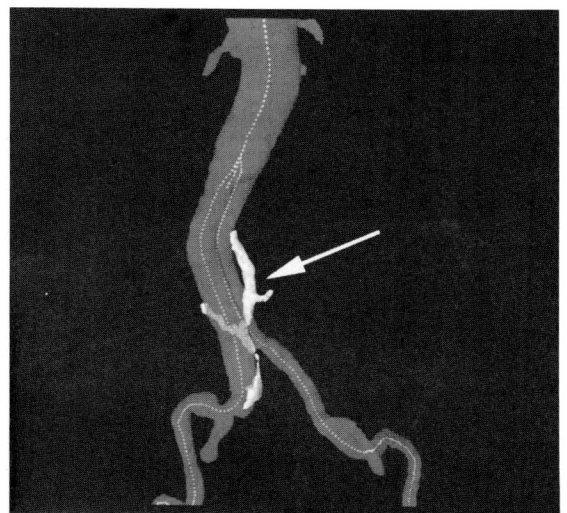
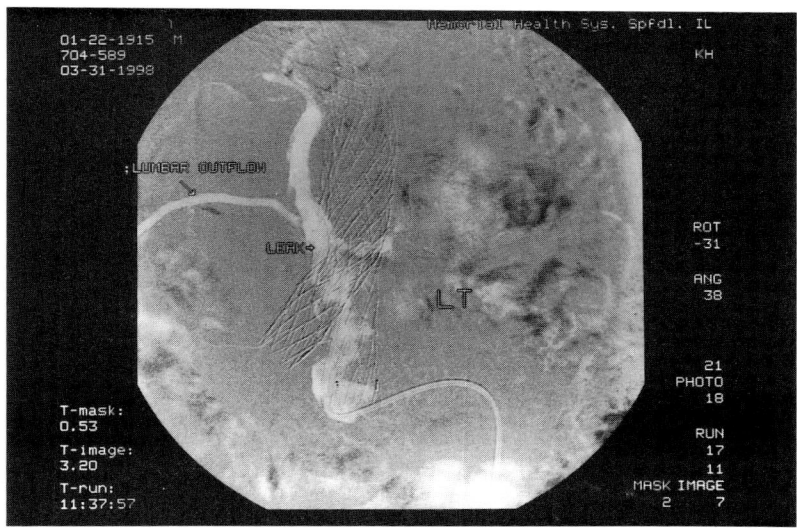
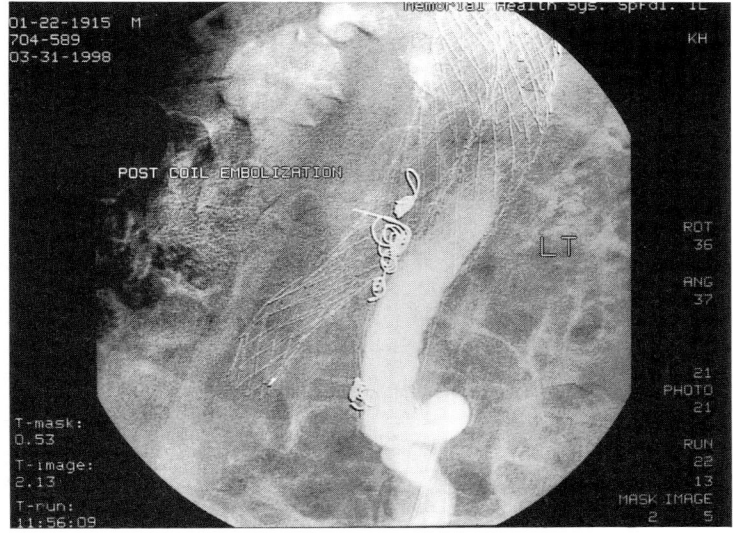

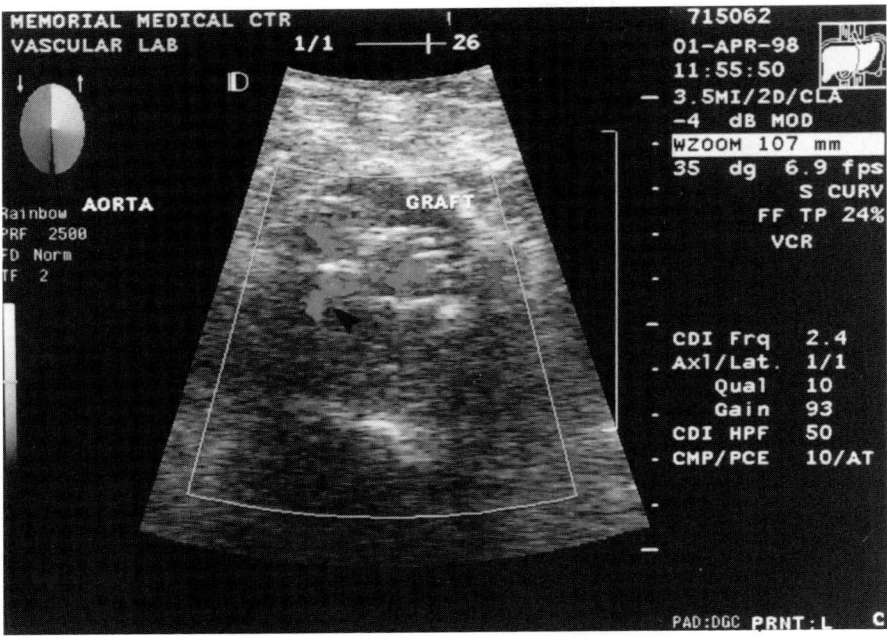

FIGURE 8–7. Color-flow duplex scan reveals flow outside the confines of an endograft, indicating the presence of an endoleak. (See color plate).

however, may be able to be traced back to their source, allowing directed angiographic confirmation.

To date, no endoluminal aortic aneurysm graft has attained US Food and Drug Administration approval. Outside the United States a number of grafts have been approved but only relatively recently. Consequently, most surveillance protocols presently in use are based on those in effect during each graft's investigational trial period[28–31] and therefore may not be consistent among the various grafts. Furthermore, as we learn more about the natural history of endografted aortic aneurysms and of the different endografts in use, the frequency and intensity of surveillance will likely change. Presently, most interventionalists recommend evaluation at 48 hours, 1 month, 6 months, and every 6 to 12 months thereafter. Though not well established, most advocate more frequent follow-up of patients with endoleaks, regardless of whether they are graft-related or non-graft-related. In the former instance corrective action is generally recommended, whereas in the latter case, once the etiology is established, careful observation is a reasonable course of action so long as the overall aneurysm sac diameter is not increasing.

Conclusion

Postintervention surveillance of endovascular interventions serves a variety of valuable functions. In the case of occlusive disease, early detection of recurrent stenoses allows timely reintervention, which can prolong the functional life of the revascularization and minimize the risk to the patient. Surveillance of endografted aneurysms serves the vital function of ensuring that aneurysm exclusion is maintained and therefore that the patient remains protected from the risk of rupture. In both scenarios, surveillance facilitates the evaluation of new modalities of treatment and the comparison of competing forms of intervention. Lastly, assessment of the results of interventions performed by different endovascular therapists serves a quality assurance and educational function that promotes optimal patient care.

Color-coded duplex ultrasonography is presently the most widely utilized surveillance modality for the carotid and mesenteric circulations and in the extremities, where it is supplemented by hemodynamic measurements and clinical evaluation. Although color-coded duplex ultrasonography can often detect endoleaks, spiral CT is the most definitive means of evaluating endografted aortic aneurysms for evidence of endoleaks; it is an absolute necessity for thoracic aneurysm surveillance where ultrasound penetration is not possible. Recommended reporting standards and definitions of success remain inexact and may be too rigid to accommodate the variety of clinical circumstances encountered when treating patients with vascular disease. Nonetheless, they do serve a valuable function when assessing new therapeutic modalities in strictly controlled trials.

References

1. Bandyk DF, Schmitt DD, Seabrook GR et al: Monitoring functional patency of in situ saphenous vein bypasses: the impact of a surveillance protocol and elective revision, *J Vasc Surg* 9:286–296, 1989.
2. Berkowitz HD, Hobbs CL, Roberts B et al: Value of routine vascular laboratory studies to identify vein graft stenosis, *Surgery* 90:971–979, 1981.
3. Turnipseed WD, Acher CW: Postoperative surveillance: an effective means of detecting correctable lesions that threaten graft patency, *Arch Surg* 120:324–328, 1985.
4. Blum U, Krumme B, Flugel P et al: Treatment of ostial renal artery stenoses with vascular endoprostheses after unsuccessful balloon angioplasty, *N Engl J Med* 336:459–465, 1997.
5. Raynaud AC, Beyssen BM, Turmel-Rodrigues LC et al: Renal artery stent placement: immediate and midterm technical and clinical results, *J Vasc Interv Radiol* 5:849–858, 1994.
6. Tullis MJ, Zierler RE, Glickerman DJ et al: Results of percutaneous transluminal angioplasty for atherosclerotic renal artery stenosis: a follow-up study with duplex ultrasonography, *J Vasc Surg* 25:46–54, 1997.
7. Rutherford RB, Becker GJ: Standards for evaluating and reporting the results of surgical and percutaneous therapy for peripheral arterial disease, *Radiology* 181:277–281, 1991.
8. Ahn SS, Rutherford RB, Becker GJ et al: Reporting standards for lower extremity arterial endovascular procedures, *J Vasc Surg* 17:1103–1107, 1993.
9. Rutherford RB, Flanigan DP, Gupta SK et al: Suggested standards for reports dealing with lower extremity ischemia, *J Vasc Surg* 4:80–94, 1986.
10. Bray A: Reporting guidelines: another perspective, *J Endovasc Surg* 2:334–340, 1995.
11. Veith FJ, Marin ML: Can there really be "uniform" reporting guidelines? *J Endovasc Surg* 2:332–333, 1995.
12. Myers KA: Reporting guidelines for open and endovascular surgery: why the current recommendations should be revised, *J Endovasc Surg* 2:321–328, 1995.
13. Rutherford RB: Revising the reporting guidelines: how far do we need to go? *J Endovasc Surg* 2:329–331, 1995.
14. Sacks D, Robinson ML, Summers TA, Marinelli DL: The value of duplex sonography after peripheral artery angioplasty in predicting subacute restenosis, *AJR* 162:179–183, 1994.
15. Sacks D, Robinson ML, Marinelli DL, Perlmutter GS: Evaluation of the peripheral arteries with duplex US after angioplasty, *Radiology* 176:39–44, 1990.
16. Nyamekye I, Sommerville K, Raphael M et al: Non-invasive assessment of arterial stenoses in angioplasty surveillance: a comparison with angiography, *Eur J Vasc Endovasc Surg* 12:471–481, 1996.
17. Mewissen MW, Kinney EV, Bandyk DF et al: The role of duplex scanning versus angiography in predicting outcome after balloon angioplasty in the femoropopliteal artery, *J Vasc Surg* 15:860–866, 1992.
18. Spijkerboer AM, Nass PC, de Valois JC et al: Evaluation of femoropopliteal arteries with duplex ultrasound after angioplasty: can we predict results at one year? *Eur J Vasc Endovasc Surg* 12:418–423, 1996.
19. Sensier Y, Hartshorne T, Thrush A et al: A prospective comparison of lower limb colour-coded duplex scanning with arteriography, *Eur J Vasc Endovasc Surg* 11:170–175, 1996.
20. Winter-Warnars HAO, van der Graaf Y, Mali WPTM: Ankle-arm index, angiography, and duplex ultrasonography after recanalization of occlusions in femoropopliteal arteries: comparison of long-term results, *Cardiovasc Intervent Radiol* 19:234–238, 1996.

21. Soulen MC, Benenati JF, Sheth S et al: Changes in renal artery Doppler indexes following renal angioplasty. *Vasc Interv Radiol* 2:457–462, 1991.
22. Hudspeth DA, Hansen KJ, Reavis SW et al: Renal duplex sonography after treatment of renovascular disease, *J Vasc Surg* 18:381–390, 1993.
23. Ahn SS, Rutherford RB, Johnston KW et al: Reporting standards for infrarenal endovascular abdominal aortic aneurysm repair, *J Vasc Surg* 25:405–410, 1997.
24. Rozenablit A, Marin ML, Veith FJ et al: Endovascular repair of abdominal aortic aneurysm: value of postoperative follow-up with helical CT, *AJR* 165:1473–1479, 1995.
25. Balm R, Kaatee R, Blankensteijn JD et al: CT-angiography of abdominal aortic aneurysms after transfemoral endovascular aneurysm management, *Eur J Vasc Endovasc Surg* 2:182–188, 1996.
26. Wain RA, Marin ML, Ohki T et al: Endoleaks after endovascular graft treatment of aortic aneurysms: classification, risk factors, and outcome, *J Vasc Surg* 27:69–80, 1998.
27. White GH, Yu W, May J et al: Endoleak as a complication of endoluminal grafting of abdominal aortic aneurysms: classification, incidence, diagnosis and management, *J Endovasc Surg* 4:152–168, 1997.
28. White RA, Donayre CE, Walot I et al: Modular bifurcation endoprosthesis for treatment of abdominal aortic aneurysms, *Ann Surg* 226:381–391, 1997.
29. Moore WS, Rutherford RB: Transfemoral endovascular repair of abdominal aortic aneurysm: results of the North American EVT phase 1 trial, *J Vasc Surg* 23:543–553, 1996.
30. Blum U, Voshage G: Abdominal aortic aneurysm repair using the Meadox/Vanguard prosthesis: indications, implantation technique, and results, *Tech Vasc Intervent Radiol* 1:19–24, 1998.
31. White GH, Yu W, May J et al: Three-year experience with the White-Yu endovascular GAD graft for transluminal repair of aortic and iliac aneurysms, *J Endovasc Surg* 4:124–136, 1997.

9
Safety Considerations for Endovascular Surgery

George E. Kopchok

The continuing evolution of endovascular techniques and instrumentation has enhanced the armamentarium available to vascular surgeons. The majority of endovascular procedures are minimally invasive with reduced risk and morbidity for the patient. However, imaging techniques, endovascular instrumentation, and delivery devices may introduce environmental safety concerns that were not present in conventional surgery. In this regard, it is essential that operating room personnel become knowledgeable about potential hazards and appropriate precautions that are necessary to create a safe work environment for themselves, as well as the patient.

As with most surgical procedures, adequate visualization allows for precise evaluation, treatment, and postprocedural assessment. For endovascular surgery, the majority of visualization and imaging is achieved through fluoroscopic radiation. Fluoroscopic imaging in the endovascular suite may introduce new or prolonged radiation exposure risks not normally associated with vascular surgery. Other hazards associated with the endovascular suite may include laser exposure and increased blood contact resulting from patient catheterization. This chapter reviews the considerations relevant to reduce risks and produce a safe utilization of endovascular suites.

Radiation Safety

History

The x-ray was first discovered, quite by accident, by Wilhelm Roentgen.[1] Roentgen was investigating the conduction of cathode rays (electrons) through a large, partially evacuated glass tube known as a Crookes' tube (Figure 9–1A). On November 8, 1895, Roentgen was working in his laboratory in Wurzburg University and had completely enclosed his Crookes' tube with black photographic paper so that he could visualize the effects of the cathode rays. A plate of fluorescent material (barium platinocyanide) was lying on a bench several feet away from the Crookes' tube. When the enclosed tube was excited, Roentgen noticed that the barium platinocyanide began to fluoresce. The intensity of the fluorescence increased as the barium platinocyanide was brought closer to the Crookes' tube, leaving little doubt as to the origin of the stimulus. Based on this initial observation, Roentgen began a feverish investigation of this "X-light" by interposing different materials, including his hand, between the Crookes' tube and the fluorescing plate. He reported his findings to the scientific community near the end of 1895. Roentgen quickly recognized the value of his discovery to medicine and produced the first medical x-ray

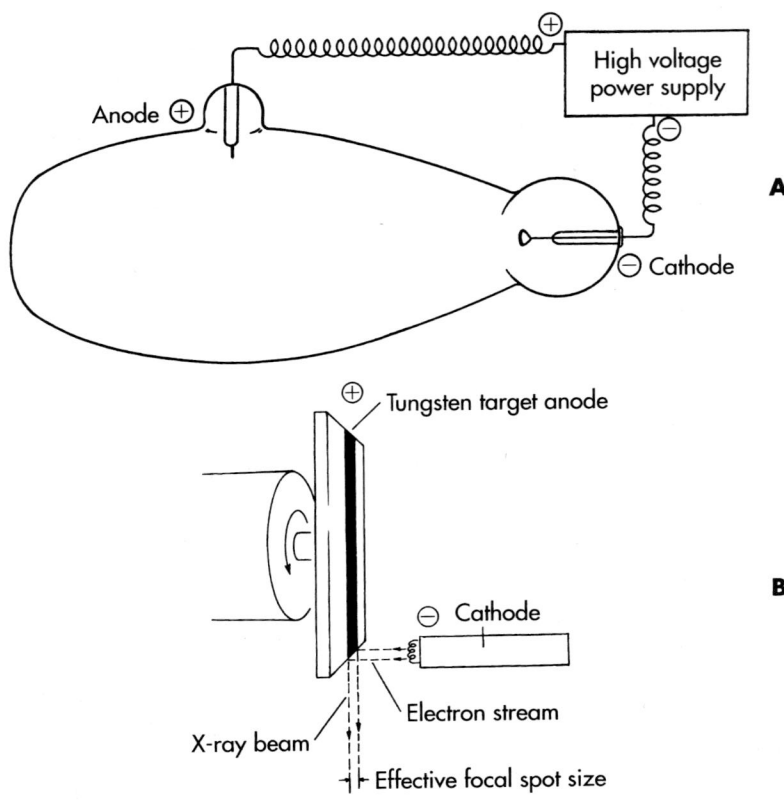

FIGURE 9–1. **A**, Original Crookes' tube used by Wilhelm Roentgen to study conduction of cathode rays (electrons). These experiments led to the accidental discovery of x-rays. **B**, Modern rotating disk used to produce x-rays. The production of x-rays from electrons is very inefficient; most of the energy loss is in the form of heat. By rotating the anode, heat is kept to a minimum.

film, one of his wife's hand. For his work he received the first Nobel prize given in physics in 1901.

The first case of human injury was reported a few months after Roentgen's original paper announcing the discovery of x-rays. The first x-ray-induced fatality in the United States was reported in 1904 by Thomas A. Edison. Edison, who invented the fluoroscope in 1898, was experimenting with new fluorescent materials, including two materials that are still used today. However, he discontinued his x-ray research when his assistant and friend, Clarence Dally, received a severe x-ray burn of both arms that eventually required amputation. Dally died in 1904 and is considered the first x-ray fatality in the United States. By 1910, x-ray exposure and safety parameters were developed. Shortly thereafter, new imaging techniques and protective wear reduced exposure, thus leading to a new emphasis for radiation control and safety.

Fluoroscopic Image Production

Fluoroscopic imaging is defined as a radiologic examination using fluorescence for observation of a transient image. The two major components of image-intensified fluoroscopy are the x-ray tube and image intensifier (Figure 9–2). The x-ray tube (much like the original Crookes' tube) contains two major parts, the cathode, which serves as the source of the electrons, and the anode, which acts as the target for the electrons. As the stream of high-velocity electrons hit the target (i.e., anode), most of their energy

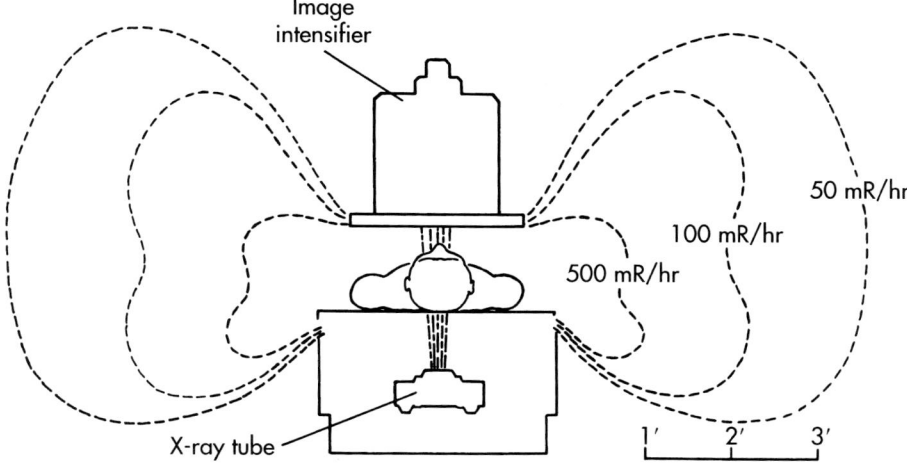

FIGURE 9-2. Fluoroscopic intensifier demonstrating the position of the x-ray tube and image intensifier. Also illustrated are the approximate x-ray exposures at 1, 2, and 3 feet. It is important to realize that x-ray exposure decreases with the square of the distance from the source.

is transformed into heat, but a small part is transformed into x-rays, which can be directed onto a patient and image intensifier (Figure 9-1B). When the x-rays are directed onto the patient, most are absorbed by the dense structures such as bone, whereas some pass through and strike the image intensifier's phosphor. This layer of fluorescent material absorbs the x-rays and converts the energy into different levels of light photons that are directly proportional to the intensity of incident energy. The light photons then impact a photocathode, causing electrons to be given off in direct proportion to the intensity of the fluorescent light. The electrons are then accelerated and focused onto a smaller electrostatic layer called an output phosphor. The output phosphor is hundreds of times brighter than the input phosphor because of its smaller size and the additional energy given to the electrons through acceleration. The output phosphor is then viewed, usually with a television camera, and displayed on a high-resolution black and white monitor.

Radiation Safety

The unit of radiation exposure from x-rays is the roentgen (R). A roentgen is defined as the amount of radiation that will produce 2.1×10^9 ion pairs in $1\,cm^3$ of air. For diagnostic imaging such as fluoroscopy, exposure rate is measured in roentgens per minute (R/min). The absorbed radiation dose is referred to as a rad, which refers to the absorption of 100 erg (10^{-5} joule) of energy per gram of mass. A more useful unit used to measure the biologic effects in humans are rem (rad equivalent in man). Rems are commonly used to record and monitor human exposure to radiation. Total annual background radiation for individuals without occupational exposure to x-rays is about 125 millirems (mrem).

The knowledge that any exposure to radiation is injurious to human tissue has led to the development of maximum permissible dose (MPD) guidelines. The MPD is defined as the maximum dose of radiation that, in light of present knowledge, would not be expected to produce significant radiation effects. The guidelines have steadily dropped in the last 60 years. In 1931 the MPD was 50 rems per year. In 1936 and 1948 the MPD was dropped to 30 and then 15 rems per year. In 1958 the MPD was again dropped to the current standard of 5 rems per year for any person over the age of 18. The whole body exposure of 5 rems per year applies to the head, neck, trunk, lens of the eye, blood-forming organs, and gonads. A higher MPD is allowed for less sensitive parts of the body such as the hands (75 rems), skin (15 rems), and forearms (30 rems).

The three major principles of radiation protection are *time*, *distance*, and *shielding*. The radiation dose to an individual is directly proportional to the duration of exposure (i.e., exposure = exposure rate × time). During fluoroscopic procedures it is important that the investigator only activate the foot pedal when the x-ray image is needed. The investigator should try to pulse the fluoroscopic foot switch to limit overall exposure. For example, many short pulses of exposure can be used to watch a balloon angioplasty while the balloon is stationary and inflated. This foot-tapping technique should be used whenever possible. Exposure should also be used only when the investigator is actually viewing the video monitor. Fluoroscopic equipment is required to have an audible 5-minute timer to remind the physician that a considerable amount of imaging time has elapsed.

The distance between the radiation source and personnel should also be kept at the maximum. As with many energy sources, radiation exposure decreases with the square of the distance (inverse square law). If a person moves from 1 foot to 3 feet from an x-ray tube, the amount of exposure will drop 9 times. Thus it is important that investigators and personnel remain as far from the fluoroscope and examining table as reasonably practical. A diagram demonstrating the scatter of radiation measured from a fluoroscopic C-arm can be seen in Figure 9–2. It demonstrates how to reduce one's exposure simply by standing one or two steps back.[2]

The level of exposure can also be reduced by placing shielding between personnel and the radiation source. The amount of shielding or "protective barrier" that reduces radiation energy by a factor of 2 is the half-value layer (HVL). The amount of protective barrier that reduces radiation exposure 10-fold is the tenth value layer (TVL). These values are used to rate the protective apparel used during radiographic imaging. Current protective aprons consist of a lead and tin mixture that optimizes energy absorption and comfort. Protective aprons come in two thicknesses, 0.25- and 0.50-mm lead equivalent.[3] Absorption of x-rays is nonlinear with respect to thickness of shielding. Overall, the 0.5-mm equivalent apron provides approximately 90% reduction in radiation exposures. The 0.25-mm apron provides only a 75% reduction and is therefore usually limited to pediatric procedures or used as a back for wraparound aprons. The exact amount of protection offered by lead aprons will vary with the kilovolts peak (kVp) used for patient imaging. The higher the kVp, the lower the protection. Protective aprons should be examined radiographically every 3 months and repaired or discarded if leakage is confirmed. Aside from lead aprons, it is also suggested that personnel wear thyroid shields and lead glasses to minimize exposure to these sensitive areas. Other protective screens such as ceiling-mounted transparent lead glass screens can be very effective at reducing exposure.

Another technique that can reduce radiation scatter and also improve image quality is collimation. Collimation is the restriction of the radiation beam by moveable lead shields. This technique, which is often underused by the investigator, minimizes the field of view (exposure to radiation) to only the area of visual importance (Figure 9–3A,B).

Personnel Monitoring

Personnel who are routinely involved with fluoroscopic procedures or other forms of radiation exposure should be monitored to determine the total amount of exposure. The most common monitoring device is the film badge. The film badge contains a film that is sensitive to ionizing radiation. Film badges must be worn on the front, outside of the protective apron, preferably at the level of the shoulders or neck. The badges should be exchanged and processed every month. State and federal regulations require that personnel be given monthly reports summarizing their monthly, quarterly, cumulative annual, and cumulative lifetime exposure. As mentioned above, adults should receive far less then the recommended MPD of 5 rems per year.

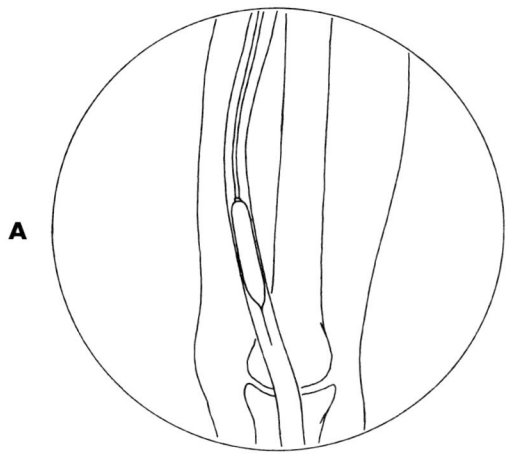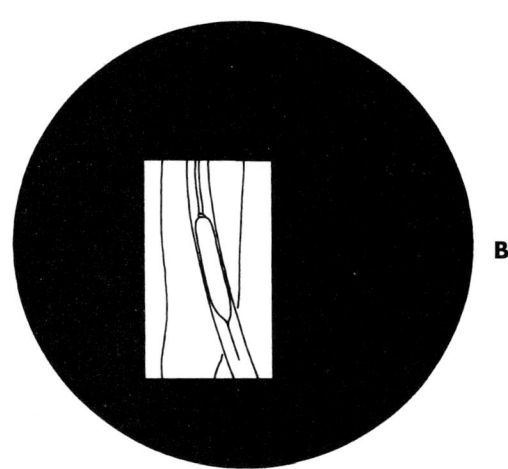

FIGURE 9–3. **A**, Typical fluoroscopic image in which collimation is not being used. **B**, Same fluoroscopic image as seen in **A**, except collimation has been used to reduce the amount of scattered radiation and improve image quality.

Pregnancy

Pregnancy can greatly alter the tolerable level for safe exposure to radiation. This is of obvious importance for personnel, as well as potential patients. When personnel become pregnant, it is important that they discuss their options with a supervisor. The MPD for a fetus is 500 mrem for the period of pregnancy. Most personnel in a fluoroscopic imaging room receive less than 500 mrem per year. Therefore, by simply reviewing the individual's records, it may be decided that she could safely continue working in an exposed area. Exposure at the waist, under a protective apron, will not normally exceed 10% of the whole body value measured outside of the apron. Pregnant personnel who decide to continue their work should wear a second monitoring badge under the protective apron at the level of the waist to further measure the fetal exposure. If possible, personnel should be offered a temporary position in a nonexposed area.

Inadvertent irradiation of a pregnant patient should be avoided if at all possible. The fetus is at greatest risk to radiation during the first month of pregnancy. It is during this first month that a patient may be unaware of pregnancy. Under normal conditions, radiographic procedures should not be performed on any pregnant patient unless the health of the mother or fetus would be directly compromised. The International Commission on Radiological Protection (ICRP) suggests that women of childbearing years only be exposed to lower abdominal or pelvic area radiographic examination during the 10-day interval after the onset of menstruation.

Lasers

Physics

Laser is an acronym for "light amplification by stimulated emission of radiation." The theoretic principles of the lasing process were first described by Albert Einstein in 1917.[4] In the paper entitled "Quantum Theory of Radiation," he described the process of stimulated emission. This theory combined with other work was the basis for awarding Einstein the Nobel prize in physics in 1921.

Before one can understand the concept of stimulated emission, an understanding of spontaneous emission is required. Under normal conditions, atoms interact with photons and absorb their energy by elevating an electron from a lower energy orbit to a higher energy orbit. This process will only occur when an atom interacts with a photon that has enough energy

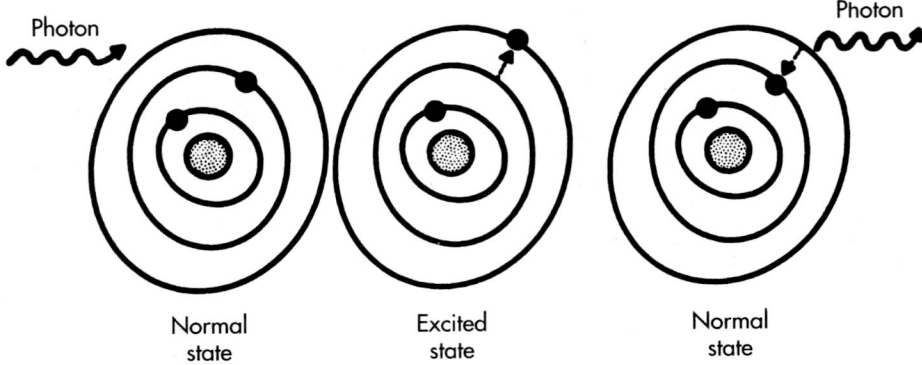

FIGURE 9–4. Spontaneous emission. An atom absorbs the energy of a photon by elevating an electron to a higher orbit and then spontaneously releases the energy as a second photon.

to elevate an electron one orbit. An atom with an electron in the elevated energy state (excited atom) quickly releases the energy in the form of a photon as the electron returns to its normal orbit. The wavelength and energy of the emitted photon corresponds to the differences between the higher and lower energy orbits. This process, because it occurs naturally in all matter, is called spontaneous emission (Figure 9–4).

Lasers work by a process known as stimulated emission. The process begins when atoms (or molecules) are excited from an external source. When one excited atom returns to its normal state, it emits a photon (Figure 9–5). This photon in turn interacts with a second excited atom. The photon is not absorbed by the second excited atom. It causes the atom to drop back to its normal state and emit two photons with identical characteristics (the incident photon and its own photon). The two photons proceed to stimulate 2 more excited atoms, which emit 4, then 8, 16, 32, etc. identical photons. The photons are identical in wavelength, phase, and amplitude. This process is called stimulated emission and is the basis for laser energy.

Laser light has three unique characteristics: the light is monochromatic, directional, and coherent. Monochromaticity means that the laser light consists of a particular wavelength or a very narrow range of wavelengths. If the wavelength of laser energy is in the visible range [i.e., wavelength between 350 to 1400 nanometers (nm)], it will have a color corresponding to its particular wavelength. Normal

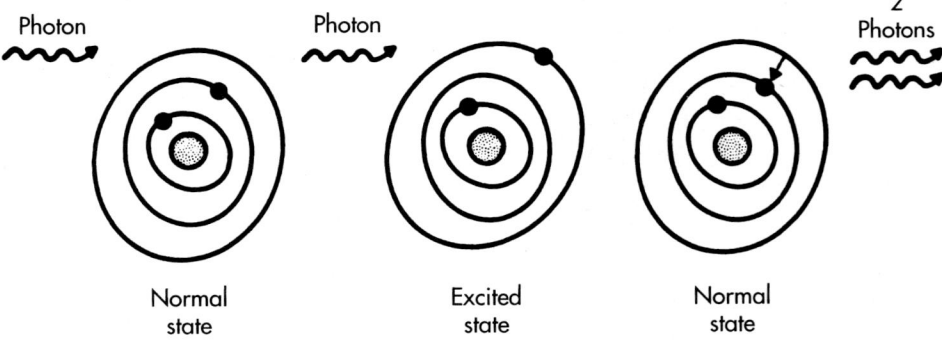

FIGURE 9–5. Stimulated emission. When an atom in the excited state is struck by a photon, it will be stimulated to return to its normal state and in the process emit two identical photons.

white light from a source such as a lamp contains the entire spectrum of wavelengths of visible light. When the light is passed through a prism, the individual wavelengths are separated to produce the characteristic colors in the pattern of a rainbow. When laser energy is passed through a prism, because of the select wavelength distribution, only one wavelength or color is visible (Figure 9–6). Lasers that operate above the visible wavelengths (>1400 nm) are known as infrared lasers. Lasers that operate below the visible spectrum (<350 nm) are called ultraviolet lasers.

Laser light is also described as directional. Directionality or collimation means that the laser energy is released in a highly concentrated, parallel beam with minimal amounts of light spread. As an example, light emitted from a light bulb is not directional and spreads so that it lights up the whole room. In contrast, laser light emitted in a dark room only illuminates a very small spot. Spread of laser energy is so minimal that a point source aimed at the moon only spreads to the extent that it would illuminate a circle approximately one-half mile in diameter on the moon's surface.[5]

The third unique property of laser energy is that it is coherent. According to the wave theory of electromagnetic radiation, the waveform of laser energy can be characterized according to the wavelength, amplitude, and frequency. Amplitude is the vertical height of the wave, wavelength (λ) is the distance between two successive wave peaks, and frequency (f) is the speed of light (c) divided by the wavelength ($f = c/\lambda$). The light waves emitted from a normal lamp are incoherent in that the waveforms have different amplitudes and different wavelengths, and they are not aligned spatially as to peaks and valleys of the waveform. Laser energy is coherent in that all of the waveform amplitudes, wavelengths, and temporal distribution of the peaks and valleys of the curves are the same (Figure 9–7).

The major advantage of lasers for endovascular surgery is the ability to precisely deliver a large amount of energy through a very small conduit. For the majority of lasers (Nd:YAG, holmium:YAG, excimer, argon) this is easily accomplished by using fiberoptic waveguides. Most fibers are made from quartz and will vary in diameter, flexibility, and shape according to the laser wavelength and clinical application. The efficiency of energy transmission through a fiber varies with wavelength of the light, the diameter, and the quality of the fiber. On transmission through the fiber, the collimated laser light bounces from side to side as it travels

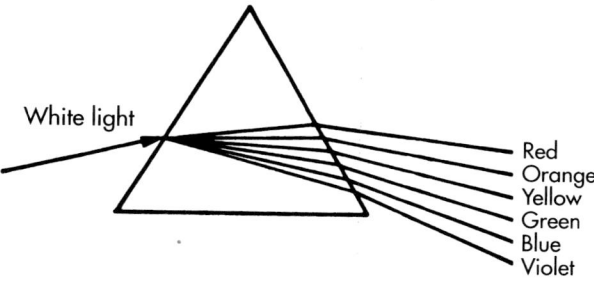

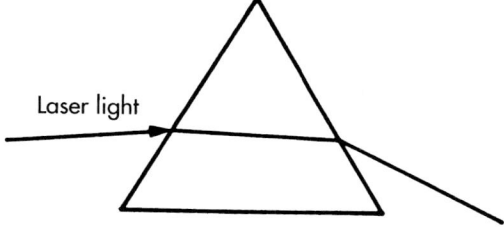

FIGURE 9–6. Monochromaticity of laser light. White light passed through a prism is separated into its component wavelengths. Laser light has a select wavelength spectrum.

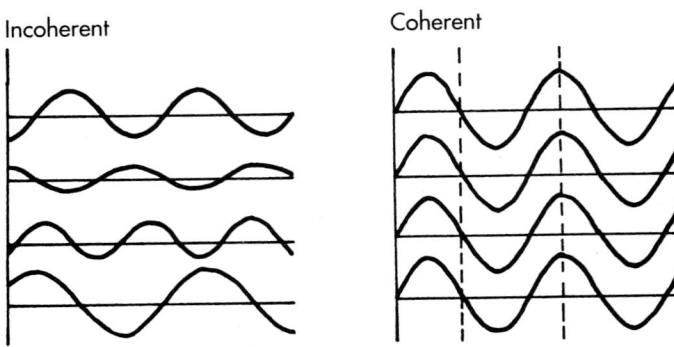

FIGURE 9-7. Incoherent waveforms of normal light vs. coherent waveforms of laser light.

through the fiber. This change of direction causes the laser light to diverge 10 to 15 degrees as it exits the fiber tip (Figure 9–8). The divergence property can be used to vary the power density (watts/area) and resultant tissue effects (cutting or coagulating) by changing the distance between the fiber tip and the tissue.

When laser energy interacts with the tissue, it may be absorbed, transmitted, scattered, or reflected. Laser-tissue interactions depend on how the laser energy is dissipated and the absorption characteristics of the tissue for the particular wavelength. When tissue absorption occurs, the laser energy produces variable effects depending on the type of interaction. These include laser photochemical effects (chemical bond disruption), laser fluorescence (reemission of photons), or photothermal changes (heat-producing vibration and collision of atoms).

Laser Safety

Establishment of a laser protocol, facility specifications, approvals, in-service training sessions, and continuing education for personnel are essential to maintain a safe environment. Personnel must be trained in operating procedures and precautions to prevent personal injury and property damage. Only laser certified personnel should be permitted to set up, use, and discontinue use of laser equipment. Although laser radiation can cause eye damage, skin burns, and combustion of flammable materials, these hazards can easily be avoided by a carefully planned program.

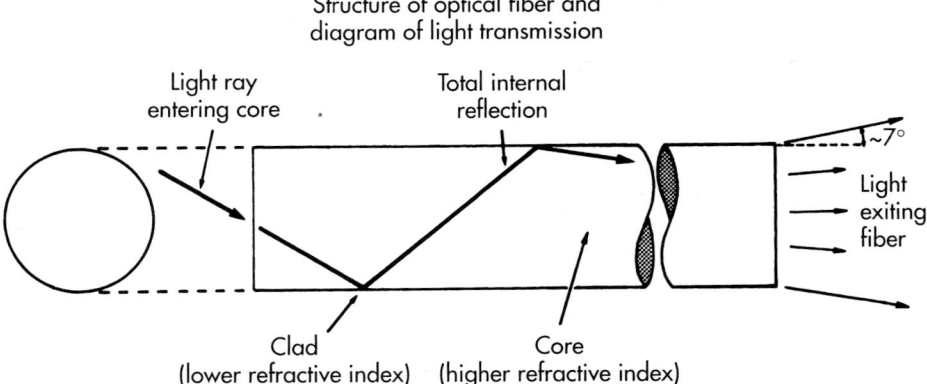

FIGURE 9-8. Transmission through the optic fiber causes the laser light to bounce from side to side, thus losing its coherent property. This also causes the light to diverge at an angle of 10 to 15 degrees from the tip of the fiber.

The physician and all key operating room personnel should be fully versed with an understanding of laser physics, appropriate nomenclature regarding laser energy, and laser-tissue interactions.[6,7] The physician user is ultimately responsible for selecting the wattage, appropriate lens or fiber, and ensuring safe laser use for each procedure. However, a laser safety officer or designee should be present at all cases.[8]

Lasers are classified according to their potential to cause biologic injury. The parameters used for laser classification are laser power, wavelength, exposure duration, and beam spot size at the area of interest. Lasers are stratified into four classes. Class I, or exempt lasers, produce no hazard under normal operating conditions. The total amount of energy produced is less than the maximum permissible exposure level established by the American National Standards Institute (ANSI), and therefore no special facility or safety precautions are needed. Class II lasers are low-power lasers that do not present a visual hazard resulting from a normal aversion response. The eye normally closes in approximately 0.25 second when exposed to a noxious stimulus. This response avoids eye damage from a class II laser. Class IIIa lasers operate with maximum power output ($<2.5\,mW/cm^2$). These lasers present a hazard if viewed through collecting optics but present no hazard if viewed momentarily with the unaided eye. Class IIIb lasers can damage the eyes if viewed directly but present no hazard to the skin. Class IV denotes high-power laser systems that are hazardous to the eyes, skin, and flammable material from a direct or diffusely reflected beam. Facility requirements vary with the class of laser being used. Generally, class IV lasers are used in surgical applications, and therefore operating facilities must be set up in accordance with requirements for this classification.[7,9]

Class IV laser procedure and operating rooms must have all windows covered with nontransparent barriers to prevent the inadvertent passage of laser light. All doors must be closed, and access to the room should be restricted while the laser is activated. Clearly visible warning signs with flashing lights to signify that the system is activated are mandatory. All persons in the room must wear eye protection while the laser is activated. Personnel should not be allowed into the room while the laser is in use unless they are wearing the appropriate safety glasses and are aware of the laser hazards. The laser should remain in the off position or with the safety shutter closed until ready for use. Control of laser emission by a foot pedal and direction of the beam by hand control greatly enhances the safety. As with the electrocautery or any active device, laser energy should be activated only when the tip of the fiber is in the field of view and/or in contact with the specific target. Reflective surgical instruments should be avoided and reflective surfaces in the laser procedure room minimized. Moist sponges in the open operating fields can prevent combustion of dry or paper materials.

Laser energy can affect different parts of the eye depending on which structure absorbs that particular wavelength. The three areas of most concern are the cornea, lens, and retina. Laser energy outside the visible range ($<350\,nm$ and $>1400\,nm$) is absorbed by the cornea and lens. Exposure to this energy can produce cataracts and corneal scarring. Laser energy in the visible wavelength is focused by the cornea and lens onto the retina and causes up to $100,000\times$ amplification of radiant exposure.[9] Careless misdirection of the laser light even at low powers can result in instantaneous burning of the retina and consequent blindness in the visual field corresponding to the burn spot. As mentioned in the preceding paragraph, everyone in the operating room, including the patient, must have appropriate eye wear during the procedures. For the CO_2 laser, clear plastic or glass lenses with side guards are adequate, and wet gauze can be used to protect an anesthetized patient's eyes. Green lenses (nontransparent to 1060 nm) are required for the Nd:YAG laser, and amber lenses (nontransparent to 488 to 515 nm) are necessary to absorb the green or blue light of the argon laser. Other lasers with different wavelengths require specific lenses for eye protection as recommended by the manufacturer.

The most frequent cause of laser injury in industrial environments is electrical accidents.

Laser systems frequently require large power supplies with the potential for fatal shock. Electrical outlets with safety switches should be carefully positioned when the laser is installed. Adequate warning signs and in-service training are essential to prevent inadvertent accidents. Maintenance is to be performed by trained technicians only. Laser use and maintenance should be recorded from the date of installation. The laser system should be stored so that components and the ignition key are secured when the laser is not being used.

Although the risk of airborne contaminants with endovascular laser applications is minimal, users should be aware that precautions must be implemented to prevent exposure and inhalation of laser plume. There is still a controversy whether laser (or electrocautery) plume contains viable cancer and/or mutagenic cells or whether laser exposure destroys these organisms. A closed-system smoke evacuator should be used if exposure to laser plume is likely to occur. Dangerous by-products may also be released from inorganic materials. Plastic bottles, drapes, instruments, polytetrafluoroethylene (PTFE) prosthetic materials, and tubing may emit poisonous gases if exposed to laser energy.

Blood Exposure

No current description of endovascular suite safety can be complete without mentioning the risk of blood exposure. Although one may dismiss blood exposure as minimal risk because of the "noninvasive" environment, the potential for blood exposure still exists. Maneuvers that reduce the risk of exposure are a benefit to both health care workers and patients.

Several studies of general surgical procedures have shown a correlation between the duration of an operation and the potential for blood contamination, as well as a strong correlation between blood loss and contamination.[10,11] Telford et al. reported on two categories of contamination: injuries and blood exposure. They found that, under stringent monitoring by a study nurse, cuts to at least one surgical team member occurred during 2.6% of the operations, and needle sticks occurred during 13% of operations. Most of the cuts in this study occurred during hand-to-hand passing of knives from surgeon to the scrub nurse, whereas most of the needle sticks occurred during suturing. The same study monitored effectiveness of double-gloving to control blood exposure to the hands. They found that 11.5% of single-gloved personnel had hand contamination, whereas only 1.2% of double-gloved personnel had contamination. During procedures that lasted more than 2 hours and resulted in more than 100 ml of blood loss, personnel who single- or double-gloved had a hand contamination of 40% and 9%, respectively.

Endovascular surgical techniques should greatly reduce blood exposure because of shorter procedure times and less blood loss. However, the use of indwelling arterial sheaths and catheters present a new exposure modality. Because of arterial pressures, the simple misdirection of a three-way stopcock or flush with a syringe can contaminate a person several feet away. Protective clothing for personnel near the operating field should include fluid-resistant gowns, eye guards or face shields, and double-gloving if the procedure lasts longer than 1 hour. Personnel who might be within 3 to 4 feet of the access site would also be advised to wear protective eye wear. Needles are routinely used for arterial access. When a needle or any sharp instrument is exchanged, care must be taken not to drop or toss the sharp object toward the scrub nurse. The safest mode of exchange is to set the needle or sharp instrument down, allowing the other person to pick it up.

References

1. Bushong SC: *Radiologic science for technologists*, St Louis, 1984, Mosby.
2. Nissen SE: Principles of radiographic imaging. In Roubin GS, Califf RM, O'Neill WW et al, editors: *Interventional cardiovascular medicine*, New York, 1994, Churchill Livingstone.
3. Geise RA, Hunter DW: Personnel exposure during fluoroscopy procedures, *Postgraduate Radiology* 8, 1988.

4. Einstein A: Zur Quantem Theorie dr Strahlung, *Phys Zeit* 18:121, 1917.
5. Hallmark C: *Lasers, the light fantastic*, Blueridge Summit, Pa, 1979, TAB Books.
6. Arndt KA, Noe JM, Northam BC: Laser therapy—basic concepts and nomenclature, *J Am Acad Dermatol* 5:649–654, 1981.
7. American National Standards Institute: *American national standard for the safe use of lasers*, [ANSI] Z 130.1, New York, 1980, the Institute.
8. American National Standards Institute: *American national standard for the safe use of lasers in health care facilities*, [ANSI] Z 136.3, New York, 1988, the Institute.
9. *A guide for the control of laser hazards*, Cincinnati, 1981, American Conference of Governmental Industrial Hygienists.
10. Telford GL, Quebbeman EJ: Assessing the risk of blood exposure in the operating room, *Am Pract Infect Cont* 6(21):351–356, 1993.
11. Quebbeman EJ, Telford GL, Wadsworth K et al: Risk of blood contamination and injury to operating room personnel, *Ann Surg* 214:614–620, 1991.

Part III
Facilities and Equipment for Endovascular Intervention

10
Endovascular Suite Design

Edward B. Diethrich

Advancements in the field of endovascular surgery have altered the treatment of vascular disease substantially over the last 20 years. Endovascular interventions now incorporate techniques that employ highly specialized imaging and monitoring equipment as well as numerous disposable devices. Balloon angioplasty, for example, requires extensive use of fluoroscopic visualization and employs low-profile sheaths, guidewires, catheters, and balloons. More recently, the introduction of stents has furthered our ability to provide lasting results with percutaneous procedures. Endoluminal graft technology, still early in its evaluation, is likely to make an even greater impact on endoluminal treatment of vascular disease.

The introduction of sophisticated imaging techniques, such as angioscopy and intravascular ultrasonography (IVUS), and the use of new endovascular techniques and more sophisticated devices has changed the requirements for designing and equipping the modern endovascular suite. High-resolution fluoroscopy and angiography equipment and IVUS capability are now essential to the success of advanced endovascular interventions. Although most hospitals in the United States currently have excellent imaging capabilities, vascular surgeons may find the equipment and environment in the radiology suite or catheterization laboratory less than ideal for endovascular interventions. It may also be difficult for vascular surgeons to work with technicians and nurses who are not well versed in endovascular surgery routines, particularly when they are unfamiliar with classic sterile technique and the environment does not adequately support its use. The renovation of an existing operating room or construction of a new one is expensive but may be cost-effective for the vascular surgery department with an adequate caseload. Some of the requirements for designing and equipping the endovascular suite are reviewed in this chapter.

Designing and Equipping the Endovascular Suite

The design of the modern endovascular suite must incorporate adequate space and sufficient electrical capacity to facilitate procedures. Optimal lead shielding is integral in ensuring the safety of patients and health care personnel, and it must comply with stringent state requirements in most locations. To accommodate the core equipment comfortably, the suite should be at least 500 square feet, with a minimum clear area of 400 square feet. A typical layout for an endovascular suite is shown in Figure 10–1.

The design of the endovascular suite should include the option of full "operative" sterile conditions, particularly for procedures that incorporate prosthetic materials, such as endoluminal grafting. Dacron, Teflon, and other graft materials are used for lining vessels during these procedures, and a sterile setting is required. Initiating a case in a "semisterile"

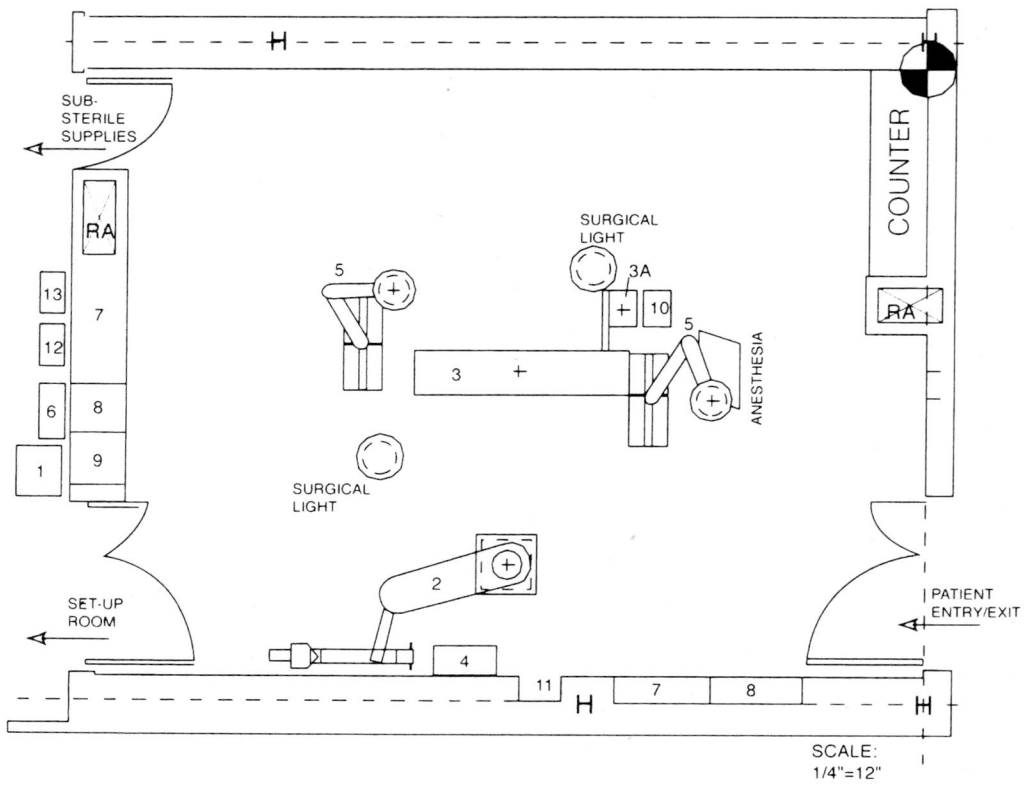

FIGURE 10-1. Endovascular surgical suite layout in the Arizona Heart Hospital in Phoenix, AZ. The room is equipped for all types of cardiovascular procedures with optimum equipment and arrangements for endovascular intervention. *1*, Generator; *2*, C-arm; *3*, table; *3A*, table base; *4*, video cart; *5*, monitors; *6*, table electronics; *7*, catheter cabinets; *8*, miscellaneous cabinet; *9*, desk unit with computer for inventory, patient records, radiologic archives; *10*, medical utility pedestal with outlets for nitrogen, oxygen, air, vacuum, electrical connections, phone, data, and video port for intravascular ultrasography (IVUS) and angioscopy; *11*, IVUS machine location; *12*, physiologic monitors; *13*, video composite monitors (outside shots, IVUS, angioscopy);

environment and then attempting to convert to strict sterile conditions if more radical intervention is called for inevitably results in unacceptable contamination. Given that it is nearly impossible to ensure that an operating room typically used as a "semisterile" environment can then be made "sterile" for special procedures, our recommendation and practice is to adhere to strict, sterile conditions at all times. Most endovascular programs in which vascular surgeons are participating have adopted this policy.

Decisions about the basic design of the endovascular suite are, perhaps, most dependent on the type of imaging equipment that will be included in the facility.

Fluoroscopy Systems

Fixed and mobile imaging systems are available, and the advantages and disadvantages of each must be weighed carefully. Generally speaking, a fixed C-arm imaging system is preferable for endovascular procedures. Fixed imaging systems (Figure 10-2, see color plate) provide excellent image quality, an adjustable source-to-intensifier distance, processing that results in immediate image availability, and fast setup and

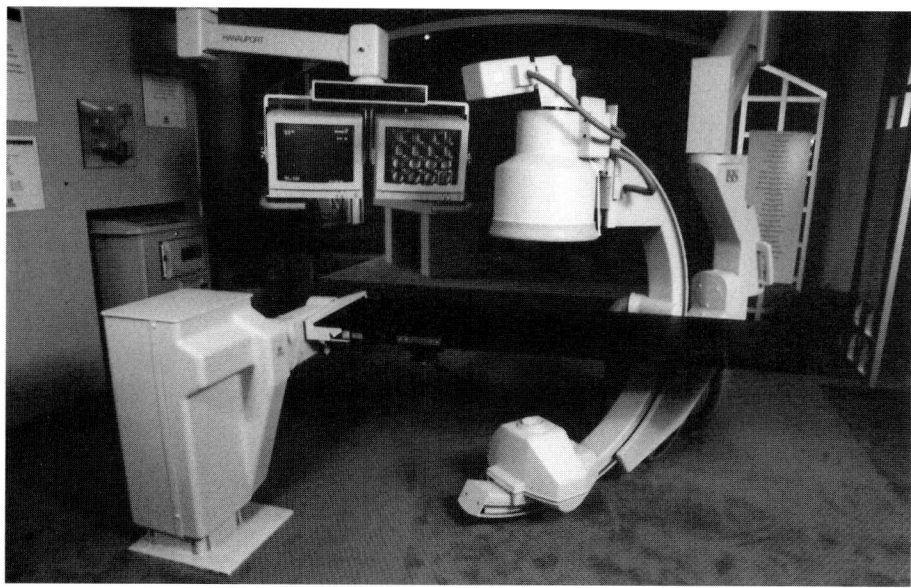

FIGURE 10–2. International Surgical Systems fixed C-arm imaging system. This system provides maximum flexibility for the operator and permits high quality imaging during complex endovascular procedures. (See color plate).

use time. Most importantly, these systems permit rapid "panning" (horizontal movement of the image intensifier along the entire course of the artery), which is an essential function during advanced endoluminal procedures. In addition, fixed systems allow the use of lower radiation doses and smaller amounts of dye than most mobile systems and are less technician-dependent because of their ease of operation. They are, however, more costly and require significant lead shielding. Mobile systems (Figure 10–3, see color plate) are less expensive than fixed systems and require no special construction. They may also be used in a variety of locations by other specialists. The disadvantages of mobile units include suboptimal image quality and resolution, a fixed source-to-intensifier distance, and a longer setup time.

The fixed, ceiling-mounted, surgical C-arm roentgenographic unit should incorporate an image enhancer that is integrated with a 0.75-inch videotape recorder and monitors for contrast injection visualization. A second monitor with a digital storage disk should also be included to provide still images of selected arteriographic segments. This technique, known as *road mapping*, is essential to complex angioplasty procedures. Hard-copy documentation is also an integral part of the imaging system, and a multiformat x-ray film camera or Polaroid film pack with adapters should be included in the setup. The unit (ISS-2000 Plus Intraoperative Imaging System; International Surgical Systems, Phoenix, AZ) in our endovascular suite at the Arizona Heart Hospital has been designed and refined under our supervision to create a system that fulfills all of our current and foreseeable requirements for endovascular surgery. It incorporates a digital system with a 1024×1024 pixel matrix coupled to a 1024-line medical television unit. The digital system has a minimum storage capacity of 4000 images and allows postprocessing before copying to the high line multiformat camera.

The endovascular surgeon may access vessels in the extremities as well as in the aortoiliac, brachiocephalic, and carotid region. For the superficial femoral, popliteal, and tibial arteries, the fluoroscopic unit must be moved in a horizontal plane from the groin along the course of the vessel. Images are obtained as the unit pans the length of the vessel, reducing the amount of time and contrast material needed to complete the procedure.

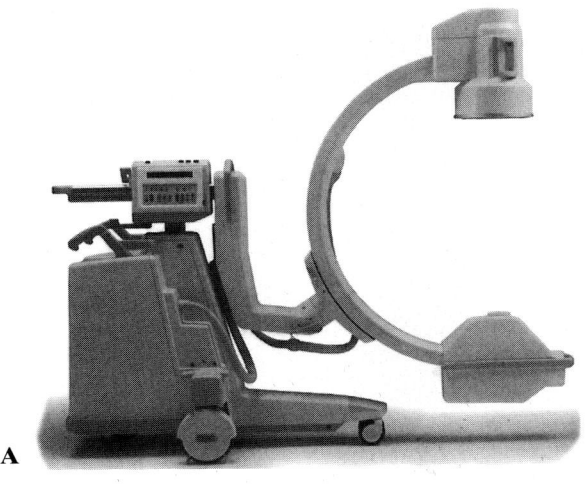

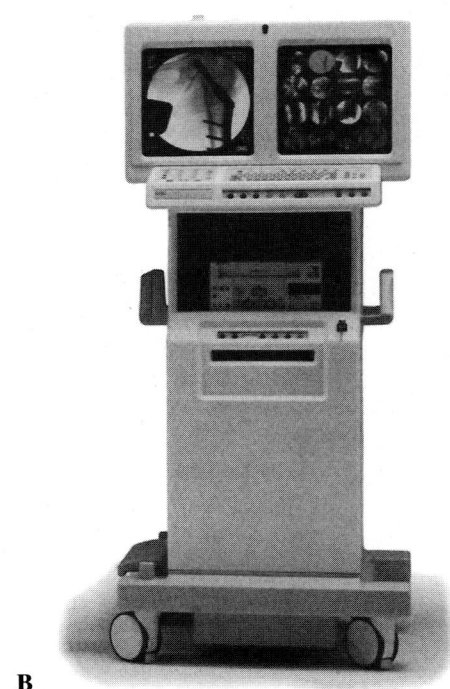

FIGURE 10–3. **A, B**, Popular mobile imaging system distributed by OMC. The unit is often used by various specialists, whereas fixed units are frequently dedicated to use by the vascular specialist. (See color plate).

In the aortoiliac region, the abdominal aorta may be visualized from the renal arteries down to the groin. Again, the fluoroscopic unit must move freely such that wire guidance and other aspects of the angioplasty procedure are not impeded. Antegrade thrombolysis or access from above to the lower aorta and the mesenteric, renal, iliac, and femoral vessels is frequently necessary; the fluoroscopic unit must move rapidly over the catheter's path. The success of these procedures may be limited if obstructions from a table or a floor-mounted portable unit prevent rapid panning. The carbon fiber table shown in Figure 10–2 is ideal for endovascular procedures because it is totally free of any metal attachments or obstructions.

Endovascular treatment of lesions in the aortic arch and cervical and intracranial arteries is becoming more prevalent. These arteries may be approached via brachial, femoral, and retrograde carotid access routes; and adequate visualization is certainly paramount to the success of the procedure.

Angioscopy

Complex percutaneous and open interventions often require imaging techniques that are complementary to angiography. Angioscopy provides direct visualization and is particularly useful for viewing the suture lines and lumens of grafts, evaluating hemorrhagic plaques, determining the flow-inhibiting potential of flaps, assessing intimal hyperplasia in stents, and estimating thrombosis volume and marking the progress of its removal. Angioscopic imaging is also valuable for establishing the etiology of restenosis after interventional therapy. Poststent dissection, bulging of tissue into the lumen at the stent articulation site, gaps between stents, and thrombus are easily visualized. Angioscopic data may motivate changes in therapy or guide the selection of treatment before and after stent deployment.

Angioscopic equipment is available from a variety of manufacturers. We use a 2.3F disposable angioscope (Intramed; Baxter Healthcare, Irvine, CA) connected to high-quality medical video color monitors with video recorders for hard copy documentation. Irrigating systems provide computer-assisted, pulsed irrigation and image storage for maximum visibility with minimal flush volume. The Baxter system allows on-demand delivery of heparinized saline under pressure at preset pulse durations via a foot pedal. Both freeze-frame and real-time imaging are possible, and the flush and image capture may be synchronized for digitized output. We have found angioscopy to be most beneficial in procedures below the inguinal ligament. Lesions above this level are more difficult to visualize as a result of the increased blood velocity in these areas.

Intravascular Ultrasonography

At the Arizona Heart Institute and Arizona Heart Hospital, we use IVUS as an adjunct to angiography in a high percentage of cases. IVUS provides baseline luminal dimensions before and after angioplasty (intraluminal cross sections and arterial circumferences) and allows precise determination of arterial architecture and lesion pathology. In most cases, the IVUS examination following balloon dilation plays a significant role in determining the need for stenting and then in assessing adequate deployment (Figure 10–4). IVUS has also become a standard tool in the endoluminal graft program for exclusion of abdominal aortic aneurysms. Exact measurements can be acquired to facilitate selection of the proper device size and assess placement after it has been deployed.

Our extensive experience in intraprocedural imaging does not indicate that IVUS and angioscopy should be used routinely for intraluminal therapy. IVUS is well suited for use in lesions above the inguinal ligament, and angioscopy is the imaging procedure of choice in small-caliber vessels. The indications for the use of these assessment modalities depends on the nature of the procedure being performed. In the most modern suites, their images appear on several video monitors, which should be positioned so all members of the endovascular team have an unobstructed view.

For our endovascular procedures, we interrogate anastomotic sites and inflow lesions using 6.2F intravascular ultrasound catheters [12.5 MHz (Medi-tech, Watertown, MA) or 20 MHz (Sonicath; Mansfield/Boston Scientific, Watertown, MA)] for two-dimensional imaging with SONOS (Hewlett Packard, Andover, MA) or Cathscanner (Endosonics, Pleasanton, CA) imaging systems. Three-dimensional reconstruction is achieved with a real-time processing system (Quinton Imaging Division, Quinton Instruments, Santa Clara, CA) that is easily integrated with the existing ultrasound equipment (Figure 10–5).

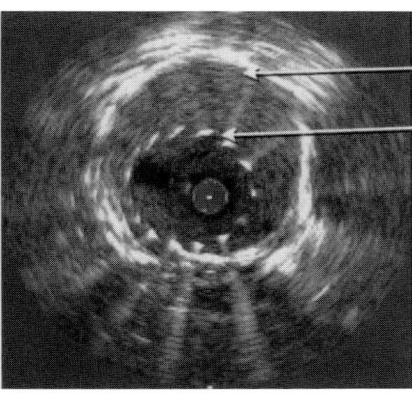

FIGURE 10–4. Intravascular ultrasonography (IVUS) image of a stent showing incomplete apposition, which that was not visible on the control angiogram. The condition was corrected by dilation with a larger balloon.

Tables

Nonmetallic, carbon fiber surgical tables are available for interventional techniques and optimize the utility of radiographic equipment. We use a table (ISS-1000 Plus, International Surgical Systems, as shown in Figure 10–2) that is supported at only one end and allows complete clearance underneath it for a panning x-ray system. This particular table incorporates a telescoping pedestal that allows vertical travel from 28 to 48 inches, 20-degree side-to-side roll, and 20-degree Trendelenburg tilt (standard and reverse). A number of other table types are available and possess specific characteristics,

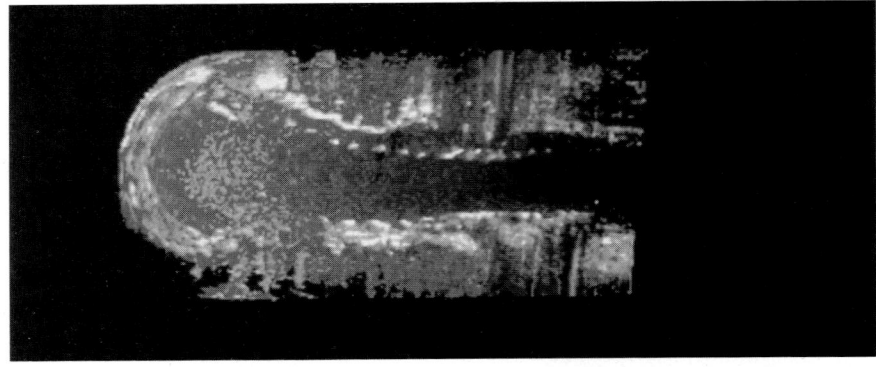

FIGURE 10-5. Three-dimensional IVUS reconstruction showing incomplete expansion of a Wallstent. The three-dimensional images provide superb assessment capabilities for endovascular techniques.

the most important of which is the unobstructed head-to-toe fluoroscopic imaging capability.

Monitoring Equipment

Accurate patient monitoring is imperative for ensuring the patient's safety during an endovascular procedure. Many patients have systemic arterial disease and coronary artery obstructions and require continuous electrocardiographic surveillance. Central venous monitoring should be provided for patients who are at high risk and undergoing complex procedures. Observation of urine output is also essential for patients in whom the intervention involves the renal arteries and the upper abdominal or thoracic aortic segments.

When pressure differentials play a role in assessing the performance of the procedure, intraarterial monitoring is useful. Precise measurement of pressure differentials can easily be accomplished with special 4F or 5F, 65-cm, wire-guided, radiopaque-tipped catheters (Medi-tech or Cook, Bloomington, IN) placed retrogradely across the lesion. The exact proximal origination point of the gradient is determined by pulling the catheter back through the lesion and noting on fluoroscopy the level at which the radial artery and catheter pressures begin to differ.

Equipment for Complementary Procedures

Thrombolysis

Technologic enhancements have greatly facilitated and optimized the delivery of lytic agents to peripheral obstructions. Most notable among them is a pulsed infusion system (Pulse Spray; AndioDynamics, Glen Falls, NY) that offers computer-controlled drug administration through a multihole catheter. This accelerated thrombolysis uses less drug to achieve results, so hospitalization is shorter and drug costs are reduced. The unit is portable; and although it is usually based in the endovascular suite, it is frequently moved into the intensive care unit for continual delivery of lytic agents. To establish thrombolysis, a guidewire is passed across the lesion, and the 5F (90 or 135 cm long) pulse spray catheter is positioned so the entire length of the occlusion is in contact with the delivery ports (the catheter comes with 10, 20, and 30 cm long infusion patterns). The injecting system can be programmed to any desired infusion cycle.

In our facility, we have found urokinase to offer therapeutic consistency with minimal side effects. Typically, 500,000 units of urokinase are delivered over a 30-minute period, but longer cycles may be preferable when treating an older thrombus. At the conclusion of the programmed infusion period, repeat angiography is performed to determine the need for a repeated cycle or longer, more classic infusions. The results with this method have been favorable, especially when the thrombus appears to be less than 30 days old. Even chronic occlusions with a significant thrombus load have been lysed sufficiently to allow further intraluminal therapy.

Lasers

The use of lasers in endovascular procedures has waned considerably since the late 1980s. The long-term results of laser therapy have not supported its use, and few institutions have laser facilities. Nonetheless, there are some endovascular specialists who continue to use "cool," lesion-specific lasers for recanalizing otherwise impassable obstructions. Today, with the newer wires and catheters, laser recanalization is seldom needed.

In general, local reimbursement practices and potential patient volume are used to assess the cost-effectiveness of acquiring a system for laser angioplasty. Because medical lasers of various types and configurations are in general use many operating rooms may already be modified to accommodate laser therapy. If this is not the case, the expense of upgrading the suite (e.g., protective eyewear, visible/audible warning lights/signs, controlled entryways, window coverings) and providing administrative support (e.g., laser safety officer) and technicians must be considered. Even with an established laser program at the hospital, cost-conscious administrators may be reluctant to purchase a new laser system to be used for only vascular applications. It is not yet known whether the use of lasers in stenting procedures might affect the rate of restenosis. If the adjunctive use of lasers with stenting does prove successful in limiting restenosis, the introduction of the technology will certainly affect endovascular suite design.

Atherectomy

Atherectomy devices have largely taken the place of lasers as an alternative mode of revascularization. When used as sole therapy or as an adjunct to another therapeutic intervention, most atherectomy devices are valuable in reducing plaque burden. The Simpson device (Atherocath; Devices for Vascular Intervention, Redwood City, CA) is a mechanical cutter that may be used to biopsy recurrent lesions to determine their histopathologic etiology. The device does not, however, extract sufficient quantities of the obstructing materials to reduce the total vessel plaque. The other two atherectomy devices currently available are rotational cutters that require a table-top drive unit to rotate the cutting head on the catheter. The transluminal endarterectomy catheter (TEC; Interventional Technologies, San Diego, CA) can provide satisfactory debulking of soft plaque stenoses and thrombotic material, but the excisions are not consistent and it does not perform well with calcified tissue. For hard plaque, rotational atherectomy with the Rotablator (Heart Technology, Bellevue, WA) works far better but can produce hemoglobinuria and distal embolization. Both of these devices require a lumen for wire guidance and adjunctive dilation in most cases. Atherectomy systems are either "single tool" devices or completely portable units; therefore other than for external connections and appropriate space, no special provisions are required for their use in endovascular suites. Because the long-term follow-up of atherectomy techniques on peripheral artery disease has not shown significant positive results, it is not likely that this modality will play an important role in the future unless more effective treatments become available.

Disposable Equipment

The rapid advances in angioplasty techniques since the 1970s has placed substantial demands on equipment manufacturers to supply sheaths, catheters, wires, and balloons in a greater variety of dimensions and to incorporate design features that address specific pathologies. There are a number of devices available for use in endovascular procedures.

Sheaths

Sheaths come in a number of lengths and diameters with assorted sideports for infusion. The "profile" of the equipment continues to be reduced, and it is now possible to perform most standard angioplasty procedures through 6F and 7F sheaths. Some sheaths (e.g., Super Flex Introducer; Arrow International, Reading, PA) are particularly useful in obese patients and those with heavy scarring from previous interventions. For stent techniques using the brachial approach (aortic arch vessels and aorta), a 7F sheath is generally used. For antegrade infrarenal aortic deployment, long sheaths (7.5F and 8F, 70cm; Daige Corporation, Minnetonka, MN) protect the stent as it is being delivered to the designated location.

Guidewires

Hydrophilic-coated guidewires (Glidewire; Boston Scientific, Watertown, MA, USA) have greatly increased the ease and safety of lesion traversal, and high-resolution fluoroscopic equipment ensures more accurate positioning of all wires. Steerable guidewires add another measure of control and cost, but in our experience the nitinol alloy core of the Glidewire resists bending and kinking, making it functionally identical to the steerable wires in all but the most circuitous vessels. "Activated" guidewires may bring us a step closer to the "wire through every lesion" ideal envisioned by many interventionists.

Catheters

Guiding catheters are not commonly used for lower limb interventions because tortuous pathways are seldom encountered. Instead, less expensive angiographic catheters are usually sufficient for lesion traversal. The new Glidecatheter (Boston Scientific), which incorporates some of the "slippery" characteristics of the Glidewire, has proven useful in many cases, and a 5F, 65-cm custom angiographic catheter with a radiopaque tip marker makes quantifying the location of pressure differentials relatively easy.

Balloons

Advances in balloon technology have been considerable, and manufacturers have succeeded in lowering the profile of their products and improving performance capabilities with new materials. Indeed, a number of designs have successfully overcome the traumatic aspects of the traditional overflagged balloon design. For peripheral interventions, catheter lengths from 65 to 150cm are commonly inventoried for a variety of balloon dimensions. Balloons of all diameters and shaft lengths are now being made by a number of manufacturers.

Stents

Stents represent an important technologic advance in endovascular surgery. These devices were introduced to treat abnormal dilation characteristics (e.g., resistance, recoil and dilation failure, persistent filling defects, dissection, intimal flaps) and have been used successfully in some anatomic regions such as the iliac artery and the abdominal aorta. Stenting has also been used to treat lesions in the brachiocephalic arteries arising from the aortic arch and more recently in the extracranial carotid arteries.

There are several stent models now being used in the peripheral vessels, from the carotids to the popliteals; and there are many more under study. All have certain advantages and varying degrees of radiopacity that make high resolution fluoroscopy mandatory.

The Palmaz balloon-expandable stent (Johnson & Johnson Interventional Systems, Warren, NJ) is a stainless steel tube designed with multiple rows of staggered rectangular slots that assume a diamond shape when expanded. Only 10% of the metal is in contact with the luminal surface. The Palmaz design is available in varying lengths from 10 to 39mm, with expansion ranges of 4 to 18mm; newer models labeled "medium" and "long" permit expansion to even longer lengths. The stent's longitudinal rigidity and large diameter make it ideally suited for straight

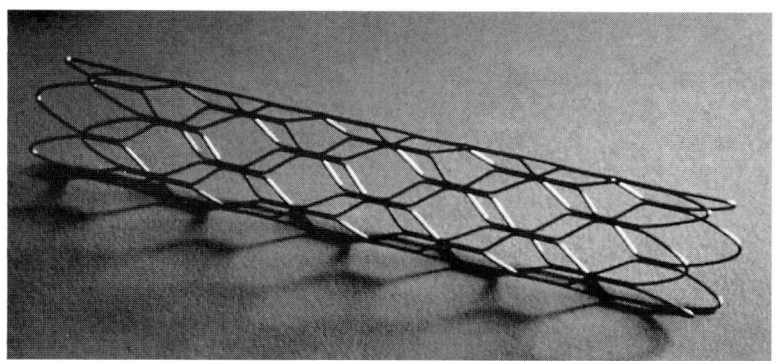

FIGURE 10–6. Symphony stent, a nitinol stent from Boston Scientific/Meadox. The flexibility of the stent makes it ideal for arterial use but it is not yet approved by the US Food and Drug Administration for arterial locations. (Courtesy of Medi-tech/Boston Scientific Corporation, Natic, MA.) (See color plate).

vessels, such as the distal aorta, and in the mesenteric, renal, and iliac arteries.

The Wallstent (Schneider, Minneapolis, MN) is a cylindrical device constructed by braiding multiple stainless steel monofilaments. Because of its spring-like structure, the Wallstent is flexible, compliant, and self-expanding, making it useful for delivery through curved arteries, for implantations overlying the graft–artery junction in end-to-side anastomoses, and for vessels subject to flexion from adjacent joints or structures, such as in the common femoral and popliteal arteries. The Wallstent comes in a variety of lengths ranging from 50 to 150 mm and in diameters from 5 to 10 mm. The Palmaz stent and Wallstent are the only two stents currently approved for arterial implantation, and the approved location is the iliac artery. Larger sizes have been approved for nonarterial applications but are available for "off label" uses.

A new generation of flexible stents has been introduced, and these devices are useful at sites of articulation where flexion and extension of the artery is common. The Symphony stent (Figure 10–6, see color plate) (Boston Scientific) and others may provide answers to the challenges presented by small external iliac arteries with diffuse calcific disease that extends to the inguinal ligament or beyond. This particular stent permits transaortic deployment, a highly useful technique in settings of diffuse disease. It has not yet been approved by the US Food and Drug Administration for arterial use.

Endoluminal Grafts

The endoluminal graft is a percutaneous interventional device that lines the diseased arterial wall with biomaterials such as Dacron or polytetrafluoroethylene, excluding contact with blood and protecting the lumen from cellular overgrowth that causes constriction and restenosis. Placement of the device effectively eliminates the conventional anastomotic junction (a site of inherent flow disturbances) and may reduce the incidence of graft thrombosis. Endoluminal grafting procedures frequently require brachiofemoral wire and catheter placement—maneuvers that can be the ultimate test of how well imaging equipment functions. In the future, endoluminal graft technology will become the most important component of an endovascular program. Aneurysm exclusion using the endoluminal graft has already shown dramatic results in both the abdominal and thoracic regions. One can only anticipate that as newer generations of devices become available a continual escalation of these procedures will lead to their use in every region of the vascular system (Figure 10–7, see color plate).

Conclusion

Optimal design of the endovascular surgical suite must take a variety of factors into consideration. Equipment choice frequently dictates the basic parameters, although adequate lead shielding and sufficient electrical supply

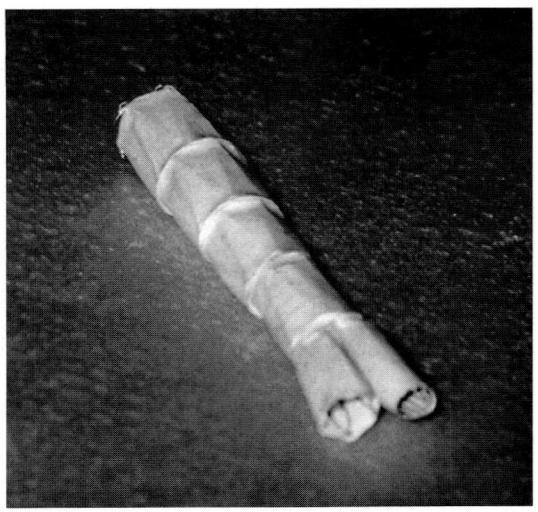

FIGURE 10–7. Prototype single-stage, bifurcated endoluminal graft (ELG). In the future, multiple ELG designs will become available, and the endovascular suite must be designed to accommodate this advancing technology. (See color plate).

are primary design considerations as well. The modern endovascular suite now incorporates a wide spectrum of imaging and monitoring equipment. It is possible to renovate existing facilities, but substantial modification is frquently required to achieve desirable results.

Changes in imaging and monitoring equipment and disposable devices have had a substantial impact on current endovascular procedures. Indeed, innovations in angiography and angioscopy and the introduction of IVUS have provided the interventionist with indispensable information about lesion morphology and appropriate device placement. Disposables such as sheaths, guidewires, and catheters have been improved significantly by reductions in profile and the use of new biomaterials. The introduction of stents has been an important breakthrough in the treatment of coronary and peripheral lesions, and the more recent use of endoluminal grafts offers yet another important percutaneous treatment alternative for the future. Successful use of any of these endovascular techniques and devices relies on the clinician's ability to access the lesion, choose the correct device for treatment, and select appropriate imaging and monitoring procedures to maximize device placement and ensure the patient's well-being. It is clear that a well-equipped and well-staffed endovascular surgery unit can facilitate providing the ultimate in patient care.

11
Image Production and Visualization Systems: Angiography, US, CT, and MRI

Suzanne M. Slonim and Lewis Wexler

The role of imaging in vascular disease and its treatment have expanded with the rapid advent of new technologies. Clinicians rely on imaging techniques for the identification of the location and morphologic features of disease. Imaging has become increasingly important in quantifying the degree of disease and following its progression. It is routinely used to monitor therapy and to evaluate results after medical, surgical, or percutaneous intervention.

Multiple vascular imaging modalities are currently available, each with specific advantages and disadvantages. These include angiography, ultrasound (US), computed tomography (CT), computed tomographic angiography (CTA), magnetic resonance imaging (MRI), and magnetic resonance angiography (MRA). Given these choices, it is important to remember that the ideal imaging modality would be very sensitive and specific, noninvasive, reproducible, and readily available. Additionally, it would carry low risk and be inexpensive. Although none of the available imaging techniques is ideal, evaluation of patients with vascular disease using the appropriate modalities provides indispensable information for planning therapeutic interventions.

Angiography

Techniques

Angiography involves imaging of the vascular system after the intravascular injection of contrast material. There are several angiographic techniques currently available.

Film-Screen Angiography

Conventional film-screen angiography remains the gold standard for the evaluation of peripheral vascular disease. After intravascular placement of an angiographic catheter, contrast material is rapidly injected and multiple x-ray images are recorded on film. Images can be reviewed after film development. The capability to simultaneously acquire images at orthogonal views (biplane imaging) can be very helpful. In addition, multiple oblique projections are often necessary to evaluate complex lesions. The most common type of rapid-sequence film changer in use today holds 30 films measuring 14 inches by 14 inches. A variable rate of filming can be programmed, with a maximum of four films per second. Contrast material is rapidly injected using a power injector that can be programmed for rate and volume of injection. To record the passage of contrast material through the vascular system from the aorta to the feet, filming can be performed at multiple levels with repeat injections or the bolus of contrast material can be followed by moving the patient over the film changer. This is achieved with a stepping table. An alternative is a "long-leg" film changer that covers the entire leg with 14-inch by 34-inch film. In this case the x-ray tube must be placed at a greater distance from the film, small vessel detail is reduced, and only six films are obtained. Film-screen studies require the use of full-strength contrast material (300 to 370 mg/ml iodine).

Digital Subtraction Angiography

Intraarterial digital subtraction angiography (IADSA or commonly DSA) is a technique in which the fluoroscopic image received by an image intensifier (II) is electronically converted into digital form and stored on a hard disk. A preliminary mask image without contrast material is obtained. The mask image is electronically subtracted from later contrast-enhanced images so that only the contrast-filled vessels are seen. The images are displayed on a screen with up to a 1024- by 1024-image matrix and are available for immediate review. DSA allows computer manipulation of the digital data for image improvement. Selected images can be laser-printed on film, and the entire study can be archived on computer disk for storage. The technique has high-contrast sensitivity, which allows the use of dilute contrast material (150 mg/ml iodine). Better contrast resolution also improves the ability to identify smaller vessels with smaller volumes of contrast material (Figure 11–1). Although multiple obliquities may still be necessary, the amount of contrast material needed is significantly reduced. Oblique filming is facilitated by mounting the x-ray tube and II on a gantry capable of complex rotation about the patient. DSA equipment is now available with stepping table or stepping gantry technology, in which the x-ray tube and II move relative to the patient, resulting in further decrease in contrast dose. The ability to immediately image without moving the equipment or patient and the ability to immediately review images greatly simplify complex interventional procedures. The primary disadvantage of DSA is its high sensitivity to motion artifact. Since the technique involves the subtraction of one image from another, any motion between the images will significantly degrade the image quality. Patient cooperation is necessary, and patient restraint (taping of the feet) is often useful. Computer manipulation of the images can usually compensate for small amounts of movement. Acquiring extra mask images before the injection of contrast material or after the contrast has passed through the area being imaged can also be helpful. Another disadvantage of DSA is that it has lower spatial resolution than direct film recording (3 line pairs per millimeter as opposed to 5 line pairs per millimeter); however, the technology is advancing. For example, modern digitized systems permit "road mapping," which uses an image obtained after contrast injection as the mask image during fluoroscopy, subtracting the real-time fluoroscopic image from the mask. This technique facilitates catheter and guidewire manipulation through the previously opacified vessel that would otherwise be devoid of contrast during the period of manipulation.

Because DSA records any change in contrast between the mask image and later images, it is possible to use an inert gas such as carbon dioxide as a contrast agent. This is particularly useful in patients with impaired renal function.

When comparing film-screen angiography and DSA for the evaluation of peripheral vascular disease in the lower extremities, the techniques were found to be equivalent for vessel visualization, identification of occlusions, and grading of stenoses.[1] Although there is no difference in diagnostic adequacy, some angiographers find the large film format subjectively better in vessel opacification, ease of reading, and overall superiority.[2] The field of view that is available with DSA depends on the size of the image intensifier. IIs of 14 inches give equivalent coverage to 14-inch film. Smaller IIs of 9 or 11 inches, which are commonly used in cardiac laboratories, provide inadequate fields to view both extremities simultaneously. Because of improving digital technology and the significant cost savings with DSA related to the decreased use of film and contrast, DSA will likely eventually replace film-screen techniques.

Other Techniques

Spot film radiography is a technique in which 100- or 105-mm film records from the II at up to 12 frames per second. The technique offers resolution similar to that of larger films but

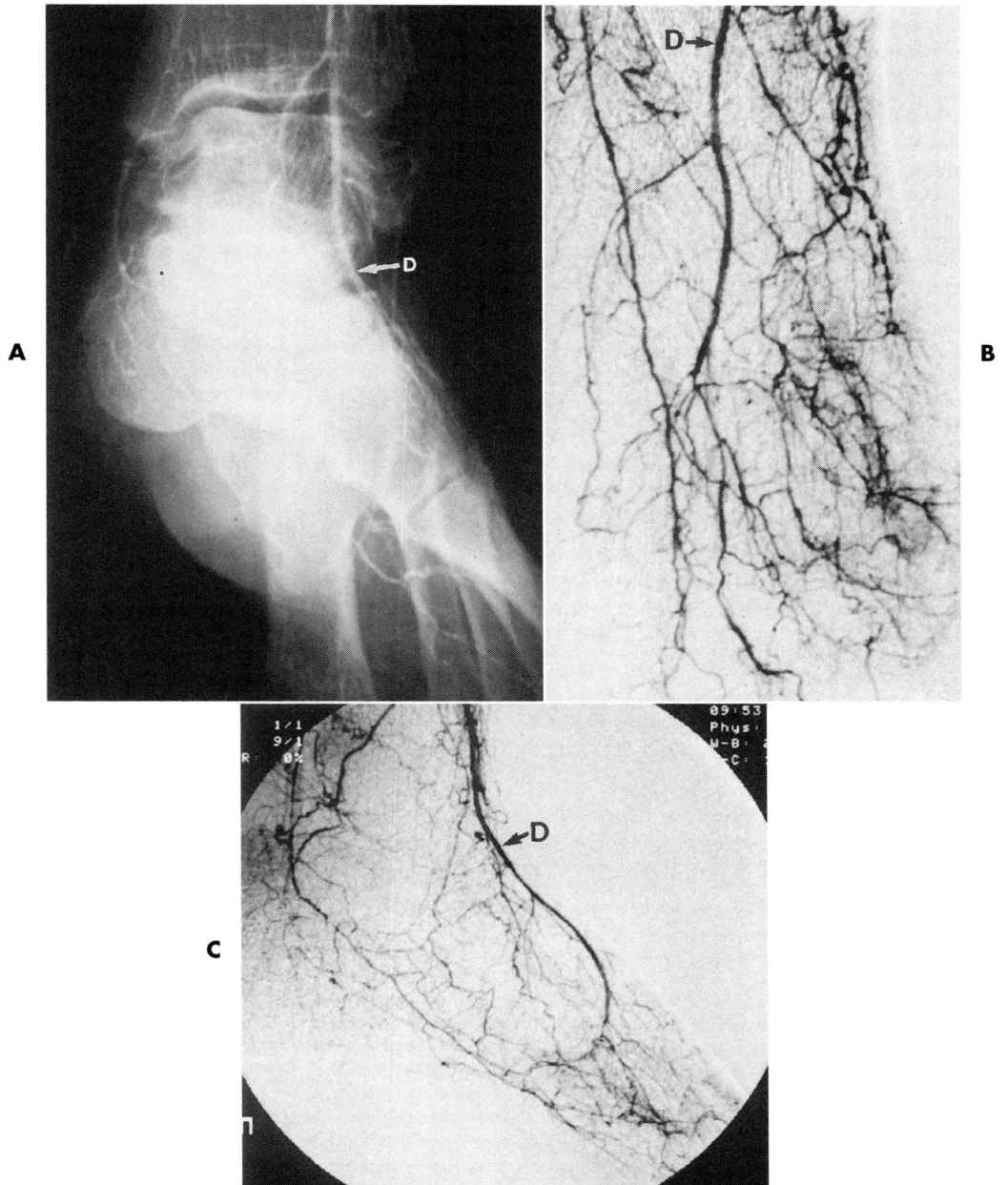

FIGURE 11–1. **A**, Film-screen angiography in this patient with a proximally occluded anterior tibial artery does not optimally demonstrate the distal extent of the reconstituted vessel. AP (**B**) and lateral (**C**) digital subtraction angiography of the same foot clearly demonstrates the arterial anatomy of the foot. *D*, dorsalis pedis artery.

requires an extremely high radiation dose and is less versatile than film-screen angiography or DSA.

Cineradiography records through the II at rates of 15 to 90 frames per second. This mode is commonly used for cardiac and coronary angiography and has a typical resolution of 2 to 3 line pairs per millimeter depending on the magnification used. Because of the limited field of view available with most cineradiography systems, it is necessary to "pan" or move the patient to follow the contrast bolus. Degradation of the image is common because of motion, and typically the cardiac catheterization table is limited in its travel so that the entire extremity cannot be visualized to the feet.

Video fluoroscopy entails coupling a video recorder to the fluoroscope and making a videotape recording of the fluoroscopic image. This technique provides insufficient resolution for accurate diagnosis and for planning of interventions.

Intravenous digital subtraction angiography (IVDSA) involves the injection of a large bolus of contrast material into the central venous circulation. After the contrast has passed through the pulmonary circulation and entered the systemic circulation, an arterial area of interest is imaged using the digital subtraction technique. Image quality is severely degraded by contrast dilution and bolus disruption during passage through the venous and pulmonary circulation. Motion artifact further degrades the images. For these reasons, IVDSA is not useful in arterial diagnosis and intervention. It is very useful, however, in venous interventions.

Iodinated Contrast Media

Vascular contrast agents are based on a triiodinated benzene ring. The degree of opacification on imaging studies is proportional to the concentration of iodine in the blood. There are four types of iodinated contrast material: ionic monomers, ionic dimers, nonionic monomers, and nonionic dimers.

An *ionic monomer* is a salt consisting of an anionic benzene ring with three iodine atoms linked to it. The side chains on the other benzene binding sites may be either diatrizoate or iothalamate. The cation of the salt may be either sodium or meglumine or a combination of both.

An *ionic dimer* is a salt consisting of an anion composed of two linked benzene rings with six bound iodine atoms. The choice of cations is the same. This structure produces twice the concentration of iodine atoms per particle in solution, or half the osmolality.

A *nonionic monomer* is a stable benzene ring with three iodine atoms bound to it. This produces the same concentration of iodine atoms with half the osmolality as can be achieved with ionic monomers.

Nonionic dimers are still being developed and investigated.[3] The structure consists of two stable linked benzene rings with six bound iodine atoms. This produces the same iodine concentration with one-fourth the osmolality as ionic monomers.

The osmolality of blood is approximately 300 (measured in mOsm/kg). The osmolality of an ionic monomer contrast medium is 1500 to 1700, that of an ionic dimer or nonionic monomer contrast medium is 580 to 880, and that of a nonionic dimer is approximately 320. The variability of osmolality is due to particle aggregation related to charge and other chemical properties of the contrast agent. The hyperosmolality of contrast media in comparison with blood contributes significantly to the adverse reactions they produce.

Systemic Adverse Reactions to Contrast Media

Systemic adverse reactions to contrast media have been categorized as minor, moderate, or severe.[4] Minor reactions require no treatment and include nausea, limited vomiting, itching, limited urticaria, and diaphoresis. Moderate reactions are non-life-threatening but require treatment, usually with antihistamines. They include fainting, severe vomiting, severe urticaria, facial or laryngeal edema, and mild bronchospasm. Severe reactions are life-threatening and include hypotensive shock, seizure, pulmonary edema, respiratory arrest, and cardiac arrest. In addition to antihistamines, epinephrine and cardiopulmonary support may be required to treat these severe reactions.

Systemic contrast reactions can be further categorized into chemotoxic or anaphylactoid types. Chemotoxic reactions are due to specific physiochemical effects of the contrast agent related to its hyperosmolality, potential for calcium binding, or the composition of its cation side chains. These reactions are related to the dose and concentration of contrast administered. They are less common but often more serious than anaphylactoid types of reactions. They include intravascular, hemodynamic, neurologic, and renal effects. Intravascular changes are related to fluid shifts across capillary and red blood cell (RBC) membranes, resulting in increased blood volume and potential pulmonary edema. Tissue anoxia develops, likely related to hemodilution and to alterations in RBC pliability. There is a possible anticoagulant effect of ionic contrast and a thrombotic effect of nonionic contrast. The common perception of pain and heat during extremity arteriography is likely due to vasodilatation and anoxia. Generalized hemodynamic effects include peripheral vasodilatation, hypotension, and tachycardia. Cardiac effects such as prolongation of atrioventricular (AV) node conduction, asystole, ventricular fibrillation, and impaired cardiac function can be seen during coronary angiography. Neurologic consequences may be related to hyperosmolar damage to the endothelial blood-brain barrier and direct neurotoxicity. Contrast can produce nausea, temperature variations, pulmonary edema, and seizure related to its neurologic effects.

In contrast to chemotoxic reactions, anaphylactoid reactions are idiosyncratic and unpredictable. They are unrelated to dose or concentration of contrast. They may be related to cell-mediated or complement-mediated immune reactions; however, their cause is uncertain.

In a very large study (300,000 people) of adverse systemic contrast reactions the overall prevalence was 12.66% with ionic contrast and 3.13% with nonionic contrast.[5] The prevalence of severe reactions (e.g., dyspnea, sudden drop in blood pressure, cardiac arrest, loss of consciousness) was 0.22% with ionic contrast and 0.04% with nonionic contrast. The prevalence of very severe reactions (i.e., severe reactions requiring the intervention of an anesthesiologist and/or hospitalization) was 0.04% with ionic and 0.004% with nonionic contrast. The most frequent symptoms of contrast reactions were nausea, urticaria, itching, and heat sensation, all of which were less prevalent with nonionic contrast. Of all reactions, including severe reactions, 70% occurred during or within 5 minutes of injection of the contrast material. Death occurred in between 1:75,000[6] and 1:150,000[5] of contrast injections.

Several risk factors for systemic adverse reactions to contrast material have been identified.[4,5] Unstable or debilitated patients are at increased risk. Patients with allergic tendencies have 2 times the relative risk of a reaction in comparison with those without allergic tendencies. Patients with asthma have 1.5 to 2.5 times the relative risk for all reactions and 5 (nonionic) to 8 (ionic) times the relative risk for severe reactions. Patients with a history of a previous adverse reaction to contrast have 5 times the relative risk for reactions. Contrast reactions are more common in patients with cardiac disease (prevalence of adverse reactions is 0.53% with ionic and 0.10% with nonionic contrast) than in patients with other diseases, including diabetes, renal, or respiratory disease. Intravenous injection carries a greater risk of producing a reaction than intraarterial injection, although the latter produces more severe reactions. Nonionic contrast decreases the overall relative risk by 5 times.

There is interest in prophylaxis regimens to prevent contrast reactions in patients at increased risk. Premedication with corticosteroids (one dose given the night preceding and one dose the morning of a contrast procedure) can reduce the incidence of all reactions occurring with ionic contrast.[7] Premedication with steroids, antihistamines, and/or sedatives only decreased the frequency of severe reactions in patients receiving ionic contrast. No benefit was seen in patients receiving nonionic contrast.[8] However, in another large study, premedication with two doses of oral corticosteroids produced a significant decrease in reactions to nonionic contrast.[9]

Renal Toxicity

Contrast-induced nephropathy can be defined as a rise in serum creatinine (Cr) of 0.5 mg/dl within 48 hours of exposure to contrast material. The pathophysiology may be related to hemodynamic alterations in renal blood flow in relation to hyperosmolality and renal artery spasm. In addition, there may be direct toxicity of contrast on renal tubular cells. Contrast-induced nephropathy usually resolves within 1 to 2 weeks; however, occasionally chronic dialysis is required. Risk factors for contrast-induced nephropathy include chronic renal insufficiency (Cr > 1.5), diabetes, and congestive heart failure.[10] Additional factors generally believed to increase the risk of renal compromise include dehydration, especially in patients with multiple myeloma or gout; large or repeated doses of contrast; and age over 60 years. Low osmolar contrast material significantly decreases nephrotoxicity in patients with prior renal impairment. This decrease in renal toxicity is seen only with intraarterial (rather than intravenous) contrast administration. There is no significant benefit from nonionic contrast with regards to nephrotoxicity in patients who have normal renal function.[11,12] In patients with chronic renal insufficiency, hydration with 0.45% saline provides better protection against contrast-induced nephrotoxicity than 0.45% saline with mannitol or 0.45% saline with furosemide.[13]

Box 11–1 shows specific indications for the use of low osmolar contrast that have been established by the American College of Radiology. In addition to these settings, it may be prudent to use low osmolar contrast in patients with renal insufficiency and in pediatric patients.

Given the remarkably increased cost of nonionic contrast and the relative safety of the ionic contrast material in most settings, economic restrictions will likely lead to self-imposed rationing of nonionic contrast.

Carbon Dioxide Contrast

Intraarterial injection of carbon dioxide with DSA and advanced imaging techniques includ-

---

Box 11–1. Indications for Low Osmolar Contrast Use

1. Patients with a history of a previous adverse reaction to contrast, with the exception of a sensation of heat, flushing, or a single episode of nausea or vomiting
2. Patients with a history of asthma or allergy
3. Patients with known cardiac dysfunction, including recent or potentially imminent cardiac decompensation, severe arrhythmias, unstable angina pectoris, recent myocardial infarction, and pulmonary hypertension
4. Patients with generalized severe debilitation
5. Any other circumstances where, after due consideration, the radiologist believes there is a specific indication for the use of low osmolar contrast. Examples of this include but are not restricted to:
    a. Sickle cell disease
    b. Patients at risk of aspiration
    c. Patients who are manifestly very anxious about the contrast procedure
    d. Patients in whom communication cannot be established in order to determine the presence or absence of risk factors
    e. Patients who request or demand the use of low osmolar contrast.

From Committee on Drugs and Contrast Media: Current criteria for the use of water soluble contrast agents for intravenous injections. In *Manual on iodinated contrast media*, Reston, VA, 1991, American College of Radiology.

ing image stacking or "maximum opacification" can produce diagnostic images of similar quality to iodinated contrast.[14] The use of carbon dioxide allows the avoidance of the potential systemic and renal toxicity of iodinated contrast material. It requires a dedicated injection technique and special positioning of the patient to fill dependent vessels. The aortic arch and great vessels cannot be studied with this technique because of the adverse effects of carbon dioxide on certain brain centers, including the center for respiratory drive. Because carbon dioxide angiography can produce ischemia related to a vapor lock phenomenon, it is important to allow time between injections for absorption of the boluses if repeated injections are performed. This technique is particularly useful for identification of arteriovenous shunts, collateral circulation, malignant tumors, and minute amounts of arterial bleeding. It has been successfully applied to renal, visceral, and extremity arteriography (Figure 11–2).

Ultrasonography

There are several features of ultrasound imaging that make it a nearly ideal screening modality. Ultrasound can provide anatomic and hemodynamic information about vessels. It can demonstrate the presence of flow, as well as its velocity and direction. Valuable information about the vessel wall can be gained. Noninvasive ultrasound is readily available. The rapidly advancing technology is likely to produce superior imaging and physiologic data in the future. The performance of a thorough vascular ultrasound examination, however, requires a well-trained dedicated vascular ultrasound technologist because the results are extremely operator-dependent. To some degree, the results are also dependent on the body habitus of the patient, with obese patients being much more challenging to image. Variability in diagnostic criteria, reporting techniques, and technical skill among institutions can make comparison of results from different vascular laboratories difficult. Despite these problems, this modality has the broadest range of vascular applications, particularly in carotid and lower extremity disease and graft surveillance.

Current vascular ultrasound imaging requires a scanner that can combine a gray scale ultrasound image, Doppler spectral waveform analysis, and color Doppler imaging. The combination of gray scale imaging with Doppler spectral waveform analysis is called a duplex scan. The gray scale image allows appropriate selection of a sample volume to be evaluated with Doppler. In addition, most current vascular studies include color Doppler imaging, which is a combination of a gray scale image with dynamic color flow information. This technique allows for simultaneous evaluation of flow throughout a long segment of the vessel

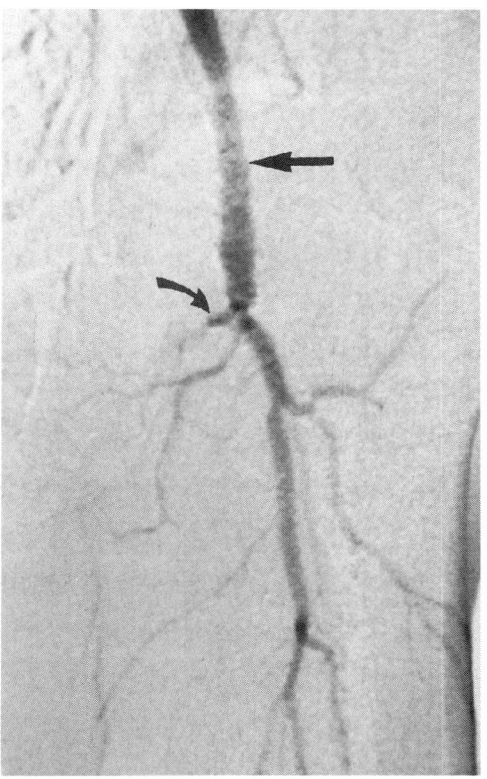

FIGURE 11–2. Carbon dioxide digital subtraction angiography demonstrates a patent left profunda femoral artery and occlusion of the left superficial femoral artery. The *straight arrow* indicates the common femoral artery. The *curved arrow* indicates the occluded origin of the superficial femoral artery.

being imaged. The color and hue overlay on the gray scale image depend on the velocity and direction of flow. Increased velocity produces increased color saturation. Color imaging significantly reduces the amount of time required to perform a study by allowing easier identification of vessels.

High-quality ultrasound imaging requires selection of the appropriate Doppler angle, wall filter, color scale, and Doppler gain by the technologist. In addition, use of the optimal ultrasound transducer is very important. The choice of transducer depends primarily on the depth of the vessel and on the available acoustic window. A high-resolution, high-frequency transducer (5.0, 7.5, 10.0 MHz) is optimal for imaging superficial vessels, 1 to 3 cm deep. Most carotid and extremity studies can be performed using one of these. A low-frequency transducer (2.0 to 3.5 MHz) provides the 10- to 15-cm depth penetration necessary to image vessels in the abdomen and pelvis; however, the resolution is not as good. In addition to frequency, transducers may be categorized as either linear array or sector scanners. A linear array transducer produces a rectangular image with a larger field of view. It produces an image of a longer segment of vessel; however, a larger area of skin surface must be available to use it. A sector scanner only requires a small area of skin surface, but it produces a smaller field of view. This becomes important when trying to image in an area of surgical bandages or open wounds. A sector scanner produces a pie- or wedge-shaped image.

Images from a vascular ultrasound study usually include several standard features. There is a gray scale image of the vessel of interest. A line across the image demonstrates the angle being used for Doppler analysis. A point or box within the vessel demonstrates which portion of the vessel is being sampled for Doppler analysis. A Doppler spectral waveform display at the sampled volume is usually present at the bottom or side of the ultrasound image. The Doppler spectral waveform demonstrates a plot of flow velocity against time. Images may also include color within the vessels, usually with arteries depicted in red and veins in blue, but this is variable.

Interpretation of the vascular ultrasound study incorporates information from the gray scale image, the color image, and the Doppler spectral waveform. For example, intraluminal echoes on the gray scale image indicate plaque, with calcification producing acoustic shadowing. The shadowing may obscure the lumen of the vessel. Color imaging can provide important information about flow turbulence in an area of stenosis. The Doppler study, however, contributes the most significant portion of the examination. Each vessel has a characteristic spectral Doppler pattern. Vessels may show high- or low-resistance waveforms, depending on the organs they supply and on the physiologic state at the time of examination. Vascular disease alters the characteristic spectral waveform. An area of stenosis creates turbulence in the flow. Turbulence is depicted as a broadening of the velocities seen on Doppler examination. Whereas the normal vessel produces a crisp line on Doppler analysis (all blood flowing at the same velocity), turbulence produces a fuzzy or widened line. This is referred to as spectral broadening. As a stenosis produces more turbulence, more velocities are represented in the waveform until the area under the Doppler waveform curve is filled in. This is referred to as loss of the spectral window. Significant stenosis produces acceleration of blood flow, similar to the effect of a finger on a garden hose. First, velocity during systole is increased; however, with more severe stenosis, velocity during diastole also increases. The highest velocity measured at a point of stenosis is used to grade the stenosis. A severe stenosis may cause decreased flow velocity distally in the vessel. Therefore the features of an area of stenosis include plaque on gray scale, turbulence on color flow, spectral broadening, loss of the spectral window, and increased peak systolic velocity and end-diastolic velocity.

Applications

Vascular ultrasound has a broad scope of vascular applications, including evaluation of carotid disease, extremity peripheral vascular disease, disease of the aorta and its major abdominal branches, graft evaluation, and evaluation for deep venous thrombosis.

The indication for carotid duplex scanning is any symptom that indicates an increased risk for a neurologic vascular event. Widely accepted indications include asymptomatic carotid bruit, transient ischemic attack, stroke with recovery, or preoperative screening for cardiac or peripheral vascular surgery.[15] Carotid endarterectomy has been found to significantly reduce neurologic symptoms in both asymptomatic[16,17] and symptomatic[18] patients with significant carotid stenosis in comparison with patients who did not have carotid endarterectomy. Duplex scanning is very effective in identifying significant stenosis of the extracranial carotid arteries.[19]

Evaluation of the abdominal aorta with vascular ultrasound can be limited by obesity and bowel gas. It can be very useful, however, in several settings. Ultrasound is an excellent method for following abdominal aortic aneurysms. It has the capability to demonstrate both the outer diameter and the luminal diameter, with good visualization of luminal thrombus. Size measurements are reliable and reproducible, although care must be taken to assure that transverse images are acquired in a plane perpendicular to the aorta at each level. Oblique transverse scans can overestimate the aneurysm diameter. Longitudinal imaging of the aorta is the plane of imaging that is least likely to overestimate the diameter.[20] Ultrasound is often unable to demonstrate the extent of the aneurysm into the chest or pelvis. Also, it is often unreliable in demonstrating involvement of renal or visceral vessels. Given these limitations, ultrasound is very good as a means of following aneurysm progression, but it is not adequate for surgical planning.

Although transesophageal ultrasound is very useful in evaluating thoracic aortic dissection, it is of limited value in abdominal aortic dissection. Aortic dissection can be confused with periaortic fibrosis on ultrasound. In some instances an intimal flap with to-and-fro motion can be identified.[21,22] Theoretically, Doppler waveform analysis could be useful in demonstrating differential flow in each lumen, but this technique is not often used in clinical practice.

Finally, ultrasound can be very useful in identifying fluid collections around aortic grafts, due either to bleeding or infection.

Vascular ultrasound can be very valuable in the evaluation of extremity peripheral vascular disease. A thorough examination may take up to 2 hours to complete; the use of color flow imaging significantly decreases this time. The study should begin at the aortic bifurcation, if this region can be visualized, with imaging of the common and external iliac arteries. The common femoral, superficial femoral, and profunda femoral arteries should be imaged, as well as the popliteal and tibial arteries. The popliteal artery in the adductor canal may be difficult to evaluate. Studies should include Doppler waveform analysis at regular intervals.

Several diagnostic criteria for significant stenosis in extremity arteries have been described.[23-25] The concepts for defining a significant lesion in the extremities are similar to those for the carotid arteries. An increase in peak systolic velocity of 100% indicates a 50% or greater stenosis. Color flow imaging increases the specificity of the examination.[8]

The ability to identify the site, length, and severity of a lesion and the status of the inflow and runoff vessels makes this modality particularly useful for planning the arteriographic approach to a lesion. It is also very helpful in planning a percutaneous or surgical intervention.[26] After an intervention, ultrasound imaging is a good means of evaluating results; however, immediate postangioplasty studies may overestimate residual stenosis.[27]

Graft surveillance with vascular ultrasound and Doppler waveform analysis significantly increases long-term graph patency because it identifies stenosis that requires surgical or percutaneous revision before thrombosis occurs.[28,29] Although color flow imaging shortens the average time per examination by approximately 50%, it does not significantly affect its accuracy.[30] The entire length of a graft must be examined, as well as the inflow and runoff vessels. Stenosis criteria are based on peak systolic and end-diastolic velocities.[31,32] Vascular ultrasound is also very useful in identifying nonlysed valve cusps, arteriovenous fistulas, and anastomotic pseudoaneurysms associated with extremity grafts.

Evaluation of the renal arteries can be technically very difficult and is extremely operator-dependent. Examinations can be degraded by obese body habitus, respiratory motion, and bowel gas. An examination can take 2 hours to perform. Criteria for significant stenosis are based on the ratio of the peak systolic velocity in the renal artery to that in the aorta[33] and on peak systolic velocity in the renal artery.[34] Vascular ultrasound can be very helpful in identifying renal artery aneurysm, but accessory renal arteries and stenotic lesions in branch vessels cannot be adequately evaluated. For these reasons, but primarily because of the extreme technical difficulty of the examination, vascular ultrasound is not considered a reliable screening test for renal artery stenosis.

The celiac axis and the superior mesenteric artery are routinely visualized on abdominal ultrasound studies. Because stenotic lesions in these vessels are often ostial, they may be detectable with duplex. The Doppler waveforms in the mesenteric vessels are dependent on the timing of the examination with respect to meals. In the postprandial state, there is a low-resistance waveform, which is high-resistance in the fasting state. The short trunk of the celiac axis and the many proximal branches alter the flow phenomena and waveform. The distal vessels are not well visualized, and the inferior mesenteric artery is usually too small to see or is obscured by bowel gas. In the evaluation of mesenteric ischemia the finding of an ostial stenosis in duplex imaging is of uncertain significance because there is usually such a rich collateral network that multiple stenoses must be present to produce ischemia. Vascular ultrasound can be very helpful, however, in identifying aneurysms of the celiac axis, superior mesenteric artery, and the splenic, hepatic, and gastroduodenal arteries. It may also be useful in postintervention follow-up in the mesenteric vessels.

A vascular ultrasound examination for deep venous thrombosis in the lower extremities should begin as far proximally as can be imaged. The examination should include Doppler examination and longitudinal and axial imaging of the entire deep venous system, as well as the greater saphenous vein. The superficial veins can also be imaged. Tests for compressibility of the vein, augmentation (increased flow with squeezing of the distal extremity), and normal respiratory variation in flow should be carried out at all levels. Color flow imaging decreases the time necessary to perform the examination. Evaluation of the calf veins is usually technically difficult and has questionable clinical significance.[35] Diagnostic criteria for deep venous thrombosis[36,37] include intraluminal echogenicity, venous distention, absence of normal compressibility, flow void in color imaging, lack of flow variations with respiratory cycle, and lack of augmentation. Response of thrombus to therapy can be easily and noninvasively followed. Vascular ultrasound is also very useful in the evaluation of venous valvular incompetence and vein mapping for graft harvest.

Vascular ultrasound can be very helpful in the evaluation of problems with dialysis fistulas. It can demonstrate and help characterize arterial or venous stenosis, arterial steal, aneurysm, pseudoaneurysm, thrombosis, and perigraft fluid collections.[38] Transplant arterial and venous anastomoses, including renal, hepatic, and pancreatic transplants, can be evaluated for occlusion, pseudoaneurysm, or arteriovenous fistula.[39] In the evaluation for portal hypertension, patency and direction of flow in the portal vein, patency of the hepatic veins, and the presence of varices can be demonstrated. Patency of surgical or percutaneous vascular shunts can be readily noninvasively followed.

Intravascular ultrasound, which can be very helpful in monitoring complex vascular interventions, particularly treatment of aortic dissection complications, is discussed in Chapter 14.

Computed Tomography

Current CT equipment allows rapid scanning and image reconstruction. These features provide images with minimal respiratory or motion artifact. The ability to acquire and reconstruct images with thin section collimation allows reliable delineation of branch vessel origins. CT routinely provides axial images; however, modern scanners with spiral or helical capabilities can produce three-dimensional reconstructions of vascular structures, a process termed CT angiography (CTA). Axial imaging and CTA are discussed separately.

Axial Imaging Applications

Computed tomography is very useful in the diagnosis of diseases of the aorta. With current technology the major branch vessels of the aorta can be routinely identified, including the great vessels, the celiac axis, the superior mesenteric artery, and the renal arteries. CT allows identification of congenital anomalies of the inferior vena cava and kidneys, which may alter the surgical approach. In addition, any other intraabdominal pathology can be detected and evaluated.

It is particularly helpful in the diagnosis of aortic dissection and in planning potential therapeutic measures. CT is as accurate as angiography in diagnosing dissection.[40] Findings include identification of two contrast-filled lumens separated by an intimal flap and displacement of mural calcification into the lumen. The intraluminal calcification may be seen even in the setting of thrombosis of the false lumen. Pleural or pericardial effusion or the presence of mediastinal fluid suggest rupture of the aorta. It is usually possible to distinguish a type A from a type B dissection on the basis of CT. The degree of compromise of the true lumen by an expanded false lumen can be assessed. It may be possible to identify which lumen supplies which branch vessels for planning of interventions (Figure 11–3). There are a few pitfalls in the use of CT to evaluate aortic dissection. CT may miss a dissection if a poor IV contrast bolus is administered or if the area of interest is not imaged before the bolus dissipates. Streak artifact across the aorta may produce the appearance of a flap when none is present. A dissection with thrombosis of the false lumen can be misinterpreted as an aneurysm with mural thrombus. Except in these unusual settings, CT is extremely helpful in the diagnosis and evaluation of aortic dissection.

Computed tomography is also useful in the evaluation of ascending and descending thoracic and abdominal aortic aneurysms. Findings include enlargement of the lumen to greater than 1.5 times normal, loss of the normal decrease in caliber from proximal to distal aorta, and abdominal aortic diameter of greater than 3.0 cm. Historically, the neck of an aneurysm often could not confidently be identified on CT in relation to branch vessels.[41] However, helical scanning with thin or variable collimation can allow depiction of the relationship of the aneurysm neck to mesenteric and renal arteries.[42] CT allows demonstration of mural thrombus and residual lumen size. More importantly, CT allows the identification of aneurysm rupture. Major hemorrhage produces

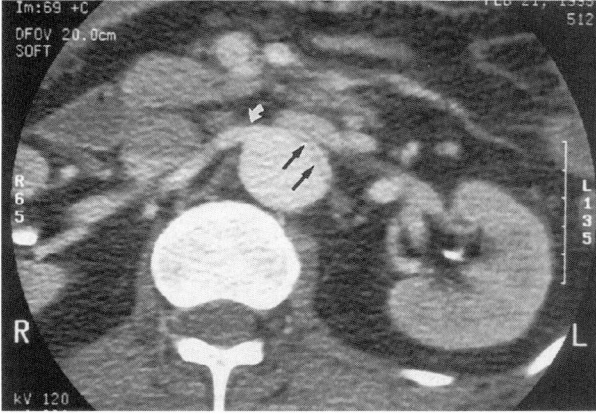

FIGURE 11–3. CT image at the level of the right renal artery in this patient with a complicated aortic dissection demonstrates the origin of the right renal artery from the larger false lumen (*curved arrow*). The *straight arrows* indicate the dissection flap compressing the true lumen anterolaterally.

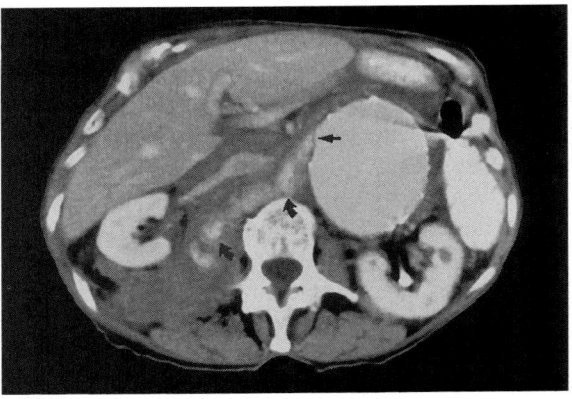

FIGURE 11-4. CT image demonstrates a massively dilated calcified aorta with extravasation of contrast material through a rupture in the right lateral wall (*straight arrow*). Contrast and blood collect along the right lateral margin of the aneurysmal aorta and in the right posterior perirenal space (*curved arrows*).

large retroperitoneal and periaortic fluid collections with discontinuity of the aortic wall (Figure 11-4). More subtle signs associated with rupture include a crescent of high attenuation within the thrombus and a focal break in a continuous calcification within the aneurysm wall.[43] Contained or chronic rupture with pseudoaneurysm or inflammatory or mycotic aneurysms can be identified. Potential problems with CT evaluation of aortic aneurysm include sometimes inadequate depiction of extension into the iliac arteries,[42] inadequate demonstration of accessory renal arteries, and inadequate evaluation of the aortic valve and coronary artery involvement in ascending aortic aneurysms. CT is helpful in the postoperative evaluation of aortic grafts. A perigraft fluid collection or infection, an anastomotic pseudoaneurysm, or aortoenteric fistula can be identified.

Computed tomography can be very helpful in the setting of suspected traumatic aortic rupture.[44] Findings can be divided into direct and indirect signs of rupture. Direct signs include a pseudoaneurysm, an intimal tear, and marginal luminal irregularity. Indirect signs include intramural, periaortic, and mediastinal hematoma. CT has a sensitivity of 100% and a specificity of 86% for traumatic aortic rupture.[45] The appropriate imaging algorithm in the setting of major trauma is variable and depends on the level of suspicion that a rupture is present. It is preferable to avoid the contrast load of performing both a CT scan and an aortogram. Certainly, unstable patients should proceed to surgery without imaging.

Visceral and renal arteries are routinely identified with current CT technology. Pathology in these vessels, including aneurysm, pseudoaneurysm, or extension of a dissection flap into the visceral or renal vessels, can be identified. Proximal occlusion can be recognized by lack of equal contrast enhancement between the vessel of interest and the aorta or an adjacent branch artery. Similar criteria can be used for diagnosis of mesenteric venous thrombosis or thrombosis of any other large venous structure. In addition, ischemic changes can be seen in the bowel or mesentery, and absence of a portion of a nephrogram is readily noted.

Currently, CT is of limited use in the evaluation of extremity peripheral vascular disease. Popliteal[46] and femoral diseases are accurately depicted with CT, but US is routinely used for these areas because of its easy availability, accuracy of diagnosis in these regions, and low cost. Extremity bypass grafts and carotid arteries are routinely imaged with US for similar reasons. CT can be useful for imaging of popliteal artery entrapment syndrome.[47]

Three-Dimensional CT Angiography Applications

Three-dimensional CT angiography (CTA) requires spiral imaging along the length of vessels of interest with narrow collimation, optimized contrast bolus administration, and optimized timing of imaging in relation to the contrast administration.[48] Image acquisition takes approximately 20 minutes, and image processing takes approximately 30 to 45 minutes. Images can be reconstructed using maximum intensity projection (MIP), producing two-dimensional images that can differentiate mural calcification from intraluminal contrast. Alternatively, a shaded surface display (SSD) rendering technique may be used, producing three-dimensional images depicting the surface of the contrast-enhanced structures. CTA then allows an infinite number of viewing angles of the three-dimensional reconstructed image.

In the abdominal aorta, CTA is useful in preoperative or preintervention planning. It allows thorough evaluation of the size and extent of an abdominal or thoracic aortic aneurysm, with reliable depiction of the neck and branch vessel involvement (Figure 11-5). Similarly, aortic dissection is well demonstrated, including flap extent and branch vessel involvement. CTA is helpful in determining which vessels are supplied by the true or false lumen, which is very important when planning intervention for ischemic sequela of dissection. It is also useful in the follow-up of grafts, stents, and stent grafts.

In the iliac arteries, CTA is useful in the evaluation of occlusive disease and identification of collateral vessels. Aneurysms, dissections, grafts, and stents are well demonstrated. CTA is sensitive (92%) and specific (83%) for the detection of hemodynamically significant renal artery stenosis with appropriate rendering techniques. It is also accurate for the detection of accessory renal arteries.[49,50] Stenoses involving mesenteric vessels and collateral vessels can be identified with CTA.[51] In the carotid arteries, CTA has good correlation with conventional angiography.[52,53] It is useful in the evaluation of the degree of stenosis, the presence of calcified plaque, the presence of ulceration, and vessel size.

Magnetic Resonance Imaging

Magnetic resonance imaging provides many benefits, including multiplanar imaging capability and the ability for three-dimensional reconstruction. Magnetic resonance angiography (MRA) is a technique of stacking the axial images of the vessels to produce angiogram-like images that can be rotated around an axis. Taking advantage of the physical properties of flowing blood in a magnetic field, the phenom-

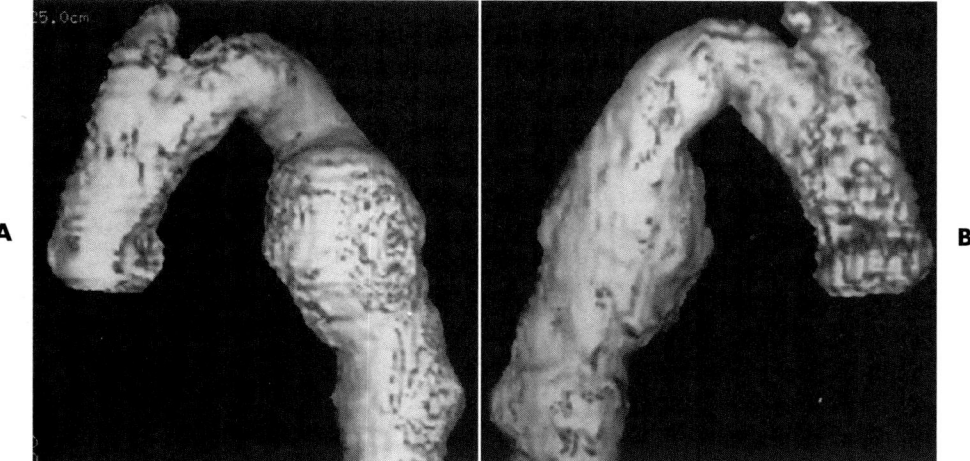

FIGURE 11-5. Left lateral (**A**) and right lateral (**B**) three-dimensional CTA with shaded surface display of a thoracic aortic aneurysm demonstrates an ample neck above the aneurysm.

ena of time-of-flight (TOF) or phase contrast imaging effects can be used to display flow. There is no need for the administration of iodinated contrast. MRI can provide information on the magnitude and direction of blood flow, and there is the potential for more detailed physiologic information in the future. One possibility includes information on oxygen saturation in the superior mesenteric vein.[54] With the continual advancement in MRI technology and postimaging software, further vascular capabilities will no doubt be on the horizon. MRI, however, does have its drawbacks. It is not always readily available. The advanced vascular applications and MRA may not be available on a particular magnet. Some patients are too claustrophobic to undergo the examination. Patients with pacemakers or recently implanted metallic devices cannot be imaged. Monitoring and resuscitation equipment cannot be taken into the room with the magnet. Finally, cardiac and respiratory motion can significantly degrade the images.

With MRI, image quality improves with increasing magnet strength to 1.5 tesla (T). Magnet strengths of 1.0 or 0.5 T can produce acceptable-quality MRA. Dedicated surface coils are required for optimal imaging of specific body parts. Coil placement by the technologist can affect the image quality.

Applications

The use of MRI and MRA to evaluate the carotid arteries is convenient because the examination is often needed in patients who require MRI of the brain. In contrast to vascular ultrasound, MRI and MRA can also readily image the intracranial vessels. Axial images are best for differentiating an occlusion from a severe stenosis. MRA is better than MRI for the depiction of stenoses. There is very good correlation between MRA and angiography for the percent of carotid stenosis.[55] MRI and MRA are useful for the identification of collateral pathways, but they are not good for the depiction of plaque morphology. Another drawback of MRA is that the origins of the great vessels from the arch are often too deep to be well seen.

Imaging of the thoracic aorta is often degraded by cardiac and respiratory motion. This problem can be improved with cardiac and respiratory gating. Multiplanar imaging is especially useful in the evaluation of thoracic aortic aneurysm size, extent, and branch vessel involvement. The anatomy of a coarctation of the aorta is well demonstrated. MRI may be inappropriate for an unstable patient in the setting of an acute aortic dissection; however, it may be the method of choice for following patients with chronic dissection (Figure 11–6). MRI has been found to be better than transesophageal echocardiography (TEE) in identifying aortic dissection,[56] but the availability of TEE at the bedside or in the intensive care unit contribute to its wide use in unstable patients with suspected aortic dissection. Involvement of branch vessels by a dissection flap is well demonstrated. Cine display techniques allow evaluation of flow phenomena in the true and false lumen.

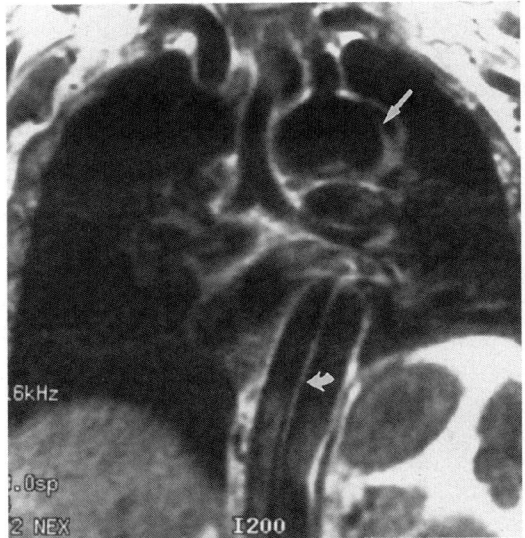

FIGURE 11–6. Coronal magnetic resonance image in the plane of the trachea and carina depicts an aortic dissection at two levels. In the arch the carotid artery arises from the true lumen with a small curvilinear dissection flap seen laterally (*straight arrow*). In the lower thoracic and upper abdominal aorta the flap is seen longitudinally (*curved arrow*).

In the abdominal aorta, MRI has the advantage over ultrasound of not being hindered by bowel gas or depth. It is very good for the evaluation of aortic aneurysm or dissection, as well as occlusive disease. MRI has good sensitivity (91%) for renal artery stenosis,[57] especially when axial and coronal planes of imaging are used. Lesions in the distal main renal artery and in the branch vessels cannot be detected, however.

In peripheral vascular disease of the extremities, MRI provides accurate identification of occlusions and the presence of adequate runoff vessels, but it is less accurate in the grading of stenoses.[58] MRA has been found to have greater sensitivity than angiography in detecting distal runoff vessels.[59] However, it currently is not widely used in evaluation of the extremities because of long imaging times required to examine the entire length of the affected vessel. Motion artifact often significantly degrades these images. MRI and MRA are very useful for the evaluation of bypass grafts and their complications, but they are less helpful for the evaluation of stents because the metallic artifact obscures the region of interest.

Magnetic resonance imaging is as sensitive and specific for deep venous thrombosis as venography,[60] but it is not widely used because US is reliable, readily available, and less costly. MRI may be useful for evaluation of deep venous thrombosis in the pelvic, subclavian, and brachiocephalic veins, which are not well seen by US.

Conclusion

There are many vascular imaging modalities that can provide invaluable information in patients with peripheral vascular disease. The choice of the appropriate imaging modality must be based on knowledge of the information each modality can provide, the risks involved, the cost, and the availability. Diagnosis of a vascular lesion, monitoring its progression, planning for its surgical or percutaneous management, and follow-up after treatment are all possible in a relatively noninvasive manner. It is incumbent on the surgeon or interventionist to have a complete understanding of the anatomic, hemodynamic, and functional circumstances of a given vascular problem before embarking on a course of therapy.

References

1. Smith TP et al: Comparison of the efficacy of digital subtraction and film-screen angiography of the lower limb: prospective study in 50 patients, *AJR Am J Roentgenol* 158:431, 1992.
2. Malden ES et al: Peripheral vascular disease: evaluation with stepping DSA and conventional screen-film angiography, *Radiology* 191:149, 1994.
3. Morris TW et al: Iotrol, iodixanol, and 2-deoxy-D-glucose effects on neural tissue CO_2 production, *AJNR Am J Neuroradiol* 10:1123, 1989.
4. Bush WH, Swanson DP: Acute reactions to intravascular contrast media: types, risk factors, recognition, and specific treatment, *AJR Am J Roentgenol* 157:1153, 1991.
5. Katayama H et al: Adverse reactions to ionic and nonionic contrast media. A report from the Japanese Committee on the Safety of Contrast Media, *Radiology* 175:621, 1990.
6. Hartman GW et al: Mortality during excretory urography: Mayo Clinic experience, *AJR Am J Roentgenol* 139:919, 1982.
7. Lasser EC et al: Pretreatment with corticosteroids to alleviate reactions to intravenous contrast material, *N Engl J Med* 317:845, 1987.
8. Cossman DV et al: Comparison of contrast arteriography to arterial mapping with colorflow duplex imaging in the lower extremities, *J Vasc Surg* 10:522, 1989.
9. Lasser EC et al: Pretreatment with corticosteroids to prevent adverse reactions to nonionic contrast media, *AJR Am J Roentgenol* 162:523, 1994.
10. Schwab SJ et al: Contrast nephrotoxicity: a randomized controlled trial of a nonionic and an ionic radiographic contrast agent, *N Engl J Med* 320:149, 1989.
11. Barrett BJ, Carlisle EJ: Metaanalysis of the relative nephrotoxicity of high- and low-osmolality iodinated contrast media, *Radiology* 188:171, 1993.

12. Rudnick MR et al: Nephrotoxicity of ionic and nonionic contrast media in 1196 patients: a randomized trial, *Kidney Int* 47:254, 1995.
13. Solomon R et al: Effects of saline, mannitol, and furosemide to prevent acute decreases in renal function induced by radiocontrast agents, *N Engl J Med* 331:1416, 1994.
14. Hawkins IF et al: CO_2 digital angiography: a safer contrast agent for renal vascular imaging?, *Am J Kidney Dis* 24:685, 1994.
15. Strandness DE et al: Vascular laboratory utilization and payment: report of the Ad Hoc Committee of the Western Vascular Society, *J Vasc Surg* 16:163, 1992
16. Moneta GL et al: Operative versus nonoperative management of asymptomatic high-grade internal carotid artery stenosis: improved results with endarterectomy, *Stroke* 18:1005, 1987.
17. Roederer GO et al: The natural history of carotid arterial disease in asymptomatic patients with cervical bruits, *Stroke* 15:605, 1984.
18. North American Symptomatic Carotid Endarterectomy Trial Collaborators: Beneficial effect of carotid endarterectomy in symptomatic patients with high-grade carotid stenosis, *N Engl J Med* 325:445, 1991.
19. Robinson ML et al: Diagnostic criteria for carotid duplex sonography, *AJR Am J Roentgenol* 151:1045, 1988.
20. Yucel EK et al: Interobserver reproducibility of measurements of the abdominal aorta, *Radiology* 177(suppl):253, 1990.
21. Conrad MR et al: Real time ultrasound in the diagnosis of acute dissecting aneurysm of the abdominal aorta, *AJR Am J Roentgenol* 132:115, 1979.
22. Kotval PS et al: Role of the intimal flap in arterial dissection: sonographic demonstration, *AJR Am J Roentgenol* 150:1181, 1988.
23. Jager KA et al: Noninvasive mapping of lower limb arterial lesions, *Ultrasound Med Biol* 11:515, 1985.
24. Kohler TR et al: Duplex scanning for diagnosis of aortoiliac and femoropopliteal disease: a prospective study, *Circulation* 76:1074, 1987.
25. Leng GC et al: Accuracy and reproducibility of duplex ultrasonography in grading femoropopliteal stenoses, *J Vasc Surg* 17:510, 1993.
26. Edwards JM et al: The role of duplex scanning in the selection of patients for transluminal angioplasty, *J Vasc Surg* 13:69, 1991.
27. Sacks D et al: Evaluation of the peripheral arteries with duplex US after angioplasty, *Radiology* 176:39, 1990.
28. Idu MM et al: Impact of a color-flow duplex surveillance program on infrainguinal vein graft patency: a five-year experience, *J Vasc Surg* 17:42, 1993.
29. Mattos MA et al: Does correction of stenoses identified with color duplex scanning improve infrainguinal graft patency?, *J Vasc Surg* 17:54, 1993.
30. Killewich LA, Fisher C, Bartlett ST: Surveillance of in situ infrainguinal bypass grafts: conventional vs. color flow duplex ultrasonography, *J Cardiovasc Surg* 31:662, 1990.
31. Buth J et al: Color-flow duplex criteria for grading stenosis in infrainguinal vein grafts, *J Vasc Surg* 14:716, 1991.
32. Green RM et al: Comparison of infrainguinal graft surveillance techniques, *J Vasc Surg* 11:207, 1990.
33. Kohler TR et al: Noninvasive diagnosis of renal artery stenosis by ultrasonic duplex scanning, *J Vasc Surg* 4:450, 1986.
34. Hoffmann U et al: Role of duplex scanning for the detection of atherosclerotic renal artery disease, *Kidney Int* 39:1232, 1991.
35. Kakkar VV et al: Natural history of postoperative deep-vein thrombosis, *Lancet* 2:230, 1969.
36. Cronan JJ et al: Deep venous thrombosis: US assessment using vein compression, *Radiology* 162:191, 1987.
37. Rose SC et al: Symptomatic lower extremity deep venous thrombosis: accuracy, limitations, and role of color duplex flow imaging in diagnosis, *Radiology* 175:639, 1990.
38. Finlay DE et al: Duplex and color Doppler sonography of hemodialysis arteriovenous fistulas and grafts, *Radiographics* 13:983, 1993.
39. Finlay DE, Letourneau JG, Longley DG: Assessment of vascular complications of renal, hepatic, and pancreatic transplantation, *Radiographics* 12:981, 1992.
40. Thorsen MK et al: Dissecting aortic aneurysms: accuracy of computed tomographic diagnosis, *Radiology* 148:773, 1983.
41. Papanicolaou N et al: Preoperative evaluation of abdominal aortic aneurysms by computed tomography, *AJR Am J Roentgenol* 146:711, 1986.
42. Zeman RK et al: Abdominal aortic aneurysms: evaluation with variable-collimation helical CT and overlapping reconstruction, *Radiology* 193:555, 1994.
43. Siegel CL et al: Abdominal aortic aneurysm morphology: CT features in patients with rup-

tured and nonruptured aneurysms, *AJR Am J Roentgenol* 163:1123, 1994.
44. Heiberg E et al: CT in aortic trauma, *AJR Am J Roentgenol* 140:1119, 1983.
45. Raptopoulos V et al: Traumatic aortic tear: screening with chest CT, *Radiology* 182:667, 1992.
46. Rizzo RJ et al: Computed tomography for evaluation of arterial disease in the popliteal fossa, *J Vasc Surg* 11:112, 1990.
47. Muller N, Morris DC, Nichols DM: Popliteal artery entrapment demonstrated by CT, *Radiology* 151:157, 1984.
48. Rubin GD: Three-dimensional helical CT angiography, *Radiographics* 14:905, 1994.
49. Galanski M et al: Renal arterial stenoses: spiral CT angiography, *Radiology* 189:185, 1993.
50. Rubin GD et al: Spiral CT of renal artery stenosis: comparison of three-dimensional rendering techniques, *Radiology* 190:181, 1994.
51. Rubin GD et al: Three-dimensional CT angiography of the splanchnic vasculature, *Radiology* 189(suppl):229, 1993.
52. Cumming MJ, Morrow IM: Carotid artery stenosis: a prospective comparison of CT angiography and conventional angiography, *AJR Am J Roentgenol* 163:517, 1994.
53. Marks MP et al: Diagnosis of carotid artery disease: preliminary experience with maximum-intensity-projection spiral CT angiography, *AJR Am J Roentgenol* 160:1267, 1993.
54. Li KC et al: Oxygen saturation of blood in the superior mesenteric vein: in vivo verification of MR imaging measurements in a canine model. Work in progress, *Radiology* 194:321, 1995.
55. De Marco JK et al: Prospective evaluation of extracranial carotid stenosis: MR angiography with maximum-intensity projections and multiplanar reformation compared with conventional angiography, *AJR Am J Roentgenol* 163:1205, 1994.
56. Laissy JP et al: Thoracic aortic dissection: diagnosis with transesophageal echocardiography versus MR imaging, *Radiology* 194:331, 1995.
57. Kent KC et al: Magnetic resonance imaging: a reliable test for the evaluation of proximal atherosclerotic renal arterial stenosis, *J Vasc Surg* 13:311, 1991.
58. Yucel EK, Dumoulin CL, Waltman AC: MR angiography of lower-extremity arterial disease: preliminary experience, *J Magn Reson Imaging* 2:303, 1992.
59. Owen RS et al: Magnetic resonance imaging of angiographically occult runoff vessels in peripheral arterial occlusive disease, *N Engl J Med* 326:1577, 1992.
60. Evans AJ et al: Detection of deep venous thrombosis: prospective comparison of MR imaging with contrast venography, *AJR Am J Roentgenol* 161:131, 1993.

12
Preoperative and Postoperative Spiral CT Evaluation of Patients Undergoing Placement of Endovascular Stent-Grafts

Irwin Walot

Endovascular stent grafts are rapidly becoming a viable alternative to open repair of many abdominal aortic aneurysms (AAAs). Therefore the development of accurate noninvasive methods for preoperative and postoperative evaluation of patients is important. Spiral computed axial tomography (spiral CT) is one alternative. Other alternatives include vascular ultrasonography and magnetic resonance angiography (MRA). Vascular ultrasonography is operator-dependent, and a complete preoperative examination is difficult and time-consuming. Even postoperative evaluation can be difficult because of the presence of intervening bowel gas. MR scanners and pulse sequences are improving daily but as yet do not yield as consistent results as does spiral CT.

Current CT Scanners

Current CT scanners are constructed so their x-ray tubes can rotate continuously around the patient during scan acquisition. Because the tube can rotate continuously and no longer has to stop its rotation for each "slice," the scanner table (and patient) can also move continuously. This innovation in scanner technology coupled with the price/performance improvements in computer equipment and the increases in x-ray tube power and heat-handling capacity, allow spiral CT scanners to acquire, process, and store large data sets from overlapping sections rapidly. Each data set represents an entire volume of interest. Spiral scanners are now widely available.

As pertains to analysis of the vascular system, this ability has several major consequences. First, the overall spatial resolution of this volume data set is better than that from similar data sets acquired by older generations of scanners. Such a data set can be reformatted and displayed accurately in various projections, utilizing different reconstruction techniques, in real time on a computer workstation or on the scanner. Second, the volume data set can be acquired rapidly enough that with an appropriate delay time between injection and the start of data acquisition a bolus of iodinated contrast agent injected intravenously is within the arterial system during the acquisition of the data set. In short, the current generation of spiral CT scanners can acquire data fast enough that a contrast bolus injected intravenously (in a safe amount at a safe rate) can be "chased" through the volume of interest while the contrast bolus is almost entirely within the arterial system. The density of the arterial system is therefore significantly increased with respect to adjacent soft tissues during the scan, allowing "subtraction" of most of the other soft tissues by simply adjusting the window and level parameters (thresholding).

Protocol

We have used the following acquisition protocol to achieve good results on our scanners for evaluating the abdominal aorta and iliac arteries:[1]

Pitch 1.5
Index 2.0
Voltage 120 kV
Amperage 250 mA
Scan time 1.0
Smooth acquisition algorithm
Sharp reconstruction algorithm
Reconstruct slices 5 mm thick 2 mm apart
Contrast, nonionic, 300 mg/ml via IV infusion in an arm vein
Scan delay of 25 seconds after starting contrast injection
Rate of 2.5 ml/s for 135 ml injected volume
Single acquisition from top of L1 vertebral body to top of femoral heads

Many other protocols (supplied by the various equipment manufacturers and well documented in the radiology literature[2-5]) can also be used to achieve good CT angiographic results in the abdomen. Protocols vary depending on the capabilities of the scanner used. We have used a set delay time and contrast dose to standardize our acquisitions, but software and hardware currently available allow some scanners to optimize delay times automatically for each patient and even to trigger a contrast injector automatically at the optimum time for injection.

After the data set is acquired, cross-sectional images are photographed at standard abdomen/pelvis window and level settings by the technologist. Although much of the information necessary for pre- and postoperative evaluation can be taken from the cross-sectional data, more accurate representations and measurements can be obtained by transferring the data set to a computer workstation. Alternatively, the data set can be reconstructed and reformatted by an outside contractor and then be returned to the referring physician on a CD-ROM for viewing and evaluation on a standard personal computer using proprietary software.

Workstations are available from each of the scanner manufacturers and from other companies specializing in medical imaging. The data set can be displayed at the workstation in several ways. Each method of data display has particular strengths and weaknesses.[3,4,6] Data can be displayed as shaded surface images that accurately depict the complex three-dimensional morphology of the aorta and iliac vasculature (Figure 12–1A). However, the surface shaded images include calcification as part of the surface but do not include soft plaque or noncalcified thrombus. Moreover, inappropriate window and level parameters can introduce artifacts or obscure important information. Making accurate distance and diameter measurements on the shaded surface images can be difficult and inaccurate. Maximum intensity projection (MIP) images (Figure 12–1B) do not have the capability of displaying the same three-dimensional relationships that surface-rendered images do and also fail to depict soft plaque, noncalcified thrombus, and arterial wall thickening. MIP images do allow calcified plaque and metallic stents to be well depicted, but overlying and underlying bone must be edited from the images before they can be assessed accurately. Finally, multiplanar reformatted images (Figure 12–1C) and axial images allow accurate measurement and depict noncalcified thrombus well, but they do not illustrate complex three-dimensional relationships or show the position or severity of calcified plaques as well as do the MIP images. For evaluation of pre- and postoperative stent-graft patients, we have chosen to use all of the reconstruction methods, utilizing each for the information it best yields.

Technique

When evaluating a patient for placement of a bifurcated stent-graft, we initially display the data set as thin cross-sectional images. The number and position of arteries supplying each kidney are identified by panning up and down through the images. If the aortic neck is tortuous, accurate length and diameter measurements from the axial images are difficult

12. Spiral CT and Stent-Graft Placement

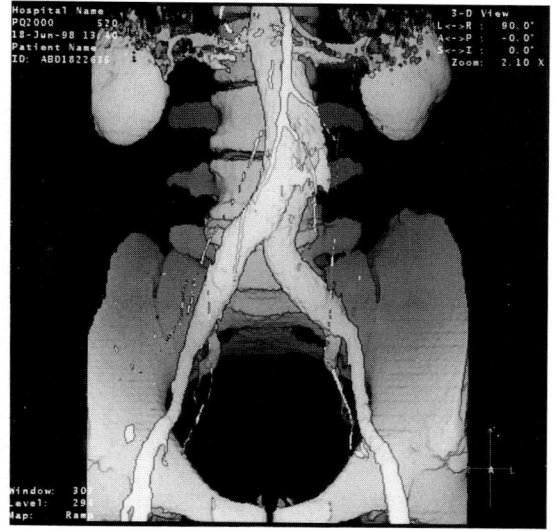
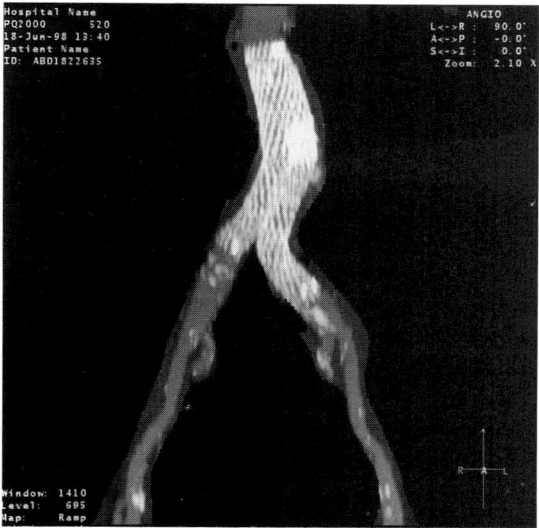
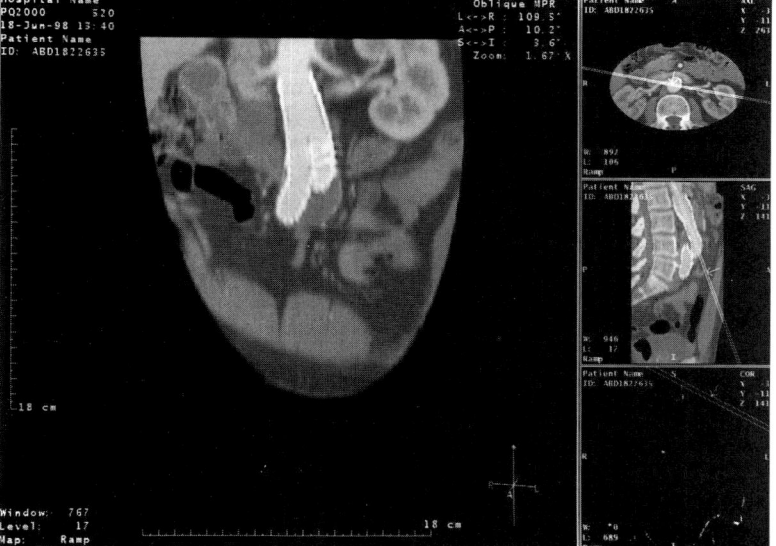

FIGURE 12–1. Patient with infrarenal abdominal aortic aneurysm following repair with an endovascular stent graft. **A**, Shaded surface reconstruction of the abdominal aorta and iliac vessels accurately depicts the three-dimensional appearance. **B**, MIP image clearly shows the position of the metallic components of the stent-graft. **C**, Planar reconstruction. Oblique coronal image demonstrates the relationship of the stent-graft to the origin of the renal arteries. The small windows to the right of the reconstructed image show the position of the plane of section on axial and sagittal sections.

(Figure 12–2A,2B). The data set is then displayed as multiplanar two-dimensional reformatted oblique coronal or sagittal images (or both). An image plane is selected that best represents a cross section orthogonal to the center line of the aortic neck (the section of relatively normal size aorta between the inferior aspect of the lowest renal artery origin and the beginning of the aneurysm) (Figure 12–2C). The interactive nature of the workstation

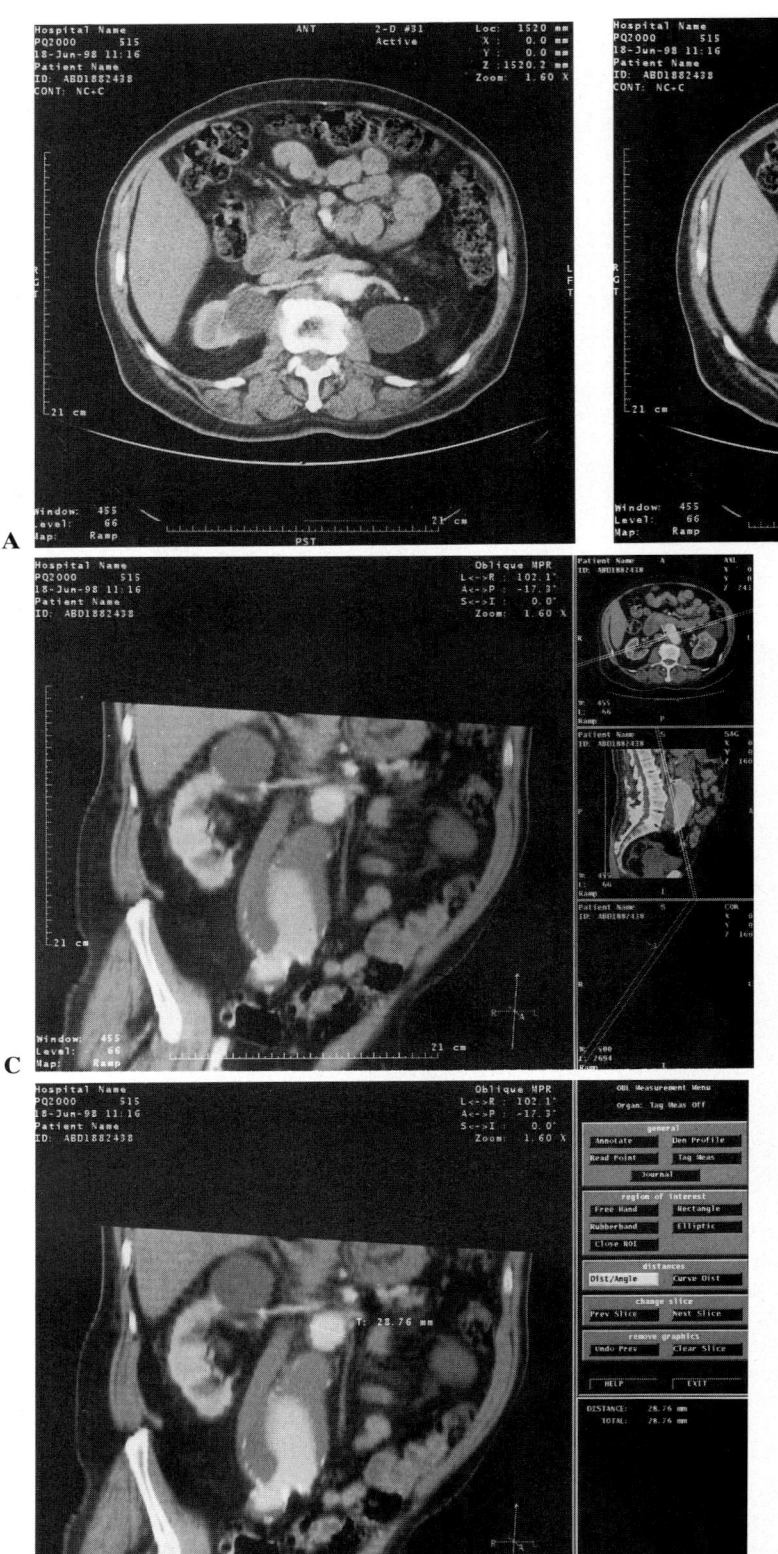

FIGURE 12–2. Preoperative evaluation of a patient with a tortuous aortic neck. **A**, **B**, Axial images make it appear as though there is a short aortic neck (segment of relatively normal diameter aorta between renal arteries and the top of the abdominal aortic aneurysm). **C**, **D**, Selection of a reconstruction plane orthogonal to the center line of the aortic neck allows the physician or technologist to make accurate diameter measurements. **E**, **F**, Selection of a reconstruction plane parallel to the center line of the aortic neck makes possible accurate measurement of the aortic neck.

FIGURE 12–2. *Continued.*

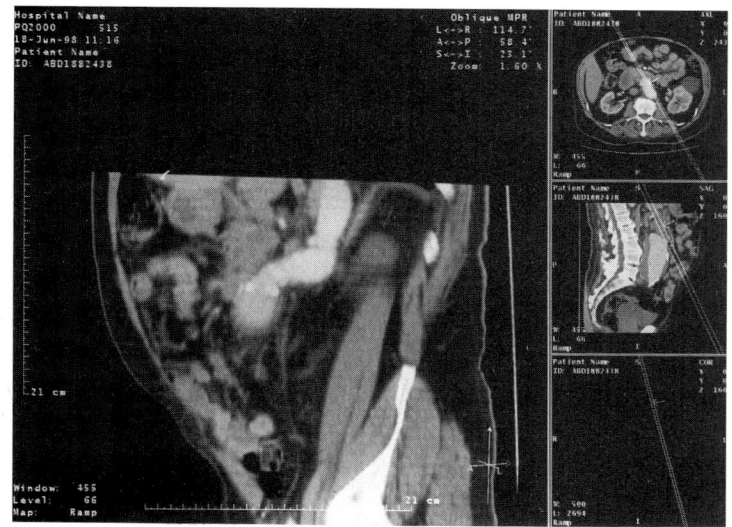

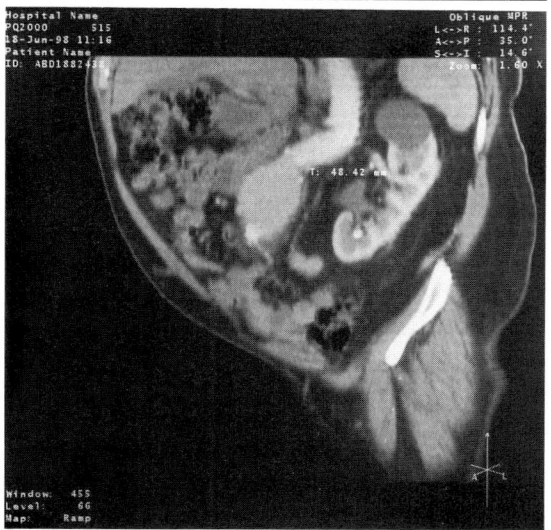

allows the physician or technologist to select accurately the best plane in which to measure. The diameter of the aortic neck is measured (Figure 12–2D) and correlated with diameters measured from the oblique coronal and sagittal reconstructions. Devices come in various diameters, and accurate measurement of the diameter of the aortic neck allows us to choose an appropriately sized component or device. A plane of section parallel to the center line of the aortic neck is then chosen (Figure 12–2E), and the length of the aortic neck is measured (Figure 12–2F). All currently available endovascular devices require a length (which varies with the device—typically 0.5 to 1.5 cm) of relatively normal-diameter aorta below the renal arteries and above the top of the aneurysm to allow the device to seal.

Although it has been suggested that aortic neck configuration (shape) is a factor in successful endovascular repair,[7] we have not in general tried to classify the shape of the aortic neck. Most devices we have placed have excellent column strength, so the shape of the aortic neck is less important for keeping the device in place. The shape of the aortic neck may be a much more important factor when deploying stent-grafts with low or moderate column strength. If necessary, the neck configuration can be assessed from the multiplanar reformatted image or shaded surface image.

The angle between the centerline of the aortic neck and the centerline of the aneurysm can also be measured easily. Some devices have restrictions on the amount of angulation of the aortic neck that is acceptable for device placement. Similar to assessing the aortic neck, the diameters of the aneurysm and the common iliac and external iliac arteries are measured (Figure 12–3A–C), and areas of stenosis are identified. The diameter of the distal aorta is also measured, as a markedly narrow distal aortic neck may preclude placement of a bifurcated device (both limbs of the stent-graft must pass through the distal neck, so a narrow distal neck results in compression of one or both limbs). Placement of a tube-type stent-graft or a single-limb aortoiliac device with a femorofemoral crossover graft and occlusion of the opposite iliac artery may be viable alternatives in such a case.

Utilizing a mid-sagittal slice oriented as closely as possible to the center line of the aorta, the distance from the origin of the lowest renal artery to the aortic bifurcation is estimated (Figure 12–4). Similarly, the lengths of the common iliac arteries are measured (and can be correlated to length measurements obtained from the shaded surface image). We also determine whether the internal iliac arteries are patent, as we try to adjust stent-graft lengths and diameters to maintain flow in at least one internal iliac artery. If the diameter of the common iliac artery is larger than the available limb diameters or it is aneurysmal, the stent-graft limb may have to be extended into the proximal external iliac artery. If a common iliac artery aneurysm is present, the internal iliac artery may have to be occluded prior to stent-graft placement.

The workstation environment provides near real-time visual feedback when the data set is manipulated. This enables the physician or technologist to rapidly choose (1) appropriate planes of section so accurate measurements can be made and (2) appropriate window and level settings. In our experience, the measurements acquired in the above manner have correlated well with intravascular ultrasonographic and angiographic measurements obtained at the time of device placement. Utilizing the workstation, decisions can be made that allow "tailoring" modular devices or the manufacture of custom devices to the individual patient's anatomy. Measuring the diameters of the external iliac arteries and identifying areas of stenosis are particularly important, as the currently available devices are large and vascular access is often a problem.

Prior to reconstructing the data set as a shaded surface image, a volume of interest can be drawn around the aorta and iliac arteries. All data outside the volume of interest are discarded to reduce the amount of data that must be manipulated. The remaining data are then rendered as shaded surfaces. With good contrast enhancement and proper window and level settings (thresholding), bone, arteries, and portions of the kidneys are usually the only rendered objects (Figure 12–5A,B). The interactive nature of the workstation allows the window and level (threshold) to be adjusted to minimize artifacts without losing important information. The images may be photographed at this time to show the relationship of the arterial system to bony landmarks. The images can then be rotated into various positions to allow the bone to be easily subtracted, leaving only the arterial system rendered (Figure 12–5C,D). The resulting images are viewed (and photographed) in various orientations to gauge the tortuosity of the aortoiliac system. Most bifurcated endovascular devices require a larger delivery device or sheath to position the body and one leg of the device than is needed to position the contralateral limb. Diameters being equal, the least tortuous iliac artery is usually the most favorable one through which to try to pass the larger sheath or device.

Finally, the data set is reconstructed as an MIP image (Figure 12–6A,B), which allows visualization and characterization of calcified plaques. The assumptions are that (1) the more heavily calcified an artery, the less flexible it is (and therefore less able to accommodate a large, relatively inflexible sheath or device); and (2) heavily calcified plaques may pose difficulty when passing large sheaths.

FIGURE 12–3. Preoperative evaluation. **A**, Aneurysm diameter is measured. **B**, Common iliac artery diameter is measured. **C**, Diameters of external iliac arteries are measured.

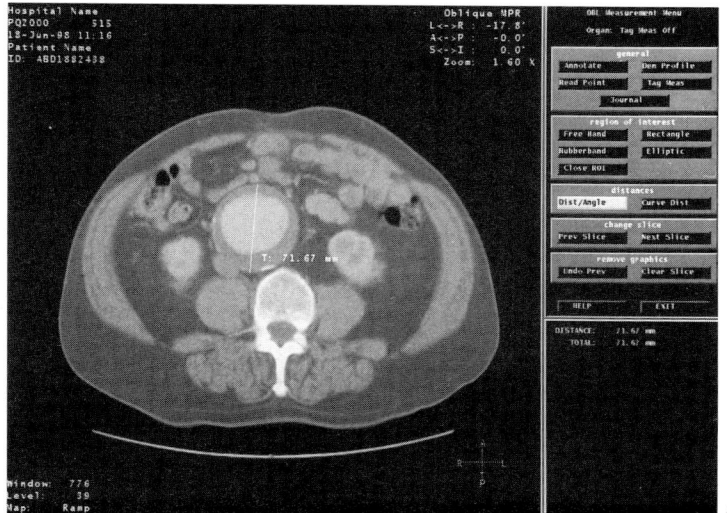

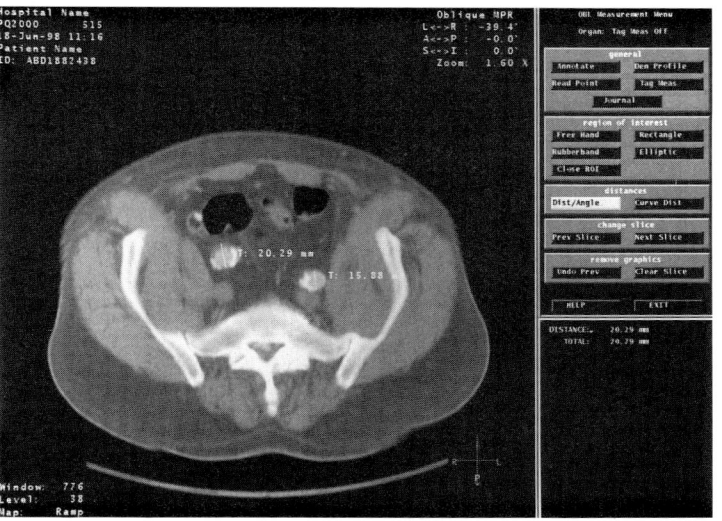

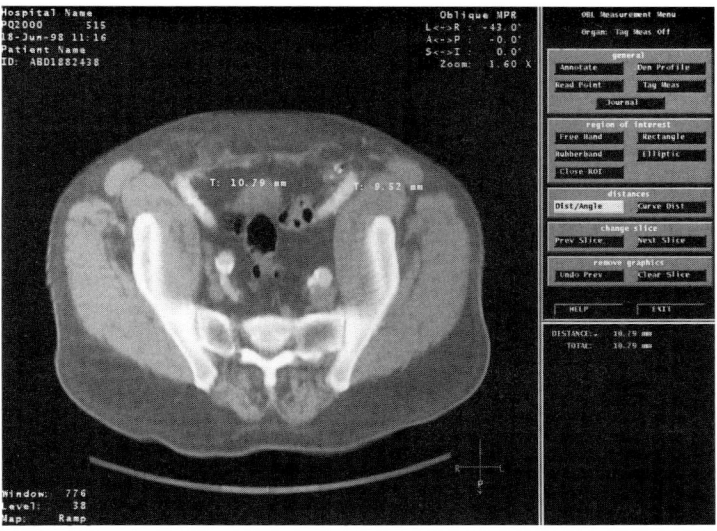

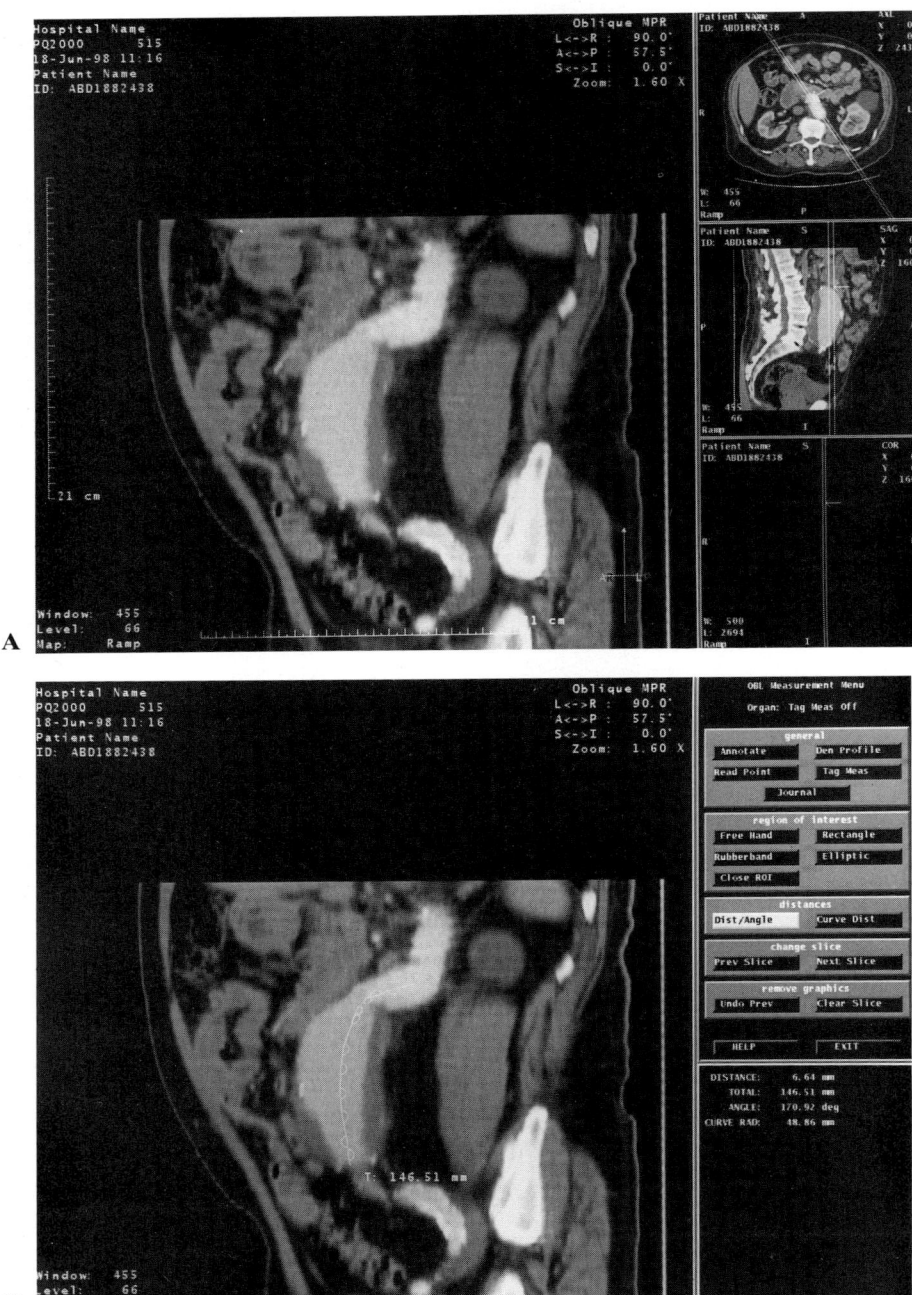

FIGURE 12–4. Preoperative evaluation. **A, B,** Utilizing a midsagittal slice oriented as closely as possible to the center line of the aorta, the distance from the projected top of the device to the aortic bifurcation is estimated (usually the distance from the lowest renal artery origin to the bifurcation).

12. Spiral CT and Stent-Graft Placement 169

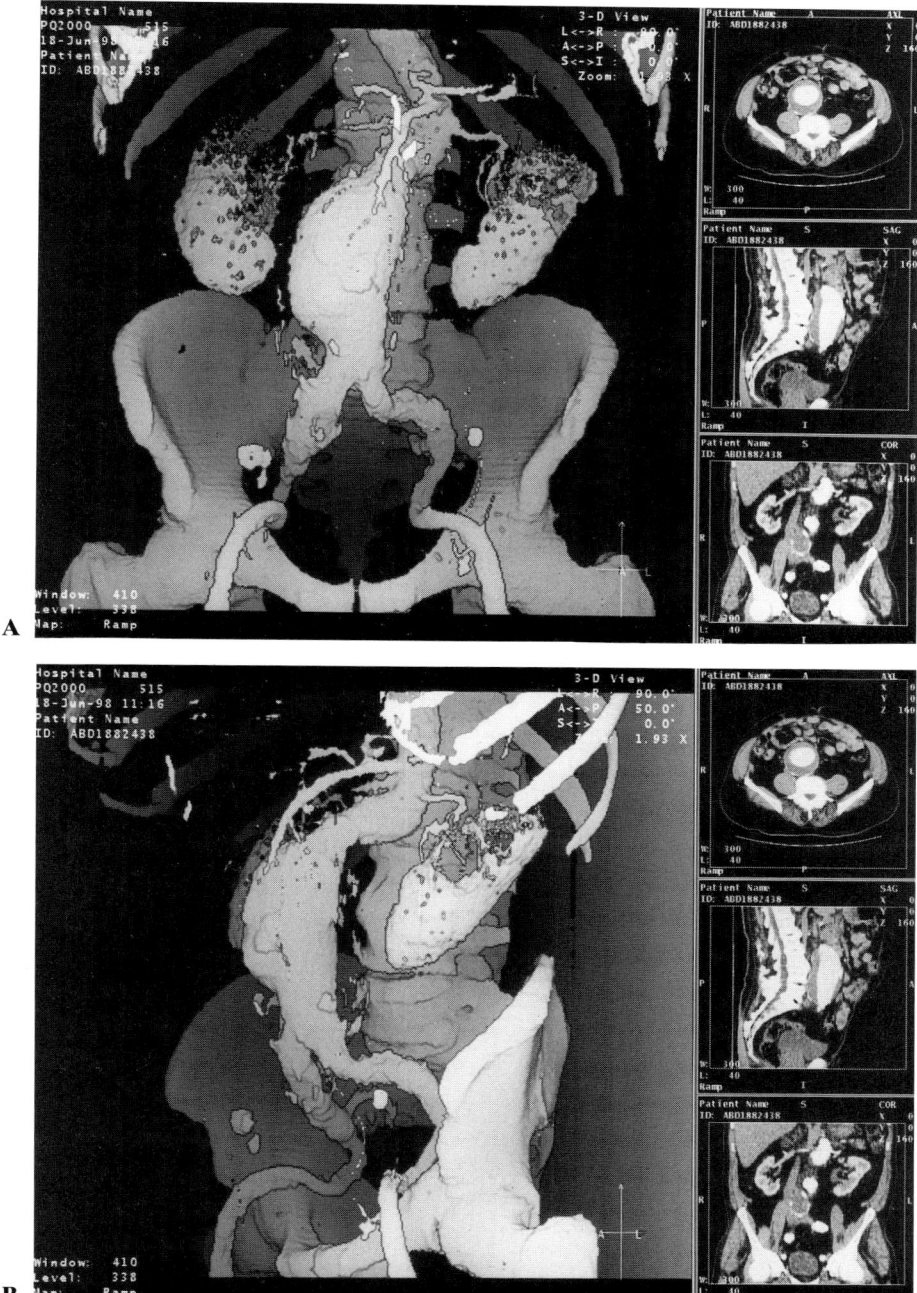

FIGURE 12–5. Preoperative evaluation. **A**, **B**, Shaded surface reconstruction shows the relationship of the vasculature to the adjacent bone. **C**, **D**, The bone can then be edited out, leaving only the vasculature.

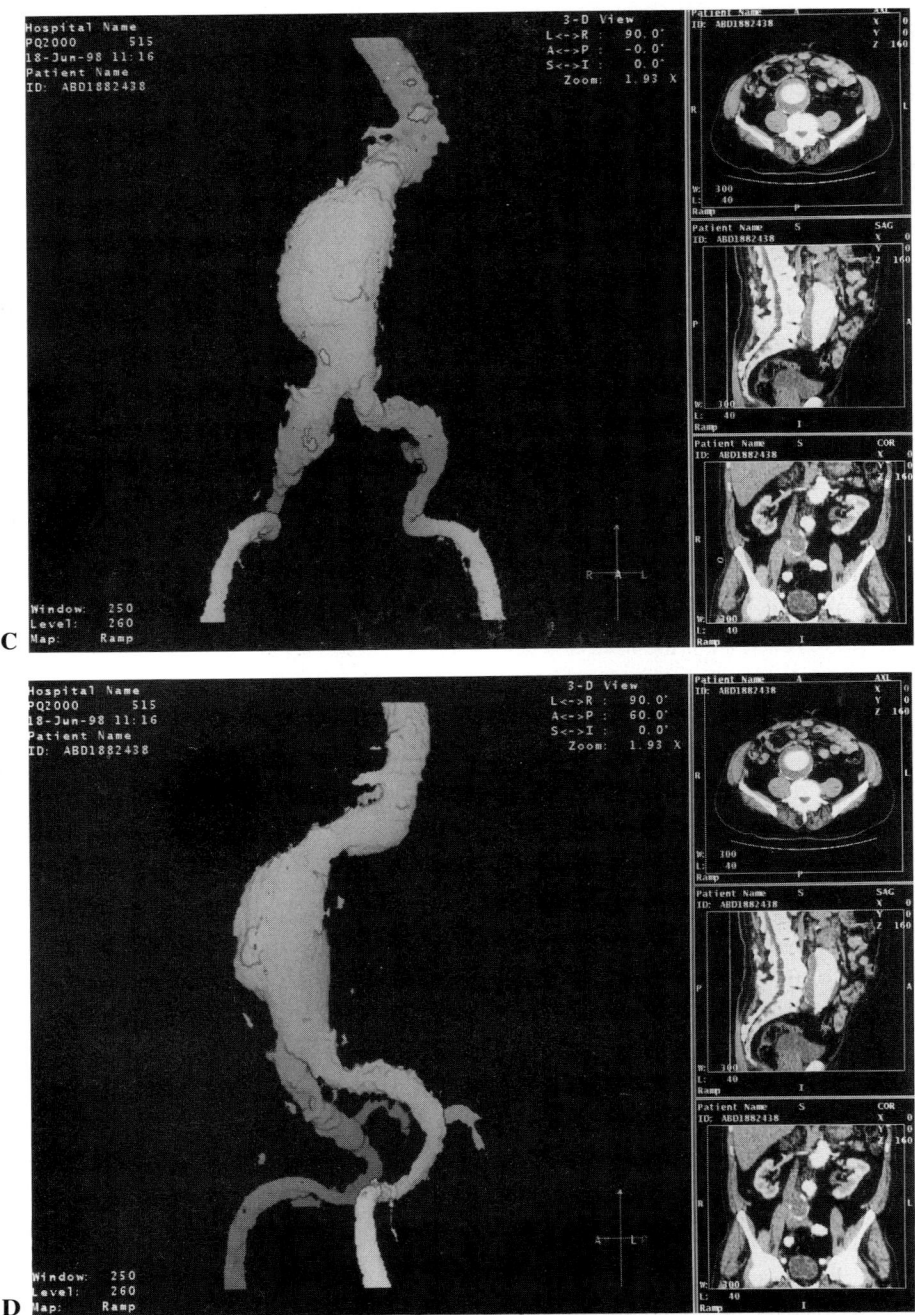

FIGURE 12–5. *Continued.*

12. Spiral CT and Stent-Graft Placement

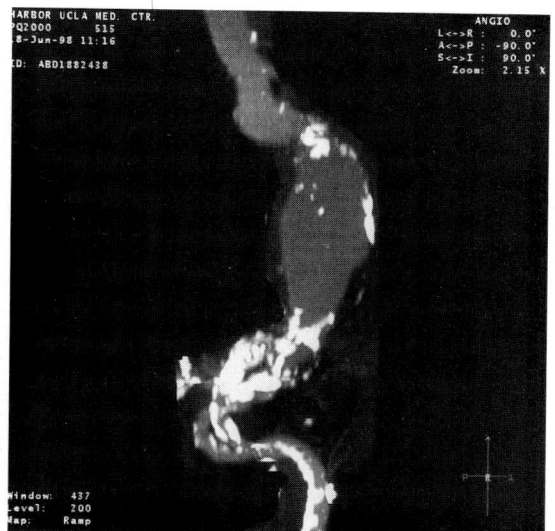

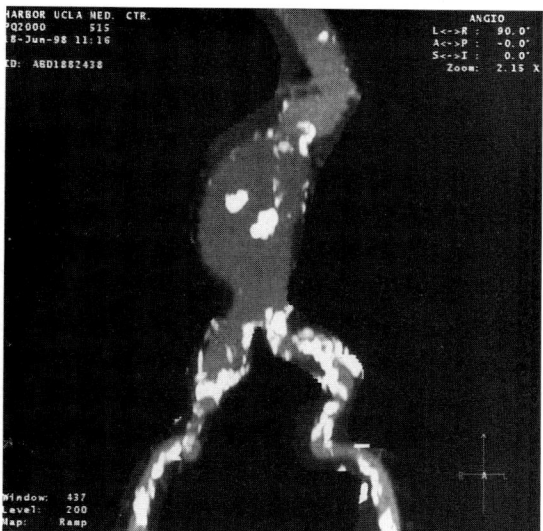

FIGURE 12-6. Preoperative evaluation. **A, B**, MIP image allows visualization and characterization of calcified plaques.

Interpretation

Generally, based on the data extracted from spiral CT, the patient is accepted or rejected as a candidate for endovascular repair. If accepted, the appropriate size and type of device is chosen to fit the patient's anatomy. Occasionally, a patient with an equivocal spiral CT scan is referred for intravascular ultrasonography (IVUS) prior to attemped device placement. As a rule, angiograms are not obtained unless specifically called for in device protocols or obtained as part of the IVUS examination.

Computed tomography is also used to evaluate patients prior to discharge and for periodic follow-up.[6] Endoleaks (leakage of contrast through or around the stent-graft into the aneurysm sac) are easily detected on axial images (Figure 12-7A,B) and multiplanar reformatted images (Figure 12-7C). Acquisition of the postoperative CT scan is somewhat different from that for the preoperative scan. Noncontrast standard axial images are acquired before spiral CT, and delayed postcontrast nonspiral images are obtained following spiral CT. Delay times are typically 3 to 5 minutes (time required for the tube to cool following spiral CT and for programming the postcontrast scan). When compared to the spiral CT images, the noncontrast image helps differentiate intrathrombus calcification and plaque calcification within the patient's aneurysm from contrast leakage through or around the stent-graft (an endoleak) (Figure 12-8A,B). The delayed postcontrast images are obtained to identify small or slow endoleaks.[8] CT scans obtained days after stent-graft placement may show gas within the aneurysm sac (Figure 12-8C). The gas probably is introduced during device placement and then trapped within the aneurysm sac following stent-graft deployment. We generally consider gas within the aneurysm sac to be a positive finding in that it seems to signify at least partial isolation of the aneurysm sac from the remainder of the circulating blood volume.

Shaded surface and oblique sagittal and coronal multiplanar reformations are also obtained and may help identify the origin of endoleaks (Figure 12-9); and MIP images illustrate the position of metallic graft components (Figure 12-10). Periodic spiral CT evaluation allows us to monitor aneurysm diameter and volume, detect endograft component migration, detect arterial stenosis, and follow up endoleaks. Evaluation of reconstructed images can help formulate a plan to repair endoleaks if they do not stop spontaneously and can clarify the relationship of graft components

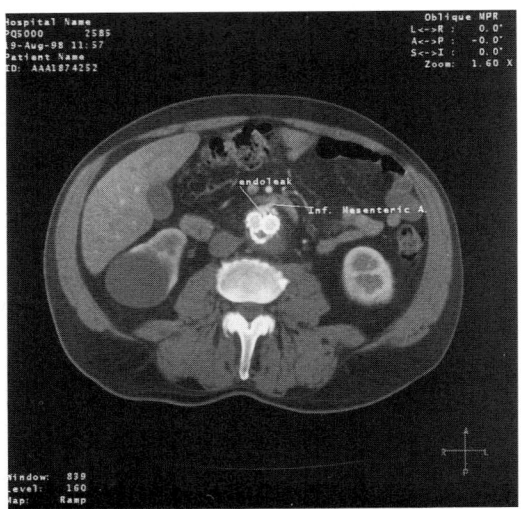

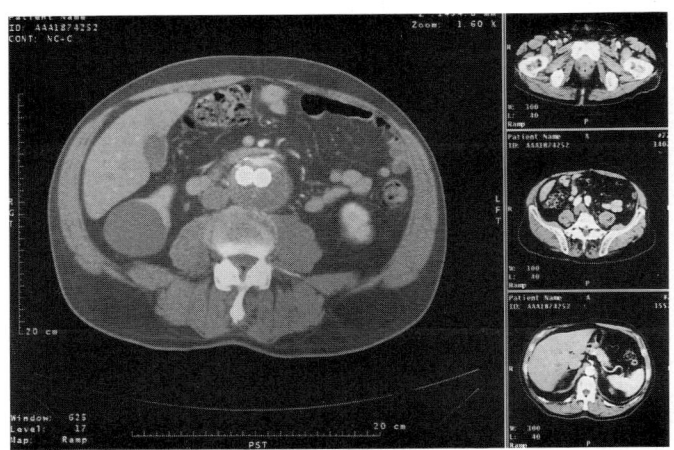

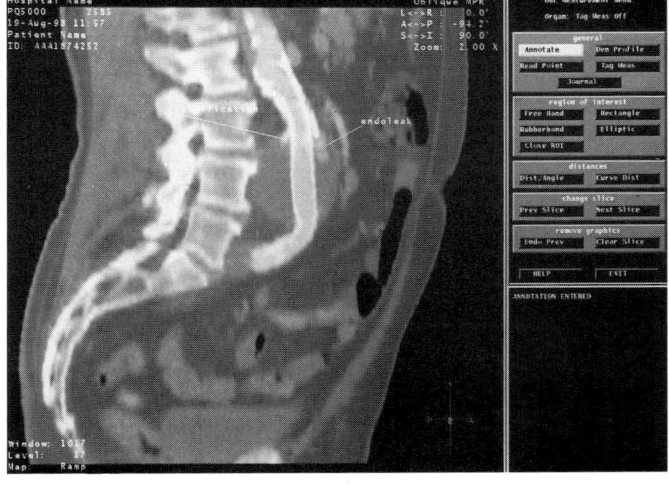

FIGURE 12–7. Postoperative evaluation. **A**, **B**, Endoleaks can easily be identified on axial images. **C**, Multiplanar reformatted images can help identify the source and extent of endoleaks.

12. Spiral CT and Stent-Graft Placement

FIGURE 12–8. Postoperative evaluation. **A**, Spiral CT axial image shows a possible endoleak. **B**, Non-contrast axial CT image shows the "endoleak" to be an intrathrombus calcification. **C**, Spiral CT axial image shows gas within the aneurysm sac several days after stent-graft placement. Gas was probably introduced during placement and then trapped within the aneurysm sac by the stent-graft.

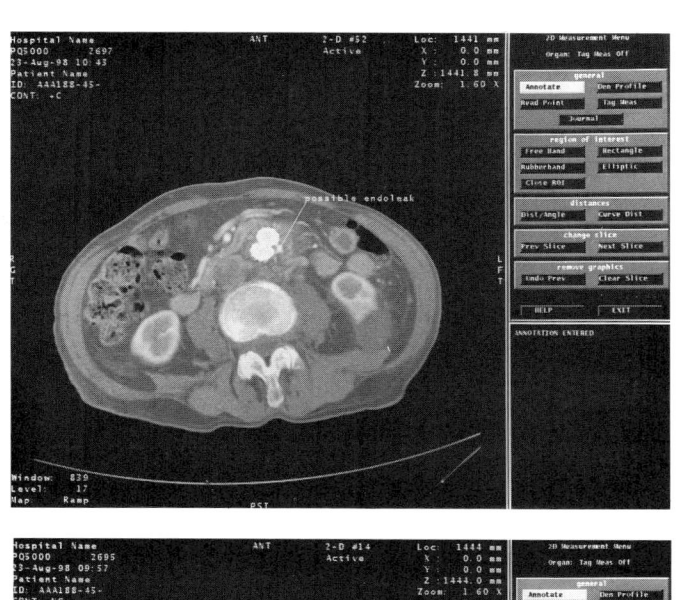

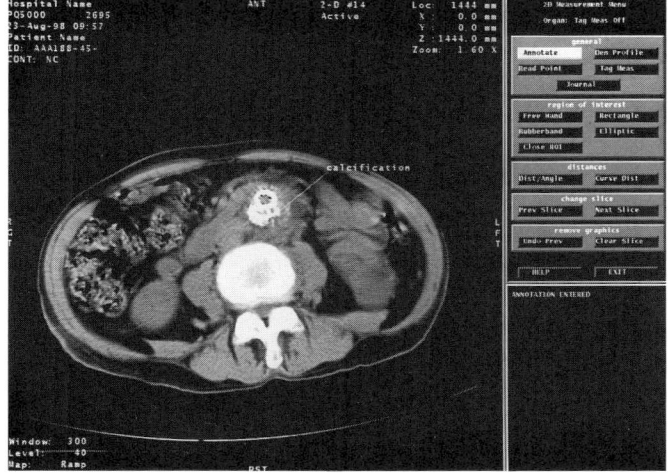

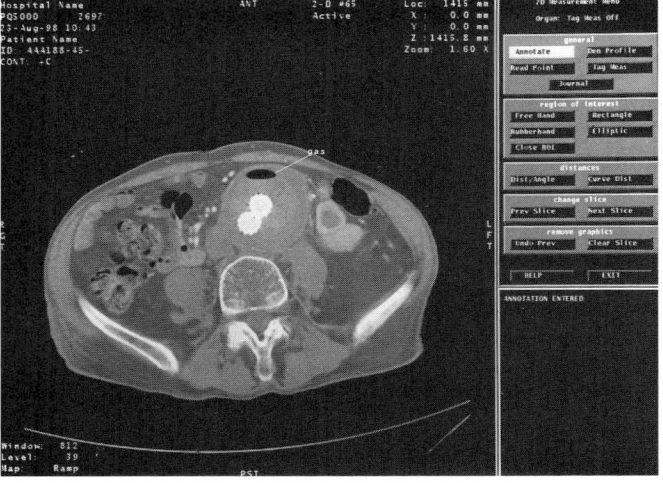

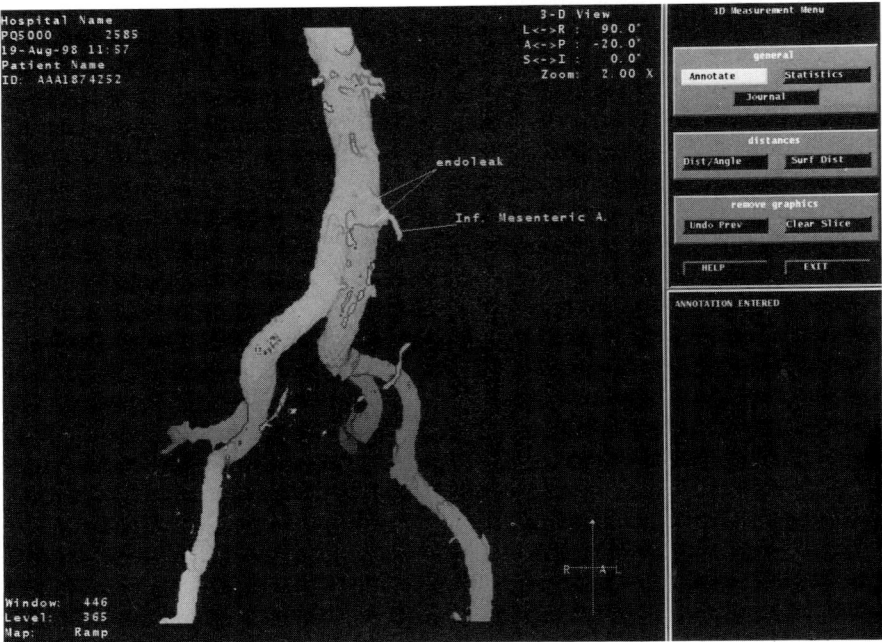

FIGURE 12–9. Postoperative evaluation. Endoleaks can also be identified on shaded surface images.

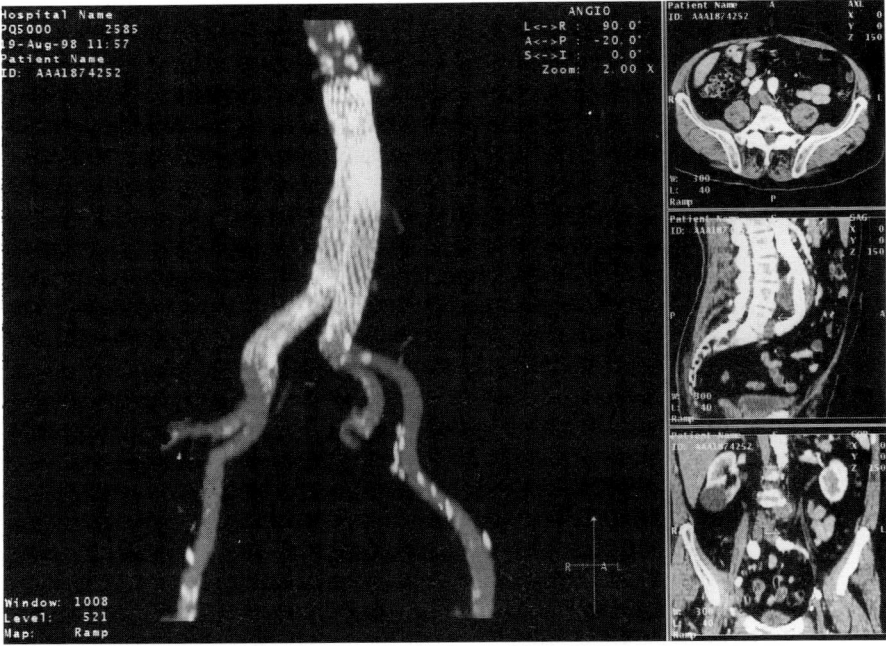

FIGURE 12–10. Postoperative evaluation. MIP images are best for demonstrating the position of stent-graft components.

12. Spiral CT and Stent-Graft Placement

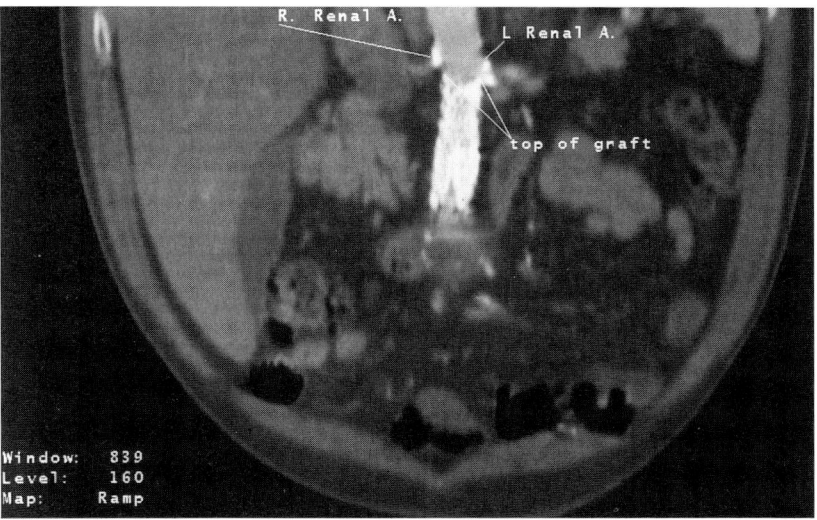

FIGURE 12-11. Multiplanar reformatted images can clarify the relationship of stent-graft components to other arterial structures (the renal arteries in this instance).

to other arterial structures (Figure 12-11). Typically, complete evaluation of pre- or post-operative spiral CT scans, including filming, take 15 to 20 minutes at the workstation.

Note: The images in this chapter were acquired on Picker PQ 2000 and 5000 spiral CT scanners and reconstructed on Picker Voxel computer workstations.

Conclusion

In experienced hands, spiral CT, when coupled with the ability to perform multiplanar reformatting and three-dimensional reconstruction, is an efficient, accurate, noninvasive method for evaluating endovascular stentgraft patients.

References

1. *Picker Computed Tomography Clinical Study Guide*, Picker International Incorporated, 1996, Cleveland.
2. Rubin GD, Dake MD, Napel SA et al: Abdominal spiral CT angiography: initial clinical experience, *Radiology* 186:147–152, 1993.
3. Rubin GD, Walker PJ, Dake MD et al: Three-dimensional spiral computed tomographic angiography: an alternative imaging modality for the abdominal aorta and its branches, *J Vasc Surg* 18:656–665, 1993.
4. Zeman RK, Silverman PM, Berman PM et al: Abdominal aortic aneurysms: findings on three-dimensional display of helical CT data, *AJR* 164:917–922, 1995.
5. Errington ML, Ferguson JM, Gillespie IN et al: Complete pre-operative imaging assessment of abdominal aortic aneurysm with spiral CT angiography, *Clin Radiol* 52:369–377, 1997.
6. Dorffner R, Thurnher S, Youssefzadeh S et al: Spiral CT angiography in the assessment of abdominal aortic aneurysms after stent grafting: value of maximum intensity projections, *J Comput Assist Tomogr* 21:472–477, 1997.
7. Balm R, Stokking R, Kaatee R et al: Computed tomographic angiographic imaging of abdominal aortic aneurysms: implications for transfemoral endovascular aneurysm management, *J Vasc Surg* 26:231–237, 1997.
8. Golzarian J, Dussaussois L, Abada HT et al: Helical CT of aorta after endoluminal stent-graft therapy: value of biphasic acquisition, *AJR* 171:329–331, 1998.

13
Angioscopy: Instrumentation, Techniques, and Applications

Arnold Miller and Juha P. Salenius

Angioscopy is the only imaging technology that allows direct in vivo visualization of the interior of blood vessels in real-life colors. This capability to detect and quantify endoluminal findings and delineate subtle variations of the different normal and abnormal endoluminal states has only begun to be appreciated. The evolution and clinical application of the endoluminal techniques in the treatment of occlusive arterial disease and the performance of the distal bypass to the tibial and pedal arteries have highlighted the deficiencies of the arteriogram in providing accurate and clinically relevant information regarding the endoluminal state.

The main obstacle to the expanding role of angioscopy in modern vascular surgery remains the necessity to remove all blood from the visual field within the lumen of the vessel to obtain good endoluminal visualization. Blood is opaque to all light. To achieve complete removal of blood is not always easy. It requires skill and an understanding of the available instrumentation and techniques required for the different procedures.

Acceptance of angioscopy as an essential part of the armamentarium of the vascular surgeon based solely on the ability to demonstrate clear "superiority" with regard to outcome ignores the obvious benefits of direct intraluminal observation in normal and diseased states. These include the recognition of new or previously unappreciated intraluminal pathologies and their correlation with clinical outcome, as well as the use of the angioscope for evaluating technical success of surgical procedures and the new interventional procedures. In addition, angioscopy has proven to be an excellent educational tool for teaching surgical technique. Most reported studies defining the role of angioscopy in the treatment of vascular disease have focused on infrainguinal bypass surgery, thromboembolectomy, carotid endarterectomy, vascular access surgery, and percutaneous coronary and peripheral arterial angioscopy.[1-16] It should be appreciated that endoscopic vascular surgery is still in its infancy and remains one of the exciting and challenging areas of exploration in vascular surgery.

Since 1987, we have attempted to explore and optimize angioscopic techniques and instrumentation and to critically assess the role of angioscopy in clinical practice. In this chapter, we describe the basic instrumentation, the principles of irrigation, and our current techniques of angioscopy for vascular surgery.

Angioscopic Equipment

Flexible angioscopes in current clinical use range in external diameter from 0.5 to 3.0mm. They consist of bundles of flexible glass fibers (3000 to as many as 30,000 or more) of various types and refractive indexes (clear glass or quartz) coherently arranged and covered by an outer coating or *cladding*, which ensures undistorted light and image transmission (Figure 13–1). The number of fiber bundles ("pixels") and the lensing systems are the main factors responsible for the resolution of the angio-

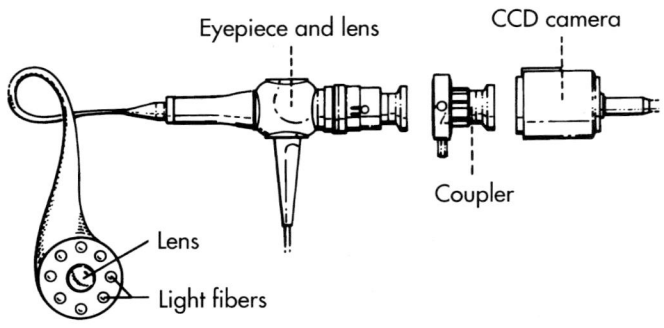

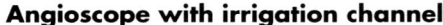

Angioscope with irrigation channel

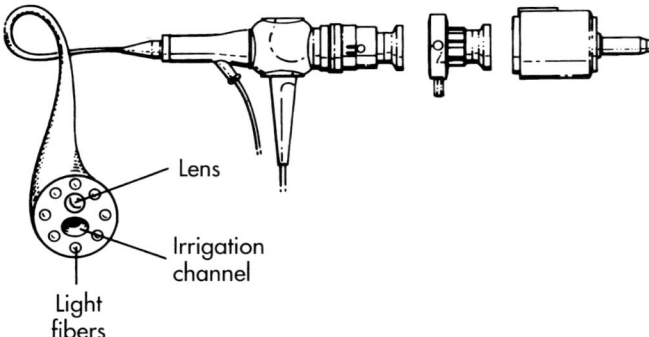

FIGURE 13–1. Anatomy of an angioscope. (From Miller A, Jepsen S: Technique of intraoperative angioscopy in lower extremity revascularization. In Bergan J, Yao J, editors: *Techniques in arterial surgery*, Philadelphia, 1990, WB Saunders.)

scopic image; the more fibers there are, the more pixels and the higher the resolution. The fiber bundles are organized into those for imaging and those conducting light. At the distal end of the angioscope a convex lens is fitted to capture the light emitted from the viewed intraluminal object and to refocus the "image" onto the mosaic of fibers of the optical bundle. (See Box 13–1 for a list of angioscopic equipment.)

Because the fiber bundles are coherently arranged, this image is faithfully reproduced at the opposite end of the optical bundle, where it may be magnified by an eyepiece and viewed directly or transmitted directly to a computer-controlled display (CCD) chip video camera and viewed as an image on a high-resolution monitor (or attached to any other camera lens system). This has been an important advance in the clinical application of angioscopy because it allows the procedure to be visualized as an enlarged image, avoiding all problems of maintaining a sterile field in the operating room or angiography suite. To inject sufficient light for transmission through the small volume of fiber bundles available in the modern angioscope for satisfactory intraluminal viewing, a very intense and focused cold light source is used, most usually derived from quartz-halogen or xenon-arc lamps with an energy of 250 to 300 watts.

The definitive clinical angioscope may consist of only the flexible light fibers or include hollow channels of 0.3 to 1.0 mm, allowing irrigation at the distal tip of the angioscope or for use as a working channel for special intraluminal instrumentation. Steering the distal tip of some special angioscopes 120° in two directions is possible. This is usually mechanical and is facilitated by thin cables that extend along the surface of the angioscope sheath. Such specialized features, hollow channels, or steering mechanisms increase the external diameter of the angioscope and the overall rigidity of the instrument. Inclusion of these special features into a particular angioscope is always a compromise between the resolution and light intensity (i.e., total number of fiberoptic bundles) and the external diameter of the angioscope.

For percutaneous applications, particularly in the coronary arteries, an occlusion balloon

> **Box 13–1. Angioscopy Equipment**
>
> Angioscopes
>   0.5- to 3.0-mm outer diameter
>   Steerability (120° in two directions)
>   Working/irrigation channel
>   Reusable/disposable
> Dedicated irrigation pump
> Light source
> Camera (chip, CCD)
> High-resolution monitor
> Documentation
>   Patient record, paperprint, slides
>   Video (VHS, U-matic) and microphone
>   Programmable character generator
>   Computerized processing and storing
> Endovascular tools
>   Valvulotome
>   Endoluminal microinstrumentation
>   Occlusion devices
> Angioscopy cart

either built-in at the distal part of the endoscope (Mitsubishi Cable Industries, Ltd, Tokyo, Japan, and Advanced Cardiovascular Systems, Santa Clara, Calif) or integrated with a guidewire catheter system (Baxter, Irvine, Calif) may allow brief periods of antegrade occlusion of the blood flow essential to successful angioscopy.

Currently, both reusable and disposable angioscopes are available for routine clinical use. In general, the optics of the reusable angioscopes have a better resolution. However, with modern fiberoptic and imaging technologies the resolution of both types of angioscope are adequate for clinical application. The choice for the individual surgeon depends on the circumstance, volume of procedures, and economics. The availability of a particular angioscope for clinical use is limited by the necessity for gas sterilization, a fairly lengthy procedure after each use. On a busy vascular service, a large number of angioscopes may be required for routine application.

Immediately after use, the reusable angioscope should be rinsed with water to remove all blood and cleaned in accordance with the manufacturer's instructions. Excessive kinking must be avoided to prevent breakage of the optical glass fibers. Gas sterilization is performed with ethylene oxide at a temperature of 55°C for a maximum of 105 minutes followed by aeration for 12 hours in a special aeration chamber. Before gas sterilization a venting cap is attached to allow escape of air from within the endoscope and to prevent sheath rupture.

The adequacy of the irrigation system is crucial to consistent high-quality endoscopic studies, with volumes of irrigation fluid safe for routine clinical use. The venous infusion bag, an inflatable pressure-cuff device, is only useful in a few special circumstances. A dedicated roller pump for irrigation, with adjustable high and low flow rates, is the cornerstone of the irrigation necessary for consistent clearing of all the blood from the relevant vessel.

Standard medical-grade video (i.e., VHS or U-matic) and audio equipment (e.g., a directional microphone) is used to record relevant parts of the angioscopy procedure, allowing repeated review of the procedure and the unique intraoperative findings. A character generator provides patient and study identification. Hard copy is useful to present the intraoperative findings. Paperprints may be included immediately in patient records or with computer technology stored in an electronic database for later processing.

Storage of the equipment on a dedicated mobile cart minimizes the complexity of all the electronic equipment, which once adjusted reduces the entire operation to a single on/off switch. It also facilitates transfer of the equipment between operating rooms or even several institutions. Finally, it reduces the required storage space and minimizes the risk of damage to the equipment.

Basic Techniques of Angioscopy

Principles of Saline Irrigation

The fundamental problem with vascular endoscopy remains the necessity to clear blood from the visual field. In the intraoperative setting, complete isolation of the vascular segment may be obtained by isolating the segment of the vasculature to be visualized between arterial clamps and removing the blood by flushing with a clear saline solution. This is standard practice during surgery for blood vessels in the suprainguinal and abdominal vasculature, during carotid surgery, and during venous thrombectomy. In the infrainguinal region, only proximal control by occluding the antegrade blood flow is necessary. The retrograde blood flow from collaterals is cleared by flushing these vessels or grafts with clear saline solution.

The intraarterial injection of CO_2[17] for blood displacement, although promising, remains an experimental technique. Unlike saline, the gas is compressible; thus the delivery of CO_2 requires a special injector that delivers a precise volume of CO_2 over a prolonged injection time. A standard angiographic contrast injector may compress the gas with an explosive delivery.

Lack of appreciation of the factors governing successful saline irrigation and the difficulty in achieving the flow rates necessary for irrigation during angioscopy have delayed the incorporation of angioscopy as a routine procedure in the practice of vascular surgery. Unlike angiography, where a sufficient concentration of contrast medium mixing with the blood allows high-quality angiograms, during angioscopy the intraluminal blood must be totally replaced by a clear column of fluid. A small volume of red cells causes blurring of the visual field, and the image appears to be out of focus. Addition of any more blood makes meaningful visualization impossible.

Certain requirements are necessary to achieve a clear column of fluid in the vessels or grafts being studied by angioscopy (summarized in Box 13–2). All antegrade blood flow, from both the main inflow vessel and collaterals, needs to be prevented; otherwise, blood flowing in the same direction as the irrigation fluid will join the irrigation fluid and a clear fluid column will never be established. At surgery this usually entails proximal clamp occlusion of the native arteries or graft.

To clear all blood and establish the clear fluid column, a bolus of fluid, injected at a high flow

---

Box 13–2. Principles of Irrigation for Intraoperative Angioscopy

Aim
- To establish and maintain a *column of clear fluid* within the vessel

Requirements
- No antegrade flow in the main vessel or collateral vessels
- Initial fluid bolus of large volume and high flow rate to establish column of clear fluid
- Subsequent small volume and low flow rate, with pressure in excess of backflow pressure, to maintain clear fluid column

---

From Miller A, Lipson W, Isaacson K et al.: Intraoperative angioscopy: principles of irrigation and description of a new dedicated irrigation pump, *Am Heart J* 118:391–399, 1989.

rate and large volume, is necessary. The more rapidly the column of fluid can be established, the less total fluid will be needed for the angioscopic study.[18] Once the column of fluid is established, it can be maintained by irrigating at a much lower flow rate and smaller volume. This prolongs the time that visualization is possible and minimizes the total volume of irrigation fluid used.

The practical problem in achieving these flow rates is the small size of the irrigation catheters necessary for intraoperative use. Inflating a standard venous transfusion pressure-cuff device to between 400 to 450 mm Hg, around a single liter of saline in a plastic container, allows a maximum flow rate of approximately 150 ml/min.[18] As the saline container empties and alters its shape, despite maintaining the pressure in the pressure cuff inflated to between 400 and 450 mm Hg, the flow rate decreases. With the addition of various irrigation catheters, there is a further decrease in the flow rate. From our experimental[18] and clinical[19–21] experience the flow rates achieved with the pressure cuff device are inadequate for routine intraoperative angioscopy except in very limited circumstances. Furthermore, there is no control over the flow rate. The flow rate cannot be varied,

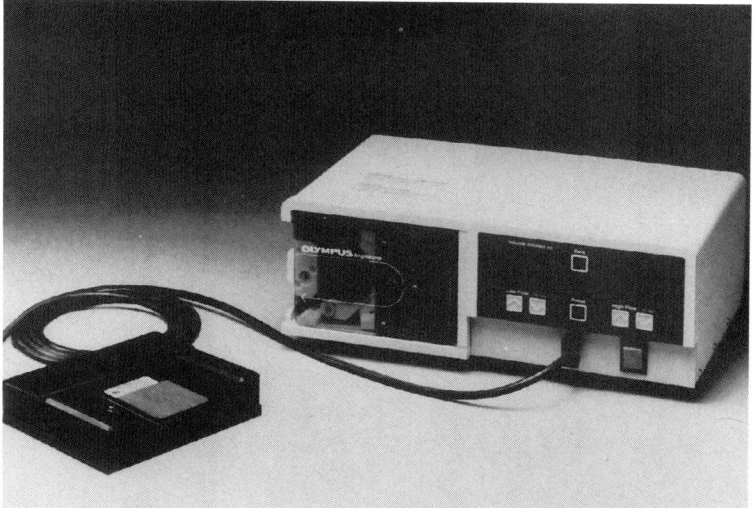

FIGURE 13–2. Dedicated irrigation pump (Angiopump, Olympus Corporation) controlled with foot pedal. High and low flow rates may be set independently. Safety features include bubble detector and monitor to measure total volume infused.

and the exact volume of fluid being injected into the patient is difficult to monitor until termination of the procedure, when the pressure cuff is removed and the saline bag examined.

Together with the Olympus Corporation (Lake Success, NY), we developed a dedicated irrigation pump (Angiopump, Figure 13–2) for angioscopy. This pump is designed to provide flow rates between 10 ml/min and 400 ml/min and to generate a maximum pressure of 2000 mm Hg at the pump head. The pump provides for the selection of two independent flow rates, a high flow rate, or *bolus*, and a low flow rate, or *maintenance*. These flow-rate settings are variable and independent of each other and may be adjusted either before or during the procedure. The flow rate is controlled remotely with a foot pedal, allowing switching back and forth from bolus to maintenance so that, after the column of clear fluid is established, it may be maintained at all times in the vessel under examination.[18]

A serious concern when infusing fluid intraarterially into a relatively restricted outflow tract at high flow rates is that excessively high intraarterial pressures may be generated, which could damage either the intimal lining or inner layer of the arterial wall even to the extent of complete rupture. In our experimental and clinical studies we have shown this not to be a problem, provided the vessel is not totally occluded or the irrigation is ceased as soon as clearing of the visual field occurs.[18–20,22]

The most significant limitation of angioscopy is the volume of irrigation fluid that can safely be infused into a particular patient. In our experience during intraoperative angioscopy the volumes of fluid routinely required for irrigation with the dedicated irrigation pump, less than a half a liter, have not been excessive[19,20,22]; and provided the patient is carefully monitored, such volumes are safe even in the elderly and ill population typically undergoing infrainguinal bypass surgery. Furthermore, no increased patient morbidity or mortality in the intraoperative, perioperative, or early postoperative (<30 days) periods could be demonstrated, even in patients with the highest preoperative cardiovascular risk status.[22] The irrigation fluid volumes necessary for successful completion angioscopy are safe, provided the anesthetist is aware that angioscopy is to be performed, runs the patient "dry" until the angioscopy is completed, and includes the irrigation fluid in the calculations of the patient's total fluid requirements.

Techniques of Angioscopy

We have previously described in detail the basic techniques for intraoperative angioscopy.[23] The standard equipment and technique for setting up in the operating room are shown in Figure

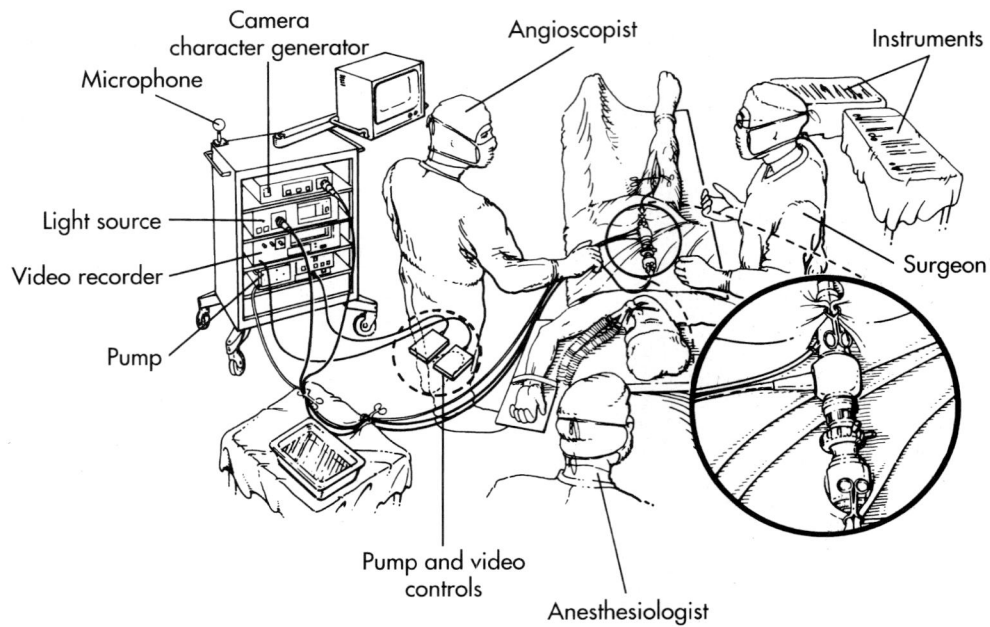

FIGURE 13–3. Angioscopy equipment and setup in the operating room. (From Miller A, Jepsen S: Technique of intraoperative angioscopy in lower extremity revascularization, In Bergan J, Yao J, editors: *Techniques in arterial surgery*, Philadelphia, 1990, WB Saunders.)

13–3. For each angioscopic application we use a standard method of angioscopic examination. The following general principles are important to achieve consistently good studies, maintain safety, and avoid complications.

1. To avoid inducing spasm in the native artery or vein, choose an angioscope for the procedure smaller than the lumen of the smallest vessel to be intubated and pass it through these vessels only in the presence of flowing blood or irrigation fluid. Passage of an angioscope occupying almost the entire lumen of the vessel or passage in a vessel emptied of all blood or irrigation fluid may result in intense, irreversible vasospasm.

2. To minimize the irrigation fluid volume and optimize the duration of angioscopic imaging, do the following:

    a. Perform angioscopy on withdrawal whenever possible.

    b. During completion angioscopy for bypass grafts, occlude the artery just proximal to the distal anastomosis whenever possible. This reduces the size of the outflow tract and the likelihood of any blood mingling with the clear column of irrigation fluid.

    c. Whenever possible, reduce the retrograde flow or prevent it from flowing into the clear fluid column. In bypass grafts, when withdrawing the angioscope from the distal artery and anastomosis and moving it into the graft, occlude the distal end of the graft between the fingers or use a fine "bulldog" clamp to trap the column of clear fluid within the graft. During thrombectomy, external compression of the inflow or outflow vessels may reduce the blood flow.

3. We perform irrigation most commonly through a separate irrigation catheter or needle inserted collateral to the angioscope or, more recently, through an irrigation sheath with a proximal hemostatic valve, coaxial with the angioscope. Even with the dedicated angioscopy pump, flow rates achieved through angioscopes with built-in irrigation channels are

usually less than 175 ml/min and are often inadequate for successful angioscopic studies during infrainguinal bypass or thrombectomy. In certain situations with limited blood flow, such as vein conduit preparation, these flow rates may be sufficient.[24] In our experience, angioscopes with an irrigation channel of 1 mm are almost always too large and rigid to be inserted through the distal anastomosis and into the distal artery, particularly in bypass grafts distal to the popliteal arteries.

4. Do not pass the angioscope through the native vessels or graft unless flowing blood or normal vessel architecture is observed on the video monitor. A "white out" of the image means that the angioscope is abutting an obstruction; insertion should be halted and the angioscope withdrawn a few centimeters. If the obstruction remains and the freely flowing blood is not seen, further insertion of the angioscope must be performed under direct vision. This avoids injury to the vessels or the anastomotic structures, even if it means using more irrigation fluid, and prevents "buckling" of the optical fibers with irreparable damage to the angioscope.

5. Visualize the entire lumen of the vessels being studied to ensure completeness of the angioscopy study. This may be achieved using a steerable angioscope or manipulating a nonsteerable angioscope. Steerable angioscopes not only enhance the quality of the angioscopic study but are much easier to manipulate intraluminally than the standard nonsteerable angioscope. Although useful in the femoropopliteal and larger tibial vessels, their large size precludes use in many of the more distal bypass grafts. For the smaller nonsteerable angioscopes, rolling or torquing the angioscope between the plantar surfaces of the thumb and index finger allows rotation of the angioscope and the entire vessel circumference to be visualized. Direct manipulation on the distal end of the angioscope through the vessel wall is another method of ensuring full visualization of the entire lumen and in particular the anastomosis. Coordinating these manipulations is best achieved by watching the images produced on the monitor and making adjustments of position accordingly, not by attempting to directly position the angioscope tip within the anastomosis or lumen of the vessel or graft. These techniques significantly enhance the value of the studies and avoid missing relevant pathologic findings.

Interpretation

The value and reliability of the angioscopic examination is enhanced with the development of interpretative skills and experience of the endoscopist. These skills may be acquired from the review of previous studies and findings but are refined with the continued critical review and evaluation of the angioscopic findings after each study. Many of the findings are new, subtle, and of uncertain clinical significance. Careful follow-up and correlation with the clinical course will eventually establish the significance of these findings.

It is especially important to appreciate that the angioscope in its current form is a qualitative instrument. The accurate assessment of size of an angioscopic image on the video monitor remains problematic. Magnification of the image changes with the distance of the angioscope lens to an object; the closer the lens to the object, the larger the image.[5] This makes much of the interpretation of the angioscopic images subjective and the significance of many of the more subtle endoluminal findings difficult to assess, even with a large amount of experience. Methods to quantitate the angioscopic image would substantially enhance the value of angioscopy.

Clinical Applications

Indications

Our current indications for angioscopy are summarized in Box 13–3. The usefulness and varied applications of angioscopy depend in the main on the ingenuity and creativity of the individual surgeon. We conceptualize and use the angioscope as an adjunctive tool to see inside vessels so that rational and informed clinical and surgical decisions can be made with "objective" findings. We do not rely simply on "experience."

> **Box 13–3. Indications for Angioscopy of Peripheral Vessels**
>
> **Diagnostic:**
> Monitoring of surgical interventional procedures
>   Bypass, endarterectomy, thrombectomy, embolectomy, vascular access, preparation of renal transplants, and valvuloplasty for venous insufficiency
>   Angioplasty, atherectomy, stenting, and endoluminal grafting
>   Lesions responsible for anginal syndromes
>   Endoscopic findings and graft failure
>
> **Therapeutic:**
> Surgical
>   Endoluminal vein graft preparation (valvulotomy and tributary occlusion)
>   Catheter-directed thrombectomy or embolectomy
> Percutaneous
>   Thrombolysis
>   Assisted interventions (angioplasty, atherectomy, stenting, and endoluminal grafting)

Initially, we used angioscopy as a simple alternative or adjunct to the operative angiogram as a means to avoid or correct technical errors. However, we soon appreciated that the rich an detailed endoluminal information not only provides a sensitive and accurate method for the detection of technical errors but allows continual assessment of technical proficiency. It has become an excellent teaching tool, improving and refining surgical technique of the surgeon and resident staff. Angioscopy has also identified new or previously unappreciated endovascular pathologies that have enhanced our understanding of the pathogenesis of graft failure[25] and fostered the development and design of new instrumentation for intraluminal manipulations such as valve cutters, tributary occluders, and various grabbing and cutting intraluminal instruments.[21,24,26,27]

Infrainguinal Bypass Grafting

Angioscopy plays a significant role in infrainguinal bypass grafting. It allows preparation of the best-quality vein conduit available, irrespective of the configuration of the vein graft or the source of the vein. We have shown that, whereas the incidence of unsuspected endoluminal pathology of the saphenous vein[20] is between 10% and 20%, in arm veins[28] it is much more frequent, between 60% and 70% of arm veins harvested for grafting. It also allows the application of the minimal surgical techniques for the in situ vein graft and monitoring of the entire bypass graft after completion of the surgery, including the conduit, distal anastomosis, and distal artery, to assess technical success of the surgery.

Vein Conduit Preparation

Reversed Vein

We monitor all reversed veins for quality control and the detection of endoluminal defects. This may be performed ex vivo or after completion of the distal anastomosis. The advantage of examining the vein ex vivo is that no irrigation fluid enters the patient's circulation.

Nonreversed Vein

After harvesting the nonreversed vein, the angioscope is introduced through an irrigation sheath into the proximal portion of the vein; and the valvulotome, a modified Mills retrograde valvulotome, is introduced from the distal end of the vein. Irrigation fluid to distend the vein is provided through the sheath. Angioscopically directed valvulotomy proceeds smoothly, coordinating the movements of the valvulotome and angioscope so that the valvulotome is visualized at all times and guided to cut each valve leaflet accurately. This is perfomed ex vivo with no irrigation fluid entering the patient's circulation.

In Situ Vein Conduit Preparation

Open Technique. Our open technique of angioscopically directed valvulotomy with variations used, depending on clinical preference or circumstance, is shown in Figure 13–4. The greatest advantage of this technique is that it allows the accurate ligation of the tributaries before valvulotomy and thereby minimizes the volume of irrigation fluid needed; it also simplifies angioscopically directed valvulotomy. In general, the greater saphenous vein is completely exposed through a single continuous incision. The inflow and outflow arteries are dissected out, and the patient is systemically heparinized in a dosage of 0.5 to 1.5 mg/kg according to the surgeon's preference. Thereafter, the proximal end of the vein is divided and the saphenofemoral junction oversewn. The saphenous vein is likewise mobilized several centimeters distal to the distal arterial anastomotic site and ligated distally. The first proximal valve is invariably located close to the saphenofemoral junction and can be identified by gentle eversion of the vein and excised with scissors under direct vision. The vein is then gently distended with warm irrigation fluid (a balanced salt solution with normalized pH containing papaverine hydrochloride, 60 mg/500 ml, and heparin sodium, 2000 IU); and the flexible shaft of the valvulotome, with the blunt bullet-shaped introducer in place, is passed from the distal end to protrude through the proximal open end of the vein graft. The introducer is removed and replaced by the appropriate-sized cutting valvulotome head, and the valvulotome is withdrawn into the proximal vein. The angioscope is then introduced into the proximal end of the vein and the valvulotome visualized. The vein is flushed clear of blood, and the fluid is allowed to escape at the end of the vein opposite to that of the irrigation catheter. The valvulotome is gradually withdrawn under constant angioscopic visualization, avoiding all tributaries, and maneuvered accurately onto the center of each valve leaflet. Ideally, each leaflet is cut by a single pull on the valvulotome shaft. The valvulotome is then repositioned on the opposite valve leaflet, and the procedure is repeated throughout the length of the vein graft.

Semiclosed Techniques. The aim of semiclosed techniques is to minimize the size of the wound necessary to harvest and prepare the vein. Various techniques have been described. Mehigan described the technique of tributary ligation through small stab incisions at the same time as endoluminal valvulotomy.[24] Others have modified the technique with preoperative vein and tributary mapping.[29,30] These mapped tributaries are then ligated before valvulotomy through small stab incisions.

Exposure and mobilization of the arteries and the greater saphenous vein at the anticipated sites of proximal and distal anastomosis is similar to the open technique described in the preceding section. Generally, location and ligation of side branches are performed concurrently with valvulotomy. This reduces the volume of irrigation fluid required for the procedure. Others complete the valvulotomy and then ligate the marked-out tributaries. Side branch visualization from the interior of the saphenous vein is readily accomplished, since on the video monitor a branch site is characterized by a dimple in the side wall of the vein, from which often a thin stream of blood exudes if the irrigation stream is set at a low flow rate or discontinued. As each side branch is visualized, the valvulotome is positioned so that it points to the exact opening. The angioscope light transilluminates the skin of the leg at that point, and a small marking on the skin is made. The side branch can also be located both visually and by palpation of a vein, inside of which the tip of the valvulotome can be felt pointing to the exact orifice of the side branch. The side branch is thereby pinpointed and can be ligated with minimal mobilization of the vein, preserving the in situ character of the operation.

When the angioscope and valvulotome have reached the most distal aspect of the vein, all valves having been incised, a completion study to ensure that all valves have been cut is performed as the angioscope is slowly withdrawn. Each valve site is again inspected for completeness of incision and for incompetence. After removal of the angioscope, the proximal and distal anastomoses are performed in the usual fashion.

Our preferred technique is a combination of the open and semiclosed techniques. The entire vein is exposed through short interrupted skin

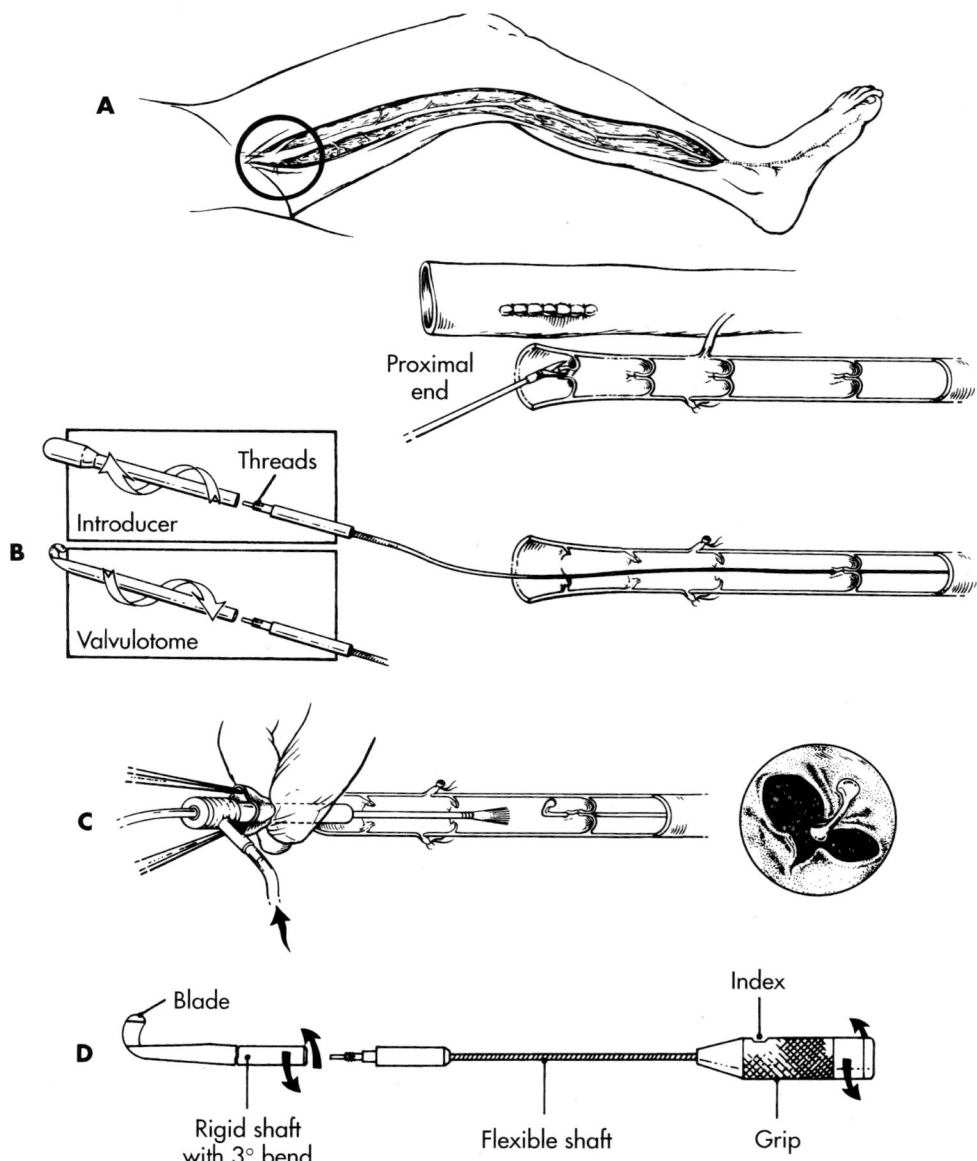

FIGURE 13–4. Angioscopically directed valvulotomy. **A,** Saphenous vein is completely exposed and tributaries ligated. Patient is heparinized and vein transected at both ends. Vein is gently distended with papaverine-heparin-saline solution, and the first proximal valve is excised with scissors. **B,** Valvulotome with introducer in place is passed through vein from distal end to protrude through proximal end of vein. Introducer is replaced with appropriately sized valvulotome. **C,** Valvulotome is withdrawn under constant angioscopic direction steering past the tributary orifices and accurately cutting each valve leaflet. **D,** Valvulotome. (From Miller A, Stonebridge P, Tsoukas A et al: Angioscopically directed valvulectomy: a new valvulotome and technique, *J Vasc Surg* 13:813–821, 1991.)

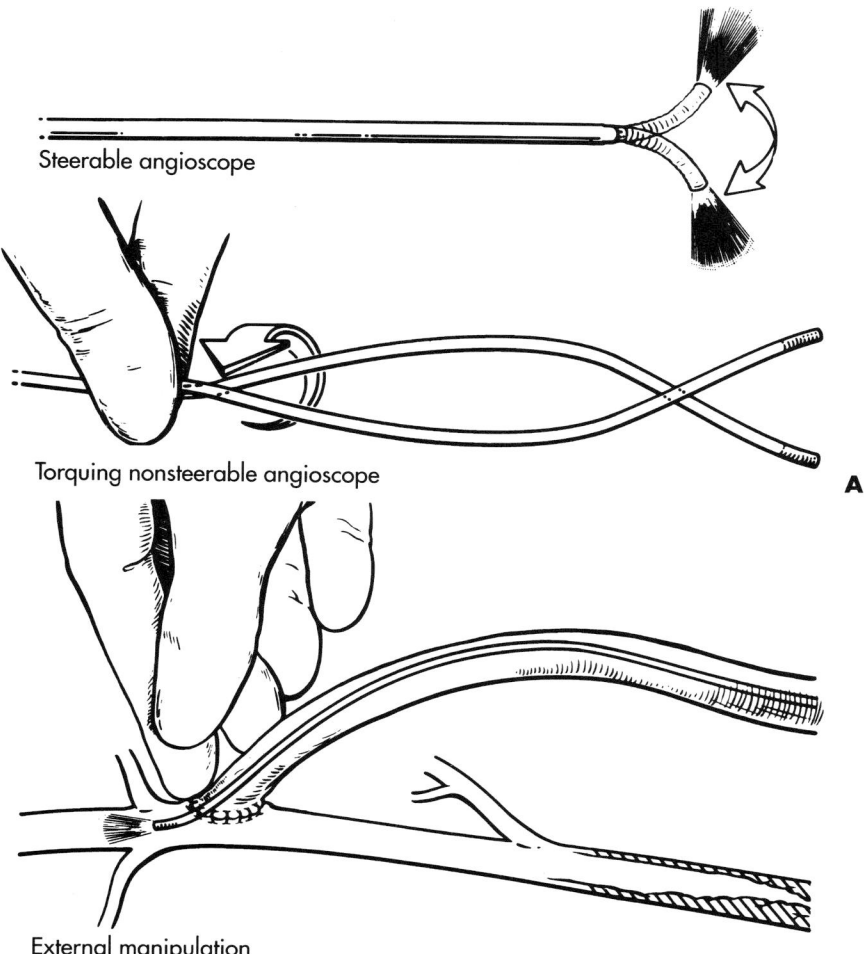

FIGURE 13–6. Technique of the completion angioscopy. **A**, Inspection of anastomotic region with distal outflow artery and methods to enhance angioscopic visualization. (From Miller A, Jepsen S: Technique of intraoperative angioscopy in lower extremity revascularization. In Bergan J, Yao J, editors: *Techniques in arterial surgery*, Philadelphia, 1990, WB Saunders.) **B**, Each valve site and ligated side branch are inspected for completeness while the angioscope is slowly withdrawn.

nous (AV) fistula. For autogenous AV fistula surgery, the angioscope is inserted through the open distal end of the outflow vein, either through an irrigation sheath or collateral to an irrigation catheter, where an in situ vein inspection is performed similarly to that described for arm vein harvesting in infrainguinal bypass grafting.[28] In the failing or occluded autogenous AV fistula, the angioscope is introduced into the vein at a site where the cause of failure is most likely, determined either by clinical examination or preoperative fistulogram. The angioscope is introduced in both antegrade and retrograde directions, allowing inspection of the runoff veins of the forearm and upper arm, as well as the proximal vein and anastomosis.[34]

In primary surgery for the synthetic bridge-graft vascular access surgery, the angioscope is inserted through the open end of the graft after completion of the venous anastomosis and tunneling of the graft. Again, irrigation is provided either with an irrigation sheath or collateral catheter. The outflow vein and the anastomosis are inspected. The techniques of angioscopy

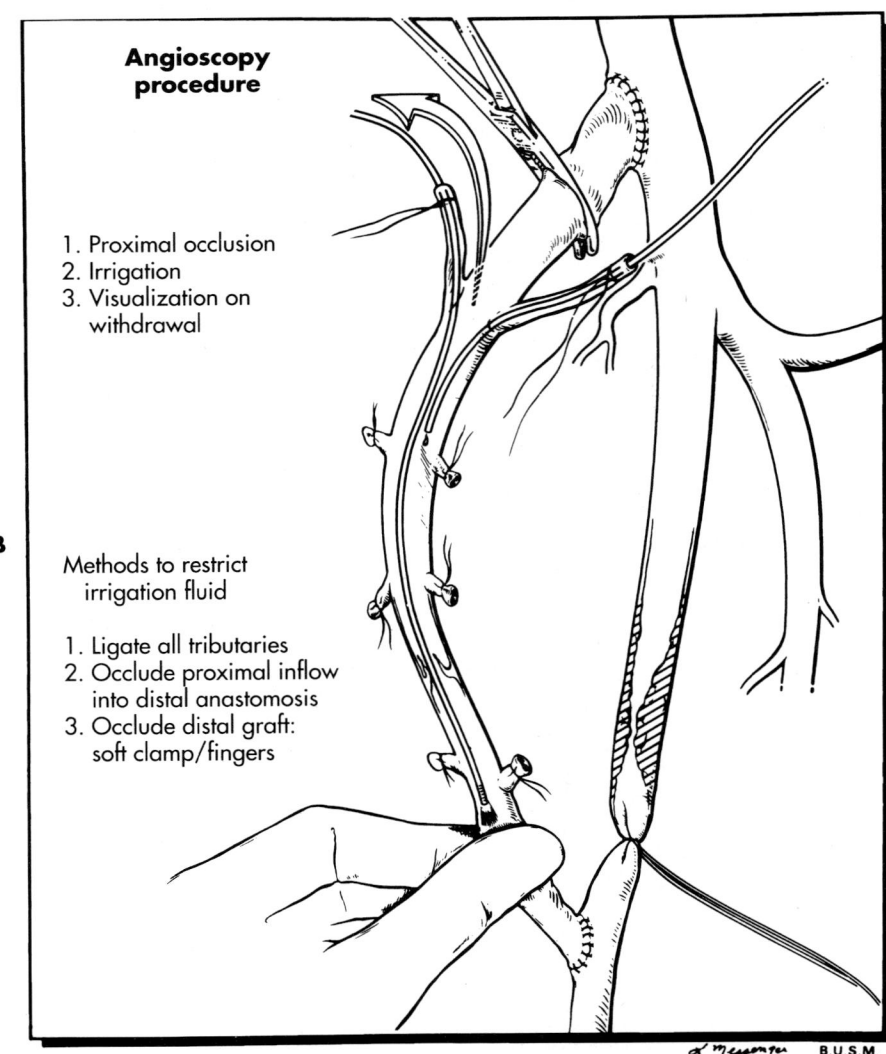

FIGURE 13–6. *Continued.*

unique for revision surgery in synthetic bridge grafts are illustrated in Figure 13–7.[35] A small skin incision is made, usually at the apex of the loop graft. A few centimeters of the synthetic graft are freed up, sufficient to allow placement of fine occluding clamps after reestablishing flow. Rummel tourniquets are placed to prevent leakage of irrigation fluid around the angioscope after insertion. A transverse incision is made in the anterior wall of the graft. Thrombectomy of the venous limb is generally performed first to take advantage of the lack of bleeding from the occluded arterial limb. The arterial limb is approached only after completion of all manipulations on the venous limb. The angioscope is then introduced through an irrigation sheath and passed through the graft, through the anastomosis, and into the runoff vein. The extent and location of any endoluminal pathology, completeness of the thrombectomy, or other endoluminal intervention are determined. Repeat angioscopic examination after each manipulation may be performed. On occasion, the light of the angioscope shining

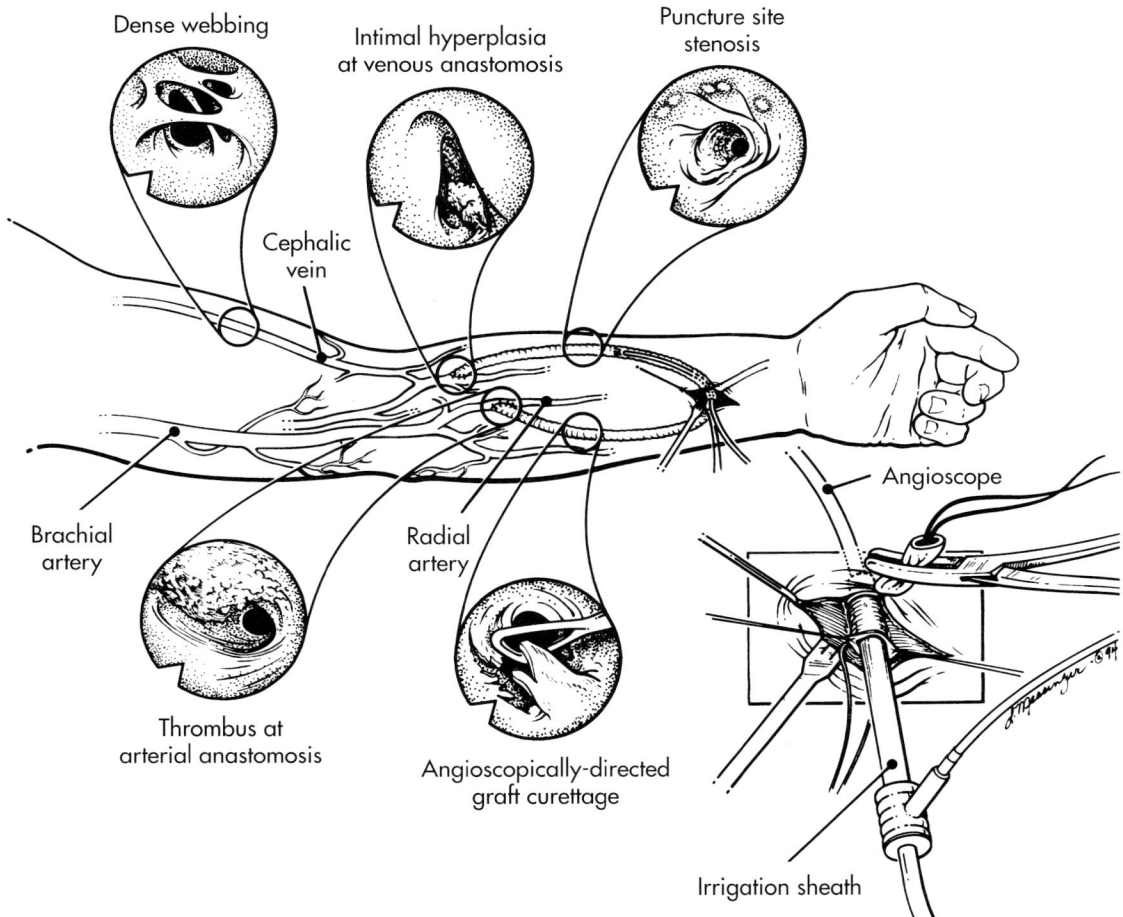

FIGURE 13–7. Technique of angioscopy to evaluate a failed vascular access graft. Angioscope, inserted through a small skin incision and a transverse graft arteriotomy, is dected toward venous and arterial anastomoses to evaluate the graft, both anastomoses, and native vessels. If additional sites of pathology are localized, direct limited exposures are facilitated by the light of the angioscope shining through the skin. Occlusive lesions can be removed under direct vision using a Kevorkian-Young curette. (From Hölzenbein T, Miller A, Gottlieb M et al.: The role of routine angioscopy in vascular access surgery, *J Endovasc Surg* 2:10–25, 1995.)

through the skin may serve as a guide to direct further exposure of the graft or autogenous vessel at the site of a particular abnormality. This allows much of the revision surgical procedure to be performed through separate small skin and graft incisions, limits surgical exposure of the graft and extent of the surgery, and eliminates the need for general anesthesia. In addition, to monitor thrombus removal with the various thrombectomy catheters, angioscopy may be used to direct removal of the excessively thickened intimal lining causing stenosis of the graft with a curette or any other interventional device.

To minimize the volume of irrigation fluid used during angioscopy, a tourniquet may be applied to the upper arm preoperatively, or simple digital pressure on the upper arm or inflow artery may be used. This may be helpful when repeated angioscopies are performed, particularly with multiple interventions.

Thromboembolectomy

After Fogarty balloon-catheter thromboembolectomy has been performed, the angioscope is introduced into the vessel or graft, usually through an irrigation sheath inserted into the arteriotomy or vein graft using the introducer guidewire system.[12] The presence and location of any residual thrombus is noted. Angioscopy can clearly differentiate between occlusive atherosclerotic plaque and residual thrombus and can assess the degree of stricture or stenosis. This information is often crucial in the clinical decision with regard to further reconstructive surgery. In the failed or failing vein graft the amount of residual thrombus after all thrombectomy interventions may aid in deciding whether salvage of the graft is worthwhile or if the vein graft conduit should be abandoned.[34] To retrieve any residual thrombus, the balloon catheter is reinserted together with the angioscope and the thrombus removed under visual control. Adherent thrombus can be removed from the vessel wall with special balloon catheters or directly with various endoluminal microforceps. Using an occlusion balloon, the occluded limb of an aortofemoral bypass graft may be safely thrombectomized and the cause of the occlusion, most commonly an anastomotic stenosis, corrected through a small groin incision.[36]

Venous Thrombectomy

Angioscopy has been used for monitoring completeness of venous thrombectomy.[37] After the disobliteration of the iliac and femoral veins via transfemoral thrombectomy, the proximal common iliac vein is isolated with a proximal occlusion catheter and large tributaries isolated and controlled. Antegrade angioscopy is performed until the occlusion catheter is observed and the venous thrombectomy completed. When indicated, the proximal femoral vein can be examined in a retrograde fashion. The angioscope can pass through the valve without injury if powerful sural compression is performed with simultaneous momentary cessation of irrigation.[38] Isolation of the venous segment is critical to limit the total volume of irrigation fluid used.

Venous Valve Repair Without Venotomy

Valvular incompetence is the most common cause of chronic venous insufficiency, with an incidence approaching 70%.[39] Valvuloplasty has shown promising results in the management of this difficult, debilitating clinical problem. The most critical part of the surgical technique is to determine the location and number of sutures required to reestablish valvular competence. Angioscopy provides direct visual and functional information on the competence of the valve repair without the necessity of a venotomy.[40,41] Exclusion of the venous segment is done by the appropriate clamp placement and temporary occlusion of the tributaries. The angioscope is inserted through a tributary. The repair of the incompetent valve is performed by external placement of 7-0 monofilament polypropylene sutures. Suture placement is facilitated by transillumination of the vein wall by the light source of the angioscope, which clearly defines the insertion lines of each valve leaflet, and needle placement is directed by the angioscope. Assessment of the valvular competence is done after placement and tying of each suture, using the irrigation fluid infused through the angioscope to oppose the valve leaflets.

Percutaneous Applications of Angioscopy

Depending on the size of angioscope, introducer sheaths from 6F to 9F can be used. Percutaneous angioscopy may be performed through a direct antegrade needle stick of the superficial femoral artery just below the bifurcation of common femoral artery using the introducer sheath[11,13,16] or a small angioscope [<1mm outer diameter (OD)] through an angioplasty catheter passed over the aortic bifurcation into the contralateral superficial femoral artery. The angioscope is guided to the endoluminal lesions identified on fluoroscopy using standard contrast studies. Placing a radiopaque marker on the tip of the angioscope is useful. Proximal occlusion can be achieved by using a sheath large enough to occlude the superficial femoral artery, external compression of the femoral artery, or an angioplasty balloon inflated proximal to the angioscope. Irrigation is through the sheath or angioplasty catheter with the variable flow of between 300 to 400 ml/min using the dedicated angioscopy irrigation pump. To minimize the irrigation fluid requirements, a tourniquet may be applied below the knee joint to reduce the collateral circulation.

Conclusion

Since performing our first clinical angioscopy, we have performed intraoperative angioscopy during more than 1500 revascularization procedures. Our clinical studies have been directed to systematically evaluate this technology and evaluate its place in the modern practice of vascular surgery. As outlined in this chapter, angioscopy is a useful clinical tool for the modern practicing vascular surgeon. It provides endoluminal information on the vasculature remote from the surgical site and exposed vessels, which enhances the intraoperative decision-making process. Angioscopy has proven a most valuable tool for monitoring the technical success of reconstructive surgery, for quality control of the graft conduit, and for providing a reliable method to assess the effectiveness of endoluminal surgery and interventions.

References

1. Vollmar J, Storz L: Vascular endoscopy, *Surg Clin North Am* 54:111–122, 1974.
2. Towne J, Bernhard V: Vascular endoscopy: an adjunct to carotid surgery, *Stroke* 8:569–571, 1977.
3. Towne J, Bernhard V: Technique of intraoperative endoscopic evaluation of occluded aortofemoral grafts following thrombectomy, *Surg Gynecol Obstet* 148:87–89, 1979.
4. Shure D, Gregoratos G, Moser K: Fiberoptic angioscopy: role in the diagnosis of chronic pulmonary artery obstruction, *Ann Intern Med* 103:844–850, 1985.
5. Spears J, Marais H, Serur J et al: In vivo coronary angioscopy, *J Am Coll Cardiol* 1:1311–1314, 1983.
6. Grundfest W, Litvack F, Sherman T et al: Delineation of peripheral and coronary detail by intraoperative angioscopy, *Ann Surg* 202:394–400, 1985.
7. Grundfest W, Litvack F, Glick D et al: Intraoperative decisions based on angioscopy in peripheral vascular surgery, *Circulation* 78(suppl I):I13–I17, 1988.
8. Sherman T, Litvack F, Grundfest W et al: Coronary angioscopy in patients with unstable angina pectoris, *N Engl J Med* 315:913–919, 1986.
9. Seeger J, Abela G: Angioscopy as an adjunct to arterial reconstructive surgery: a preliminary report, *J Vasc Surg* 4:315–320, 1986.
10. Mehigan J, Olcott C: Videoangioscopy as an alternative to intraoperative arteriography, *Am J Surg* 152:139–145, 1986.
11. Beck A: Percutaneous angioscopy. First reports on percutaneous transluminal angioplasty and local lysis under angioscopic conditions, *Radiologe* 27:555–559, 1987.
12. White G, White R, Kopchok B et al: Angioscopic thromboembolectomy: preliminary observations with a recent techique, *J Vasc Surg* 7:318–325, 1988.
13. Lee G, Morelli R, Long J et al: Combined laser-thermal and atherectomy treatment of peripheral arterial occlusion: documentation by angioscopy and angiography, *Am Heart J* 118:1324–1327, 1989.
14. Mehigan J, DeCampli W: Angioscopic control of carotid endarterectomy. In Ahn SS. Moore WS, editors: *Endovascular surgery*, ed 2, Philadelphia, 1992, WB Saunders.
15. Raithel D, Kasprzak P: Angioscopy after carotid endarterectomy, *Ann Chir Gynaecol* 81:192–195, 1992.
16. Dietrich E, Yoffe B, Kiessling J et al: Angioscopy in endovascular surgery: recent technical advances to enhance intervention selection and failure analysis, *Angiology* 43:1–10, 1992.
17. Silverman S, Mladinich C, Hawkins I et al: The use of carbon dioxide gas to displace flowing blood during angioscopy, *J Vasc Surg* 10:313–317, 1989.
18. Miller A, Lipson W, Isaacsohn J et al: Intraoperative angioscopy: principles of irrigation and description of a new dedicated irrigation pump, *Am Heart J* 118:391–399, 1989.
19. Miller A, Campbell D, Gibbons G et al: Routine intraoperative angioscopy in lower extremity revascularization, *Arch Surg* 124:604–608, 1989.

20. Miller A, Stonebridge P, Jepsen S et al: Continued experience with intraoperative angioscopy for monitoring infrainguinal bypass grafting, *Surgery* 109:286-293, 1991.
21. Miller A, Stonebridge P, Tsoukas A et al: Angioscopically directed valvulotomy: a new valvulotome and technique, *J Vasc Surg* 13:813-821, 1991.
22. Kwolek C, Miller A, Stonebridge P et al: Safety of saline irrigation for angioscopy: results of a prospective randomized trial, *Ann Vasc Surg* 6:62-68, 1992.
23. Miller A, Jepsen S: Technique of intraoperative angioscopy in lower extremity revascularization. In Bergan J, Yao J, editors: *Techniques in arterial surgery*, Philadelphia, 1990, WB Saunders.
24. Mehigan J: Angioscopic preparation of the in situ saphenous vein for arterial bypass technical considerations. In White G, White R, editors: Angioscopy: vascular and coronary applications, St Louis, 1989, Mosby.
25. Miller A, Jepsen S, Stonebridge P et al: New angioscopic findings in graft failure after infrainguinal bypass grafting, *Arch Surg* 125:749-755, 1990.
26. Stierli P, Aeberhard P: Angioscopy-guided semiclosed technique for in site bypass with a novel flushing valvulotome: early results, *J Vasc Surg* 15:546-548, 1992.
27. White G, White R, Kopock G et al: Endoscopic intravascular surgery removes intraluminal flaps, dissections, and thrombus, *J Vasc Surg* 11:280-288, 1990.
28. Marcaccio E, Miller A, Tannenbaum G et al: Angioscopically directed interventions improve arm vein bypass grafts, *J Vasc Surg* 17:994-1004, 1993.
29. La Muraglia G, Cambria R, Brewster D et al.: Angioscopy facilitates a closed technique for in-situ vein bypass, *J Vasc Surg* 12:601-604, 1990.
30. Maini B, Andrews L, Salimi T et al: A modified, angioscopically assisted technique for in situ saphenous vein bypass: impact on patency, complications, and length of stay, *J Vasc Surg* 17:1041-1049, 1993.
31. Rosenthal D, Cickson C, Rodriguez FL et al: Infrainguinal endovascular in situ saphenous vein bypass: ongoing results. *J Vasc Surg* 20:389-395, 1994.
32. Miller A, Marcaccio E, Tannenbaum G et al.: Comparison of angioscopy and angiography for monitoring infrainguinal bypass grafts: results of a prospective randomized trial, *J Vasc Surg* 17:382-398, 1992.
33. Gaunt M, Naylor A, Ratliff D et al.: Role of completion angioscopy in detecting technical error after carotid endarterectomy, *Br J Surg* 81:42-44, 1994.
34. Hölzenbein T, Miller A, Tannenbaum G et al: Role of angioscopy in reoperation for the failing or failed infrainguinal vein bypass graft, *Ann Vasc Surg* 8:74-91, 1994.
35. Hölzenbein T, Miller A, Gottlieb M et al: The role of routine angioscopy in vascular access surgery, *J Endovasc Surg* 2:10-25, 1995.
36. White J, Haas K, Comerota A: An alternative method of salvaging occluded suprainguinal bypass grafts with operative angioscopy and endovascular intervention, *J Vasc Surg* 18:922-931, 1993.
37. Vollmar J, Hutschenreiter S: Vascular endoscopy for venous thrombectomy, In Ahn SS, Moore WS, editors: Endovascular surgery, ed 2, Philadephia, 1992, WB Saunders.
38. Woelfle K, Bruijnen H, Zuegel N et al.: Technique and results of vascular endoscopy in arterial and venous reconstructions, *Ann Vasc Surg* 6:347-356, 1992.
39. Raju S, Fredericks R: Valve reconstruction procedures for nonobstructive venous insufficiency: rationale, techniques, and results in 107 procedures with two- to eight-year follow-up, *J Vasc Surg* 7:301-310, 1988.
40. Gloviczki P, Merrell S, Bower T: Femoral vein valve repair under direct vision without venotomy: a modified technique with use of angioscopy, *J Vasc Surg* 14:645-648, 1991.
41. Welch H, McLaughlin R, O'Donnell T Jr: Femoral vein valvuloplasty: intraoperative angioscopic evaluation and hemodynamic improvement, *J Vasc Surg* 16:694-700, 1992.

14
Intravascular Ultrasound Imaging

Martin R. Back, George E. Kopchok, and Rodney A. White

Development of miniaturized piezoelectric transducers positioned at the end of intraluminal catheters has allowed high-resolution, ultrasonic imaging of various cardiac, vascular, and hollow organ structures. Current intravascular ultrasound (IVUS) catheters provide real-time, luminal, and transmural cross-sectional imaging in large vessels with dimensional accuracy. IVUS can also delineate wall morphology, lesion shape, volume, length, and branch configuration. Concomitant rapid expansion of minimally invasive endovascular therapies in coronary and peripheral vasculature have added new roles for IVUS. In addition to diagnostic information, IVUS enables choice of appropriate angioplasty technique, endovascular device guidance, and controlled assessment of the efficacy of interventions. Real-time IVUS imaging can only be used during invasive diagnostic and therapeutic procedures after vascular access is established. Further acceptance and implementation relies on the effectiveness of IVUS in improving endovascular outcomes and minimizing periprocedural complications as compared with alternative imaging modalities. This chapter reviews the design and function of available IVUS catheters, imaging techniques, and interpretation and the present and future clinical utility in peripheral endovascular interventions.

Device Design and Function

The first IVUS prototypes were used to measure intracardiac dimensions and cardiac motion in the 1950s, utilizing A-mode transducers fixed to large intraluminal catheters.[1,2] Various devices (A-, B-, and M-mode) were developed for both intravascular and transesophageal imaging of vascular structures, but it was not until the early 1970s that intraluminal, cross-sectional imaging of vessels was reported using a multielement array transducer.[3-6] To obtain a 360° cross-sectional image, the ultrasound beam must be scanned through a full circle and the beam direction and deflection on the display synchronized. This can be achieved by mechanically rotating the imaging element or by using electronically switched (or phased) arrays (Figure 14–1).

Current multiple-element IVUS catheters use frequencies in the range of 15 to 25 MHz. The plane of imaging is perpendicular to the long axis of the catheter and provides a full 360° image of the blood vessel. A problem of the early phased array devices was the electronic noise caused by the multiple wires within the catheter itself, since each of the elements was an independent minitransducer needing its own connections. This problem was later overcome by the incorporation of a miniature integrated circuit at the tip of the catheter, which provided sequenced transmission and reception without the need for numerous electrical circuits traveling the full length of the catheter. In addition to reducing the electronic noise, this modification simplified the manufacturing complexity and improved the flexibility of the catheter. A problem of these imaging catheters, common to all high-frequency ultrasound

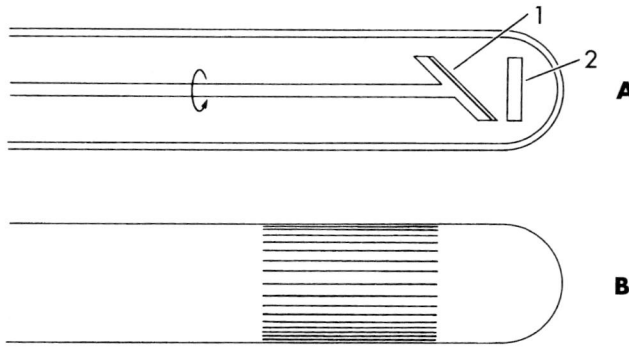

FIGURE 14–1. **A**, Mechanical ultrasound device with rotating (*1*) and fixed (*2*) elements. Either the transducer or the mirror may be fixed with the other element in a rotating position. **B**, Phased-array device with the elements arranged circumferentially around the tip of the catheter. (From White RA: Indications for fiberoptic angioscopy and intraluminal ultrasound, *Compr Ther* 16:23–30, 1990.)

devices to some extent, is the inability to image structures in the immediate vicinity of the transducer (i.e., in the "near field"). Because the imaging crystals in a phased array configuration are in almost direct contact with the structure being imaged, a bright circumferential artifact known as the *ring down* surrounds the catheter. The ring-down artifact can be electronically removed, but structures within the masked region will not be imaged.

Mechanical transducers are the most frequently used type of IVUS catheters and are of two basic configurations. Either the transducer itself or an acoustic mirror is rotated at the tip of the catheter using a flexible, high-torque cable that extends the length of the device (Figure 14–2). Catheters using a rotating transducer that is directed at less than 90° from the catheter's long axis produces a cone-shaped ultrasound image of the vessel slightly forward in front of the transducer assembly. In the rotating mirror devices, the ultrasound energy produced by the fixed transducer at the distal tip of the catheter is directed toward an angled mirror placed a short distance proximally. The mirror is set at a 45° angle to the rotating shaft, producing an image that is exactly perpendicular to the axis of the catheter. In both rotating transducer and rotating mirror devices, ultrasound frequencies between 10 and 30 MHz are generally used, although some experimental devices using frequencies up to 45 MHz have produced excellent images of human arteries in vitro.[7]

In addition to avoiding the necessity for rotating the transducer, an advantage of the rotating mirror configuration is afforded by the necessary distance between the transducer and the mirror, partially eliminating the ring-down image artifact and the poor near-field resolution. Both of these problems are substantially reduced by allowing the ultrasound energy to travel a short distance in the imaging chamber filled with saline. The scan converter in the image processing unit compensates for this nonimaging portion of the beam and generates images beginning at the surface of the catheter. In the rotating transducer and multiple array devices, a part of the ring-down region and near-field zone of the beam occurs outside the catheter so it is not possible to image clearly in this area. However, both types of mechanical imaging catheters suffer from less image loss resulting from these problems than do the phased array transducers.[8] In devices with a distally placed transducer and proximal rotating mirror, it is necessary for an electrical connecting wire to pass along the side of the imaging assembly. This wire produces an artifact that occupies approximately 15° of the image cross section. An interesting modification of the mechanical catheter design involves rotation of both the transducer and the mirror, offering the advantage of no electrical wire artifact. Current disposable mechanical catheters use a saline- or water-filled imaging chamber that must be maintained bubble-free to allow adequate imaging.

Necessary miniaturization of the moving parts of the rotating mechanical systems is a challenge to their utility in smaller-caliber vessels. On the other hand, as phased array catheters are used in progressively smaller vessels, the problems of ring-down and near-

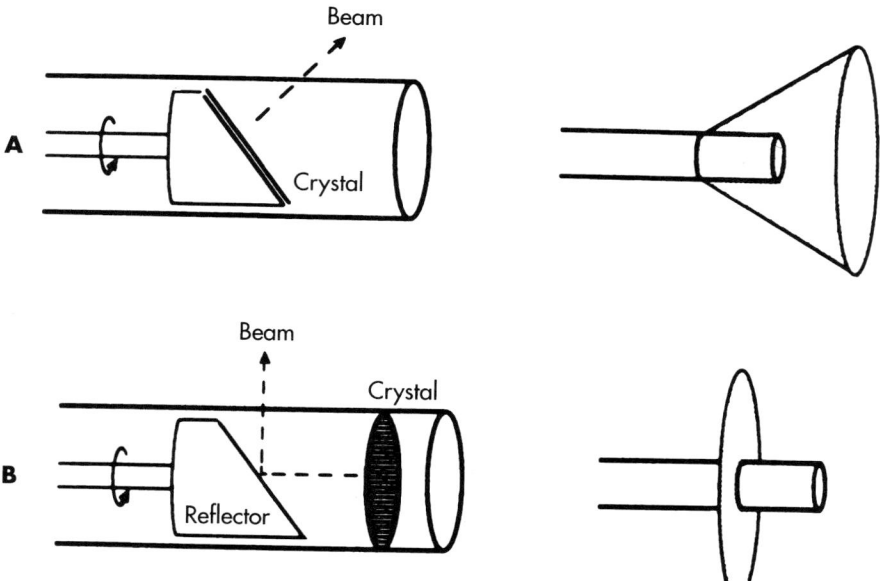

FIGURE 14–2. **A**, Rotating element device (*left*) where the ultrasound beam is directed forward of perpendicular with respect to the catheter long axis, producing a cone-shaped imaging plane (*right*). **B**, Rotating mirror configuration (*left*) where the ultrasound beam is directed at a 90° angle to the catheter axis, producing a true cross-sectional imaging plane (*right*). (From Yock PG et al: Two-dimensional intravascular ultrasound: technical development and initial clinical experience, *J Am Soc Echocardiogr* 2:296–304, 1989.)

field imaging become more appreciable. The smallest currently available mechanical catheters (2.9F or 0.9mm diameter) approximate the size of diseased coronary arteries; and, when used with higher frequency ultrasound, they may prove to be superior in most applications. Newer prototype catheters are 0.035 inch in diameter and will pass through the lumen of devices that will accommodate this size guidewire.

Imaging Techniques

Access

The IVUS catheters can be introduced either percutaneously through a standard vascular access sheath (5F to 10F) or via an arteriotomy or venotomy during an open procedure. If large vessels proximal to the arteriotomy are imaged (e.g., iliac artery imaging via a femoral cutdown), a hemostatic access device should be used to reduce blood loss and prevent catheter damage during insertion. In most situations, a retrograde femoral puncture provides access to the entire aorta and aortoiliac segments, since IVUS catheters are available in lengths up to 125cm and are flexible. It is possible to pass some currently available IVUS catheters over a guidewire across the aortic bifurcation from a femoral artery puncture to the contralateral iliac or femoral artery, but orientation of the image can be difficult in this setting. Antegrade femoral artery puncture is used to image the infrainguinal vessels, particularly if an endovascular intervention such as atherectomy is planned. A retrograde popliteal approach can be used to provide access to a patent distal superficial femoral artery when there is occlusion at the origin of that vessel. Percutaneous brachial or axillary puncture provides access to upper limb vessels and may be more convenient for imaging the thoracic aorta in cases of major aortic dissection.

Image Acquisition

Mechanical and phased array IVUS catheters are available in the range of 2.9F to 12F diameter. Smaller-diameter catheters use higher ultrasound transducer frequencies with greater resolution but decreased depth of beam penetration into adjacent tissues. Phased array devices are generally more flexible and do not require careful flushing. When using mechanical devices, the catheter lumen and guidewire channel must be flushed manually with saline or water to ensure a bubble-free fluid medium within the imaging chamber. Repeated, low-pressure manual irrigations may be necessary to clear all bubbles from the system, and care must be taken not to overdistend the device, which can cause damage to the imaging chamber.

Several IVUS devices can be passed over a guidewire (0.009 to 0.038 inch in diameter), which allows more controlled maneuvering of the device within the lumen of the vessel from a remote introduction site, particularly in tortuous or tightly stenotic vessels. Because of the configuration of mechanical rotating catheters, a central guidewire channel is not possible, and these catheters have a variety of monorail and coaxial lumen options for over-the-wire applications. Multielement array devices use a central guidewire channel, which offers potential advantages if the IVUS images are to be used for angioplasty device guidance. When IVUS is used to image vessels before and after interventions such as balloon angioplasty or stent deployment, a guidewire is essential to allow manipulation of the catheters and repeated crossing of the lesion without further disruption of the angioplasty or stent site.

It is important to orient the IVUS catheter within the vessel so that anteroposterior accuracy can be achieved. One method to maintain proper alignment involves the use of the image artifact produced by the mechanical transducer connecting wire and establishing correct initial positioning during catheter insertion. The image artifact can be rotationally aligned with both an external longitudinal mark on the catheter and the vessel lumen being imaged (Figure 14–3). When imaging the aortoiliac segments via a femoral puncture site, rotational accuracy can also be confirmed by the relative position of constant anatomic landmarks. For example, as the catheter crosses the aortic bifurcation, the common iliac arteries should be positioned side by side horizontally on the screen. Occasionally this anatomic arrangement is not true, especially in tortuous, dilated vessels, and the alignment must be checked against other parameters. The posteromedial position of the internal iliac artery orifices and the known position of the catheter at the site of insertion are used in combination to also provide the best possible rotational alignment of the device. Because the catheters are easily torqued, there is very little loss of orientation with rotation and manipulation during imaging.

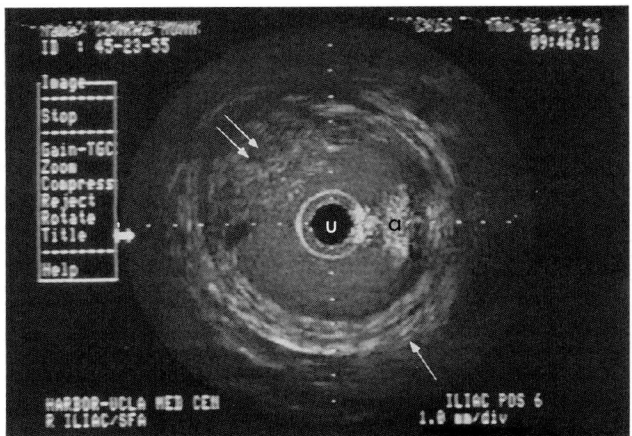

FIGURE 14–3. IVUS image of human iliac artery. *u*, void from ultrasound probe; *single arrow*, normal vessel wall; *double arrow*, soft, fibrous plaque; *a*, artifact produced by transducer electrical wire. (From Tabbara, M, White RA, Cavaye DM et al: In-vivo human comparison of intravascular ultrasound and angiography, *J Vasc Surg* 14:496–504, 1991.)

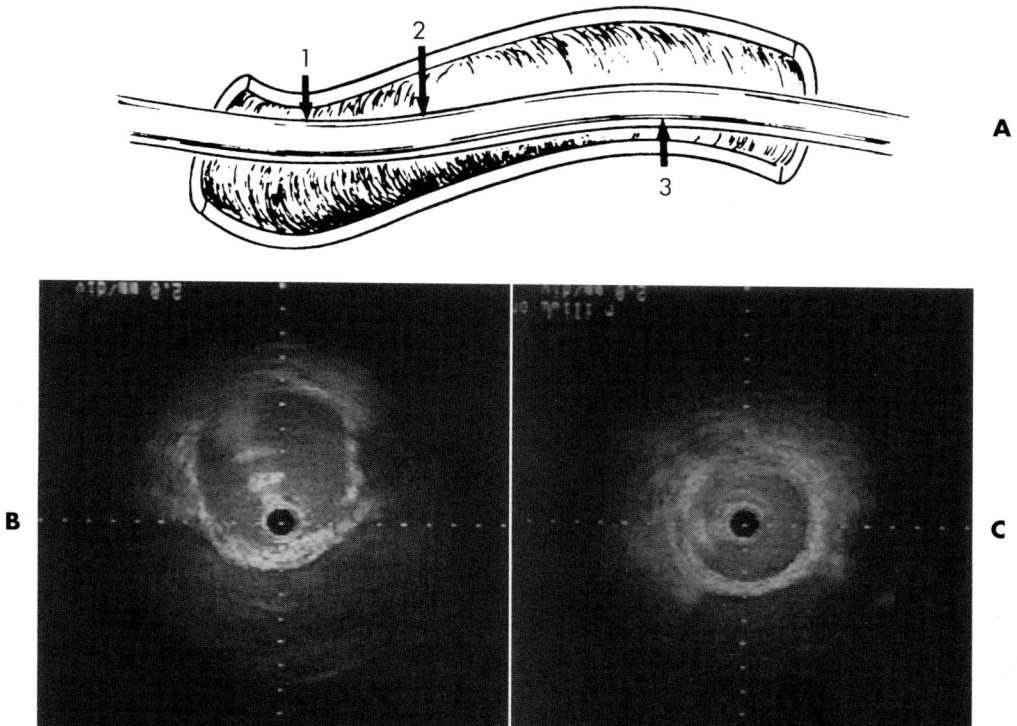

FIGURE 14-4. **A**, Schematic representation of an IVUS catheter within a tortuous vessel. The tip of the catheter lies within the lumen in the same position as the shaft, resulting in images of varying eccentricity. At positions *1* and *3*, the catheter lies against the vessel wall, and at position *2* the catheter is centered within the lumen. **B**, Eccentric image produced at positions *1* or *3* showing highly echogenic near wall and hypoechoic distant wall. **C**, Concentric image produced at position *2* showing relatively equal echogenicity of the wall at all locations. (From Cavaye DM, White RA: *Intravascular ultrasound imaging*, New York, 1993, Raven Press.)

Careful positioning of the catheter tip within the vessel and appropriate size matching of the device to the artery caliber are essential to optimizing visualization. Image quality is best when the catheter is parallel to the vessel wall (i.e., the ultrasound beam is directed at 90° to the luminal surface), although minor angulations may affect the luminal shape and dimensional accuracy. Eccentric positioning of the catheter within the vessel cross section causes the wall nearer the imaging chamber to appear more hyperechoic than the distant wall, resulting in an artifactual difference in wall thicknesses (Figure 14-4). Although the off-center position may not be an immediate problem during standard two-dimensional IVUS imaging, the differences in mural echogenicity produced by eccentric catheter positioning may greatly affect the results of three-dimensional image reconstructions. Catheter centering is especially difficult in tortuous vessels, and rotational alignment may also be partly lost as the catheter meanders through the vessel. The best-quality images are generally obtained as the catheter is withdrawn through the lumen rather than during advancement. In tortuous segments within a limb, manual pressure applied to skin overlying the vessel may aid in centering the catheter within the lumen.

With the use of higher-frequency ultrasound transducers and shorter imaging distances in small-caliber vessels, the echogenic character of

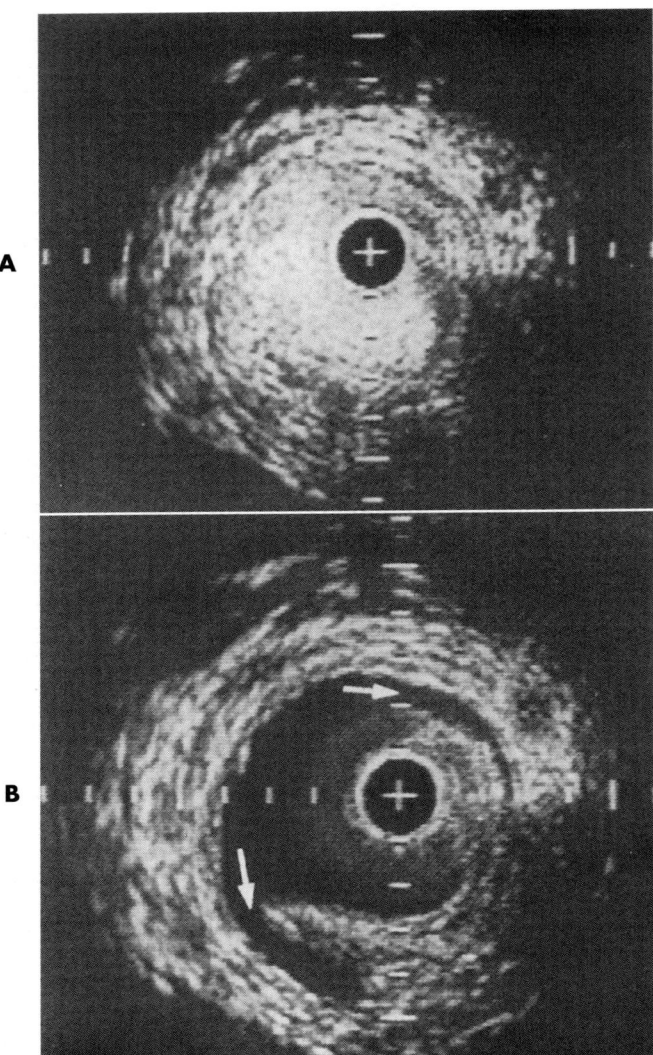

FIGURE 14-5. IVUS images of the superficial femoral artery showing the advantage of saline flushing. **A**, Echogenicity of blood obscures the intimal detail. **B**, After saline irrigation of the imaged vessel, the lumen/intima interface is enhanced showing plaque dissection (*arrow*). (From van Urk H, Gussenhoven WJ, Gerritsen GP et al: Assessment of arterial disease and arterial reconstructions by intravascular ultrasound, *Int J Card Imaging* 6:157–164, 1991.)

blood surrounding the catheter is amplified. Although this problem can be partly overcome by adjustments of overall gain and use of image processing techniques such as time-gain-compensation and suppression, the echogenic blood may still obscure the interface between the lumen and vessel wall. Manual flushing of the catheter lumen with saline during imaging displaces blood and results in an echolucent lumen. This technique can improve the delineation of acoustic interfaces in lower flow, small, and medium-sized vessels (Figure 14–5).[9] Alternatively, radiographic or ultrasound contrast agents can be injected into the vessel being imaged to alter luminal echogenicity and allow interface enhancement at the wall.[10]

Computerized Image Reconstruction

Three-dimensional (3D) IVUS imaging has developed as a result of advances in digital computer graphics technology and mass data storage capabilities of personal computers. 3D image reconstruction involves either surface- or volume-rendering algorithms. Currently available 3D IVUS imaging uses surface rendering where object surfaces are assembled within computer memory and the image depicted on a 2D screen using techniques such as hidden-part removal, shading, translucency, dynamic rotation, and stereo projection.[11] With this technology, a longitudinally aligned set (up to 300 images per set) of consecutive 2D images obtained during a "pullback" through a vessel segment is assembled in sequence to produce the 3D image (Image Comm, Inc., Santa Clara, Calif) (Figure 14–6).[12] The "pullback" is performed by withdrawing the IVUS catheter at a uniform rate using a mechanical device at a rate of 1 cm every 4 seconds. The 2D IVUS data set from a 5-cm vessel segment is therefore gathered during a 20-second "pullback," which can be recorded on videotape or reconstructed on-line. The images are then sampled in digital format (i.e., "stacked") after analogue-to-digital conversion at rates of up to 7.5 frames per second (150 frames for a 20-second "pullback"). Preacquisition of these data provides the advantage of selection of the most suitable segments for reconstruction and allows the user to adjust screen cropping parameters to electronically eliminate the artifact of the IVUS catheter and other unwanted image data.

Computer processing time of approximately 12 seconds is required for the initial reconstruction of a high-resolution gray scale longitudinal 2D view of the vessel segment (Figure 14–7). This image represents a user-defined hemisection of the vessel for viewing luminal and transmural morphology in true multiple gray scale. Before final 3D reconstruction, the image density threshold is adjusted to optimize differentiation of structures. This step is particularly important when it is necessary to separate tissues of similar echodensity, such as soft plaque and thrombus. The 3D image is then displayed in multiple orientations to allow inspection of the arterial segment in all possible projections, both from within the lumen and from the adventitial surface (Figure 14–8). Other parameters such as image sharpness, contrast, and ambient light can be altered to improve the resolution of particular features being examined in the reconstructions. Images of the luminal volume alone can also be produced by removing vessel wall signals.

Although it has been shown that 2D cross-sectional IVUS and longitudinal gray scale reconstructions provide accurate luminal and transmural dimensions, the accuracy of currently available 3D imaging has not been established. By viewing all three image formats simultaneously on a screen, however, the location of the 2D image site along the length of the 3D image can be identified using a linear cursor and dimensions of a site on the 3D image can be estimated. A continuing problem associated with many 3D imaging techniques is the near-field effect of IVUS transducer frequencies of 20 to 30 MHz, which result in bright echoes of blood immediately surrounding the catheter. With improvement in 3D imaging software, data manipulation can partially reduce the blood artifact.

Current Clinical Utility

Diagnostic Capabilities

Two-dimensional images produced by IVUS catheters not only outline the luminal and adventitial surfaces of vessel segments but also can discriminate between normal and diseased components within the wall. In muscular arteries, distinct sonographic layers are visible, with the media appearing as an echolucent layer sandwiched between the more echodense intima and adventitia (Figure 14–3). The precise correlation between the ultrasound image and the histology of the muscular artery wall is still uncertain. The internal and external elastic laminae and adventitia are considered to be the backscatter substrates for the inner and outer echodense zones.[13,14] Precise measurements of adventitial thickness may be difficult to obtain unless the vessel is surrounded by tissues of differing echogenicity, such as echolucent fat. Even small lesions such as intimal flaps or tears are well visualized because of their high fibrous tissue content and the contrasting echoic properties of surrounding blood. The three-layer appearance of medium-sized muscular arteries is lost in smaller distal vasculature

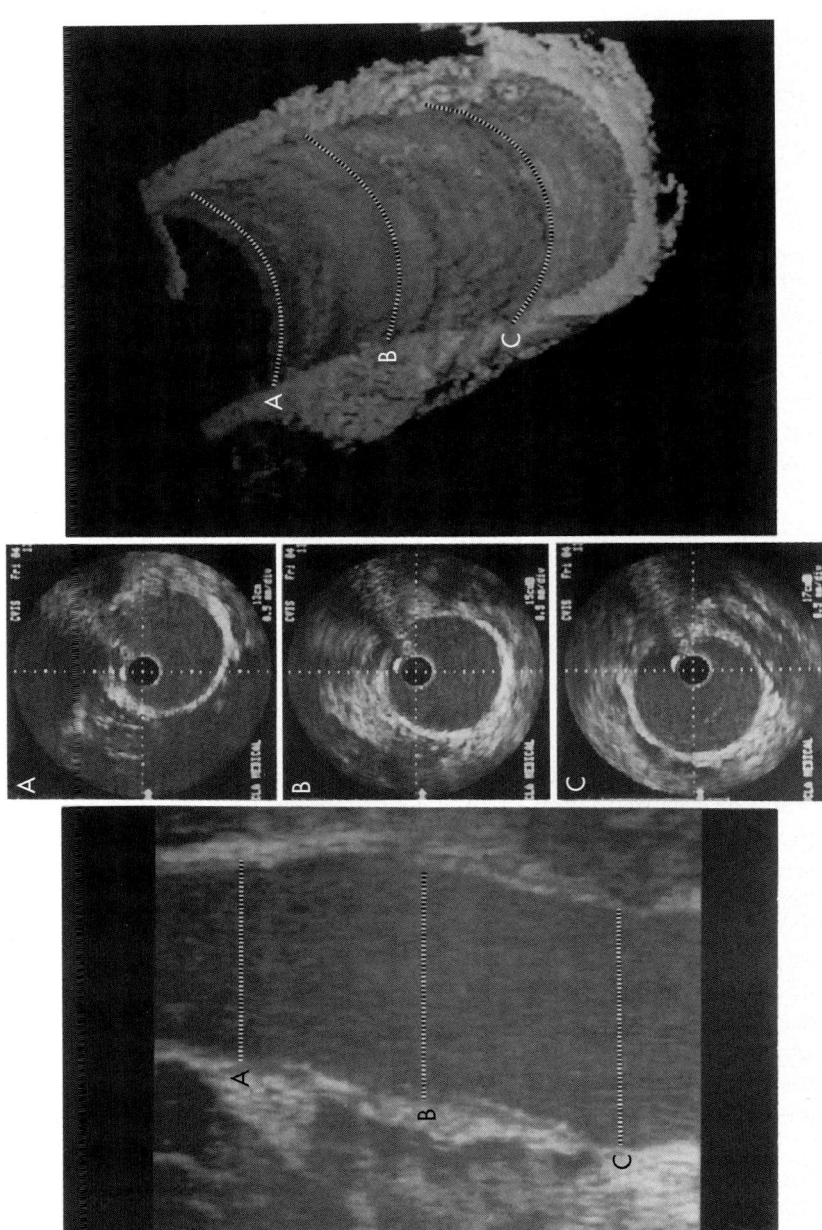

FIGURE 14–6. The 2D images labeled A, B, and C (*center panel*) are representative of those "stacked" by the computer and correspond to the sites labeled with the same letters on the 3D image (*right*) and longitudinal section of the 3D image (*left*). The longitudinal section of the 3D image is displayed on the computer monitor to allow optimal adjustments of the image density threshold and viewing orientation. (From Cavaye DM, Tabbarra MR, Kopchok GE et al: Three dimensional vascular ultrasound imaging, *Am Surg* 57:751–756, 1991.)

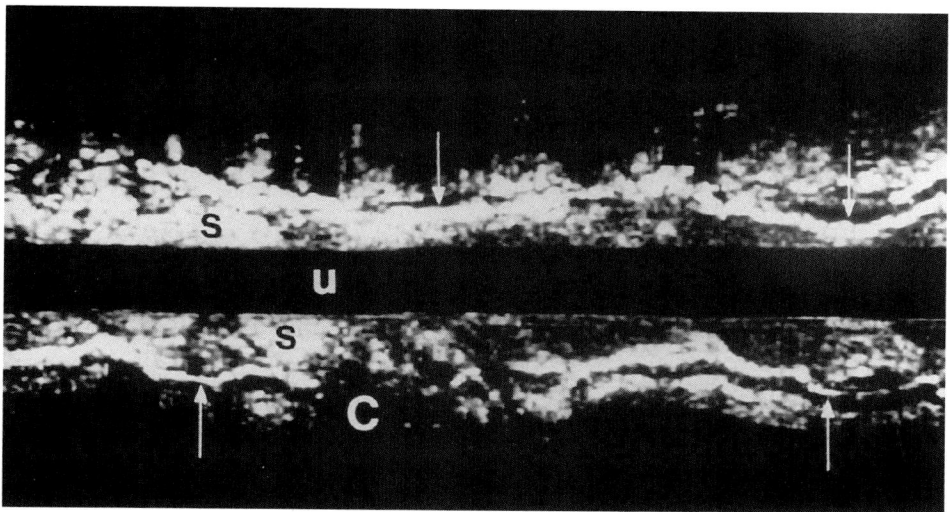

FIGURE 14–7. High-resolution, gray scale, longitudinal 2D view of an atherosclerotic human superficial femoral artery. The ultrasound catheter void (*u*) is seen within the lumen and abuts soft plaque (*s*) at left. C, calcific plaque; *single arrows*, hypoechoic media. (From Cavaye DM et al: Three dimensional intravascular ultrasound imaging of normal and diseased, human and canine arteries, *J Vasc Surg* 16:509–519, 1992.)

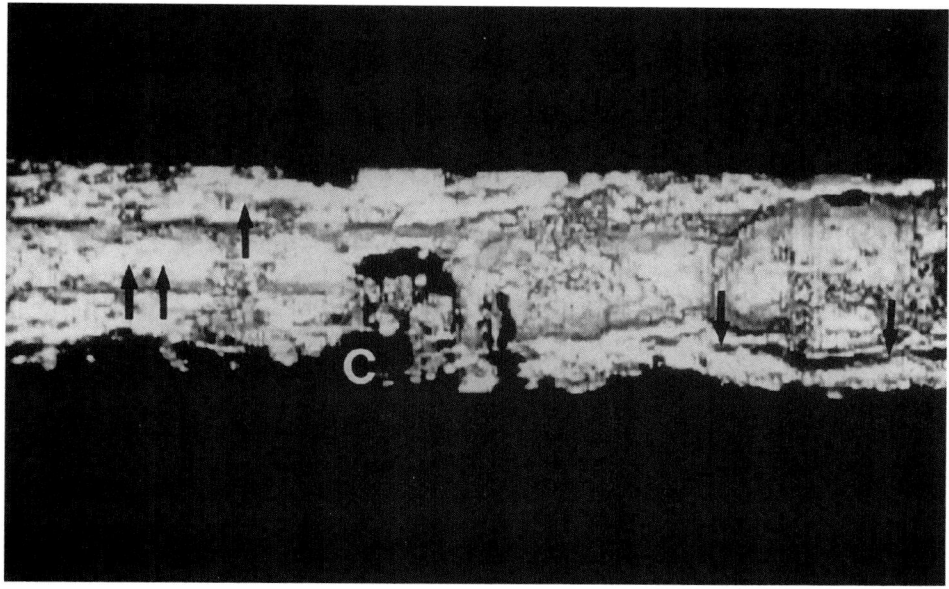

FIGURE 14–8. 3D image of the vessel in Figure 13–7. The reconstructed image is viewed in a longitudinal hemisection to allow complete examination of the luminal surface in this projection. Image dropout occurs at the site of maximal calcific stenosis (*C*). Smooth luminal surface (*double arrow*) upstream of plaque. Hypoechoic media is evident (*single arrows*). (From Cavaye DM et al: Three-dimensional intravascular ultrasound imaging of normal and diseased, human and canine arteries, *J Vasc Surg* 16:509–519, 1992.)

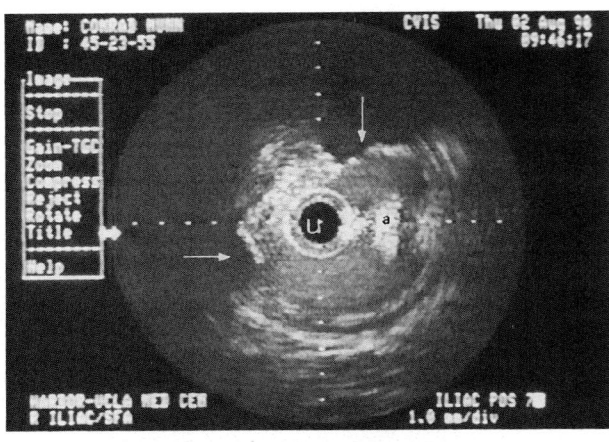

FIGURE 14–9. IVUS image of atherosclerotic human iliac artery. A large calcified plaque (*arrows*) produces a bright luminal line with acoustic shadowing behind it. u, ultrasound catheter void; a, imaging artifact. (From Tabbara M, White RA, Cavaye M et al: In-vivo human comparison of intravascular ultrasound and angiography, *J Vasc Surg* 14:496–504, 1991.)

and larger elastic vessels such as aorta because of the increased elastin content in the media. Fresh intraluminal thrombus can be distinguished from underlying vessel wall. It typically appears as a highly echogenic, homogeneous mass with varying image attenuation beyond its location.

IVUS devices are sensitive in differentiating calcified and noncalcified vascular lesions. Because the ultrasound energy is strongly reflected by calcific plaque, it appears as a bright image with dense acoustic shadowing behind it (Figures 14–7 to 14–9). For this reason, the exact location of the media and adventitia cannot be seen in segments of vessels containing heavily calcific disease, and dimensions must be estimated by interpolation of adjacent size data. Gussenhoven et al. have described four basic plaque components that can be distinguished using 40-MHz IVUS in vitro.[14] Hypoechoic images denote significant lipid deposits. Soft echoes represent fibromuscular tissue or intimal proliferation with varying amounts of dispersed lipid. Bright echoes denote collagen-rich fibrous tissue, whereas bright echoes with acoustic shadowing beyond the lesion represent calcified tissue.

Luminal dimensions and wall thickness determined by IVUS of normal and minimally diseased arteries both in vitro and in vivo are accurate to within 0.05 mm.[13,15–19] Determination of outer vessel diameter may be less accurate, with error up to 0.5 mm. Additional studies have compared contrast angiography and IVUS for determining luminal dimensions of normal and moderately atherosclerotic human arteries.[19–21] The luminal cross-sectional areas calculated from biplanar angiograms and measured from IVUS correlate well for normal or minimally diseased peripheral arteries in vivo. Uniplanar and biplanar angiography and IVUS also correlate well when used to image mildly elliptical lumens. In severely diseased vessels with elliptical lumens, angiography is less accurate in calculating luminal cross-sectional area and tends to underestimate the severity of atherosclerosis in the wall compared with IVUS.

Evaluating the extent of atherosclerotic disease in the arterial wall is as important as measuring reductions in luminal dimensions by plaque for successful lesion debulking or displacement during an endovascular intervention. 2D IVUS is superior to angiography and other vascular imaging modalities in this regard. Lesion volume is measurable using 3D IVUS imaging, but data regarding its accuracy are not currently available. Plaque volume estimation is based on the concept of differing cylindric volumes, where the inner (smaller) cylinder is represented by the vessel lumen and the outer (larger) cylinder is confined by the adventitia. By creating a surface-rendered luminal image and a complete cylindrical adventitial reconstruction of a vascular segment, these two volumes can be displayed (Figure 14–10). The difference between the two cylinders represents the "volume" occupied by

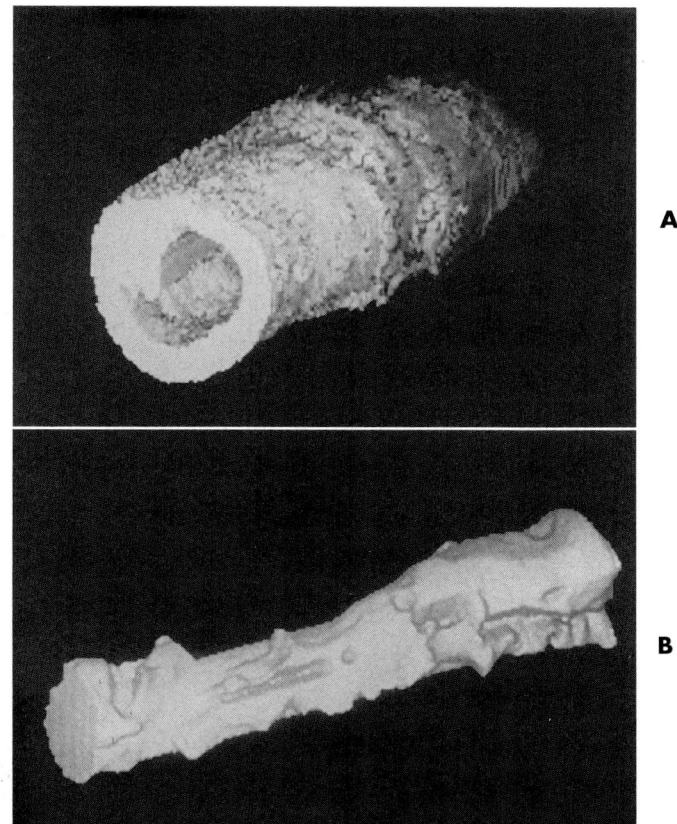

FIGURE 14–10. **A**, Complete cylindrical vessel reconstruction, with the outer boundary formed by the adventitia. **B**, Luminal reconstruction from the same vessel. By subtracting the volume of the luminal cylinder from the volume of the complete vessel cylinder, the volume of the vessel wall (pathologic or normal) can be derived. (From Cavaye DM et al: Three-dimensional vascular ultrasound imaging. In Cavaye DM, White RA, editors: *A text and atlas of arterial imaging: modern and developing technologies*, London, 1993, Chapman & Hall.)

the arterial wall elements, either normal or pathologic. If this volume is measured before and after an intervention such as atherectomy, the difference in the volumes represents the amount of actual lesion removed. This information is required to delineate the mechanisms of angioplasty failure, since the roles of residual stenosis and recurrent stenosis have not been adequately defined using currently available angiographically determined data.

IVUS is capable of identifying intimal flaps and arterial wall dissections and determining the size, location, and extent of these lesions (Figure 14–11).[22,23] Because IVUS imaging is a dynamic, real-time imaging modality, the movement of arterial flaps with pulsatile blood flow variation can be seen. The precise location and orientation of the flap is important, since it may determine the need for excision and grafting, stenting, or repair. IVUS may enable endovascular assessment and treatment alone.[24,25] 3D IVUS imaging is especially useful in this role, since aortic dissection commonly results in a spiral or complex-shaped flap that is diffcult to appreciate in three dimensions using alternative imaging modalities. 3D reconstruction allows identification of the dissection entry site, extent of the flap, and relation of the false lumen to major visceral branches and plays a vital role in experimental endoluminal stenting of aortic dissections.

One study compared 2D and 3D IVUS with angiography and 3D computed tomography (CT) for imaging abdominal aortic aneurysms.[26] Each modality provides unique information regarding the anatomy of the aorta and the distribution of components of the aneurysm (Figure 14–12). In the illustrated case, aortography confirmed that the aneurysm was confined to the infrarenal aorta but under-

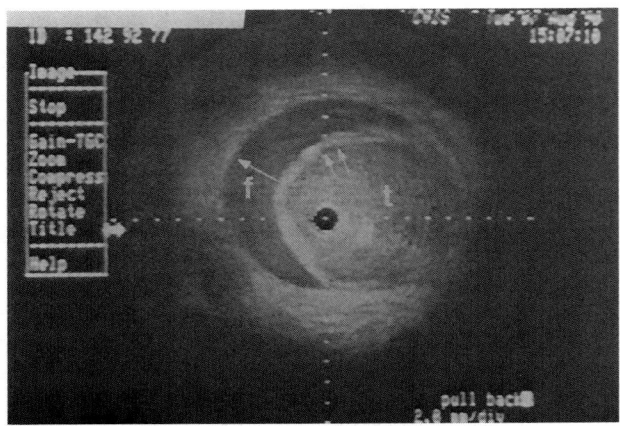

FIGURE 14–11. IVUS image of the distal abdominal aorta in a patient with an acute dissecting aortic aneurysm confirms dissection extending to this level. Dissection flap (*double arrows*), aortic wall (*single arrow*), true (*t*), and false (*f*) lumens are seen. (From Cavaye DM, French WJ, White RA et al: Intravascular ultrasound imaging of an acute dissecting aortic aneurysm: a case report, *J Vasc Surg* 13:510–512, 1991.)

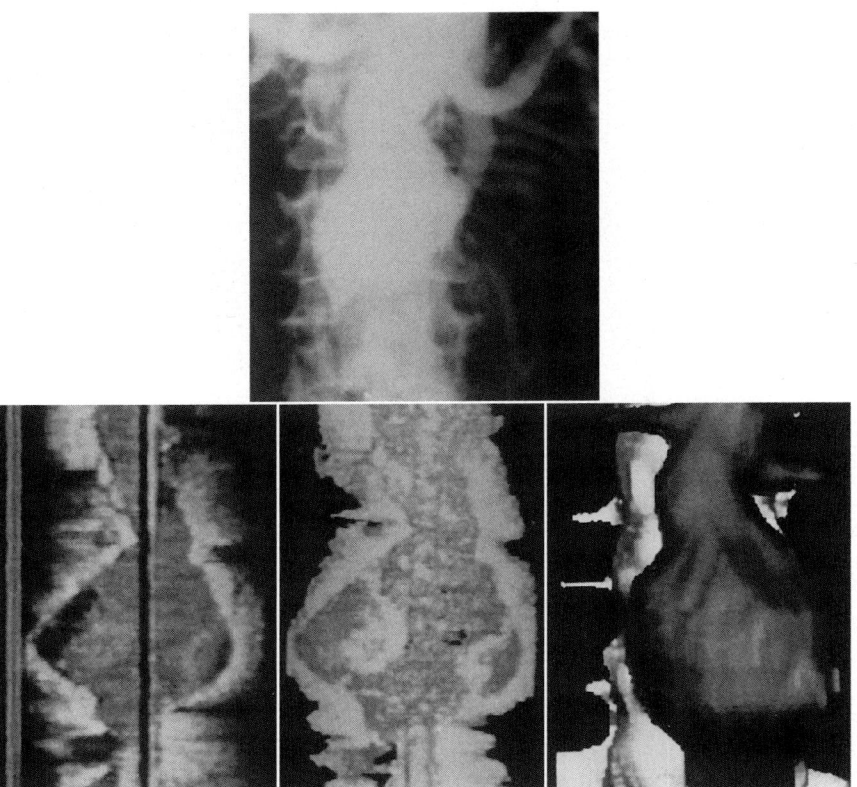

FIGURE 14–12. Counterclockwise from top: Aortogram, longitudinal gray-scale IVUS, surface rendered 3D IVUS, and 3D CT of the external surface of the aortic aneurysm. The images are of comparable lengths of the aorta with similar magnification to enable comparison of the methods. (From White RA, Scoccianti M, Back M et al: Innovations in vascular imaging: angiography, 3D CT and 2D and 3D intravascular ultrasound of an abdominal aortic aneurysm, *Ann Vasc Surg* 8:285–289, 1994.)

estimated the size of the aneurysm. Angiography does not provide precise cross-sectional and volumetric data regarding the dimensions of the neck of the aneurysm, quantity of thrombus, and aortic wall characteristics that are apparent by CT and IVUS imaging. Accurate sizing of luminal and wall dimensions along the aneurysm are obtained with cross-sectional images acquired by either CT or IVUS (Figure 14–13). 3D CT reconstructions outline only the external surface of the aneurysm, whereas 2D and 3D IVUS visualize luminal and transmural wall characteristics including inner and outer surface topography. Calcification of the aortic wall is more evident by IVUS than by angiography or CT.

IVUS has been used in diagnostic assessment of a number of other pathologic vascular scenarios. Accelerated intimal thickening in the coronary arteries of cardiac transplant recipients has been documented by IVUS when angiograms appear normal.[27,28] Ricou et al. used

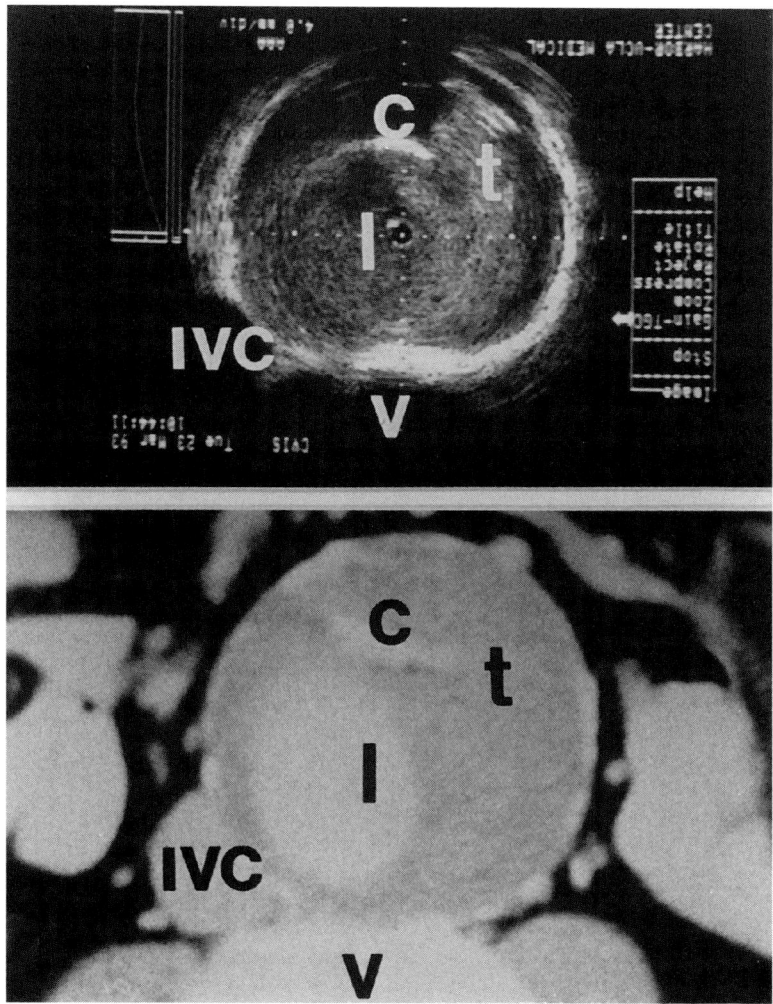

FIGURE 14–13. Comparison of tomographic views by IVUS (*top*) and CT (*bottom*) of the aneurysm at the same location. Aortic lumen (*l*), thrombus in the aneurysm (*t*), calcification (*c*), inferior vena cava (*IVC*), and vertebral body (*v*). (From White RA, Scoccianti M, Back M et al: Innovations in vascular imaging: angiography, 3D CT and 2D and 3D intravascular ultrasound of an abdominal aortic aneurysm, *Ann Vasc Surg* 8:285–289, 1994.)

IVUS to determine candidacy for pulmonary thromboendarterectomy as treatment for pulmonary hypertension in patients with chronic pulmonary thromboembolic disease.[29] Intravascular tumors such as vena caval extensions of renal cell carcinoma can be localized by IVUS to aid in planning resection.[30]

Therapeutic Interventions

Long-term success of endovascular procedures requires restoration of near-normal hemodynamic conditions (i.e., brisk flow rates with minimal local flow disturbances) across diseased vessel segments as a result of adequate enlargement of luminal diameters (i.e., minimized residual stenosis) and smooth wall surfaces (i.e., without deep intimal flaps or medial dissections). Conventional angiography has been unable to provide sensitive data regarding the effects of endovascular therapies. For meaningful critical assessment of these minimally invasive methods, plaque extent and the consistency and distribution of residual lesions after an intervention must be known. The advantage afforded by IVUS in evaluating lesion morphology involves accurate assessment of not only luminal dimensions but also transmural lesion characteristics (Box 14–1).[31] Uniplanar or biplanar angiography, by providing only a luminal "silhouette," is limited in this regard. Delineation by IVUS of the spatial distribution of the lesion in a concentric or eccentric pattern and the presence of a soft (fibrous) or hard (calcific) plaque may influence choice of endovascular therapy and predict the risk of immediate or late complications (e.g., perforation, thrombosis, restenosis).[32,33] Evaluation of lesion volume before and after the procedure by IVUS provides a method to quantitate the amount of lesion debulking or displacement by the intervention and a reference point from which to assess lesion recurrence or restenosis. IVUS fulfills many of the necessary requirements of an ideal guidance system for endovascular procedures, including precise delivery and positioning of devices within target lesions (Box 14–2).[31]

Box 14–1. Lesion Morphology: Data Acquired by IVUS

1. Lumen diameters and cross-sectional area
2. Wall thickness
3. Lesion length, shape, and volume
4. Lesion position within the lumen: concentric vs. eccentric
5. Lesion type: fibrous (soft) vs. calcific (hard)
6. Presence and extent of flap, dissection, or ulceration
7. Presence and volume of thrombus

From Scoccianti M, Verbin CS, Kopchok GE et al: IVUS guidance for peripheral vascular interventions, *J Endovasc Surg* 1:71–80, 1994.

Box 14–2. Ideal Guiding System for Endovascular Procedures

1. Expedite passage through tight stenoses and obstructions.
2. Identify the target lesion in a diffusely diseased vessel.
3. Define lesion shape, dimensions, and morphology.
4. Provide useful data to choose the appropriate therapeutic modality.
5. Guide the therapeutic device to the target site.
6. Provide on-line information during the endovascular procedure with a sensitivity equivalent to the thickness of the lesion or of the treated vessel.
7. Evaluate the effects of various endovascular procedures and provide useful data to establish prognostic factors of success and of early or late recurrence of lesions.

From Scoccianti M, Verbin CS, Kopchok GE et al: IVUS guidance for peripheral vascular interventions, *J Endovasc Surg* 1:70–80, 1994.

Percutaneous Transluminal Angioplasty

Adjunctive use of IVUS has allowed description of the mechanism of percutaneous transluminal angioplasty (PTA) in treating coronary and peripheral arterial occlusive disease and helped to define the factors associated with restenosis. The et al. studied 16 patients with superficial femoral artery lesions before and after PTA.[34] IVUS accurately detected the presence of dissections, plaque fractures, and internal elastic lamina ruptures with thinning of the media. This study demonstrated that increased luminal dimensions occurring after PTA are due to overstretching of the arterial wall while the volume of the lesion remained relatively constant. Embolization of thrombotic material adherent to the lesion was also observed during balloon angioplasty. Losordo et al. performed a similar study in 40 patients with iliac artery lesions.[35] IVUS evaluation showed plaque fracture and displacement contributing to 72% of the final luminal cross-sectional area after PTA, with wall stretching providing an additional 18% increase.

Honye et al. found a correlation between the morphometric characteristics of the plaque, the mechanism of percutaneous transluminal coronary angioplasty (PTCA), and the risk of restenosis.[36] In this study, calcified plaques (detected in 83% of cases by IVUS but only in 14% by angiography) were more prone to dissection and were associated with larger post-procedural residual lumens than fibrous plaques. Lesions at high risk of late restenosis were those fibrous and concentric lesions that did not show signs of fracture or dissection after PTCA. The study demonstrated that fibrous lesions are more likely to undergo elastic recoil if the vessel wall remains intact after PTA. Tobis et al. have confirmed these findings and have suggested that, when IVUS detects this type of lesion, directional atherectomy or stenting should be considered as an alternative or as an adjunct to PTCA.[32]

Studies have indicated that balloon size for PTA is often underestimated when selection is made using quantitative angiography alone and that optimal balloon size is more accurately determined by IVUS.[37,38] In addition to specific plaque characteristics, several variables including oversized and undersized balloons have been associated with an increased risk of early or late restenosis (Box 14–3).[36–48] All of these factors are identifiable by IVUS and allow periprocedural decisions regarding additional interventions to be made. Detection and correction of residual stenosis, extensive postprocedural dissections, or luminal thrombus may improve outcomes after PTA.

A balloon ultrasound imaging catheter (BUIC, Boston Scientific, Watertown, Mass) has been used clinically with promising results.[49,50] Single-plane images can be obtained through the midsection of the angioplasty balloon during inflation. Luminal features before, during, and after inflation, such as plaque fracture and elastic recoil, can be monitored in real time with this new IVUS device, thereby eliminating the need to exchange individual balloon and IVUS catheters.

Intravascular Stents

Intravascular stents have been used in various applications including post-PTA situations. Common indications for stent deployment after angioplasty are deep arterial wall dissections, elastic recoil, residual stenosis, the presence of a significant residual pressure gradient across the lesion, or plaque ulceration with local thrombus accumulation. Proper stent selection and deployment are critical for salvage of the angioplasty procedure and improving chances of long-term patency. It has been shown that inadequate stent expansion can lead to early thrombosis or stent migration, whereas overexpansion can result in excessive intimal hyperplasia or vessel perforation.[51] IVUS is effective in assessing the result of the primary intervention, establishing the need for stenting, and guiding stent deployment.[31,52,53]

IVUS has been useful in stent deployment for both coronary and peripheral lesions. In some studies, IVUS has demonstrated adequate stent expansion in only 13% of treated coronary lesions and enabled subsequent further stent expansion in 73% of patients.[32,33] Katzen et al. reported that angiography-guided stent deployment in peripheral lesions resulted in incorrect positioning or expansion in 20% of cases that were evaluated by IVUS.[54] Residual lumen area is known to be an important variable in predicting the long-term patency of

> **Box 14–3. Risk of Restenosis after PTA**
>
> **Early:**
> 1. Luminal thrombus[a–c]
> 2. Extensive dissection[a,c]
> 3. Oversized balloon[d,e]
>
> **Late:**
> 1. Residual stenosis >30%[f–h]
> 2. Small residual lumen[h,i]
> 3. Undersized balloon[j]
> 4. Concentric fibrous plaque[k,l]
> 5. Absence of dissection[k,l]
> 6. Absence of calcification[k,l]

From Landau C, Lange RA, Hillis LD: Percutaneous transluminal angioplasty, *N Engl J Med* 330(14):981–983, 1994.
[a] Ellis SG, Roubin GS, King SB III et al: Angiographic and clinical predictors of acute closure after native vessel coronary angioplasty, *Circulation* 77:372–379, 1988.
[b] Mabin TA, Holmes DR Jr, Smith HC et al: Intracoronary thrombus: role in coronary occlusion complicating percutaneous transluminal coronary angioplasty, *J Am Coll Cardiol* 5:198–202, 1985.
[c] Detre KM, Holmes DR Jr, Holubkov R et al: Incidence and consequences of periprocedural occlusion: the 1985–1986 N.H.L.B.I. Percutaneous Transluminal Coronary Angioplasty Registry, *Circulation* 82:739–750, 1990.
[d] Roubin GS, Douglas JS Jr, King SB III et al: Influence of balloon size on initial success, acute complications, and restenosis after percutaneous transluminal coronary angioplasty: a prospective randomized study, *Circulation* 78:557–565, 1988.
[e] Colombo A: *Coronary stenting without anticoagulation*, abstract presented at International Congress VII—Endovascular Interventions, Phoenix, Feb 13–17, 1994.
[f] Lambert M, Bonan R, Cote G et al: Multiple coronary angioplasty: a model to discriminate systemic and procedural factors related to restenosis, *J Am Coll Cardiol* 12:310–314, 1988.
[g] Leimgruber PP, Roubin GS, Hollman J et al: Restenosis after successful coronary angioplasty in patients with single-vessel disease, *Circulation* 73:710–717, 1986.
[h] Hirshfeld JW Jr, Schwartz JS, Jugo R et al: Restenosis after coronary angioplasty: a multivariate statistical model to relate lesion and procedure variables to restenosis, *J Am Coll Cardiol* 18:647–656, 1991.
[i] Kuntz RE, Gibson CM, Nobuyoshi M et al: Generalized model of restenosis after conventional balloon angioplasty, stenting and directional atherectomy, *J Am Coll Cardiol* 21:15–25, 1993.
[j] Nichols AB, Smith R, Berke AD et al: Importance of balloon size in coronary angioplasty, *J Am Coll Cardiol* 13:1094–1100, 1989.
[k] Honye J, Mahon DJ, Jain A et al: Morphological effects of coronary balloon angioplasty in vivo assessed by intravascular ultrasound imaging, *Circulation* 85:1012–1025, 1992.
[l] Farb A, Virmani R, Atkinson JB et al: Plaque morphology and pathologic changes in arteries from patients dying after coronary balloon angioplasty, *J Am Coll Cardiol* 16:1421–1429, 1990.

endovascular procedures, and optimizing luminal dimensions by stenting is crucial. Early thrombosis after PTCA and stenting occurs in up to 25% of patients and has required the use of anticoagulation after stent deployment. Colombo demonstrated that this complication is usually related to inadequate stent expansion. By assuring proper deployment, IVUS can decrease the incidence of thrombosis and eliminate the need for long-term anticoagulation.[42]

Precise measurement of the arterial diameters permits selection of the appropriate stent size, whereas visualization of the lesion and of the stent-wall interface allows exact stent positioning and expansion (Figure 14–14). 3D reconstruction can be particularly useful because incomplete stent deployment is visualized as a "lattice" pattern independent of the arterial wall surface on the reconstructed images of the stented vessel.[53] In the near future, the incorporation of an IVUS transducer into the stent delivery system will permit simultaneous imaging at the time of stent deployment, enhancing the precision of the procedure.

Atherectomy

The effects of several atherectomy devices have been discerned by IVUS. Significant plaque burden remains after both directional and high-speed rotational atherectomy. Although cineangiography reveals a satisfactory result with both types of devices, IVUS evaluations

FIGURE 14–14. **A**, IVUS image of a stent in an artery that appeared fully deployed by fluoroscopic examination. **B**, After further balloon inflation, IVUS demonstrates full deployment. *Single arrow*, stent struts; *double arrow*, artery wall.

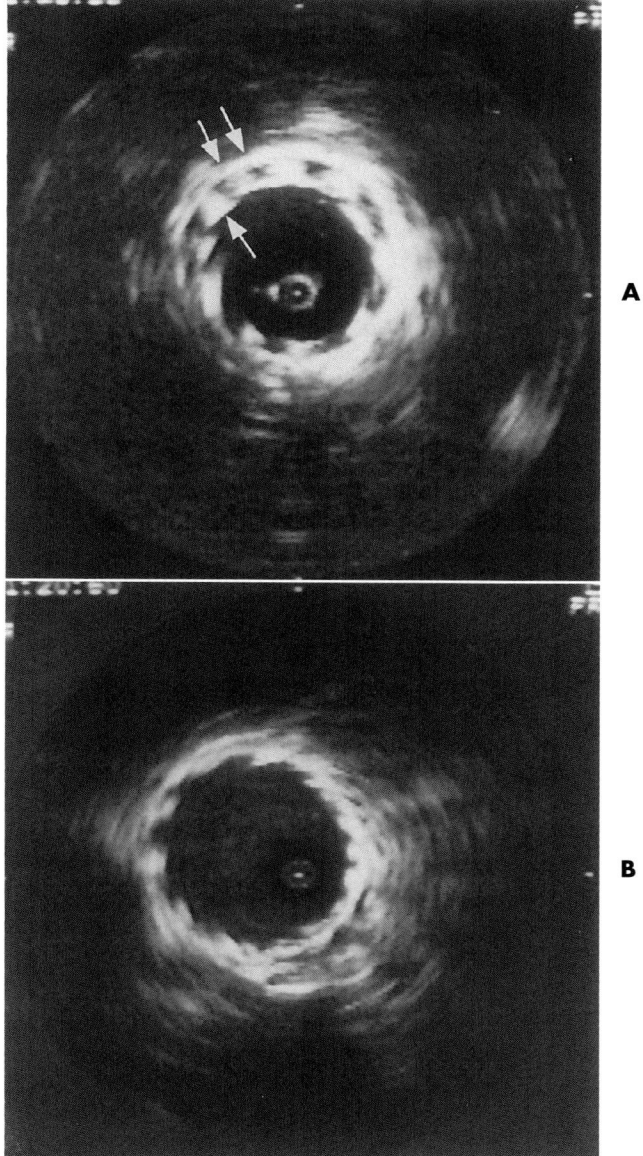

after the intervention demonstrate residual plaque volumes of 48% and 74%, respectively.[33,55]

IVUS has demonstrated that directional atherectomy, in addition to plaque ablation, causes stretching of the arterial wall and that this Dotter effect contributes an additional 18% cross-sectional area to the immediate postprocedural arterial lumen. Schnitt et al.[56] and Serruys et al.[57] have shown that directional atherectomy removes normal arterial tissue in 26% to 61% of cases and that removal of tissue is frequently too deep in the arterial wall. It is conceivable that IVUS examination before and during the procedure might help to orient the cutting blade with relation to the lesion, enabling adequate removal of the plaque and reduction of the incidence of both inadequate debulking and vessel perforation.

Mintz et al.[58] and Kovach et al.[55] have studied the effect of high-speed rotational atherectomy (Rotablator, Heart Technology, Redmond,

Wash) on coronary lesions. They confirmed that this device causes an increase of the vessel lumen by selective ablation of the calcific portion of the plaque. The residual lumen is usually circular and homogeneous, with dissections in 26% of treated lesions confined locally to the calcified plaque. These studies demonstrate that rotational atherectomy's mechanism of lesion reduction differs from that of PTA, where dissections at the junction of the plaque with the normal wall occur in 77% of treated lesions.[55] The studies also show the inaccuracy of cineangiography in the evaluation of postprocedural morphology and the mechanisms of restenosis. In vessels where angiography displayed adequate results, IVUS documented residual plaque occupying a significant percentage of the cross-sectional area of the vessel.

Fitzgerald et al. underscored the importance of calcium location within a lesion and atherectomy effects.[59] Superficial calcific plaques respond well to high-speed rotational atherectomy and are relatively resistant to both PTA and directional atherectomy. With deeper calcifications, directional atherectomy appears to be a suitable therapeutic modality. IVUS may be used to select the appropriate therapy based on specific plaque morphology and predict the result of each specific intervention.

The impact of IVUS in coronary revascularization has been well illustrated by the GUIDE (Guidance by Ultrasound Imaging for Decision Endpoints) study, in which IVUS influenced the choice of therapy in 48% of revascularization procedures.[60] In angioplasty cases, this resulted in the decision to perform more dilations or to use larger balloons. In atherectomy procedures, the decision to perform more tissue removal, to treat different segments, or to use larger devices was also made based on IVUS interpretations.

Endovascular Grafts

A novel and important application of IVUS is in endoluminal grafting for the exclusion of aneurysms or arteriovenous fistulas and bypass of occlusive peripheral lesions (Figure 14–15). The success of such procedures is closely related to an accurate knowledge of critical parameters of the lesion to be treated and a knowledge of proper deployment of the device.

Experimental laboratory studies have shown that IVUS is useful for choosing the site of endovascular stent-graft deployment and determining the appropriate-size device by accurately measuring the luminal dimensions of the aorta.[61] IVUS interrogation of the aortic lumen before device deployment enables accurate identification of the branch arteries and selection of the appropriate site for proximal stent placement. During placement of an intraluminal graft IVUS is the most accurate way to determine full stent expansion and to obtain information regarding the continuity and alignment of the graft material in the aortic lumen. Using certain devices, it is possible to place prostheses by IVUS guidance alone. Although cinefluoroscopy and IVUS are complementary in terms of enabling expedient placement of intraluminal grafts, an additional important aspect supporting the use of IVUS in this application is that the fluoroscopy time can be significantly reduced during the procedures, minimizing the exposure of both personnel and the patient.

In an experimental series, incomplete proximal stent expansion in approximately 20% of graft deployments was determined by IVUS when there was no apparent abnormality on angiography.[61] This information is important, as it averts potential migration of the devices by enabling further expansion of the stent before completing the procedure. The implications of secure proximal stent positioning are obvious. The improved accuracy of IVUS to determine stent deployment has been confirmed by other investigators, who have documented that IVUS examination leads to repositioning the intravascular stent devices in approximately 20% to 30% of cases after cinefluoroscopy suggested that the deployment was adequate.[62,63]

Other studies have compared 2D and 3D IVUS to angiography, 3D computed tomography (CT), and IVUS imaging of abdominal aortic aneurysms.[64] Each modality provides unique information regarding the anatomy of the aorta and the distribution of the aneurysm components. In our series of endoluminal vascular prostheses placed for a variety of indica-

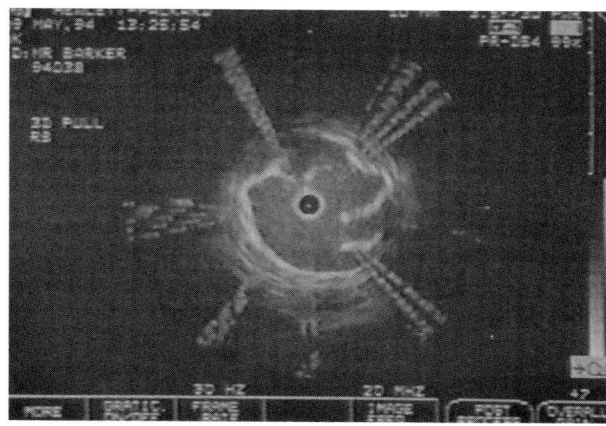

FIGURE 14–15. IVUS imaging of an endoluminal graft (*arrows*) with multiple folds and kinks that move with arterial pulsations. A completion angiogram performed at the same interval appeared to have no significant abnormalities. (From Scoccianti M, Verbin CS, Kopchok GE et al: IVUS guidance for peripheral vascular interventions, *J Endovasc Surg* 1:71–80, 1994.)

tions, including aortic and iliac aneurysms and traumatic AV fistulas, IVUS was the most accurate method for choosing the location and determining the dimensions of the fixation sites.[65–67] IVUS was also the most accurate way to determine the morphology of vascular structures (i.e., calcium, thrombus) and allowed "real-time" observation of the expansion of stent devices to ensure firm fixation of balloon-expanded stents before the procedures were completed. The implications of these observations on the development of future deployment devices and the effect IVUS can have on enhancing the success of procedures is yet to be determined, although the preliminary evidence strongly supports the utility of IVUS in peripheral and aortic endovascular interventions.[67,68]

Future Developments

Implementation of IVUS involves both diagnostic applications when used during invasive studies such as peripheral angiography or cardiac catheterization or use as a guidance method during therapeutic procedures including angioplasty, atherectomy, and stent deployment. Information obtained by IVUS allows selection of an appropriate ablation method for particular plaque types or distributions. Further miniaturization and cost-effective manufacturing of IVUS devices are needed for continued adjunctive use during vascular interventions. Development of combined endovascular devices with an interventional component and an ultrasound transducer capable of real-time imaging during a procedure will simplify catheter exchanges, techniques, and assessment. Such a device has been proposed for guided laser recanalization of arterial occlusions.[69] 3D, real-time reconstructions of IVUS images of complex vascular lesions can also enhance the practicality of endovascular interventions by providing more easily interpretable vessel images. Refinements in computer software and hardware will further reduce processing times and improve 3D image quality.

The recent development of a forward-looking IVUS catheter may provide new and unique imaging capabilities for guidance of devices in treating occlusive vascular lesions. This system (Echoeye, EchoCath Inc., Princeton, NJ) uses a mechanically rotated acoustic beam from a 25.5-MHz transducer to generate 64 axially aligned, cross-sectional images in the shape of a truncated cone in front of the 7.5F catheter. Preliminary in vitro experience with the device has demonstrated accurate imaging of various configurations within diseased arterial segments.[70]

References

1. Bom N, ten Hoff H, Lancee CT et al: Early and recent intraluminal ultrasound devices, *Int J Card Imaging* 4:79–88, 1989.
2. Cieszynski T: Intracardiac method for the investigation of structure of the heart with the aid of

ultrasonics, *Arch Immunol Ter Dow* 8:551–557, 1960.
3. Kossof G: Diagnostic applications of ultrasound in cardiology, *Australas Radiol* X:101–106, 1966.
4. Carleton RA, Sessions RW, Graettinger JS: Diameter of heart measured by intracavitary ultrasound, *Med Res Engng* 28–32, May 1969.
5. Frazin L, Talano JV, Stephanides L et al: Esophageal echocardiography, *Circulation* 54:168–171, 1976.
6. Bom N, Lancee CT, Van Egmond FC: An ultrasonic intracardiac scanner, *Ultrasonics* 10:72–76, 1972.
7. Lockwood GR, Ryan LK, Foster FS: High frequency intravascular ultrasound imaging. In Cavaye DM, White RA, editors: *A text and atlas of arterial imaging: modern and developing technologies*, London, 1993, Chapman & Hall.
8. Yock PG, Linker DT, Angelsen BAJ: Two-dimensional intravascular ultrasound: technical development and initial clinical experience, *J Am Soc Echocardiogr* 2(4):296–304, 1989.
9. van Urk H, Gussenhoven WJ, Gerritsen GP et al: Assessment of arterial disease and arterial reconstructions by intravascular ultrasound, *Int J Cardiac Imaging* 6:157–164, 1991.
10. Burns PN, Goldberg BB: Ultrasound contrast agents for vascular imaging. In Cavaye DM, White RA, editors: *A text and atlas of arterial imaging: modern and developing technologies*, London, 1993, Chapman & Hall.
11. Heffernan PB, Robb RA: A new method for shaded surface display of biological and medical images, *IEEE Transactions on Medical Imaging* MI-4:26–38, 1985.
12. Cavaye DM, Tabbara MR, Kopchok GE et al: Three dimensional vascular ultrasound imaging, *Am Surg* 57:751–755, 1991.
13. Gussenhoven WJ, Essed CE, Lancee CT: Arterial wall characteristics determined by intravascular ultrasound imaging: an in-vitro study, *J Am Coll Cardiol* 14:947–952, 1989.
14. Gussenhoven WJ, Essed CE, Frietman P et al: Intravascular echographic assessment of vessel wall characteristics: a correlation with histology, *Int J Cardiac Imaging* 4:105–116, 1989.
15. Kopchok GE, White RA, Guthrie C et al: Intraluminal vascular ultrasound: preliminary report of dimensional and morphologic accuracy, *Ann Vasc Surg* 4:291–296, 1990.
16. Kopchok GE, White RA, White G: Intravascular ultrasound: a new potential modality for angioplasty guidance, *Angiology* 41:785–792, 1990.
17. Mallery JA, Tobis JM, Griffith J et al: Assessment of normal and atherosclerotic arterial wall thickness with an intravascular ultrasound imaging catheter, *Am Heart J* 119:1392–1400, 1990.
18. Nissen SE, Grines CL, Gurley JC et al: Application of new phased-array ultrasound imaging catheter in the assessment of vascular dimensions, *Circulation* 81:660–666, 1990.
19. Nissen SE, Gurley JC, Grines CL et al: Intravascular ultrasound assessing of lumen size and wall morphology in normal subjects and patients with coronary artery disease, *Circulation* 1087–1099, 1993.
20. Tabbara MR, White RA, Cavaye DM et al: In-vivo human comparison of intravascular ultrasound and angiography, *J Vasc Surg* 14:496–504, 1991.
21. Tobis JM, Mahon D, Lehmann K et al: The sensitivity of ultrasound imaging compared to angiography for diagnosing coronary atherosclerosis, *Circulation* 82(suppl III):439, 1990 (abstract).
22. Cavaye DM, French WJ, White RA et al: Intravascular ultrasound imaging of an acute dissecting aortic aneurysm: a case report, *J Vasc Surg* 13:510–512, 1991.
23. Pandian NG, Fries A, Broadway B et al: Intravascular high frequency two-dimension detection of arterial dissection and intimal flaps, *Am J Cardiol* 65:1278–1280, 1990.
24. Neville RF, Yasuhara H, Watanabe BI et al: Endovascular management of arterial intimal defects: an experimental comparison by arteriography, angioscopy and intravascular ultrasonography, *J Vasc Surg* 13:496–502, 1991.
25. Cavaye DM, White RA, Lerman RD et al: Usefulness of intravascular ultrasound for detecting experimentally induced aortic dissection in dogs and for determining the effectiveness of endoluminal stenting, *Am J Cardiol* 69:705–707, 1992.
26. White RA, Scoccianti M, Back M et al: Innovations in vascular imaging: angiography, 3D CT and 2D and 3D intravascular ultrasound of an abdominal aortic aneurysm, *Ann Vasc Surg* 8:285–289, 1994.
27. St Goar FG, Pinto FJ, Aldermann EL et al: Intracoronary ultrasound in cardiac transplant recipients: in-vivo evaluation of angiographically silent intimal thickening, *J Am Coll Cardiol* 17:103A, 1994 (abstract).
28. Pinto FJ, St Goar FG, Chaign M et al: Intracoronary ultrasound evaluation of intimal thickening in cardiac transplant recipients: correlation with clinical characteristics, *J Am Coll Cardiol* 17:103A, 1994 (abstract).
29. Ricou FJ, Nicod PH, Moser KM: Intravascular ultrasound imaging of chronic pulmonary

thromboembolic disease: correlation with surgical results, *Circulation* 82(suppl 3):441, 1990 (abstract).
30. Barone GW, Kahn MB, Cook JM et al: Recurrent intracaval renal cell carcinoma: the role of intravascular ultrasonography, *J Vasc Surg* 13:506–509, 1991.
31. Scoccianti M, Verbin CS, Kopchok GE et al: Intravascular ultrasound guidance for peripheral vascular interventions, *J Endovasc Surg* 1:71–80, 1994.
32. Tobis JM, Mahon DJ, Goldberg SL et al: Lessons from intravascular ultrasonography: observations during interventional angioplasty procedures, *J Clin Ultrasound* 21:589–607, 1993.
33. Fitzgerald PJ, Yock PG: Mechanisms and outcomes of angioplasty and atherectomy assessed by intravascular ultrasound imaging, *J Clin Ultrasound* 21:579–588, 1993.
34. The SHK, Gussenhoven WJ, Zhong Y et al: Effect of balloon angioplasty on femoral artery evaluated with intravascular ultrasound imaging, *Circulation* 86:483–493, 1992.
35. Losordo DW, Rosenfield K, Pieczek A et al: How does angioplasty work? Serial analysis of human iliac arteries using intravascular ultrasound, *Circulation* 86:1845–1858, 1992.
36. Honye J, Mahon DJ, Jain A et al: Morphological effects of coronary balloon angioplasty in vivo assessed by intravascular ultrasound imaging, *Circulation* 85:1012–1025, 1992.
37. Roubin GS, Douglas JS Jr, King SB III et al: Influence of balloon size on initial success, acute complications, and restenosis after percutaneous transluminal coronary angioplasty: a prospective randomized study, *Circulation* 78:557–565, 1988.
38. Nichols AB, Smith R, Berke AD et al: Importance of balloon size in coronary angioplasty, *J Am Coll Cardiol* 13:1094–1100, 1989.
39. Ellis SG, Roubin GS, King SB III et al: Angiographic and clinical predictors of acute closure after native vessel coronary angioplasty, *Circulation* 77:372–379, 1988.
40. Mabin TA, Holmes DR Jr, Smith HC et al: Intracoronary thrombus: role in coronary occlusion complicating percutaneus transluminal coronary angioplasty, *J Am Coll Cardiol* 5:198–202, 1985.
41. Detre KM, Holmes DR Jr, Holubkov R et al: Incidence and consequences of periprocedural occlusion: the 1985–1986 N.H.L.B.I. Percutaneous Transluminal Coronary Angioplasty Registry, *Circulation* 82:739–750, 1990.
42. Colombo A: *Coronary stenting without anticoagulation*. Abstract presented at International Congress VII—Endovascular Interventions. Phoenix, Feb 13–17, 1994.
43. Lambert M, Bonan R, Cote G et al: Multiple coronary angioplasty: a model to discriminate systemic and procedural factors related to restenosis, *J Am Coll Cardiol* 12:310–314, 1988.
44. Leimgruber PP, Roubin GS, Hollman J et al: Restenosis after successful coronary angioplasty in patients with single-vessel disease, *Circulation* 73:710–717, 1986.
45. Hirshfeld JW Jr, Schwartz JS, Jugo R et al: Restenosis after coronary angioplasty: a multivariate statistical model to relate lesion and procedure variables to restenosis, *J Am Coll Cardiol* 18:647–656, 1991.
46. Kuntz RE, Gibson CM, Nobuyoshi M et al: Generalized model of restenosis after conventional balloon angioplasty, stenting and directional atherectomy, *J Am Coll Cardiol* 21:15–25, 1993.
47. Farb A, Virmani R, Atkinson JB et al: Plaque morphology and pathologic changes in arteries from patients dying after coronary balloon angioplasty, *J Am Coll Cardiol* 16:1421–1429, 1990.
48. Landau C, Lange RA, Hillis LD: Percutaneous transluminal angioplasty, *N Engl J Med* 330,14:981–993, 1994.
49. Crowley RJ, Hamm MA, Joshi SH et al: Ultrasound guided therapeutic catheters: recent developments and clinical results, *Int J Card Imaging* 6:145–156, 1991.
50. Isner JM, Rosenfield K, Losordo DW et al: Combination balloon-ultrasound imaging catheter for percutaneous transluminal angioplasty, *Circulation* 84:739–754, 1991.
51. Busquet J: The current role of vascular stents, *Int Angiol* 12(3):206–213, 1993.
52. Diethrich EB: Endovascular treatment of abdominal aortic occlusive disease: the impact of stents and intravascular ultrasound imaging, *Eur J Vasc Surg* 7:228–236, 1993.
53. Cavaye DM, Diethrich EB, Santiago OJ et al: Intravascular ultrasound imaging: an essential component of angioplasty assessment and vascular stent deployment, *Int Angiol* 12:212–220, 1993.
54. Katzen BT, Benenati JF, Becker GJ et al: Role of intravascular ultrasound in peripheral atherectomy and stent deployment, *Circulation* 84(suppl II):2152, 1991 (Abstract).
55. Kovach JA, Mintz GS, Pichard AD et al: Sequential intravascular ultrasound characterization of the mechanisms of rotational atherectomy and

adjunct balloon angioplasty, *J Am Coll Cardiol* 22:1024–1032, 1993.
56. Schnitt SJ, Safian RD, Kuntz RE et al: Histologic findings in specimens obtained by percutaneous directional coronary atherectomy, *Hum Pathol* 23:415–420, 1992.
57. Serruys PW, Umans VA, Strauss BM et al: Quantitative angiography after directional coronary atherectomy, *Br Heart J* 66:122–129, 1991.
58. Mintz GS, Potkin BN, Keren G et al: Intravascular ultrasound evaluation of the effect of rotational atherectomy in obstructive atherosclerotic coronary artery disease, *Circulation* 86:1383–1393, 1992.
59. Fitzgerald PJ, Muhlberger VA, Moes NY et al: Calcium location within plaque as a predictor of atherectomy tissue retrieval: an intravascular ultrasound study, *Circulation* (Suppl 1), 86(4):I-516, 1992 (abstract).
60. The GUIDE trial investigators: impact of intravascular ultrasound on device selection and end-point assessment of intervention: phase I of the GUIDE trial, *J Am Coll Cardiol* 21:134A, 1993 (abstract).
61. White RA, Verbin C, Scoccianti M et al: Role of cinefluoroscopy and intravascular ultrasound in evaluating the deployment of experimental endovascular prostheses, *J Vasc Surg* 21:365–374, 1995.
62. Katzen BT, Benenati JF, Becker GJ, Zemel G: Role of intravascular ultrasound in peripheral atherectomy and stent deployment, *Circulation* 84(suppl II):2152, 1991.
63. Colombo A, Hall P, Nakamura S et al: Intracoronary stents without anticoagulation accomplished with intravascular ultrasound guidance, *Circulation* 91:1676, 1995.
64. White RA, Donayre C, Kopchok G et al: Vascular imaging prior to, during and following endovascular repair, *World J Surg* 20:622–629, 1996.
65. White RA, Donayre CE, Walot I et al: Preliminary clinical outcome and imaging criterion for endovascular prosthesis deployment in high risk patients with aortoiliac and traumatic arterial lesions, *J Vasc Surg* 24:556–571, 1996.
66. White RA, Donayre CE, Walot I et al: Modular bifurcation endoprosthesis for treatment of abdominal aortic aneurysms, *Ann Surg* 226:381–391, 1997.
67. White RA, Donayre CE, Kopchok G et al: Intravascular ultrasound: the ultimate tool for abdominal aortic aneurysm endovascular graft assessment and delivery, *J Endovasc Surg* 4:45–55, 1997.
68. White RA, Donayre C, Kopchok G et al: Utility of intravascular ultrasound in peripheral interventions, *Tex Heart Inst J* 24:28–34, 1997.
69. White RA, Kopchok GE, Tabbara MR et al: Intravascular ultrasound guided holmium:YAG laser recanalization of occluded arteries, *Lasers Surg Med* 12:239–245, 1992.
70. Back MR, Kopchok GE, White RA et al: Forward-looking intravascular ultrasonography: in-vitro imaging of normal and atherosclerotic human arteries, *Am Surg* 60:738–743, 1994.

Part IV
Endovascular Instrumentation and Devices

15
Biomaterials: Considerations for Endovascular Devices

Martin R. Back and Rodney A. White

Rapidly evolving catheter-based technology has stimulated increasing application of endovascular therapy for the treatment of atherosclerotic coronary arteries and more recently peripheral vascular disease. Research and development advances have affected metal, textile, and polymer biomaterials and have facilitated refinements in design and construction of endovascular devices. As a result, the performance of these devices has improved, complications have been reduced, and the uses of minimally invasive applications have expanded. This chapter reviews the biomaterial properties and design characteristics of existing guidewires, angioplasty balloons and catheters, and metallic intravascular stents and filters with reference to their implementation and function. Design and biomaterial considerations for newly developed endoluminal grafts and their applications are also discussed.

Guidewires

Few balloon or other angioplasty catheters are sufficiently steerable and so require advancement through the vascular lumen over guidewires. Guidewires serve to find and secure a pathway through the vascular system from an entrance site and across a target lesion. Proper guidewire selection is as important as the choice of angioplasty device and catheters during endovascular interventions. Ideal guidewire characteristics include strength (to track across lesions and transmit torque), softness at the tip (atraumatic to vessel wall), steerability, and slipperiness (to minimize friction between wire, lesion, and catheter).

Standard guidewires are composed of a stiff inner core wire and an outer spring coil (Figure 15–1). The central core wire usually does not extend to the tip and is tapered distally to allow a gradual decrease in stiffness. Guidewires contain a safety wire anchored to the end of the inner core and welded to the distal end of the outer coil to prevent separation of these components and allow shaping of the tip.

The mechanical properties of guidewires determine their performance. The stiffness of a guidewire in its shaft portion varies directly with the fourth power of the inner core wire diameter.[1] Torsional strength and resistance to kinking are also dependent on the fourth power of the core diameter. The outer spring coil does not provide stiffness or torsional strength along the guidewire shaft but does influence function at the tip. Variation in construction at the guidewire tip affects its distal stiffness, which is generally less than that in the shaft (Figure 15–2). Guidewires composed of stainless steel for an equivalent diameter are four times stiffer than titanium alloy wires (Figure 15–3). Steel core wires are also more kink resistant and are the chief component of most available guidewires.[2] Frictional resistance of a guidewire is determined by the stiffness of the wire and a coefficient of friction that depends on the surface characteristics (Figure 15–4). Tetrafluoroethylene (Teflon) coating reduces the coefficient of friction by 50% for both steel

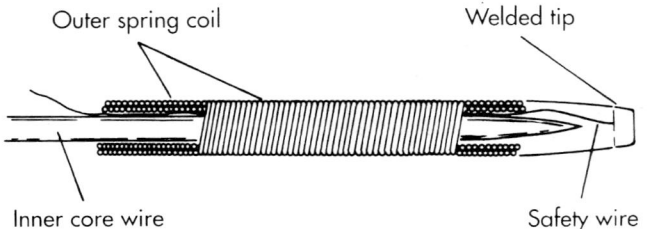

FIGURE 15–1. Components of standard stainless steel guidewire.

solid wires and guidewires with an outer spring coil.[3] Addition of a hydrophilic polymer (silicone) decreases the coefficient of friction to one-sixth the value for uncoated steel guidewires. Most guidewires have surface coating to facilitate passage through long catheters and across narrow, tortuous vessels.

Most standard steel guidewires have adequate strength and slipperiness for positioning and catheter exchanges yet lack steerability. Straight wires are relatively traumatic and are rarely used. J-shaped guidewires have tapered, softer distal ends that can be straightened or curled by moving the inner core relative to the

Type of construction of the wire tip	Mean stiffness of the tip.$10^{-6}/Nm^2/°$
Short safety wire welded onto the core at the front	0.04
Core shorter than safety wire	0.08
Core extends up to the tip (at the side of the safety wire)	0.15
No safety wire, tip fixed on the core	0.26
Moveable core without tapering of the tip Tapered at the tip	0.07
Titanium wire, hydrophilic plastic cast around the core	0.03

FIGURE 15–2. Effect of construction at the guidewire tip on average tip stiffness. (Modified from Schroder J: The mechanical properties of guidewire. Part I. Stiffness and torsional strength, *Cardiovasc Intervent Radiol* 16:43–46, 1993.)

15. Biomaterials: Considerations for Endovascular Devices

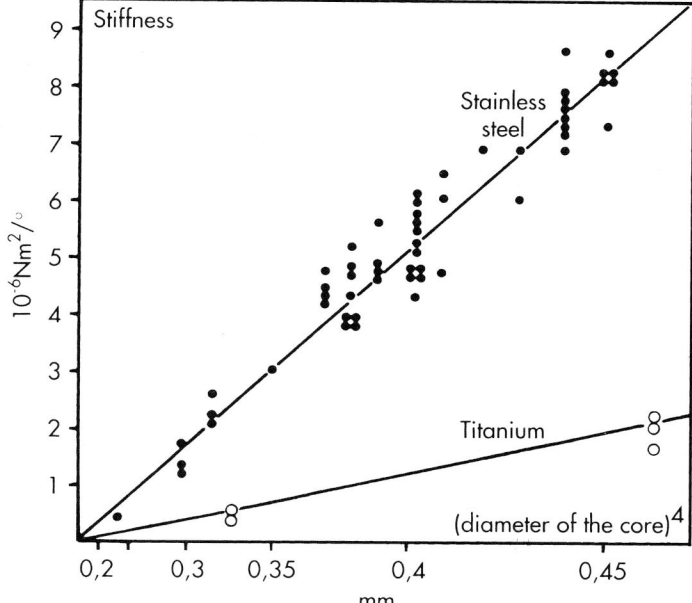

FIGURE 15–3. Dependence of guidewire stiffness on the fourth power of the inner core diameter. (Modified from Schroder J: The mechanical properties of guidewire. Part I. Stiffness and torsional strength, *Cardiovasc Intervent Radiol* 16:43–46, 1993.)

outer coil. Floppy-tip guidewires have no core wire in their distal 10 to 15 cm and are maximally flexible. Long exchange wires ranging from 145 to 260 cm in length allow shorter catheters to be withdrawn and new ones to be loaded over the wire without moving the distal tip from its position across a lesion.

Steerable guidewires are required when the diseased vessel lumen is tortuous, is nearly occluded, or has branches that are difficult to

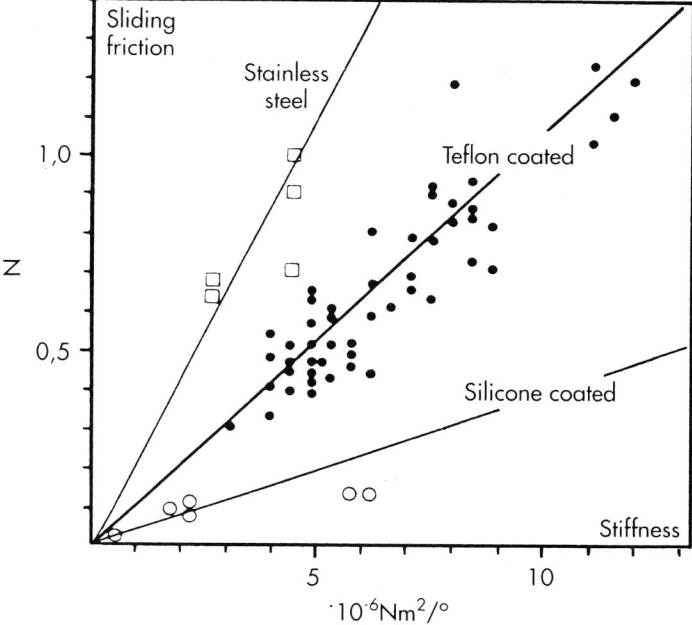

FIGURE 15–4. Dependence of sliding friction on guidewire stiffness and material surface. (Modified from Schroder J: The mechanical properties of guidewires. Part III. Sliding friction, *Cardiovasc Intervent Radiol* 16:93–97, 1993.)

cannulate owing to acute angulation. They contain a relatively long, tapered, distal segment with gradual reductions in the stainless steel core wire diameter to provide a maneuverable leading end. The proximal shaft must be relatively stiff to transmit torque and steer the distal tip. The guidewire tip may be steered by bending the proximal shaft and rotating it or applying a torque device over the proximal shaft to facilitate rotation. Standard-size steerable guidewires range from 0.028 to 0.038 inch in diameter and have variable distal tip curvatures and degrees of floppiness. Smaller balloon catheters for coronary and distal lower extremity arterial applications require smaller steerable guidewires 0.015 to 0.018 inch in diameter. These small guidewires are fragile and deform easily. Slippery guidewires are frequently coated with layers of silicone, creating a low friction surface when wetted. A slippery guidewire distributed as the GlideWire (Medi-Tech, Watertown, MA) has several unique features. Its core wire is composed of minimally elastic nickel-titanium alloy, is tapered at its distal end, and has an outer surface of polyurethane rather than spring coil. This "eel" wire is easily pliable yet kink resistant, and it is able to cross occluded arterial segments by virtue of its minimal frictional properties.

Angioplasty Balloons and Catheters

Treatment of symptomatic, focal atherosclerotic lesions in coronary arteries presently relies on percutaneous transluminal angioplasty (PTA) techniques with balloon-tipped catheters. The success of balloon angioplasty in coronary and peripheral arterial applications is related to improved balloon catheter materials and design beginning in 1974 with Gruntzig's development of a more constant volume balloon.[4] A better understanding of how balloon angioplasty dilates a stenotic lesion may also contribute to further catheter refinements. Description of the mechanism of lesion alteration by balloon dilatation has been elucidated.[5,6] There appears to be little remodeling or compaction of plaque as a result of balloon inflation. Instead, the force exerted by the balloon causes formation of cracks and tears along the luminal surface of the plaque and arterial wall. The intimal plaque is circumferentially separated from underlying media for variable distances, and less diseased arterial wall is radially stretched. The resultant increase in luminal dimensions at both the narrowest stenotic site and along adjacent vessel generally creates noncircular luminal cross sections (Figure 15–5). Because thin portions of the plaque are more easily cracked than thick atheroma, eccentrically positioned lesions are generally easier to balloon-dilate than concentric stenoses. Eccentric stenoses account for roughly two-thirds of atherosclerotic lesions found in coronary and peripheral arteries.[7] Most cracks and tears occur longitudinally along the vessel. Tears in this orientation are less apt to be lifted and produce local dissections in the wall following restoration of blood flow. This accounts for the relatively infrequent observation of significant intimal flap formation and early thrombotic occlusion after balloon angioplasty.

Balloon Mechanics

Adequate luminal enlargement within a stenotic lesion depends on the radial dilating force generated by the inflated angioplasty balloon. This dilating force is influenced by a number of factors including balloon diameter and length, inflation pressure, compliance of the balloon, and the length and degree of stenosis. If the balloon surface is indented by a localized

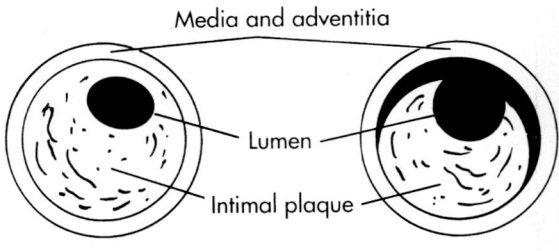

FIGURE 15–5. Mechanism of dilatation of an atherosclerotic stenosis by transluminal balloon angioplasty with a resulting noncircular luminal cross section.

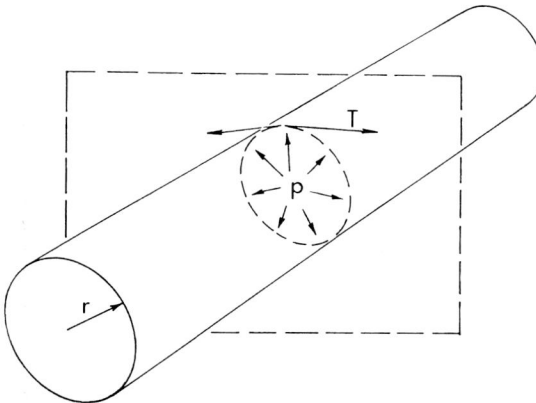

FIGURE 15–6. Circumferential tension directed tangentially at the surface is known as hoop stress (T) for thin-walled cylindrical structures. According to Laplace's law, hoop stress is equal to the product of internal pressure (p) and the radius (r).

stenosis, the dilating force is the sum of radial forces generated by the hydrostatic pressure of fluid within the balloon and the radial component of tangential stress along the balloon membrane as it expands.[8] According to Laplace's law for cylindrical thin wall structures, this tangential membrane tension or hoop stress is equal to the product of the internal pressure and the radius (Figure 15–6). Large-diameter balloons generate more hoop stress at their surface for the same applied internal pressure and thus more dilating force on a stenotic lesion. The radial force component of the hoop stress generated at the balloon membrane is greatest when the balloon is most "hourglass" in shape as occurs with large balloons and in discrete stenotic lesions with steep constriction angles. The "clothesline effect" describes the diminishing radial force component of hoop stress as the balloon fully expands and loses its "waist" as the stenosis dilates (Figure 15–7).[9]

These mechanical relationships have several important clinical implications. Large-diameter balloons generate greater dilatation force for two reasons. For a given inflation pressure in large balloons, not only is hoop stress greater within a stenotic lesion, more internal surface area exists over which hydrostatic fluid pressure acts. Large balloons therefore require less distending pressure to generate an equivalent dilating force than small-diameter balloons. Conversely, small-diameter balloons require higher inflation pressures to generate adequate dilatation. For a distended balloon with a fixed balloon and lesion diameter, the dilating force linearly increases with inflation pressure. Applying more pressure to eliminate a small dent in the balloon produces little additional dilating force owing to the "clothesline" effect and is more likely to rupture the balloon. Hoop stress exists in the vessel wall as well. In general, large-diameter vessels require less pressure to dilate and potentially to rupture. In addition to the dilating force generated by the balloon, the composition of the stenotic lesion influences the degree of luminal enlargement. Diffusely calcified plaques may resist displacement despite use of large-diameter balloons and high inflation pressures. However, because wall stresses tend to concentrate within calcific regions, balloon angioplasty more effectively cracks plaque adjacent to focal calcifications.

The relation between balloon stretch and inflation pressure (i.e., compliance) determines how effective the balloon is in terms of generating dilating force. If yield strength (i.e., the force causing permanent deformation) of the material approximates its ultimate tensile strength (i.e., the force required for material breakage), the diameter changes little with increasing inflation pressure. Inelastic balloons with low compliance provide more dilating force for a given inflation pressure at the stenosis and more predictable diameter and shape, and they resist inefficient overexpansion at the ends of the balloon (Figure 15–8). With nonstretch balloons the dilating force is not affected by balloon length. In an eccentric lesion, however, where the vessel opposite the lesion is relatively elastic, a longer balloon provides more surface area to anchor the balloon during attempted displacement of the plaque.

Balloon Materials

Several polymers have been utilized in constant-volume balloons of low compliance.[10] Early balloons and several current designs are constructed of polyvinyl chloride (PVC).

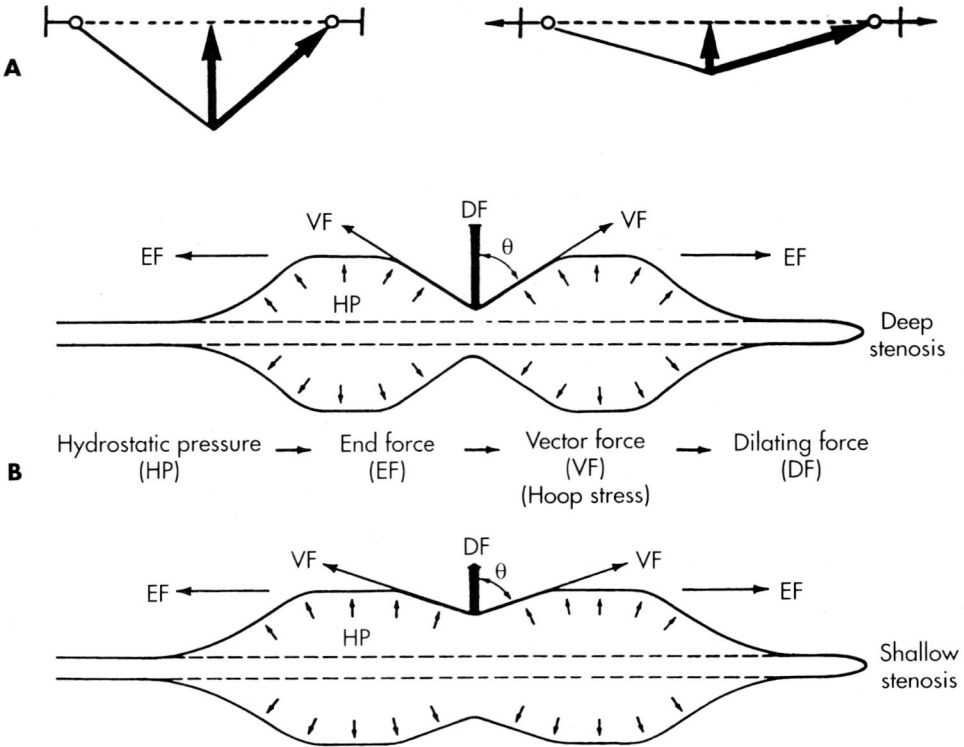

FIGURE 15–7. Dilating force and clothesline effect. **A**, When weight hanging at the center of the clothesline is lifted by pulling on each end of the line, the force vector pushing upward decreases as the line straightens. **B**, Same principle applies to balloon dilatation. If the balloon surface is indented by localized stenosis, the radial force component force pushing outward is the dilating force. With progressive balloon expansion or dilatation of the stenosis, the dilating force decreases. (From Abele JE: Balloon engineering and materials. In Vliestra RE, Holmes DR, editors: *Coronary balloon angioplasty*, Boston, 1994, Blackwell Scientific, pp 292–304.)

Because PVC balloons are more compliant than those made of other available materials, they continue to elongate and are prone to rupture with increasing inflation pressures. Large-diameter PVC balloons are more compliant than small ones. Polyethylene (PE) balloons are generally less compliant, generate greater dilating force, and have higher burst pressure than equivalent-sized PVC balloons (Figure 15–9). Diameter changes of less than 2% occur with standard PE balloons during working inflation pressures. Thin-walled PE balloons used with low-profile catheters are more compliant with 5% to 10% increases in diameter at maximum inflation pressures. Polyethylene can be chemically treated to alter its expansile properties, and these balloons are relatively "scratch resistant" within hard calcified lesions.

Newer polyethylene terephthalate (PET) balloons have low compliance and can withstand inflation pressures above 15 atm. The balloons have thin walls and low profiles and are used in small-diameter applications. They are more prone to rupture than PE balloons in calcified lesions. Balloons of composite nylon derivatives (Duralyn, Nydex) have variable compliance characteristics depending on the individual composition. Polyurethane balloons reinforced with nylon mesh (Olbert design, Meadox Medicals, Oakland, NJ) are relatively noncompliant (less than 2.5% diameter change) and have high burst pressures (more than 12 atm).

15. Biomaterials: Considerations for Endovascular Devices

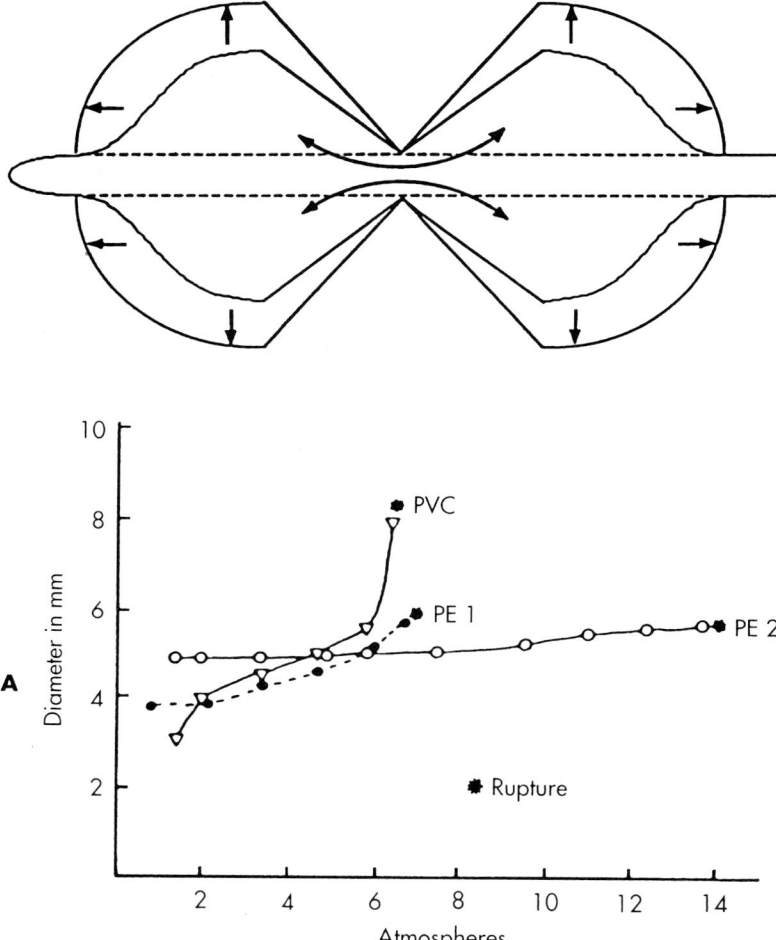

FIGURE 15-8. Overdistention of a compliant balloon, which stretches longitudinally and outward around the stenosis. (From Abele JE: Balloon catheters and transluminal dilatation: technical considerations, *Am J Radiol* 135:901–906, 1980.)

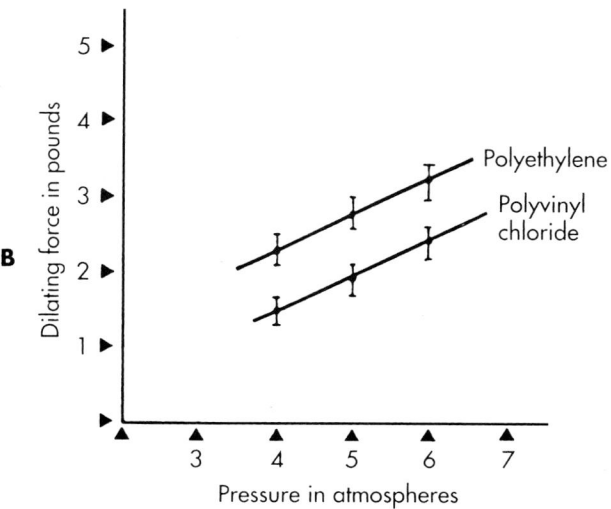

FIGURE 15-9. Comparison of balloon materials. **A**, Diameter vs. inflation pressure for polyvinyl chloride (*PVC*) and polyethylene (PE) balloons. *PE1* and *PE2* balloons have been treated differently. PE2 is almost noncompliant compared to the more elastic PVC. **B**, Dilating force for a given inflation pressure is greater for low compliance PE than for a PVC balloon. (From Abele JE: Balloon catheters and transluminal dilatation: technical considerations, *Am J Radiol* 135:901–906, 1980.)

Angioplasty Catheters

Catheters used during angioplasty procedures have varying function depending on their length, diameter, and construction. Guiding catheters provide a low-friction, large-bore channel for delivery of endovascular devices to remote target lesion sites. Although less important for interventions of iliac or femoral arteries from a transfemoral approach, guiding catheters are required for selective cannulation of coronary ostia, extracranial cerebral arteries, visceral branches, and distal extremity vasculature. In addition, these catheters must deliver contrast agents to visualize the distal vessel bed adequately and measure the pressure accurately while not occluding arterial inflow.

Traditional femoral guiding catheters range from 7F to 9F in outer diameter, whereas the newer, smaller catheters have diameters of 5F to 6F. The shaft is relatively stiff compared to the tapered, preshaped softer catheter tip. Stiff catheters provide more support for positioning and catheter exchanges and a faster torque response, but they are more difficult to advance into distal vessels. The catheter shaft is constructed in three layers.[11] An outer layer of polyethylene or polyurethane provides stiffness and a preformed shape. A middle layer permits torque control and is composed of epoxy and fiber braid or a wire braid. Inner coating with Teflon reduces frictional resistance during guidewire or catheter manipulations through the guiding catheter.

Depending on lesion location and character, angioplasty catheters are designed with differing pushability, trackability, and crossability.[12] *Pushability* refers to how application of axial force to the proximal end of the catheter translates into advantageous movement of the tip. This property depends on column strength along the catheter and resistance to buckling or kinking under an axial compressive load. *Trackability* describes the ability of a catheter to follow over a guidewire through a tortuous vessel. A number of characteristics influence trackability, including shaft diameter and length, column strength, lateral flexibility (opposite of catheter stiffness), and frictional resistance between the inner guidewire, catheter, and vessel wall. What small-diameter catheters gain in flexibility they tend to lack in column strength. To minimize the outer diameter for small-vessel applications and preserve inner diameters, the catheter wall thickness is reduced necessitating stronger shaft materials, reinforcement with braids, coils, metallic stylets, or stiffening wires, and distal catheter tapering. Current catheter shafts are constructed from polyester, polyethylene, nylon, or polyamide derivatives. *Crossability* defines how easily the distal end of the catheter traverses the lesion to be treated. The development of low profile angioplasty catheters with small-diameter, tapered distal tips, and deflated balloon segments facilitate placement across high grade stenoses. Balloons with high expansion ratios (inflated/deflated diameters) are ideal. Polymeric surface coatings on angioplasty balloons reduce frictional forces and improve crossability. Application of silicone or similar materials can reduce friction by 30% in vitro.[13] Balloons are attached to catheter shafts by adhesives or thermal bonding. This region tends to be relatively stiff and can hinder catheter tracking. Gradual transitions in catheter stiffness in the distal balloon segment and "matching" the properties of catheters and guidewires optimize lesion crossing and tracking performance.

There are three basic types of balloon angioplasty catheter: over-the-wire, fixed-wire, and monorail (Table 15–1).[13] Most balloon catheters employ an over-the-wire system and have two or more channels in their shaft: one for inflation of the balloon and one for guidewire passage, pressure measurement, or dye injection. Early catheters had coaxial shaft lumens. Current catheters have a separate dual-lumen design and allow independent movement of the balloon and the guidewire, thereby facilitating tracking and positioning in tortuous vessels and across difficult lesions. The newer fixed-wire catheters use a balloon in a guidewire design that reduces shaft diameter. The lower profile and greater flexibility of these catheters provide access to distal vessel lesions and use of smaller-bore guiding catheters. Monorail catheters have an exit port for the guidewire 20 to 40 cm from the distal balloon. The more proximal catheter shaft has a smaller

TABLE 15–1. Advantages and Disadvantages of Various Balloon Catheter Systems

Over-the-wire systems
  Advantages
    Large selection of balloons
    Exchange easy
    Can measure pressure gradient
    Distal contrast injection possible
    Can use a variety of guidewires
  Disadvantages
    Large profile
    Poor visualization
    More complicated to use than fixed wire
Fixed-wire systems
  Advantages
    Small profile
    Excellent visualization
    Conform well to bends
    Easy to use
  Disadvantages
    Cannot easily exchange
    Fixed guidewire at tip
    Wire movement less responsive than independent wires
Monorail systems
  Advantages
    Rapid lesion access
    Rapid exchange
    Improved visualization
    Improved pushability
  Disadvantages
    Back-bleeding
    Wire and balloon can tangle

From Faxon DP: Selection of balloon catheters and guidewires. In Faxon DP, editor: *Practical angioplasty*, New York, 1993, Raven Press, pp 53–70.

diameter and allows contrast injection during angioplasty. Rapid balloon catheter exchange and lesion access are provided by monorail systems.

Newer alternative catheter designs exist for balloon angioplasty, including catheters with passive perfusion sideports, porous drug delivery balloons, Olbert-type sliding coaxial catheters, the Stealth single-lumen dilation catheter, no-tip dilatation balloons, and the Fogarty-Chin extrusion balloon. For iliac and femoral arteries 5 to 10 mm diameter balloons with stiffer (5F to 8F) catheter shafts are utilized. For small coronary and infrapopliteal arteries, balloons 2 to 4 mm in diameter on 3.1F to 4.8F shafts are compatible with the necessary small-diameter guidewires.

Metallic Intravascular Stents and Caval Filters

Several metallic devices are available for endovascular applications, including stents for treatment of difficult arterial and venous stenoses, inferior vena cava filters employed to prevent pulmonary embolism, and coils used to embolize bleeding vessels, arterial true or false aneurysms, and arteriovenous fistulas. Biocompatibility (corrosion resistance, thrombogenicity, toxicity) and the mechanical and physical properties of the commonly utilized metals affect the function and healing characteristics of various stent and filter designs.

Biocompatibility

Metallic devices should not undergo significant change in their mechanical, physical, or chemical properties during the period of implantation (corrosion and fatigue resistant) and should not induce any untoward clinically significant local or systemic changes in the body (nontoxic). Ideally, cardiovascular implants are thromboresistant, easy to produce, manufactured with consistent dimensional accuracy, of good quality without impurities or contaminants, easy to sterilize, and inexpensive, and they have an appropriate surface finish.[14]

Corrosion Resistance

All available metallic endovascular devices (stents, filters, coils) are susceptible to corrosion. Because metals have high surface energy compared to that of their core, they tend to reach stability by absorbing elements from the environment. In contact with air they absorb oxygen, forming a thin layer of oxide on their surface. Such a surface is said to be "passive." It is protective for the metal by acting as a physical barrier that separates the metal core from its corrosive environment and prevents the transport of metal cations into solution. Corrosion takes place when this film is removed. The ideal corrosion-resistant metal has the ability to form a thin (1.0 to 1.5 nm), self-limiting, uniform oxide layer.[15] Corrosion of a vascular implant occurs in the presence of a saline environment by electrochemical mechanisms where the difference between electrical potential of the metal and blood determines how corrosion resistant the metal is. Metals forming a good protective film are aluminum, titanium, tantalum, and chromium, whereas stainless steel is relatively prone to corrosion.[16] Noble metals such as platinum, gold, and titanium are passive and extremely corrosion resistant but have limited use because of their excessive ductility and low tensile strength.[16]

Several additional factors influence the overall corrosion resistance of a metallic device including its bulk state, surface state, and design and processing and its handling at the time of implantation. Stainless steel (SS) in its austenitic and annealed forms is more corrosion resistant than the martensitic and work-hardened structures; and electropolished surfaces are more resistant than those mechanically polished. The sterilization method also affects the state of the final surface. Sterilization of SS by steam is superior to that by dry heat, moist ethylene oxide, or 24-hour immersion in benzalkonium chloride.[15] Corrosion can be limited by avoiding heterogeneities in the material, eliminating crevices or sharp corners, and abolishing friction between metal struts, which can produce fretting corrosion.[16]

Wallstents (Schneider USA, Plymouth, MN) and Strecker stents (MediTech/Boston Scientific, Watertown, MA) have woven and knitted configurations that are potentially more susceptible to fretting corrosion than Palmaz stents (Cordis/Johnson & Johnson, Miami Lakes, FL), which are made from a single piece of SS tube. Coating the implant with metallic plating (chromium, nickel, cadmium) or with organic or inorganic nonmetallic agents can increase corrosion resistance.[17,18] Scratching, bending, or surface contamination during handling may accelerate corrosion and produce mechanical failure.[16]

Several types of localized corrosion have been described.[15,16] Interface corrosion develops between two opposing surfaces owing to incomplete physical contact, creating electrolyte exchange (crevice corrosion), or because of two metals with different corrosion potentials exchanging electrons in a common electrolyte solution (galvanic corrosion). Pitting corrosion is the formation of small holes on the metal surface that tend to grow and can cause fracture and fatigue failure of the device. Pitting corrosion can occur with SS but is rare with vitallium and nonexistent with titanium. Intergranular corrosion, which occurs with SS, is characterized by carbide precipitation and depletion of chromium; and it is usually the result of improper manufacturing. Corrosion fatigue is due to repeated cyclic stress, causing disruption of the protective film, thereby promoting pitting corrosion and eventual fatigue cracks. Fatigue corrosion can occur with SS but not with titanium or cobalt-chromium alloys.

Toxicity

Localized or systemic toxicity can result from metal surface corrosion or by element dissolution in the medium. Local signs of biodegradation are common and are manifested by the presence of intracellular particulate matter or areas of discoloration in the tissues adjacent to the implant. Biodegradation of metals in vivo is typically less than that seen in vitro owing to the protective coating of implants by adsorbed proteins that in some cases (e.g., nickel) are metal-specific. Few data are available concerning the systemic toxicity of metals commonly used in human implants. In general, no toxicity has been associated with iron, nitinol, tantalum, or titanium compounds, whereas cobalt, chromium, molybdenum, and nickel are potentially toxic.[16] Copper, mercury, chromium, and vanadium can form biopolymer complexes that cross the cell membranes and interrupt nutrient or respiratory pathways.[19] There are also reports of severe allergic reactions to nickel and cobalt-chromium alloys present in fracture plates, joint prostheses,[15,16,20,21] cardiac pacemakers,[22] and cardiac valves[23,24] with such reactions often requiring removal of the implant.

Thromboresistance

The thrombogenic activity of a metal implant depends on its chemical and physical parameters, such as the surface charge, surface energy, and texture. The electrical charge of the surface influences the "wettability" (surface area occupied by a drop of blood) of the metal, with greater wettability increasing thrombogenicity.[25] Surfaces that are highly electronegative and donate electrons to blood (e.g., aluminum) are more thromboresistant whereas those that absorb electrons (e.g., copper) are relatively thrombogenic.[26] Increased thromboresistance is unfortunately associated with decreased corrosion resistance. DePalma et al.[27] studied type 316 SS, tantalum, nickel, and stellite 21 (Co, Cr, Mo, C) but did not find a correlation between preimplantation surface charge and thrombogenicity. A direct correlation did exist between the degree of passivation of the metal by proteinaceous deposits on its surface and thromboresistance. Surface roughness (inhomogeneities more than 1 µm in height) creates steep electrical potential gradients that hinder surface passivation and contribute to local thrombus formation.[28] This phenomenon can be limited by electropolishing and generation of smooth, homogeneous surfaces with uniform surface potential.

Thrombogenicity in vivo also depends on rheologic and hemodynamic factors (blood coagulability, blood flow patterns, shear stress). All cardiovascular devices should ultimately be evaluated in the configuration in which they are going to be used clinically, as flow abnormalities and blood hypercoagulability can lead to failure of an otherwise satisfactory material or device.[29] Available metallic stents are thrombogenic and perform best in high flow locations with adjuvant administration of antiplatelet agents. The amount of thrombus deposition is proportional to the total metal surface area of the stent,[17] so optimal thrombogenicity is gained with low profile stents with thin struts and large expansion ratios matched to the vessel diameter and lesion length to be treated. These design considerations must be balanced against the degree of mechanical support required of the expanded stent to maximize the luminal cross-sectional area after angioplasty.

Healing

The early and late events reported during the healing around metallic stents deployed in arteries and vena caval filters are derived mainly from animal investigations.[30-34] Metal composition, surface characteristics, thrombogenicity, and device design may each independently influence healing, but similar luminal and vessel wall responses occur after implantation of different stent types.

Immediately after stent implantation, fibrinogen and other blood proteins adhere to the oxide film and form a thin (5 to 20 nm) proteinaceous layer over exposed metal struts. This layer passivates the metal surface and creates a substrate for platelet and other blood element deposition.[30] After several minutes an amorphous, heterogeneous clot rich in platelets attaches to the protein layer. The early platelet-rich clot tends to fragment and slough but slowly stabilizes as the underlying protein layer thickens. After 24 hours the clot becomes less cellular and consists mainly of fibrin strands oriented in the direction of flow[30] (Figure 15–10). Within 3 to 4 weeks this thrombotic layer is replaced by a neointima of fibromuscular cells and extracellular matrix. Endothelial coverage over the neointima occurs, although several histologic and ultrastructural abnormalities suggest phenotypic heterogeneity or a cell origin different from that of native vascular endothelium.[31] Thinning of the neointima after 8 weeks is associated with resorption of cellular elements below the endothelium, leaving residual extracellular matrix and scattered fibrocytes.

Maximal neointimal thickness ranges from 50 to 400 µm and varies with the animal model and the stent used. A direct association has been found between the area of metal exposed to blood flow, the amount of initial thrombus formation, and the resulting thickness of the neointima. Stent-induced thrombosis and intimal thickening may be reduced by periprocedural anticoagulation and proper embedding of the stent struts into the arterial wall. Adequate stent deployment in a noncompliant vessel can

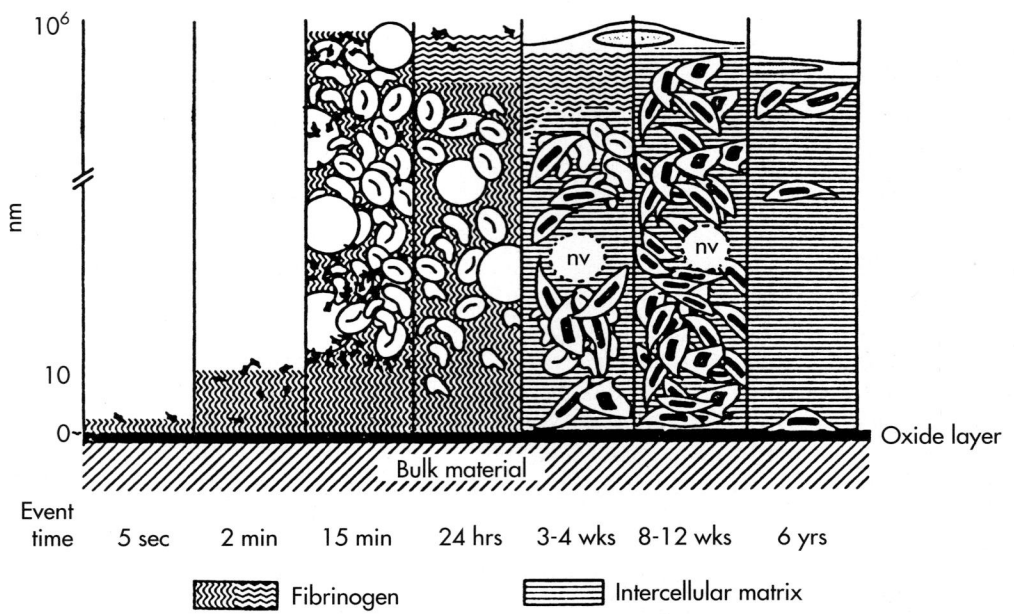

FIGURE 15–10. Deposition along the luminal surface of a stent within a vessel. Layer height is in nanometers. NV, neovessels. *Vertical undulating lines* represent randomly oriented fibrinogen strands, and *horizontal undulating lines* are fibrinogen oriented in the direction of flow. *Parallel lines* represent extracellular matrix. (From Palmaz JC: Intravascular stents: tissue-stent interactions and design considerations, *AJR* 160:613, 1993.)

usually be accomplished by dilating the stent to 10% to 15% larger than the native arterial diameter, whereas in compliant vessels a 1:1 stent/artery diameter ratio is appropriate.[30]

Periadventitial fibrosis occurs around arterial stents implanted clinically and in animal models[34] and may represent an inflammatory response to a metallic foreign body. Alternatively, altered wall stresses imparted by expanded stents may induce local tissue remodeling and inflammatory changes. Thinning of the media under expanded stent struts has been observed with Palmaz stents,[35] Wallstents,[32,34,36,37] Strecker stents,[38,39] nitinol stents,[40] Gianturco-Roubin "Bookbinder" stents (Cook, Bloomington, IN),[41] and Gianturco Z-stents (Cook).[42] Medial thinning may be due to mechanical compression of the arterial wall by oversized stents or a result of smooth muscle atrophy caused by diminished pulsatile wall stresses and motion under relatively rigid stents.[34]

Mechanical and Physical Properties of Specific Metals

Stainless Steel

Austenitic stainless steel (SS) is the most widely used metal in endovascular implants. Type 304 (Fe 70%, Cr 18% to 20%, Ni 8% to 12%, Mn < 2%, silicone < 1%, C < 0.08%) is the constituent of Gianturco Z-stents, Gianturco-Roubin "Bookbinder" stents, several vena caval filters, and Gianturco embolization coils. Type 316 (Fe 70%, Cr 16% to 18%, Ni 10% to 14%, Mn < 2%, Mo 2% to 3%, silicone < 1%, C < 0.03%) is the component of Palmaz stents and Greenfield filters (MediTech/Boston Scientific). Wallstents are made of a variant of 316 SS called Elgiloy.

The various elements present in SS provide specific properties. Chromium is a ferriteformer and stabilizes iron in a body-centered cube (bcc) crystalline state that is corrosion resistant. Nickel maintains the iron in a fully austenitic crystal structure at room temperature; and at concentrations of more than 8% it decreases ferrite production, thereby improving corrosion resistance. Molybdenum is a ferrite stabilizer and at concentrations of 3% confers special resistance against pitting corrosion. Carbon is an austenite former and strengthening agent, but low concentrations are necessary to prevent precipitation in the form of chromium carbide, which decreases the corrosion resistance of the alloy. Silicone favors surface passivation, thereby increasing corrosion resistance.[15]

Stainless steel is easy to fabricate and has adequate mechanical properties for use in vascular devices (Table 15–2). High ultimate tensile strength, low yield stress, and high ductility allow the plastic deformation necessary for construction of balloon-expandable stents. Although 316 SS is less prone to corrosion than other types of SS, its resistance to interface (crevice) corrosion and fatigue is inferior to that of other metals. Stainless steel is generally biocompatible, but several adverse reactions have been reported potentially due to liberation of a nickel derivative or iron deposits.[15,43]

Tantalum

Strecker and Viktor stents (Medtronic) are made of tantalum. This metal has a bcc structure and resists corrosion by forming a stable surface film of tantalum pentoxide. In addition to favorable corrosion resistance and biocompatibility,[44–46] tantalum is dense and highly radiopaque.[14] Despite its low tensile strength, tantalum has a relatively high elastic modulus and fatigue resistance, making it a suitable metal for balloon-expandable but not self-expanding stents.[36] Tantalum and SS stents knitted in the same pattern have demonstrated equivalent resistance to compression.[44] Despite in vitro studies showing tantalum's electronegative surface to be more thromboresistant than that of titanium, SS, or copper,[47] in vivo evaluation has revealed similar thrombogenicity.[48] Diminished platelet adhesion to tantalum stents has been achieved with polyurethane coating,[49] whereas plasma treatment has not decreased the thrombogenicity but has increased the elasticity and flexibility of Strecker stents.[18]

Titanium

Titanium has been widely used in orthopedic and oral implants, artificial heart valves, and the newer Greenfield caval filters. Titanium has a crystalline structure that varies with temperature. At low temperatures it has a hexagonal form; but if it is worked above 900°C, beta-titanium in a bcc form is produced.[38] Vanadium added to titanium stabilizes the beta form at lower temperatures. The tensile strength of titanium varies with its oxygen content, and

TABLE 15–2. Properties of Metals Used in Endovascular Implants[a]

Property	SS (annealed)	Tantalum (annealed)	Beta-titanium (F67)	Nitinol 55–45	Co-Cr alloy (wrought)
Specific gravity (g/cm^3)	7.9	16.6	4.5	4.5	9.2
Elastic modulus (Young's) (MPa)	2.0×10^5	1.0×10^5	1.0×10^5 to 1.2×10^5	0.8×10^5	2.1×10^5 to 2.5×10^5
Yield strength (0.2% strain) (MPa)	2.8×10^2	—	1.6×10^2 to 5.5×10^2	7.6×10^2	4.5×10^2 to 4.9×10^2
Ultimate tensile strength (MPa)	5.5×10^2	0.3×10^2 to 1.3×10^2	4.0×10^2 to 6.2×10^2	1.1×10^3	6.5×10^2 to 6.9×10^2
% Elongation	50	40	30	8	8
Fatigue endurance limit (MPa)	2.3×10^2 to 2.8×10^2	—	—	—	2.4×10^2 to 2.8×10^2

[a] Data were extracted from Keller et al.[46] and Castleman and Motzkin.[54]
MPa, megapascals.

high oxygen concentrations increase strength but compromise ductility. Titanium is flexible, having an elastic modulus roughly one-half that of SS, tantalum, and cobalt-chromium alloy.[50] Titanium's surface readily passivates and is resistant to pitting and crevice and stress corrosion (cracking).[50] Titanium does have a tendency to gall or seize when in sliding contact with itself or other metals, contributing to relatively poor wear resistance.[14] Greenfield and Savin compared titanium and SS vena caval filters and demonstrated more flexibility, allowing downsizing of titanium devices into 12.5F delivery sheaths from the 19F sheaths required for SS filters.[33] In vitro testing revealed greater resistance to fatigue and less corrosion of titanium filters than for SS devices. Titanium's low specific gravity allows construction of lightweight devices but hinders radiographic visualization of implants. Titanium is relatively biologically inert[51] and thromboresistant.

Nitinol

Devices constructed of nitinol (45% to 50% titanium, 50% to 55% nickel) have found increasing endovascular applications and include the Cragg stent (Mintec), Simon caval filter (Nitinol Medical Technologies, Woburn, MA), and several investigational endoluminal stent-graft devices. Nitinol is an acronym for nickel titanium Naval Ordinance Laboratory; the properties of this alloy were discovered by William Buehler.[52] The unique characteristics of this alloy are its shape memory (Marmen) effect and its superelasticity. If plastically deformed at a low temperature, it recovers its original shape when raised to a higher temperature. To possess this shape memory effect, an alloy must have a crystal structure that can shift to a martensitic (ordered, bcc superlattice) configuration when subjected to certain thermal or mechanical stresses and then revert to an austenitic (disordered bcc) structure when the stress is removed. Nitinol wires can be shaped at room temperature; and when cooled quickly with saline irrigation they assume straighter, lower profile configurations. Exposure to body temperatures at deployment allows return to its expanded, deformed shape.

To achieve full shape recovery, however, the initial deformation must not exceed an internal strain of 3% to 9%.

Superelasticity is due to the martensitic transformation induced by mechanical stress. The stress-strain relation for nitinol is linear up to a plastic deformation threshold, which is normally an irreversible process where it reverts from the austenitic to the martensitic structure and continues to deform plastically under further stress loading. When the load is removed nitinol can return to its original unstressed dimensions and austenitic structure, as occurs after an elastic deformation. Superelasticity confers to nitinol an elasticity about 10 times greater than for any other metal alloy[52] and increases the effective expansion ratio of stents by allowing greater initial compression and packaging within smaller introducer catheters. The tensile strength of nitinol is comparable to that of 316 SS, and the Cragg stent has demonstrated a hoop strength double that of the Wallstent.[53] Nitinol also has excellent fatigue resistance and corrosion resistance comparable to that of titanium.[54] Biocompatibility of nitinol is not completely known, but concern exists because of the potential allergenic and toxic effects of nickel. It has been estimated that 0.1% of the population is allergic to nickel, and of these patients 0.1% have some reaction to nitinol.[55] However, orthopedic devices and endovascular stents implanted in animals were not associated with local or systemic toxicity.[53,56,57] Inflammatory responses to implants were not different from those found around other metals despite the presence of small amounts of free nickel and titanium elements in surrounding tissue.

Cobalt-Chromium Alloys

Several cardiovascular devices are made of cobalt-chromium-based alloys and include the Vena-Tech (LG Medical, Chasseneuil, France) caval filter (Co 42%, Cr 21.5%, Ni 18%, Fe 8.85%, Mo 7.5%, Mn 2%) and several heart valves and rings. These alloys exhibit good wear and corrosion resistance and have a high elastic modulus and ductility. Carbon impurities can lead to the formation of carbides that may induce brittle behavior of the alloy. Cobalt-chromium alloys are biocompatible, but the presence of nickel and chromium have the potential to cause adverse systemic effects.[58]

Radiologic Considerations

Endovascular devices ideally are easily visible under fluoroscopy to aid deployment and do not produce artifacts when imaged by computed tomography (CT) or magnetic resonance imaging (MRI). MRI studies may be contraindicated in patients with metallic implants because of concern over potential device displacement generated by the induced electromagnetic field during the procedure. Distortion and artifact on MRI images depends on the magnetic susceptibility of the metal, its specific gravity, its shape, its position and orientation in the body, and the type of image processing.[59] The risk of device displacement is related to the strength of the magnetic field and the length of time since implantation. Endovascular device movement is unlikely after approximately 6 weeks of healing even with ferromagnetic metals.

Few studies have been performed comparing the behavior of endovascular devices when examined by CT or MRI.[45,59–61] Because of its high density, tantalum implants are easily visible under fluoroscopy but produce significant artifacts on CT images. Titanium devices are relatively radiolucent but produce little CT artifact owing to their lower specific gravity. MRI imaging artifacts, ferromagnetism, and magnetic torque of several endovascular devices have been investigated by Teitelbaum et al.[60] Although 304 and 316SS are both austenitic and therefore nonmagnetic, the type of cold working required to fabricate devices can induce significant ferromagnetism. The 316SS has a higher nickel content than the 304 type, which better stabilizes iron in a nonmagnetic state. However, all SS devices generate marked "black hole" artifacts and MRI image distortion. Elgiloy and nitinol devices create mild MRI artifacts. Titanium devices have little ferromagnetism in fields up to 4.7 tesla and do not generate MRI artifacts. MRI images of tantalum-constructed Strecker stents implanted in dogs showed few artifacts and provided clear visualization of the stented arterial lumen.[61]

Design Characteristics

Stents

Three general types of intravascular stent have been developed: balloon-expandable, self-expanding, and thermal memory (nitinol) stents (Table 15–3). Available stents are currently made of acceptable biocompatible materials. Performance of a given stent is influenced by the biomaterial properties and the stent design. Characteristics of an ideal intravascular stent have been described by Becker (Table 15–4).[62]

The invitro mechanical properties of Palmaz stents,[63] Wallstents,[37,64] Gianturco Z-stents,[65] and Cragg stents[53] have been reported. Overall stent stiffness is related to the metal used, strut caliber, the length of the stent, and the ratio between the compressed and expanded diameter.[32] In vitro, the Palmaz stent is three times more rigid and has a higher radial strength than the Wallstent.[63] Cragg et al. reported nitinol spiral stents to have a hoop strength twofold that of Wallstents.[53] However, after expansion invivo, the adequacy of radial stiffness of the stent for optimizing luminal diameter is more dependent on matching stent and artery size, plaque distribution, and morphology than on stent material. Strut thickness of available stents varies with stent diameter but differs among designs. Nitinol's superelastic properties potentially facilitate construction of stents with small struts while maintaining radial strength. Currently, Wallstents and Strecker stents have the smallest caliber struts. Although the surface area occupied by exposed struts in an expanded stent may influence stent thrombogenicity, most available stents have similar metal surface areas. Gianturco Z-stents and Viktor and Cragg spiral stents have the least metal surface area, and Strecker stents have the largest area. Palmaz stents have a metal surface area of 31% when collapsed and 12% at 6mm diameter expansion[35]; expanded Wallstents have 20% exposed metal surface area.[32]

TABLE 15–3. Characteristics of Current Vascular Stents

Characteristic	Palmaz	Strecker	Viktor	Gianturco Roubin	Wallstent	Gianturco Z-Stent	Cragg
Manufacturer	Cordis/ J & J	MediTech/ Boston Scientific	Medtronic	Cook	Schneider (USA)	Cook	Mintec
Expansion mode	Balloon exp	Balloon exp	Balloon exp	Balloon exp	Self-exp	Self-exp	Thermal memory
Configuration	Slotted	Knitted mesh	Helical coil	Bookbinder coil	Woven mesh	Zigzag pattern	Spiral
Composition	316SS	Tantalum	Tantalum	304SS	Elgiloy	304SS	Nitinol
Strut thickness (mm)	0.12	0.07–0.10	0.13	0.15	0.07–0.17	—	0.27
Delivery sheath (F)	6–9	10	8	—	7–9	—	8–10
Expanded diameter (mm)	3–18	2–14	2.5–3.5	2–4	2.5–15.0	—	8–10
Expansion ratio	High	High	High	Low	High	High	High
Foreshortening	++	++	+	++	+++	0	+
Metal surface	++	+++	+	++	++	+	+
Longitudinal flexibility	0	+++	++	+++	+++	0	++
Radial flexibility	0	+++	+	+	+++	+	+
Retrievable when deployed	No	No	?	No	No	?	Yes
Biocompatibility	+	+	+	+	+	+	+
Radiopacity	+	+++	+++	+	+	+	+
MRI artifacts	++	0	0	+++	++	+++	+

exp, expandable; MRI, magnetic resonance imaging.

TABLE 15–4. Characteristics of Ideal Intravascular Stents

Biocompatible (thromboresistant, corrosion resistant, fatigue resistant)
Induce minimal intimal hyperplasia
High expansion ratio
Low profile
High hoop strength
Longitudinal flexibility
Minimal foreshortening when deployed
Sufficient compliance
Easy to deliver
Reliable expansion
Retrievable if maldeployed
Does not migrate
Highly radiopaque
No artifact when imaged by CT or MRI
Inexpensive

From Becker GJ: Intravascular stents: general principles and status of lower extremity arterial applications. *Circulation* 83 (suppl I): 122, 1991.

Although all available stents have an expansion ratio of approximately 6:1, their degree of foreshortening at full expansion varies. Little foreshortening exists with nitinol spiral stents (about 7%)[53] but increases to between 13% and 25% for Palmaz stents and up to 40% for Wallstents.[64] Significant foreshortening makes precise positioning of the stent difficult, necessitates the use of longer stents for proper lesion treatment, and potentially increases the thrombogenic potential of the stent because of the larger exposed metal surface areas. Whereas expansion is more predictable with balloon- and self-expandable stents, thermal memory stents are dependent on a critical change in temperature for expansion. Deployment of nitinol stents requires constant infusion of cold saline prior to delivery and precise matching of the expanded stent to the target artery diameter to avoid undersizing the stents. The nitinol stent is the only stent potentially retrievable after deployment.

Some stent flexibility is required to cross tortuous vessels and is desirable if positioning is required within vessels near flexing joints. Wallstents and Strecker stents have both longitudinal and radial flexibility,[37,38] whereas Cragg spiral stents have only longitudinal flexibility and Palmaz stents are relatively rigid. Some radial flexibility may decrease the compliance mismatch between the stented and unstented portions of the vessel and potentially reduce intimal hyperplasia and restenosis phenomena.[66] However, radial flexibility of Wallstents deployed in normal canine arteries is lost within weeks after stenting due to progressive fibrous encapsulation.[34] Recurrent intimal trauma caused by the cyclic motion of flexible stents has been proposed to contribute to a neointimal reaction,[30,32,36,62] but no significant differences in neointimal thickness have been found between self-expanding (Wallstent) and balloon-expandable (Palmaz) stents deployed in animals.[32,37] Strecker stents produce some retraction at the ends of the struts (i.e., flaring), which may protrude into the lumen[38,48,68,69] and potentially contribute to increased intimal thickening, irregular surface contour, and an occasional marked inflammatory reaction around the metal struts.[69]

Vena Caval Filters

Several inferior vena cava filters have been developed to prevent pulmonary embolism, and their characteristics have been extensively reviewed.[70] With the exception of the Simon nitinol filter, they are all self-expandable. Greenfield SS filters have been used for more than 12 years and have a filter patency rate of 98%, an inferior vena caval (IVC) patency rate of 95%, and a low incidence of recurrent pulmonary embolism (4%), moreover, only a few cases of migration or perforation have been reported. Hampered by its large delivery system (24F) insertion site, venous thrombosis unfortunately occurs with significant frequency (41%).[70] Newer models of the Greenfield filter have been constructed of beta-titanium and have modified attachment hooks. The greater elasticity of titanium has facilitated downsizing of the device and delivery through a 12F carrier system (14F sheath), and it has reduced the incidence of insertion site thrombosis to 8% while maintaining comparable efficacy (recurrent pulmonary embolism rate 3.5%, IVC patency rate 99%).[71] The greater elasticity of titanium may be responsible for the 10% incidence of filter limb asymmetry[71] and potential perforation of the IVC due to excessive limb splaying.[72]

The Gianturco-Roehm Bird's Nest filter made of 304 SS can be delivered through a 12F sheath and can expand up to 4 cm, making it ideal for deployment into large IVCs. Although its use is associated with an IVC patency rate of 97%, a filter patency rate of 81% and an incidence of recurrent embolism of only 2.7%, cases of filter migration have been reported.[70]

The Vena-Tech/LGM filter is conposed of a cobalt-chromium alloy, can potentially self-center when deployed, and is delivered through a 12F sheath. It has been evaluated in a multi-center clinical trial in Europe. Although the incidence of recurrent pulmonary embolism has been low (2%), the incidence of complications is high (migration 13%, IVC thrombosis 8%, tilting 8%).[73]

The Simon nitinol filter has the lowest profile available, is delivered through a 9F sheath, and requires cold saline irrigation during its deployment. Its use has not been fully evaluated clinically, but a high incidence of IVC thrombosis (20%) has been reported. This poor patency rate may be due to filter design the thrombogenicity of the nitinol alloy, or both.[70,74]

Endoluminal Grafts

Great interest has been generated by the early animal and clinical experience with catheter-based delivery of endoluminal prostheses to exclude infrarenal abdominal aortic aneurysms.[75-87] Various combinations of anchoring stents attached to prosthetic grafts have also been used selectively to treat peripheral aneurysms,[88-90] arterial occlusive disease involving aortoiliac and femoropopliteal segments,[90-94] and traumatic arterial pseudoaneurysms and arteriovenous fistulas.[80,86,95] Little comparative information exists regarding early and long-term healing and performance of the various endoluminal graft designs. The clinical success and acceptance of these devices will depend on careful controlled examination of their endovascular deployment, function, modes of failure, and associated complications. Only from such data can optimal design characteristics be discerned.

Prosthetic Materials

Most endoluminal prostheses are constructed from currently available graft materials and metallic stents. Various polyester (Dacron) grafts have generally been used for placement within aortic aneurysms,[76,78-87,92] and polytetrafluoroethylene (PTFE) grafts have been utilized in peripheral arterial applications.[88-91,93-96] Although endoluminal graft designs under evaluation differ significantly, the choice of prosthetic material may influence device performance.

Dacron grafts have been the mainstay of aortic reconstruction since the early 1960s, and PTFE found application as an arterial conduit during the 1970s. Dacron grafts are soft and pliable yet relatively inelastic; they demonstrate minimal dilatation after implantation, with a 6% to 12% increase in cross-sectional area observed during extended in vitro testing.[97] At physiologic arterial pressures Dacron and PTFE vascular grafts have radial compliances much less than that of normal or diseased arteries (Table 15-5).[98-100] Compliance of synthetic grafts tends to decrease further after implantation owing to necessary fibrous tissue ingrowth and encapsulation. Strength in the polyester fabric structure is cumulatively determined by basic polymer, individual fiber, and yarn structure properties (Figures 15-11, 15-12, 15-13).[101] Tensile yield strengths range from nearly 100 times that of native aorta for woven Dacron and standard wall PTFE grafts to 10-fold greater for double velour knits (Table 15-6).[99] Radial burst strengths are 110 to 120 pounds per square inch (psi) for double velour knitted Dacron grafts and 30 psi for thin-walled PTFE grafts—considerably more than the maximal arterial pressure (250 mm Hg = 4.8 psi).[97,102] Small-caliber, thin-walled, nonreinforced PTFE sleeves used for endoluminal grafting allow low profile device delivery and can be balloon-expanded to 3 to 5 times their original diameters.[103] Significant microscopic structural deformation may occur in material dilated beyond this elastic limit, generating concern over the long-term stability and strength of PTFE endografts used with large expansion ratios. Adequate short-term (less than 1 year) structural integrity of PTFE endoluminal grafts within experimental aortic aneurysms has been demonstrated by Palmaz et al.,[104] but long-term evaluation is needed.

TABLE 15-5. Radial Compliance of Human Artery and Synthetic Grafts

Graft	Conduit time after implantation	Species	Compliance (% diameter change/ mm Hg × 10^{-2})
Thoracic aorta[98]		Human	
		(Age 20 years)	27
		(Age 40 years)	20
		(Age 60 years)	14
Femoral artery[99]		Human (age > 50 years)	6-11
Woven Dacron[100]	0	Human	0.16
Knitted Dacron[99,100]	0	Human	1.5-1.9
	8 mo		0.8
Double velour Dacron[100]	0	Human	3.4
Standard PTFE[99]	0	Human	1.6

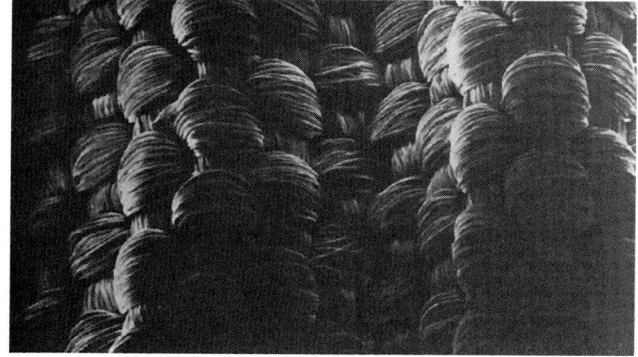

FIGURE 15–11. Scanning electron micrography (SEM) of the outer surface of a DeBakey woven Dacron vascular graft. ×37. (From Snyder RW, Botzko KM: Woven, knitted and externally supported Dacron vascular prostheses. In Stanley JC, editor: *Biologic and synthetic vascular prostheses*, Orlando, 1982, Grune & Stratton, pp 485–494.)

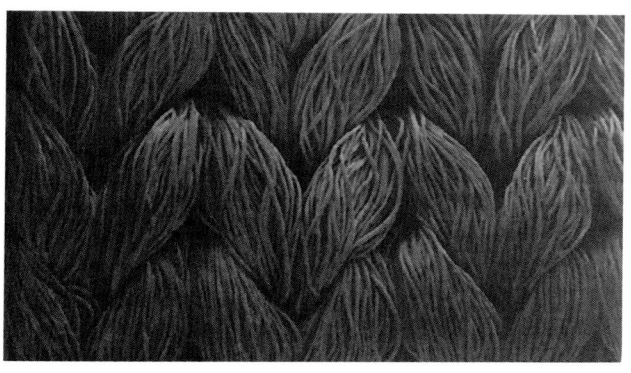

FIGURE 15–12. SEM of the outer surface of a DeBakey standard knit Dacron vascular graft. ×37. (From Snyder RW, Botzko KM: Woven, knitted and externally supported Dacron vascular prostheses. In Stanley JC, editor: *Biologic and synthetic vascular prostheses*, Orlando, 1982, Grune & Stratton, pp 485–494.)

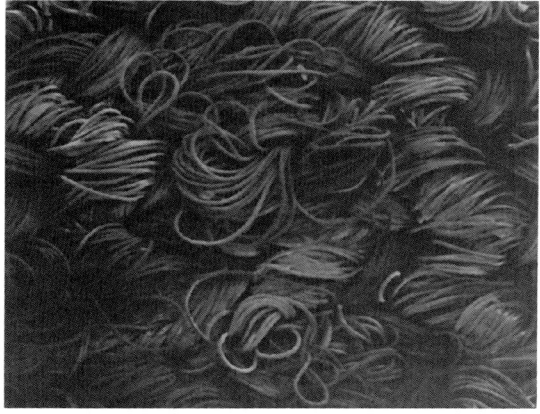

FIGURE 15–13. SEM of the inner, luminal surface of a Dacron velour graft. ×37. (From Turner RJ, Hoffman HL, Weinberg SL: Knitted Dacron double velour grafts. In Stanley JC, editor: *Biologic and synthetic vascular prostheses*, Orlando, 1982, Grune & Stratton, pp 509–522.)

TABLE 15–6. Tensile Yield Strength of Native Artery and Synthetic Grafts

Material	Yield strength (dynes/cm^2)
Thoracic aorta	3.8×10^7
Woven Dacron	2.2×10^9
Knitted Dacron	0.8×10^9
Double velour knitted Dacron	0.3×10^9
Standard wall reinforced PTFE	3.3×10^9

Modified from Kinley CE, Marble AE: Compliance: a continuing problem with vascular grafts, *J Cardiovasc Surg* 21:163–170, 1980.

Porosity is an essential component for the function of synthetic vascular prostheses. For textile grafts this parameter is difficult to describe quantitatively. Wesolowski et al. assessed the porosity of fabric grafts in terms of their permeability by measuring the volumetric flow of water through the material at a pressure differential of 120 mm Hg (ml H$_2$0/cm^2/min).[105] Early studies in pigs and dogs advocated the use of Dacron grafts, with the permeability approaching 5000 ml/cm^2/min for optimal healing (Gossamer theory).[105] These porous, ultrathin-wall, knitted grafts were associated with significant dilatation and hemorrhage clinically, however.[106] Current Dacron grafts have lower porosity, thicker walls, greater strength, and improved healing characteristics (Figure 15–14). Connective tissue penetration is not essential for genesis of a pseudointima, but connective tissue support is critical to its long-term existence. This statement is based on the observation that a pseudointima is not formed in areas where tissue incorporation is completely absent, although it is frequently present in areas where adjacent connective tissue is minimal.[107] Extensive proliferation of fibrous tissue as observed in Gossamer grafts in animals may not be desirable but some degree of ingrowth is necessary. Higher-porosity (60 μm fibril length) PTFE grafts have shown improved healing and luminal surface endothelialization in animals,[108] but clinical evaluation did not demonstrate differences in the healing response compared to standard-wall (20 to 30 μm fibril length) PTFE grafts.[109]

Whereas heavy polyester fabric with greater wall thickness potentially reduces the risk of graft dilatation or aneurysm rupture, the lightweight, thin-walled grafts facilitate reduction of the delivery catheter diameter and associated vessel trauma during their insertion and positioning. The ideal balance for endoluminal graft applications between material strength, porosity, pliability, distensibility, and thickness remains to be determined.

In general, more porous, thinner-walled polyester grafts have greater distensibility (Figure 15–15).[94] Velour Dacron grafts were developed initially to improve healing along luminal and external surfaces (Figure 15–13). Early velour

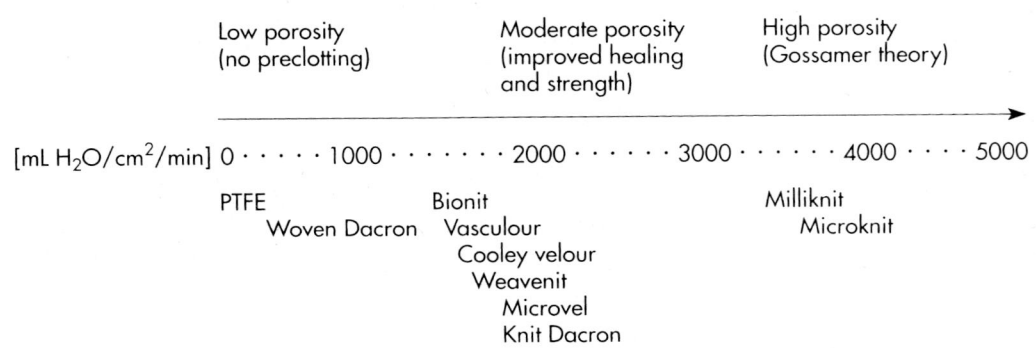

FIGURE 15–14. Range of permeabilities and corresponding porosity for available polyester and PTFE vascular prostheses (in milliliters of water per square centimeter per minute) at a 120 mm Hg pressure differential. (Modified from Snyder RW, Botzko KM: Woven, knitted and externally supported Dacron vascular prostheses. In Stanley JC, editor: *Biologic and synthetic vascular prostheses*, Orlando, 1982, Grune & Stratton, pp 485–494.)

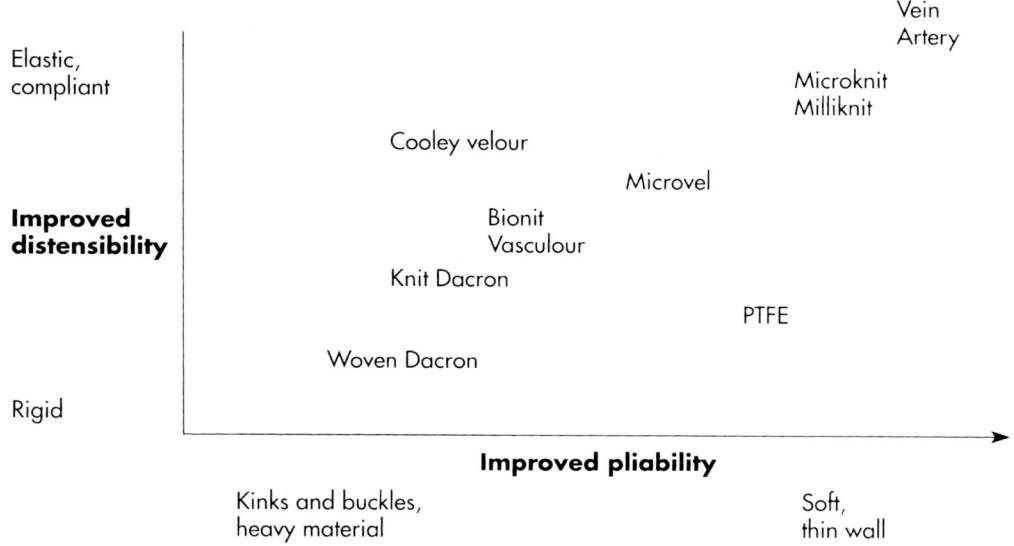

FIGURE 15-15. Range of qualitative handling characteristics of available polyester and PTFE vascular graft materials compared to those of native vessels. With a thinner wall, the lighter-weight Dacron prostheses tend to be more elastic. (From Snyder RW, Botzko KM: Woven, knitted and externally supported Dacron vascular prostheses. In Stanley JC, editor: *Biologic and synthetic vascular prostheses*, Orlando, 1982, Grune & Stratton, pp 485-494.)

grafts (Sauvage Bionit, DeBakey Vasculour) had intermediate porosity compared to woven and knit Dacron but improved handling characteristics. The newer double velour grafts (Microvel and Cooley knit) have permeability similar to that of knit Dacron and are more elastic. The wall thickness of double velour grafts is increased by the inner and outer layers (pile heights 180 and about 400 μm, respectively) of perpendicular yarn loops.[90] Thin-walled knitted Dacron (Weavenit) has a wall thickness of 380 μm by comparison. The fine porous surface within the velour pile increases the tissue bond between graft and perigraft tissues and improves the rate of tissue incorporation in Dacron grafts implanted in experimental animals. These studies utilized mechanical peel tests to document more complete and adherent tissue layers along luminal and external surfaces of velour grafts.[99] Lindenauer described enhanced healing of double-velour Dacron grafts compared with either internal or external velour surfaces alone.[100] Other studies have noted a more adherent outer fibrous layer with double velour fabrics but no difference in luminal surface healing.[101] Clagett reported reduced platelet survival and less pseudointimal development on double-velour grafts compared with knitted surfaces for 42 weeks following surgery.[102] At present, improved healing characteristics of velour Dacron fabrics, especially in humans, have not been adequately documented.

The healing characteristics of various endoluminal grafts used for arterial aneurysmal and occlusive disease applications and how they differ from responses to standard, open prosthetic reconstructions are largely unknown. Prosthetic coating over stents has been proposed to inhibit the neointimal ingrowth that limits long-term patency rates following angioplasty and stenting of occlusive lesions, but clinical and experimental evidence of this benefit is lacking. Preliminary studies of endoluminal prostheses constructed from PTFE grafts and Palmaz stents deployed in nondiseased canine iliac arteries showed more neointimal development but a preserved luminal cross-sectional area compared to that of the anastomotic regions of interposition PTFE grafts.[114] Interestingly, more complete endothelial cell coverage of endoluminal PTFE/Palmaz stented grafts has been observed in dogs than occurred on the inner surface of interposition PTFE grafts.[114,115] Descriptions of clinical endoluminal graft healing are limited to several brief reports.[116-118] Detection of endothelial cell coverage up to 7cm into an endoluminal graft by factor VIII staining was noted 5 months after device deployment for arterial occlusive disease.[116] In that series, a local inflammatory response to endoluminal grafting appeared to be related to the presence or absence of a reinforcing wrap on the PTFE used and the layer within the wall in which the device recanalized. It remains to be seen whether reendothelialization is facilitated by intraluminal positioning of stent-graft devices compared to the pseudointima developing after standard prosthetic reconstructions that remain devoid of endothelial cells. The healing characteristics of prosthetic materials deployed within thrombus-filled aneurysmal arteries also have not been fully elucidated.

A pronounced, early, systemic inflammatory response to endoluminal grafts has been observed in several clinical series, manifested by fever and leukocytosis. Elevated levels of various serum markers of inflammation were noted by Hayoz et al.[119] in patients after deployment of Cragg Endopro System 1 devices (Mintec Minimally Invasive Technologies SARL, La Ciotat, France) when compared to nitinol stents implanted for occlusive disease and by Norgren and Swartbol[120] after endoluminal grafting of aortic aneurysms compared to conventional open repairs. Despite significant proinflammatory cytokine and leukocyte adhesion molecule responses after endoluminal grafting, no correlation was found between inflammatory mediator levels and the presence of patient symptoms.[119] Interestingly, in vitro neutrophil activation could be elicited only by exposure to complete endoluminal devices but not to individual biomaterial components of the endografts.[119] The clinical importance of systemic inflammatory responses and their specific cause as related to device construction and deployment are unknown.

Device Design

Endoluminal grafts under evaluation are constructed of various prosthetic graft and stent devices and have varying designs that differ beyond their intended application (Table 15–7). Devices developed for exclusion of infrarenal aorta and iliac artery aneurysms have evolved from (1) single piece, tubular grafts that are anatomically appropriate in fewer than 10% of abdominal aortic aneurysms (AAAs) to (2) bifurcated modular designs. Because of the need for precise device size specifications (e.g., aortic and iliac limb diameters and lengths) necessary for successful aneurysm exclusion and to avoid the inefficiency of manufacturer customization for each case, "telescoping," or "trombone," designs have been proposed that require sequential deployment and overlap of multiple individual components. These devices remain in the developmental stage, although several modular designs are under early controlled clinical evaluation.

Both woven and knitted polyester coverings have been utilized in endoluminal graft designs to exclude aortic aneurysms. Conventional, thicker-walled Dacron grafts were used in several initial clinical series and required ironing to eliminate crimps and allow catheter packaging and device delivery.[83,86] The straight, aortoaortic EVT (Endovascular Technologies, Menlo Park, CA) device used in the North American phase I trial[85] and the modified bifurcated endograft of Chuter et al.[82] were constructed of lightweight, thin-walled, uncrimped woven Dacron. Woven material was chosen to optimize graft strength and minimize the porosity and potentially continued perfusion of the aneurysm sac through the graft interstices. The AneuRx (Medtronic AneuRx, Cupertino, CA) and Vanguard (Meadox/Boston Scientific, Oakland, NJ) bifurcated modular prostheses currently in phase II trials utilize seamless, ultrathin, low porosity, woven Dacron coverings. Knitted Dacron materials have desirable handling characteristics (pliability, distensibility) but are more permeable and potentially may not seal as effectively as woven grafts. However, thin-walled (200 μm thick), knitted

TABLE 15-7. Endoluminal Graft Designs

Device	Application	Configuration	Graft material	Support
Parodi[79,80]	AAA	Aortomonoiliac	Dacron (ultrathin, knit)	Palmaz stent (prox, distal)
White[86]	AAA	Aortomonoiliac	Dacron (thin, knit)	Palmaz stent (prox, distal)
Chuter[82] (Cook/Meadox)	AAA	Singular, bifurcated	Dacron (thin, woven)	Gianturco Z (prox, distal, barbed)
EVT[85]	AAA	Tubular, aortoaortic	Dacron (thin, woven)	Self-expanding (prox, distal, barbed)
White-Yu GAD[84]	AAA	Modular, "trombone"	Dacron (thin, woven)	Elgiloy scaffold (balloon exp)
Vanguard (Meadox)/Boston Scientific)	AAA	Modular, bifurcated	Dacron (ultrathin, woven)	Nitinol scaffold (self-exp)
AneuRx[87] (Medtronic)	AAA	Modular, bifurcated	Dacron (ultrathin, woven)	Nitinol scaffold (self-exp)
Talent (World Medical Manufacturing)	AAA	Modular, bifurcated	Dacron ± PTFE (contralat limb)	Nitinol scaffold (self-exp)
Cragg/Dake[91]	Occl dz	Straight	6mm PTFE (thin wall)	Nitinol/Palmaz/Wallstent
Cragg Endopro System 1[92] (Mintec)	Occl dz	Straight	Dacron (thin, woven) + LMW heparin bonding	Nitinol scaffold (self-exp)
Marin[93]	Aortoiliac occl dz	Singular	6mm PTFE (thin wall)	Palmaz stent (prox)
Diethrich[90]	SFA occl/aneurysm dz)	Singular	2-3mm PTFE (ultrathin wall)	Palmaz stent (prox, distal)

AAA, abdominal aortic aneurysm; occl dz, occlusive disease; SFA, superior femoral artery; LMW, low molecular weight; prox, proximal; exp, expandable.

Dacron endovascular grafts used clinically by Parodi have not been associated with bleeding complications, endoleaks, or aneurysm rupture.[80] These relatively elastic grafts have a midshaft radial compliance of 15% and a proximal end overlying a Palmaz stent capable of nearly 45% diameter expansion. Progressive dilatation has not been observed clinically in these knitted grafts during a mean follow-up of 17 months.

As prosthetic covering used in endoluminal grafts has evolved from thick conventional materials to thinner, unsupported prototypes, the need for stent reinforcement along the entire length of the device has become apparent. Initial clinical series of endoluminal grafts for AAA exclusion employed individual balloon- or self-expandable stents (Palmaz, Gianturco Z-stents) at aortic and iliac device fixation sites.[79-83,85,86] Intravascular ultrasonography (IVUS) during and after endoluminal graft deployment in dogs has provided insight into device performance.[120] In unsupported segments between proximal and distal anchoring stents, thinner-walled, uncrimped knitted polyester moved away from the vessel wall during arterial pulsations. The longitudinal folding that occurred during decelerated systolic and diastolic flow phases diminished graft luminal diameter and is due to elastic instability causing buckling along the unsupported cylindrical tube subjected to variation in external and internal pressures. Thrombus accumulation between the prosthesis and the aortic wall occurred in these grafts after implantation. Fibrous tissue reaction was enhanced in areas of excessive graft motion and resulted in luminal narrowing.[121,122] Transverse and longitudinal folding was also observed in thin-walled, uncrimped, knitted grafts and thin-walled PTFE stented grafts when they were inadequately extended to full length during deployment.[121,122] In contrast, crimped Dacron endoluminal grafts had greater radial support, did not buckle with arterial pulsation, and conformed better to the vessel wall.[121] A fibrotic reaction was minimized along crimped grafts and in stented regions. Based on these findings, firm apposition of graft material to adjacent vessel wall (or aneurysm clot) appears to promote healing, preserve luminal diameter, and optimize graft flow characteristics.

More complete graft support has been accomplished with self-expanding stent designs utilizing attachment of material to metallic struts at multiple sites or incorporation of metallic scaffolding within the prosthetic material. Self-expanding nitinol wire in a zigzag configuration provides column strength and radial support along the full length of a Dacron graft in the Vanguard, Talent (World Medical Manufacturing, Sunrise, FL), and AneuRx devices; the wire is present on the outer surface of the prosthetic material in the latter device to diminish potential thrombogenicity associated with metal exposure. The strength of proximal aortic neck fixation for various expanded endoluminal grafts has not been comparatively evaluated but appears adequate for the unbarbed stent designs that comprise most current devices.

References

1. Schroder J: The mechanical properties of guidewires. Part I. Stiffness and torsional strength, *Cardiovasc Intervent Radiol* 16:43–46, 1993.
2. Schroder J: The mechanical properties of guidewires. Part II. Kinking resistance, *Cardiovasc Intervent Radiol* 16:47–48, 1993.
3. Schroder J: The mechanical properties of guidewires. Part III. Sliding friction, *Cardiovasc Intervent Radiol* 16:93–97, 1993.
4. Gruntzig A, Hopff H: Percutane Rekanalisation chronischer arterieller Verschlusse mit einem neuen Dilatationskatheter: Modification der Dotter-Technik, *Dtsch Med Wochenschr* 99:2502–2505, 1974.
5. Castaneda-Zuniga WR, Formanek A, Tadaverthy M et al: The mechanism of balloon angioplasty, *Radiology* 135:565–571, 1980.
6. Chin AK, Kinney TB, Rurik GW et al: A physical measurement of the mechanisms of transluminal angioplasty, *Surgery* 95:196–200, 1983.
7. Waller BF: The eccentric coronary atherosclerotic plaque: morphologic observations and clinical relevance, *Clin Cardiol* 12:14–20, 1989.
8. Abele JE: Balloon catheters and transluminal dilatation: technical considerations, *Am J Radiol* 135:901–906, 1980.
9. Abele JE: Balloon catheter technology. In: Castaneda-Zuniga WR, Tadavarthy SM, editors: *Interventional radiology*, Baltimore, 1992, Williams & Wilkins, pp 345–350.
10. Matsumoto AH, Barth KH, Selby JB, Tegtmeyer CJ: Peripheral angioplasty balloon technology, *Cardiovasc Intervent Radiol* 16:135–143, 1993.
11. Jacobs AK: Selection of guiding catheters. In Faxon DP, editor: *Practical angioplasty*, New York, 1993, Raven Press, pp 43–52.
12. Abele JE: Balloon engineering and materials. In Vlietstra RE, Holmes DR, editors: *Coronary balloon angioplasty*, Boston, 1994, Blackwell Scientific, pp 292–304.
13. Faxon DP: Selection of balloon catheters and guidewires. In Faxon DP, editor: *Practical angioplasty*, New York, 1993, Raven Press, pp 53–70.
14. Williams DF: The selection of implant materials. In Williams DF, Roaf R, editors: *Implants in surgery*, London, 1973, Saunders, chap 6.
15. Sutow EJ, Pollack SR: The biocompatibility of certain stainless steels. In Williams DF, editor: *Biocompatibility of clinical implants materials*, vol 1, Boca Raton, 1981, CRC Press, chap 3.
16. Williams DF: The deterioration of materials in use. In Williams DF, Roaf R, editors: *Implants in surgery*, London, 1973, Saunders, chap 4.
17. Palmaz JC: Balloon expandable intravascular stent, *AJR* 150:1263–1269, 1988.
18. Crochet D et al: Plasma treatment effects on the tantalum Strecker stent implanted in femoral arteries of sheep, *Cardiovasc Intervent Radiol* 17:285–291, 1994.
19. Lemons JE: Corrosion and biodegradation. In von Recum A, editor: *Handbook of biomaterials evaluation*, New York, Macmillan, 1986, chap 9.
20. Fisher AA: Safety of stainless steel in nickel sensitivity, *JAMA* 221:1282, 1972.

21. Fisher AA: Allergic dermatitis presumably due to metallic bodies containing nickel or cobalt, *Cutis* 19:285, 1977.
22. Samitz MH, Katz SA: Nickel dermatitis hazards from prostheses: in vivo and in vitro solubility studies, *Br J Dermatol* 92:287, 1975.
23. Lyell A, Bain WH: Nickel allergy and valve replacement, *Lancet* 1:408, 1974.
24. Pegum JS: Nickel allergy, *Lancet* 1:674, 1974.
25. Williams DF: The response of the body environment to implants. In Williams DF, Roaf R, editors: *Implants in surgery*, London, 1973, Saunders, chap 5.
26. Sawyer PN et al: Electrochemical precipitation of blood cells on metal electrodes: an aid in the selection of vascular prostheses, *Natl Acad Sci* 53:294, 1965.
27. De Palma VA et al: Investigation of three-surface properties of several metals and their relation to blood compatibility, *J Biomed Mater Res Symp* 3:37, 1972.
28. Sawyer PN et al: Electron microscopy and physical chemistry of healing in prosthetic heart valves, skirts and struts, *J Thorac Cardiovasc Surg* 67(1):24, 1974.
29. Sawyer PN, Sophie Z, O'Shaughnessy AM: Hemocompatibility assessment. In von Recum A, editor: *Handbook of biomaterials evaluation*, New York, 1986, Macmillan, chap 26.
30. Palmaz JC: Intravascular stents: tissue–stent interactions and design considerations, *AJR* 160:613, 1993.
31. Robinson KA et al: Correlated microscopic observations of arterial responses to intravascular stenting, *Scanning Microsc* 3:665, 1989.
32. Rousseau H et al: Self-expanding endovascular prosthesis: an experimental study, *Radiology* 164:709, 1987.
33. Greenfield LJ, Savin MA: Comparison of titanium and stainless steel Greenfield vena caval filters, *Surgery* 106:820, 1989.
34. Back M, Kopchok G, Mueller M et al: Changes in arterial wall compliance after endovascular stenting, *J Vasc Surg* 19:905–911, 1994.
35. Palmaz JC et al: Normal and stenotic renal arteries: experimental balloon-expandable intraluminal stenting, *Radiology* 164:705, 1987.
36. Schatz RA: A view of vascular stents, *Circulation* 79:445, 1989.
37. Vorwerk D et al: Neointima formation following arterial placement of self-expanding stents of different radial force: experimental results, *Cardiovasc Intervent Radiol* 17:27, 1994.
38. Barth KH et al: Flexible tantalum stents implanted in aortas and iliac arteries: effects in normal canines, *Radiology* 175:91, 1990.
39. White CJ et al: A new balloon-expandable tantalum coil stent: angiographic patency and histologic findings in an atherogenic swine model, *J Am Coll Cardiol* 19:870, 1992.
40. Sutton CS et al: Titanium-nickel intravascular endoprosthesis: a 2-year study in dogs, *AJR* 151:597, 1988.
41. Roubin G et al: Early and late results of intracoronary arterial stenting after coronary angioplasty in the dog, *Circulation* 76:891, 1987.
42. Rollins N et al: Self-expanding metallic stents: preliminary evaluation in an atherosclerotic model, *Radiology* 163:739, 1987.
43. Den Otter G: Total prosthetic replacement of atrioventricular valves in the dog, *Thorax* 27:105, 1972.
44. Strecker EP et al: Expandable tubular stents for treatment of arterial occlusive diseases: experimental and clinical results, *Radiology* 175:97, 1990.
45. Von Holst H, Collins P, Steiner L: Titanium, silver and tantalum clips in brain tissue, *Acta Neurochir (Wien)* 56:239, 1981.
46. Keller JC, Lautenschlager EP: Metal and alloys. In von Recum A, editor: *Handbook of biomaterials evaluation*, New York, 1986, Macmillan, chap 1.
47. Hearn JA, Robinson KA, Roubin GS: In vitro thrombus formation of stent wires: role of metallic composition and heparin coating [abstract], *J Am Coll Cardiol* 17:302A, 1991.
48. Ribeiro PA et al: A new expandable intracoronary tantalum (Strecker) stent: early experimental results and follow-up to twelve months, *Am Heart J* 125:501, 1993.
49. Fontaine AB et al: Decreased platelets adherence of polymer-coated tantalum stents, *J Vasc Intervent Radiol* 5:567, 1994.
50. Williams DF: Titanium and titanium alloys. In Williams DF, editor: *Biocompatibility of clinical implant materials*, vol 1, Boca Raton, 1981, CRC Press, chap 2.
51. Williams DF: Titanium as a metal for implantation. Part 2. Biological properties and clinical applications, *J Med Eng Technol* Sept: 266, 1977.
52. Schetky LM: Shape-memory alloys, *Sci Am* 241:74, 1979.
53. Cragg AH et al: Nitinol intravascular stents: results of preclinical evaluation, *Radiology* 189:775, 1993.

54. Castleman LS, Motzkin SM: The biocompatibility of nitinol. In Williams DF, editor: *Biocompatibility of clinical implant materials*, vol 1, Boca Raton, 1981, CRC Press, chap 5.
55. Haasters J, Bensmann G, Baumgart F: Memory alloys: a new material for implantation in orthopedic surgery. Part II. In: Uhthoff HK, editor: *Current concepts of internal fixation of fractures*. New York, 1980, Springer-Verlag.
56. Castleman LS et al: Biocompatibility of nitinol alloy as an implant material, *J Biomed Mater Res* 10:695, 1976.
57. Oonishi H et al: Biological reaction of Ni in Ti-Ni shape memory alloy, *Trans Soc Biomater* 7:183, 1984.
58. Williams DF: The properties and clinical uses of cobalt-chromium alloys. In Williams DF, editor: *Biocompatibility of clinical implant materials*, vol I, Boca Raton, 1981, CRC Press, chap 4.
59. Shellock FG, Kanal E: MR procedures and patients with biomedical implants, materials, and devices. In Shellock FG, Kanal E, editors: *Magnetic resonance: bioeffects, safety and patient management*, New York, 1994, Raven Press, chap 10.
60. Teitelbaum GP, Bradley WG, Klein BD: MR imaging artifacts, ferromagnetism and magnetic torque of intravascular filters, stents and coils, *Radiology* 166:657, 1988.
61. Matsumoto AH et al: Tantalum vascular stents: in vivo evaluation with MR imaging, *Radiology* 170:753, 1989.
62. Becker GJ: Intravascular stents, general principles and status of lower extremity arterial applications, *Circulation* 83(suppl I):122, 1991.
63. Fluckiger F et al: Firmness, elasticity and deformation characteristics of metal stents [abstract], *Cardiovasc Intervent Radiol* 16(suppl):19, 1993.
64. Jedwab MR, Clerc CO: A study of the geometrical and mechanical properties of a self-expanding metallic stent—theory and experiment, *J Appl Biomater* 4:77, 1993.
65. Fallone BG, Wallace S, Gianturco C: Elastic characteristics of self-expanding metallic stents, *Invest Radiol* 23:370, 1988.
66. Abbott WM et al: Effect of compliance mismatch on vascular graft patency, *J Vasc Surg* 5:376, 1987.
67. Hausegger KA et al: Iliac artery stent placement: clinical experience with a nitinol stent, *Radiology* 190:199, 1994.
68. Laird JR et al: Placement and angiographic patency of the Strecker coronary stent, *Cathet Cardiovasc Diagn* 31:322, 1994.
69. Santoian EC, King S: Intravascular stents, intimal proliferation and restenosis [editorial comment], *J Am Coll Cardiol* 19:877, 1992.
70. Greenfield LJ, DeLucia A: Endovascular therapy of venous thromboembolic disease, *Surg Clin North Am* 72:969, 1992.
71. Greenfield LJ et al: Extended evaluation of the titanium Greenfield vena caval filter, *J Vasc Surg* 20:458, 1994.
72. Teitelbaum GP et al: Vena caval filter splaying: potential complication of use of the titanium Greenfield filter, *Radiology* 173:809, 1989.
73. Ricco JB et al: Percutaneous transvenous caval interruption with the "LGM" filter: early results of a multicenter trial, *Ann Vasc Surg* 3:242, 1988.
74. Dorfman GS: Percutaneous inferior vena cava filters, *Radiology* 174:987, 1990.
75. Balko A, Piasecki GJ, Shah DM et al: Transfemoral placement of intraluminal polyurethane prosthesis for abdominal aortic aneurysm, *J Surg Res* 40:305–309, 1986.
76. Lawrence DD, Charnsanngavej C, Wright KC et al: Percutaneous endovascular graft: experimental evaluation, *Radiology* 163:357–360, 1987.
77. Mirich D, Wright KC, Wallace S et al: Percutaneously placed endovascular grafts for aortic aneurysms: feasibility study, *Radiology* 170:1033–1037, 1989.
78. Laborde JC, Parodi JC, Clem MF et al: Intraluminal bypass of abdominal aortic aneurysm: feasibility study, *Radiology* 184:185–190, 1992.
79. Parodi JC, Palmaz JC, Barone HD: Transfemoral intraluminal graft implantation for abdominal aortic aneurysms, *Ann Vasc Surg* 5:491–499, 1991.
80. Parodi JC: Endovascular repair of abdominal aortic aneurysms and other arterial lesions, *J Vasc Surg* 21:549–557, 1995.
81. Chuter TAM, Green RM, Ouriel K et al: Transfemoral endovascular aortic graft placement. *J Vasc Surg* 18:185–197, 1993.
82. Chuter TAM, Wendt G, Hopkinson BR et al: European experience with a system for bifurcated stent-graft insertion, *J Endovasc Surg* 4:13–22, 1997.
83. May J, White G, Waugh R et al: Treatment of complex abdominal aortic aneurysms by a combination of endoluminal and extraluminal

aortofemoral grafts, *J Vasc Surg* 19:924–933, 1994.
84. White GH, Yu W, May J et al: Three-year experience with the White-Yu endovascular GAD graft for transluminal repair of aortic and iliac aneurysms. *J Endovasc Surg* 4:124–136, 1997.
85. Moore WS, Rutherford RB: Transluminal endovascular repair of abdominal aortic aneurysm: results of the North American EVT phase I trial. *J Vasc Surg* 23:543–553, 1996.
86. White RA, Donayre CE, Walot I et al: Preliminary clinical outcome and imaging criterion for endovascular prosthesis development on high-risk patients who have aortoiliac and traumatic arterial lesions. *J Vasc Surg* 24:556–571, 1996.
87. White RA, Fogarty TJ, Kopchok GE et al: Evaluation of a modular endovascular bifurcation prosthesis in a canine aortic aneurysm model. *J Vasc Surg* 24:1034–1042, 1996.
88. May J, White G, Waugh R et al: Transluminal placement of a prosthetic graft-stent device for treatment of subclavian artery aneurysm. *J Vasc Surg* 18:1056–1059, 1993.
89. Marin ML, Veith FJ, Panetta TF et al: Transfemoral endoluminal stented graft repair of a popliteal artery aneurysm. *J Vasc Surg* 19:754–757, 1994.
90. Diethrich EB, Papazoglon K: Endoluminal grafting for aneurysmal and occlusive disease in the superficial femoral artery: early experience. *J Endovasc Surg* 2:225–239, 1995.
91. Cragg AH, Dake MD: Percutaneous femoropopliteal graft placement. *Radiology* 187; 643–646, 1993.
92. Henry M, Amar M, Ethernenot G et al: Initial experience with the Cragg Endopro System 1 in the interventional treatment of peripheral vascular disease. *J Endovasc Surg* 1: 31–43, 1994.
93. Marin ML, Veith FJ, Sanchez LA et al: Endovascular aortoiliac grafts in combination with standard infrainguinal arterial bypasses in the management of limb-threatening ischemia: preliminary report, *J Vasc Surg* 22:316–325, 1995.
94. Ohki T, Marin ML, Veith FJ et al: Endovascular aortounifemoral grafts and femorofemoral bypass for bilateral limb-threatening ischemia, *J Vasc Surg* 24:984–997, 1996.
95. Marin ML, Veith FJ, Panetta TF et al: Transluminally placed endovascular stented graft repair for arterial trauma, *J Vasc Surg* 20:466–473, 1994.
96. Back MR, Kopchok GE, White RA et al: Endoluminal placement of PTFE graft-stent devices in a canine model. *Vasc Surg* 28:441–448, 1994.
97. Turner RJ, Hoffman HL, Weinberg SL: Knitted Dacron double velour grafts. In Stanley JC, editor: *Biologic and synthetic vascular prostheses*, Orlando, 1982, Grune & Stratton, 509–522.
98. Gonza ER, Marble AE, Shaw A, Holland JG: Age related changes in mechanics of the aorta and pulmonary artery in man, *J Appl Physiol* 36:407, 1974.
99. Kinley CE, Marble AE: Compliance: a continuing problem with vascular grafts, *J Cardiovasc Surg* 21:163–170, 1980.
100. Walden R, L'Italien GJ, Megerman J, Abbott WM: Matched elastic properties and successful arterial grafting, *Arch Surg* 115:1166–1169, 1980.
101. Snyder RW, Botzko KM: Woven, knitted and externally supported Dacron vascular prostheses. In Stanley JC, editor: *Biologic and synthetic vascular prostheses*, Orlando, 1982, Grune & Stratton, pp 485–494.
102. Diethrich EB: Initial experience with in vivo expansion of PTFE in the treatment of occlusive and aneurysmal disease [abstract], *J Endovasc Surg* 2:308–309, 1995.
103. Bergeron P, Henric A, Bonnet C, Reim R: Tensile characteristics of expanded PTFE for use in endoluminal grafting [abstract], *J Endovasc Surg* 2:302–303, 1995.
104. Palmaz JC, Tio FO, Laborde JC et al: Use of stents covered with PTFE in experimental abdominal aortic aneurysm, *J Vasc Intervent Radiol* 6:879–885, 1995.
105. Wesolowski SA, Fries CC, Karlson KE et al: Porosity, primary determinant of ultimate fate of synthetic grafts, *Surgery* 50:91–101, 1961.
106. Ottinger LW, Darling RC, Werthlin LS et al: Failure of ultra light weight knitted Dacron grafts in arterial reconstruction, *Arch Surg* 111:146–149, 1976.
107. Szilagyi E, Pfeifer JR, DeRusso FJ: Long-term evaluation of plastic arterial substitutes: an experimental study, *Surgery* 55:165–183, 1964.
108. Golden MA, Hanson SR, Kirkman TR et al: Healing of PTFE arterial grafts is influenced by graft porosity, *J Vasc Surg* 11:838–845, 1990.
109. Kohler TR, Stratton JR, Kirkman TR et al: Conventional versus high-porosity PTFE grafts: clinical evaluation, *Surgery* 112:901–907, 1992.
110. Bennett JG, Trono R, Norman JC et al: Experimental comparisons of vascular grafts,

111. Lindenauer SM, Weber TR, Miller TA et al: Velour vascular prostheses, *Trans Am Soc Artif Intern Organs* 20:314–319, 1974.
112. Guidoin R, Gosselin C, Martin L et al: Polyester prostheses as substitutes in the thoracic aorta of dogs. I. Evaluation of commercial prostheses, *J Biomed Mater Res* 17:1049–1077, 1988.
113. Claggett PC: In vivo evaluation of platelet reactivity with vascular prostheses. In Stanley JC, editor: *Biologic and synthetic vascular prostheses*, Orlando, 1982, Grune & Stratton, pp 131–152.
114. Ohki T, Marin ML, Veith FJ et al: Anastomotic intimal hyperplasia: a comparison between conventional and endovascular stent graft techniques, *J Surg Res* 69:255–267, 1997.
115. Ombrellaro MP, Stevens SL, Freeman MB, Goldman MH: Reendothelialization and platelet derived growth factor activity associated with intraarterial stented grafts, *Vasc Surg* 31:631–637, 1997.
116. Marin ML, Veith FJ, Cynamon J et al: Human transluminally placed endovascular stented grafts: preliminary histopathologic analysis of healing grafts in aortoiliac and femoral artery occlusive disease, *J Vasc Surg* 21:595–604, 1995.
117. White RA, Donayre CE, deVirgilio C et al: Deployment technique and histopathological evaluation of an endoluminal vascular prosthesis used to repair an iliac artery aneurysm, *J Endovasc Surg* 3:262–269, 1996.
118. McGahan TJ, Barry GA, McGahan SL et al: Results of autopsy 7 months after successful endoluminal treatment of an infrarenal abdominal aortic aneurysm, *J Endovasc Surg* 2:348–355, 1995.
119. Hayoz D, Do-Dai D, Mahler F et al: Aortic inflammatory reaction associated with endoluminal bypass grafts, *J Endovasc Surg* 4:354–360, 1997.
120. Norgren L, Swartbol P: Biological responses to endovascular treatment of abdominal aortic aneurysms, *J Endovasc Surg* 4:169–173, 1997.
121. White RA, Verbin C, Kopchok G et al: The role of cinefluoroscopy and intravascular ultrasonography in evaluating the deployment of experimental endovascular prostheses, *J Vasc Surg* 21:365–374, 1995.
122. Matlaga BF, Yasenchak LP, Salthouse TN: Tissue response to implanted polymers: the significance of sample shape, *J Biomed Mater Res* 10:391–397, 1976.
123. White RA, Kopchok G, Zalewski M et al: Comparison of the deployment and healing of thin walled expanded PTFE stented grafts and covered stents, *Ann Vasc Surg* 10:336–346, 1996.

16
Catheter Skills

Edward V. Kinney, Thomas J. Fogarty, and Christine E. Newman

Catheter-based therapies have had a profound effect on the practice of medicine and surgery. Use of these treatment modalities continues to increase each year. High doctor and patient acceptance is primarily attributable to the low morbidity and low incidence of complications that accompany catheter use. In fact, the efficacy and durability of some catheter-based therapies is marginal. If complication rates were higher, the risk/benefit balance might be shifted against endovascular intervention. Avoiding complications depends on understanding when and why they occur. A discussion of proper catheter skills should start with a discussion of wire/catheter complications. Subsequently, we discuss the various specialty guidewires and preformed angiographic catheters that are available and their proper usage. Finally, we use some clinically relevant situations to illustrate proper wire/catheter skills.

Not all vascular surgeons routinely perform percutaneous arterial puncture. Increasing numbers of surgeons are recognizing the need and value of becoming proficient in the application of all endovascular techniques. It is obvious that a large number of endovascular procedures can and should be handled via percutaneous access. The importance of cleanly accessing the vasculature should not be underestimated. Situations in which percutaneous arterial puncture is or will be useful include stent placement, contrast injection from a superiorly placed catheter to localize the renal arteries during aortic stent-graft placement, contrast injection and pressure measurement via the contralateral femoral artery during retrograde iliac stent placement, and thrombolytic therapy. Percutaneous arterial puncture may be complicated by hematoma formation, pseudoaneourysm formation, arteriovenous fistula formation, or arterial thrombosis. Selective catheterization may be complicated by dissection, perforation, embolization, catheter occlusion, or arterial occlusion.

Hematoma formation is relatively frequent after arterial puncture. Most hematomas are small and without clinical significance. Large, tense hematomas may result in skin gangrene. Retroperitoneal hematoma may be fatal. Brachial plexus hematoma after axillary artery catheterization may result in compressive neuropathy. Surgical intervention for hematoma is necessary for 0.25% to 0.50% of arterial catheterizations.[1] Surgical intervention for hematoma is necessary after 3% of axillary artery punctures. Factors that increase the likelihood of hematoma formation include improper puncture site; multiple puncture attempts; use of large-bore arterial catheters and sheaths; multiple catheter exchanges without a sheath resulting in arterial laceration; improper or inadequate postcatheterization compression; preexisting coagulopathy; and antiplatelet or anticoagulant therapy.

The femoral artery is the most common site for percutaneous puncture. This site is chosen in part because it is easy to monitor and because postcatheterization compression against the femoral head reliably produces hemostasis. Puncture sites that are significantly above or below the inguinal ligament may be difficult or impossible to compress adequately after catheterization, thereby increasing the likelihood of hematoma formation (Figure 16–1). With the exception of translumbar aortic puncture, arterial catheterization should always be performed at a site where the artery may be directly compressed against a bony structure after catheter removal.

Hematoma formation resulting from the use of large-bore sheaths percutaneously is best avoided by performing a cutdown and repairing the artery directly. Direct arterial exposure involves minimal morbidity and should probably be used more frequently. The other advantage of direct suture closure is that anticoagulants may be safely continued postoperatively. This practice is also advisable if arterial catheterization must be performed on a patient with preexisting coagulopathy.

Devices that allow percutaneous arterial closure either by collagen plug or suture are commercially available. The early experience with these devices suggests that their use will decrease hematoma formation, decrease compression time, and allow earlier ambulation.

Pseudoaneurysms occur in 0.03% to 0.05% of arterial catheterizations.[1] Pseudoaneurysms result from significant arterial injury combined with inadequate compression. The same factors that increase the likelihood of hematoma formation are also associated with pseudoaneurysm formation: improper puncture site, multiple arterial punctures, large-bore sheaths, and preexisting coagulopathy or the use of anticoagulants. Pseudoaneurysms have generally been treated surgically, although there is increasing use of the nonoperative technique of ultrasound-guided compression. The best treatment is avoidance, either by changes in technique or cutdown or by direct arterial repair in high-risk situations.

Arterial laceration as a result of guidewire-catheter mismatch or dilator-sheath mismatch can also play a role in hematoma or pseudoaneurysm formation. Guidewire-catheter mismatch refers to a wire with an outside diameter that is significantly smaller than the catheter end-hole inside diameter. Dilators and sheaths are designed to present a minimal sheath edge step-up. If sheaths are reused or used with the wrong dilator, the leading edge of the sheath will not fit smoothly against the dilator. Arter-

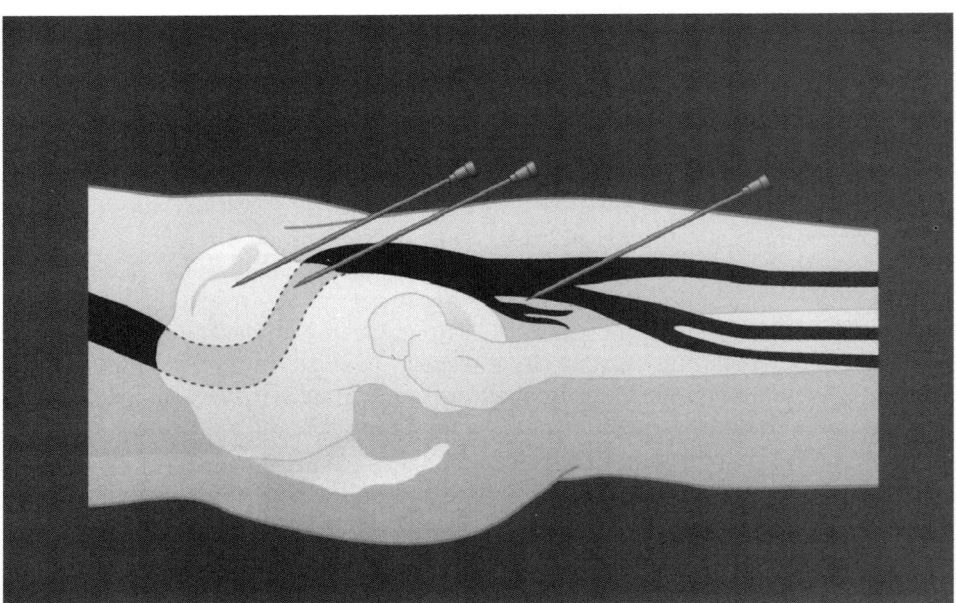

FIGURE 16–1. Retrograde puncture of common femoral artery.

ial wall laceration or intimal injury from guidewire-catheter mismatch or dilator-sheath mismatch are best treated by avoidance.

Arterial thrombosis as a complication of catheterization occurs in 0.1% to 0.7% of cases.[1] Factors contributing to puncture-site thrombosis include dissection of the arterial wall, intimal injury as a result of guidewire-catheter or dilator-sheath mismatch, or sheath or catheter thrombosis as a result of infrequent flushing. Guidewires, catheters, and sheaths are all thrombogenic. Guidewires should not be left naked in the artery because clots will begin to form immediately. Catheters and sheaths must be aspirated at frequent intervals and then flushed with heparinized saline. When wires and catheters are removed from the body, they must be flushed and the blood wiped from the outside surface.

Arterial dissection can occur either at or remote from the puncture site. Puncture-site dissections occur with wire advancement when the tip of the needle is not completely in the lumen. Wires should not be advanced through the needle unless brisk, pulsatile back-bleeding has been seen. If the wire does not pass easily, it should be withdrawn. Contrast should then be injected to obtain a road map and to verify that the needle tip is within the true lumen. Once the wire is within the true lumen, it should be passed under fluoroscopic control. If the wire does not pass easily, a road map should be obtained. An arterial sheath should then be placed and the wire, typically a Bentson (Cook, Bloomington, Ind) or a flexible J-tip, exchanged for a steerable guidewire.

Acute arterial occlusion after selective catheterization or balloon dilatation may be caused by thrombosis, dissection, or spasm. An assumption by the operator that the occlusion is probably a spasm and will therefore improve on its own is a recipe for failure. If a spasm is suspected, tolazoline (Priscoline) or nitroglycerin should be injected until the spasm resolves. If a thrombus is suspected or if there is no response to intraarterial vasodilators, then urokinase should be injected intraarterially. Failure to respond to either vasodilators or thrombolytic agents suggests that acute arterial occlusion is secondary to dissection. Arterial dissection should be treated by repeat balloon dilatation and/or stent placement.

Catheters that become occluded either because they are twisted or because of a clot may be exchanged by one of three methods. The catheter hub may be cut off and a sheath advanced over the catheter, or the catheter may be nearly pulled out, divided near the tip, and the clot aspirated with a syringe and needle. The third method involves partially removing the catheter, making a side hole in the catheter, introducing a wire into the new side hole, passing the catheter and wire back into the artery, withdrawing the wire tip out of the side hole, removing the occluded catheter, and finally, passing a new catheter over the wire.

Do's and Don'ts, Principles, and Axioms

1. Never pass a wire through the arterial puncture needle unless the back-bleeding is brisk and pulsatile.

2. Never pass or advance any wire, catheter, or sheath unless a guidewire has already been passed and the wire tip is freely movable (intraluminal).

3. Wires, catheters, and sheaths are all thrombogenic. Wires should never be left exposed within the artery. Catheters and sheaths must be frequently aspirated and then flushed with heparinized saline.

4. Be sure that the catheter and guidewire are a good size match so that the wire-catheter transition zone is smooth. The same consideration should be given to dilator-sheath matching.

5. Never pass a coated wire—such as Glidewire (Medi-tech/Boston Scientific, Natick, Mass)—through a needle. The needle tip will shear the coating and form emboli.

6. Always use test (hand) injections of contrast medium after catheter placement to detect a possible subintimal position or a catheter that is wedged into the artery.

7. When exchanging a larger-diameter catheter for a smaller-diameter catheter or when performing multiple catheter exchanges, always use an artery sheath to prevent

hematoma formation and avoid arterial laceration.

8. When using mechanical injectors and end-hole catheters, be sure that the end-hole is not against the arterial wall. The contrast jet is forceful enough to dissect the artery.

9. Catheters with multiple side holes are useful for mechanical contrast injection in large arteries. They should not be used for contrast injection in small arteries because of the risk of dissection. Clots form very rapidly in side holes. Therefore, when using multiple side-hole catheters, forceful aspiration and subsequent flushing with heparinized saline must be performed at frequent (1 to 2 minute) intervals. When performing arterial catheterization and/or intervention, choose the shortest, straightest, most direct route to the artery or lesion of interest. All wires and catheters become less torquable and less pushable as they are advanced farther into the arterial tree. Choosing the most direct route also minimizes the chance of injuring other uninvolved arteries.

10. Never give up wire position across a lesion until the intervention has been proven to be satisfactory by angiography and ultrasound. Recrossing a dilated arterial segment or stent is possible, but the possibility of dissection is increased.

Specialty Guidewires and Preformed Catheters

Standard guidewires have a stainless-steel core and a coiled-spring outer wall. The coiled spring makes the wire flexible, whereas the core lends column strength and makes the wire pushable. The distal end of the core can be tapered to increase the flexibility at the tip. This increased flexibility allows the tip to buckle when a plaque is encountered rather than dissect beneath it. When the tip is in a buckled configuration, it will generally pass atraumatically through tortuous vessels. The distal tip may also be formed into a J configuration to achieve this same atraumatic profile. Standard guidewires are available in diameters ranging from 0.010 to 0.045 inch. Flexible tips ranging from 10 to 20 cm in length (e.g., Bentson wire, LT wire, LLT wire) and preformed J-tips ranging from 1.5 to 15 mm in radius are also available. Standard lengths range from 100 to 150 cm. Exchange wires range from 260 to 300 cm.

Steerable guidewires are very useful for traversing tortuous, stenotic vessels or for accomplishing selective or subselective catheter placement. To be steerable, a guidewire must be torquable and must have a preformed, angled tip. There are steerable guidewires available in a range of diameters, with and without floppy tips. Steerability may be obtained from non-steerable guidewires by using them in combination with preformed angiographic catheters [e.g., Bentson wire (Cook) and Berenstein catheter (Medi-tech/Boston Scientific)].

Another feature available in specialty guidewires is a hydrophilic coating, which makes the wire extremely slippery in the bloodstream. This slippery feature makes the wire very atraumatic and greatly increases the wire's ability to cross stenoses.

Angiographic Catheters

Angiographic catheters are available in a variety of materials, including polyethylene, polyurethane, Teflon, and nylon. The catheters are impregnated with barium, bismuth, or lead salts to make them radiopaque. Each material has some, but not all, desirable characteristics. Polyethylene, the most commonly used catheter material, is quite flexible—which means that catheters made of it will follow guidewires well. The column strength (pushability and torquability) of polyethylene may be inadequate for some applications. Polyurethane catheters are quite flexible but have little column strength and undesirable frictional characteristics. Consequently, polyurethane catheters are frequently stiffened by incorporating stainless-steel mesh or coils into their walls. Frictional characteristics are improved by coating the catheter with friction-reducing agents. Teflon catheters have low friction but are quite stiff. These characteristics make Teflon a particularly suitable material for sheaths and dilators. Nylon catheters are intermediate between polyethylene and Teflon in terms of stiffness. Nylon also has a relatively low coefficient of friction; catheters made of nylon are therefore quite pushable and quite torquable. They are also flexible enough to follow a wire for selective and subselective catheter placement. An example of a currently available nylon catheter is the Imager line of catheters (Medi-tech).

Preformed angiographic catheters are available in a variety of shapes and sizes. A preformed shape, combined with good torque characteristics, makes a catheter steerable. Commonly used preshaped catheters include the standard straight catheter, the hockey-stick catheter (Berenstein, DAV, Cook) the cobra-head catheter, and the Simmons catheter (Medi-tech) (Figure 16–2). Preformed catheters may be used with or without steerable guidewires. A very effective wire-catheter combination for traversing tortuous vessels or eccentric lumens would be an angled Glidewire (Medi-tech) and a Berenstein hockey-stick catheter (Medi-tech) (Figure 16–3). The Berenstein catheter is made of nylon and thus has a low coefficient of friction and is quite torquable.

Catheters such as the pigtail, cobra-head, or Simmons catheter are typically introduced over a floppy tip wire such as the Bentson wire (Cook). The catheter is able to assume its preformed shape when the floppy portion of the wire is withdrawn into the distal end of the catheter. Secondarily curved catheters such as the Simmons catheter usually require further reshaping by catching the tip in an aortic branch vessel (visceral or left subclavian) and advancing or rotating the catheter slightly. A suture technique for reshaping the Simmons catheter has also been described.[2]

Selective catheterization is usually performed after a midstream aortic contrast injection. This allows road mapping, if desired, but more importantly, it allows one to determine the angle of vessel take-off from the aorta. Knowing the angle of vessel take-off from the aorta aids in selecting the correct preformed catheter. Generally, within the abdominal aorta, the angle of the primary curve of the catheter should be similar to the angle of vessel take-off. The primary curve of the catheter is the curve that is closest to the tip. The distance from the primary curve to the tip of the catheter should be less than the diameter of the aorta. The secondary curve of the catheter will push the tip of the catheter farther into the vessel of interest once its origin has been engaged. Obviously, the angle of vessel take-off from the aorta varies with the site of arterial puncture. That is, an acute angle of take-off from a femoral approach will become an obtuse

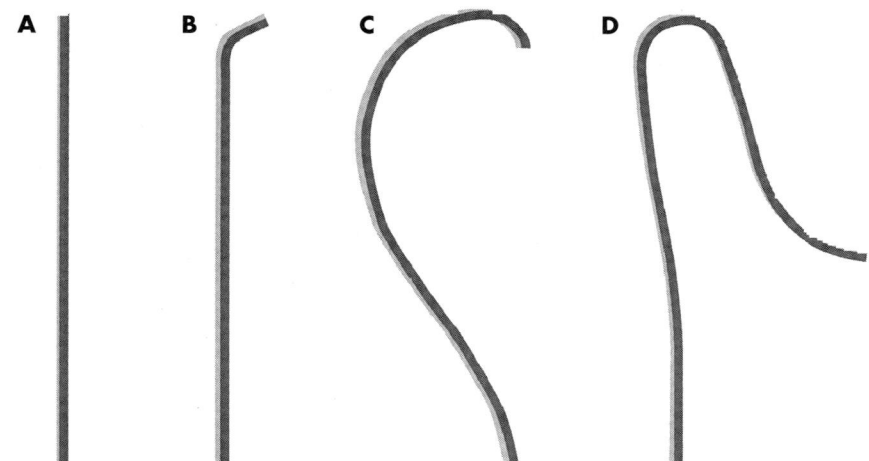

FIGURE 16–2. Standard preformed catheter shapes: **A**, straight; **B**, Berenstein; **C**, Cobra; **D**, Simmons.

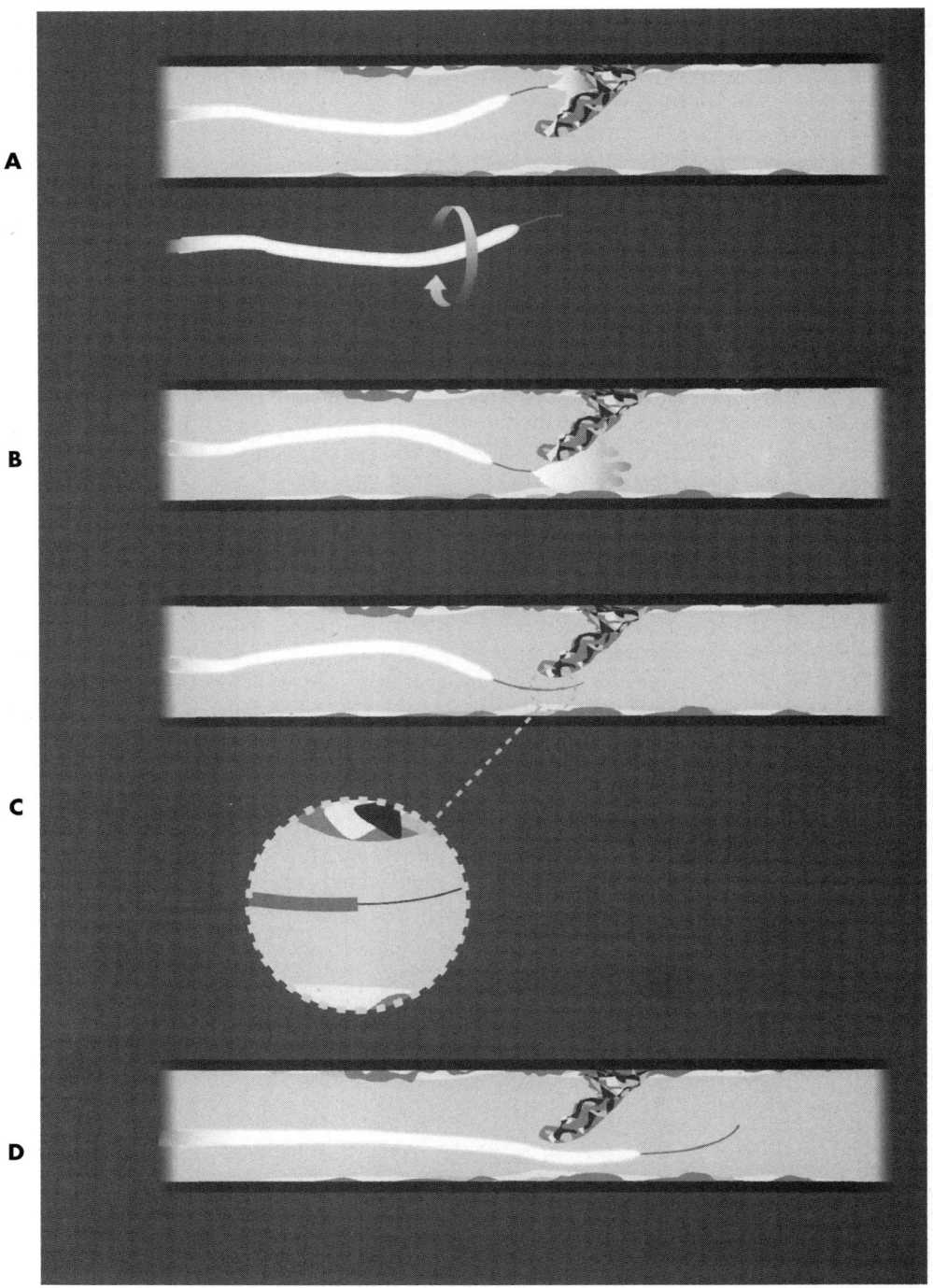

FIGURE 16–3. A steerable catheter and injectable guidewire may be used as follows: **A**, Contrast is injected to identify obstructive lesion or intimal flap. The steerable catheter is then torqued away from the obstruction. **B**, Additional contrast confirms correct catheter position beyond obstruction. **C**, A 0.018-inch guidewire is then advanced through the injectable guidewire. **C**, Enlarged detail shows guidewire advanced through injectable wire. **D**, After exchanging the injectable guidewire for an angled glidewire to more easily traverse the obstruction, the catheter is advanced along the glidewire crossing the flap or obstruction.

16. Catheter Skills

angle of take-off from an axillary approach. In general, hockey-stick or cobrahead catheters are more useful for vessels with an obtuse angle of take-off, whereas the pigtail or Simmons type of catheter is more useful for vessels with an acute angle of take-off (Figure 16–4).

The general technique for selective aortic branch catheterization from a femoral approach is described in Figure 16–5. A flexible-tip guidewire is introduced into the aorta and positioned upstream of the vessel of interest. A pigtail catheter is passed over the wire. The wire is then removed and a flush aortogram obtained. The aortogram will reveal the angle of vessel take-off and the size of the aorta. This information will guide selection of a preformed angiographic catheter. The floppy-tip wire is then replaced and the pigtail removed. The preformed catheter is passed over the wire to a position upstream of the vessel of interest (Figure 16–5A). The floppy tip of the wire is then withdrawn into the distal end of the catheter, and the catheter is reformed.

The catheter tip is torqued until the tip rests against the lateral aortic wall above the vessel to be catheterized (Figure 16–5B). While maintaining the torque, the catheter tip is dragged back (Figure 16–5C) until the tip engages the orifice of the vessel of interest (Figure 16–5D). A hand injection of 2 to 3 ml of contrast is made to verify the correct position of the catheter tip. A steerable guidewire is advanced out into the catheterized vessel as far as possible (Figure 15–5E). If the steerable catheter has a flexible tip, it must be advanced such that the stiff portion is within the vessel. (Do not attempt to advance the catheter when only the floppy portion is in the vessel because the wire will kink and the catheter position may be lost or the vessel injured.) The preformed catheter may then be advanced or exchanged for a more flexible end-hole catheter.

If the catheter will not advance, it may be necessary to exchange the wire for one that is stiffer. If the catheter still will not advance, it may be necessary to remove the catheter and place a larger-diameter, stiffer guiding catheter. The guiding catheter will decrease the friction against the smaller angiographic catheter, thus improving the smaller catheter's torque

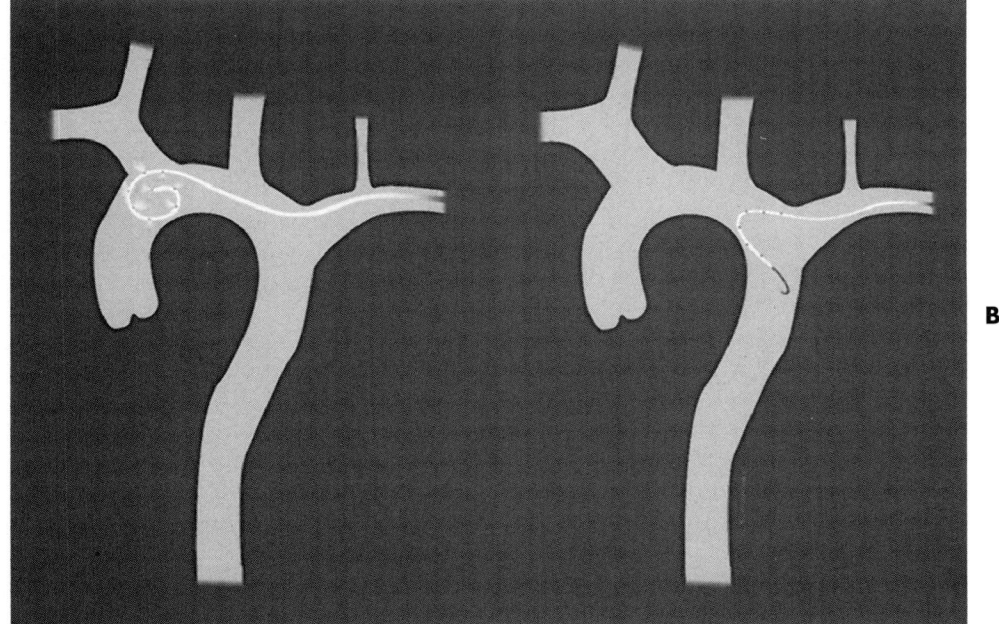

FIGURE 16–4. **A**, A pigtail catheter is inserted via the left subclavian artery to ascertain vessel orientation. **B**, Insertion of guidewire effects slight straightening of the catheter, allowing angulation into the descending aorta.

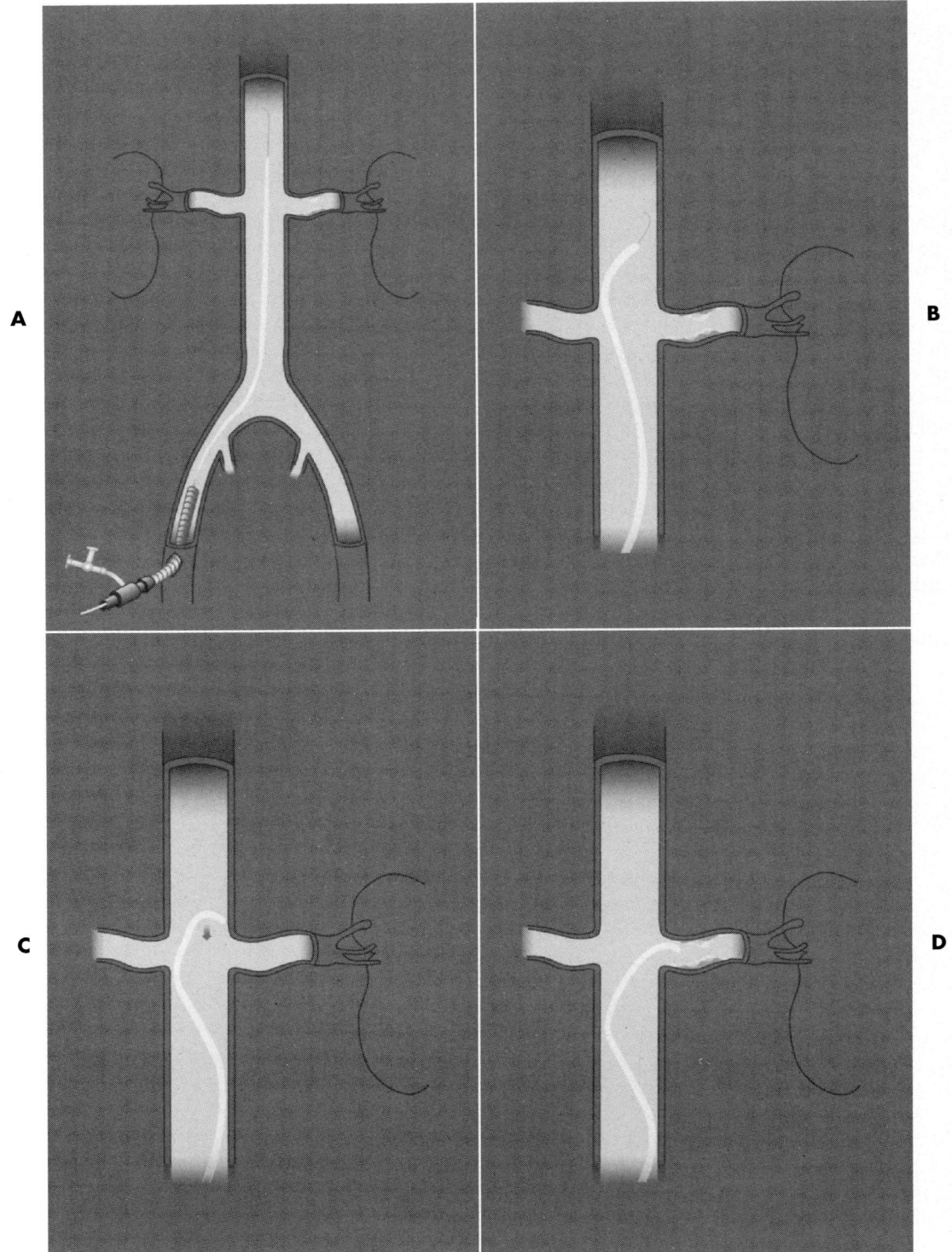

FIGURE 16–5. **A–F**, Procedural steps for selective aortic branch catheterization to access renal arteries or visceral vessels.

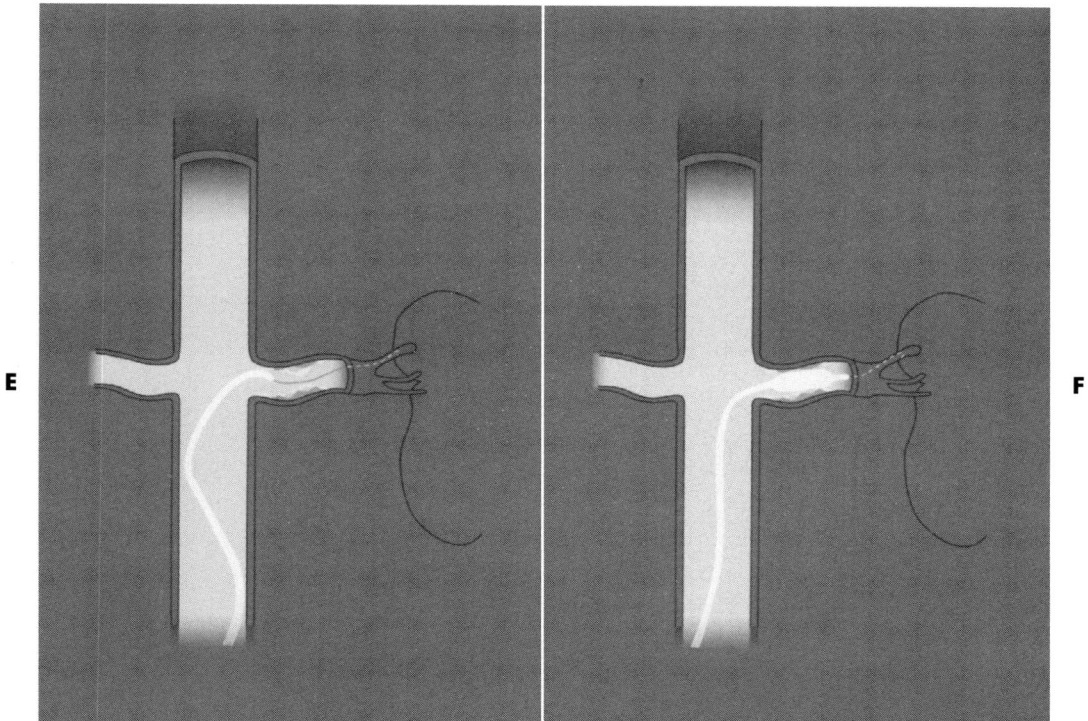

FIGURE 16–5. *Continued.*

characteristics. The support that the guiding catheter lends to the angiographic catheter will improve the column strength and pushability of the smaller catheter. An angioplasty catheter may then be either exchanged for the angiographic catheter or passed through a guiding catheter (Figure 16–5F).

Another technique is to stiffen the wire by passing a 3F catheter inside the angiographic catheter. The combined stiffness of the wire and the 3F catheter may allow advancement of the angiographic catheter. A modification of this technique is to replace the wire with a 2F or 3F Fogarty balloon catheter (Baxter Healthcare, Vascular Systems, Irvine, Calif), inflate the balloon, and allow the catheter to float well out into the vessel. The Fogarty balloon does not have an end-hole, but when the obturator wire is replaced, the Fogarty balloon-obturator wire may be stiff enough to allow advancement of the 6F angiographic catheter. The Fogarty balloon and obturator can then be removed and, if further advancement is necessary, replaced with a steerable guidewire.

Relevant Clinical Examples

Crossiliac Catheter Placement

Crossiliac catheter placement is frequently required for arterial intervention. For instance, attempted retrograde recanalization of an occluded common iliac artery is complicated by subintimal passage of the wire (Figure 16–6A). To complete the intervention, it will be necessary to perform crossiliac wire placement. First, an arterial sheath is placed retrograde in the contralateral common femoral artery. A Bentson wire or J-tipped wire is then passed into the infrarenal aorta. A pigtail catheter is advanced over the wire, and the wire is removed (Figure 16–6B). A flush aortogram is obtained to act as a road map and to determine

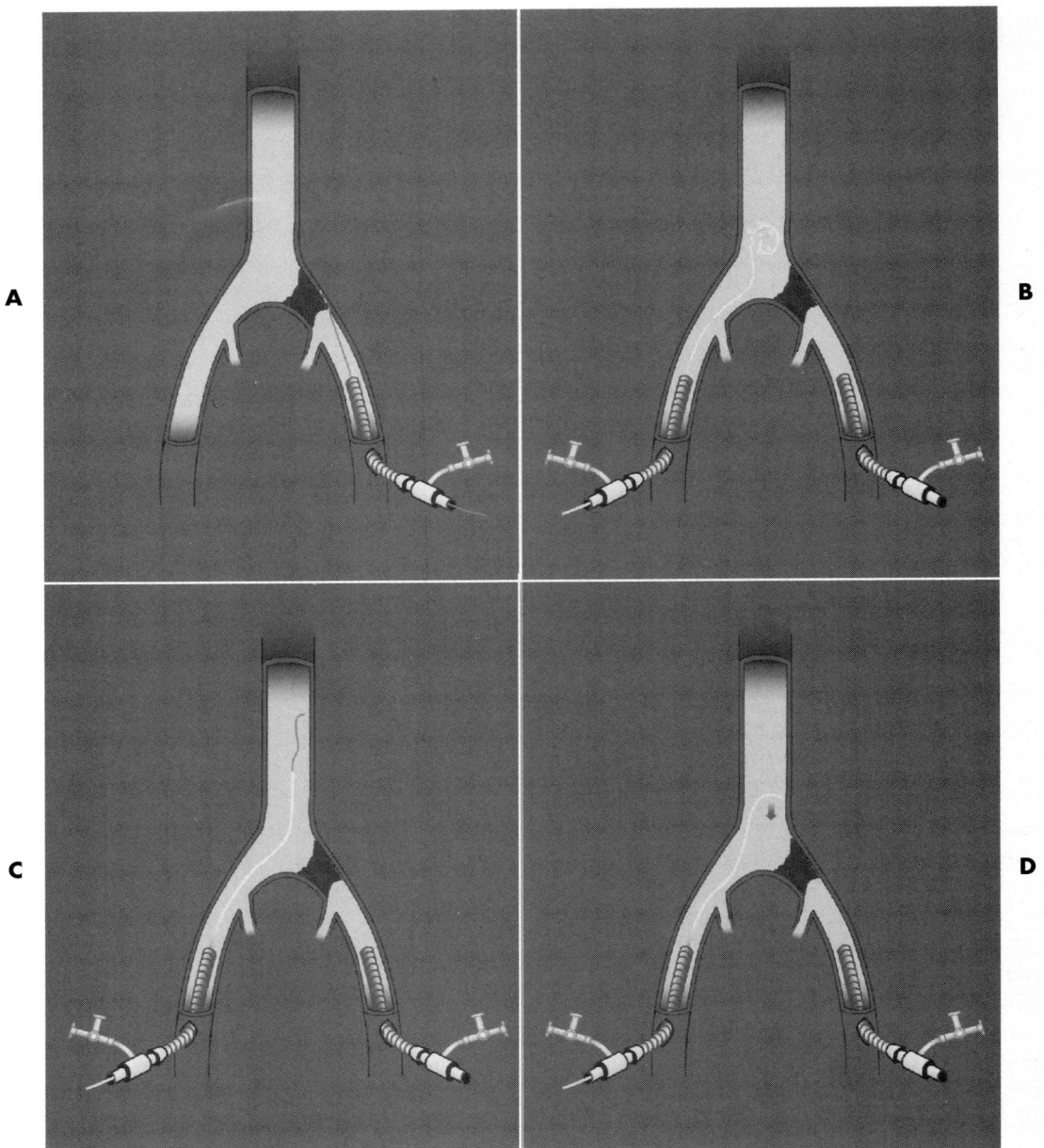

FIGURE 16–6. **A–G**, Procedures for crossiliac catheter placement, described in text under Relevant Clinical Examples.

the size of the vessels, the degree of ectasia, and the angle between the aorta and the common iliac artery. With this information, an appropriately sized and shaped preformed catheter can be chosen. If the angle is acute and the vessels are not particularly ectatic, the pigtail catheter or a Simmons catheter may be used. If the vessels are ectatic or the vessel angle is obtuse, a cobra-head catheter will be more appropriate.

The floppy-tip guidewire is replaced and passed upstream of the contralateral iliac orifice. The preformed catheter is then passed

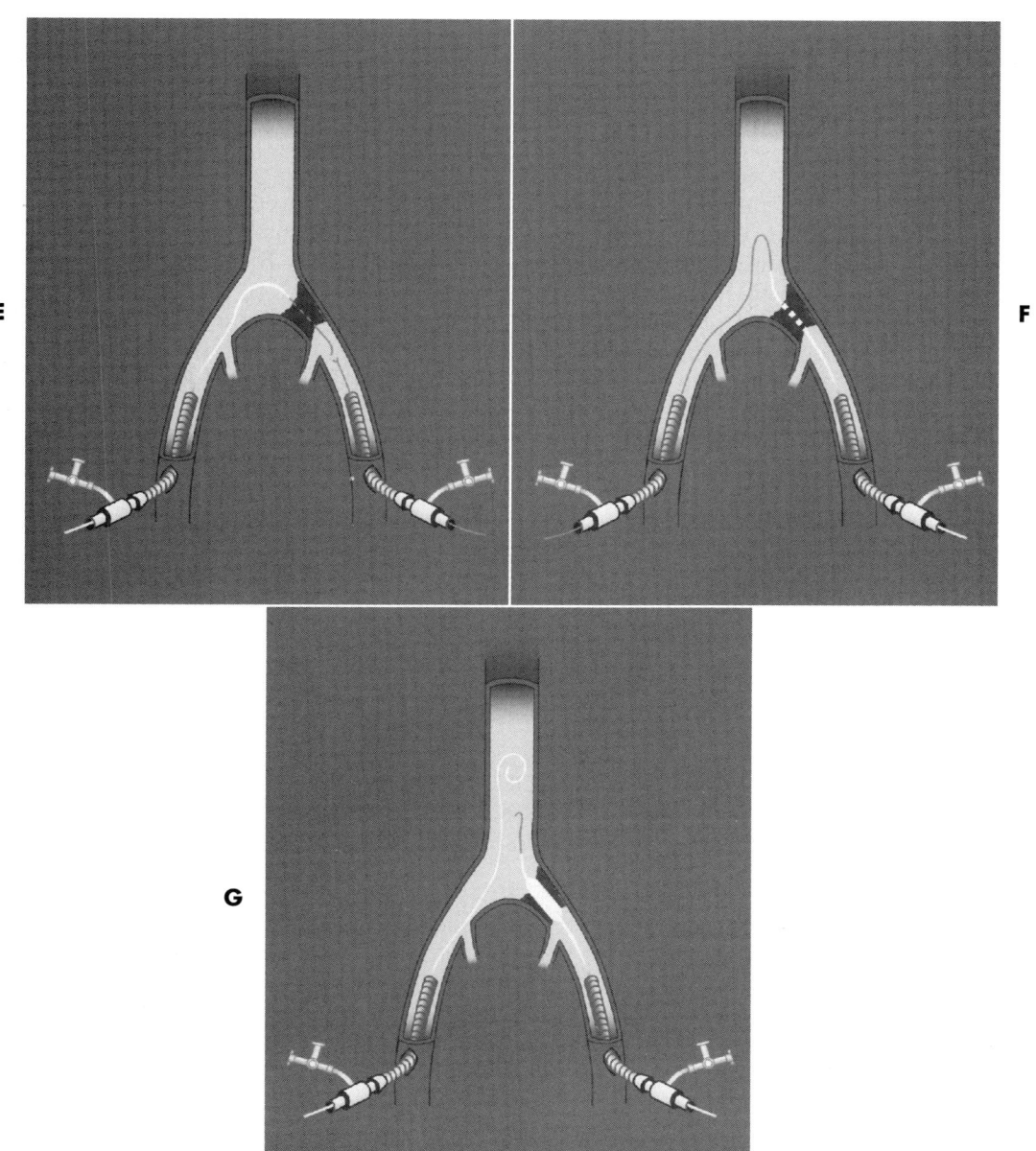

FIGURE 16–6. *Continued.*

until the tip is upstream of the iliac orifice (Figure 16–6C). The floppy tip of the guidewire is withdrawn into the distal end of the catheter and the catheter is reformed. The catheter is then torqued until the tip is against the lateral aortic wall cephalad to the iliac orifice (Figure 16–6D). Then, while maintaining the torque, the catheter is withdrawn until the iliac orifice is engaged. The wire is removed, and a hand injection of 2 to 3 ml of contrast is made to verify proper tip position. Next, a steerable guidewire is introduced and the lesion is traversed. The wire is then passed into the external iliac artery. A cardiac biopsy forceps or snare is used to grab the wire and pull it out of the sheath (Figure 16–6E).

There is now a crossiliac wire and true-lumen wire placement across the lesion. An end-hole catheter can now be passed over the wire, crossing the lesion in a retrograde manner. The guidewire can then be withdrawn into the aorta and a second guidewire passed retrograde through the end-hole catheter (Figure 16–6F). Now the iliac lesion can be dilated and stented from a retrograde femoral approach, as originally planned (Figure 16–6G). The contralateral wire can be used to position a catheter for contrast injection and aortic pressure measurements.

Crossing a Superficial Femoral Artery Occlusion

Another clinical example of wire-catheter techniques is crossing of a superficial femoral artery (SFA) occlusion. Initially, antegrade crossing with a floppy-tip straight LLT (extra long tapered) or straight Glidewire (Medi-tech) may be attempted. The catheter tip should be well above the lesion, and minimum force should be applied so that (hopefully) the wire will not go subintimally. If this technique is unsuccessful, a 1.5-mm J-wire can be placed with the J-tip right at the end of a straight end-hole catheter. The wire and the catheter are both advanced through the lesion as a unit. The J-tip generally prevents subintimal passage. If this technique is unsuccessful, the balloon-centering technique may be tried. This technique involves inflation of an angioplasty balloon just proximal to the lesion followed by passage of a straight LLT wire. The final option for crossing the lesion involves a retrograde popliteal puncture. When the lesion has been crossed from the retrograde popliteal puncture, the wire can be grasped with a snare or cardiac biopsy forceps and pulled through the femoral sheath. Wire exchange can then be performed through the femoral sheath, and the lesion can be recanalized as originally planned. If the popliteal artery is punctured, nothing larger than a 7F sheath should be used. Popliteal puncture should be a last resort because postcatheterization compression at this site is more difficult, and therefore hematoma formation is more likely.

References

1. Dyer R: *Handbook of basic vascular and interventional radiology*, New York, 1993, Churchill Livingstone.
2. Cope C, Burke DR, Meranze S: *Atlas of interventional radiology*, Philadelphia, 1990, JP Lippincott. New York, Gower Medical Publishing.

Suggested Reading

Johnsrude IS, Jackson DC, Dunnick NR: *A practical approach to angiography*, ed 2, Boston, 1987, Little, Brown.

Kadir S: Angioplasty of superficial femoral artery stenoses and occlusions. In Kadir S, editor: *Current practice of interventional radiology*, Philadelphia, 1991, BC Decker.

17
Devices and Techniques for Vascular Access: Utility and Limitations of Current Methods

Rodney A. White and Thomas J. Fogarty

Intravascular surgical procedures may be performed by either percutaneous or open-incision surgical techniques. Percutaneous insertion of devices is used both in the radiology and cardiology suites and in the operating room. Outside of the operating room the percutaneous route is used in the majority of procedures, whereas in the operating room a higher percentage of the interventions are done through an open surgical incision to accommodate the introduction of larger devices or to combine an intravascular procedure with a conventional operation.[1] Aside from balloon angioplasty catheters, many intravascular devices are difficult to use percutaneously because of size limitations. As interventional devices develop, percutaneous adaption occurs after miniaturization of the instruments.

Passing devices along the lumen of a vessel theoretically enhances the thrombogenicity of the vessel wall by endothelial denudation and can predispose the vessel to the long-term development of hyperplastic lesions caused by commitment fracture of the internal elastic lamina of the artery.[2] During endovascular procedures, multiple insertions and withdrawals of devices compound the potential of this risk. Fluid overload is possible during procedures where repeated contrast dye examinations and anticoagulant fluid irrigations are used to avert thrombogenesis and to clear the field of view for angioscopic examinations. Contrast media volumes should be minimized during difficult procedures where repeated imaging is required. Blood loss must also be closely monitored in prolonged cases, particularly if an open approach is used or in cases where undetected bleeding can occur. Introducer sheaths that have a hemostatic valve at the instrument introduction port and additional ports for infusion of fluids and contrast dyes are extremely useful in reducing the trauma to vessel walls and in controlling blood loss (Figure 17–1).

After proximal clamping, a small arteriotomy is made and the sheath is introduced over a guidewire. Distal occlusion is accomplished by a double-loop tape over the sheath. The distal end of the sheath should be placed near the pathologic structure. Therapeutic or diagnostic devices used to interrogate the structure can then be exchanged quickly and without danger to the arterial wall. Intraluminal access devices for use during both percutaneous and open-incision approaches are being developed to decrease vessel trauma, provide better hemostasis, and facilitate removal of intravascular material (Figure 17–2). An access sheath that combines directional control of a guidewire through a side port has great utility in accessing side branches, bifurcations, and areas of tortuosity and angulation (Figure 17–3).

Percutaneous Procedures

The percutaneous procedures are limited to those that can be performed using low-profile catheters (less than 8F to 10F in diameter) and procedures that have a suitable vessel segment for introduction of the instruments. Introduc-

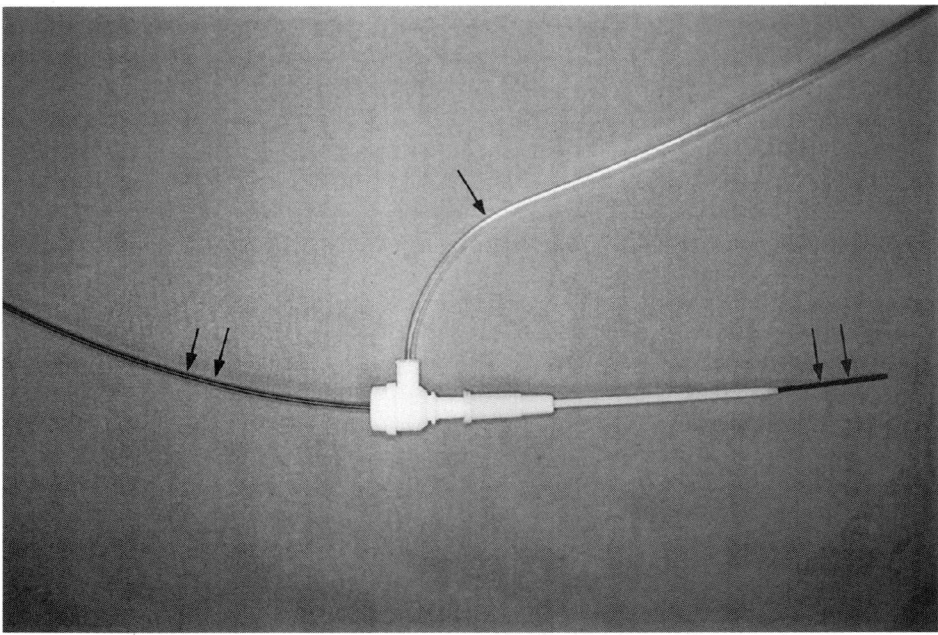

FIGURE 17–1. Hemostatic 8F introducer sheath with side port (*single arrow*) for infusion of fluids or contrast media. A 1-mm diameter angioscope is passed through the introduction port (*double arrows*).

tion of percutaneous devices is usually accomplished using the conventional Seldinger technique.[3] The percutaneous vascular access is performed using one of several techniques depending on the arterial anatomy and vessels being evaluated or treated. Percutaneous arterial puncture under local anesthesia (lidocaine 1% without epinephrine, 2 to 10 ml subcutaneously) is accomplished after appropriate skin preparation and draping. This is required unless a general or regional anesthetic has been instituted. The anatomic surface landmarks of the relevant target vessel are noted, and pulsation is detected by palpation. It is often helpful to make a small (2 to 4 mm) skin incision before insertion of the vascular needle. Alternatively,

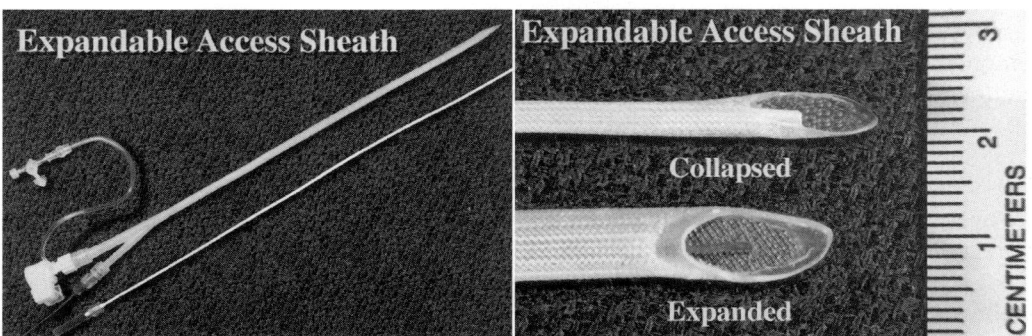

FIGURE 17–2. Expandable-access sheath that combines low profile diameter for percutaneous access and expansion of the lumen after placement to enable introduction of larger devices and to protect the vessel wall during interventions.

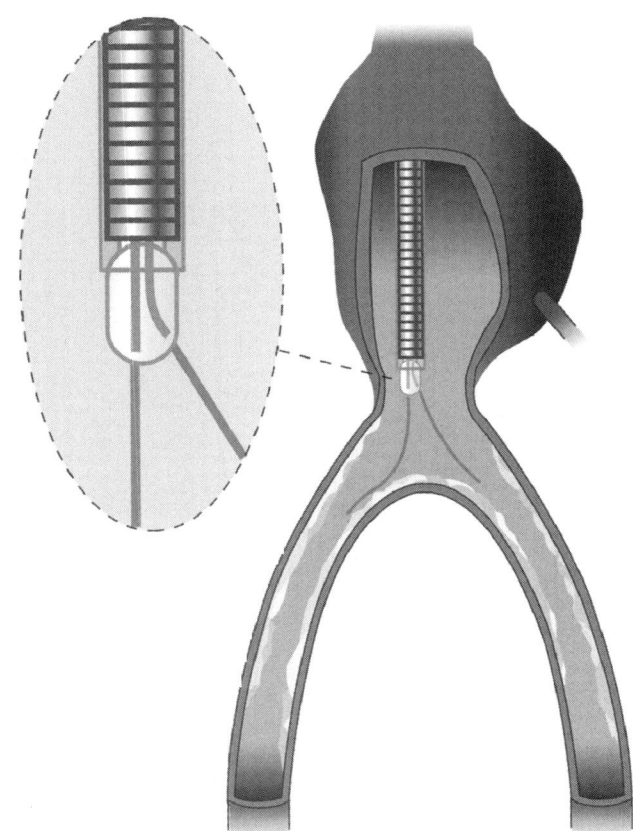

FIGURE 17–3. Deflector-guiding catheter inserted through sheath with guidewires directed into iliac arteries from tip of catheter and angled from side port.

the skin stab can be performed after the guidewire is in place and before dilator or sheath introduction. Constant palpation of the arterial pulse serves to guide the direction of the needle. The technique of arterial puncture varies according to the vessel to be imaged, patient's body habitus, and extent and type of vascular pathology.

Double-wall arterial puncture is the most commonly used type of arterial access (Figure 17–4). The needle is inserted at a 45° angle to the skin surface and advanced slowly until arterial pulsation is felt (Figure 17–4A). It is then advanced through the artery in a single forward thrust, and the stylet is removed (Figure 17–4B). The needle is then withdrawn gradually; appearance of a pulsatile jet of blood indicates free intraluminal positioning (Figure 17–4C). A guidewire is then inserted to allow sheath introduction (Figure 17–4D–G).

Single-wall arterial puncture is indicated for a high femoral puncture (to avoid a retroperitoneal hematoma), in patients with coagulation abnormalities, and for puncture of synthetic grafts. The maneuvers are identical to double-wall puncture except that a stylet is not used during initial needle insertion into the artery. As the needle point is felt to be near the anterior wall of the artery, the stylet is removed. The needle is then slowly inserted into the artery until a jet of blood is encountered, indicating luminal entry. The guidewire is then passed, followed by sheath introduction. At all times the passage of wires and devices should be monitored with cinefluoroscopy to assure introduction without causing trauma and to assure cannulation of desired vessels. The length of introduced devices must also be carefully assessed to prevent inadvertent complications such as producing cardiac arrythmias by introduction of devices into the heart or by

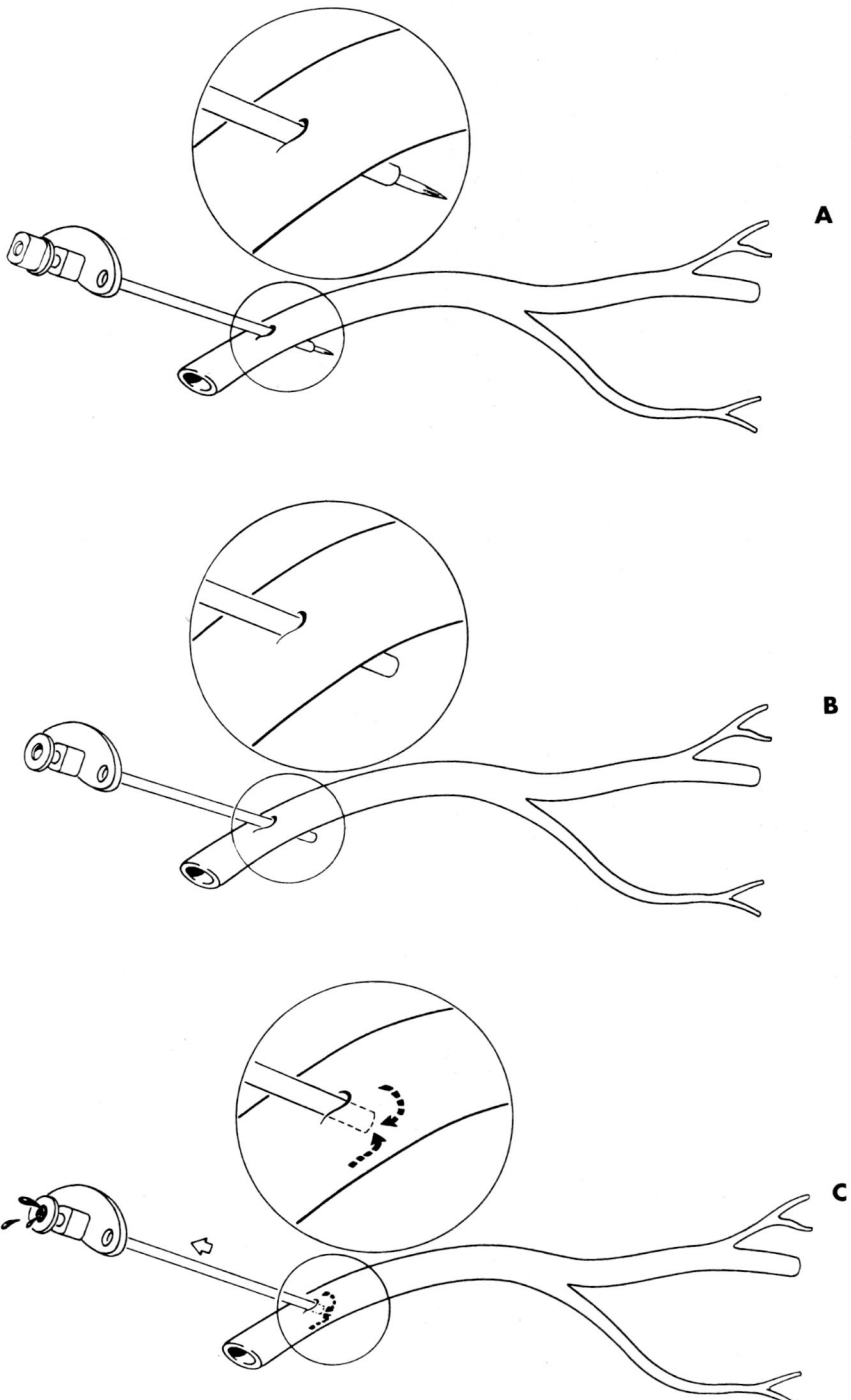

FIGURE 17–4. **A–G**, Double-wall arterial puncture technique.

17. Devices and Techniques for Vascular Access: Utility and Limitations of Current Methods 263

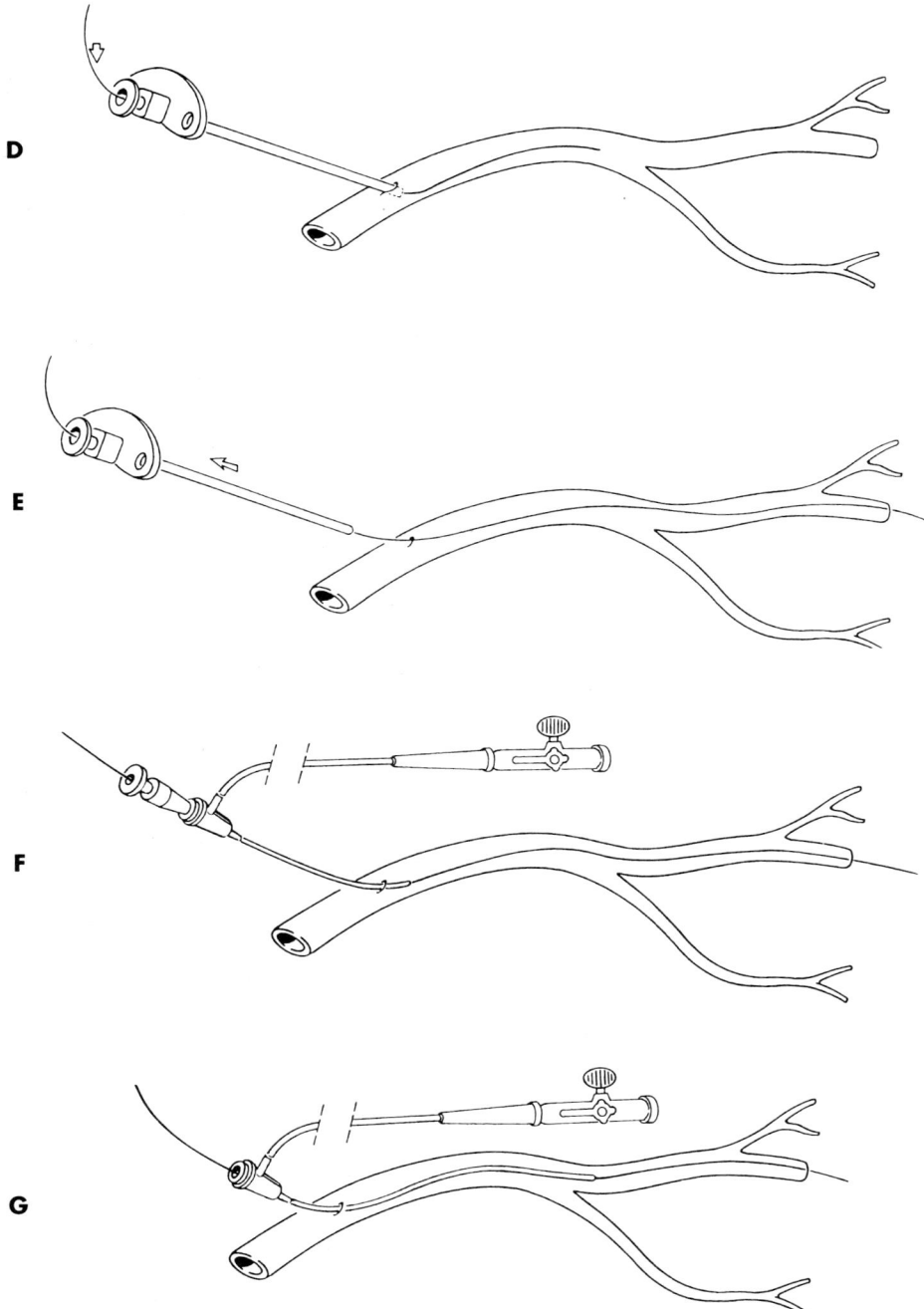

FIGURE 17–4. *Continued.*

perforation of renal parenchyma by excessive length of guidewires through the renal vasculature.

A pulsatile jet of blood may not be encountered in vessels with diminished or absent pulses, and blood return may be very slow. In this case a transparent extension tubing can be attached to the needle hub for injection of radiographic contrast to assess the positioning by fluoroscopy. Duplex scanning can also provide excellent guidance of the initial puncture. Occasionally a nonpulsatile, hard calcified artery can be palpated in thin patients.

Several methods of percutaneous introduction are used for various applications. For example, a retrograde femoral puncture provides access to the entire aorta and aortoiliac segments. It is also possible to pass some currently available guidewires and catheters across the aortic bifurcation from a femoral artery puncture to the contralateral iliac or femoral artery. Antegrade femoral artery puncture is used to access infrainguinal vessels if an adequate segment of patent proximal artery is available for access. A retrograde popliteal approach can be used to provide access to a patent distal superficial femoral artery when there is flush occlusion of the origin of that vessel. Percutaneous brachial or axillary puncture provides access to upper limb vessels and may be more convenient for imaging and treating the thoracic aorta and brachiocephalic vessels. An additional innovative method of access to aortoiliac and femoral vessels via the subclavian artery has been described (Figure 17–5).[4]

After accomplishing vascular access, a guidewire is then introduced through the lumen of the needle and positioned using fluoroscopy control. For many procedures an introducer sheath is threaded over the guidewire after passage of a vascular dilator. The diameter of the sheath is determined by the size of the device that will be passed through the sheath lumen into the artery.

Passage of needles, introducers, and instruments through the arterial wall predisposes the wall to dissection and formation of intimal flaps.[5] Acute arterial occlusion may occur from dislodged or embolized intimal lesions. Perforations of vessels that occur using smaller-diameter interventional devices usually do not require repair, particularly if they occur in previously occluded or thrombosed vessels. In this case there is usually little blood loss, and the perforation seals by rethrombosis of the segment. In addition, arteriovenous fistulas usually close spontaneously after reversal of anticoagulation. Rarely, perforations may continue to bleed, requiring surgical control. The most frequent site where this occurs is in intraperitoneal vessels or with punctures to the external iliac artery above the inguinal ligament to facilitate antegrade access to the femoral vessels. This approach is associated with a risk of hemorrhage into the retroperitoneum.

Intimal flaps usually require operative repair if they produce flow restriction. Microembolization of thrombus or atheromatous material is usually of no consequence if it is limited and there is no evidence of distal ischemia. If larger artery occlusion develops, percutaneous aspiration thrombectomy or open surgical embolectomy is required to restore flow.[6] Intraarterial infusion of thrombolytic therapy may also be effective in dissolving fresh thrombus. Massive embolization of small (20 to 200 μm diameter) particles can cause diffuse necrosis of tissues, producing devastating clinical consequences such as a "trash limb."

The majority of complications of percutaneous procedures associated with long-term failures, particularly recurrence of lesions, are common to all endovascular devices. False aneurysms or pseudoaneurysms at the puncture site in the arterial wall are unique to the percutaneous introduction sites, and the frequency increases as the size of the cannulas and endovascular instruments increase. False aneurysms frequently become apparent at relatively short intervals after procedures and require surgical repair to prevent bleeding or embolization. Pulsating hematomas often require intervention. An improved technique of ultrasound-guided compression with distal continuous pulse amplitude monitoring can help in avoiding direct surgery in 80% of those cases with pulsating hematomas.[7]

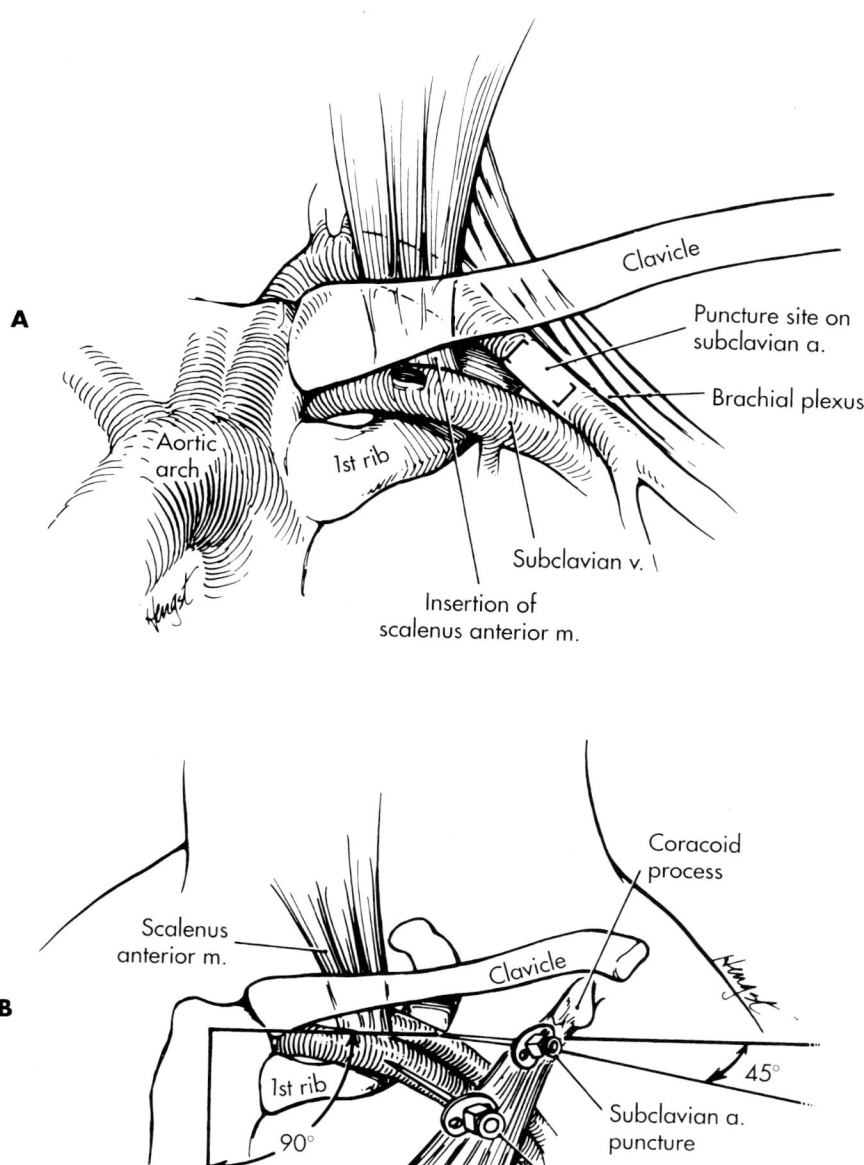

FIGURE 17–5. **A**, Anatomy of the point of entry for the subclavian artery. **B**, Insertion technique. (From Andros G, Harris RW, Delawa LB et al: Subclavian artery catheterization: a new approach for endovascular procedures, *J Vasc Surg* 20:566–576, 1994.)

Intraoperative Applications of Endovascular Devices

Intraoperative application of endovascular devices permits use of a large variety of instruments as either primary therapy or adjunctive to another vascular procedure. A key factor in accomplishing successful angioplasty in the operating room is adequate radiologic imaging. High-resolution images significantly enhance the precision of procedures; lack of this capability is a limiting factor in many institutions. Digital subtraction techniques have increased contrast imaging sensitivity, allowing detection of low levels of iodinated materials. Many digital units have freeze-frame and road-mapping features that permit superimposition of a subtracted contrast image of a vessel on a live fluoroscopic visualization. The quality of equipment available for radiologic imaging of procedures varies from conventional C-arm fluoroscopes to sophisticated image intensifiers and TV monitoring systems. Immediate image-replay systems can improve the accuracy of information and enhance the safety of interventions. Advances in computerized image processing systems extends the advantages of digital imaging technology to C-arm fluoroscopy by enabling modular addition of contrast enhancement, image holding, and road mapping during angiographic procedures.

Intraoperative percutaneous use of devices is accomplished by the methods described in the previous section. Many patients have significant vascular occlusive disease near a possible insertion site, which precludes safe passage of a percutaneous introducer. In these cases, surgical incisions provide the best access to the vessel. Introduction of intravascular instruments through an open surgical incision has several advantages compared with percutaneous methods. Open incisions permit inspection of intravascular anatomy such as the orifices of adjacent branch vessels and helps to decrease the incidence of vessel-wall dissection during device introduction. Control of blood flow from collateral vessels by conventional operative methods also expedites intraluminal visualization.

Once an arteriotomy has been fashioned, it is advantageous to work through a hemostatic introducer sheath with a side port similar to ones used for percutaneous procedures. This side port can help to prevent trauma to the blood vessel wall by repeated introduction and withdrawal of devices, provide hemostasis at the introduction port, and provide a port for injection of contrast dye. Introducer sheaths must be used very carefully because it is quite easy to injure the luminal surface of the artery during placement of the sheath, particularly when it is introduced for some distance into an artery. If a vessel is too diseased to accommodate an introducer sheath, hemostasis can be maintained with Roumel tourniquets with the endoluminal devices passed carefully through the controlled area.

Surgical incisions also permit continuation of anticoagulation throughout the procedure and postoperatively if the wound is drained to prevent hematoma formation. Continuation of anticoagulation may help to prevent acute thrombosis of difficult recanalizations in comparison with percutaneous procedures, where anticoagulation is reversed and pressure applied to the wound after removal of the intraluminal device to assure hemostasis. An obvious liability of the open-incision technique is the risk of wound infection, particularly if a patch material or prosthetic is used in the repair. The incidence of wound infection has been shown to be higher using the open technique during endovascular procedures.[8]

Device-Related Complications

A variety of introducers are used to provide access to the vascular lumen for guidewires and angioplasty devices. The main complications of the introducers are disruption of the vascular surface, production of intimal flaps or embolization, and formation of thrombus on catheter surfaces when they are positioned in low blood-flow areas without anticoagulation. Some catheters incorporate anticoagulants in the catheter surface to decrease thrombogenicity, but systemic anticoagulation is required in most instances to prevent thrombosis.

The complications related to introducer-sheath placement can be reduced by accurately judging the appropriate diameter and length of the device for the vascular segment being treated. Many diseased vessels have segmental narrowings or friable luminal surfaces that can easily be disrupted. If intimal flaps result, a localized endarterectomy can sometimes be performed, although an otherwise successful angioplasty procedure can be disrupted by introducer complications, which frequently require a vascular reconstruction to bypass the segment.

Guidewires are extremely useful for introducing intravascular devices and helping to maintain intraluminal guidance. Stiffer wires with less flexible tips have a greater tendency to produce intimal lesions, dissections, and perforations. Some of the newer flexible-tip wires and catheters have a hydrophilic polymer coating, which aids in atraumatic passage through stenotic or occluded vessel segments. Although introduction of angioplasty devices over guidewires can be used to help prevent complications, the obligatory off-center positioning of the guidewire through eccentric atherosclerotic obstructions prevents complete debulking of lesions without affecting adjacent vessel walls that have minimal or no involvement. Improved guidance systems that would provide concentric alignment of the device within the arterial lumen need to be developed to alleviate this problem. Combined intraluminal ultrasound- and angioscopy-guided angioplasty catheter-delivery systems are promising in this regard. A description of guidewire mechanisms and materials is found in Chapter 15.

References

1. Fogarty TJ, Chin AK, Shoor PM et al: Adjunctive arterial dilation: simplified instrumentation technique, *Arch Surg* 16:1391–1398, 1983. Presented at SVS/ISCVS Meeting, Dallas, Texas, June 1981.
2. Clowes A: Theories of atherogenesis. In White RA, editor: *Atherosclerosis and arteriosclerosis: human pathology and experimental animal methods and models*, Boca Raton, Fl, 1989, CRC Press.
3. Seldinger SI: Catheter placement of the needle in percutaneous arteriography, *Acta Radiol* 39:368–376, 1953.
4. Andros GA, Harris RW, Delawa LB et al: Subclavian artery catherization: a new approach for endovascular procedures. *J Vasc Surg* 20:566–576, 1994.
5. Fogarty TJ, Krippaehne WW: Vascular occlusion following arterial catheterization, *Surg Gynecol Obstet* 122:1269, 1966.
6. White RA, White GH: Percutaneous aspiration thromboembolectomy. In Ernst CB, Stanley JC, editors: *Current therapy in vascular surgery*, Philadelphia, 1990, BC Decker.
7. Fellmeth BD, Roberts AC, Bookstein JJ et al: Postangiographic femoral artery injuries: nonsurgical repair with US-guided compression, *Radiology* 178:671–675, 1991.
8. White RA, White GH, Mehringer CM et al: A clinical trial of laser thermal angioplasty in patients with advanced peripheral vascular disease, *Ann Surg* 212:257–265, 1990.

18
Balloon Angioplasty

John V. White, Ibrahim G. Eid, Amit Kharod, and Sherry Scovell

Transluminal angioplasty was initially conceived by Dotter and Judkins in 1964.[1] Unfortunately, the technical limitations of their stiff, coaxial, Teflon catheters prevented widespread acceptance and use of their technique. When Gruntzig and Hopff introduced the flexible, polyvinyl double-lumen balloon catheter in 1974, they revolutionized angioplasty and set the stage for its extensive use to treat coronary and peripheral vascular occlusive disease.[2] Percutaneous transluminal angioplasty (PTA) is undeniably associated with lower morbidity and cost than conventional open bypass surgery. However, the vascular interventionist (i.e., radiologist, cardiologist, or surgeon) must understand the clinical indications, lasting benefit, and complications of PTA to use this therapy appropriately.

Mechanism

Early investigators believed that balloon angioplasty dilated stenotic vessels by exerting pressure and compressing the atherosclerotic plaque.[3] Experimental and cadaver studies, however, showed that atherosclerotic plaques are minimally compressible, frequently calcified lesions.[4] It is now known that angioplasty fractures the atherosclerotic media along with stretching and rupturing the muscle fibers.[5,6] Plaque compression therefore plays only a minor role in vessel dilation. The adventitia of the artery is also stretched irreversibly, thereby expanding the outer diameter of the vessel.

Remodeling of the angioplasty site, or luminal injury, begins immediately and continues indefinitely. The formation of plaque fissures and damage to the internal elastic membrane expose subendothelial collagen to blood elements, resulting in platelet deposition and the release of a variety of platelet and white blood cell mediators. These vasoactive substances can induce distal spasm and may initiate the process of intimal hyperplasia. Prevention or control of this fibrotic restenosis is currently the target of intense scientific investigation.

Indications

Patient selection is critical for effective application of balloon angioplasty. The clinical indications for balloon angioplasty are similar to those for vascular surgical intervention in the extremities. Angioplasty should be considered for patients with a life style inhibiting claudication, rest pain, ischemic ulceration, or poor surgical wound healing distal to the arterial lesion. Generally, asymptomatic stenoses should not be dilated. PTA may also be used as an adjunct to surgery to dilate a stenosis proximal to a planned surgical bypass and save a failing graft.[7]

Balloon angioplasty is ideally suited for patients who have symptomatic short-segment concentric stenoses, rather than occlusions, of a major artery. Complete occlusions have a higher complication rate and a lower long-term patency rate than stenoses. Acceptable long-term results can be expected when short-segment concentric stenoses are dilated in the presence of good distal runoff and there is an immediate return of distal pulses.

Lesion

The arterial lesion best suited for balloon angioplasty is a concentric plaque located at least 5 mm beyond the origin of a medium to large artery. The length of the stenosis should be less than 5 cm. Maintaining contact with normal proximal and distal arterial wall minimizes extension of the fissuring process beyond the stenotic area. Longer lesions can be dilated by centering the balloon near the proximal end of the lesion and then advancing the balloon after each successful dilation. Orificial lesions yield poor results because of the inability to maintain balloon contact with normal proximal arterial wall. Dilating an eccentric plaque may lead to differential distribution of lateral wall stress, resulting in subplaque hemorrhage and dissection. PTA of an anatomically or morphologically unfavorable lesion may be considered in a poor risk patient with limb-threatening ischemia.

Balloon Angioplasty Equipment

Introducer Sheaths

The introducer sheath provides a hemostatic connection between the surface of the skin and the lumen of the artery. In its simplest form, it is a thin-walled, hollow tube with a hemostatic valve on the external end. There are many types of sheath with a wide variety of features now available, including those with an internal wire to prevent kinking, a hydrophilic coating to ease introduction, and a variable diameter. Most of them are available with a side arm for the administration of fluids and medications or the monitoring of pressures. The introducer sheath is packaged with a dilator that extends beyond the end of the sheath and is tapered so the arterial puncture site can be gently expanded to accommodate the introducer. The device is sized by length and internal diameter, and various combinations are available. It is generally best to choose a sheath that is at least 0.5F larger in diameter than the largest catheter to be used. For the performance of angioplasty, a small introducer can be inserted initially to permit contrast angiography with a small catheter, such as one with a 4F diameter. Once the decision is made to perform an angioplasty and the size of the balloon catheter is established, the smaller sheath can be exchanged for a larger one. Though short sheaths are most commonly used for the performance of diagnostic angiography or simple angioplasty, longer sheaths are frequently placed across a lesion to be stented to prevent the stent from becoming dislodged while traversing the lesion (Figure 18–1).

Guidewires

Guidewires are the basic guidance tools for PTA. They are essential for safe navigation of the arterial tree and for minimizing subintimal dissection. The ideal wire is frictionless and atraumatic, resists kinking and fraying, and has good torque response. Wires are available in a variety of lengths and diameters. They are made of a stiff inner core that is wrapped in a more flexible outer layer coated by agents to reduce friction. They are also available in different tip configurations, including J, angled, straight, or deformable distal tips (Figure 18–2). Wires with a soft or J tip cause the least trauma to fragile surfaces during manipulation. Stiff wires are used to steer large balloon catheters through tortuous vessels without buckling. Wires coated with hydrophilic materials are the best choice to pass across a long, tortuous channel of disease.[8]

Standard 0.038- or 0.035-inch guidewires are useful for guiding most diagnostic and balloon catheters; however, 0.010- to 0.028-inch guidewires are available for use with miniballoons in small vessels. Guidewires 100 to 150 cm long are used for most vascular procedures. Longer wires (150 to 260 cm in length) are used

18. Balloon Angioplasty

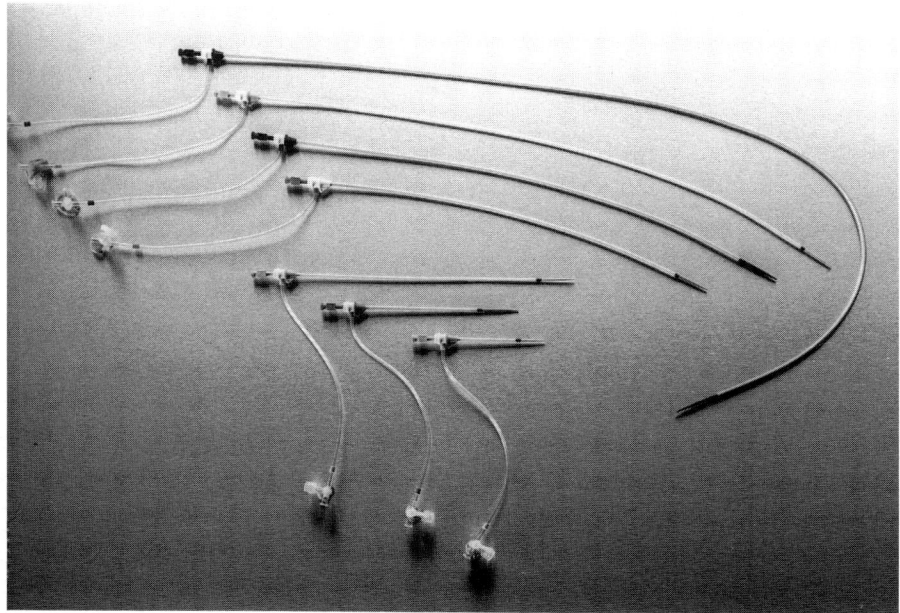

FIGURE 18–1. Introducer sheaths come in different sizes and lengths that target different sites. (Courtesy of Cordis Corporation.)

for contralateral approaches and distal catheter exchanges. Surgeons can use shorter (40 to 80 cm), more maneuverable wires intraoperatively. A variety of specialty wires are also available. Some wires contain radiopaque markers and can be used for length and diameter measurements during angioplasty procedures. There are also guidewires containing intravas-

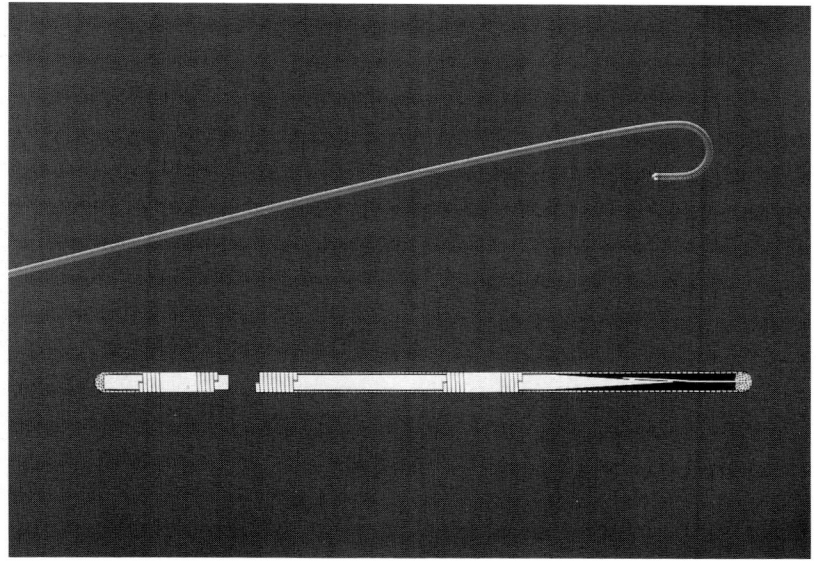

FIGURE 18–2. Anatomy of a stiff guidewire. (Courtesy of Cook Incorporated, Bloomington, IN.)

cular Doppler probes for intravascular ultrasonography during the performance of angioplasty.[9]

Catheters

Catheters are used to perform angiography, direct balloon angioplasty catheters and stents, and help position a wire or a smaller catheter into difficult locations. The large number of available catheters differ in diameter, length, distal shape, and material (Figure 18–3). The choice depends on the intended use of the catheter. Catheter length depends on the location of the target area, and the preconfigured distal shape of a catheter is selected based on the specific branch to be cannulated or lesion to be crossed. The material of the catheter determines its behavior during the procedure, but all shaped guide catheters track in a linear manner over the stiff portion of the guidewire and resume their preformed shapes as they track over the softer end of the wire. Polyethylene catheters have good shape memory and are pliable, which makes them suitable for selective catheterization of branch vessels. Polyurethane catheters have a higher coefficient of friction but are softer and more pliable and thus easier to slide over wires. Nylon catheters are the stiffest and tolerate high flow rates, a characteristic useful during aortography. The most common catheter diameter for routine angiography is a 4F or 5F pigtail or tennis racket catheter that tracks over a 0.035-inch guidewire (Figure 18–4A,B). This catheter is straightened when tracking over the stiff portion of the wire but resumes its curved head over the softer part of the wire or after the wire is withdrawn. This ability enables it to pass through tortuous vessels, navigate the aortic bifurcation, rapidly deliver contrast, and record pre- and postangioplasty pressures.

Balloons

The balloon angioplasty catheter has two lumens: The lumen through which the guidewire passes is coaxial, allowing the catheter to track along the wire; the other lumen, which is connected to the balloon, permits inflation. Angioplasty balloons have changed and improved over the years, and it is important for the interventionist to understand the various balloon characteristics and their optimal uses. The most useful catheters have a low profile and high trackability. Low-profile catheters are designed to be as thin as possible in the deflated state, thereby minimizing entry-site complications and optimizing the interventionist's ability to negotiate tight, tortuous stenoses. Trackability refers to the tendency of the balloon catheter to follow a previously placed wire without pulling the wire out of the desired position. Angioplasty balloons are selected by length, diameter, and bursting pressure. The length is defined as the portion of the

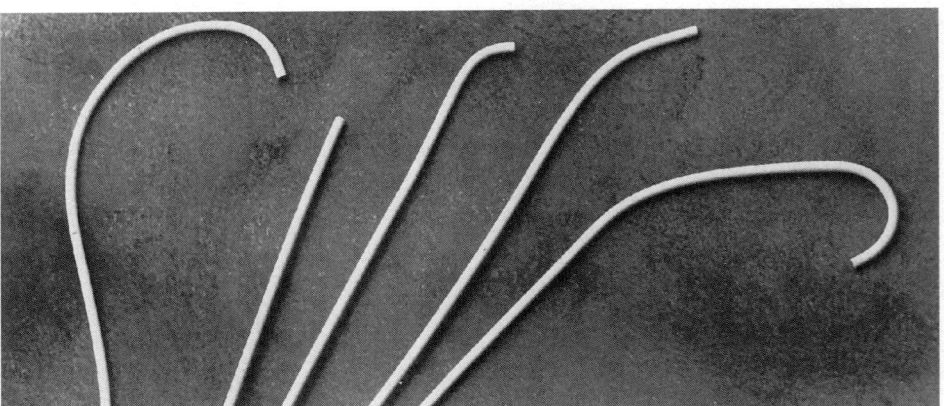

FIGURE 18–3. Guiding catheters with variable tip designs provide enhanced torque control when advancing through tortuous lesions. (Courtesy Medi-65 tech/Boston Scientific. Co., Watertown, Mass.)

18. Balloon Angioplasty

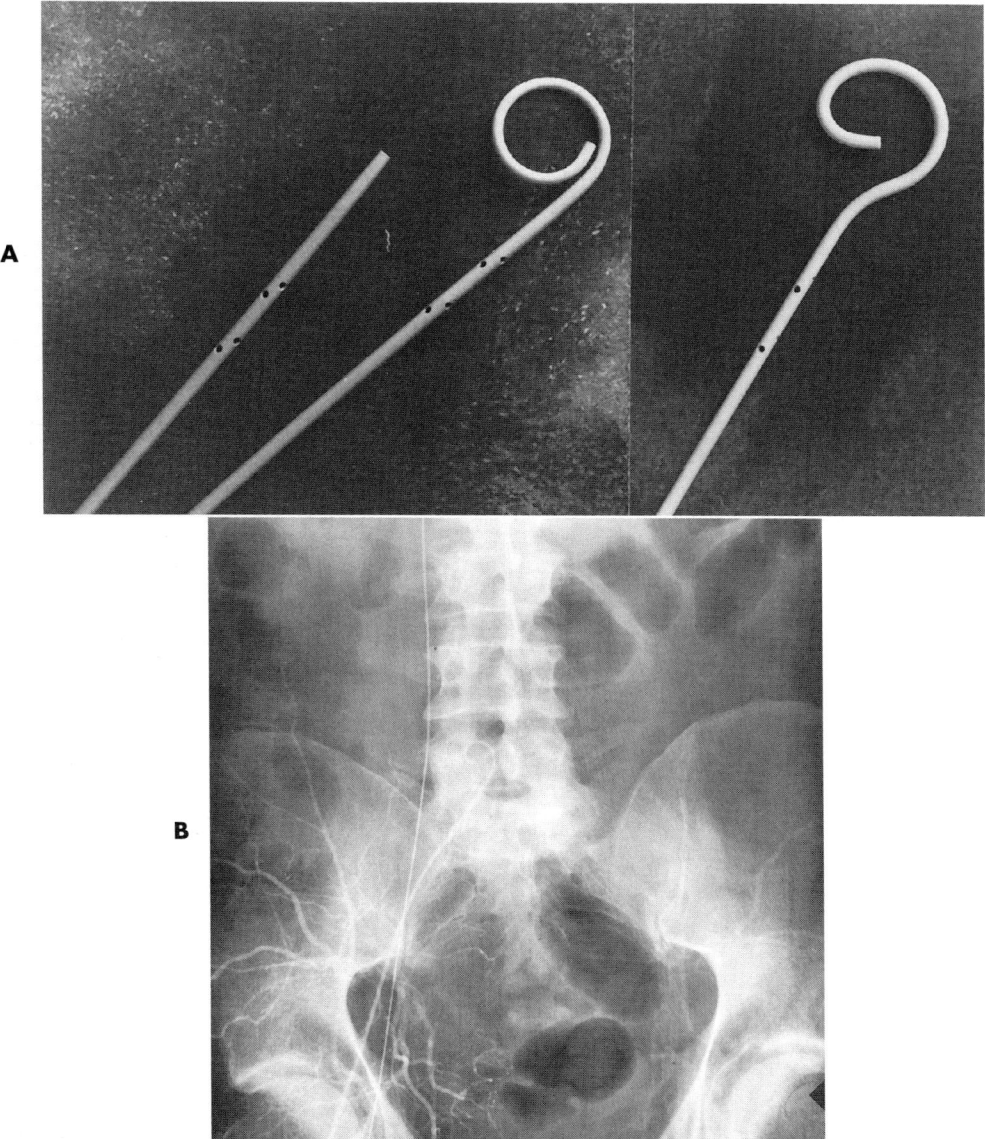

FIGURE 18–4. **A**, Pigtail and tennis racket 4F diagnostic catheters with multiple side holes for accurate pressure measurements. **B**, Pigtail catheter can be visualized in the distal aorta. (Courtesy Meditech/Boston Scientific Co., Watertown, Mass.)

balloon that has parallel walls when completely inflated. Bursting pressure is the level of pressure at which the balloon material begins to split and pressure is lost. With the current standards of construction, balloon rupture rarely results in shredding and the loss of material within the blood vessel. The dilating balloons now available are constructed with low-compliance, high-strength materials that are able to exert sufficient dilating force without becoming distorted or rupturing.

Most current balloons are made from polyethylene terephthalate or other low-complaint, strong plastic polymers. These balloons inflate

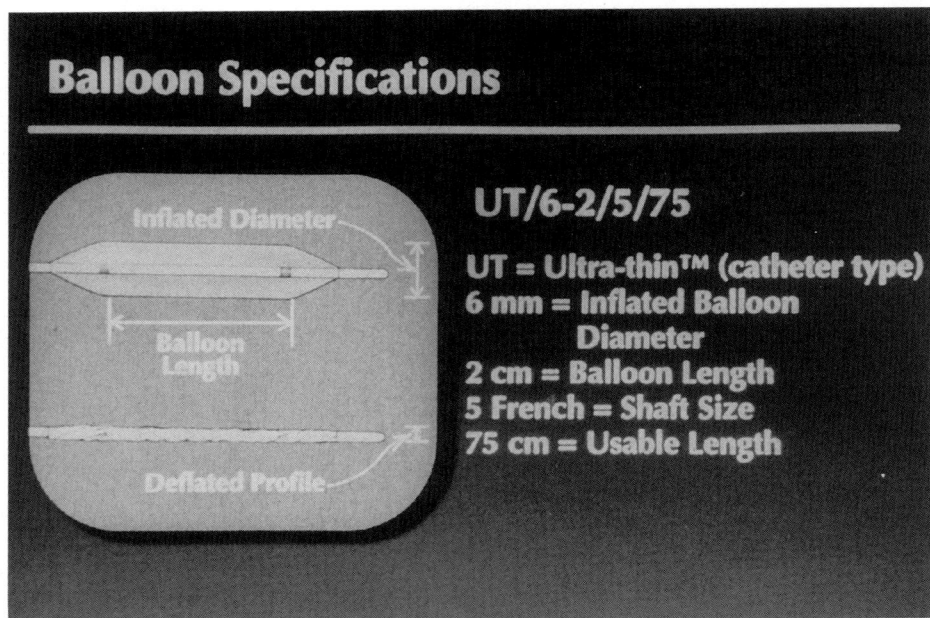

FIGURE 18–5. Angioplasty balloon specifications. (Courtesy Medi-tech/Boston Scientific Co., Watertown, Mass.)

to various preset diameters and pressures (Figure 18–5). Standard peripheral angioplasty balloons track smoothly over a 0.035-inch guidewire and have a safe operating range of 4 to 12 atm of dilating pressure (Figure 18–6). They are available in inflated balloon diameters of 3 to 10 mm, balloon lengths of 2 to 10 mm, and hydrophilic coating to enhance performance. Balloons constructed of stiffer materials such as woven nylon have higher burst pressures (more than 17 atm) and are used to cross and dilate tight, calcific stenoses. To dilate infrapopliteal vessels, balloons are available that accept 0.018-inch guidewires and are mounted on 3.8F catheter shafts. There are also balloons mounted directly on guidewires that can be used in coaxial fashion (Figure 18–7). These lowest-profile balloons are ideal for intraoperative angioplasty and can be placed through a 4F introducer sheath. The balloon should be inflated with a device that monitors pressure inside the balloon (Figure 18–8).

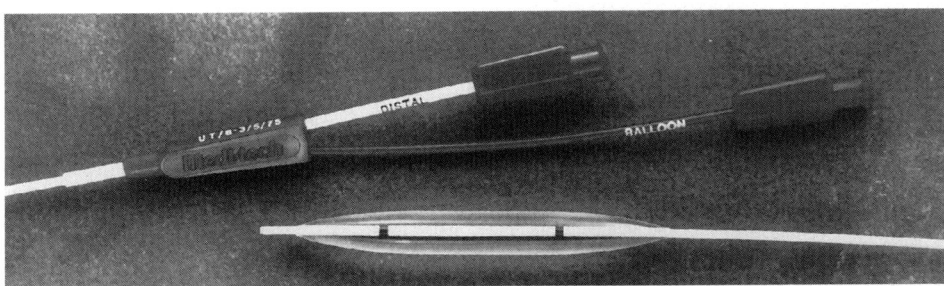

FIGURE 18–6. Ultrathin polyethylene terephthalate balloon dilation catheter (Courtesy Medi-tech/Boston Scientific Co., Watertown, Mass.)

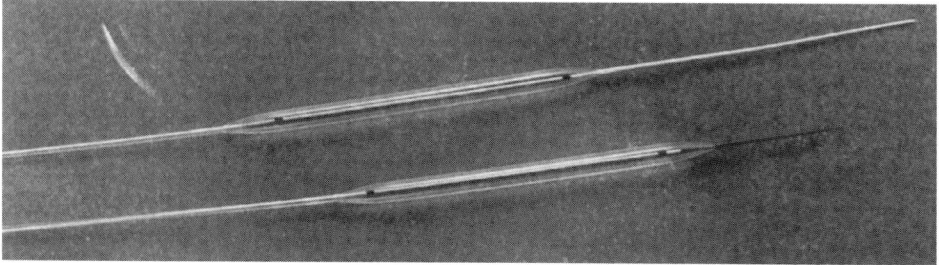

FIGURE 18–7. TEGwire balloon dilation catheters mounted on 0.035-inch wires. (Courtesy Medi-tech/Boston Scientific Co., Watertown, Mass.)

Technique

The patient is placed in the supine position on the imaging table so the arterial segments, from the cannulation point to a few centimeters beyond the region to be dilated, can be easily visualized. The patient is sedated, and a vasodilator such as nifedipine may be given 30 minutes before the procedure to help prevent vessel spasm. All patients should undergo cardiac rhythm and blood pressure monitoring throughout the procedure.

Once the appropriate site is chosen, the selected groin is prepared and infiltrated with lidocaine. A Seldinger needle is advanced into the artery; and when pulsatile backflow is visualized, a standard short 0.035-inch guidewire is advanced through the needle into the common femoral artery. Typically, a 5F introducer sheath is advanced over the guidewire and positioned to protect the insertion site without crossing the lesion. The short guidewire is then replaced by a torquable, soft-tipped guidewire that is advanced with the assistance of fluoroscopy to the level of the stenosis or occlusion and then continued a reasonable distance beyond the lesion. An exchange of guidewires may be necessary to cross the lesion. A specialized adapter with a hemostatic valve such as the Tuohy-Borst Y adapter can be connected to the introducer sheath to facilitate contrast injections through a rotating side port (Figure 18–9). Additional vasodilators may also be required (Table 18–1). When the guidewire is in the correct position, a diagnostic catheter is advanced along the guidewire proximal to the lesion to record arterial pressures above and below the lesion.

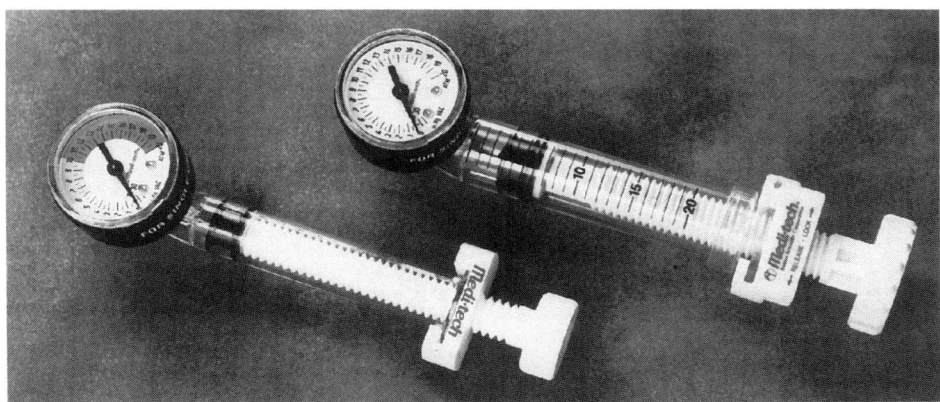

FIGURE 18–8. Leveen inflators with pressure gauge. (Courtesy Medi-tech/Boston Scientific Co., Watertown, Mass.)

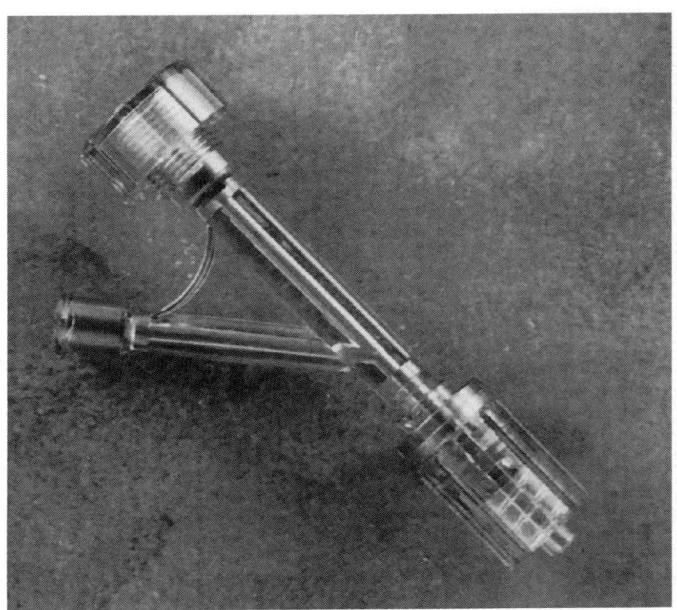

FIGURE 18–9. Tuohy-Borst Y adapter. (Courtesy Medi-tech/Boston Scientific Co., Watertown, Mass.)

A diagnostic angiogram that provides road mapping capabilities is obtained to help select the approach and size of the angioplasty balloon. An arterial puncture site is chosen that is most appropriate for the lesion being treated. In most cases the preferred entry site for balloon angioplasty is the common femoral artery below the inguinal crease. Typically, an ipsilateral approach is used to prevent injury to the less diseased extremity. A contralateral route that directs the guidewire and catheter across the aortic bifurcation can be employed, but it makes guidewire manipulation more difficult. An antegrade approach is usually used in patients with superficial femoral artery lesions, and a retrograde approach is used for more proximal stenoses.

After traversing the stenosis, the patient is heparinized. The diagnostic catheter is then removed, and a balloon catheter with a diameter that matches the outflow vessel beyond the lesion as determined by angiogram is inserted (Table 18–2). The balloon length should be greater than that of the lesion. The balloon is centered on the lesion and inflated slowly via an inflation device that also measures the intraballoon pressures (Figure 18–10). The balloon is inflated using dilute contrast so the dilation can be monitored fluoroscopically. When the balloon contacts the lesion, the contrast is pushed to the polar ends of the balloon, creating an hourglass configuration. As the pressure within the balloon increases, the waist of the balloon widens and eventually disappears (Figure 18–11A,B). Inflation is maintained for 30 to 60 seconds from the time the waist disappears. The balloon is then deflated and withdrawn several centimeters from the lesion site so contrast can be injected and the results evaluated (Figure 18–12).

TABLE 18–1. Vasodilators for Balloon Angioplasty

Drug	Dose	Method of administration
Nitroglycerin	100–200 µg	Intraarterial
Nitroglycerin	1/150 grain	Sublingual
Nifedipine	10 mg	Sublingual
Lidocaine	50–100 mg	Intraarterial
Priscoline	25 mg	Intraarterial

TABLE 18–2. Typical Balloon Sizes

Artery	Diameter (mm)	Length (cm)
Iliac	8–12	3–8
Superior femoral artery	4–7	4–10
Popliteal	3–6	2–10
Trifurcation	2–4	2–4
Renal	4–8	2

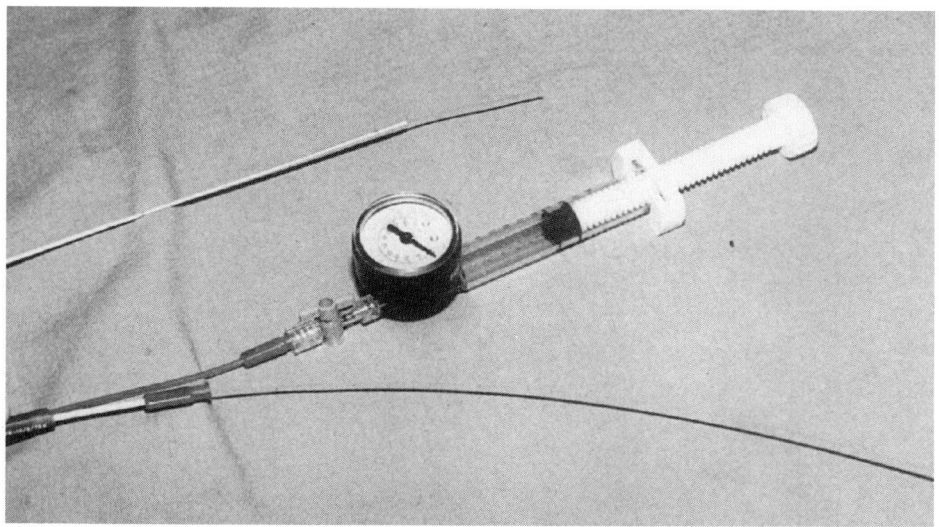

FIGURE 18–10. Complete angioplasty system with guidewire and inflation syringe with pressure gauge. (Courtesy Medi-tech/Boston Scientific Co., Watertown, Mass.)

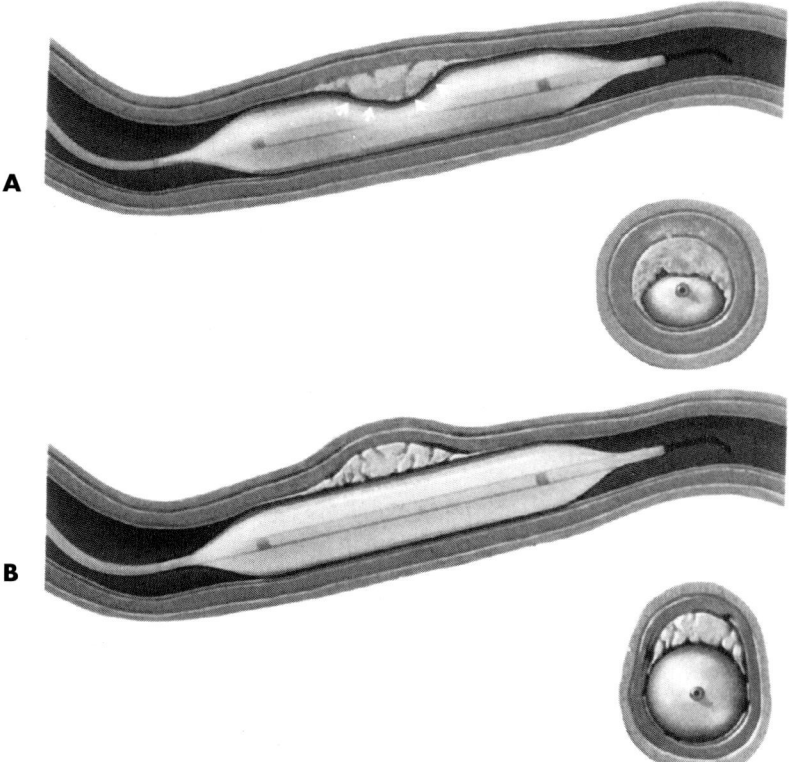

FIGURE 18–11. **A**, Once balloon inflation begins, a "waist" forms where the lesion is most resistant. **B**, As inflation progresses, the "waist" disappears. The media and adventitia are stretched, and the plaque is cracked. (Courtesy Medi-tech/Boston Scientific Co., Watertown, Mass.)

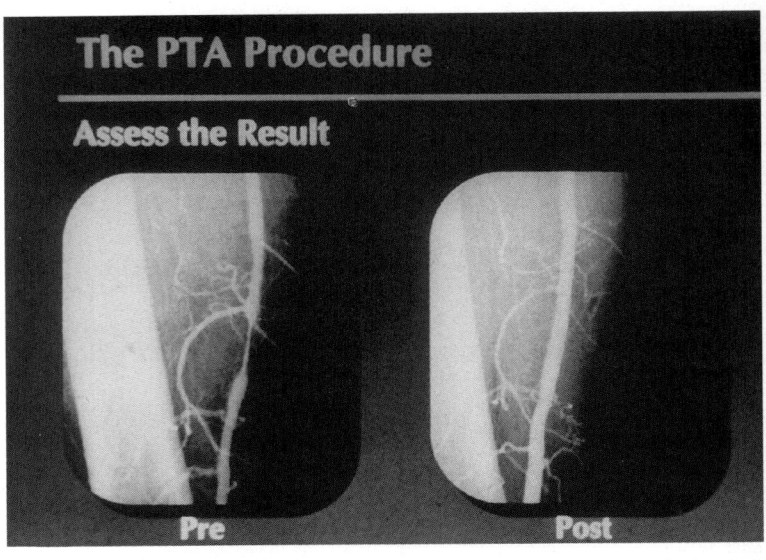

FIGURE 18–12. Contrast can be injected through the sheath side port or distal lumen of the balloon catheter to visualize the results. Postdilation angiogram demonstrates a patent, smooth lumen.

A technically successful procedure leaves a residual stenosis of 30% or less at the angioplasty site. If a significant stenosis remains or a small dissection is evident after balloon inflation, the process is repeated. Because successful angioplasty does produce small, local wall dissections, postangioplasty injections should not be made within the dilated segment and guidewires should not be advanced across dilated vessels. On completion of the procedure, the arterial pressures above and below the site of the lesion is measured to quantify the new arterial hemodynamic profile. The sheath can be removed immediately after completion of the procedure or after a period of time to allow heparin metabolism. Local compression is used to obtain hemostasis.

Patients are required to remain at bed rest for 8 hours after the procedure. Heparin infusion is maintained for 24 hours, and patients are continued on antiplatelet medication. Baseline noninvasive ankle-brachial pressure measurements are obtained shortly after angioplasty.

Site-Specific Interventions

Aortic Angioplasty

Aortobifemoral bypass grafting is generally indicated for diffuse, multifocal aortoiliac occlusive disease. Angioplasty can be effectively performed on concentric, focal, distal abdominal aortic stenoses. When the stenosis is proximal to the bifurcation, a single 15- to 20-mm balloon is used. Initial success rates are greater than 90%, with 5-year patency rates reported at 70%.[10,11] One would expect a low restenosis rate in this large, high-flow vessel. Experience is limited, however, because isolated aortic flow-restricting lesions are rare. Disease that involves the iliac arteries is more common. Lesions associated with aortic aneurysms should not be dilated.

Atherosclerosis of the aortic bifurcation involves both iliac arteries and requires a bilateral femoral artery approach using the "kissing balloon" technique described by Tegtmeyer et al.[12] With this technique, two 8- to 12-mm balloons can be simultaneously inflated within the aortoiliac region without the risk of iliac rupture. In a combined series of 52 patients with distal aortic disease, 92% of the vessels were successfully dilated with less than a 6% restenosis rate after a mean follow-up of 13 months.[10,12,13] Stent placement has improved immediate success, increasing the benefit of this minimally invasive procedure for the treatment of aortoiliac occlusive disease.[11,14,15]

Iliac Artery Angioplasty

The common iliac artery is ideally suited for balloon angioplasty. It is a large, high-flow vessel that responds well to dilation and offers the highest initial and long-term success rates. Indications for balloon dilation include circumferential high-grade stenoses of the common iliac artery located beyond the origin but proximal to the bifurcation of the iliac artery. PTA of the iliac artery has also been effective in increasing inflow in patients for whom distal bypass grafting is being considered.[16] Ulcerated lesions or lesions associated with thrombus are not usually considered for angioplasty because of the likelihood of distal embolization. Similarly, long or multiple stenoses are less likely to have a good long-term result using PTA, in contrast to that with bypass surgery.[17]

Immediate technical success can be expected in 90% to 97% of patients with iliac stenoses.[18-22] In a review of 2697 iliac artery angioplasties, Becker et al. found a mean 2-year patency rate of 81% and a 5-year rate of 72%.[23] Treatment of tandem stenoses of long-segment stenoses did not yield such promising results. Distal disease negatively influences the long-term benefit. In a series of 984 angioplasties, Johnston reported 65% and a 52% five-year patency rates for common iliac stenoses with good and poor runoff, respectively.[21] In one of the few randomized prospective studies comparing bypass surgery and iliac angioplasty, Wilson et al. found no statistical significance in long-term patency rates between these two modes of therapy.[24] Stent placement has improved the immediate results of angioplasty of the iliac arteries.[25]

The role of transluminal balloon angioplasty in the treatment of total common iliac artery occlusion is limited. Total occlusion of the common iliac artery makes accurate identification of the true lumen difficult and increases the chances of vessel dissection and perforation. Older series report a 20% to 40% technical failure rate for long-segment angioplasty of this vessel.[26] Angioplasty has proved to be beneficial in patients with short-segment occlusions that can be traversed with modern guidewires and low-profile balloon catheters. The immediate success rates for balloon angioplasty of iliac occlusions have been documented at 92% for occlusions less than 5 cm in length but only 70% in occlusions longer than 5 cm.[27] Johnston reported a 48% 3-year patency rate in an analysis of 82 patients with iliac artery occlusions. Not surprisingly, patients with long-segment occlusions and multiple stenoses had a 3-year patency rate of only 17%.[21] In this study the results of balloon angioplasty of external iliac artery stenoses were not as successful as those for the common iliac artery. Although immediate success rates were better than 90%, the 3-year patency rate was 51%. Interestingly, gender has been described as a prognosticator of long-term success, with men having a 57% three-year patency rate compared with a 34% rate for women. More recent studies combining angioplasty with stent placement have reported an improvement in immediate success and short-term patency exceeding 70% at 2 years.[28]

Femoral and Popliteal Artery Angioplasty

Dilation of distal extremity lesions has become technically possible and relatively safe with the development of lower-profile angioplasty balloons and steerable, hydrophilic guidewires. An ipsilateral approach provides the interventionist with the greatest wire and catheter maneuverability. The contralateral femoral artery approach is effective and necessary in proximal common femoral artery lesions. Because these distal vessels are prone to spasm, the use of vasodilators is more important than with balloon angioplasty of aortoiliac disease.

Regardless of the technical feasibility of femoral and popliteal angioplasty, there is significant controversy about which patients should undergo PTA and which should proceed directly to surgical bypass.[20,29-31] Lesions that respond best to PTA are mild to moderate focal stenoses causing mild or disabling claudication, especially in the presence of good distal runoff.[20,32,33] Stenoses that are eccentric, longer than 5 cm, or present in diabetic patients are more likely to have a poor long-term result after balloon angioplasty. Although some studies of superficial femoral artery angioplasty have reported technical failure rates as high as 33%, some studies describe less than a 10% initial failure rate.[23,34,35] Mean 3-year patency rates are better for stenoses (averaging 70%), compared with 55% for complete occlusions.[24] Interestingly, some studies have shown that occlusions that can be crossed with a guidewire have an equal or better long-term patency rate than stenoses. Comparing 193 femoropopliteal angioplasties (116 stenoses, 77 occlusions), Murray et al. described a 4.5-year patency rate of 54.4% for 116 stenoses and 72.9% for 77 occlusions. Stenotic lesions larger than 7 cm demonstrated the worst patency rate: only 23.1% at 6 months.[36]

More important than patency rate is the lasting clinical benefit. A study of 117 patients with critical limb ischemia who underwent femoropopliteal angioplasty as their primary form of treatment reported primary technical success rates of 92% for stenoses and 80% for occlusions, with 1-, 2-, and 3-year limb salvage rates of only 56%, 49%, and 49%, respectively. Becquemin and colleagues compared 4-year patency rates of angioplasty and surgery for the treatment of femoropopliteal disease and found 44% of those treated with angioplasty still patent but 65% of those treated with bypass grafting patent.[37]

Infrapopliteal Angioplasty

With the application of coronary angioplasty techniques, there has been increased enthusiasm for PTA of the infrapopliteal vessels. Balloon angioplasty of the tibioperoneal vessels is usually performed in poor-risk patients for limb salvage. The most common indications at this time are acute ischemia, rest pain, and tissue loss in patients whose vessels are otherwise unreconstructible by surgery.[38] The procedure requires an antegrade common femoral artery puncture and insertion of a 5.5F to 6F vascular sheath. Generally, a steerable platinum-tipped guidewire along with a small-vessel (4F) angioplasty balloon are advanced together across the lesion. Spasm and thrombosis must be treated aggressively with intraarterial vasodilators, thrombolytic agents, and intravenous heparin. Systemic heparinization should be continued for 48 to 72 hours.

The best results for infrapopliteal angioplasty are achieved in short-segment focal stenoses (less than 2 cm). Technical success rates of 75% to 100% have been reported.[39,40] Clinical benefit, as determined by an increased ankle-brachial index or limb salvage, ranges from 44% and 83% at 2 years.[38-46] Several factors have been implicated as adversely influencing the outcome, including the presence of diabetes, distal gangrene, more than six stenoses, occlusions more than 5 cm in length, and significant proximal or distal disease.[38]

Balloon angioplasty of infrapopliteal vessels requires manipulation of fine guidewires and should be attempted only by highly experienced interventionists. In most cases, patients with limb-threatening ischemia resulting from infrapopliteal disease require femoropedal bypass surgery.

Renal and Mesenteric Angioplasty

Compared with peripheral vascular procedures, angioplasty of the branches of the abdominal aorta is technically more demanding. Stenoses of these vessels should be treated only by skilled interventionists. These lesions are usually caused by atherosclerosis, fibromuscular dysplasia, extrinsic compression, or vasculitis. Generally, a femoral artery approach is used, although a left brachial or axillary artery approach is recommended when there is an abdominal aortic aneurysm or an acute angle between the diseased artery and aorta. Most renal and mesenteric arteries can be cannulated with a cobra-shaped catheter. Torquable guidewires used to cross tight stenoses may need to be exchanged for stiffer wires before advancing the balloon across the lesion. Heparin and nitroglycerin should be used before balloon inflation. When dilating renal arteries, it is important to use balloon catheters with the shortest length of catheter distal to the balloon to minimize trauma to the branch vessels.

Percutaneous transluminal renal angioplasty is most commonly indicated for the treatment of hypertension or ischemic nephropathy resulting from renal artery stenosis. Angioplasty of nonorificial lesions has an immediate technical success rate of 85% to 90%.[47-50] In a review of more than 1000 percutaneous transluminal renal angioplasties, Becker et al. found an initial success rate of 90.7% and a 2-year patency rate of 74.3%.[23] Cure and improvement rates for hypertension and ischemic nephropathy are reported to be 0% to 55% and 37% to 52%, respectively.[47,49,51,52] Restenosis is common, affecting more than 35% of vessels treated.[50] Angioplasty is more effective treatment for stenoses caused by fibromuscular dysplasia than those secondary to atherosclerosis. In a series of 55 renal angioplasty patients, Beebe et al. documented a 33% total cure rate and 50% improvement rate in patients with fibromuscular dysplasia but showed only a 10% cure rate and 42% improvement rate in patients with atherosclerotic plaques.[53] Cluzel and colleagues aggressively pursued angioplasty of renal branch vessels for the treatment of fibromuscular dysplasia and noted alleviation of hypertension in 92% of patients.[54] Bilateral stenoses have lower success rates than do unilateral stenoses. Lesions involving the origin of the renal artery respond especially poorly to PTA.[55] These plaques are actually aortic plaques that encroach on the renal artery and are thus difficult to fracture. Symptomatic atherosclerotic orificial lesions are currently better treated by surgical bypass, especially in the presence of diffuse atherosclerotic aortic disease or abdominal aortic aneurysm.[55]

Percutaneous transluminal angioplasty of renal artery stenosis in a transplant is effective and can obviate the need for difficult reoperations to salvage failing kidney transplants.[55] Indications for angioplasty are progressive hypertension and graft dysfunction.[56] These lesions are most frequently located at the anastomosis and respond well to balloon dilation. Some studies have reported technical success rates of 75% to 93%, with an excellent 2-year benefit.[57-61]

Angioplasty of the celiac or mesenteric arteries may be appropriate in poor-risk patients with intestinal angina who have nonostial occlusive lesions. Odurny et al. reported 19 mesenteric dilations in 10 patients, with an initial technical success rate of 90%.[62] Symptoms recurred within 2 years in five patients, but three of the five underwent successful retreatment. Surgical bypass or endarterectomy should remain the treatment of choice for mesenteric ischemia until long-term benefit is documented in large numbers of patients treated with angioplasty.[63] Patients with aortic aneurysms, celiac axis syndrome, or other causes of extrinsic vascular compression should not be treated by PTA.

Brachiocephalic Vessels

Subclavian and Innominate Arteries

Balloon dilation of the subclavian and innominate arteries is effective in treating some patients with subclavian steal syndrome and upper extremity ischemia. Because open surgical techniques are associated with significant morbidity and mortality, angioplasty of the aortic arch vessels should be considered in patients with focal, hemodynamically significant stenoses that do not involve the origin of the vessel. Indications include upper limb ischemia, posterior fossa ischemia, or reduced flow to an internal mammary artery used for coronary artery bypass grafting.[64] Immediate technical success has been reported in 96% to 100% of patients with stenoses; and the 1-, 2-, and 3-year patency rates are 92%, 92%, and 97%, respectively.[49,65,66] Motarjeme and colleagues have reported an initial technical success of 100% and only a 4.5% reocclusion rate at 5 years. Success rates are significantly lower for short-segment occlusions of the subclavian artery.[67] Motarjeme was able to open only 46% of totally occluded subclavian arteries; and one-fourth of the successfully treated patients were found to have restenosis at the 6-month follow-up examination.[68] Although few neurologic complications have been reported, the risk of cerebral embolization must be considered when manipulating these vessels. The risk of this procedure is minimized if the vertebral artery is also occluded.

Vertebral Artery

Balloon angioplasty represents a valuable alternative to surgical reconstruction of the vertebral artery, whose exposure can be technically difficult. Although there are reports describing the success of vertebral artery angioplasty, the data are insufficient to establish the proper role of this therapy.[69] Plaque within this vessel is typically calcified and ulcerated and can be difficult to treat.[70] Angioplasty should be reserved for patients with vertebrobasilar symptomatology who have no significant occlusive disease of the carotid arteries limiting flow through the circle of Willis. The technical success rate of vertebral angioplasty has been reported to be 92%.[71] Doppler flow studies and symptom relief have been used to document long-term success.[69]

Carotid Artery

Carotid artery angioplasty has become the source of much controversy over the past few years. This technique has been used successfully in some patients with proximal common carotid artery lesions and in fewer patients with lesions of the carotid bifurcation.[72] The initial studies involving carotid artery angioplasty revealed significantly higher stroke and death rates than those established for open endarterectomy, leading many prominent vascular specialists to support a prospective, randomized clinical trial to determine the safety and efficacy of carotid angioplasty and stenting.[71,73] Though there are still no current, accepted criteria applicable to patients who have carotid stenosis amenable to angioplasty, trials such as the Carotid and Vertebral Transluminal Angioplasty Study are underway.[74]

The risk of distal embolization is a major concern with endovascular carotid artery interventions.[75] For this reason, angioplasty has been employed for stenoses resulting from fibromuscular dysplasia, arteritides, or short, focal atheromatous lesions that contain little embolic debris.[68,76] Therefore ulcerated bifurcation lesions associated with thrombus constitute a relative contraindication for angioplasty. Stents are thought to minimize the risk of embolization and maintain patency of the carotid lumen. In a follow-up study of carotid angioplasties with and without stents, Crawley and colleagues found that if the initial reduction in stenosis is more than 20% stent placement should be performed.[77] Because some authors have reported low complication rates with carotid angioplasty, the procedure is an option in high risk patients and those with surgically inaccessible lesions.[76]

At this time, conventional carotid endarterectomy remains the gold standard for symptomatic stenoses of more than 70% and for asymptomatic lesions with more than 60% stenosis.[78] Carotid angioplasty must be regarded as still experimental and should be employed only in controlled, investigational settings.

Bypass Graft Stenosis

Angioplasty has been used to dilate vein graft stenoses and prolong graft patency.[79] Stenoses most amenable to balloon dilation are located within the body of the graft, commonly at valve sites. Stenoses that occur at the anastomosis require high pressures to dilate and are more difficult to treat successfully.

Complications

Although less invasive than surgery, angioplasty is an invasive procedure with well recognized complications (Table 18-3). A review of

TABLE 18-3. Common Complications of Balloon Angioplasty

Occurs in more than 5%
  Puncture site infection
  Blood loss during and after procedure
  Postprocedural hematoma
  Acute occlusion
  Technical failure
  Dissection with intimal flap

Occurs in 1% to 5%
  False aneurysm at puncture site
  Transient renal insufficiency
  Distal embolization

Occurs in less than 1%
  Arterial perforation or rupture
  Arteriovenous fistula formation
  Femoral/axillary nerve injury
  Angioplasty balloon rupture
  Myocardial infarction
  Retroperitoneal hemorrhage

Modified from White JV: Balloon angioplasty. In Kernstein MD, White JV, editors: *Alternatives to open vascular surgery*, Philadelphia, 1994, Lippincott.

the literature reveals an overall complication rate of 7.9% to 26.0%.[34,80-84] Most of these complications are minor and resolve without additional therapy, but surgical management is required in 2% to 3%.[85] The most common complications occur at the puncture site. Other problems can occur at or distal to the angioplasty site. Still other adverse effects have systemic sequelae.

Fruhwirth and colleagues reviewed 15,460 femoral punctures and identified 81 vascular complications.[86] They noted 65 pseudoaneurysms, 8 acute arterial occlusions, 7 profusely bleeding arteries, and 1 arteriovenous fistula. Hematoma is the most common puncture site complication. Significant bleeding at the arterial entrance site occurs in 0.2% to 4.6% of patients. Risk factors include obesity, hypertension, large balloon size, overly aggressive anticoagulation, severe atherosclerosis at the puncture site, and inadequate postprocedural groin compression. Although these groin hematomas rarely require surgical evacuation, they do increase the possibility of infection. Pseudoaneurysm at the cannulation site occurs in 0.1% to 1.5% of patients.[80] Duplex imaging can quickly confirm this diagnosis. The false aneurysm cavity of small pseudoaneurysms (less than 1.5 cm in greatest diameter) can be thrombosed by ultrasound-guided compression.[87] Large pseudoaneurysms should be treated surgically. A more disastrous puncture-site complication is retroperitoneal hemorrhage or hematoma, occurring in fewer than 0.1% of patients.[80] This complication is usually caused by attempting to puncture the common femoral artery above the inguinal ligament but instead entering the distal external iliac artery. Profuse bleeding into the retroperitoneal space can ensue without the development of a groin hematoma. Careful monitoring of the patient after angioplasty along with prompt surgical attention can avert hemorrhagic shock and death.

Other important complications associated with the angioplasty site include subintimal dissection (4.4%), acute arterial occlusion (1% to 7%), and arterial perforation or rupture (0.1%).[34,80-84,88] Subintimal dissections, along with intimal flaps, usually occur when crossing the lesion with a guidewire or catheter or when dilating the stenosis (Figure 18-13). This intimal trauma may result in acute occlusion and the need for emergent endovascular manipulation

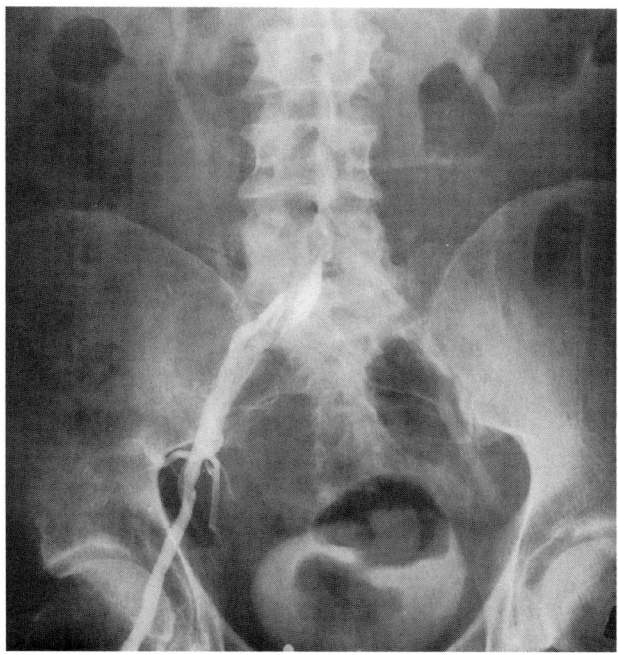

FIGURE 18-13. Extensive common iliac dissection after balloon dilation resulted in acute vessel occlusion.

(i.e., angioscopy, stenting) or bypass surgery. Small dissections or flaps usually heal within 4 to 6 weeks. Vessel occlusion resulting from thrombosis can be treated with thrombolytic therapy. Balloon dilation occasionally causes vessel rupture.[88] This serious complication results from overdistending the vessel with an oversized balloon and should be anticipated if the patient experiences more than the usual discomfort during balloon inflation. Bleeding can be controlled by reinflating the angioplasty balloon at the injury site while the patient is prepared for surgery.

Clinically significant distal embolization is seen in fewer than 1% of patients, although clinically silent microemboli occur more frequently.[82] Long-standing occlusions or lesions associated with fresh thrombus are prone to showering debris and should not be dilated before first receiving a trial of lytic therapy. If the embolic debris leads to significant distal vessel occlusion, surgical embolectomy or bypass may be required. Distal vessel spasm can be treated pharmacologically.

Renal insufficiency is the most significant systemic complication after angioplasty, occurring in 1.5% of all patients.[80,84] Worsening renal function occurs most often in the subset of patients undergoing renal angioplasty (6% of patients) and can be minimized by keeping patients well hydrated.[89] Other systemic complications include stroke (0.1%), myocardial infarction (0.1% to 0.8%), and congestive heart failure (1.9%). The direct mortality associated with angioplasty is between 0.2% and 2.2%.[80,83]

Conclusion

As technologic advances continue, more patients suffering from peripheral vascular disease are treated with balloon angioplasty. Medications to prevent myointimal hyperplasia, which causes restenosis, are being developed. Stenting devices are currently available to help prevent dissection, elastic recoil, and rapid reocclusion after balloon dilation. Techniques such as thermal, radiofrequency, and laser balloons are also being used in investigational settings to "weld" acute dissections and reduce elastic recoil. The endovascular industry has created a multitude of devices such as atherectomy catheters, intravascular ultrasound instruments, and angioscopes, which can be used as adjuncts to balloon angioplasty. As in all medical procedures, long-term patient benefit from balloon angioplasty depends on proper patient selection and close surveillance.

References

1. Dotter CT, Judkins MP: Transluminal treatment of arteriosclerotic obstruction: description of a new technique and a preliminary report of its application, *Circulation* 30:654–670, 1964.
2. Gruntzig A, Hopff H: Perkutane Rekanalisation chronischer arterieller Verschlusse mit einem neuen Dilatationskather: Modification der Dotter-Technik, *Dtsch Med Wochenschr* 99:2502–2505, 1974.
3. Dotter CT, Judkins MP, Rosch J: Nonoperative treatment of arterial occlusive disease: a radiologically facilitated technique, *Radiol Clin North Am* 5:531–542, 1967.
4. Chin AK, Kinney TB, Rurik GW et al: A physical measurement of the mechanisms of transluminal angioplasty, *Surgery* 95:196–200, 1984.
5. Block PC, Baughman KL, Pasternak RC et al: Transluminal angioplasty: correlation of morphologic and angiographic findings in an experimental model, *Circulation* 61:778, 1980.
6. Zarins CK, Lu CT, Gewertz BL et al: Arterial disruption and remodeling following balloon dilatation, *Surgery* 92:1086–1095, 1982.
7. Brewster DC, Cambria RP, Darling RC et al: Long-term results of combined iliac balloon angioplasty and distal surgical revascularization, *Ann Surg* 210:324, 1989.
8. Schneider PA: Guidewire-catheter skills. In Schneider PA, editor: *Endovascular skills*, St Louis, 1998, Quality Medical Publishing, pp 3–21.
9. Hoppe M, Wagner HJ, Klose KJ: Assessment of the hemodynamic result of PTA with a Doppler guide wire: initial experience, *J Vasc Intervent Radiol* 7:89–93, 1996.
10. Charlebois N, Saint-Georges G, Hudson G: Percutaneous transluminal angioplasty of the lower abdominal aorta, *AJR* 146:369–371, 1986.

11. Odurny A, Colapinto RF, Sniderman KW, Johnston KW: Percutaneous transluminal angioplasty of abdominal aortic stenoses. *Cardiovasc Intervent Radiol* 12:1–6, 1989.
12. Tegtmeyer CJ, Kellum CD, Kron IL, Mentzer RM Jr: Percutaneous transluminal angioplasty in the region of the aortic bifurcation, *Radiology* 157:661–665, 1985.
13. Heeney D, Bookstein J, Daniels E et al: Transluminal angioplasty of the abdominal aorta, *Radiology* 148:81–83, 1983.
14. Silva MB Jr, Hobson RW II, Jamil Z et al: A program of operative angioplasty: endovascular intervention and the vascular surgeon, *J Vasc Surg* 24:963–971, 1996.
15. Bosch JL, Hunink MGM: Meta-analysis of the results of percutaneous transluminal angioplasty and stent placement for aortoiliac disease, *Radiology* 204:87–96, 1997.
16. Wilson SE, White GH, Wolf G et al: Proximal percutaneous balloon angioplasty and distal bypass for multilevel arterial occlusion, *Ann Vasc Surg* 4:351–355, 1990.
17. Becquemin JP, Cavillon A, Allaire E et al: Iliac and femoropopliteal lesions: evaluation of balloon angioplasty and classical surgery, *J Endovasc Surg* 2(1):42–50, 1995.
18. Cambria RP, Faust G, Gusberg R et al: Percutaneous angioplasty for peripheral arterial occlusive disease, *Arch Surg* 122:283, 1987.
19. Freiman DB, Spence R, Gatenby R et al: Transluminal angioplasty of the iliac and femoral arteries: follow-up results without anticoagulation, *Radiology* 141:347, 1981.
20. Gallino A, Mahler F, Probst P, Nachbur B: Percutaneous transluminal angioplasty of the arteries of the lower limbs: a 5 year follow up. *Circulation* 70:619–623, 1984.
21. Johnston KW: Iliac arteries: reanalysis of results of balloon angioplasty, *Radiology* 186:207–212, 1993.
22. Van Andel GJ, Van Erp WFM, Krepel VM et al: Percutaneous transluminal dilatation of the iliac artery: long-term results, *Radiology* 156:321, 1985.
23. Becker GJ, Katzen BT, Dake MD: Noncoronary angioplasty, *Radiology* 170:921–940, 1989.
24. Wilson SE, Wolf GL, Cross AP et al: Percutaneous transluminal angioplasty versus operation for peripheral arteriosclerosis. *J Vasc Surg* 9:1–9, 1989.
25. Sullivan TM, Childs MB, Bacharach JM et al: Percutaneous transluminal angioplasty and primary stenting of the iliac arteries in 288 patients, *J Vasc Surg* 25:829–838, 1997.
26. Colapinto RF, Harries-Jones EP, Johnston KW. Percutaneous transluminal recanalization of complete iliac occlusions, *Arch Surg* 116:277–281, 1981.
27. Colapinto RF, Stronell RD, Johnston WK: Transluminal angioplasty of complete iliac obstructions, *Am J Radiol* 146:859–862, 1986.
28. Reyes R, Maynar M, Lopera J et al: Treatment of chronic iliac artery occlusions with guide wire recanalization and primary stent placement, *J Vasc Intervent Radiol* 8:1049–1055, 1997.
29. Blair JM, Gewertz BL, Moosa H et al: Percutaneous transluminal angioplasty versus surgery for limb-threatening ischemia, *J Vasc Surg* 9:698, 1989.
30. Krepel VM, van Andel GJ, van Erp WFM et al: Percutaneous transluminal angioplasty of the femoropopliteal artery: initial and long-term results, *Radiology* 156:325, 1985.
31. Milford MA, Weaver FA, Lundell CJ et al: Femoropopliteal percutaneous transluminal angioplasty for limb salvage, *J Vasc Surg* 8:292, 1988.
32. Dalsing MC, Cockerill E, Deupree R et al: Outcome predictors in selection of balloon angioplasty or surgery for peripheral arterial occlusive disease, *Surgery* 110:636, 1991.
33. Zeitler E, Richter EI, Roth FJ et al: Results of percutaneous transluminal angioplasty, *Radiology* 146:57, 1983.
34. El-Bayar H, Roberts A, Hye R et al: Determinants of failure in superficial femoral artery angioplasty, *Angiology* 43:877–885, 1992.
35. Matsi PJ, Manninen HI, Suhonen MT et al: Chronic critical lower-limb ischemia: prospective trial of angioplasty with 1–36 month follow up. *Radiology* 188:381–387, 1993.
36. Murray RR Jr, Hewes RC, White RI Jr et al: Long-segment femoropopliteal stenoses: is angioplasty a boon or bust? *Radiology* 162:473–476, 1987.
37. Becquemin JP, Cavillon A, Allaire E et al: Iliac and femoropopliteal lesions: evaluation of balloon angioplasty and classical surgery. *J Endovasc Surg* 2:42–50, 1995.
38. Bull PG, Mendel H, Hold M et al: Distal popliteal and tibioperoneal transluminal angioplasty: long term follow up, *J Vasc Intervent Radiol* 3:45–53, 1992.
39. Brown KT, Moore ED, Getrajdman GI et al: Infrapopliteal angioplasty: long term follow up, *J Vasc Intervent Radiol* 4:139–144, 1993.
40. Dorros G, Lewin RF, Jamnadas P, Mathiak LM: Below-the-knee angioplasty: tibioperoneal

vessels, the acute outcome, *Cathet Cardiovasc Diagn* 19:170–178, 1990.
41. Saab MII, Smith DC, Aka PK et al: Percutaneous transluminal angioplasty of tibial arteries for limb salvage, *Cardiovasc Intervent Radiol* 15:211, 1992.
42. Bakal CW, Sprayregen S, Scheinbaum K et al: Percutaneous transluminal angioplasty of the infrapopliteal arteries: results in 53 patients, *AJR* 154:171, 1990.
43. Brown KT, Moore ED, Getrajdam GI et al: Infrapopliteal angioplasty: long-term follow-up, *J Vasc Intervent Radiol* 4:139, 1993.
44. Brown KT, Schoenberg NJ, Moore ED et al: Percutaneous transluminal angioplasty of infrapopliteal vessels: preliminary results and technical considerations, *Radiology* 169:75, 1988.
45. Dorros G, Lewin RF, Jamnadas P et al: Below-the-knee angioplasty: tibioperoneal vessels, the acute outcome, *Cathet Cardiovasc Diagn* 19:170, 1990.
46. Schwarten DE: Clinical and anatomical considerations for nonoperative therapy in tibial disease and the results of angioplasty, *Circulation* 83(suppl I):86, 1991.
47. O'Donovan RM, Gutierrez OH, Izzo JL Jr: Preservation of renal function by percutaneous renal angioplasty in high-risk elderly patients: short-term outcome, *Nephron* 60:187, 1992.
48. Weibull H, Bergqvist D, Jendteg S et al: Clinical outcome and health care costs in renal revascularization-percutaneous transluminal renal angioplasty versus reconstructive surgery, *Br J Surg* 78:620, 1991.
49. Weibull H, Bergqvist D, Jonsson K et al: Long-term results after percutaneous transluminal angioplasty of atherosclerotic renal artery stenosis–the importance of intensive follow-up, *Eur J Vasc Surg* 5:291, 1991.
50. Ramsay LE, Waller PC: Blood pressure response to percutaneous transluminal angioplasty for renovascular hypertension: an overview of published series. *BMJ* 300:569–572, 1990.
51. Englund R, Brown MA: Renal angioplasty for renovascular disease: a reappraisal, *J Cardiovasc Surg* 32:76, 1991.
52. Martinez-Amenos A, Rama H, Sarrias X et al: Percutaneous transluminal angioplasty in the treatment of renovascular hypertension, *J Hum Hypertens* 5:97, 1991.
53. Beebe HG, Chesebro K, Merchant F et al: Results of renal artery balloon angioplasty limit its indications, *J Vasc Surg* 8:300, 1988.
54. Cluzel P, Raynaud A, Beyssen B et al: Stenoses of renal branch arteries in fibromuscular dysplasia: results of percutaneous transluminal angioplasty, *Radiology* 193:227–232, 1994.
55. Plouin PF, Darne B, Chatellier G et al: Restenosis after a first percutaneous transluminal renal angioplasty, *Hypertension* 21:89, 1993.
56. Matalon TA, Thompson MJ, Patel SK et al: Percutaneous transluminal angioplasty for transplant renal artery stenosis, *J Vasc Intervent Radiol* 3:55–58, 1992.
57. Fauchald P, Vatne K, Paulsen D et al: Long-term clinical results of percutaneous transluminal angioplasty in transplant renal artery stenosis, *Nephrol Dial Transplant* 7:256, 1992.
58. Matalon TA, Thompson MJ, Patel SK et al: Percutaneous transluminal angioplasty for transplant renal artery stenosis, *J Vasc Intervent Radiol* 3:55, 1992.
59. Thomas CP, Riad H, Johnson BF et al: Percutaneous transluminal angioplasty in transplant renal arterial stenoses: a long-term follow-up, *Transpl Int* 5:129, 1992.
60. Thomas CP, Riad H, Johnson BF, Cumberland DC: Percutaneous transluminal angioplasty in transplant renal arterial stenoses: a long term follow up, *Transpl Int* 5:129–132, 1992.
61. Fauchald P, Vatne K, Paulsen D et al: Long term clinical results of percutaneous transluminal angioplasty in transplant renal artery stenosis, *Nephrol Dial Transplant* 7:256–259, 1992.
62. Odurny A, Sniderman KW, Colapinto RF: Intestinal angina: percutaneous transluminal angioplasty of the celiac and superior mesenteric arteries, *Radiology* 167:59, 1988.
63. Rose SC, Quigley TM, Raker EJ: Revascularization for chronic mesenteric ischemia: comparison of operative arterial bypass grafting and percutaneous transluminal angioplasty, *J Vasc Intervent Radiol* 6:339–349, 1995.
64. Wilms G, Baert A, Dewaele D et al: Percutaneous transluminal angioplasty of the subclavian artery: early and late results, *Cardiovasc Intervent Radiol* 10:123–128, 1987.
65. Jaschke W, Menges HW, Ockert D et al: PTA of the subclavian and innominate artery: short- and long-term results, *Ann Radiol (Paris)* 32:29, 1989.
66. Selby JB Jr, Matsumoto AH, Tegtmeyer CJ et al: Balloon angioplasty above the aortic arch: immediate and long-term results, *AJR* 160:631, 1993.

67. Motarjeme A, Keifer JW, Zuska AJ et al: Percutaneous transluminal angioplasty for treatment for subclavian steal, *Radiology* 155:611, 1985.
68. Motarjeme A: Percutaneous transluminal angioplasty of supraaortic vessels, *J Endovasc Surg* 3:171–181, 1996.
69. Courtheoux P, Tournade A, Theron J et al: Transcutaneous angioplasty of vertebral artery atheromatous ostial stricture, *Neuroradiology* 27:259–264, 1985.
70. Strandness DE: Extracranial cerebrovascular arterial disease. In Young JR, Graor RA, Olin JW et al, editors: *Peripheral vascular disease*, St Louis, 1991 Mosby Year Book, pp 241–252.
71. Brown MM, Clifton A, Taylor RS: Concern about safety of carotid angioplasty, *Stroke* 27:1435, 1996.
72. Derauf BJ, Hunter DW, Erickson DL: "Washout" technique for brachycephalic angioplasty, *AJR* 146:849, 1986.
73. Anonymous. Statement regarding carotid angioplasty and stenting, *J Vasc Surg* 24:900, 1996.
74. Major ongoing stroke trials: carotid and vertebral artery transluminal angioplasty study (CAVATAS), *Stroke* 27:358, 1996.
75. Becquemin JP, Qvarfordt P, Castier Y et al: Carotid angioplasty: is it safe? *J Endovasc Surg* 3:35–41, 1996.
76. Kachel R: Results of balloon angioplasty in the carotid arteries, *J Endovasc Surg* 3:22–30, 1996.
77. Crawley F, Clifton A, Markus H et al: Delayed improvement in carotid artery diameters after carotid angioplasty, *Stroke* 28:574–579, 1997.
78. Zarins CK: Carotid endarterectomy: the gold standard, *J Endovasc Surg* 3:10–15, 1996.
79. Berkowitz HD, Fox AD, Deaton DH: Reversed vein graft stenosis: early diagnosis and management, *J Vasc Surg* 15:130, 1992.
80. Belli AM, Cumberland DC, Knox AM et al: The complication rate of percutaneous peripheral balloon angioplasty, *Clin Radiol* 41:380, 1990.
81. Johnston KW, Rae M, Hogg-Johnston SA et al: Five-year results of a prospective study of percutaneous transluminal angioplasty, *Ann Surg* 206:403, 1987.
82. O'Keeffe ST, Woods BO, Beckmann CF: Percutaneous transluminal angioplasty of the peripheral arteries, *Cardiol Clin* 9:515, 1991.
83. Samson RH, Sprayregen S, Veith FJ et al: Management of angioplasty complications, unsuccessful procedures, and early and late failures, *Ann Surg* 199:234, 1984.
84. Weibull II, Bergqvist D, Jonsson K et al: Complications after percutaneous transluminal angioplasty in the iliac, femoral, and popliteal arteries, *J Vasc Surg* 5:681, 1987.
85. Tegtmeyer CJ: Percutaneous transluminal angioplasty, *Curr Probl Diagn Radiol* 16:75–139, 1987.
86. Fruhwirth J, Pascher O, Hauser H et al: Locale Gefasskomplikationen nach iatrogener femoralarterienpunktion, *Wien Klin Wochenschr* 108:196–200, 1996.
87. Feld R, Patton GM, Carabasi A et al: Treatment of iatrogenic femoral artery injuries with ultrasound-guided compression, *J Vasc Surg* 16:832–840, 1992.
88. Chong WK, Cross FW, Rapheal MJ: Case report: iliac artery rupture during percutaneous angioplasty, *Clin Radiol* 41:358–359, 1990.
89. Cope C, Burke DR, Meranze S: *Atlas of interventional radiology*, Philadelphia, 1990, Lippincott.

19
Catheter Thromboembolectomy

Thomas J. Fogarty, Amitava Biswas, and Christine E. Newman

An embolus (from the Greek *embolos*, meaning "projectile") is a blood-borne detached mass in the vascular space that lodges at a site distant from its point of origin. Although technically emboli can be solid, liquid, or gaseous, over 99% of observed emboli originate from thrombi. Much rarer forms of emboli originate from bone fragments or marrow, ruptured atheromatous plaque debris, fat droplets, pieces of tumor, foreign bodies, or gas bubbles. Unless otherwise specified, the term *embolus* in this chapter implies "thromboembolus." Once in the circulation, emboli are carried in the blood flow until they reach a vessel that is too narrow to permit passage. At this point the embolus lodges in the vessel, causing a partial or total occlusion that can lead to potentially serious consequences for the distal tissue served by the occluded vessel.

As early as 1628, Harvey recognized the ischemic consequences of acute arterial occlusion. However, the first successful arterial embolectomy was not accomplished until nearly three centuries later, when Labey first removed an arterial thrombus in 1911. Labey's procedure required extensive dissection to properly remove the entire embolus and its distally propagated thrombus, resulting in substantial associated mortality and morbidity and a relatively subdued interest in the procedure. Despite the availability of heparin to prevent thrombus formation, both the mortality and morbidity rates for this procedure remained in the 50% range throughout the 1950s and early 1960s.

A significant improvement in the mortality and morbidity rates for arterial embolectomy occurred in 1963, when the balloon catheter technique was introduced. As the technique and instrumentation became standardized, balloon embolectomy proved to be a safe, simple, and effective method for removing arterial emboli. To this day, it remains the treatment of choice for acute embolic arterial occlusion.

Pathophysiology of Arterial Occlusion

Systemic arterial emboli may originate from a variety of sites, but in practice about 80% to 85% arise in the heart—usually as a consequence of atherosclerotic heart disease. The left ventricle in the setting of myocardial infarction is the single most common source, accounting for 60% to 65% of all systemic emboli. An additional 5% to 10% originate from atrial thrombi in rheumatic heart disease, and 5% are associated with cardiomyopathies. Cardiac arrhythmias such as atrial fibrillation, in association with any of the above disease entities, significantly increase the risk of embolism. Emboli have been known to result from thrombosis around atheromatous plaque and are also associated with aortic aneurysms, infectious endocarditis, and valvular or aortic prostheses. Very rarely, a "paradoxical" embolus arising in the venous system can enter the systemic arterial circulation through an atrial or ventricular septal defect and a right-to-left pressure gradient in the heart. In about 10% to 15% of cases, the cause remains unknown. Regardless of origin, these emboli can occlude systemic arteries and cause serious end-organ damage.

There is a relatively consistent distribution of acute arterial occlusion (Figure 19–1). Most often, emboli tend to travel to the lower extremities, with 75% to 79% lodging in the iliac, femoral, and popliteal arteries. One in ten travel to the brain and result in a cerebrovascular accident. Another 16% will occur in the aorta, whereas 2% will occur in the visceral arteries, including the mesenteric, renal, or splenic vessels. Relatively few emboli are found in the upper extremities, with only about 3% occurring in the arms. It is noteworthy that 10% of all embolic events occur at multiple sites and that there are often no clinical indications of embolism. In general, the embolus follows the vascular pathway and eventually lodges in a

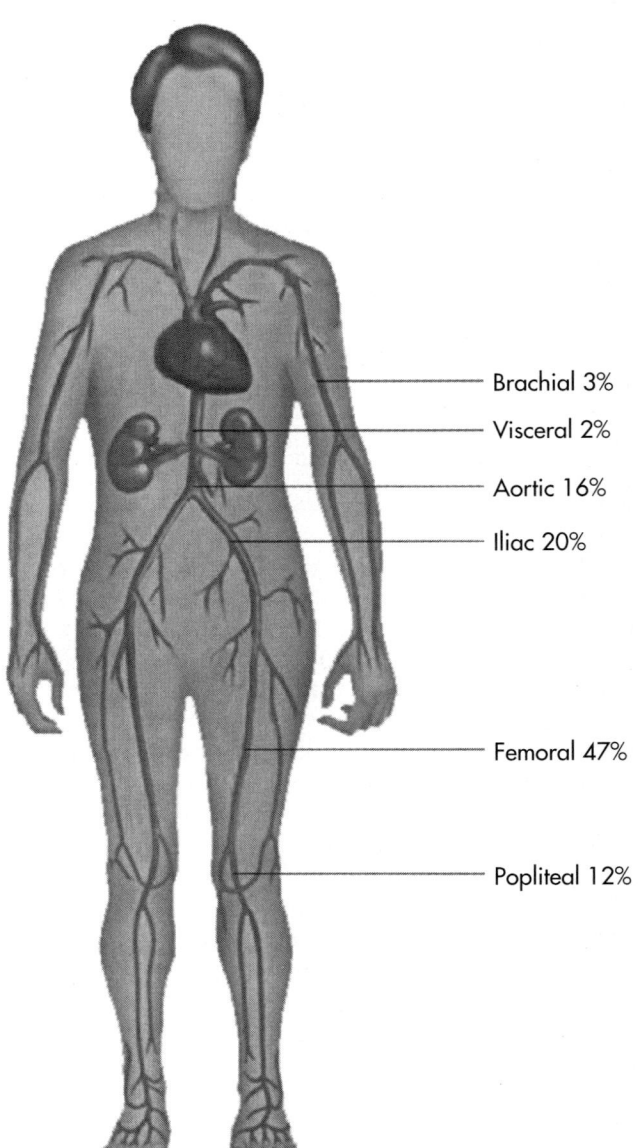

FIGURE 19–1. Anatomic distribution of embolic occlusions. (Data from Fogarty and associates' series of 500 patients.)

vessel whose diameter is smaller than that of the embolus itself.

Although historically, acute arterial occlusion was most likely to be caused by embolic events, the etiology has changed considerably in the last few decades. Because of factors such as the decline of rheumatic heart disease, the advancement of cardiac surgery, and the longer life expectancy of the general population, peripheral arterial occlusions today are more likely to result from in situ thrombotic events secondary to generalized atherosclerosis than from emboli. At a critical point of narrowing, turbulent flow and stasis result in a soft thrombus that completes the occlusion. The freshly propagated thrombus is primarily made up of red cell mass; the underlying chronic material is composed of fibrin and platelets, a substance that is more dense and adherent to the arterial wall.

Although not a "true" embolus, an occlusion-forming clot of this type, arising from atherosclerosis-associated thrombus, has many characteristics in common with occlusive emboli. Indeed, the first principle for acute intervention in the case of thrombotic occlusion is basically the same as for embolectomy. Thus, when we refer to "embolectomy," it should be understood that the procedure also applies to the initial intervention for thrombotic clot—even though in the latter case the entity causing the obstruction is not strictly an embolus.

Both embolic and thrombotic occlusion may be asymptomatic, but when such occlusions become clinically apparent, the consequences can be severe. The presence of the embolus can cause cellular death and, ultimately, gross tissue necrosis. In addition, there may be ischemic neural damage; and despite preservation of tissue, there may be chronic disabling pain. It is therefore critical to treat embolic occlusion quickly and definitively to avoid such significant morbidity.

Clinical Presentation

Clinically, arterial occlusion presents most commonly in elderly patients, particularly those who are seriously ill with multisystem disease. The presenting symptoms will vary depending on the location of the occlusion, the length of time that the blockage has been present, and the severity of the obstruction (Box 19–1). The affected tissue is usually painful, although the patient may also report numbness. There is usually paresthesia distal to the occlusion; and if an extremity is involved, it may feel cold to the touch. If the occlusion is severe, there may be some degree of paralysis.

The initial physical examination is extremely useful in identifying the location of the occlusion. The patient may exhibit cyanosis or pallor at the affected site. Decreased skin temperature, stiff muscles, loss of strength and sensation, and absent deep tendon reflexes may also be observed. If sufficient collaterals have developed around the compromised vessel, the signs and symptoms may be more subtle. The patient may experience a shorter walking dis-

---

Box 19–1. Clinical Presentation of Acute Arterial Occlusion

History	Physical Examination
Pain	Cyanosis
Numbness	Pallor
Paresthesias	Stiff muscles
Loss of sensation and proprioception[a]	Loss of strength[a]
Decreased skin temperature	Absent DTR
Paralysis[a]	Early rigor[a]

[a] Indicates need for emergent surgical intervention.
DTR, deep tendon reflexes.

tance to claudication, modest pain, or paresthesias with preservation of sensory and motor function.

Preoperative Management, Workup, and Evaluation

It is important to bear in mind that patients whose symptoms include acute arterial occlusion often have some other underlying disease process, of which cardiac pathology is the most frequent. Patients should be assumed to have significant heart disease, and its severity should be properly evaluated. Cardiac evaluation should occur concurrently with workup of the peripheral vasculature and need not delay surgical intervention. Basic cardiac agents such as digitalis, antiarrhythmics, morphine, diuretics, and heparin should be used as indicated. The primary objective in management of an ischemic limb must be the assurance of patient survival.

The chief determinant of operability is the condition of the extremity at the time of presentation—not simply the duration of the occlusion. Emergent surgical intervention is indicated when the patient's symptoms include loss of sensation and proprioception in the affected limb, loss of motor function, or early rigor. Without these signs, operation for acute occlusion may be considered urgent or perhaps even elective. Table 19–1 indicates that successful surgical intervention is possible even after prolonged periods of occlusion. Even in the presence of gangrene, a lower-level amputation can often be achieved after successful embolectomy. It is therefore imperative to prepare for emergent operation if the aforementioned signs and symptoms are present.

TABLE 19–1. Time Interval in Relation to Advanced Ischemia[a]

Age of embolus	Advanced ischemia (%)	Amputations (%)
1–24 hours	12	1.5
24–48 hours	37	5.3
2–90 days	49	12.5

[a] Patients: 500; embolectomy procedures: 570.

While emergency preparation is underway, appropriate therapy for the patient's underlying condition must be initiated. Intensive care unit monitoring is required for patients with congestive heart failure, cardiogenic shock, or significant arrhythmias. Most of these patients will benefit from central venous catheter placement, which will facilitate rapid administration of drugs and fluid, monitoring of central venous pressures, and convenient intravenous administration of heparin.

Immediate anticoagulation in conjunction with early operative embolectomy is the most common treatment for acute arterial occlusion. A loading dose of 5000 to 10,000 units of heparin given intravenously, along with constant infusion sufficient to raise the partial thromboplastin time (PTT) to about 2.5 times the control levels, should be given to prevent further embolization and propagation of the clot.

Although diagnosis and localization of the occlusion can usually be accomplished by patient history and physical examination alone, arterial blood flow may also be evaluated and recorded by Doppler ultrasound techniques. Pressure and waveform measurements can be taken noninvasively in 5 to 10 minutes. These measurements are useful to provide a preoperative benchmark for postoperative evaluation of the revascularization procedure.

The use of a continuous-pulse amplitude monitor placed directly over the pedal vessels has demonstrated significant utility in the management of acute arterial occlusion (Figure 19–2). The sensors of the device are placed over the distal vessels before beginning the procedure. The completion of the revascularization (or lack thereof) can be immediately documented at operation. The sensors are left in place until the patient is ambulatory. Hardcopy documentation of pulse amplitude becomes part of the patient record.

The possibility of simultaneous embolism to the renal or mesenteric arteries should always be considered. In these cases, preoperative arteriography of the renal and visceral vasculature is indicated. Arteriography is also useful to document the presence of atherosclerotic disease. Although additional studies may be desirable,

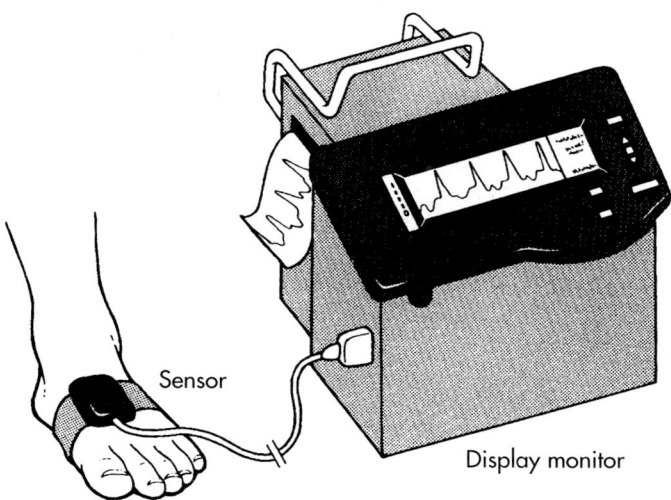

FIGURE 19-2. Continuous-pulse amplitude monitor, featuring continuous display; hard-copy printout on demand.

it is wise to avoid compromising an ischemic limb with lengthy nonessential diagnostic workups.

Once properly evaluated and stabilized, the patient is taken to the operating room. If the procedure is initiated under local anesthesia, an anesthesiologist should stand by.

Instrumentation

The critical instrumentation for the embolectomy procedure is the Fogarty balloon embolectomy catheter (Figure 19-3A). Since its introduction in 1961, the device has undergone minor modifications, but the general concept behind its use has remained constant. It was originally designed with specific adaptations to ensure safe, effective extraction of arterial emboli. The catheter consists of a hollow pliable body with a soft distensible balloon situated at the distal end. Inflation and deflation of the distal latex balloon is controlled through a proximal syringe. The device is available in graduated sizes from 2F to 7F (Figure 19-3B). The routine catheter inflation medium is saline, but air is more appropriate for the 2F and 3F catheters. There is a calibrated optimal level of balloon distension for each size of catheter. Advances in catheter technology now allow thru-lumen catheter capability for infusion of solutions or for guidewire passage (Figure 19-3C).

In use, the deflated tip of the catheter is threaded into the affected artery past the occlusion, either through the thrombus or between the thrombus and the intima (Figure 19-4). The deflated catheter has never been shown to "push" an embolus or associated thrombus. Sometimes, tortuosity or angulations at vessel bifurcation points hinder easy passage of the catheter, even when there are not large amounts of atherosclerotic plaque. In these cases, preforming the catheter tip at an angle and then rotating the catheter at the difficult site is helpful. Progressive flexion of a nearby joint to redirect the angle of the catheter tip is also useful, as is the introduction of more than one catheter. To pass an eccentric plaque, we have found it useful to gently inflate the balloon and then carefully advance the balloon while deflating. Our experience is that this brings the catheter tip away from the wall and closer to the residual lumen.

Once past the occlusion, the surgeon inflates the balloon during the process of withdrawal and exerts only minimal traction on the arterial wall. Fluid displacement within the balloon allows uniform, even contact with the vessel wall as it passes through stenotic areas. As the catheter is withdrawn, the surgeon controls the level of balloon inflation by feel to ensure

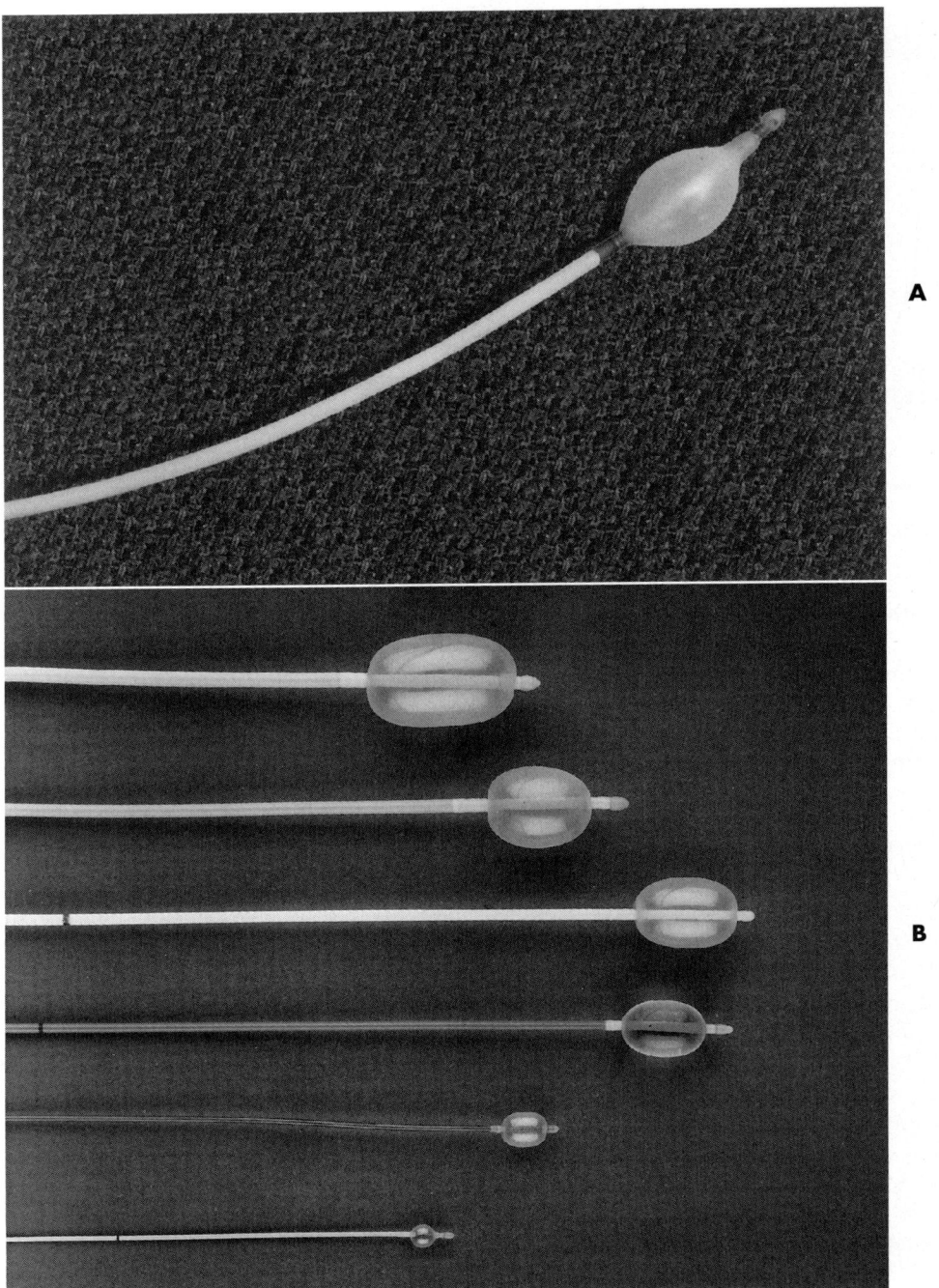

FIGURE 19–3. **A**, Original Fogarty balloon embolectomy catheter: custom-made latex balloon, hand-tied with silk suture on polyvinyl catheter body. **B**, Present-day family of embolectomy catheters in a range of sizes to accommodate differing vessel diameters. **C**, Thru-lumen embolectomy catheters, which permit infusion of contrast and therapeutic solutions and guidewire usage.

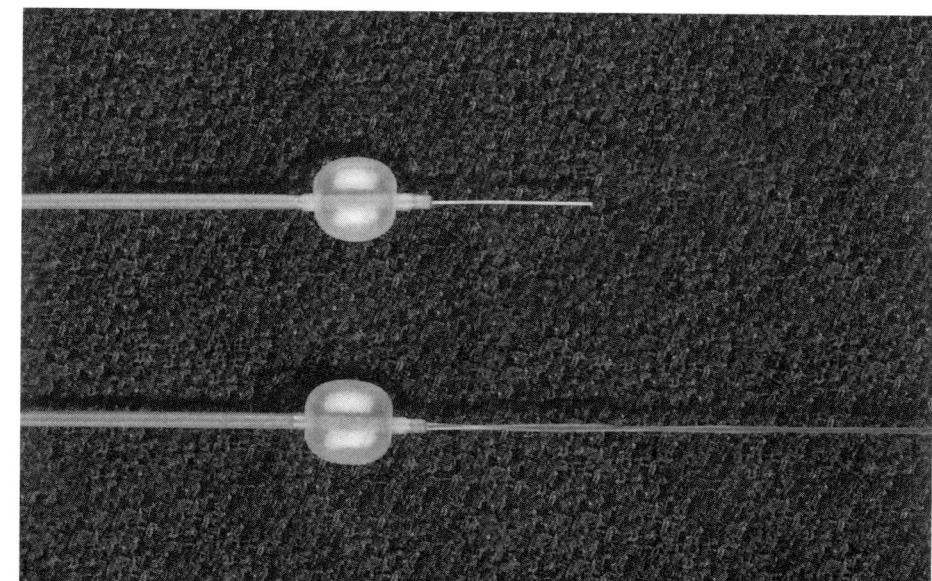

C

FIGURE 19–3. *Continued.*

maintenance of gentle wall contact. Additional fluid may be injected if it is needed, or the balloon may be slightly deflated when there is too much traction, as in segments of atherosclerotic vessel narrowing. To reduce the possibility of intimal damage or arterial perforation in smaller vessels, the smaller-caliber catheters contain a flexible spring tip.

As mentioned previously, the characteristics of the patient population with acute arterial occlusions have changed significantly, with the incidence of thrombotic clot now more prevalent than embolic occlusion. The more adherent nature of in situ thrombosis calls for a more aggressive tool than the standard balloon catheter. To meet this need, an adherent clot catheter has been designed to remove residual thrombi that the standard embolectomy catheter has difficulty retrieving (Figure 19–5). The catheter body is 6F and has a distal flexible cable coiled around a center core. The loosely spiraled outer cable is covered by an elastomeric latex membrane, which assumes a corkscrew shape because of the structure of the coiled outer wire. The spiral cable is attached to the central core wire at the distal tip. This inner wire runs the length of the catheter to a knob on the proximal control handle, which is used to expand or contract the active portion. Pulling on the control knob deploys the system into a tight-pitch 10-mm corkscrew. Pushing on the control knob and locking it in place results in a 2-mm–diameter straight catheter system (Figure 19–6).

The technique for using this catheter is similar to that used in the balloon embolectomy procedure. The initial exploration is carried out with the standard balloon catheter. Use of the adherent clot catheter always follows initial balloon catheter exploration. In the low-profile position, the tip is advanced through the vessel beyond the thrombus. The pitch of the spiral wire is then expanded to reach the proper diameter, and material is engaged within the coiled sections of the device. The surgeon then slowly draws the catheter back through the vessel, removing the material through the arteriotomy. The diameter of the instrument tip can be continuously adjusted by feel during withdrawal to accommodate variations in vessel diameter and resistance. The spiral region provides a larger contact area than the traditional balloon and thus facilitates removal of more adherent thrombus. Figure 19–7 shows the

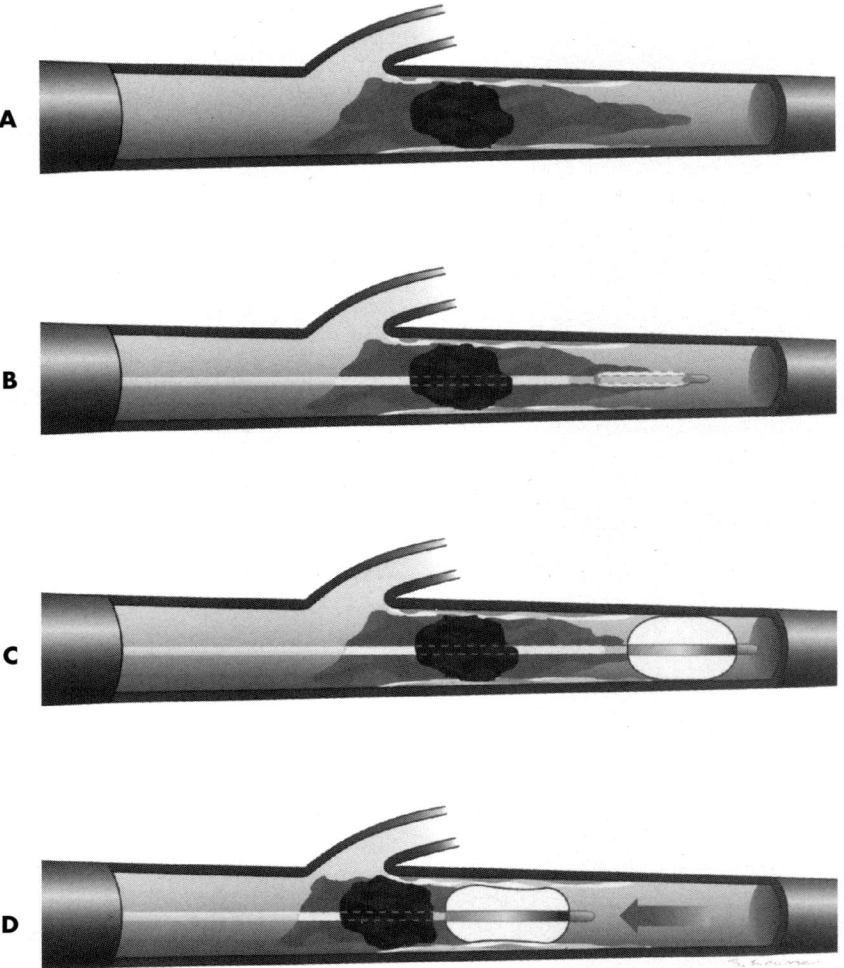

FIGURE 19–4. Embolectomy catheter removing arterial obstruction: **A**, Thrombus formation. **B**, Catheter insertion. **C**, Balloon inflation. **D**, Thromboembolism removal.

adherent clot catheter with material removed subsequent to balloon embolectomy. There is more of a well-defined structural edge in the outer surface of the fully retracted corkscrew unit, which renders it more aggressive than the conventional embolectomy catheter.

A similar device without the latex covering over the distal spiral helix is available for use in synthetic grafts (Figure 19–8). The graft thrombectomy catheter is even more aggressive than the adherent clot catheter. The technique for its use in synthetic grafts is similar to that for the procedure described on the preceding pages. The graft thrombectomy catheter functions as a ringed endarterectomy instrument. Unlike the ringed endarterectomy device, the diameter of the graft thrombectomy catheter can be varied during use and the body is pliable. The densely adherent pannus material associated with graft healing is stripped out as illustrated in Figure 19–9.

Operative Procedure

Aortic and Iliac Occlusions

The initial approach to an aortic occlusion is through bilateral vertical groin incisions. The

19. Catheter Thromboembolectomy

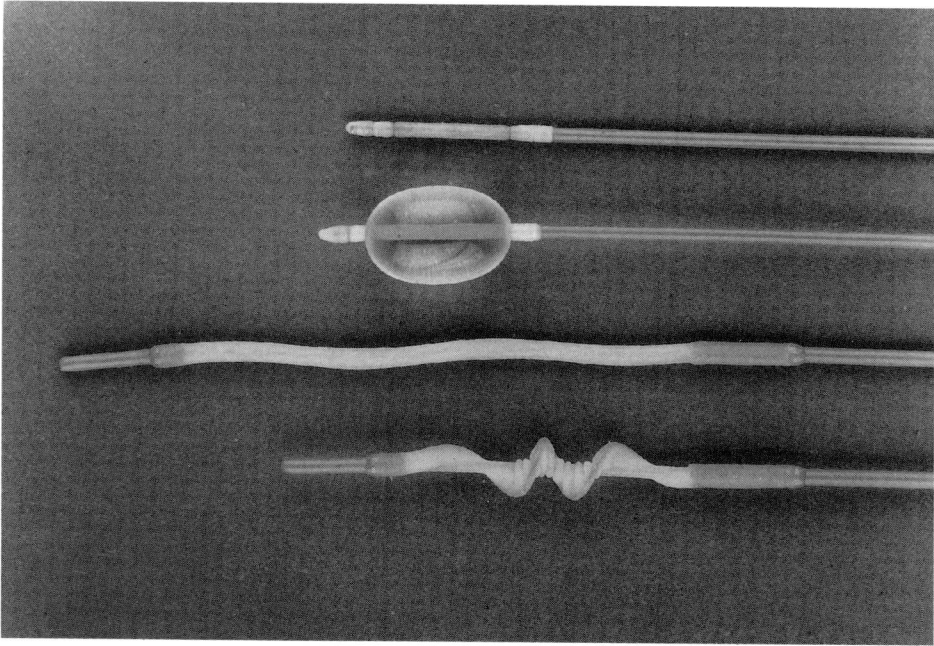

FIGURE 19-5. Balloon embolectomy catheter, designed to remove fresh emboli, and adherent clot catheter, designed to remove more adherent thrombus from native vessel.

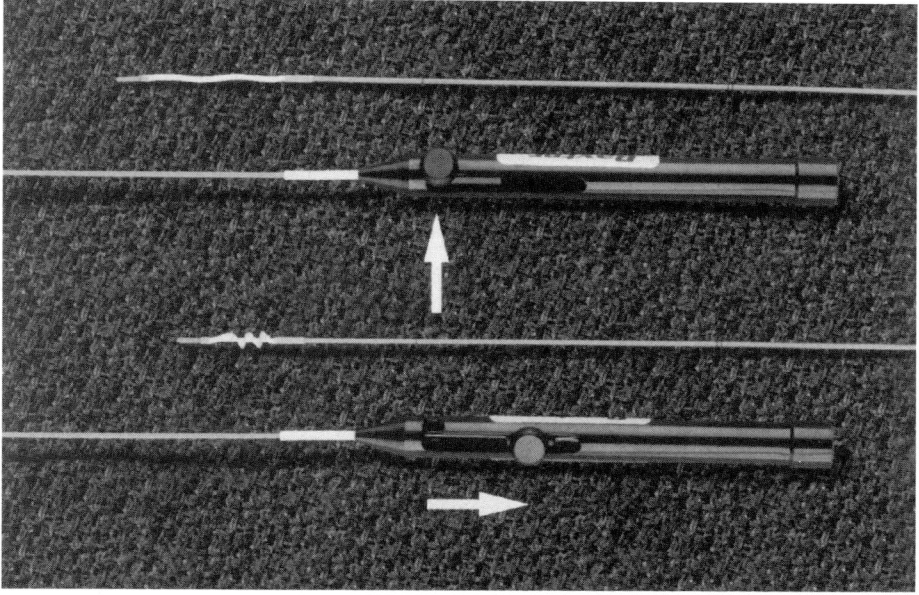

FIGURE 19-6. Knob controlling diameter and pitch of corkscrew element on adherent clot catheter.

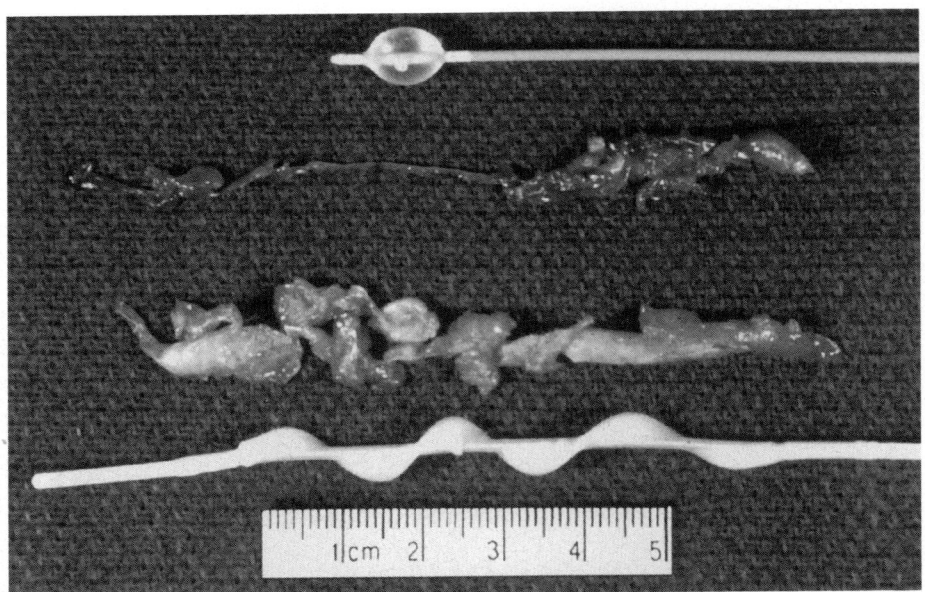

FIGURE 19–7. **TOP** Fresh gelatinous thrombus is shown removed with balloon catheter. **Bottom** Dense adherent mature thrombus is shown removed with adherent clot catheter.

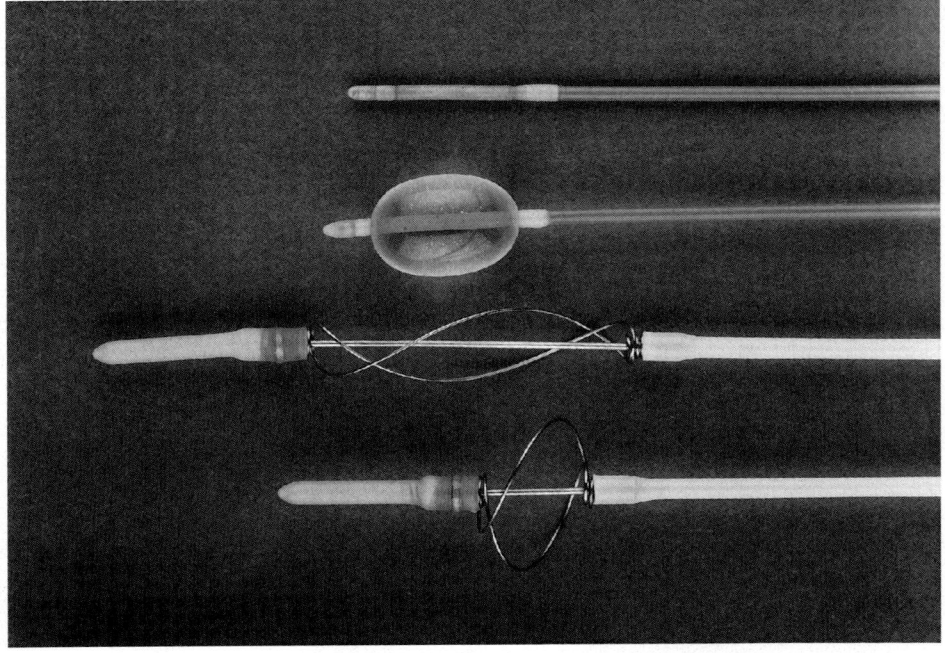

FIGURE 19–8. Balloon embolectomy catheter, used for initial removal of soft thrombotic material, above bare-wire graft thrombectomy catheter.

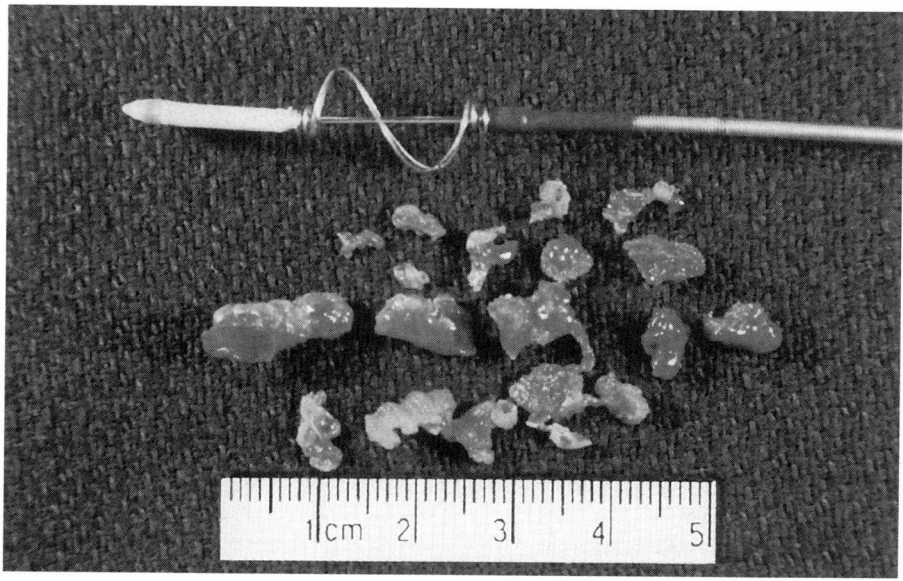

FIGURE 19–9. Graft thrombectomy catheter, shown with residual adherent thrombus unextractable with initial balloon catheter (corrugations from the graft observable in removed clot).

common, superficial, and deep femoral (profunda femoris) arteries are isolated and looped with Silastic (polymeric silicone) tapes. The arteriotomy is made in the common femoral artery proximal to the bifurcation to allow cannulation of the superficial and deep femoral orifices under direct vision. The vessel is carefully palpated, and the location of plaque is noted. A transverse arteriotomy is preferable to avoid narrowing during closure, but the presence and location of plaque may dictate tangential or even vertical incisions. If primary closure results in luminal narrowing, one should not hesitate to perform patch angioplasty.

The distal exploration is initially carried out with a 3F or 4F balloon catheter, depending on the size of the vessel. The instrument is gently introduced into the superficial femoral artery as far distally as possible and inflated until the arterial wall presents mild resistance. The catheter is then extracted while the balloon is gently inflated. Initially, only a small quantity of fluid is needed as the catheter is extracted, but as the diameter of the vessel increases, additional volume may be required. Only mild traction is required for the removal of embolic material or a soft thrombus. The deep femoral artery is explored in a similar manner. Care must be taken that the catheter is introduced into the deep femoral artery and not into one of the large circumflex branches, which may have an early origin from this vessel. If the circumflex branch is explored, it should be realized that the catheter can be introduced for only a short distance, and the 2F or 3F catheter should be used for this purpose.

After successful exploration of the distal bed, heparinized solution is injected into the distal artery via a thru-lumen balloon or irrigating catheter, and the vessels are occluded with the balloon. A 6F embolectomy catheter is placed into the common femoral artery and threaded into the aorta. The balloon is inflated with the appropriate amount of fluid and extracted in the inflated position. During the process of extraction, deflating the balloon accommodates the narrowing vessel. Significant, even somewhat pulsatile, bleeding may occur from the proximal common femoral artery in the presence of partial continued obstruction. Repeated passes should be made until one is confident that all obstructing thrombi have been removed. A similar procedure is performed on the opposite limb after adequate extraction of the clot from one side. When bilateral simultaneous pulsatile flow is ensured, both arteriotomies are closed. If one is uncertain about adequate thrombus removal, the adherent clot catheter should follow balloon catheter use.

It is important to understand that the presence of backbleeding is no assurance that distal patency has been established. Collateral circulation may result in vigorous backbleeding, even in the presence of distal arterial thrombus. Regardless of the presence or absence of backbleeding from the superficial femoral artery, distal catheter exploration is mandatory because discontinuous distal thrombosis is present in more than one-third of all instances of acute embolic occlusion. If there is uncertainty regarding the state of the distal arterial tree, angioscopy is extremely useful. Angioscopy is more expedient, less expensive, less time-consuming, and more easily repeatable than completion arteriography.

Femoral and Popliteal Occlusions

At one time, occlusions below the inguinal ligament required incisions over the presumed site of the occlusion. A more satisfactory approach for occlusions at the level of the adductor tendon and the popliteal areas is through an incision in the distal common femoral artery. This proximal approach has several advantages. First, manipulation of larger vessels reduces the possibility of rethrombosis; it also allows for exploration of the deep femoral system. Second, the proximal approach is less time-consuming than exposing the popliteal fossa. Angioscopy can be used to guide catheters into the anterior tibial and posterior tibial vessels.

Upper Extremity Occlusions

The management of upper extremity occlusions is essentially identical to that described for those in the lower extremities. Emboli in the proximal subclavian artery can be removed simply under local anesthesia by retrograde extraction. The possible morbidity associated with upper extremity emboli should not be underestimated. If the occlusion appears to be close to the origin of the cranial vessels, fragmentation during withdrawal can cause central nervous system ischemia. Although this morbidity has not occurred in our experience, the possibility should be anticipated. If there is any doubt as to the exact location of the embolus in relation to the orifices of the carotid and vertebral vessels, preoperative radiographic visualization must be performed.

Renal, Mesenteric, and Carotid Occlusions

The principles of management of renal, mesenteric, and carotid occlusions are similar to those described for management of peripheral occlusions. The major difference is that the external support provided by adjacent tissue is significantly less with vessels supplying the viscera and the brain than with vessels of the peripheral vasculature. Because of this, considerable care must be taken in introducing a catheter into these conduits. Smaller catheters such as the 2F and 3F models are appropriate sizes for distal exploration of these vessels. These catheters are provided with a very flexible tip, which significantly diminishes the possibility of vessel perforation. Only gentle inflation and traction should be used to remove emboli located in these areas.

Surgical intervention should not be considered in the internal carotid system unless emboli are observed within the first few hours of onset. Hemorrhagic infarction is a frequent and often fatal complication when attempts are made to remove cerebral occlusions, especially when they are undertaken after a considerable time lapse.

Evaluation of Procedure

Regardless of the site of the occlusion, the surgeon must recognize and atraumatically remove any distally propagated thrombus to achieve a complete restoration of circulation. Visual examination of the removed thrombus can provide valuable information regarding completeness of clot removal. A sharp cutoff usually indicates that additional thrombotic material remains, whereas a smooth taper indicates adequate clot removal.

A finding that is cause for considerable concern after an apparently successful embolectomy is a water-hammer type of pulse. A pulse that is apparently stronger than normal has been associated with obstruction at the small artery and arteriolar level. Reexploration of the vessel in these cases should include copious distal irrigation in conjunction with venous exploration. The adjunctive use of fibrinolytic agents is beneficial in such clinical situations.

The aim of surgical intervention for arterial occlusions is to restore the peripheral circulation to its preocclusive state. Evaluation of results is based on restoration of pulses, relief of symptoms, and return of normal color and temperature. It may be difficult to accurately assess results in patients whose physical status and history before the acute occlusion are unknown. Evaluation of therapy is ultimately best determined by the mortality and amputation rate.

Additional Considerations

Thrombectomy and Reconstruction

The status of the peripheral circulation before the acute episode must be ascertained; this can usually be done with a careful history and physical examination. The immediate objective of the surgical procedure is only to return the circulation to its preocclusive state, and thus the complexity of the procedure will be determined by the patient's general condition, prior level of activity, and the extent of the pathologic change encountered at the time of operation. If the general condition of the patient is favorable on initial presentation, definitive procedures may be performed if required. Otherwise, these procedures are delayed until a more complete evaluation and stabilization can be carried out. Elderly patients in poor general health are not good candidates for major reconstructive procedures.

If thromboembolectomy alone fails to restore flow, local angioplasty or end-arterectomy of the deep femoral system and femorofemoral jump grafts are simple, expedient procedures and can be done under local anesthesia. Adjunctive endovascular procedures such as balloon dilatation and atherectomy are being used with increasing frequency. In critically ill and very elderly patients, endovascular procedures serve to decrease the magnitude of the operation. These lesser interventions and procedures often provide the margin necessary to maintain viability.

Advanced Ischemia

Advanced ischemia is defined as loss of motor movement or rigor. Revascularization in the presence of advanced ischemia can lead to significant complications and possible death if not handled properly. Mortality and morbidity can be ameliorated by recognition and appropriate management of the revascularization syndrome. Components of this syndrome include both local and systemic phenomena.

The local effects include venous thrombosis and the development of significant edema. Acute venous thrombosis in the presence of acute arterial occlusion was present in 27% of patients who had advanced ischemia and in 8% of those who exhibited major venous occlusion. The operative technique employed in the presence of advanced ischemia includes venous exploration. The common femoral, deep femoral, and superficial femoral veins are isolated and encircled with Silastic tapes. A clamp is placed on the common femoral vein. The artery is explored, and flow is reestablished. With the common femoral venous clamp in place, venous hypertension is created by dorsiflexion and extension of the foot. A venotomy is made at the confluence of the superficial femoral vein with the common femoral vein. Approximately 250 to 300 ml of blood is shed. Gross thrombus is sometimes present, and microthrombi in varying amounts are present in all patients with advanced ischemia. If catheter exploration is required, venous catheters should be used.

Massive edema occurs after successful revascularization in the presence of advanced ischemia. The swelling is caused by loss of capillary integrity, resulting in fluid leakage into the surrounding ischemic tissue. The condition is aggravated by venous obstruction. Failure to control massive swelling may result in compression of the arterial inflow and subsequent reocclusion. If manometric pressure readings exceed 30 mm Hg, fasciotomy is indicated. Initial fascial decompression should be a limited subcutaneous approach. If immediate improvement is not observed, the skin incision should be extended and all deeper fascial compartments opened.

The systemic effects of arterial revascularization in the presence of early rigor can lead to death. Pooled blood in ischemic limbs is acidotic and has a high potassium content. When this blood is restored to the systemic circulation, hypotension and significant cardiac arrhythmias can occur. These symptoms can be minimized by phlebotomy of the affected limb, as previously described. The need for the use of buffering agents, volume loading, and antiarrhythmic agents should be anticipated and begun before clamp release. Electrolytes and acid-base balance must be closely monitored in the postrevascularization period. With early recognition and proper treatment, adverse occurrences can be avoided and a favorable outcome achieved.

Rhabdomyolysis occurs in situations of advanced ischemia. Restoration of arterial blood flow results in systemic myoglobinuria. Myoglobin is cleared by the kidney; precipitation in the tubules severely impairs renal function. A positive urine guaiac test in conjunction with the absence of red cells in the urine on microscopic examination is indicative of myoglobinuria. Alkalinization of the urine, hydration, and diuresis at 100 ml/hr is the required treatment. Temporary renal dialysis may also be required.

Adjunctive Procedures

Approximately 60% of patients sustaining an acute arterial occlusion require an additional operative procedure either at the time of thrombectomy or within 1 month of the original procedure. The additional peripheral reconstructive procedures performed in a series of 500 patients are listed in Box 19–2. Associated catheter-mediated procedures such as dilatation are increasing, whereas major standard surgical procedures are being done less often.

Marginal viability or thrombosis in the immediate postprocedure period requires emergency reexploration. If there is a cardiac source for the embolus, this pathology should be corrected early. Major cardiac pathology can be corrected soon after balloon thrombectomy without major limb loss or death. Box 19–3 lists the number and type of cardiac procedures done simultaneously with or within 1 month of thromboembolectomy.

Lytic Treatment

Systemic lytic therapy has largely been replaced by catheter approaches. A variety of catheter systems are available that allow the lytic agent to be directly placed in the occluding thrombus. Multihole catheters and pulsed spray systems serve to improve the rapidity of

Box 19–2. Peripheral Reconstructions Associated with Thromboembolectomy[a]	
Common and deep femoral endarterectomy	24
Femorofemoral graft	14
Proximal endarterectomy	9
Aortofemoral graft	5
Adjunctive dilatation	22
Adjunctive atherectomy	17

[a] 91 Reconstructions/570 thromboembolectomies = 16%.

Box 19–3. Cardiac Procedures Performed in Association with Thromboembolectomy[a]	
Replacement of prosthetic valve	
Aortic	2
Mitral	7
Replacement of mitral valve	
Ruptured papillary	8
Rheumatic	13
Triple valve	1
Resection of ventricular aneurysm and/or CABG	27
Repair of infarct VSD	2

[a] 60 Cardiac procedures/500 patients = 12%.
CABG, coronary artery bypass graft; VSD, ventricular septal defect.

lysis. Lytic therapy is rarely a primary therapeutic modality. The advantages and disadvantages of lysis as a sole intervention versus mechanical or surgical intervention are illustrated in Table 19–2.

Lytic therapy should be considered a preamble to a therapy that treats the underlying cause of the occlusion. The more definitive therapy can be catheter-mediated (dilatation), stent placement, or direct surgical intervention. We find lytic therapy to be most useful in failed autogenous vein grafts below the inguinal ligament. After successful lysis, the underlying pathology is identified, which usually allows a less extensive operation to be undertaken and preservation of the good portion of the conduit.

A second area in which lytic treatment has utility is in situations of advanced ischemia. Distal thrombosis occurs in vessels too small or too distant to be accessed by balloon catheters.

After removal of as much thrombus as can be taken out with the mechanical catheter system, the arteriotomy is closed around a 4F thru-lumen balloon catheter. Distal placement of the catheter should be above the knee joint but beyond the adductor tendon. The balloon is inflated to occlude the artery, and 250,000 to 300,000 units urokinase in 200 ml saline solution is hand-pulsed into a targeted area over a 10- to 15-minute period. Subsequently, the balloon is deflated but left in place. Urokinase is administered continuously for 24 to 48 hours through the indwelling thru-lumen catheter; concurrently, the patient is systematically heparinized. Arteriograms can be obtained after dye injection via the thru-lumen embolectomy catheter. On completion of therapy, the catheter is removed by pulling it out through the arteriotomy. The wound should be observed for hematoma formation. Significant hematomas require exploration and drainage.

TABLE 19–2. Relative Merits of Therapies: Mechanical vs. Lytic[a]

Parameter	Mechanical	Lytic
Safe	3	2
Simple	4	2
Secure	4	2
Predictable	4	2
Durable	4	1
Cost	3	1
Total	22	10

[a] Relative merits: 1 = least value, 4 = most value.

Emerging Thrombectomy Technologies

In 1990 Fogarty et al. first described a technique for performing thrombectomy with a thru-lumen embolectomy catheter introduced over a guidewire through a variable-diameter, Expandable Access Sheath (Applied Vascular Devices, Laguna Hills, CA).[1] Figure 19–10 (see color plate) shows the catheter components and features of the expandable tip. The thromboem-

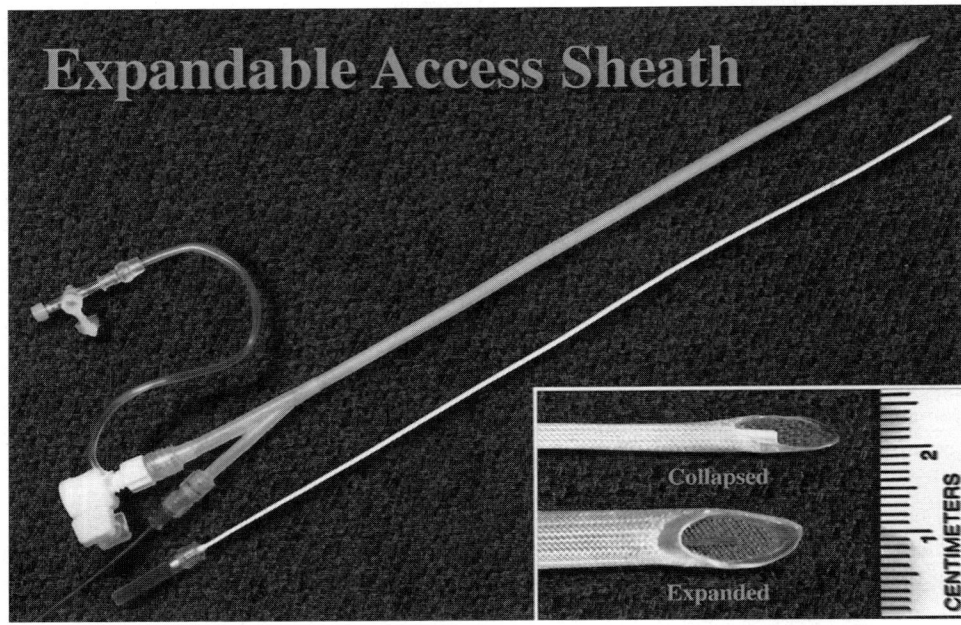

FIGURE 19–10. Variable-diameter sheath allows perctaneous thrombectomy. **Inset**, enlarged detail of the tip. (See color plate).

bolectomy was performed to remove soft gelatinous clot prior to initiating atherectomy utilizing the Simpson Athrocath (Devices for Vascular Intervention, Redwood City, CA). This early percutaneous balloon thrombectomy demonstrated the feasibility of achieving successful declotting of vessels through a percutaneous port of entry. Today, a resurgence of interest in percutaneous disobliteration of embolic and thrombotic material from the vasculature has prompted the development of new devices for this application. Most devices are undergoing clinical investigation under US Food and Drug Administration (FDA) protocols. Currently the systems are being tested for arterial and venous applications. A few have received approval from the FDA for specific applications, but clinical usage is not widespread. The basic premise employed in the design of these devices involves fragmentation of thromboembolic material followed by aspiration and removal of the contents by some mechanical means.

More than 30 devices have been developed for these applications. It appears that many have specific applications because of their design characteristics, which render them more effective in occlusions or in nontortuous vessels; or they have application in particular anatomic sites. Most devices can be categorized according to their method of mechanical operation. Broad thrombectomy categories include aspiration, pull-back entrapment devices, recirculation ablation devices, nonrecirculation maceration without aspiration, acoustic lysing with and without pharmacologic agent devices, and laser- or radiofrequency-assisted lysing devices. A brief description of each of these device catagories follows.

Aspiration thrombectomy instrumentation allows passage of an aspiration catheter over a guidewire that traverses the thrombus. After passage, the clot is aspirated via syringe suction. If dense clot plugs the tip it can be removed by withdrawing the catheter and the process repeated with additional catheter introductions until all clot is extracted. These devices are usually more effective when used in conjunction with other thrombectomy techniques, such as cutting, brushing, lysing with pharmacologic agents, or other types of mechanical instrumentation. The advantages of this system include reduction in the cost of the procedure and less risk of embolization and vessel damage. The cost may increase if adjunctive methods are required to perform the thrombectomy adequately and expeditiously.

Pull-back and *entrapment thrombectomy* consists of removing the thrombus via suction and withdrawing the material through a sheath, This is accomplished by trapping the clot via balloon pull-back of the offending thrombus into a specially designed cup, funnel, or bag or engaging mural thrombus in a mesh basket; it is then removed through the entry access sheath. Limitations of this thrombectomy modality are related to the ability of the trapping device to envelop or ensnare the entire clot completely without fragmentation (resulting in embolization) or damage to the vessel walls. Further studies are needed to provide data that can answer questions regarding these all-important embolization concerns.

Thrombectomy utilizing *recirculation techniques* to effect the therapeutic response basically involves high speed rotation of a mechanical component—a blunt-tipped cam or coaxial impeller blades housed in a protective capsule. The rotation of these elements draws the thrombus into a recirculation vortex and subsequently into the pulverization mechanism at the leading catheter tip, which creates a vortex to entrap clot and macerate it into minute particles. These systems offer the advantage of being able to open occluded peripheral arteries and clotted hemodialysis grafts. The drawbacks lie in the inability of the instrumentation to be used in tortuous, thin-walled, or small-diameter vessels due to the real potential for vessel injury from the rotational cam. Limited steerability of these devices also creates a deterrent to use, as the high-speed mechanical rotation can generate excessive heat. Unless adequately controlled by the introduction of cooling solutions, the cable can break if the device becomes kinked in highly angulated grafts or vessels. This potential for vessel wall perforation has been minimized in some of the newer system designs that house the pulverization elements in a protective capsule or basket. Although attempts have been made to center the devices within the vessel using guidewires and the like, steerability remains a problem.

Other recirculation systems incorporate hydraulic elements combined with active aspiration of fragmented thrombus through exit ports posterior to the pulverization mechanism to accomplish thrombectomy. The AngioJet system (Possis Medical, Minneapolis, MN) is an example of this type of hydrolyzer device.

Nonrecirculation mechanical thrombectomy devices can be used with or without suction. Among the devices without suction, one system's primary mode of operation consists of removing the offending thrombus by homogenizing the clot via high speed rotating basket fragmentation (Trerotola Percutaneous Thrombectomy Device; Arrow International, Reading, PA) Another uses mechanical brush cleanout with simultaneous lytic agent infusion (Cragg Thrombolytic Brush Catheter; Micro Therapeutics, Aliso Viego, CA) to effect thrombectomy. Yet another device using this mechanical methodology without suction employs a rotational wire(s) that winds fibrin around the exposed wire tip to clear the conduit. Another variation of this thrombectomy device uses high pressure fluid pulses to fragment the thrombus surrounding its high speed pulsatile side-port jets. One of the more frequently utilized nonsuction devices is the Simpson Atherectomy Catheter (Atherotrac; Mallinckrodt Medical, St. Louis, MO), which achieves its therapeutic result by entrapping, slicing, and removing atheroma through a unique catheter side window housing a cutting blade. Once the atheroma is sliced within the housing, the window is closed and the atheromatous cutting is withdrawn through the access sheath. Figure 19–11 (see color plate) shows two devices in this category and illustrates their different mechanisms of action.

Within the larger category of mechanical maceration thrombectomy devices several systems have been developed that couple suction of the fragmented material with the fragmentation process. The idea is similar: maceration of clot by mechanical means using a propeller (Gunther Thrombectomy Catheter), rotating torque tube/cutting blade

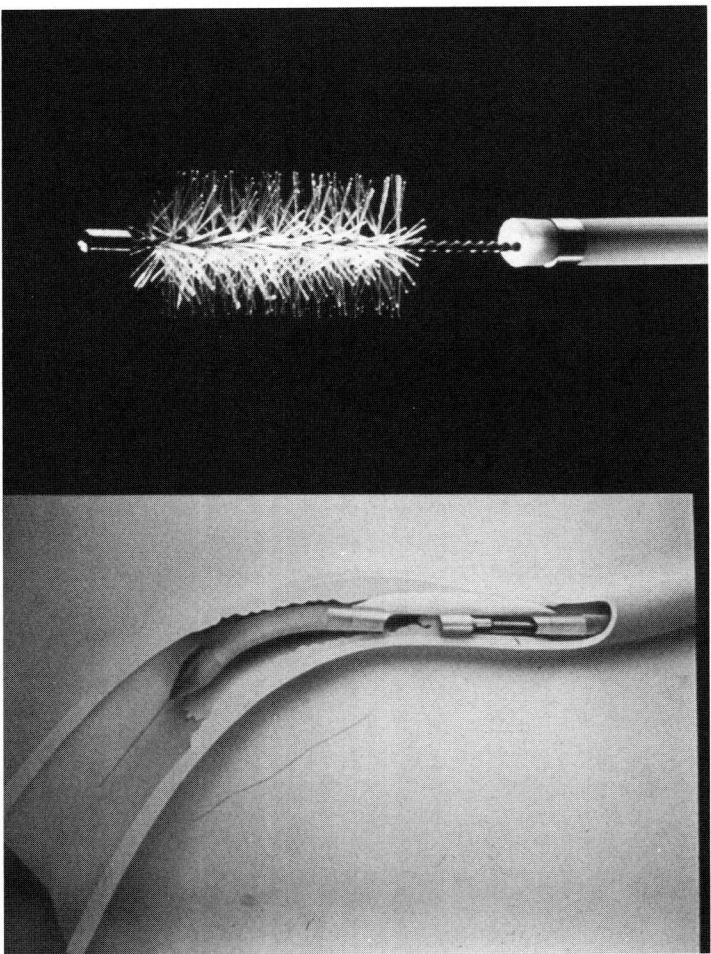

FIGURE 19-11. Two examples of nonrecirculation thrombectomy devices. **Top**, Cragg Thrombolytic Brush (Micro Therapeutics, Aliso Veijo, CA). **Bottom**, Simpson Atherotrac device (Mallinckrodt Medical, St. Louis, MO). Both devices operate by essentially scraping or cutting atheroma from vessel walls and removing it via percutaneous access site. (See color plate).

combination (Transluminal Extraction Catheter, or TEC), coaxial oscillating probe stimulated by ultrasound or an electric motor (Oscillation Aspiration Thrombectomy Device), or a manual reciprocating clot scoop or spoon (Gelbfish Endo-Vac System) combined with dynamic irrigation or suction to aspirate fragmented material. An example of this technology is shown in Figure 19-12 (see color plate). The cost-effectiveness of these systems must be considered when contemplating usage, as their multicomponent action—maceration via mechanical modality, suction aspiration, and in some instances combined standard balloon catheter embolectomy—may contribute to a high cost for achieving thrombectomy.

Clinicians, independent of their specialty background training, appear to have acknowledged the potential advantages of mechanical thrombectomy over lytic therapy. However, the *combined* use of percutaneous mechanical systems with lysing therapeutic agents may offer the significant benefit of being able to reduce the amount of lytic agent used, thereby reducing the duration of therapy and lessening the chance of hemorrhagic complications. In addition, several devices are being evaluated that attempt to maximize the effect of thrombolytic agents by combining with indirect ultrasound or laser photothermo energy to potentiate an enhanced therapeutic result. The work is promising but requires

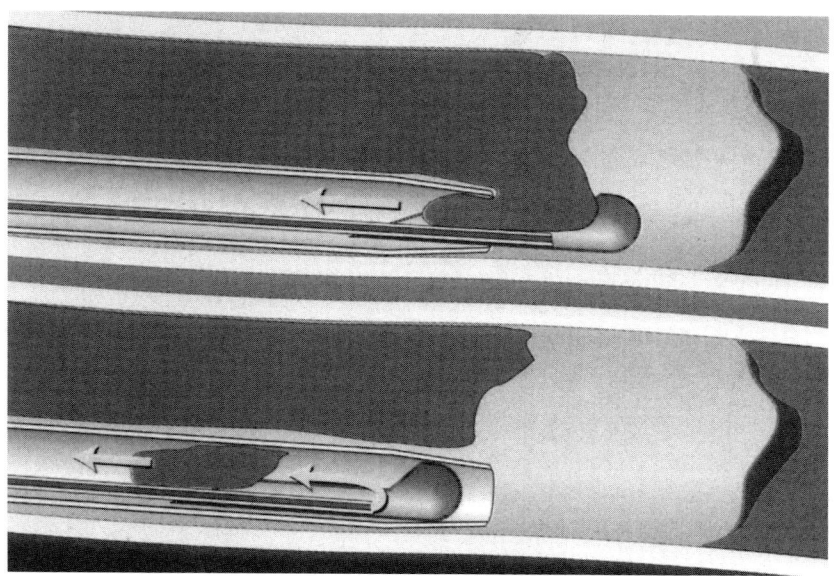

FIGURE 19–12. Gelbfish Endo Vac Device (Neovascular Technologies, Brooklyn, NY) performs thrombectomy by combining thrombus maceration, utilizing a reciprocating "clot spoon", with simultaneous or concomitant suction. (See color plate).

additional study to ascertain long-term patency rates.

All devices discussed have particular advantages and limitations. None is perfect, so we must choose carefully the modality we wish to employ, taking into consideration the individual pathology we wish to treat and matching the appropriate device to the task. Clearly it is important to have a flexible system capable of traversing angulated and tortuous vessels or grafts, one that is steerable to ensure safety, and a device or combination of devices that is simple to use, cost-effective, and durable in material and result.

Visually Assisted Thromboembolectomy

The blind passage of balloon catheters for embolectomy represented an improvement at the time of initial introduction for the management of emboli and distally propagated thrombus. The relatively disease-free arteries in a young patient with rheumatic heart disease were the most common candidates. The current acute occlusions are thrombotic and occur in elderly patients with significant atherosclerosis; stenosis and significant tortuosity are common accompaniments. Visualization for the purpose of catheter guidance for access is important and necessary in this environment. Documentation of the state of restoration of flow in the operating room is critical when determining management during the postprocedural period. Real-time visualization is accomplished by two simple means, both of which are available to the surgeon in the operating room environment. The efficiency and improvement in patient outcomes is obvious to those who have learned the techniques. The importance of angioscopy has been documented by Miller and Sacks.[2] The needs and specific applications of embolectomy have been outlined by others. The second visualization technique of fluoroscopy has been outlined by Marin's group.[3] These two techniques should become part of the routine technology utilized by the vascular surgeon when indicated.

Conclusion

The pathology of acute arterial occlusion has significantly changed over the last 30 years. In situ thromboses now account for 80% of acute arterial occlusions, and these lesions are densely adherent to the arterial wall. The patients are elderly, have systemic atherosclerosis, and often have significant multiorgan disease. Despite this difficult and advanced pathology, the development of instruments designed specifically to remove adherent thrombus has resulted in improved limb salvage rates. The quality of care and mortality rates have improved for multiple reasons, including decreasing the magnitude of the operation, the ability to treat the underlying cardiac disorder better, improved anesthesia, improved postoperative care, and a better understanding and management of the pathophysiology associated with advanced ischemia.

References

1. Fogarty TJ, Hermann GD: The role of atherectomy devices in the management of infrainguinal occlusive disease. In Ernst CB, editor: *Current therapy in vascular surgery*, 2nd edition, Toronto, 1991, Decker, pp 533–535.
2. Miller A, Sacks BA: Angioscopy in interventional surgery: diagnostic use and therapeutic application in endovascular procedures. In Yao JST, Pearce WH, editors: *Techniques in vascular and endovascular surgery*, Stamford, CT, 1998, Appleton & Lange, pp 47–57.
3. Parsons RE, Marin ML, Veith FJ et al: Fluoroscopically assisted thromboembolectomy: an improved method for treating acute arterial occlusions, *Ann Vasc Surg* 10:201–210, 1996.

20
Disobliteration Techniques

Gwan H. Ho and Frans L. Moll

Endovascular surgical procedures have become an integral part of the treatment of arterial occlusive disease in the femoropopliteal segment—an adjunct to conventional peripheral arterial reconstructions.[1-3] Additionally, new percutaneous arterial disobliteration devices have been designed. Catheter-based therapies such as percutaneous transluminal balloon angioplasty (PTA) have been effective for short and solitary lesions in the femoropopliteal segment. However, the long-term patency results of PTA or laser-assisted balloon angioplasty are discouraging for long (more than 10cm) occlusive lesions.[4-7] The use of stents in the femoropopliteal artery in combination with angioplasty has not truly altered these results despite close surveillance and reintervention.[8-10] Alternative techniques to recanalize chronic occlusions of the superficial femoral artery are based on plaque removal rather than stretching and remodeling the arterial wall. These methods can be divided into two categories: "going through" and 'going around" the occlusion. Common to both methods is the ability to remove the occlusive atheroma using a mechanical atherectomy device or performing endarterectomy. Atherectomy devices were developed to improve the results of lesions that were unfavorable for PTA and to decrease the incidence of acute arterial thrombosis. Transluminal endarterectomy has a history of more than 50 years, the first case being reported in 1947 by the Portugese surgeon J. Cid Dos Santos.[11,12] Also, endarterectomy has shown far better long-term patency results than PTA for long lesions because of a high incidence of recurrent stenoses after balloon angioplasty that require repeated intervention.[13]

Atherectomy

The basic concept of atherectomy is the removal of atheroma from the obstructed arterial vessel. The procedure can be performed percutaneously or through a small arteriotomy. Hypothetically, atherectomy was expected to be superior to PTA, as arterial segments appeared to be smoother angiographically than after PTA. The risk of subintimal dissection and subsequent thrombosis would thus be smaller. Although in theory smooth-muscle injury was expected to be minimal owing to the removal of plaque only, histopathologic studies have identified medial elements in up to 64% of atherectomy samples.[14,15]

There are currently four atherectomy devices approved by the US Food and Drug Administration (FDA) for which clinical data are available: Simpson AtheroCath, transluminal extraction cathether, Theratec recanalization arterial catheter (Trac-Wright, formerly Kensey atherectomy catheter), and Auth Rotablator (Figure 20–1). These devices either cut and remove or pulverize the atheroma plaque.

The Simpson AtheroCath (DVI, Redwood City, CA) was the first atherectomy device, developed by John B. Simpson in 1985. In contrast to other atherectomy devices, the cutting element is *directionally* exposed to the arterial

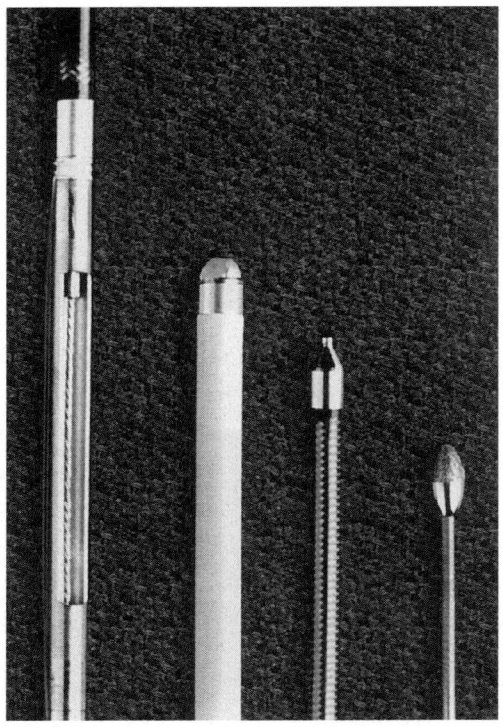

FIGURE 20–1. Enlarged view of "working ends" of four atherectomy devices used to remove atheromatous plaques (left to right): Simpson AtheroCath, Trac-Wright system, TEC system, and Auth Rotablator.

wall over one-third of its circumference (120°). Atheroma protruding into the window is excised and pushed into the collection chamber (Figure 20–2). As soon as this collection chamber is full, it must be emptied. The Transluminal Extraction Cathether (TEC) (Interventional Technologies, San Diego, CA) system consists of an over-the-wire *nondirectional* cutter mounted on the distal end of a torque tube (Figure 20–3). The excised atheroma is simultaneously removed by aspiration through the torque tube into a 125-ml vacuum bottle, which can be changed without removing the catheter. The Theratec recanalization arterial catheter (Trac-Wright, formerly Kensey atherectomy catheter) is a *nondirectional*, noncoaxial, atheroablative device (Figure 20–4). The rotating cam mechanically pulverizes the atheromatous lesion with 60,000 to 100,000 rpm. As this system is not over-the-wire, perforations have been reported in up to 37% of the cases.[16] The Auth Rotablator (Heart Technologies, Redmond, WA) is a *nondirectional*, coaxial, atheroablative device with a metal burr embedded with fine diamond chips. The tip is available in diameters ranging from 1.25 to 4.50 mm (Figure 20–5). As the burr size is the limiting factor, this device is often used in combination with PTA. The inability to burn through soft thrombus or rubbery atherosclerotic lesions limits the use of the Auth Rotablator. Despite the promising reported early technical and clinical success in some studies, the mid- and long-term results have been disappointing for all atherectomy devices owing to the high incidence of restenoses.[17–19]

Semiclosed Endarterectomy

Wylie and Cannon in the United States and Vollmar in Europe have popularized the technique of semiclosed endarterectomy for long segments of the iliac and femoral arteries. Different arterial wire loop ring dissectors have been introduced with the ring placed at various angles with the metal shaft, ranging from 90° (De Bakey 1954), to 105° (Cannon), to 135° (Vollmar 1967) with blunted edges and with an ellipse-shaped ring instead of a circular ring.[20–22] Despite promising results in early studies, endarterectomy was abandoned after several reports suggested that it was inferior to femoropopliteal venous bypass grafting.[23,24] However, publications by vascular surgeons who still perform semiclosed endarterectomy in the superficial femoral artery (SFA) have reported similar long-term cumulative patency rates, approaching that of saphenous femoropopliteal bypass grafting.[25–29] The developments in endovascular techniques have resulted in endoluminal stent implantation and minimally invasive surgical endarterectomy devices. Based on removal of the atheromatous plaque from the vessel percutaneously or through a small single arteriotomy remote from the diseased site, thereby increasing the intraluminal size, five theoretic advantages of endarterectomy over PTA and arterial bypass surgery could be postulated: (1) a higher immediate success rate with less subintimal dissec-

20. Disobliteration Techniques

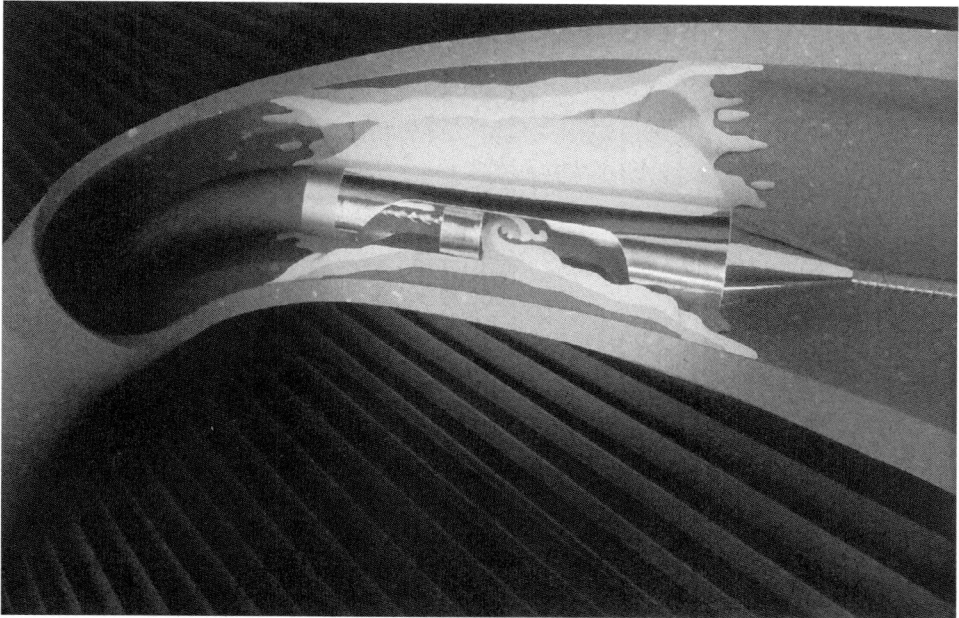

FIGURE 20–2. Simpson AtheroCath cutting element, shown shaving an atheroma and collecting it in the distal collection chamber.

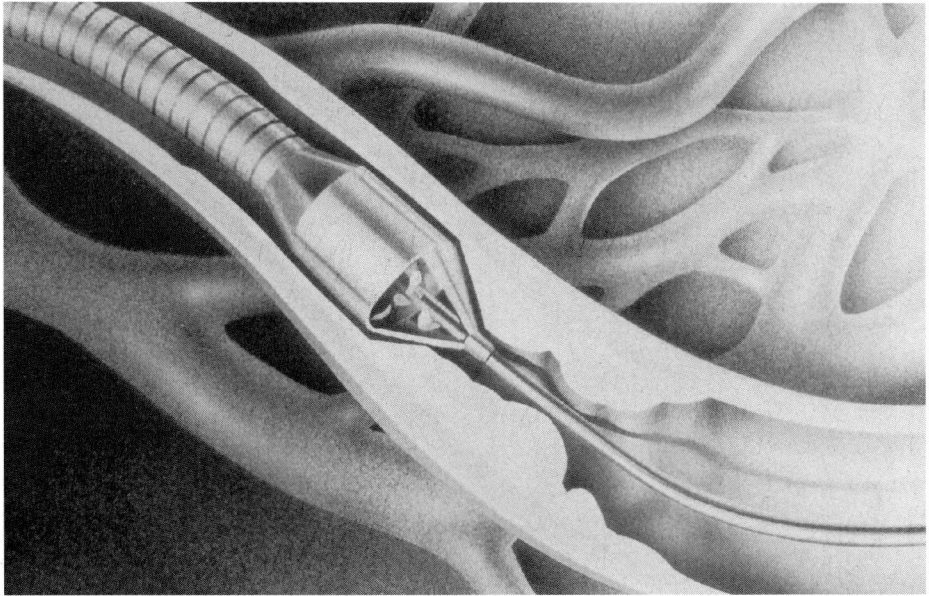

FIGURE 20–3. Rotational technique employed with the TEC system's cutting element, followed by vacuum aspiration of the shaved atheroma.

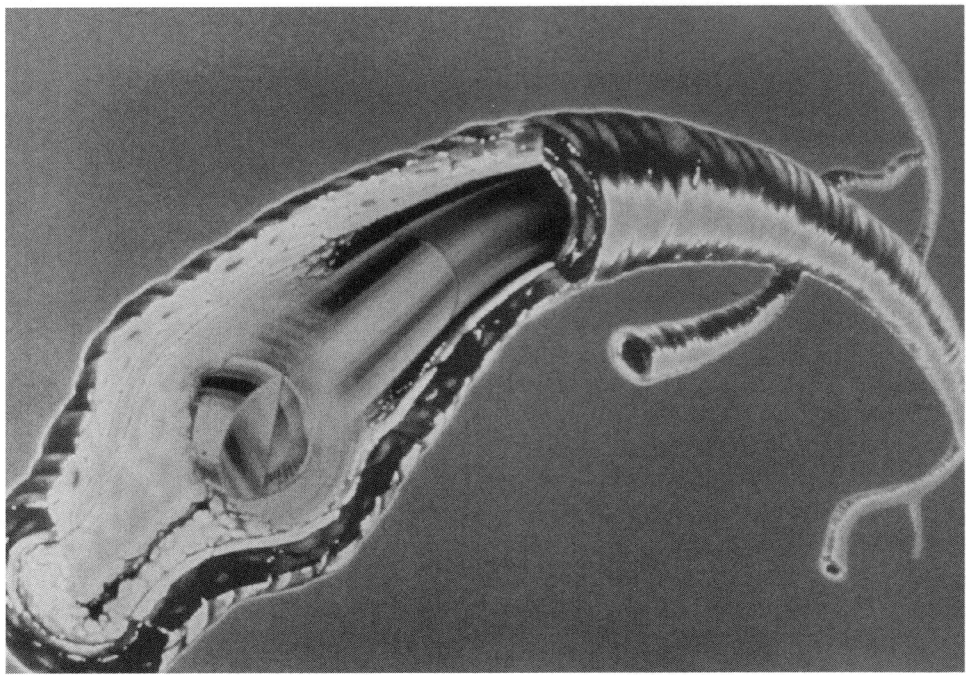

FIGURE 20-4. Enhanced detail of a rotating cam tip pulverizing the atheromatous lesion into minute particles using the Trac-Wright sytem atherectomy device.

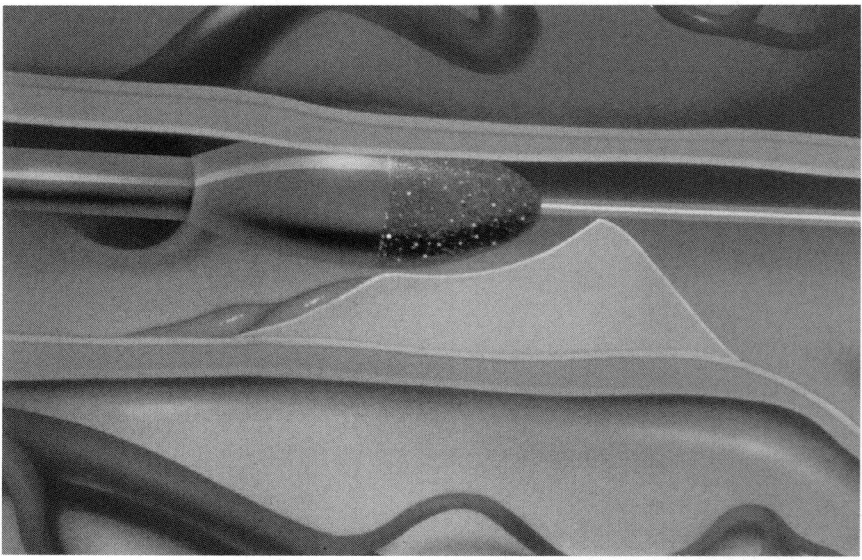

FIGURE 20-5. Detail of the catheter-guided rotating burr tip of the Auth Rotablator that is used to accomplish ablation of an obstructive atheroma.

tion and subsequent occlusion; (2) wider therapeutic options for lesions currently not amenable to angioplasty alone (diffusely diseased or totally occluded lesions); (3) reduction of the restenosis rate by removing or debulking the affected thickened intimal layer from the artery; (4) minimally invasive surgery without the harvesting and use of autologous venous material, which could be saved for later cardiac or peripheral reconstructions; and (5) the option to perform a bypass operation in case of failure after endarterectomy.

Technique

The common femoral artery, proximal profunda, and proximal few inches of the SFA are exposed through an 8-cm vertical groin incision. The terminal portion of the SFA and proximal popliteal artery is exposed through a medial low-thigh incision. The adductor canal is fully released and is not reapproximated so there is better exposure, facilitating passage of the arterial stripper. After administration of 25 to 50mg heparin intravenously, a vascular clamp is applied to the most proximal part of the SFA in the groin, permitting flow to continue into the usually patent profunda femoris artery. Longitudinal arteriotomy (3cm) of the proximal SFA permits development of a cleavage plane between the diseased plaque and media or preferably between the media and adventitia. The former is recognizable from the circular fibers of the media, the latter from its featureless smooth appearance. After dissecting the intimal core from the remaining arterial wall, the endarterectomy core is cut, and a suitable ring stripper is passed over the core and advanced distally into the SFA with a gentle rotating movement. If passage of the ring stripper is not possible, a different-caliber ring stripper can be used or an additional arteriotomy can be performed. After reaching the patent distal SFA or proximal popliteal artery, a second arteriotomy is needed to cut the intimal core distally. The entire intimal core can then be removed through the proximal arteriotomy by slight traction and pulling the ring stripper back simultaneously. The ring stripper can also be inserted from the distal site and advanced toward the femoral bifurcation, as originally described by Vollmar, but the proximal site of the endarterectomy should always be visualized to ensure the completeness of the procedure. Blind removal of the intimal core through the distal arteriotomy might leave some intimal flaps behind, which could develop as a source of emboli, restenosis, or both. The distal intimal flaps must be fixed with 6-0 tacking sutures to ensure a smooth distal transitional zone to normal intima. This maneuver also prevents dissection and subsequent occlusion of the artery after restoring the blood flow. At the proximal site, the endarterectomy usually must be extended into the common femoral artery. The ostium of the profunda femoris artery can be inspected; it permits better inflow into both the superficial and deep femoral artery.

At the completion of the procedure, the proximal and distal arteriotomies are closed by a venous or prosthetic patch. Finally, intraoperative angiography is performed to detect residual intimal flaps and visualize the runoff vessels. Usually, intravenous heparin is administered continuously. Patients should commence warfarin (Coumadin) medication on the first day postoperatively and continue it for at least 3 months and sometimes indefinitely.

Results

The results of using this technique were reported by van der Heijden and Eikelboom in 1993.[25] Between 1980 and 1990 a total of 231 successfully performed endarterectomies of the SFA were studied. Presenting symptoms were disabling intermittent claudication (grade I, category 1 to 3, Rutherford) in 186 (80%), rest pain (grade II, category 4, Rutherford) in 21 (9%), and ischemic ulceration or gangrene (grade III, category 5) in 24 patients (11%). A 5-year overall cumulative patency rate of 71% was achieved at a single institution, with a complication rate of 10% and mortality less than 1%. The SFA lesions consisted of a 1- to 10cm occlusion in 52 cases (23%), less than 10-cm occlusion in 96 (41%), single stenosis in 21

(9%), multiple stenoses in 28 (12%), and unknown in 34 (15%). No difference in 5-year cumulative patency was seen between treatment for stenosis and that for occlusion (74% or 70%). Multivariate analysis found a statistically significant difference in increased failure rate in regard to age (less than 64 years), preoperative stage (grades II and III, categories 4 and 5 vs. grade I, categories 1 to 3), and extent of the SFA abnormality (multiple vs. single stenosis). Earlier studies by other authors have shown similar results with 5-year cumulative patency rates of 64% to 70%.[3,28,30] Nevertheless, several reports have favored venous bypass instead of endarterectomy as the treatment for femoropopliteal occlusive disease. These studies compared the patency results of venous bypass with those after endarterectomy.[23,24,31] However, all studies have been retrospective, often with historical control groups; and several important variables, such as arterial runoff and reasons a particular procedure was chosen, which could have influenced patency rates, were not routinely evaluated. Therefore these comparative studies should be interpreted with caution. It is also important to emphasize that venous bypass is not always possible, and that prosthetic bypass grafting may have a worse outcome than venous bypass or endarterectomy.[32] Abbott et al. reported 58% and 62% three-year primary patency rates for polytetrat fluoroethylene (PTFE) and Dacron femoropopliteal above-knee bypasses.[32]

Recurrent stenosis is one of the major prognostic factors that influence the patency of endarterectomy or bypass procedures.[33,34] Brücke et al. reported in 1973 that even after technically successful endarterectomy recurrent occlusions were reported in 40% after 4 years with no preceding clinical symptoms.[35] It is clear now that technical failure and especially neointimal hyperplasia is probably the most important cause of reocclusion within the first 2 years, as it is in venous bypass reconstructions. It was only a few years ago that repeated clinical evaluation and arterial ankle pressure measurements were found insufficient for detecting all recurrent stenoses. This situation led to routine surveillance programs by noninvasive duplex scanning after arterial bypass reconstructions to prevent recurrent occlusion by earlier detection and correction of significant hemodynamic stenoses.[34,36] Arterial surveillance using duplex scanning after endarterectomy should be performed routinely as well. It might improve future results, as impending SFA occlusions resulting from progressive stenoses can be corrected by, for example, PTA.

Mollring Cutter Remote Endarterectomy

Modifications of the classic Cannon/Vollmar ring stripper with a double-ring construction instead of one ring and sharpened cutting inside edges have resulted into the development of a ring strip cutter (Mollring Cutter; Aspect Medical/NC, Portola Valley) (Figure 20–6). This device makes it possible to perform endarterectomy in an entirely occluded SFA through a single, limited surgical exposure at the groin, thereby cutting the distal intimal core at a specific endpoint remote from the site of entry.[37] Both rings are able to shear along each other. They have sharpened cutting edges on the inner side, thereby mimicking a cutting pair of scissors, as the lower ring is moved with the proximal handle. The operative technique is similar to that of semiclosed endarterectomy in that an arteriotomy of the proximal SFA is performed. After meticulously dissecting the intimal core, a ring stripper is passed around the intimal core and advanced distally, reaching the patent popliteal artery under fluoroscopic control. The ring stripper is replaced by the Mollring Cutter, which cuts the distal part of the atheroma core endoluminally (Figures 20–7, 20–8). The entire intimal core and the Mollring Cutter are then removed simultaneously. After radiologic examination of the reopened artery and the distal runoff vessels, an additional part of the intimal core can be dissected if necessary and cut and removed with the Mollring Cutter. Endoluminal stenting of the distal intimal flap with a short balloon-expandable Palmaz stent (Johnson and Johnson, Interventional Systems,

20. Disobliteration Techniques

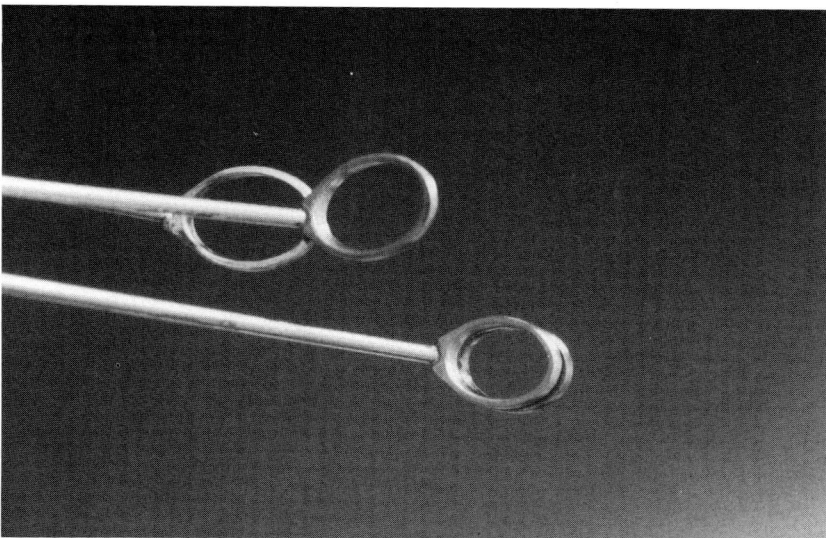

FIGURE 20–6. Double-ring construction of the Mollring Cutter is able to transect the distal end of the intima core endoluminally. It is performed by advancing the cutting component across the lesion after the device has been passed along the length of the vessel to the chosen distal endpoint.

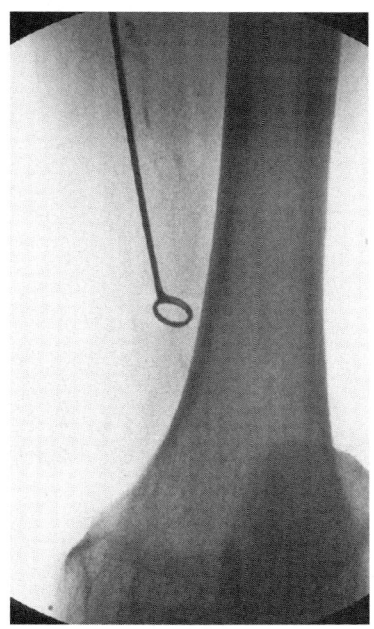

FIGURE 20–7. Fluoroscopic positioning of the Mollring Cutter beyond the occluded segment and into the distal SFA, which was patent at preoperative angiography.

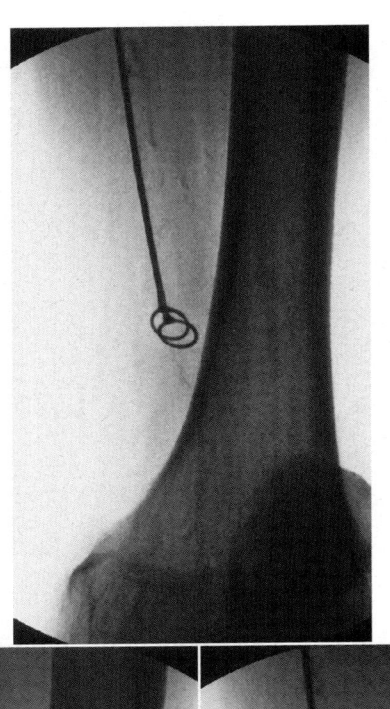
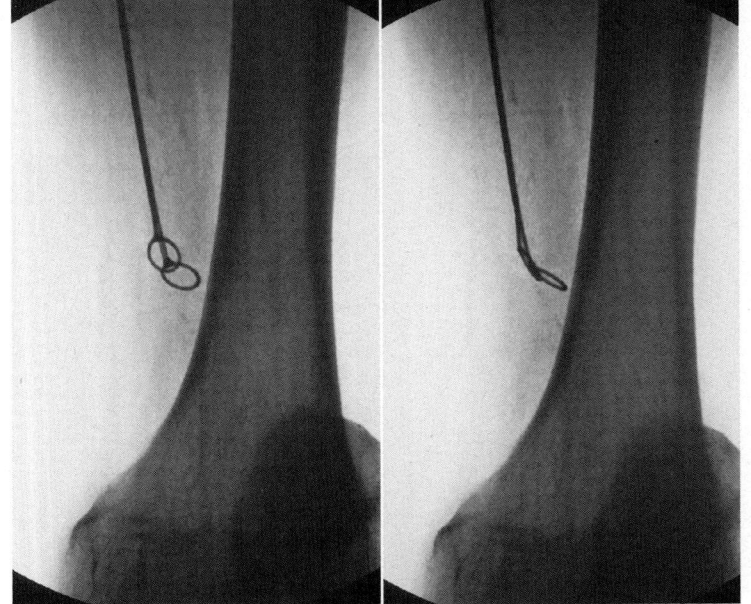

FIGURE 20-8. Intimal core is transected at the distal endpoint using the Mollring Cutter.

FIGURE 20-9. Angiographic view of the distal endpoint after endoluminal "remote" cutting and extracting the intimal core from the SFA. The distal intimal flap is secured with a balloon-expandable stent, which is positioned to prevent further dissection or occlusion after restoring normal blood flow.

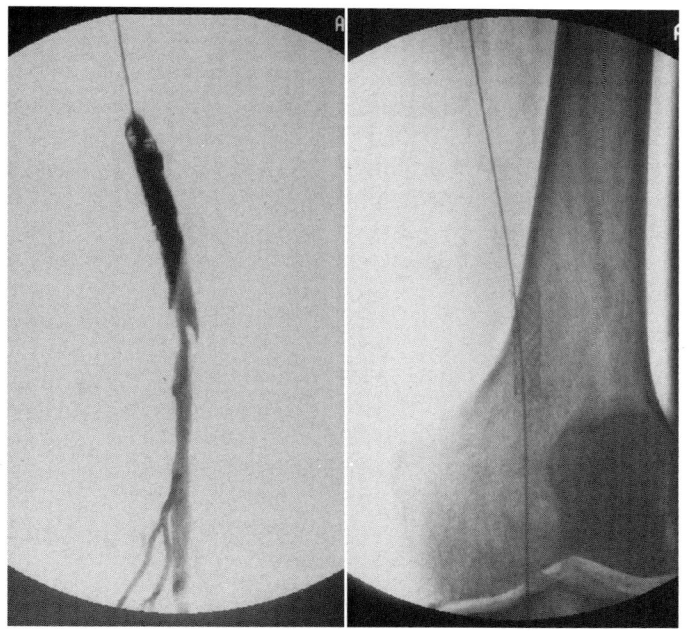

Warren, NJ) prevents further dissection and provides a smooth transitional zone to normal intima (Figures 20–9, 20–10). In addition, the minimal loss of compliance and concentric overpass would further resemble normal flow characteristics.

The minimally invasive nature of this method does not require a second distal incision and dissection of the popliteal artery. Less operative trauma and reduction of postoperative discomfort lead to earlier recovery and discharge of the patient. The procedure can be done by the vascular surgeon alone or in cooperation with the interventional radiologist. The operation is safe. Conversion into a regular semiclosed endarterectomy through an additional second incision remains possible. Currently, more than 100 remote endarterectomy procedures have been performed. The indication for surgical intervention was disabling claudication (grade I, categories 1 to 3, Rutherford) in 70% of the patients and rest pain, gangrene (grades II and III, categories 4 and 5), or both in the remaining 30%, sometimes with single vessel runoff. In 95% of cases the SFA was occluded, whereas in 65% the occlusion extended over more than half of the

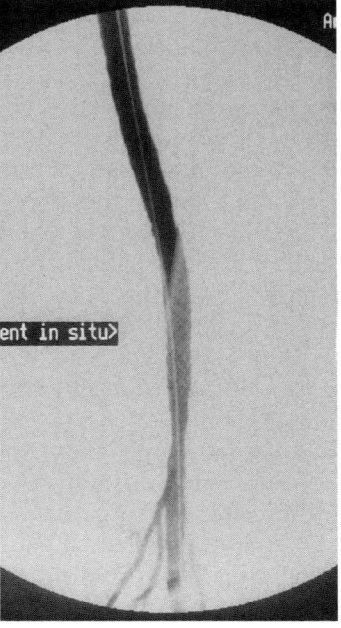

FIGURE 20–10. Completion angiogram of the distal endpoint after remote endarterectomy with a stent in situ, showing complete SFA recanalization without residual lesions and a smooth transition zone.

femoropopliteal segment. The mean length of the endarterectomized segment was 33 cm (range 10 to 45 cm). Conversion to a semiclosed endarterectomy was necessary in 10%. Clinical and hemodynamic success was obtained in all cases, except for one patient who underwent conventional femoropopliteal bypass surgery. The cumulative 2-year primary, primary assisted, and secondary patency rates were 73%, 86%, and 86%, respectively.

Surveillance and Medication

As mentioned previously, routine postoperative surveillance of the disobstructed SFA is mandatory. History has proved that recurrent occlusions after endarterectomy were not preceded by clinical deterioration or a decrease in ankle/brachial indices. Currently, all patients treated by the remote endarterectomy device in the femoropopliteal artery are entering a duplex scanning surveillance program, consisting of duplex scanning within 6 weeks postoperatively and after 3, 6, 9, and 12 months. In our series, only 25% of all recurrent stenoses after remote endarterectomy were associated with deterioration of clinical symptoms or a decrease in the ankle/brachial indices. For 82% of the restenoses the time of onset was within the first year. The location of these restenoses were equally distributed within the SFA and not restricted to the stent or distal SFA region. Preliminary studies on the results of revision indicate that early restenoses may be treated succesfully with PTA. Recurrent stenoses developing after 1 year seem to have a different natural history and do not require intervention.

There is still controversy about the use of antiplatelet drugs and warfarin (Coumadin). We give all patients warfarin postoperatively for at least 6 months. Thereafter, we prescribe an antiplatelet drug (aspirin 100 mg daily).

Future Perspectives

The preliminary results using the Mollring Cutter remote endarterectomy device show excellent immediate and early patency in the SFA. However, the enthusiasm after the introduction of several atherectomy devices has already been tempered because the high rate of restenosis has led to disappointing long-term results. The use of intravascular stents, angioscopy, and intravascular ultrasonography, which have shown their usefulness in various situations, may enhance the long-term results of transluminal endarterectomy. To overcome the problem of recurrent stenosis, endovascular grafting by a thin-walled PTFE graft has been proposed.[38] Further randomized studies should be undertaken first to reestablish the role of endarterectomy for treatment of peripheral occlusive disease.

Conclusion

Depending on the clinical status, the presence of solitary or diffuse lesions, the length of occlusion, the runoff status, and the availability of suitable veins, PTA, surgical endarterectomy, and bypass are good treatment options. Endarterectomy is being reappraised for treatment of SFA occlusive disease. The atherectomy devices may have a place in selected patients; but based on current clinical available data, their role seems to be limited.

Advances in endovascular stent implantation, improved guidewires, and better insight into the development, early detection, and treatment of recurrent stenoses in disobliterated segments may result in even better long-term results. With minimally invasive transluminal Mollring Cutter remote endarterectomy, a durable operation for SFA occlusive disease is introduced and should be in the armamentarium of every vascular surgeon.

References

1. Ahn SS: Endovascular surgery: current concepts and its importance to the vascular surgeon, *Eur J Vasc Surg* 6:1–3, 1992.
2. Bergquist D, Karacagil S: Femoral artery disease, *Lancet* 343:773–778, 1994.
3. Inahara T, Scott CM: Endarterectomy for segmental occlusive disease of the superficial femoral artery, *Arch Surg* 116:1547–1553, 1981.

4. Becquemin J-P, Cavillon A, Haiduc F: Surgical transluminal femoropopliteal angioplasty: multivariate analysis outcome, *J Vasc Surg* 19:495–502, 1994.
5. Capek P, McLean GK, Berkowitz HD: Femoropopliteal angioplasty: factors influencing long-term success, *Circulation* 83(suppl I):70–80, 1991.
6. Isner JM, Rosenfield K: Redefining the treatment of peripheral artery disease: role of percutaneous revascularisation, *Circulation* 88:1534–1557, 1993.
7. Johnston KW: Femoral and popliteal arteries: reanalysis of results of balloon angioplasty, *Radiology* 183:767–771, 1992.
8. Vroegindeweij D, Vos LD, Tielbeek AV et al: Balloon angioplasty combined with primary stenting versus balloon angioplasty alone in femoropopliteal obstructions: a comparative randomized study, *Cardiovasc Intervent Radiol* 20:420–425, 1997.
9. Do DD, Triller J, Walpoth BH et al: A comparison study of self expandable stents vs balloon angioplasty alone in femoropopliteal artery occlusions, *Cardiovasc Intervent Radiol* 15:306–312, 1992.
10. Gray BH, Sullivan TM, Childs MB et al: High incidence of restenosis/reocclusion of stents in the percutaneous treatment of long-segment superficial femoral artery disease after suboptimal angioplasty, *J Vasc Surg* 25:74–83, 1997.
11. Dos Santos JC: Sur la desobstruction des thromboses arterielles anciennes, *Mem Acad Chir* 73:409–411, 1947.
12. Dos Santos JC: Leriche memorial lecture: from embolectomy to endarterectomy or the fall of a myth, *J Cardiovasc Surg* 17:113–128, 1976.
13. Vroegindeweij D, Idu MM, Buth J et al: The cost-effectiveness of treatment of short occlusive lesions in the femoropopliteal artery: balloon angioplasty versus endarterectomy, *Eur J Vasc Endovasc Surg* 10:40–50, 1995.
14. Holfing B, Polnitz AV, Backa D et al: Percutaneous removal of atheromatous plaques in peripheral arteries, *Lancet* 1:384–386, 1988.
15. Johnson DE, Selmon MR, Simpson JB: Primary stenoses and restenoses excised by peripheral atherectomy: a histologic study, *J Am Coll Cardiol* 11:173A, 1988.
16. Snyder SO Jr, Wheeler JR, Gregory RT et al: The Trac-Wright atherectomy device. In Ahn SS, Moore WS, editors: *Endovascular surgery*, ed 2, Philadelphia, 1992, Saunders, pp 287–294.
17. Ahn SS, Eton D, Yeatman LR et al: Intraoperative peripheral rotary atherectomy: early and late clinical results, *Ann Vasc Surg* 6:272–280, 1992.
18. Fogarty TJ, Biswas A, Hermann GD et al: Atherectomy: a review of current devices and methods. In Kerstein MD, White JV, editors: *Alternatives to open vascular surgery*, Philadelphia, 1995, Lippincott, pp 247–264.
19. Collaborative Rotablator Atherectomy Group (CRAG): Peripheral atherectomy with the rotablator: a multicenter report, *J Vasc Surg* 19:509–515, 1994.
20. Cannon JA, Barker WF: Successful management of obstructive femoral arteriosclerosis by endarterectomy: experience with a semiclosed technique in selected cases, *Surgery* 38:48–59, 1955.
21. Cannon JA, Barker WF, Kawakami IG: Femoral popliteal endarterectomy in the treatment of obliterative atherosclerotic disease, *Surgery* 43:76–93, 1958.
22. Vollmar J: *Rekonstruktive Chirurgie der Arterien*, Stuttgart, 1967, Georg Thieme Verlag.
23. Darling RC, Linton RR: Durability of femoropopliteal reconstructions, *Am J Surg* 123:472–479, 1972.
24. DeWeese JA, Barner HB, Mahoney EB et al: Autogenous venous bypass grafts and thromboendarterectomies for atherosclerotic lesions of the femoropopliteal arteries, *Ann Surg* 163:205–214, 1966.
25. Van der Heijden FHWM, Eikelboom BC, van Reedt Dortland RWH et al: Long-term results of semi-closed endarterectomy of the superficial femoral artery and the outcome of failed reconstruction, *J Vasc Surg* 18:271–279, 1993.
26. Imparato AM, Bracco A, Kim GE: Comparison of three technics for femoral-popliteal arterial reconstruction, *Ann Surg* 177:375–380, 1973.
27. Mukherjee D, Inahara T: Endarterectomy as the procedure of choice for atherosclerotic occlusive lesions of the common femoral artery, *Am J Surg* 157:498–500, 1989.
28. Vercellio G, Castelli P, Coletti M et al: Semiclosed thromboendarterectomy on femoropopliteal-tract revisited after fourteen years experience on 595 cases, *Int Surg* 71:59–61, 1986.
29. Walker PM, Imparato AM, Riles TS et al: Long-term results in superficial femoral artery endarterectomy, *Surgery* 89:23–30, 1981.
30. Ouriel K, Smith CR, DeWeese JA: Endarterectomy for localized lesions of the superficial femoral artery at the adductor canal, *J Vasc Surg* 3:531–534, 1986.

31. Kouchoukos NT, Levy JF, Balfour MD et al: Operative therapy for femoral-popliteal arterial occlusive disease, *Circulation* 35(suppl I):174–182, 1967.
32. Abbott WM, Green RM, Matsomoto T et al: Prosthetic above-knee femoropopliteal bypasss grafting: results of a multicenter randomized prospective trial, *J Vasc Surg* 25:19–28, 1997.
33. Van der Heijden FHWM, Legemate DA, van Leeuwen MS et al: *Duplex scanning, ankle/brachial index and clinical symptoms to detect restenosis in the superficial femoral artery after endarterectomy*, Thesis, Universiteit Utrecht, 1994.
34. Taylor PR, Wolfe JHN, Tyrrell MR et al: Graft stenosis: justification for 1-year surveillance, *Br J Surg* 77:1125–1128, 1990.
35. Brücke, Lechner G, Piza F et al: Ursachen von früh- und spätverschlüssen nach Thromboendarteriektomie und Venenrekonstruktion im femoro-poplitealen Abschnitt, *Vasa* 2:24–27, 1973.
36. Idu MM, Blankenstein JD, de Gier P et al: Impact of a color-flow duplex surveillance program on infrainguinal vein graft patency: a five-year experience, *J Vasc Surg* 17:42–53, 1993.
37. Ho GH, Moll FL, Hedeman Joosten PPA et al: The Mollring Cutter remote endarterectomy: preliminary experience with a new endovascular technique for treatment of occlusive superficial femoral artery disease, *J Endovasc Surg* 2:278–287, 1995.
38. Cragg AH, Drake MD: Percutaneous femoropopliteal graft placement, *Radiology* 187:643–648, 1993.

21
Intravascular Stents

Vimal Murthy, Himanshu Shah, and Michael C. Dalsing

Percutaneous transluminal angioplasty (PTA) has become an accepted treatment for atherosclerotic arterial occlusive disease in properly selected patients. Delivery systems and balloon designs have matured over the last three decades, resulting in improved PTA results and fewer procedural complications.[1] However, this technique does have its limitations. Our personal experience with early technical failures and postprocedural restenosis forced a reevaluation of the technique and a consideration of methods that might improve results in areas of difficulty.[2,3] The use of supportive endoskeletons (stents), although suggested by Dotter during the late 1960s, was not pursued until the limitations of PTA were widely recognized.[4] Since the mid-1980s, various stent designs have been studied and clinical trials undertaken.

Indications for Stent Use

There were initially two situations where stent use was theoretically appealing. The primary indication was the potential salvage of an unacceptable angioplasty result. Among PTA attempts, 10% to 15% are early technical failures, but 25% to 50% of these involve cases in which a guidewire could be manipulated past the lesion but PTA could not maintain a functional channel.[2,3,5] Such cases might benefit from a device that could mechanically support the lumen until healing could take place. The underlying causes of early balloon failure are many.[1,2,5,6] The desired effect of an arterial balloon dilatation, a controlled dissection, can go awry resulting in a *spiral dissection* that narrows or occludes the lumen. The PTA may expose sufficient subintimal collagen to cause an *acute thrombosis* or *spasm* (or both) that, if sufficiently severe, predisposes the vessel to a similar event. One portion of the wall may be essentially normal, whereas the opposite wall is a hard atherosclerotic plaque. When PTA is attempted in such a case, the normal wall may easily expand but then quickly recoil once the intraluminal pressure exerted by the balloon is removed. This is called *elastic recoil*. Furthermore, any of these potential events may combine to result in an early technical failure. So long as a guidewire crosses the arterial narrowing, the procedure might be salvaged with an endoskeletal support (stent) to tack the dissection down or to maintain an intraluminal radial force sufficient to prevent elastic recoil, constrictive spasm, or constrictive thrombosis. In practice, a PTA failure is documented by a residual stenosis on angiography of 30% or more or a systolic pressure gradient at rest of 5 mm Hg or higher.

The other situation considered potentially amenable to stent use was an early PTA restenosis. Several factors, including site of stenosis, degree of narrowing, length of stenosis, and other patient factors, affect the incidence of PTA restenosis and generally occur within 6 months to 1 year of follow-up with a more gradual failure rate thereafter.[2,3,5,7–9] Restenosis can and does occur at the original site of PTA.[2,5,7] It can be caused by fibromuscular hyperplasia or rapid progression of the atherosclerotic process.[10] If a stent can prevent such rapid restenosis, its use would be ideal for this particular patient problem.

The primary use of stenting, rather than an attempt at PTA alone, has more recently been considered an option for the treatment of certain difficult clinical situations. It may be especially appropriate in the totally occluded artery where PTA results have been less than optimal owing to distal embolization and poor long-term patency rates.[5,7,9,11] Localized ulcerative plaques, thought to be a source of emboli, may also be appropriate lesions for primary stent placement to prevent dislodgment of plaque debris during PTA. Furthermore, when used intraoperatively in conjunction with a planned distal bypass, it might provide the hemodynamic support thought beneficial for maintaining inflow patency while outflow is being reconstructed.[12] Others have considered primary stent use as a plausible option for all PTA attempts if it can be proven to improve long-term patency rates without increased risk.

Stent Designs

A number of stent designs have been proposed; some have been studied only experimentally, but others have made their way into clinical trials.[13–15] A few have made a significant clinical impact in the peripheral arterial system. Still others proposed mainly for coronary use are currently under investigation for peripheral use. These designs have included the use of absorbable construction materials, antiproliferative coatings, removable designs, and other inventive concepts that may ultimately materialize into usable stents.[16–19] Currently there are two types of stent suitable for clinical use that are distinguished by the method of deployment: balloon-expandable and self-expanding. The balloon-expandable Palmaz stent and self-expanding Wallstent are both approved by the US Food and Drug Administration (FDA) for intraarterial use but only in the iliac arterial system. However, their clinical use in many other areas of the arterial tree is well accepted and has become standard practice.

The Palmaz balloon-expandable stent is a simple stainless steel tube that is available in various diameters and lengths (Figure 21–1).

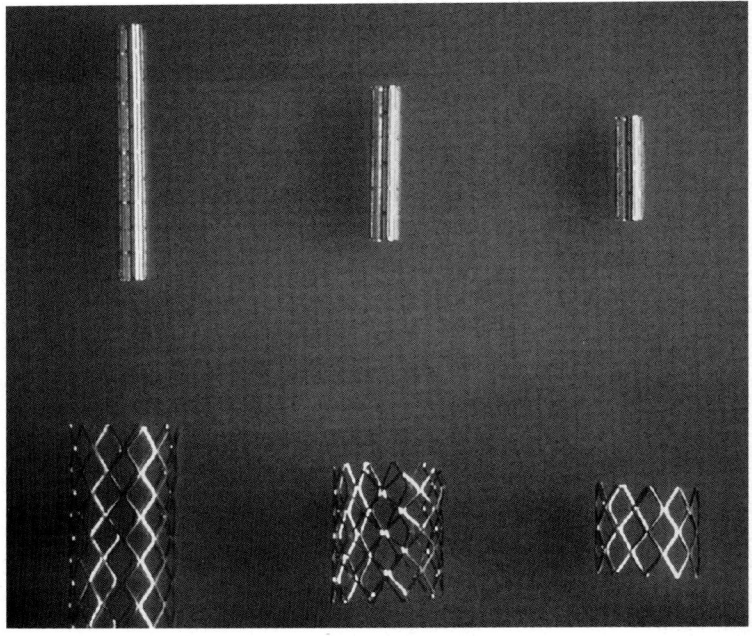

FIGURE 21–1. Various diameters and lengths of the commercially available Palmaz stent demonstrating the collapsed and expanded conditions. Note the staggered slits in the collapsed version, which allow expansion when a PTA balloon is dilated within the stent lumen.

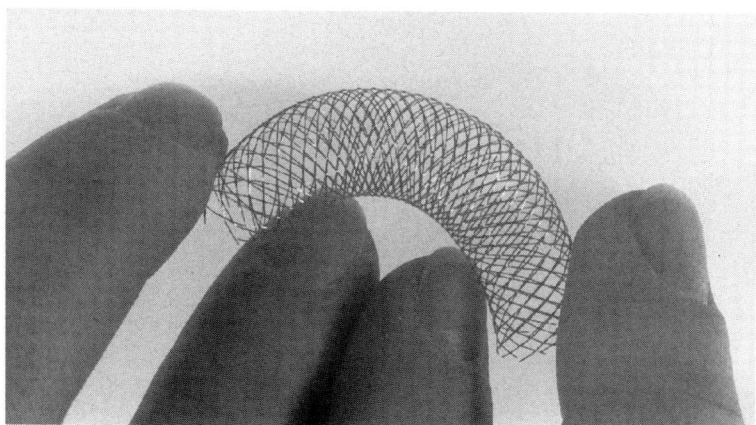

FIGURE 21–2. Wallstent demonstrating the braided filament design and flexibility of the stent.

The walls are etched into multiple rows of staggered rectangles that, like a split-thickness skin graft, allow expansion to a larger area or, in this case, diameter when dilated (Figure 21–1) (Johnson and Johnson, Interventional Systems, Warren, NJ). Its wall thickness is in the 0.12-mm range. It can be obtained from the manufacturer premounted on a balloon or alone in a sterile vial, which can then be placed on a variety of balloon catheters. Most stents are available in a wide variety of lengths up to 3 cm and may be dilated to a recommended diameter of 12 mm. The stent may be overdilated if necessary. The small stents can be delivered through a 7F sheath, whereas larger ones require a 10F delivery port. The Palmaz-Schatz long medium stent (available in lengths of 4.2 to 7.8 cm) has shown promise for eliminating the need to implant multiple overlapping stents for coverage of long lesions. What the Palmaz stent provides in terms of excellent resistance to radial recoil, it relinquishes in overall flexibility. Its biocompatibility, general ease of delivery, and reliable expansion without migration were proven in early experimental studies.[20] Intimal thickening after placement of this stent was observed in this experimental model (approximately 100 μm at 6 months) but was a much more gradual process after the initial 2 months of follow-up.[20]

The Wallstent (Schneider Peripheral Division, Minneapolis, MN) is made of 16 to 20 surgical-grade stainless steel alloy filaments braided into a flexible tubular structure (Figure 21–2). The filament's diameter can range from 0.075 to 0.170 mm, providing a thin-walled device, Because the filaments are bound together only at the ends, there is great accommodation for flexibility in all directions. The stent is manufactured in various lengths from 2.0 to 9.4 cm and diameters ranging from 5 to 24 mm. The stents commonly used in the iliac arterial system are deployed through a 7F to 8F sheath. What the Wallstent sacrifices in radial strength is compensated for by its flexibility and the ability to accommodate bends in the arterial lumen. Its biocompatibility is similar to that of all stainless steel devices and incites an intimal response with some thickening of the lumen wall.[21,22]

Another balloon-expandable device (Strecker; Meditech, Watertown, Ma) made of tantalum, a radiopaque material, has more flexibility than the Palmaz stent but less radial strength and therefore is more like the Wallstent in that aspect of its design. A third type of balloon-expandable stent is too small in diameter for practical use in the large artery peripheral vascular system (e.g., Gianturco Roubin Stent; Cook, Bloomington, In).[23] The Gianturco (Z-stent) (Cook), a unique zigzag configuration of bent stainless steel wire (Figure 21–3), is still under investigation. The new nitinol Symphony Stent (Boston Scientific, Natick, MA) is flexible and easy to deploy but has yet to be approved for clinical use in the arterial system. Nitinol stents made of a nickel-titanium alloy with thermal memory have been approved for

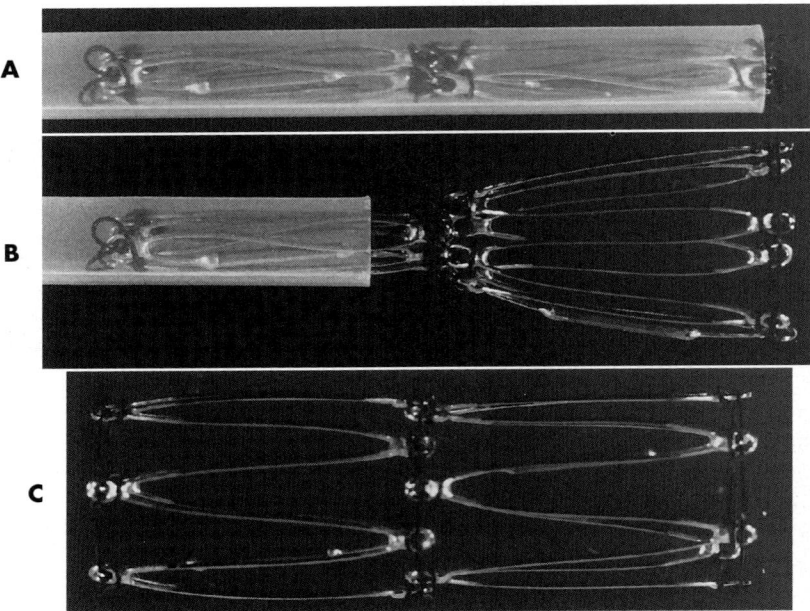

FIGURE 21–3. Gianturco stent used in the biliary system presented here to demonstrate the design of the stent (**C**) and how it expands from a sheath (**A–C**). A variation on this design has been used clinically in the arterial system in Japan.

biliary but not arterial use (e.g., Memotherm; Bard Radiology, Covington, GA).

Stent Deployment

Palmaz Stent Deployment

The common femoral artery is most often used for arterial access, utilizing either the Seldinger technique or an arterial cutdown. The vessel of importance is often the ipsilateral iliac artery, but any vessel accessible by a guidewire and that allows placement of the rather stiff stent/sheath arrangement could be a candidate for Palmaz stent placement. In those cases where prior PTA was attempted (Figure 21–4A,B), the balloon angioplasty catheter is removed while maintaining the guidewire access across the lesion. In cases where primary stenting is planned, predilatation of the lesion is performed and the balloon removed over an exchange-length wire. A vascular sheath of appropriate length and diameter is placed so the sheath crosses the lesion and is of sufficient size to accommodate the desired stent-balloon combination (7F to 10F) (Figure 21–4C). A stainless steel introducer device (Johnson and Johnson, Interventional Systems) is placed over the wire and through the hemostatic valve of the sheath to protect the stent as it is advanced through the sheath (Figure 21–4D). As soon as the stent is placed through the valve, the introducer is withdrawn from the sheath to prevent excessive blood loss. A premounted stent-balloon assembly may be used, or stents may be crimped onto the balloon catheter using a crimping tool or by hand compression. Care must be taken to ensure that the stent is securely affixed to the balloon catheter without tearing the fragile balloon material. The stent-balloon assembly is then advanced through the sheath under fluoroscopy in juxtaposition to the target lesion (Figure 21–4E). When the stent is in position, the sheath is retracted to fully expose the stent-balloon assembly. The balloon is inflated to a diameter slightly larger than the optimal luminal diameter as measured by arteriography (Figure 21–4F).

21. Intravascular Stents

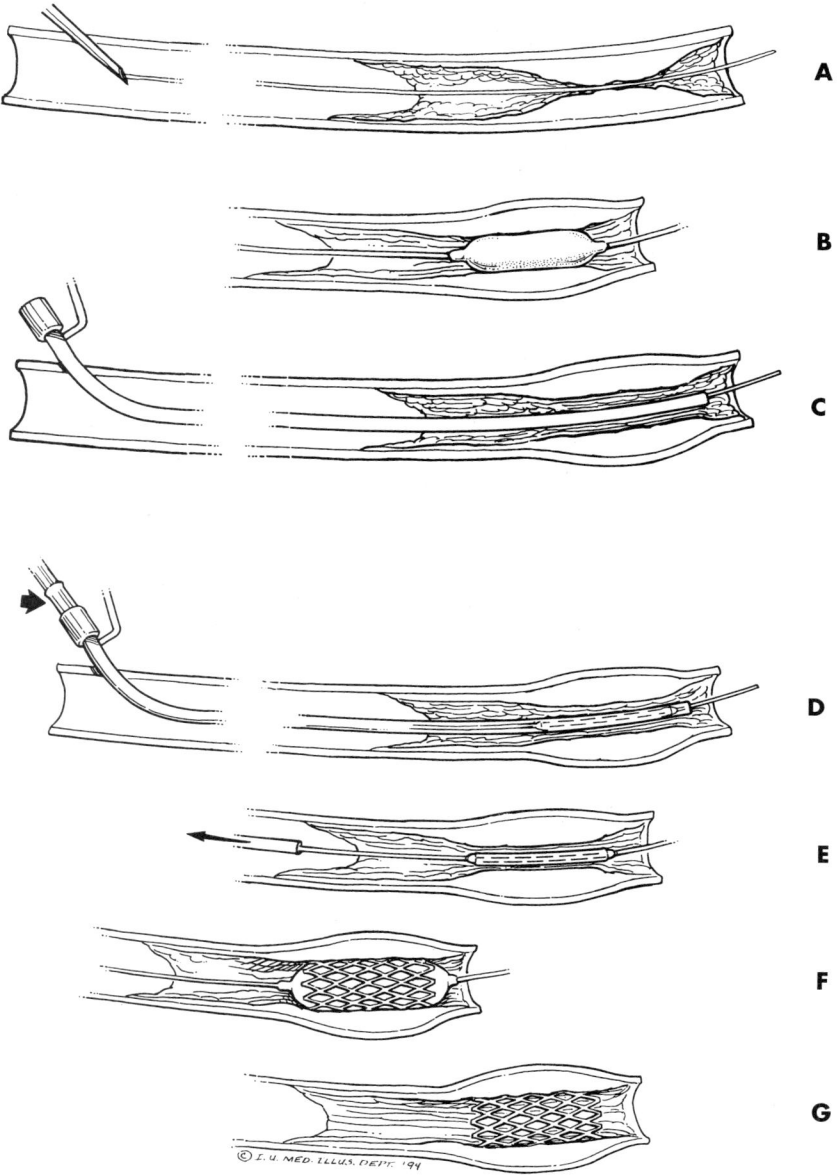

FIGURE 21–4. Technique used for placement of a Palmaz balloon-expandable stent. Access is obtained (**A**) and a PTA attempted (**B**), but in this case it did not maintain an acceptable lumen. Balloon catheter is removed, and an introducer and sheath of size sufficient for the balloon-stent assembly is placed (**C**). Specially designed metallic tube (*arrow in* **D**) allows placement of the balloon-stent assembly without dislodgement of the latter. Assembly is positioned adjacent to the vessel narrowing (**E**), and the sheath is retracted. Balloon is inflated, driving the stent into its location against the vessel wall (**F**). Stent is often deliberately embedded into the atherosclerotic plaque to hasten the process of endothelial coverage (**G**).

Figure 21–5 chronicles a case to highlight points of the technique required to provide an optimal result. After adequate stent deployment, the balloon is deflated, gently rotated to make sure the stent is free of the balloon, and removed. Overlapping sequential stents may be placed to accommodate longer areas of stenosis by simply repeating the above steps. Finally,

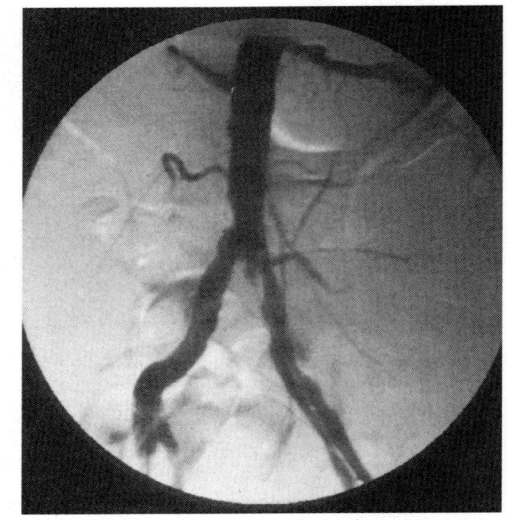

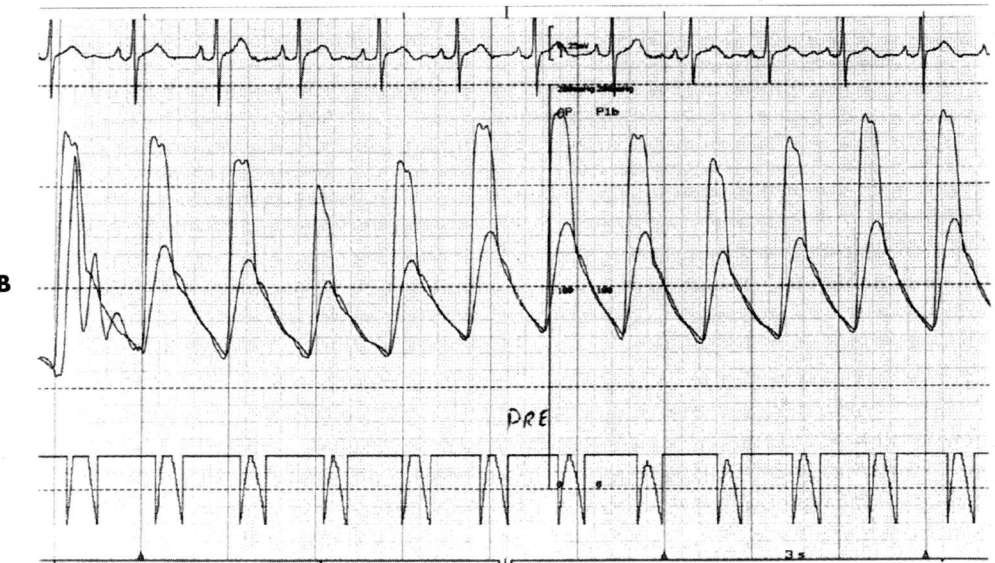

FIGURE 21-5. This patient presented 2 months after a failed left common iliac artery angioplasty with left thigh and buttock claudication at 100 steps. An arteriogram demonstrated an eccentric left common iliac artery stenosis (**A**) with a 62 mm Hg gradient at rest (**B**). A 9F sheath was advanced across the lesion, and a 308 Palmaz stent on an 8-mm balloon was advanced across the area of stenosis (**C**) and centered using guidance from an aortic catheter placed from the contralateral side (**C, D**). The sheath was pulled below the lesion and the stent deployed to 8 mm (**F, G**). An arteriogram showed that the stent was centered well but not embedded in the vessel wall (**H**). Pressure measurements demonstrated a 3 mm Hg residual gradient (**I**). After dilating the stent to 10 mm, there is good apposition of the stent to the iliac artery wall (**J**) and no residual gradient after Priscoline challenge (**K**).

if the percutaneous approach is used, the sheath and guidewire are removed, and the puncture site is compressed to prevent hemorrhage. If the cutdown method is used, vessel closure or distal reconstruction is now completed and the wound is closed. Many patients are placed on 325 mg of acetyl salicylic acid (ASA) daily after the procedure and are maintained on this

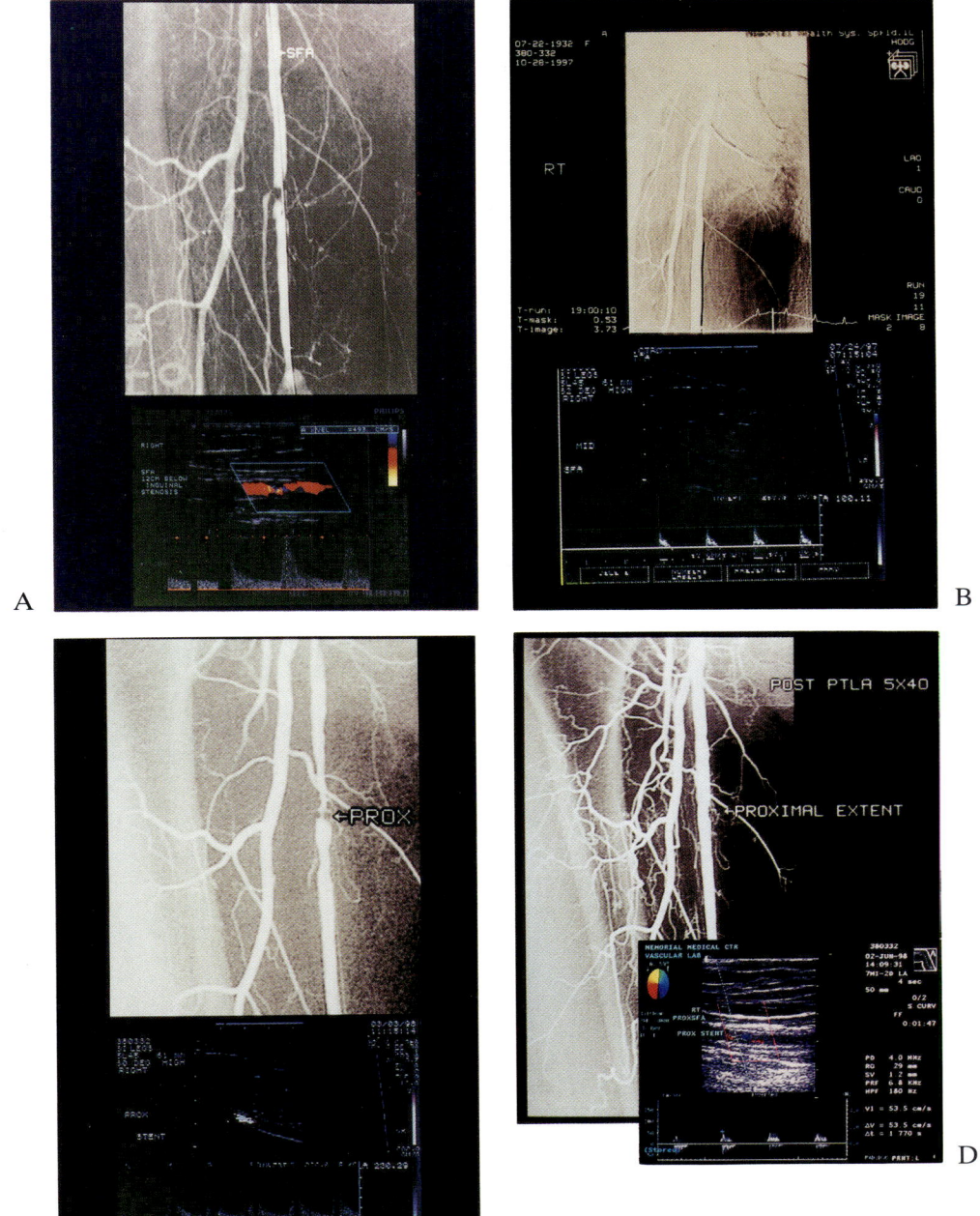

FIGURE 8–1. **A**, Angiogram and corresponding color-flow duplex scan of a high grade stenosis of the superficial femoral artery (*SFA*) proximal to the origin of an SFA–popliteal bypass graft detected on routine graft surveillance. Peak systolic velocity within the stenosis measured 493 cm/s. **B**, After PTA and Wallstent treatment of the SFA stenosis with a successful anatomic result shown by angiography and color-flow duplex scanning, which revealed a peak systolic velocity of 100 cm/s in the stented region. **C**, Stenosis of the SFA just proximal to the previously treated region detected at 8 months by a color-flow duplex scan, revealing peak systolic velocities of 230 cm/s. **D**, Early identification of the graft-threatening SFA stenosis allowed treatment with balloon angioplasty, with an excellent angiographic result. It maintained patency of the bypass graft without recurrent stenosis, seen by color-flow duplex scanning at 3 months.

Color Plate

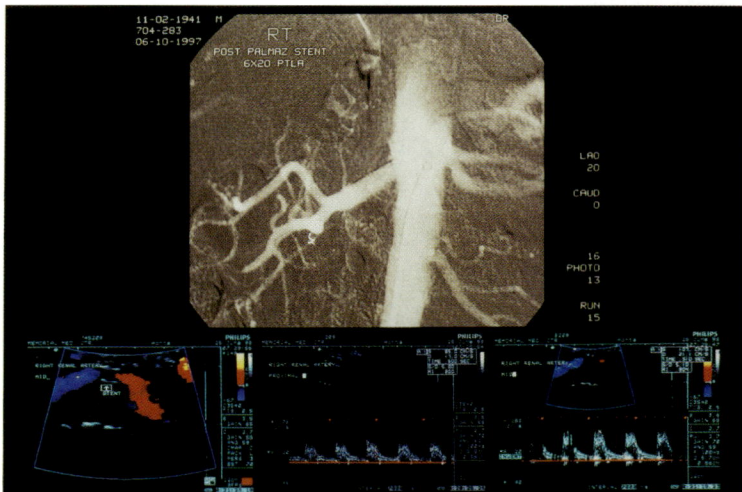

FIGURE 8–2. **B**, After angioplasty and Palmaz stenting with an excellent angiographic result. Subsequent color-flow duplex scanning at 1 year demonstrates continued anatomic success with no elevation of flow velocity in the renal artery.

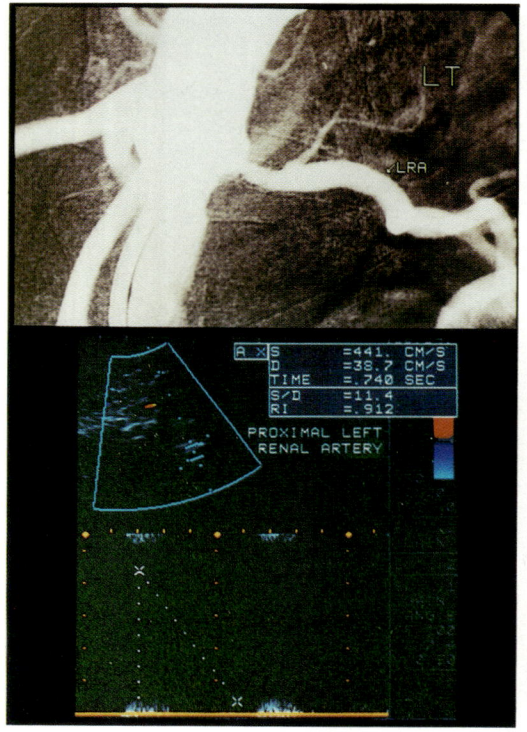

A

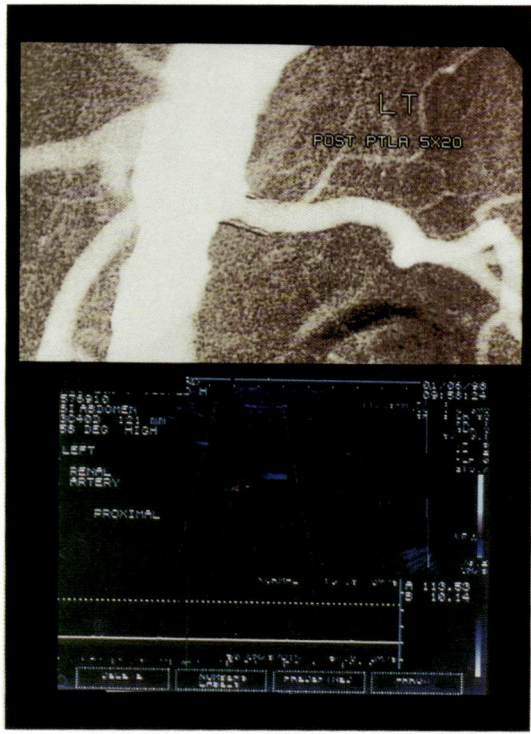

B

FIGURE 8–3. **A**, Surveillance color-duplex scanning of a dilated and stented left renal artery (*LRA*) revealed peak systolic velocities of 441 cm/s. Neointimal hyperplasia is apparent within the stent. **B**, Although complete recanalization of the left renal artery could not be achieved, leaving a 20% residual stenosis, the subsequent velocity dropped to 113 cm/s.

Color Plate

FIGURE 8–4. **C**, Color-flow duplex Doppler evaluation of the bifurcated region of an endograft demonstrating continued patency without apparent flow signals outside the endograft.

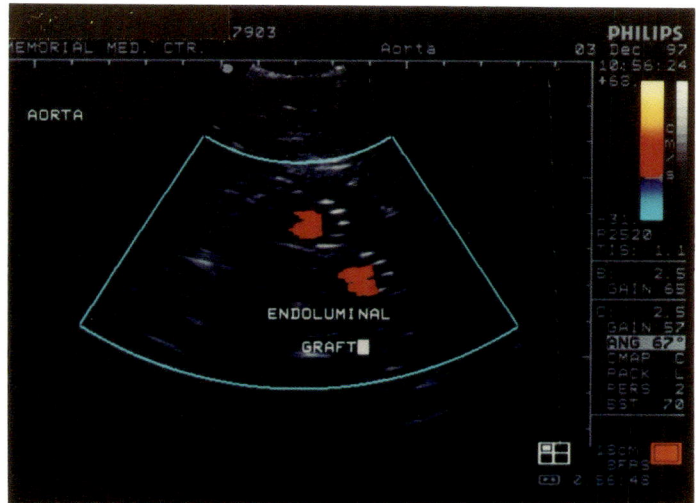

FIGURE 8–6. **B**, Three-dimensional CT reconstruction indicates that the source of the endoleak is the endograft–iliac artery junction (*arrow*).

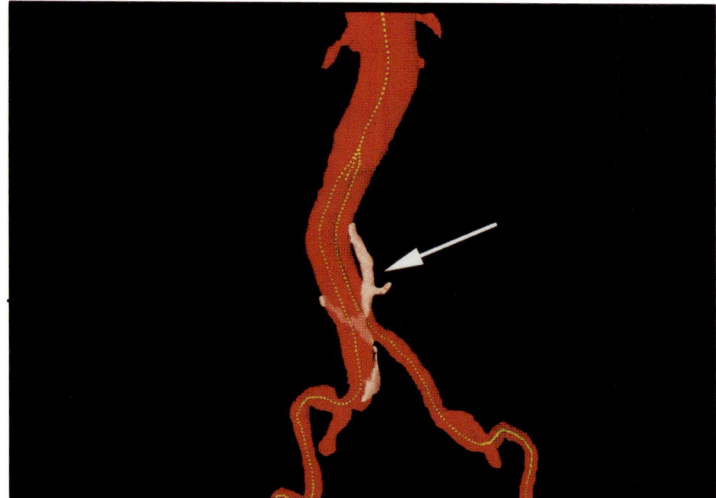

FIGURE 8–7. Color-flow duplex scan reveals flow outside the confines of an endograft, indicating the presence of an endoleak.

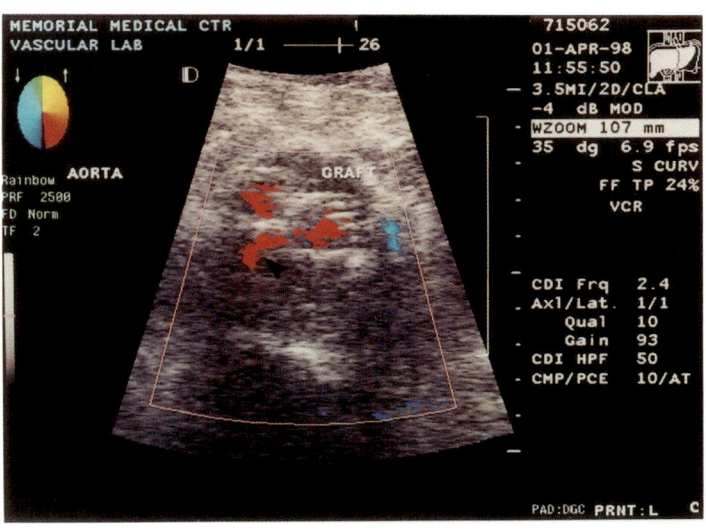

Color Plate

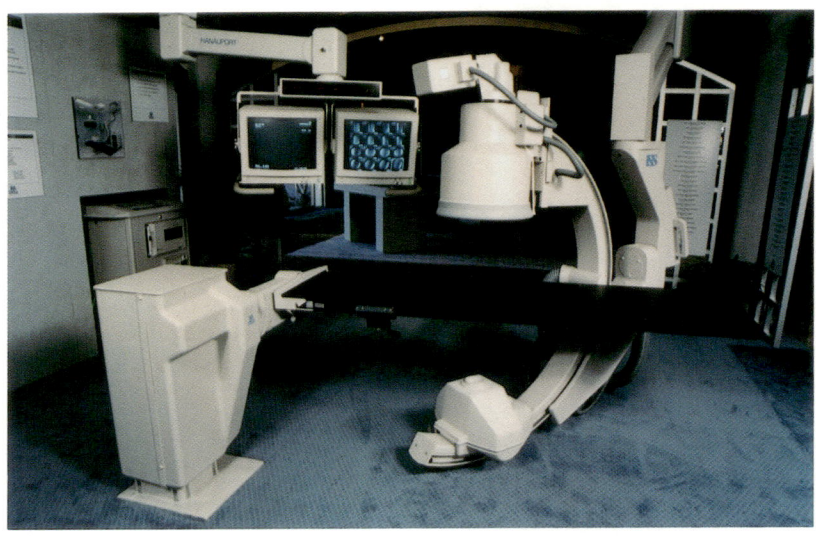

FIGURE 10–2. International Surgical Systems fixed C-arm imaging system. This system provides maximum flexibility for the operator and permits high quality imaging during complex endovascular procedures.

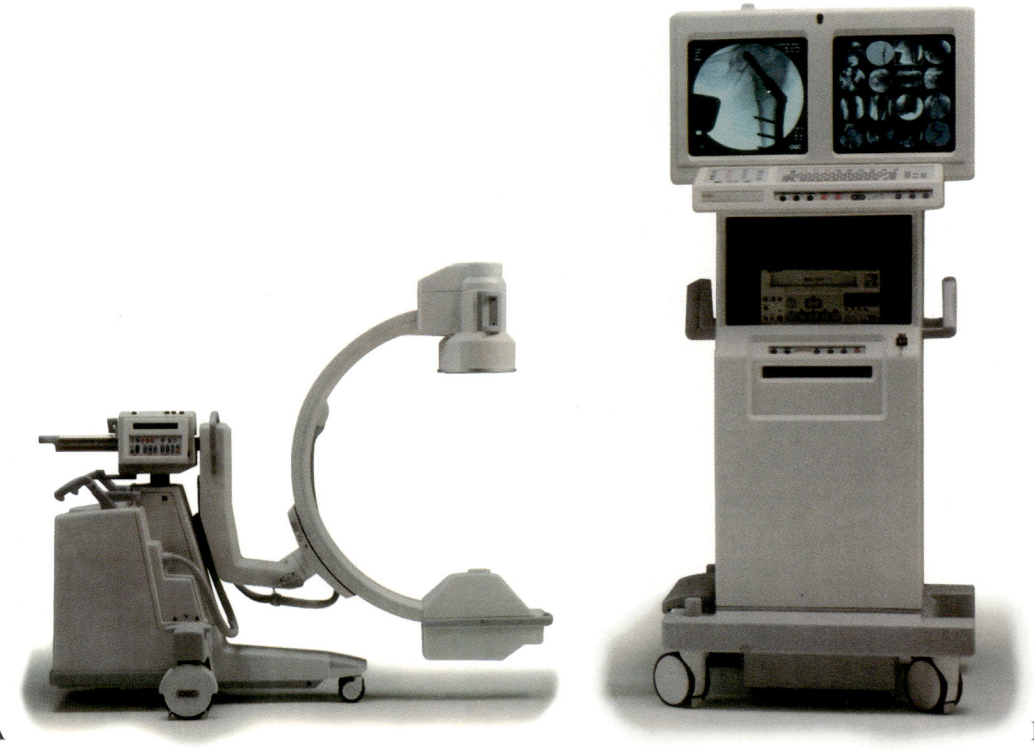

A B

FIGURE 10–3. **A**, **B**, Popular mobile imaging system distributed by OMC. The unit is often used by various specialists, whereas fixed units are frequently dedicated to use by the vascular specialist.

Color Plate

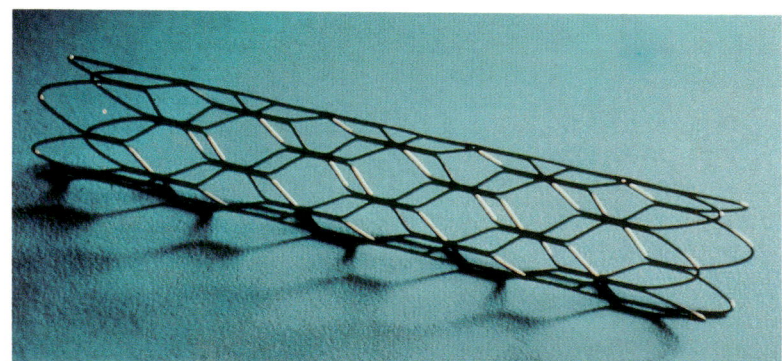

FIGURE 10–6. Symphony stent, a nitinol stent from Boston Scientific/Meadox. The flexibility of the stent makes it ideal for arterial use but it is not yet approved by the US Food and Drug Administration for arterial locations. (Courtesy of Medi-tech/Boston Scientific Corporation, Natic, MA.)

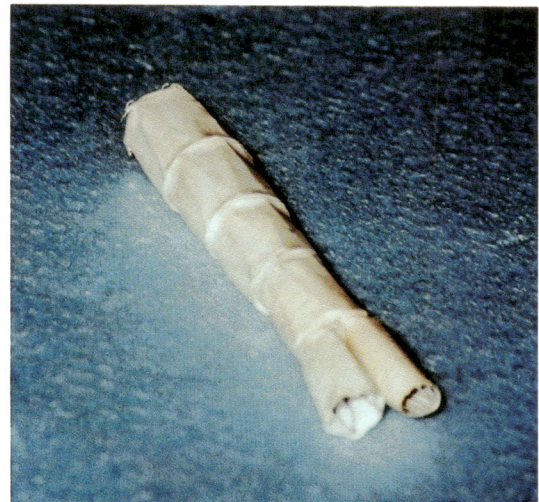

FIGURE 10–7. Prototype single-stage, bifurcated endoluminal graft (ELG). In the future, multiple ELG designs will become available, and the endovascular suite must be designed to accommodate this advancing technology.

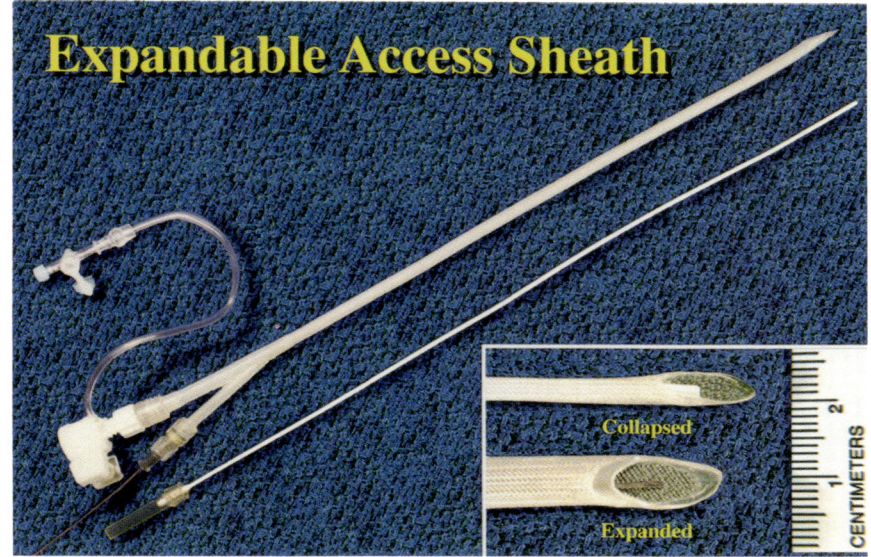

FIGURE 19–10. Variable-diameter sheath allows percutaneous thrombectomy. **Inset**, enlarged detail of the tip.

Color Plate

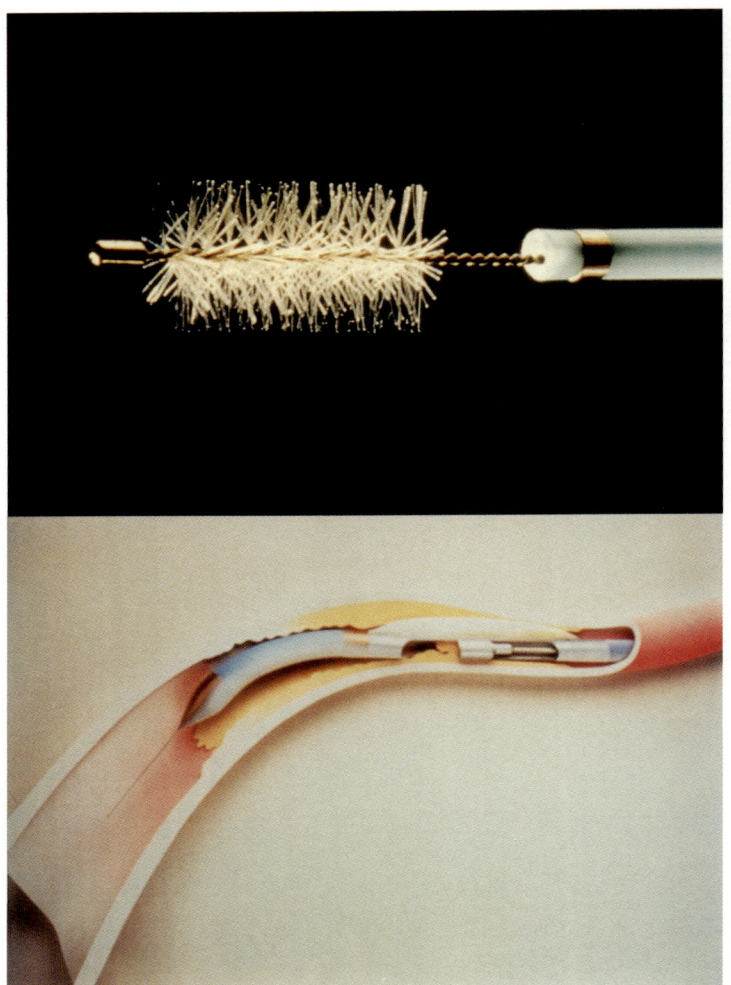

FIGURE 19–11. Two examples of nonrecirculation thrombectomy devices. **Top**, Cragg Thrombolytic Brush (Micro Therapeutics, Aliso Veijo, CA). **Bottom**, Simpson Atherotrac device (Mallinckrodt Medical, St. Louis, MO). Both devices operate by essentially scraping or cutting atheroma from vessel walls and removing it via percutaneous access site.

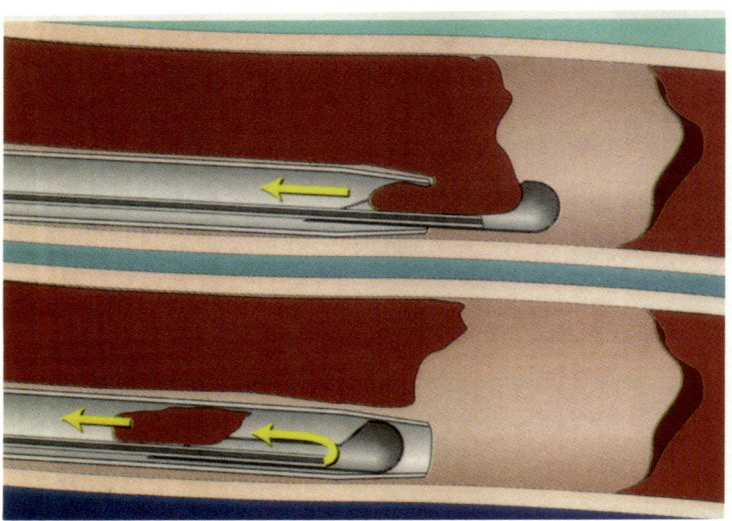

FIGURE 19–12. Gelbfish Endo Vac Device (Neovascular Technologies, Brooklyn, NY) performs thrombectomy by combining thrombus maceration, utilizing a reciprocating "clot spoon", with simultaneous or concomitant suction.

Color Plate

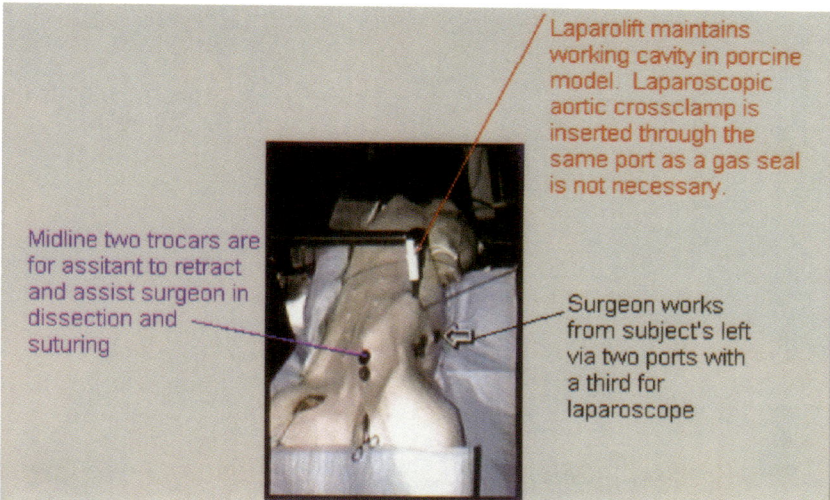

FIGURE 34–1. Porcine model as described by Dion and Gracia[24] depicting the ability to work in the retroperitoneum with the subject supine. This is in contrast to previous reported models of retroperitoneal exposure requiring the subject to be lateral. The latter is not ideal for vascular bypass, as it does not allow simultaneous access to groins and proximal aortic control.

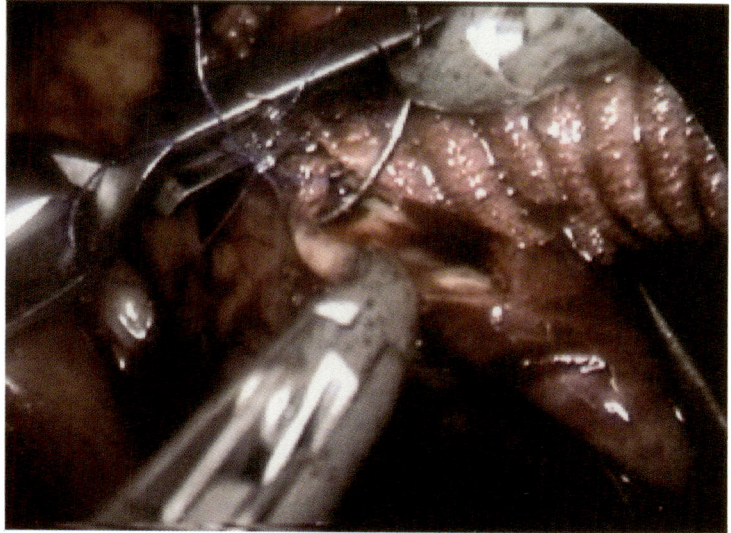

FIGURE 34–2. Laparoscopic view of intracorporeal suturing to anastomose the right common iliac artery to a prosthetic Dacron graft for a right iliofemoral bypass graft. This type of bypass could be performed via an entirely retroperitoneal dissection and space. When applied to the infrarenal aorta, this approach becomes more problematic without a peritoneal "apron."

Color Plate

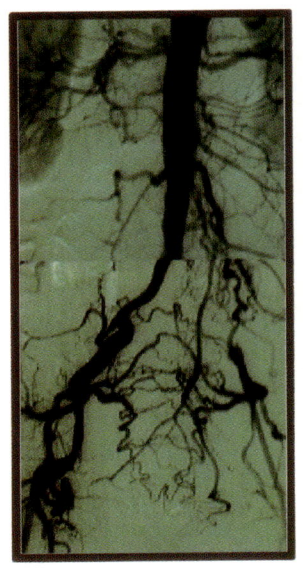
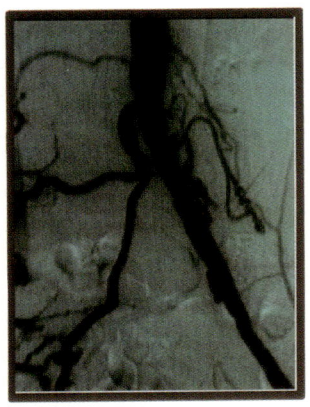

FIGURE 34–3. Preoperative arteriograms of patients with aortoiliac occlusive disease. **A**, A 61-year-old woman had diffuse bilateral iliac disease of both external and internal iliac arteries. **B**, A 57-year-old male patient had an occluded right iliac system and contralateral disease. **C-1**, A 61-year-old man had bilateral common iliac artery stenosis. **C-2**, Same patient after successful placement of bilateral common iliac artery stents following angioplasty. **C-3**, Same patient about 14 months after stent placement with recurrent disease and symptoms. He elected to not have any further endoluminal procedures but to have aortobifemoral bypass. A laparoscopic approach was then discussed with the patient.

A

B

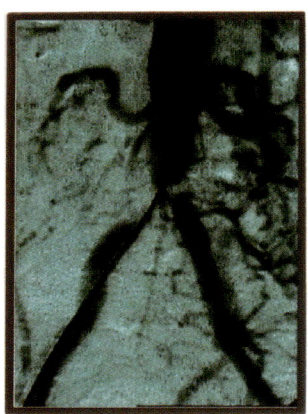
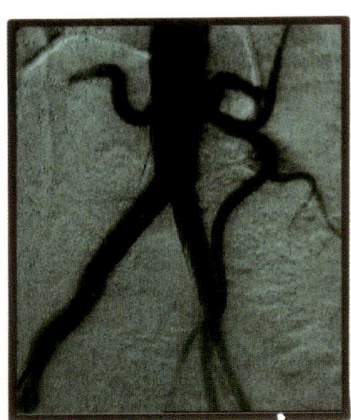
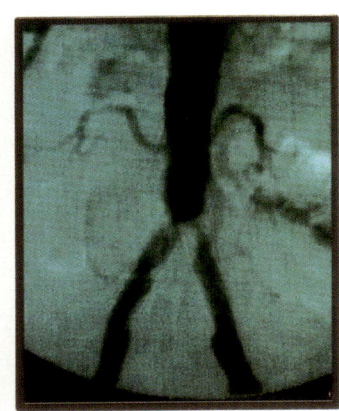

C1

C2, 3

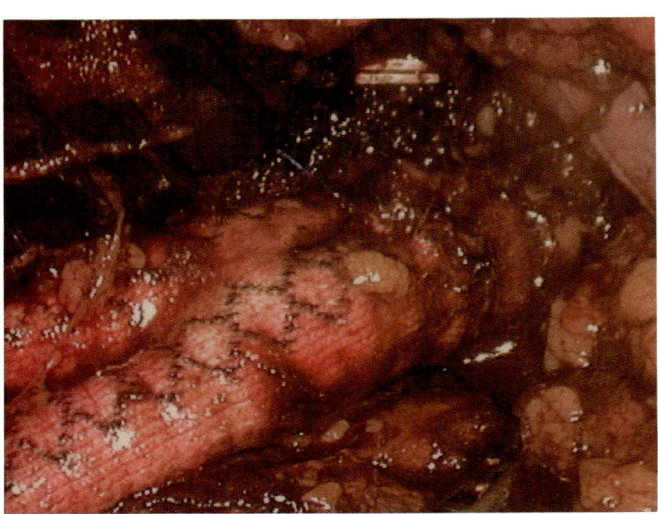

FIGURE 34–4. Laparoscopic view of the aortoprosthetic anastomosis completed in end-to-end fashion.

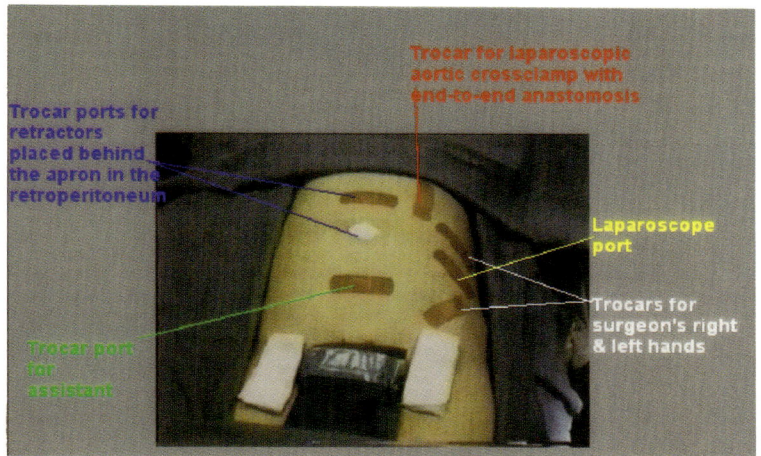

FIGURE 34–5. Patient position with identification of trocar sites for totally laparoscopic aortobifemoral bypass, not requiring minilaparotomy. If minilaparotomy were necessary, connecting the two superior midline trocars (in blue) would provide ready access to the retroperitoneum with the use of renal vein retractors. They are placed behind the retroperitoneal "apron" facilitating exposure of the infrarenal arorta up to the renal vein without difficulty from the small intestine.

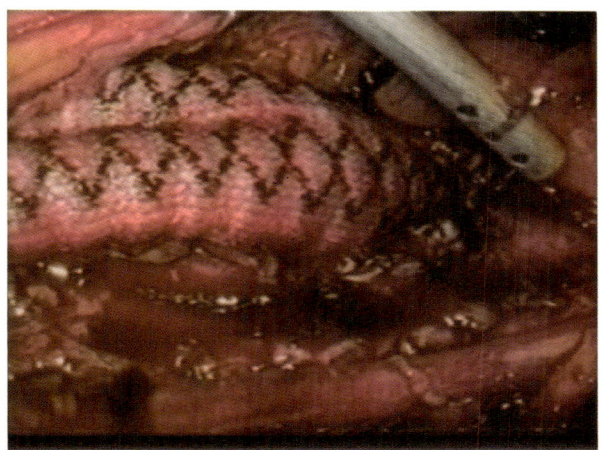

FIGURE 34–6. Laparoscopic view of the aortoprosthetic anastomosis completed in end-to-side fashion.

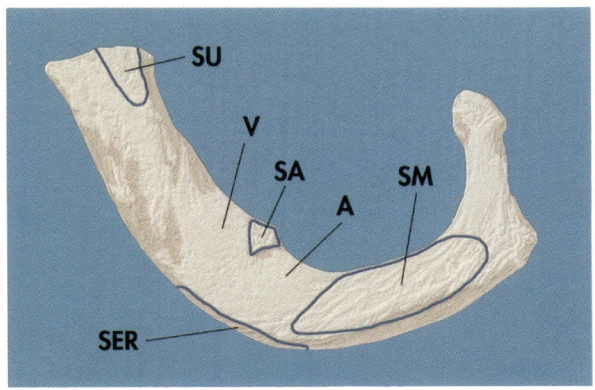

FIGURE 36–1. The left first rib shows its muscular insertions. *SU*, subclavius; *V*, venous space; *SA*, scalenus anterior; *A*, arterial space; *SER*, serratus anterior; *SM*, scalenus medius.

Color Plate

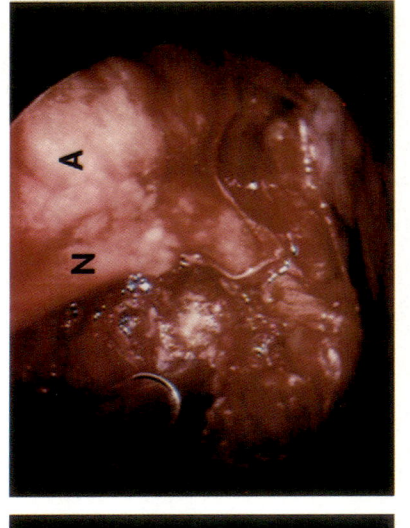

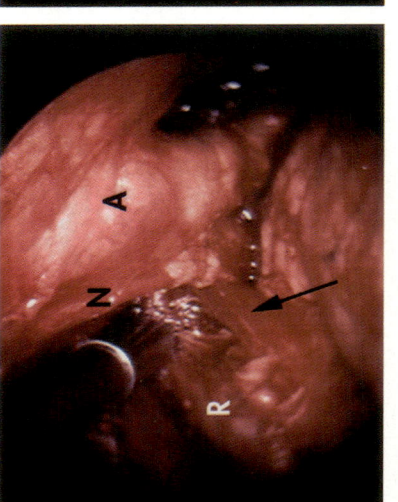

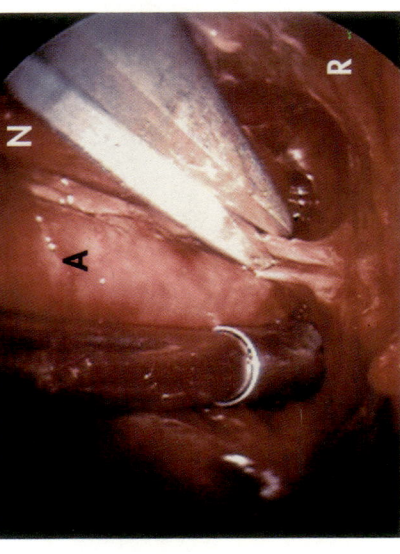

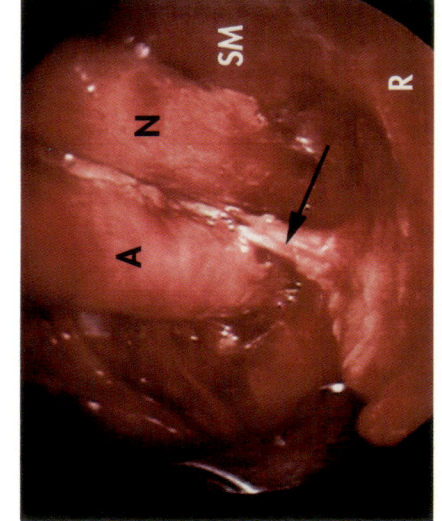

FIGURE 36–2. Right transaxillary approach. *Arrow* shows area of the compression of the nerve by a type 3 band. *SM*, scalenus medius; *N*, nerve; *A*, artery; *R*, rib; *SA*, scalenus anterior; *V*, vein.

FIGURE 36–3. Right transaxillary approach. *Arrow* shows type 3 band and compression to the nerve. The suction device shows the first rib. *N*, nerve; *A*, artery; *R*, rib.

FIGURE 36–4. Completion of the transaxillary first rib resection. Suction device shows cartilaginous surface of the transverse process of thoracic I vertebra. *N*, nerve; *A*, artery.

FIGURE 36–5. Left transaxillary approach. *Arrow* shows type 5 band between the artery and the nerve. *A*, artery; *N*, nerve; *SM*, scalenus medius; *R*, rib.

FIGURE 36–6. Left transaxillary approach. Scissor is cutting a type 5 band. *A*, artery; *N*, nerve; *R*, rib.

Color Plate

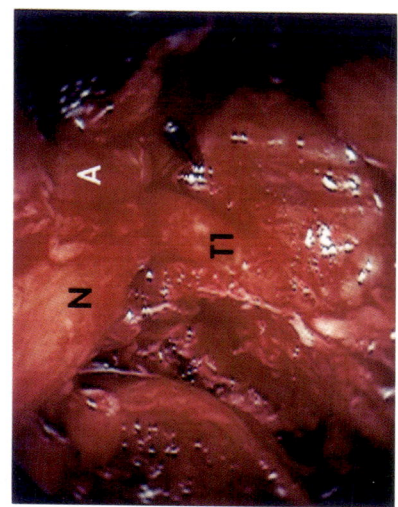

FIGURE 36–7. Right transaxillary approach. *Arrow* shows critical compression of the nerve and the artery by a type 4 band. *N*, nerve; *A*, artery; *SM*, scalenus medius; *SA*, scalenus anterior; *R*, rib.

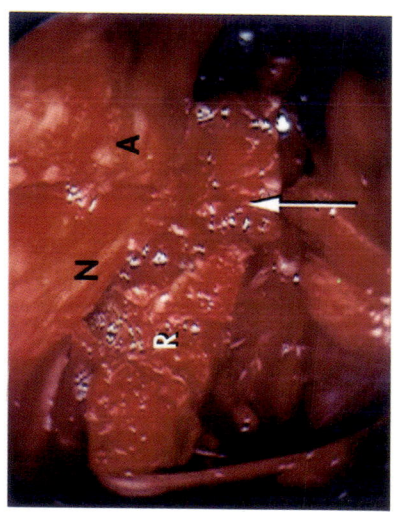

FIGURE 36–8. Right transaxillary approach. Anterior and middle third of the first rib is already excised. *Arrow* shows that abundant muscle fibers (type 4) are still compressing the nerve and artery. *R*, rib; *N*, nerve; *A*, artery.

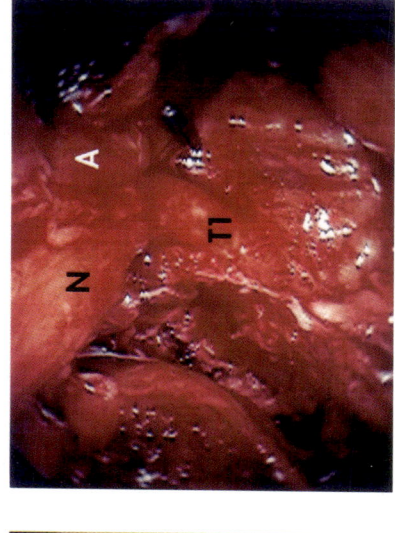

FIGURE 36–9. Completed right first rib resection. The nerve and the artery are decompressed. *N*, nerve; *T1*, lower branch of brachial plexus; *A*, artery.

Color Plate

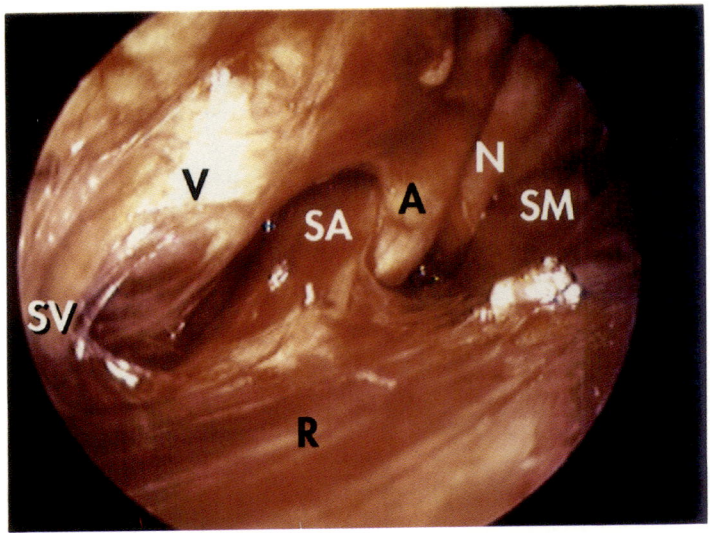

FIGURE 36–10. Left transaxillary approach, overall view. SV, subclavius; V, vein; SA, scalenus anterior; A, artery; N, nerve; SM, scalenus medius; R, rib.

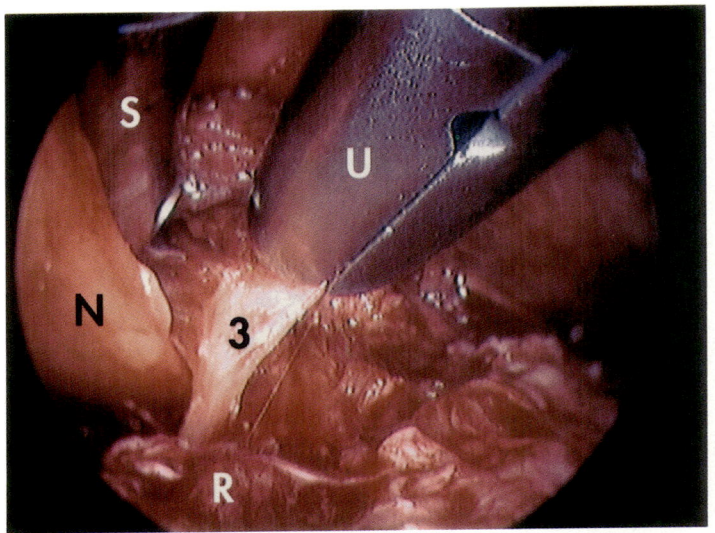

FIGURE 36–12. Left transaxillary approach. Urschel instrument is excising residual muscular fibers of a type 3 band in close proximity to the nerve. N, nerve; U, Urschel rongeur; 3, type 3 residual fibers; S, suction device; R, rib.

Color Plate

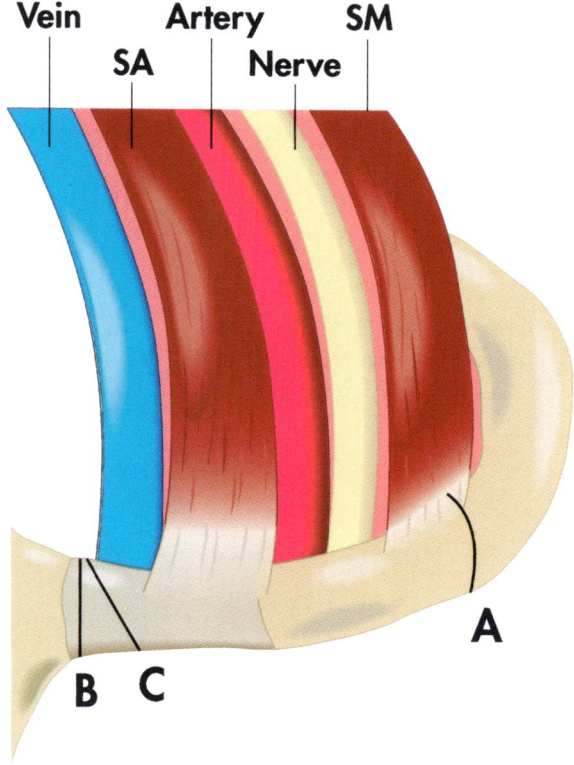

FIGURE 36–13. Left transaxillary first rib resection. Placement of the rib cutter instrument: *A*, posterior to the nerve; *B*, anterior to the vein; *C*, wedge diagonal cut to ensure a safe margin toward the vein. *SA*, scalenus anterior; *SM*, scalenus medius.

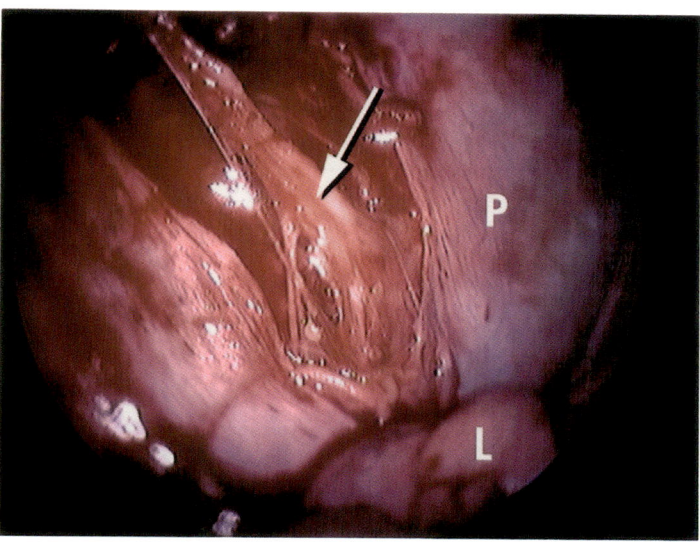

FIGURE 36–14. Left endoscopic thoracodorsal sympathectomy view. *Arrow* indicates thoracic ganglia (T2). *P*, pleura; *L*, lung.

Color Plate

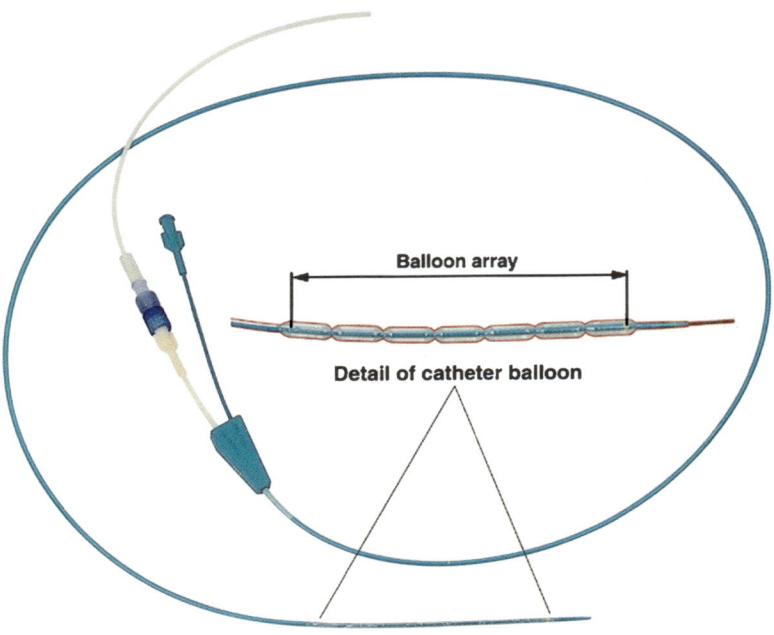

FIGURE 38–2. Centering balloon catheter from Nucletron.

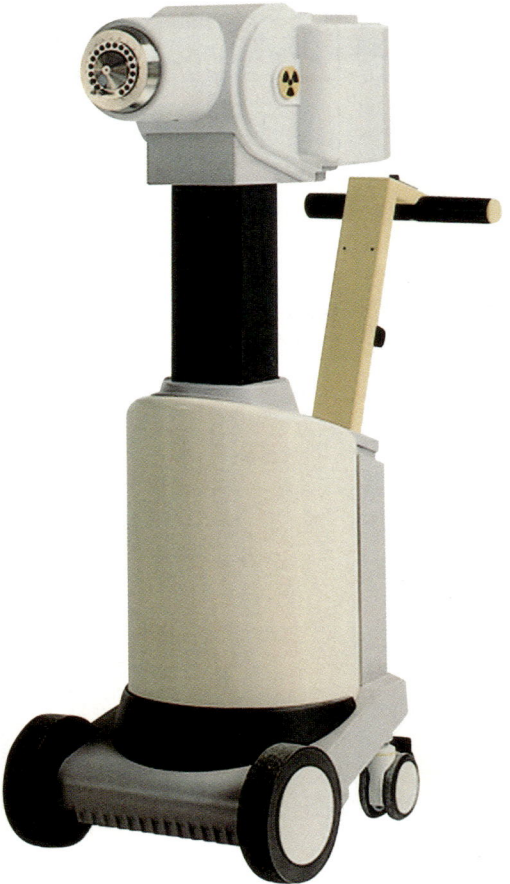

FIGURE 38–5. Nucletron HDR afterloader.

Color Plate

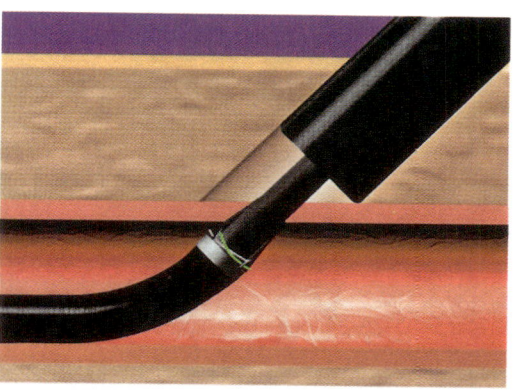

Figure 40–1. Correct position of the device prevents bleeding by occlusion of the puncture orifice.

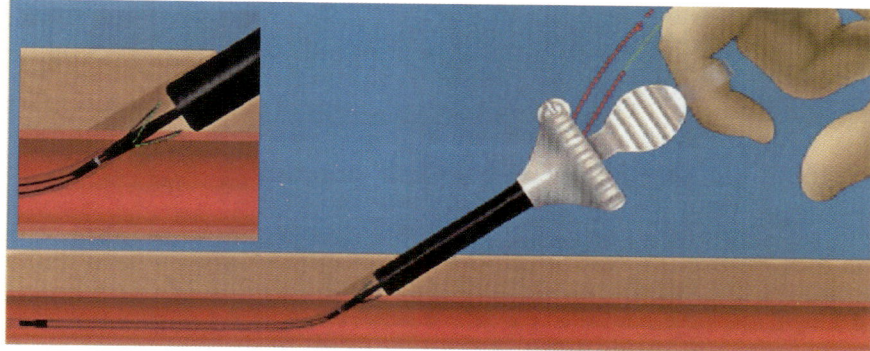

Figure 40–2. Confirm that the Interlocks are reengaged and correctly aligned with the locking indents in the hub. Then, unlock the pull handle (90° counterclockwise) and pull the needles fully back. Pull the first few millimeters very slowly.

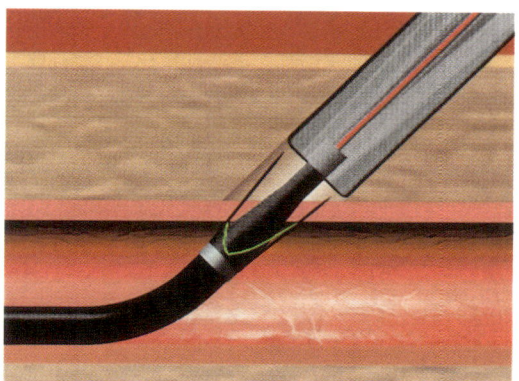

Figure 40–3. Backbleeding via the marker port confirms that needle tips will correctly puncture the arterial wall from within.

Color Plate

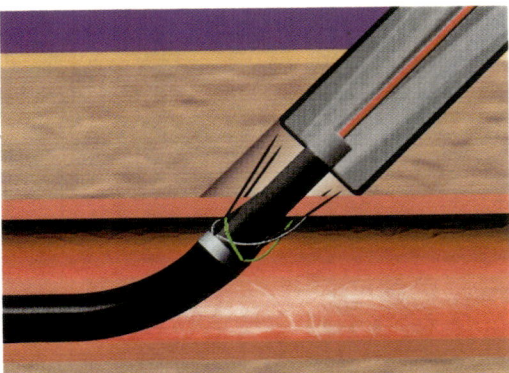

Figure 40–4. Needle tips carry sutures through the vascular wall. They also puncture the wall at a precisely controlled distance from the of orifice edge.

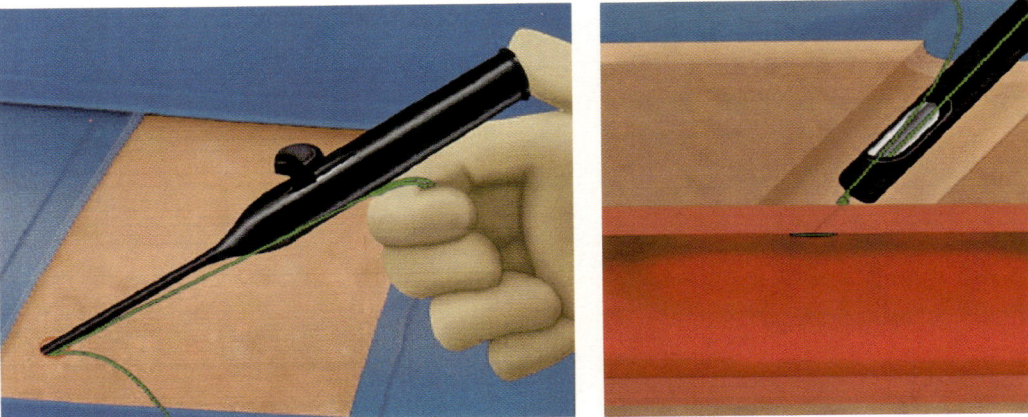

Figure 40–5. (A) To avoid an "air knot," apply tension to the suture while advancing the knot. (B) Tension must be applied to remove slack in the suture while advancing the knot.

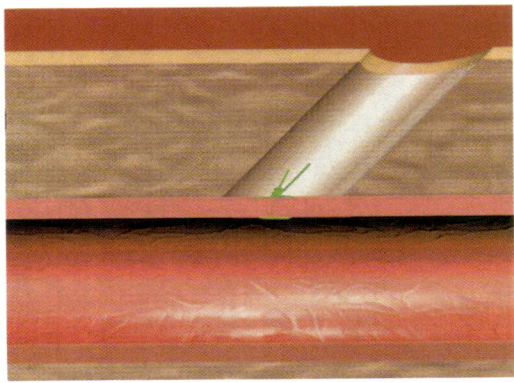

Figure 40–6. Completed knot resulting in secure closure of the vascular puncture orifice. The suture each are trimmed close to the knot allowing minimal residual material.

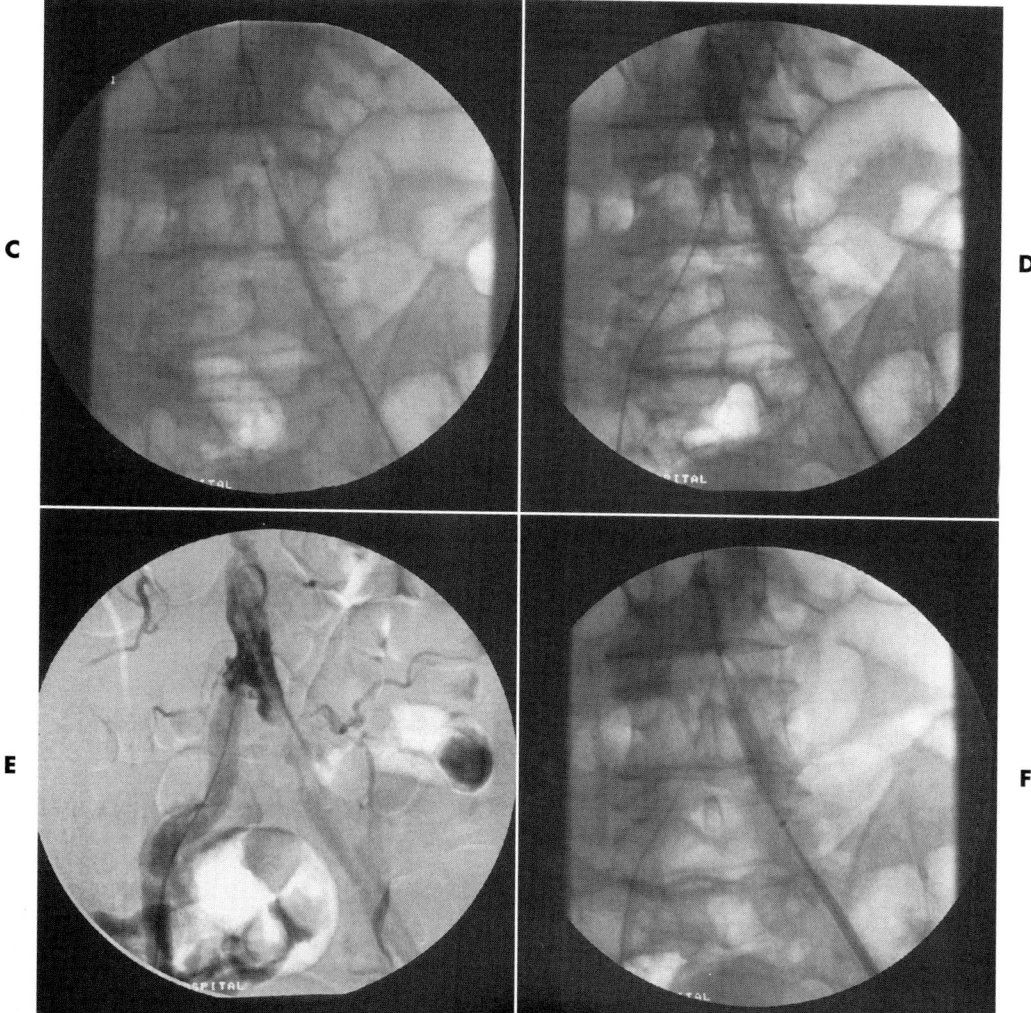

FIGURE 21–5. *Continued.*

medication for at least 3 months. The use of intraprocedural heparin is not uniform. Generally, the patient is heparinized [about 100 units/kg to result in an activated clotting time (ACT) of 200 or greater] when crossing iliac occlusions or treating small-caliber vessels [renal artery, superficial femoral artery (SFA), popliteal artery].

Wallstent Deployment

Vascular access for placement of the Wallstent is obtained as previously described. A 7F to 8F sheath is used for iliac Wallstents. Unlike the Palmaz stent, this one may be deployed from a contralateral approach or into an area of vessel tortuosity because of its flexible construction (Figure 21–6). The proper stent diameter is 1 to 2 mm larger than the angiographically measured diameter of an adjacent proximal or contralateral normal vessel. The length of the stenosis and therefore the desired stent length can be measured likewise. The target lesion (stenosis or occlusion) must be crossed with a 0.035- or 0.038-inch guidewire. Again, the use of intraprocedural heparin is not uniform. Gener-

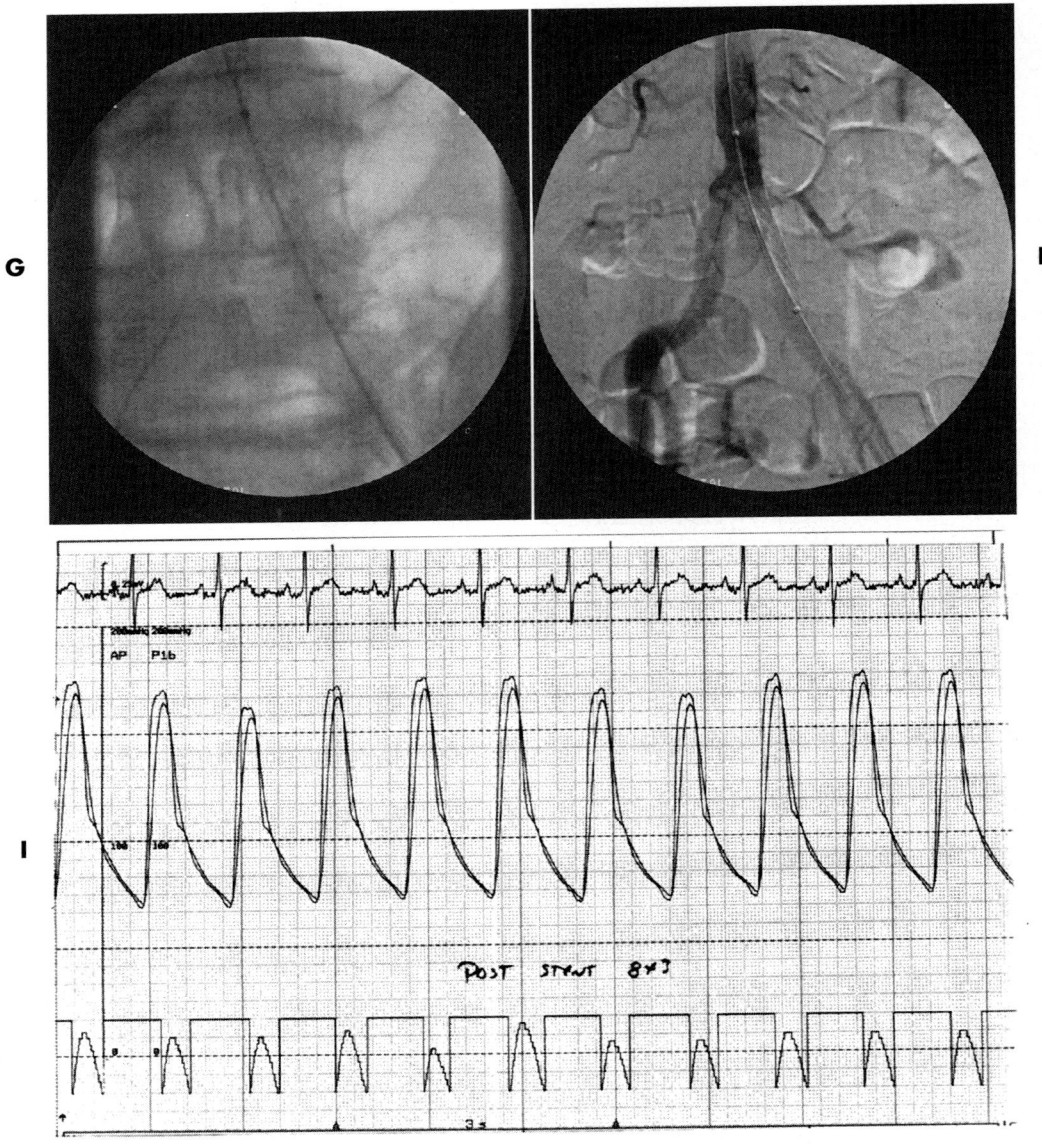

FIGURE 21-5. Continued.

ally, the patient is heparinized (about 100 units/kg to result in an ACT of 200 or more) when crossing iliac occlusions or treating small-caliber vessels. The lesion may be predilated using standard balloon angioplasty technique to facilitate passage of the Wallstent delivery system. Stenoses are initially underdilated to 2 mm less than the optimal measured diameter to allow better gripping of the stent and to decrease the likelihood of migration. The balloon catheter is removed. Optionally, the Wallstent may be deployed without predilatation.

The Wallstent assembly catheter (Figure 21-7A,B,C) is placed over the guidewire and positioned within the target lesion. A separate side port allows lubrication of the contracting membrane. As the contracting membrane is retracted (Figure 21-7D,E,F), the stent is exposed and starts to expand. Complete

21. Intravascular Stents

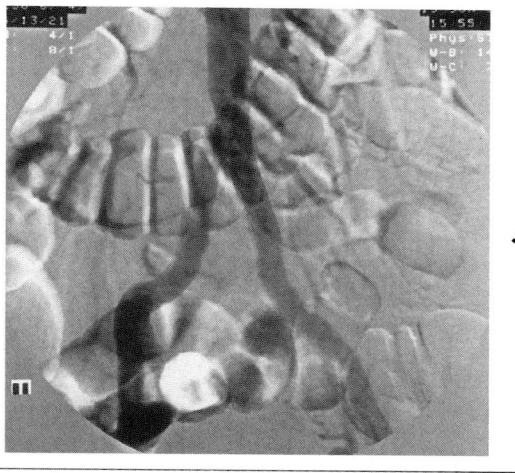

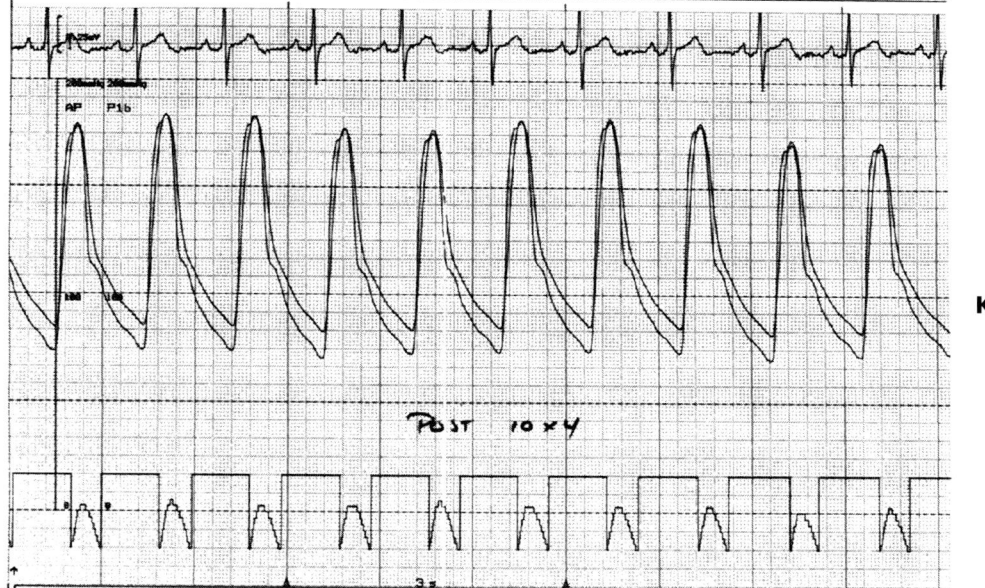

FIGURE 21-5. *Continued.*

retraction allows the stent to spring into position against the vessel wall (Figure 21-7G,H). If the stent does not expand to the desired final diameter, it may be assisted by further balloon dilatation after an appropriate balloon exchange for the stent catheter. The stent may be moved back after beginning deployment. The original Wallstent could not be advanced after beginning deployment, but a reconstrainable version is now available that allows complete recapture of the partially deployed stent. If more than one stent must be used, simple overlapping of the ends is required. After stent deployment and a good hemodynamic result, all catheters, sheaths, and guidewires are removed; and groin hemostasis is obtained. Patients are then generally placed on an appropriate antiplatelet regimen, such as ASA 325 mg daily.

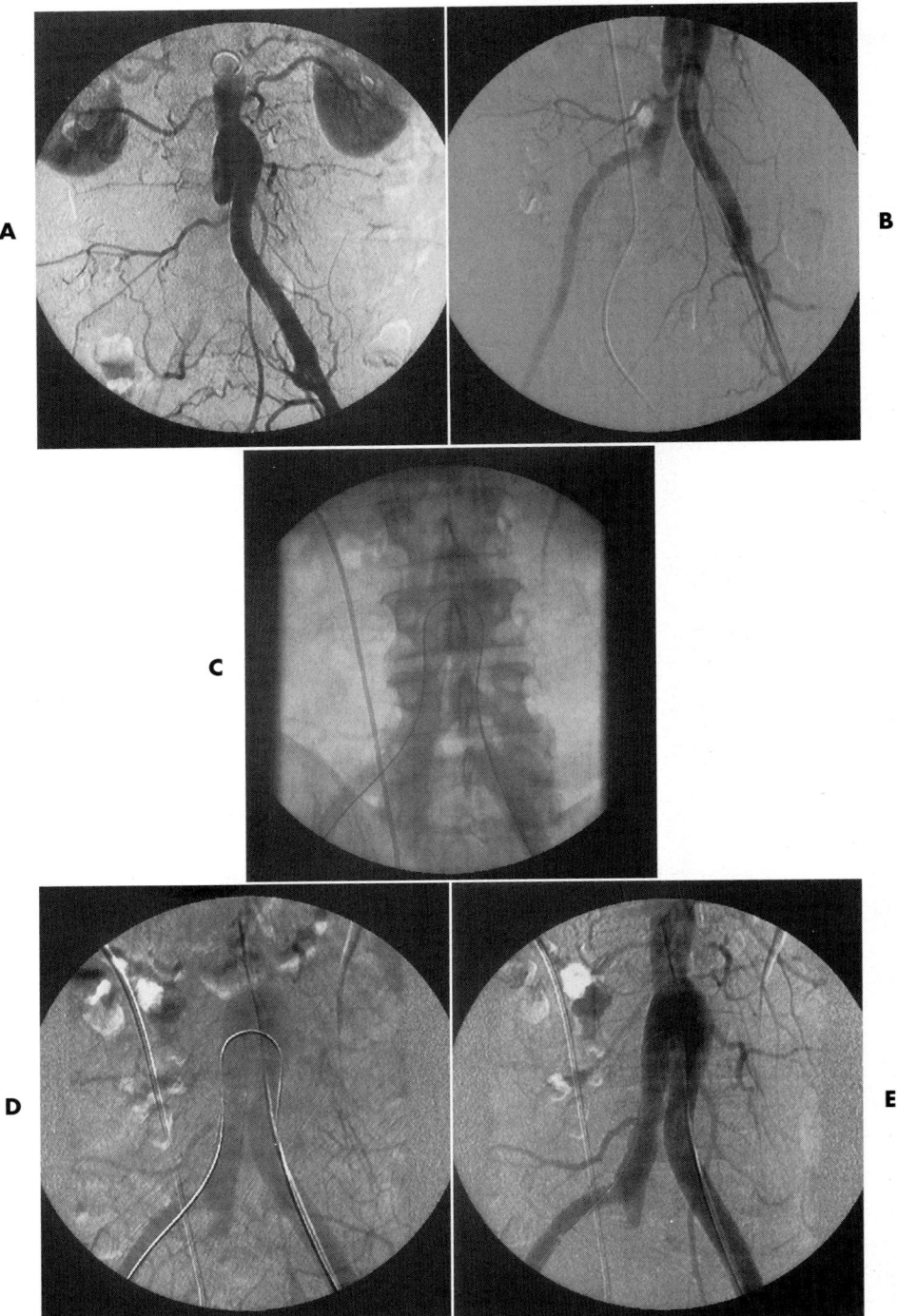

FIGURE 21–6. This patient had previously undergone aortobifemoral bypass grafting with subsequent revision of the right limb of the graft. He had acute graft occlusion (**A**). After surgical thrombectomy of the right limb, there was an intimal disruption (**B**). Because there was a fresh incision in the right groin, the retrograde placement of a Palmaz stent in the radiology suite was not deemed appropriate. Therefore a Wallstent was placed from a contralateral approach. A hydrophilic-coated Simmons catheter and hydrophilic wire were used to negotiate the lesion from a left common femoral artery access (**C**). Next, a 10 mm diameter by 20 mm length Wallstent was deployed across the flap and dilated with a 10-mm balloon. A poststent arteriogram showed excellent flow through the area without residual stenosis (**D**, **E**).

21. Intravascular Stents

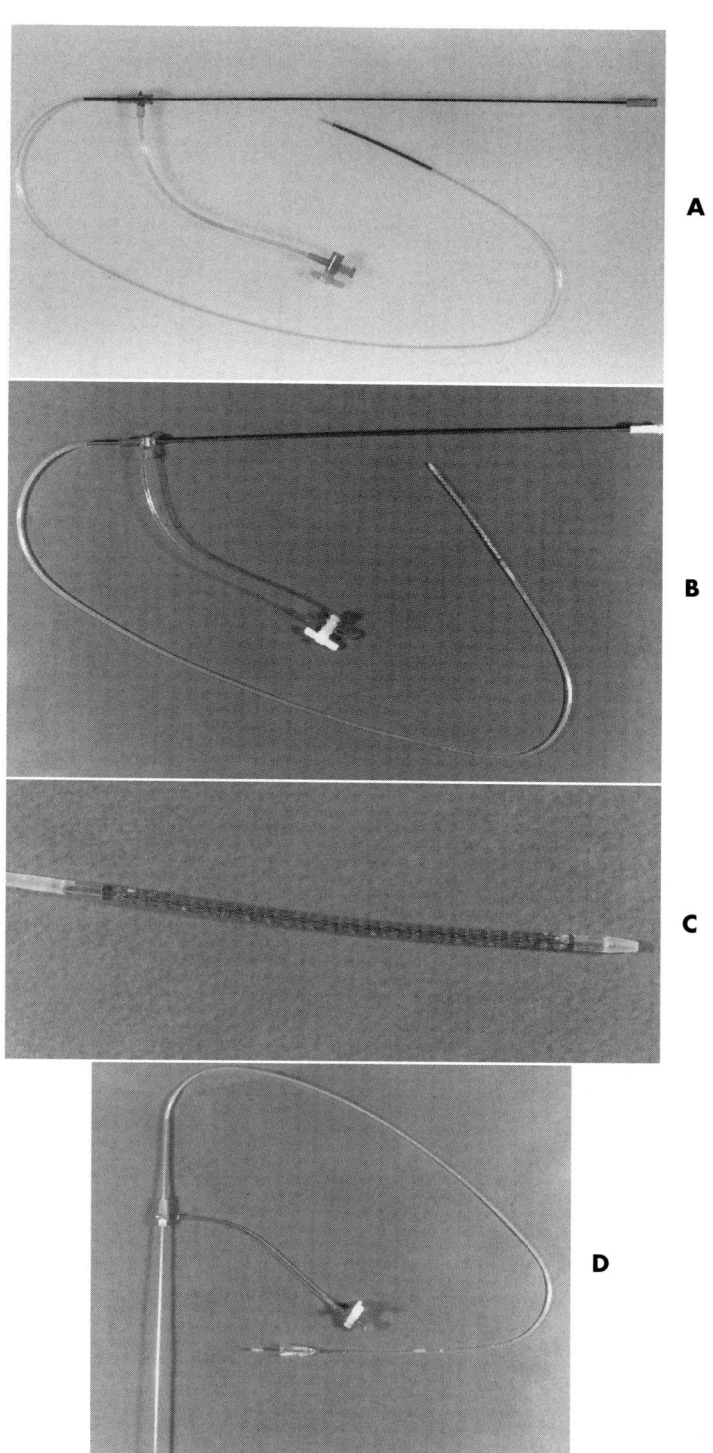

FIGURE 21–7. Small (**A**) and large (**B**) Wallstent introducer catheter with stent in place. **C**, Close-up view of the Wallstent within its retractable sheath and mounted on a smaller inner catheter. **D**, Wallstent is partially deployed. **E**, A closer view of **D**. **F**, Demonstrating how the inner sheath must be held stationary while the outer rolling membrane is pulled back to allow the Wallstent to expand. **G**, Stent is fully deployed with the inner catheter still in place. **H**, Close-up of how the stent would appear fully deployed within the vessel lumen.

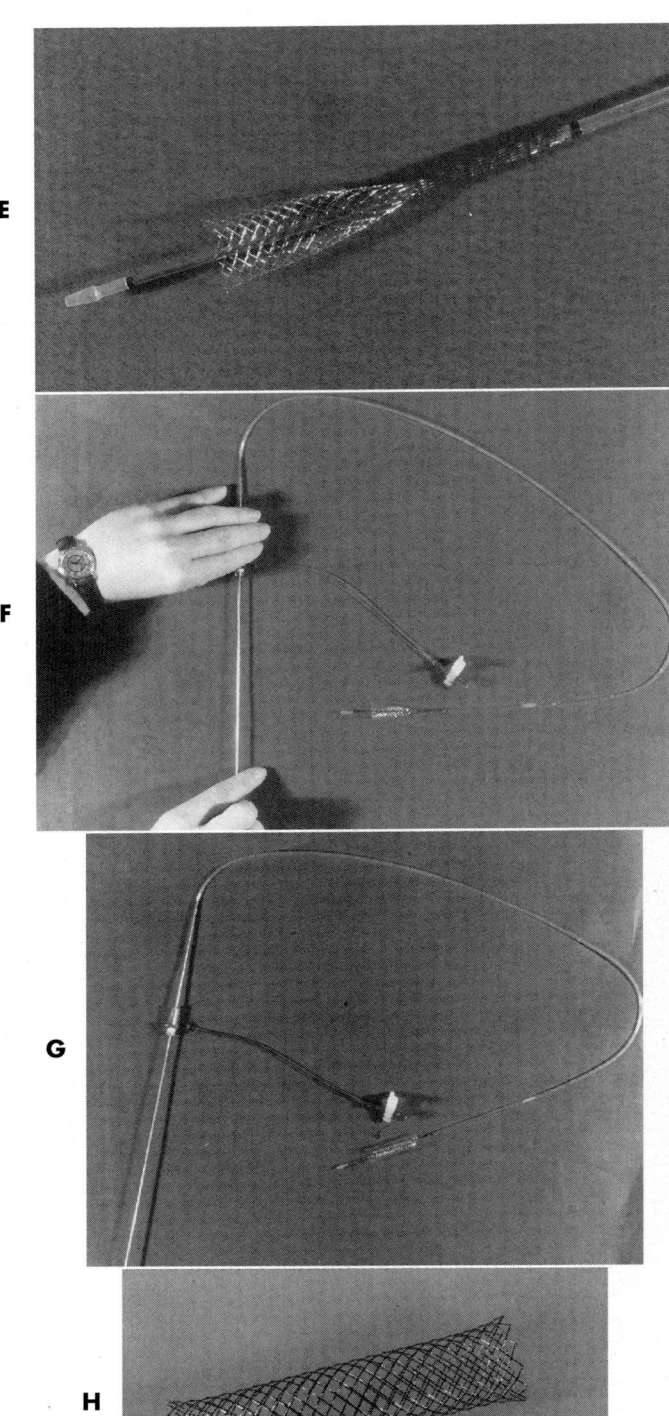

FIGURE 21–7. *Continued.*

Results

Aortic Stents

True isolated midabdominal aortic stenosis (i.e., infrarenal lesions sparing the iliac distribution) are rare but may be amenable to treatment with PTA or stent placement (Figure 21-8). Hallisey and colleagues treated 15 focal infrarenal abdominal aortic stenoses with PTA in 14 patients over a 10-year period.[24] The initial technical success rate was 100%. Clinical patency, as defined by continued absence or alleviation of symptoms, was achieved with 93% of the procedures. Mean follow-up was 4.3 years (range 0.6 to 9.8 years). Sheeran et al. deployed Palmaz stents in six patients and Wallstents in three patients with focal midabdominal stenoses not involving the aortic bifurcation.[25] One patient had undergone remote aortic endarterectomy, and aortic narrowing in another patient developed at the proximal anastomosis of an aortobifemoral graft performed 4 years prior to presentation. Technical success of stent placement was 100%. Follow-up (mean 1.6 years) demonstrated some degree of clinical improvement in all patients treated with Wallstents (100%) and in five patients treated with Palmaz stents (83%). No early or late complications were noted.

Iliac Artery Stents

Iliac artery occlusive disease treated by PTA is quite successful for localized disease, with 1-year patency rates of 50% to 93%.[3,5,7,8,26,27] Five-year results are less well reported but range from approximately 20% to 76%,[7,8] depending on the indications for angioplasty, runoff, occlusion versus stenosis, and other variables. Initial failure in those cases with guidewire-accessible lesions occurs in about 1.5% to 7.5% of all iliac PTAs,[2,3,5] and restenosis (3% to 17%)[3,8,9,28] or locally progressive disease accounts for most of the chronic failures.[2-4,7-9] PTA for a totally occluded iliac artery is technically less rewarding than PTA performed for stenosis, and the complication rate appears to be higher.[5,7,9,11]

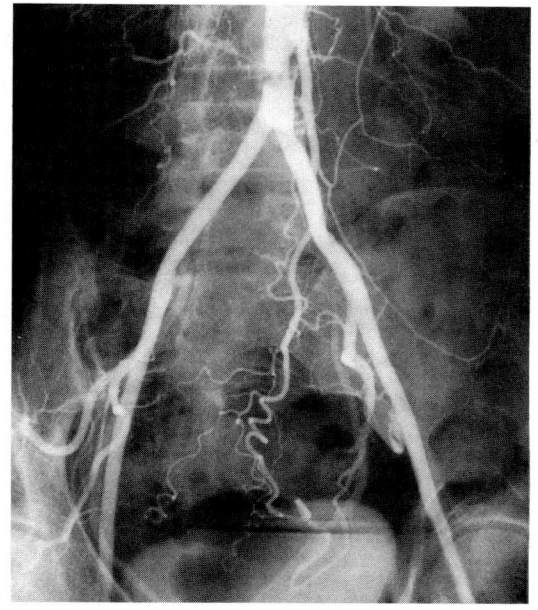 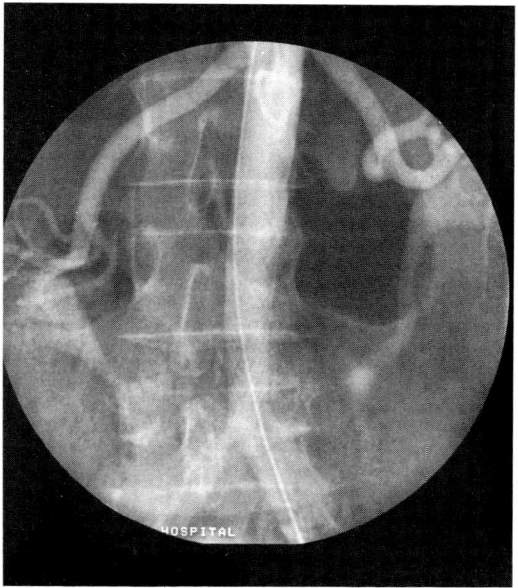

FIGURE 21-8. This patient presented with bilateral blue toes and claudication. **A**, Abdominal aortogram demonstrates a severe focal aortic stenosis just above the bifurcation. **B**, After placement of a 16 × 40 mm Wallstent dilated to 14 mm, an arteriogram shows a good cosmetic result.

Provided optimal patient selection were always addressed, these studies suggest that there is room for stent technology to improve the long-term results of iliac PTA.

Palmaz Stent

The Palmaz stent has been studied in the United States via a multicenter trial, with indications for stent placement being an immediate inadequate postangioplasty response (Figure 21-9), PTA restenosis, or total iliac occlusion.[29-31] The results were generally not segregated precisely by these categories but were combined to provide an overall success rate. When results were categorized by indication for placement, the findings were consistent with the following generalizations.[32] The findings from this group of patients treated with stents were clinical benefit rates of 90.9% at 1 year and 68.6% at 43 months, the benefit defined as at least a one-stage improvement in the ischemic rating system used.[31] The mean ankle-brachial index (ABI) remained approximately 0.18 above the pretreatment mean of 0.62, corresponding with the fact that approximately 67% of the patients were treated for claudication and only 33% for limb-threatening ischemia. Approximately one-fifth of the participants agreed to a postprocedural angiogram 1 to 35 months after treatment, and it demonstrated a mean loss of luminal diameter of 15% and a restenosis rate of 2.7% (50% or less of the original stent diameter). Probably more interesting was the approximately 5.0% per year progression of significant atherosclerotic disease at a site distant from the stent. The 30-day procedural mortality was 1.9%, with a 9.9% rate of complications, of which 1.9% were related to the stent itself. These results suffered from short follow-up (only about 20% were more than 2 years) but constitute a dedicated effort to report all aspects of stent placement.

Wolf et al. placed stents in a group of 37 patients (50 stenoses, 6 occlusions: 128 stents).[33] Resolution of symptoms was noted in 27 patients. One death and four complications (treated nonoperatively) occurred. Follow-up was not lengthy (range 6 to 21 months). Routine 6-month arteriograms obtained for 19 patients revealed 6 patients with mild to moderate stenoses (9% to 43% diameter reduction). Of these six, only two had recurrence of symptoms. These results are comparable to the 17.8% mean stenosis at 6 months reported by Murphy et al.,[34] who observed no correlation between outcome and the presence of hypertension, coronary artery disease, obesity, age, or length of stenosis. They did, however, demonstrate a statistically significant difference in maintaining improved symptomatology at 4 years in nondiabetics.[34]

Henry et al. stented 230 arteries in 184 patients.[35] The 6-month angiographic restenosis rate was 0.5% with a mean follow-up of 35 months. Life-table analysis of their data revealed a 4-year primary patency rate of 86.0 ± 4.1%, with successful treatment of most restenotic lesions by repeat angioplasty resulting in a 4-year secondary patency rate of 94.0 ± 2.8%.

The use of stents in cases of total iliac artery occlusion may have found a viable application. An early report by Rees et al. demonstrated its success in 12 patients, but the embolic risk was high (16%).[36] The most recent multicenter study results from this same group found an 87.8% success rate at 40 months in this select group; and although it was not statistically different from the stenosis-only group (66.6%), there was a tendency for improved outcome.[30] Surgical exposure to prevent the risk of procedure-induced emboli is a possible solution to a continuing problem of distal embolus.[30,36]

Primary stenting based on the theoretic advantages of a smooth flow surface, optimal resolution of pressure gradients, and reduced subintimal collagen exposure has been an active area of research.[37] Bonn et al. reported a feasibility study and concluded that early stent results were acceptable and did not significantly increase the complication rate of iliac PTA.[38] Williams and colleagues in 1994 confirmed these results but reported a 13% complication rate; but there was also an initial cost saving of 25% to 66% compared with surgical interventions.[39] Long-term durability could not be confirmed. A randomized trial of PTA versus

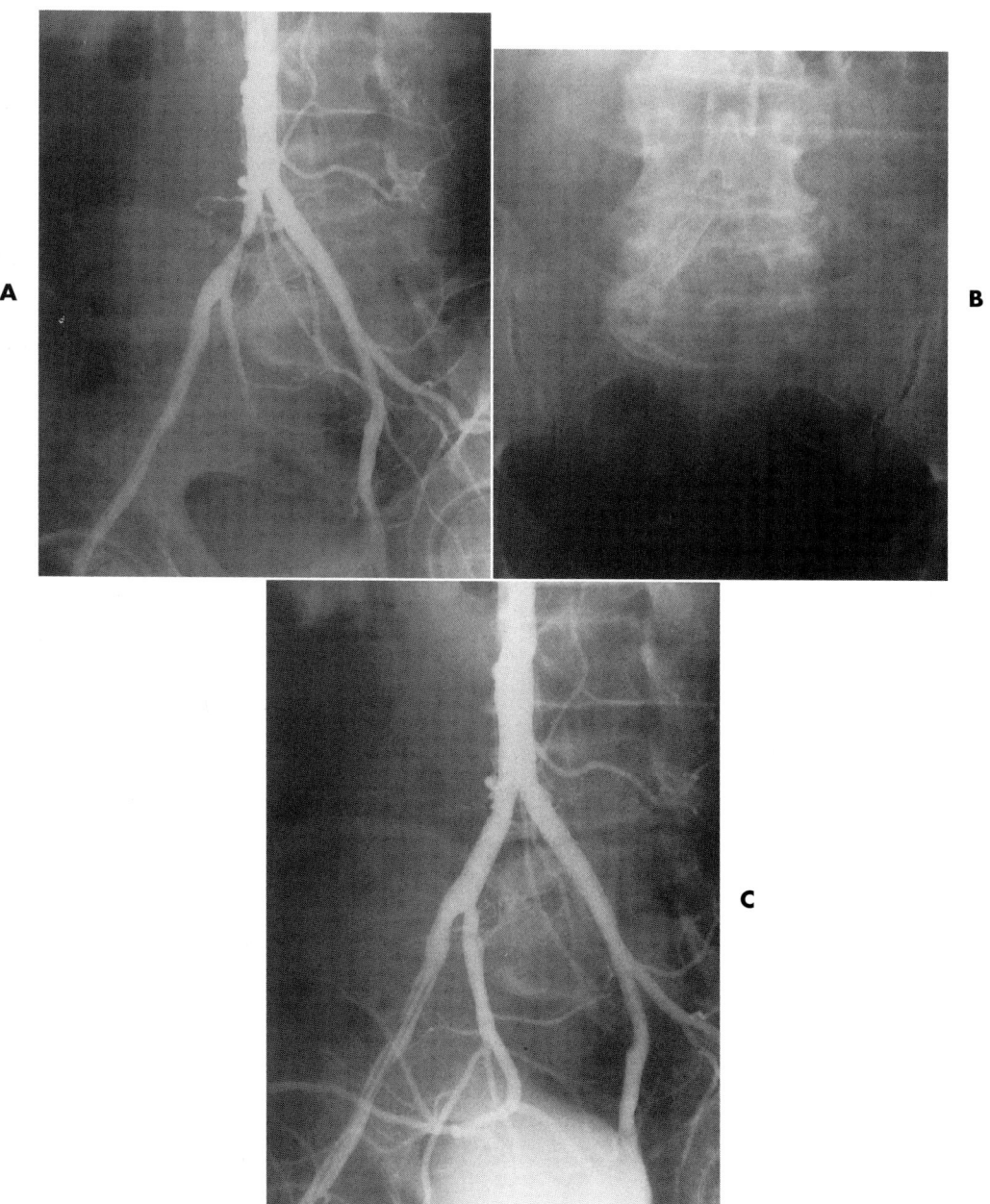

FIGURE 21–9. This patient developed recurrent right lower extremity claudication 1 year after a successful right common iliac artery angioplasty. **A**, Arteriogram demonstrates a significant stenosis in the area of prior angioplasty with a 35 mm Hg gradient. **B, C**, A 308 Palmaz stent was deployed primarily to 10 mm with good cosmetic results and no residual gradient.

primary stenting demonstrated a primary patency rate of 93.6% with stents versus a 64.6% rate with PTA alone.[40] To our knowledge, no confirmatory data have been published to substantiate this claim.

Wallstent

The Wallstent has been studied most extensively in Europe as part of the European Wallstent Peripheral Artery Implant Study. Indications for stent placement were a complex lesion—e.g., occlusion (Figure 21–10), long-segment stenosis with an irregular surface, aneurysm formation, markedly ulcerated plaques, eccentric stenosis, or ostial lesions extending into the aorta—or an acute complication during PTA.[41] The reports generally did not separate the results by indication but did provide an overall estimate of success.

An early report of this experience included 31 iliac lesions (16 occlusions), all but one of which were performed for claudication. Warfarin (Coumadin) was used in 11 early cases but was then deemed unnecessary. At a mean of 5.5 months, one occlusion had occurred and one case of significant restenosis secondary to pseudointimal hyperplasia was reported.[42] In 1991 there were 100 cases available for analysis.[43] Most of the patients (90%) were claudicants, 97% were primary technical stent successes, and thrombosis occurred immediately after stent placement in two patients. In general, the stent dramatically reduced the average degree of residual stenosis by about

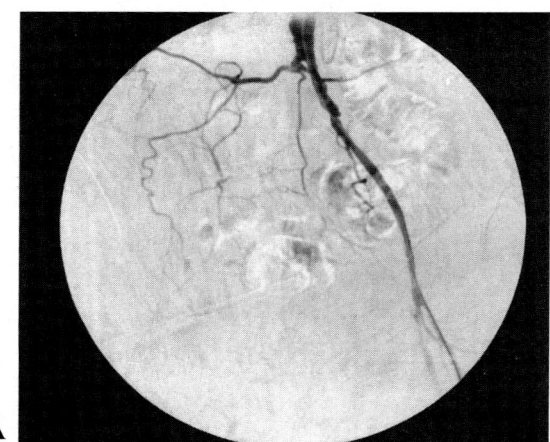
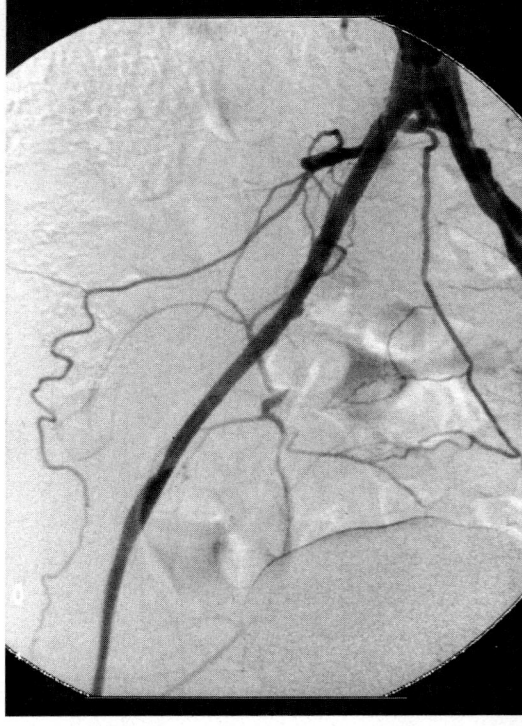

FIGURE 21–10. This patient had a history of chronic right lower extremity claudication. **A**, Arteriogram demonstrated occlusion of the right common and external iliac artery. The patient was given 5000 units of heparin. The right iliac occlusion was then negotiated with a hydrophilic wire from a contralateral approach. Without predilatation, two overlapping 8 × 60 mm Wallstents were deployed and dilated to 8 mm in the common iliac artery and 7 mm in the external iliac artery. **B**, Postprocedural arteriogram demonstrated a patent channel through the previously occluded right iliac artery. There was no pressure gradient across the system at the termination of the procedure.

30% to 50% in the patients in whom stents were used. Within the first month, six other stents occluded and were associated with uncorrected inflow disease not completely covered by the original stent in three cases. Two others failed within 3 months, which is a rate of failure similar to that reported by Hausegger et al.[44] All symptomatic patients and several asymptomatic patients underwent postprocedural angiography. The prevalence of clinically relevant restenosis was 5%. The angiographic prevalence of restenosis was 16% (10 of 62); three of the stenoses were immediately adjacent to the stent. Angiographic restenosis was defined as a more than 20% decrease from the original postintervention luminal diameter, and the results stated were for a mean follow-up of 1 year. In 10 of 14 cases, angiographic restenosis was related to the implant, and in four cases it represented a new lesion. A later report covers a 3-year clinical experience with 125 iliac stents.[41] Eliminating the 22 cases of total iliac occlusion not guidewire-accessible, the 1-year cumulative patency was 94.6% and the 2-year patency 86.5%. The procedural mortality was 0%. There was a total complication rate of 4%, but only a 1.6% major complication rate if this was defined as the patient requiring some type of reintervention. Reobstruction (resulting from lesions inside or adjacent to the stented segment) occurred in 6.5% of cases during follow-up, generally more than 6 months after the Wallstent had been placed.

Regarding complex lesions, Vowerk et al. stented 13 ulcerated plaques and 5 aneurysms with a mean length of 3.5 ± 1.0 cm.[45] Follow-up angiography demonstrated lesion ablation in 94% of cases at 3 months and in all cases at 9 months. No embolization occurred. Follow-up revealed a 4-year cumulative patency rate of 82%. Obstruction recurred in two patients. One patient developed a thrombotic occlusion at the site of stent deployment after 17 months but underwent successful percutaneous recanalization that was still patent after 46 months. The other patient underwent successful balloon dilatation for a restenosis within the stent at 26 months, then returned 12 months later with an occlusion of the stent that was also successfully recanalized.

Long et al. reported a 3-year experience of Wallstent use in 47 iliac artery lesions (15 occlusions) in 49 patients; 7 Strecker stents were used in the remaining cases.[46] Follow-up averaged 15 months, and postprocedural angiography was undertaken in an impressive 47 cases. The procedural mortality was 2%. Thrombosis occurred in 7.7% of all cases. Significant intrastent hyperplasia was observed in 13.5% of cases (50% or more recurrent luminal narrowing) in addition to a 5.8% incidence of stenosis in adjacent areas where the stent just missed covering an offending lesion. Six of these patients required intervention for symptomatic relief. Long et al. also observed that overlapping the hypogastric artery lumen was not without consequence, as 2 of 18 (11%) occluded and 33% had documented ostial degradation in luminal size over time.

Raillat et al., studying 16 symptomatic iliac lesions treated by PTA and stent placement, noted that no stenosis occurred in the stent itself but usually occurred in an area of PTA dissection not covered by the stent, which then resulted in early occlusion.[47] Zollikofer and colleagues treated 24 iliac stenoses in 18 patients; they reported one acute occlusion and two cases of restenosis secondary to intimal hyperplasia at approximately 4 months. At a mean follow-up of 16 months, no clinical or angiographic evidence of restenosis had been observed in any of the other patients.[48]

Sapoval et al. stented 101 arteries in 95 patients,[49] with a mean follow-up of 29 months. They reported a 4-year primary patency rate of 61% and a secondary rate of 86%, similar to those reported by Murphy et al.[50]

Sapoval et al. identified the following five factors associated with long-term angiographic failure: SFA occlusion, stent diameter less than 8 mm, two or more stents implanted, current tobacco use, and, interestingly enough, the lack of hypertension. They postulated that the presence of hypertension may have caused more frequent visits to the physician and thus better general management.[48] The 1-year patency rates were $95.2 \pm 4.8\%$, $88.6 \pm 6.2\%$, $78.2 \pm 8.7\%$, and $54.9 \pm 17.2\%$ for patients with no, one, two, or three risk factors. No patient with four risk factors had a patent stent at 1 year.[48]

Martin and colleagues reported the results of an FDA phase II, multicenter trial.[51] Iliac stents were placed in 140 patients. The 6-month angiographic patency rate was 93%. The 1-year primary patency was 81% and secondary patency 91%; and the 2-year primary patency was 71% and secondary patency 86%. The major complication rate was 4.3%. Three patients died during the first 30 days after the procedure, but no death was directly related to stent deployment.

Totally occluded iliac arteries have been treated with the Wallstent. Vorwerk and Gunther reported on the European Wallstent Peripheral Artery Implant Study noting that 48 of 68 total occlusions were successfully recanalized (70.6%).[52] Once accomplished, there were two early reocclusions (less than 6 months) probably resulting from incomplete stent coverage of a coexisting common iliac artery orificial stenosis. Restenosis developed in two others; one was found at 1 month and corrected by placement of a second stent at a proximal location not previously included in the stenting procedure. The second demonstrated intimal hyperplasia within and proximal to the stent within 6 months. The distal embolus rate was 2.1%, and no thrombolysis had been used in any of these cases. Post-stent/PTA emboli after treatment of total iliac artery occlusions continued to be a problem during the course of this investigation, as noted by the 4.7% incidence reported during an extended period of follow-up.[41] A more current study by this group noted a 5.1% embolization rate.[53] Long et al. also reported a significant problem with emboli after stent treatment for total occlusions (20%).[46] Long-term follow-up of the European Wallstent study demonstrated early recurrences from incomplete stenting of the occluded segment in 3.2% of all cases.[41] Clinically relevant late reocclusions occurred 9 to 30 months (mean 16.4 months) after the procedure and developed in 10 of 123 patients. Interestingly, the rate of late reobstruction was higher for preprocedure iliac stenoses (9.6%) than for iliac occlusions (6.5%).[41]

The most recent study involving primary Wallstent deployment without thrombolysis involved 61 iliac artery occlusions. The mean length of the occluded segment was 10 cm. The technical success rate was 92%. The 2-year primary and secondary patency rates were 73.0% and 88.0%, respectively. Embolization rates were comparable to those of other studies.[54]

Miscellaneous Iliac Artery Stents

The Gianturco self-expanding metallic stent has been used in Japan for iliac artery stenosis and occlusion.[55] Early animal studies were encouraging,[15] but the device never reached clinical trial in the United States. Ten patients were treated in the clinical series; one-half had total occlusions. The technical success rate was 100%. At an average follow-up of 10.3 months no migration or occlusion was noted, and the mean ABI was significantly improved over the preintervention value. Postprocedural angiograms demonstrated mild neointimal thickening. It should be noted that the device used clinically was made of a smaller-diameter wire (0.01 inch) than that used in earlier U.S. experimental reports. The authors believed that the small amount of wire present in terms of thickness and overall bulk may help improve endothelial coverage, decrease its thrombogenicity, and allow side-branch interventions if required at a later date. Because of its rigidity, which is similar to that of the Palmaz device, acutely angulated vessels or vessels near bend areas of the body are not candidates for intervention with this device.

The Strecker stent has been used in Europe.[44,55–58] The number of totally occluding lesions ranged from 22.7% to 47.3%. The indications for stent placement were PTA failures or early restenosis following PTA. Additionally, long iliac occlusions were indications for primary stenting.[57] The patency rates ranged from 98% to 100% after 9 months. Three-year patency rates were significantly higher in short (88%) versus long (63%) lesions (using 4 cm as the line of demarcation) and in stenoses (92%) versus occlusions (63%).[58] The stent's flexibility, ease of delivery, and ability to be imaged by magnetic resonance imaging (MRI) may be clinically advantageous.

The design of nitinol stents has matured from an early spiral coil used experimentally[13] to a zigzag configuration used in ongoing clinical evaluations following renewed experimental work.[59,60] The clinical work has involved 14 patients with nine iliac stenoses and five total occlusions after unsuccessful PTA.[59] In the 13 patients available for long-term follow-up (average 12.7 months), the ABI was still more than 0.15 above preinterventional levels and no clinical deterioration had occurred. Eight patients had follow-up angiography; only minimal intimal hyperplasia involving the entire length of the stent(s) was noted.

Femoral Artery Stents

The need for adjuvants to improve femoropopliteal PTA may be more critical than in the iliac system. The initial success rate for femoropopliteal PTA averaged 80% to 98%, depending on the type of lesion and the experience and technical skill of the interventionalist.[1,3,5,7–9,28,61] The 1-year patency rate was 36% to 80%.[3,5,7,8,28] At 5 years the results continued to show a gradual decline, with rates between 13% and 70%.[3,7,8,28,61] The variety of lesions treated (e.g., length, degree of stenosis) in addition to the variable methods of reporting results account for the wide variation in long-term results observed. Restenosis was a perplexing problem, obviously more common at this site as exemplified by the poorer long-term patency rates than in the larger iliac vessels.[62,63] Total occlusions fared poorly.[7,9,28] Stents were considered a possible solution to these problems.

Palmaz Stent

One of the first to evaluate femoropoliteal deployment of the Palmaz stent were Henry et al.[35] They placed 188 stents in 126 patients. No arteries were primarily stented. In all, 63% of patients had a single stent, and a maximum of five stents was placed in one patient. The lesions were located in the common femoral artery (6 patients), the upper third of the SFA (19 patients), the middle third of the SFA (62 patients), the lower third of the SFA (29 patients), and the popliteal artery (10 patients). Immediate clinical success was achieved in 73 femoral artery stenoses (97%) and 8 popliteal stenoses (80%). Two distal emboli occurred after femoral recanalization and responded to thromboaspiration. Four patients developed stent thromboses within the first 24 hours after stent placement, but flow was restored in all by fibrinolytic therapy. The average restenosis rate at 6 months increased as interventional procedures descended within the arterial system: upper femoral artery lesions (4%), middle femoral artery lesions (10%), lower femoral artery lesions (18%), and popliteal artery lesions (20%). The 4-year primary patency rates for femoropolitreal interventions were 80.0 ± 7.4% for stenotic disease and 39.0 ± 11.5% for occlusive disease. Repeat angioplasty improved the secondary patency rates to 94.0 ± 4.3% for stenotic lesions and 86.0 ± 6.7% for occlusive lesions. Henry et al. concluded that for lower SFA and popliteal lesions, and especially for total occlusions, the relative merits of stent placement may not compare favorably with other methods of treatment.[35]

Chatelard et al. reviewed a series of 26 cases of stent deployment of SFA stenosis and 9 cases of deployment for popliteal artery stenosis.[64] Their initial success rate of insertion was 100%. Mean follow-up was 32 months. During the first 6 months after the procedure two patients developed acute thrombosis, and five developed restenosis. Of note in this study is that the restenosis rates in the popliteal artery were not significantly greater than in the SFA. The extrapolated 4-year primary patency rate of 75.7 ± 8.0% is comparable to that noted by Henry et al.[35]

Bergeron and colleagues analyzed retrospectively a series of 55 Palmaz stents placed exclusively for SFA lesions in 39 patients. In contrast to other studies, most of the lesions (57%) were occlusions. Two acute thromboses (4.8%) developed within 48 hours after the procedure; these particular patients had long segments of occlusion and poor runoff. At 2 years the primary and secondary patencies were 77%

and 89%, respectively.[65] Preprocedure occluded lesions were not statistically more likely to become restenotic when compared to preprocedure stenosis-only lesions.

Wallstent

The European Wallstent study analyzed the results of Wallstent placement for atherosclerotic narrowing of the femoral artery. Treatment of 4 stenotic and 10 occlusive femoral arteries were described in an early report from this experience.[42] Most of these patients were anticoagulated for 6 months with sodium warfarin. One acute thrombosis and two cases (14.3%) of distal emboli, which resolved on heparin therapy, were the observed procedural complications. Significant intrastent intimal hyperplasia occurred in three patients (21.4%) in less than 12 months and was most pronounced at the distal end of the stent.

Rousseau and colleagues reported a midterm analysis of Wallstent deployment for the treatment of femoropopliteal stenosis.[66] Forty implants were performed, and follow-up in all cases was more than 6 months. A 12-months angiogram was performed in 32 cases. Oral anticoagulation (acenocoumarol) was utilized in the last nine cases for a 2-month period. Claudication (78%) was the most common presenting symptom. No stent migration or traumatic dissection during stent deployment was observed, and major collateral vessels crossed by the stent remained open. Nine thromboses occurred within the first month in the subset of patients not undergoing anticoagulation. Four restenoses (10% of cases) of more than 50% narrowing were observed 3 to 6 months after stent placement and were generally most pronounced at either end of the stent.

A Swiss paper reported on 15 femoropoliteal Wallstent placements; 11 were available for follow-up. Six occlusions occurred within the first month, and only six of the stents were patent at a mean of 20 months.[48] Even in these six, one to three secondary interventions were required for continued patency. Of the six patients available for angiography more than 3 months after stent placement, two had recurrent stenosis outside the stent with moderate intrastent hyperplasia (less than 40% reduction in stent diameter), two demonstrated severe intrastent intimal proliferation, and two others had moderate intrastent hyperplasia.

Sapoval et al. followed 21 patients prospectively who underwent femoropopliteal PTA followed by Wallstent insertion for a mean of 17.6 months with angiography, Doppler ultrasonography, and clinical examinations.[67] Nine occlusions occurred: four during the first 30 days and five during the first 1 to 5 months after PTA. Three patients developed intrastent intimal hyperplasia requiring additional percutaneous intervention. The 12-month patency rates were 49% (primary) and 67% (secondary). These authors believed that stenting did not decrease the rate of reocclusion after PTA alone, and that its use may be indicated only for treatment of acute closure complicating PTA.[67]

As part of the FDA phase II multicenter Wallstent trial, Martin et al. placed stents in the femoral systems of 90 patients.[51] The 6-month angiographic patency was 80%. The 1-year clinical patencies were 61% (primary) and 84% (secondary), and the 2-year patencies were 49% (primary) and 72% (secondary). Their results were comparable to those for femoral angioplasty use alone.[51]

One investigator compared the results of primary Wallstent placement versus simple balloon angioplasty in the treatment of femoropopliteal artery occlusive disease.[68] There were 26 patients treated in each group. Warfarin therapy was substituted for aspirin (300 mg) and dipyridamole (25 mg b.i.d.) after three early occlusions occurred in the first 11 stent cases. Of 26 stented lesions, 5 (19%) occluded during the first 10 days. Eight others demonstrated severe neointimal hyperplasia within 12 months, and one occlusion at the distal end of a stent was noted. Taking into account 10 successful reinterventions, a secondary patency rate of 69% was reported. In the PTA-only group, there were six stenoses or occlusions within 6 months and four additional ones during the following 6 months. No reintervention was undertaken, and the primary patency rate was therefore 65%.

Strecker Stent

The Strecker stent was thought sufficiently flexible to be used in this location, and 58 were deployed in one study.[56] At a mean follow-up at 19 months, there were 14 restenoses or reocclusions (29.2%). Within the first 6 to 9 months after deployment, intimal hyperplasia was generally the cause of arterial narrowing. Redilation was done successfully by PTA, but the problem recurred even more quickly (within 4 to 6 months). In 10 of the cases, several redilations were required to maintain a stable clinical condition. There were some problems with stent delivery in early cases, but no major complications requiring invasive procedures were reported. Two other studies identified important risks for restenosis: distal SFA or popliteal stent placement and an area of placement longer than 4 cm.[57,69]

Problems with restenosis after the use of the Strecker stent have taken an interesting twist in the treatment of SFA disease. In four early cases, endovascular irradiation with a surface dose of 12 cGy provided encouraging results in that all irradiated stents remained patent at short-term follow-ups.[56] Long-term follow-up (23 to 30 months) demonstrated no recurrent obstructions in these patients.[70,71] A larger series ($n = 13$) is showing a similar freedom from restenosis as demonstrated by digital subtraction angiography and magnetic resonance angiography (MRA) with follow-up of 3 to 27 months.[70,71] More recently, Schopohl et al. reviewed 6 years of experience with SFA restenosis following stent/intravascular brachytherapy with a 10-Ci ^{192}Ir source. Stent length ranged from 5 to 16 cm. Of the 25 patients available with sufficient follow-up (range 8 to 71 months), 21 patients (84%) had patent treated vessel segments.[72]

Miscellaneous Femoropopliteal Stents

Data concerning a nitinol stent has been reported. SFA lesions (39 stenoses, 6 occlusions) and popliteal lesions (9 stenoses, 7 occlusions) were stented. The stent length was approximately 4 cm, and stent diameter varied from 5 to 8 mm. The respective primary and secondary patency rates at 18 months were 85% and 88% for SFA lesions and 87% and 100% for popliteal lesions. The 4.1% failure rate within 24 hours was comparable to that in other studies.[73]

Renal Artery Stents

Percentaneous transluminal angiography has not proved to be a panacea for occlusive disease of the renal artery. Ostial renal artery PTA has an immediate technical success rate in the range of 25% to 35%.[74-76] Recurrence rates of 5% to 42% have been reported for atherosclerotic stenosis, more pronounced within the first year with a more gradual decline thereafter.[74,77-80] The clinical response, which is apparently independent of gender, has been reported to be 0% to 40% in a number of series.[74,75,81-83] Nonostial fibromuscular lesions fare much better.[71,75,77,78] Moreover, most series reporting renal PTA results do not demonstrate a major improvement in renal function.[84] Dilated atherosclerotic lesions with a residual stenosis of 30% or more or most certainly those with more than 50% residual stenosis are more likely to recur or to fail clinically.[74,85] Based on this information, seeking adjunctive measures to improve renal PTA was a fruitful ground for stent investigations.

Palmaz Stent

Palmaz stent use in the renal arteries has been evaluated by many studies, the indications being an inadequate post-PTA result (Figure 21-11), ostial lesions, or PTA restenosis. Rees and colleagues reported on the multicenter trial of the Palmaz stent in 1991. Twenty-eight ostial renal artery stenoses were stented.[86] Technical success defined as less than 30% residual stenosis was achieved in 96%. At 6 months the cure or improvement rate was 64%, and angiography performed in 18 patients (average 7.5 ± 4.4 months) demonstrated restenosis (50% or more diameter narrowing) in seven cases (39%). The stenosis involved the proximal portion and midportion rather than the distal portion of the stent. Even in those without

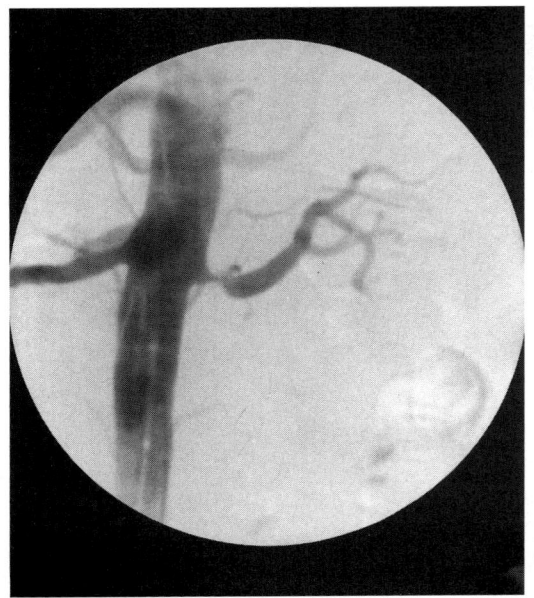
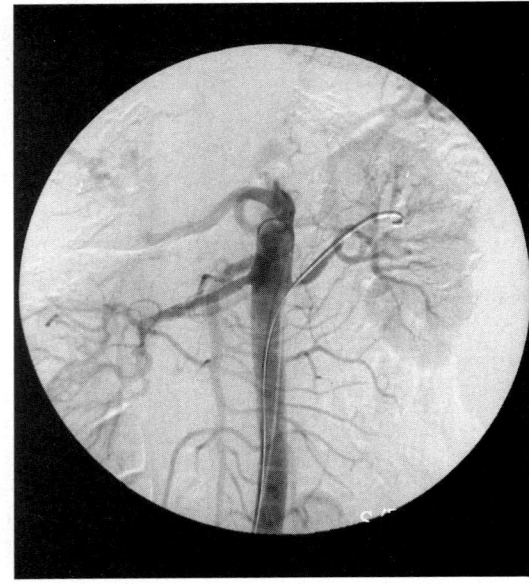
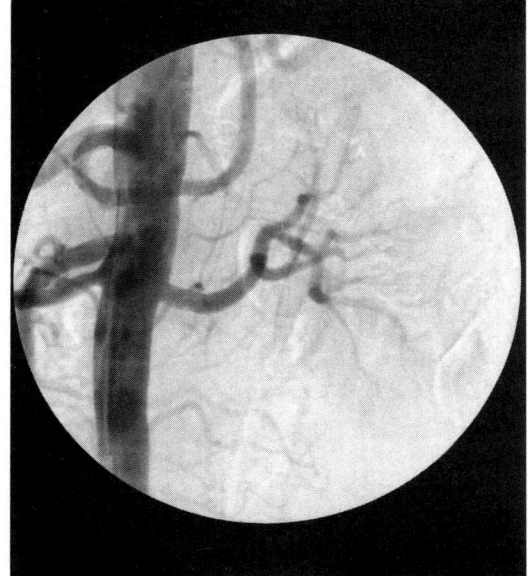

FIGURE 21–11. This patient presented with poorly controlled hypertension (bp 220/110 mm Hg) despite a multiple-drug regimen. Renal scintigraphy showed a normal right kidney but decreased size and function of the left kidney. **A**, Flush renal arteriogram demonstrates severe stenosis of the proximal left renal artery. **B**, After PTA to 5 mm there is considerable residual stenosis secondary to elastic recoil. **C**, After placement of a Palmaz 154 stent dilated to 6 mm, an arteriogram shows no residual stenosis.

restenosis, there was deposition of tissue to a thickness of 1 mm or more in all cases. The procedural mortality was 3.6%; there were two cases of renal failure, three cases of sepsis, one occlusion of a branch renal artery, and one dissection of an iliac artery. These investigators suggested that oversizing the dilatation may help compensate for the neointimal proliferation noted.

Boisclair et al. reported midterm technical and clinical results for 35 Palmaz renal artery stents in 33 patients.[87] Among these patients, 29 arteries were stented for immediate PTA failures and the remainder for recurrent stenosis after PTA. No residual stenosis was found immediately after stenting. Seven patients developed complications, including one renal artery thrombosis, four renal artery emboli, one cholesterol embolization to the lower extremities, and one femoral hematoma requiring operative intervention. Sixty-six percent of patients were either cured or had relief of their hypertension. Additionally, Boisclair and colleagues stratified their patients in terms of baseline renal function. Among their patients, 17 (52%) had a preprocedure serum creatinine of at least 1.5 mg/dl; of these patients, 7 (41%) showed improvement of their mean serum creatinine, but 4 experienced deteriorated renal function.[87] The improvement reported in their study[87] is the highest currently reported in the literature.[87-91] The least impressive results were observed by MacLeod's group,[88] but this poor showing likely reflects inclusion of patients with more advanced renal failure. The renal function improvement noted in other sutdies[89-96] ranged from 28% to 33%, but these studies also varied in their use of primary versus secondary stening[89,90] and in the use of a modified Palmaz-Schatz stent.[89,91] Of the 16 patients in the Boisclair et al. study with a serum creatinine of less than 1.5 mg/dl, all but one patient maintained stable renal function.[87] Although few data are provided, Graor reported on 47 renal artery stents and noted a 6-month patency of 88%. He suggested that expansion of the artery to more than 6 mm may improve long-term results.[97]

Wallstent

An early experience with renal artery PTA and Wallstent placement was reported for 12 renal arteries.[98] Two patients had renal failure after the procedure (16.7%), one from massive cholesterol emboli. There were no procedural deaths. Seven patients underwent repeat angiography 6 to 12 months after stent deployment. Two of these angiograms were normal, three had definite tissue buildup without stenosis, and two others were occluded. The lack of visibility of the stent during deployment was considered a problem.

Joffre and colleagues reported midterm results for Wallstent renal artery stenting.[99] Seventeen cases of stent placement for inadequate renal artery PTA were presented. The anticoagulant regimen included heparin and then acenocoumarol for 2 weeks in addition to antiplatelet agents before intervention and for 6 months after stent placement. Complications included one misplacement secondary to low radiopacity, one perirenal hematoma, and one branch renal artery thrombosis (17.6% complication rate). One case (5.9%) of more than 50% restenosis secondary to intimal hyperplasia was noted with a mean follow-up of approximately 16 months. Another midterm report by Raynaud et al.[100] evaluated deployment of 25 Wallstents into 18 renal arteries. Technical success was achieved in all patients with a residual stenosis rate of less than 20%. However, five stents were slightly misplaced, and a second stent was implanted in each of these cases to fully cover the offending lesion. Postprocedure angiography (mean 11 months after stent placement) demonstrated that in 89% of patients there was a normal patent renal artery and that this finding correlated well with a decrease in both systolic and diastolic blood pressures.[100]

Long-term results involving 25 Wallstent renal artery placements were reported in 1994.[101] At the time of follow-up angiography (29 ± 15 months), 20% of cases showed stent restenosis. The 15-month primary patency rate was 77%. No restenosis was seen in 16 other patients, but all had a thin layer of intimal hyperplasia present that covered the inner surface of the stent. Four complications (20%) were reported, two of which involved renal failure: one from cholesterol emboli and one from a clot embolus. These authors considered it important to select a stent diameter 10% to 15% larger than the normal renal artery to prevent stent migration and to compensate for neointimal growth.

Strecker Stent

Kuhn's group offered a preliminary report on the use of the Strecker stent for renal artery stenosis[102] and followed this paper with an abstract reporting their 3-year experience.[103] Restenosis or immediate PTA complications were the indications for placement in 10 patients.[102] Technical success (less than 20% residual stenosis) was observed in 80%. One acute thrombosis required immediate transaortic thromboendarterectomy, and one stent could not be successfully deployed. Six-month follow-up angiography demonstrated a restenosis (more than 50% diameter reduction) in two cases. The average maximal intimal thickness ($n = 8$, including one case of restenosis) in the proximal part of the stent was 0.97 ± 0.67 mm, with somewhat less buildup in the middle and distal areas of the stents. The 3-year experience involved 18 stent placements with an immediate technical success of 77.8%.[103] At a mean follow-up of 12 to 13 months, restenosis was reported in 18.2% of 11 cases studied.[103]

Visceral Artery Stents

Elective surgical treatment of chronic visceral ischemia, by bypass or endarterectomy, is associated with significant morbidity and mortality.[104] PTA is a lower-risk alternative but is less effective for ostial stenoses. Few patients with ostial stenoses have had patency restored with PTA alone,[105] and only one case of superior mesenteric artery (SMA) occlusion successfully treated with PTA has been reported.[106] The current literature consists of anecdotal evidence of successful Palmaz stent deployment in an occlusion of the SMA with short follow-up.[105,107] Low-dose postprocedure aspirin therapy was recommended.[105]

Infectious Complications

Infection at the site of Palmaz iliac stent placement, as reported anecdotally in the current literature, can have devastating consequences including multisystem organ failure and death.[108–111] In the four cases reviewed, patients manifested infectious complications within 10 days of stent placement. In two cases the infection appeared to complicate a pseudoaneurysm.[108,109] All patients required stent removal and extraanatomic bypass. Stent cultures grew *Staphylococcus aureus* most commonly,[109–111] and a *Staphylococcus epidermidis* infection has been reported.[110]

An unusual case of infection after renal artery Palmaz stent deployment was reported by Gordon et al.[112] A small right femoral artery pseudoaneurysm developed during the first 24 hours; it responded to ultrasound compression, and the patient was discharged 5 days later on therapeutic levels of warfarin. After some intermittent flank pain and nocturia, the patient became febrile about 3.5 weeks after stent deployment. Blood cultures were positive for group B β-hemolytic streptococci, and a computed tomography (CT) scan demonstrated peristent infiltration. The patient was normotensive and had normal renal function at that time. She was treated with 6 weeks of intravenous antibiotics followed by 6 months of oral amoxicillin therapy. The patient continued to be normotensive and asymptomatic 5 months after discontinuation of antibiotic therapy and 14 months after stent placement.

To date, there have been no randomized prospective trials to evaluate the efficacy of antibiotic prophylaxis during stent placement. Some groups do recommend use of prophylaxis before deployment and consider antibiotics while indwelling/intravascular sheaths/catheters are in place or around the time of a prolonged urokinase infusion.[111]

Comments

Stents have been designed to improve the results of PTA, especially concentrating on perceived problem areas. One can therefore expect the complication rate of stenting to be that associated with PTA plus any problems associated with the more frequent catheter exchanges required and the deployment of the stent. In general, this translates into a procedural mortality of 0% to 4% and complication rate of 5% to 20%, depending on the indication for stent placement.[31,36,41,46,86,99]

The indications for stent deployment have been adequately enumerated in the text, but the contraindications have not been mentioned. Patients who are not considered candidates are usually refused stent therapy because of the possibility of doing harm. Vessel rupture after PTA may be made worse by stenting open the defect, as it is known that branches originating from major vessels often stay open after a stent has been placed across them. The design stiffness of the Palmaz and possibly the Gianturco stent makes them less than ideal for use in tortuous vessels. The entrance vessel must be of sufficient diameter to allow sheath placement; otherwise, there is significant damage to the luminal surface of the vessel. Aneurysmal disease is considered a relative contraindication to stent placement because of the risk of rupture, thrombus, or embolus. The risk of embolization must be weighed against the potential benefits of recanalization when treating long occlusions. Finally, calcified lesions not amenable to dilation at the pressures used for PTA should not be expected to be treated with a stent because the basic technique requires a similar physical force to be applied to the atherosclerotic lesion.

The following generalizations on the placement of stents for treatment of patients with peripheral vascular arterial disease must be prefaced with the following comment. Now, more than 15 years after the introduction of stents to this field, patient numbers remain small. Furthermore, there are still concerns that the follow-up at 5 years seldom involves sufficient patients to provide meaningful long-term results. The reported data are simply insufficient to provide the final word on clinical stent use, although practice standards are becoming clearer.

A variety of stents have been found useful for salvage of unsuccessful iliac PTA. Because complications of PTA leave unresolved pressure gradients or unacceptable degrees of stenosis on the angiogram, the resolution of these deficiencies by stent placement has improved the early technical success of PTA to more than 90% in such cases.[31,41–43,46–48,55] Even with the 1 mm or more intimal hyperplasia likely to be noted on the intraluminal surface of these stents, the occurrence of significant restenosis (50% or more diameter reduction) is quite low (about 5% at 12 months).[31,41,43,55,56] The occurrence of progressive atherosclerotic disease distant to the stent may be of more concern (about 5% per year)[31,41] and may help to explain the approximately 85% two-year and 70% four-year clinical benefit rates reported.[31,41] These data rival overall PTA results in a markedly disadvantaged group of patients. Therefore if one is willing to accept PTA as a good treatment for isolated iliac occlusive disease, stent use for iliac PTA salvage should also be deemed appropriate.

Totally occluded iliac arteries are a problem for standard PTA. The use of stents has improved the success rate to about 80% at 3 years, with a late occlusion rate no different than that for treatment of stenotic lesions.[36,41] The problem with distal emboli after this type of intervention has not been completely solved, as the embolic rate remains 5% to 20%.[36,41,46] Operative exposure for the treatment of these lesions may help solve this problem.[36]

Primary stenting of iliac lesions based on theoretic advantages is reasonable and is championed by at least one investigator.[40] A 5-year angiographic patency of 93.6% would rival aortic surgical constructions and therefore would be worthwhile; however, it is yet unproven in the literature, as no full manuscript exists to confirm abstract reports. Better defining those patients not optimally served by PTA alone should be more cost-effective. Approximately 65% of patients are served well for 5 years without a stent; and the additional risk, intravascular hardware, and cost to improve the results in only one-third of patients seems excessive. Sullivan et al. identified patency of the SFA as the most important variable associated with both early and late success of primary iliac artery stent placement. Those patients with infrainguinal disease may be best served with immediate distal reconstruction because they are not likely to derive significant benefit from iliac stenting alone.[37]

As the diameter of the artery decreases, so does the long-term success of PTA. Stent deployment in the femoral artery was undertaken to improve long-term patency (i.e., prevent restenosis). Even with stringent anticoagulation regimens, it has not accomplished this goal. Significant intimal hyperplasia, often occurring within the first 12 months after deployment, has been demonstrated in more than 20% of cases[42,48,56,66] if one eliminates the 20% to 40% rate of early occlusive events.[48,68] In a prospective study comparing stent use to simple PTA, comparable patency rates could be obtained only after extensive reinterventions in the stent group.[68] Proper anticoagulation to decrease early thrombosis and some method of controlling intimal hyperplasia may be required to salvage stent use at this site.[42,56,66,70,71] There are data to suggest that the larger-diameter proximal SFA fares better than the smaller-diameter distal SFA and popliteal artery, but even so the clinical utility is questionable.[57,69] Some investigators[62,69] have postulated that in patients with long-segment SFA disease (15 cm or more) poorer patency rates may be secondary to incomplete apposition of the stent(s) to the vessel wall, a small postdeployment luminal diameter, or decreasing flow velocity through the SFA. Moreover, intrinsic stent characteristics, including composition and thrombogenicity, may promote myointimal hyperplasia, restenosis, and thrombosis.

The guidelines defined by the FDA phase II multicenter Wallstent trial called for 6 months of warfarin therapy to maintain the prothrombin time at 1.5 times control, but currently the need for long-term anticoagulation for femoropopliteal stent deployment is challenged. In a nonrandomized retrospective study, White et al. reported acceptable early and intermediate patency rates without the need for long-term anticoagulation.[63] One criticism of this study was the failure to provide a group of patients for comparison. Also, the segment length targeted for stent deployment was relatively short, at 2.7 cm.

The renal artery also suffers from diameter restrictions. Attempts to improve the initial results of ostial renal artery atherosclerotic stenosis by stenting have been limited by the occurrence of intimal hyperplasia and restenosis (range of 18% to 39%) within approximately 1 year.[86,101,103] Placing a stent 10% to 15% larger in diameter than the normal renal artery diameter or limiting the placement of stents to renal arteries more than 6 mm in diameter appears to decrease the clinical significance of tissue buildup within the stents.[86,97,101,103] Blum and colleagues suggested that the most important factor promoting long-term patency is an endoprosthesis length of only 10 to 15 mm; this is more likely to ensure rapid, undisturbed arterial flow to counter the potential shear stress generated because of the angle of departure off the aorta.[95] However, even in the presence of all potentially favorable factors for long-term patency, the effect of renal artery stent placement on renal function itself has been unpredictable.

Potential areas of investigation to improve stent results have been reviewed by Palmaz.[17] Better methods to manage the inherent thrombogenicity of the stent are critical, especially in small-diameter arteries.[16,17,19] Inhibiting unwanted tissue proliferation is an active area of research critical not only to this device but to essentially all vascular interventions.[16,17,54,70,71,113,114] Eliminating the offending device might be an alternate approach; the use of absorbable materials or stent removal when the job at hand is accomplished are two options.[16,17,18] Until more work is accomplished in these areas, the use of stents will be confined to large-diameter vessels (probably more than 6 mm in diameter) and to cases of PTA salvage where the risk/benefit ratio of the procedure favors stent use.

It remains to be seen how often endoprosthesis infection occurs. Catastrophic complications may be prevented by the use of prophylactic antibiotics, especially when stent deployment is via the femoral route.[111] However, without a randomized prospective study to prove its benefit, routine antibiotic prophylaxis is likely to be deferred until additional reports of infections mandate their use. A French group assessed all stent infections for elective revascularization of the lower limbs from 1985 to 1994. Based on their cost-analysis data, they concluded that a reasonable site-specific indication for using antibiotic-impregnated stents would be femorotibial disease.[115]

Conclusion

One should not view this summary of stent results as a condemnation of the procedure. In fact, stents have had reasonable success in providing a scaffold to maintain arterial structure and patency. Rather, it is hoped that the review brings into perspective the data available, highlights areas of concern, and provides a basis for the research now underway to correct the deficiencies inherent in a "first generation" attempt to treat vascular occlusive disease by a new modality. Modification of the design materials used, coverings on the stents, improved methods of deployment, and adjuvant medical therapy will likely propel "second generation" stents into an even more favorable clinical light.

References

1. Becker GJ, Katzen BT, Dake MD: Noncoronary angioplasty, *Radiology* 170:921–940, 1989.
2. Glover JL, Bendick PJ, Dilley RS et al: Efficacy of balloon catheter dilation for lower extremity atherosclerosis, *Surgery* 91:560–565, 1982.
3. Wilson SE, Wolf GL, Cross AP: Percutaneous transluminal angioplasty versus operation for peripheral arteriosclerosis, *J Vasc Surg* 9:1–9, 1989.
4. Dotter CT: Transluminally-placed coilspring endarterial tube grafts, *Invest Radiol* 4:329–332, 1969.
5. Spence RK, Frieman DB, Gatenby R et al: Long-term results of transluminal angioplasty of the iliac and femoral arteries, *Arch Surg* 116:1377–1386, 1981.
6. Lu C, Zarins CK, Yang C et al: Percutaneous transluminal angioplasty for limb salvage, *Radiology* 142:337–341, 1982.
7. Johnston KW, Rae M, Hogg-Johnston SA et al: Five-year results of a prospective study of percutaneous transluminal angioplasty, *Ann Surg* 4:403–413, 1987.
8. Stokes KR, Strunk HM, Campbell DR et al: Five-year results of iliac and femoropopliteal angioplasty in diabetic patients, *Radiology* 174:977–982, 1990.
9. Cambria RP, Faust G, Gusberg R et al: Percutaneous angioplasty for peripheral arterial occlusive disease. *Arch Surg* 122:238–287, 1987.
10. Simpsom JB, Selmon MR, Robertson GC et al: Transluminal atherectomy for occlusive peripheral vascular disease, *Am J Cardiol* 61:96G–101G, 1988.
11. Colapinto RF, Stronell RD, Johnston WK: Transluminal angioplasty of complete iliac obstructions. *AJR* 146:859–862, 1986.
12. Andros G: Interventional technology: intraoperative strategies and techniques. In Yao JST, Pearce WH, editors: *Technologies in vascular surgery*, Philadelphia, 1992, Saunders, pp 412–423.
13. Cragg AH, Lund G, Rysavy JA et al: Percutaneous arterial grafting, *Radiology* 150:45–49, 1984.
14. Maass D, Zollikofer CL, Largiader F et al: Radiological follow-up of transluminally-inserted vascular endoprostheses: an experimental study using expanding spirals, *Radiology* 152:659–663, 1984.
15. Wright KC, Wallace S, Charnasangavej C et al: Percutaneous endovascular stents: an experimental evaluation, *Radiology* 156:69–72, 1985.
16. DeJaegere PP, de Feyter PJ: Endovascular stents: preliminary clinical results and future developments, *Clin Cardiol* 16:369–378, 1993.
17. Palmaz JC: Intravascular stents: tissue-stent interactions and design considerations, *AJR* 160:613–618, 1993.
18. Irie T, Furui S, Yamauchi T et al: Relocatable Gianturco expandable metallic stents, *Radiology* 178:575–578, 1991.
19. Dichek DA, Neville RF, Zwiebel JA et al: Seeding of intravascular stents with genetically engineered endothelial cells, *Circulation* 80:1347–1355, 1989.
20. Palmaz JC, Windeler SA, Garcia F et al: Atherosclerotic rabbit aortas: expandable intraluminal grafting, *Radiology* 160:723–726, 1986.
21. Rousseau H, Joffre F, Raillat C et al: Self-expanding endovascular stent in experimental atherosclerosis. *Radiology* 170:773–778, 1989.
22. Vorwerk D, Redha F, Neuerburg J et al: Neointima formation following arterial placement of self-expanding stents of different radial force: experimental results, *Cardiovasc Intervent Radiol* 17:27–32, 1994.
23. Duprat G Jr, Wright KC, Charnsangavej C et al: Flexible balloon-expanded stent for small vessels, *Radiology* 162:276–278, 1987.
24. Hallisey MJ, Meranze SG, Parker BC et al: Percutaneous transluminal angioplasty of the abdominal aorta, *J Vasc Intervent Radiol* 5:679–687, 1994.
25. Sheeran SR, Hallisey MJ, Ferguson D: Percutaneous stent placement in the abdominal aorta, *J Vasc Intervent Radiol* 8:55–60, 1997.
26. Kadir S, White RI, Kaufman SL et al: Long-term results of aortoiliac angioplasty, *Surgery* 94:10–14, 1983.
27. Walden R, Siegel Y, Rubinstein ZJ et al: Percutaneous transluminal angioplasty, *J Vasc Surg* 3:583–590, 1986.
28. Gallino A, Mahler F, Probst P et al: Percutaneous transluminal angioplasty of the arteries of the lower limbs: a 5-year follow-up, *Circulation* 4:619–623, 1984.

29. Palmaz JC, Richter GM, Noeldge G et al: Intraluminal stents in atherosclerotic iliac artery stenosis: preliminary report of a multicenter study, *Radiology* 168:727–731, 1988.
30. Palmaz JC, Garcia OJ, Schatz RA et al: Placement of balloon-expandable intraluminal stents in iliac arteries: first 171 procedures, *Radiology* 174:969–975, 1990.
31. Palmaz JC, Laborde JC, Rivera FJ et al: Stenting of the iliac arteries with the Palmaz stent: experience from a multicenter trial, *Cardiovasc Intervent Radiol* 15:291–297, 1992.
32. Dalsing MC, Ehrman KO, Cikrit DF et al: Iliac artery angioplasty and stents: a current experience. In Yao JST, Pearce WH, editors: *Technologies in vascular surgery*, Philadelphia, 1992, Saunders, pp 373–387.
33. Wolf YG, Schatz RA, Knowles HJ et al: Initial experience with the Palmaz stent for aortoiliac stenoses, *Ann Vasc Surg* 7:254–261, 1993.
34. Murphy KD, Encarnacion CE, Le VA et al: Iliac artery stent placement with the Palmaz stent: follow-up study, *J Vasc Intervent Radiol* 6:321–329, 1995.
35. Henry M, Amor M, Ethevenot G et al: Palmaz stent placement in iliac and femoropopliteal arteries: primary and secondary patency in 310 patients with 2–4-year follow-up, *Radiology* 197:167–174, 1995.
36. Rees CR, Palmaz JC, Garcia O et al: Angioplasty and stenting of completely occluded iliac arteries, *Radiology* 172:953–959, 1989.
37. Sullivan TM, Childs MB, Bacharach JM et al: Percutaneous transluminal angioplasty and primary stenting of the iliac arteries in 288 patients, *J Vasc Surg* 25:829–839, 1997.
38. Bonn J, Gardiner GA, Shapiro MJ et al: Palmaz vascular stent: initial clinical experience, *Radiology* 174:741–745, 1990.
39. Williams JB, Watts PW, Nguyen VA et al: Balloon angioplasty with intraluminal stenting as the initial treatment modality in aortoiliac occlusive disease, *Am J Surg* 168:202–204, 1994.
40. Richter GM, Roeren T, Brado M et al: Results of randomized trial of PTA vs. primary stenting, *Radiology* 180:105, 1991.
41. Vorwerk D, Gunther RW: Stent placement in iliac arterial lesions: three years of clinical experience with the Wallstent, *Cardiovasc Intervent Radiol* 15:285–290, 1992.
42. Gunther RW, Vorwerk D, Bohndorf K et al: Iliac and femoral artery stenoses and occlusions: treatment with intravascular stents, *Radiology* 172:725–730, 1989.
43. Gunther RW, Vorwerk D, Antonucci F et al: Iliac artery stenosis or obstruction after unsuccessful balloon angioplasty: treatment with a self-expandable stent, *AJR* 156:389–393, 1991.
44. Hausegger KA, Lammer J, Fluckiger F et al: Iliac artery stenting—clinical experience with the Palmaz stent, the Wallstent, and the Strecker stent, *Acta Radiol* 33:292–296, 1992.
45. Vowerk D, Gunther RW, Wendt G et al: Ulcerated plaques and focal aneurysms of iliac arteries: treatment with noncovered, self-expanding stents, *AJR* 162:1421–1424, 1994.
46. Long AL, Page PE, Raynaud AC et al: Percutaneous iliac artery stent: angiographic long-term follow-up, *Radiology* 180:771–778, 1991.
47. Raillat C, Rousseau H, Joffre F et al: Treatment of iliac artery stenoses with the Wallstent endoprosthesis, *AJR* 154:613–616, 1990.
48. Zollikofer CL, Antonucci F, Pfyffer M et al: Arterial stent placement with use of the Wallstent: midterm results of clinical experience, *Radiology* 179:449–456, 1991.
49. Sapoval MR, Chatellier G, Long AL et al: Self-expandable stents for the treatment of iliac artery obstructive lesions: long-term success and prognostic factors, *AJR* 166:1173–1179, 1995.
50. Murphy TP, Webb MS, Lambiase RE et al: Percutaneous revascularization of complex iliac artery stenoses and occlusions with use of Wallstents: three-year experience, *J Vasc Intervent Radiol* 7:21–27, 1996.
51. Martin EC, Katzen BT, Benenati JF et al: Multicenter trial of the Wallstent in the iliac and femoral arteries, *J Vasc Intervent Radiol* 6:843–848, 1995.
52. Vorwerk D, Gunther RW: Mechanical revascularization of occluded iliac arteries with use of self-expandable endoprostheses, *Radiology* 175:411–415, 1990.
53. Vowerk D, Guenther RW, Schurmann K et al: Primary stent placement for chronic iliac artery occlusions: follow-up results in 103 patients, *Radiology* 194:745–749, 1995.
54. Reyes R, Maynar M, Lopera J et al: Treatment of chronic iliac artery occlusions with guide wire recanalization and primary stent placement, *J Vasc Intervent Radiol* 8:1049–1055, 1997.
55. Kichikawa K, Uchida H, Yoshioka T et al: Iliac artery stenosis and occlusion: preliminary results of treatment with Gianturco expandable metallic stents, *Radiology* 177:799–802, 1990.
56. Liermann D, Strecker EP, Peters J: The Strecker stent: indications and results in iliac and

femoropopliteal arteries, *Cardiovasc Intervent Radiol* 15:298–305, 1992.
57. Strecker EP, Hagen B, Liermann D et al: Iliac and femoropopliteal vascular occlusive disease treated with flexible tantalum stents, *Cardiovasc Intervent Radiol* 16:158–164, 1993.
58. Strecker EP, Boos IB, Hagen B: Flexible tantalum stents for the treatment of iliac artery lesions: long-term patency, complications, and risk factors, *Radiology* 199:641–647, 1996.
59. Cragg AH, DeJong SC, Barnhart WH et al: Nitinol intravascular stent: results of preclinical evaluation, *Radiology* 189:775–778, 1993.
60. Hausegger KA, Cragg AH, Lammer J et al: Iliac artery stent placement: clinical experience with a nitinol stent, *Radiology* 190:199–202, 1994.
61. Krepel VM, van Andel GJ, van Erp, WF et al: Percutaneous transluminal angioplasty of the femoropopliteal artery: initial and long-term results, *Radiology* 156:325–328, 1985.
62. Gray BH, Sullivan TM, Childs MB et al: High incidence of restenosis/reocclusion of stents in the percutaneous treatment of long-segment superficial femoral artery disease after suboptimal angioplasty, *J Vasc Surg* 25:74–83, 1997.
63. White GH, Liew SC, Waugh RC et al: Early outcome and intermediate follow-up of vascular stents in the femoral and popliteal arteries without long-term anticoagulation, *J Vasc Surg* 21:270–279, 1995.
64. Chatelard P, Guibourt C: Long-term results with a Palmaz stent in the femoropopliteal arteries, *J Cardiovasc Surg* 37(suppl 1):67–72, 1996.
65. Bergeron P, Pinot JJ, Poyen V et al: Long-term results with the Palmaz stent in the superficial femoral artery, *J Endovasc Surg* 2:161–167, 1995.
66. Rousseau HP, Raillat CR, Joffre FG et al: Treatment of femoropopliteal stenoses by means of self-expandable endoprostheses: midterm results, *Radiology* 172:961–964, 1989.
67. Sapoval MR, Long AL, Raynaud AC et al: Femoropopliteal stent placement: long-term results, *Radiology* 184:833–839, 1992.
68. Do-dai-Do, Triller J, Walpoth BH et al: A comparison study of self-expandable stents vs balloon angioplasty alone in femoropopliteal artery occlusion, *Cardiovasc Intervent Radiol* 15:306–312, 1992.
69. Strecker EP, Boos IB, Gottmann MD: Femoropoliteal artery stent placement: evaluation of long-term success, *Radiology* 205:375–383, 1997.
70. Liermann D, Bottcher HD, Kollath J et al: Prophylactic endovascular radiotherapy to prevent intimal hyperplasia after stent implantation in femoropopliteal arteries, *Cardiovasc Intervent Radiol* 17:12–16, 1994.
71. Bottcher HD, Schopohl B, Liermann D et al: Endovascular irradiation—a new method to avoid recurrent stenosis after stent implantation in peripheral arteries: technique and preliminary results, *Int J Radiat Oncol Biol Phys* 29:183–186, 1994.
72. Schopohl B, Leirmann D, Pohlit LJ et al: ^{192}Ir Endovascular brachytherapy for avoidance of intimal hyperplasia after percutaneous transluminal angioplasty and stent implantation in peripheral vessels: 6 years of experience, *Int J Radiat Oncol Biol Phys* 36:835–840, 1996.
73. Henry M, Amor M, Beyar R et al: Clinical experience with a new nitinol self-expanding stent in peripheral arteries. *J Endovasc Surg* 3:369–379, 1996.
74. Canzanello VJ, Millan VG, Spiegel JE et al: Percutaneous transluminal renal angioplasty in management of atherosclerotic renovascular hypertension: results in 100 patients, *Hypertension* 13:163–172, 1989.
75. Sos TA, Pickering TG, Phil D et al: Percutaneous transluminal renal angioplasty in renovascular hypertension due to atheroma or fibromuscular dysplasia, *N Engl J Med* 309:274–279, 1983.
76. Martin LG, Cork RD, Kaufman SL: Long-term results of angioplasty in 110 patients with renal artery stenosis, *J Vasc Intervent Radiol* 3:619–626, 1992.
77. Cicuto KP, McLean GK, Oleaga JA et al: Renal artery stenosis: anatomic classification for percutaneous transluminal angioplasty, *AJR* 137:599–601, 1984.
78. Hovinga TKK, deJong PE, deZeeuw D et al: Restenosis prevalence and long-term effects on renal function after percutaneous transluminal renal angioplasty, *Nephron* 44:64–67, 1986.
79. Klinge J, Mali WPTM, Puijlaert CBAJ et al: Percutaneous transluminal renal angioplasty: initial and long-term results, *Radiology* 171:501–506, 1989.
80. Baert AL: Renal artery stent placement. *Radiology* 191:619–621, 1994.
81. Martin LG, Price RB, Casrella WJ et al: Percutaneous angioplasty in clinical management of renovascular hypertension: initial and long-term results, *Radiology* 155:629–633, 1985.

82. Harjai K, Khosla S, Shaw D et al: Effect of gender on outcomes following renal artery stent placement for renovascular hypertension, *Cathet Cardiovasc Diagn* 42:381–386, 1997.
83. Miller GA, Ford KK, Braun SD et al: Percutaneous transluminal angioplasty vs. surgery for renovascular hypertension, *AJR* 144:447–450, 1985.
84. Losinno F, Zuccala A, Busato F et al: Renal artery angioplasty for renovascular hypertension and preservation of renal function: long-term angiographic and clinical follow-up, *AJR* 162:853–857, 1994.
85. Tegtmeyer CJ, Kofler TJ, Ayers CA: Renal angioplasty: current status, *AJR* 142:17–21, 1984.
86. Rees CR, Palmaz JC, Becker GJ et al: Palmaz stent in atherosclerotic stenoses involving the ostia of the renal arteries: preliminary report of a multicenter study, *Radiology* 181:507–514, 1991.
87. Boisclair C, Therasse E, Oliva VL et al: Treatment of renal angioplasty failure by percutaneous renal artery stenting with Palmaz stents: midterm technical and clinical results, *AJR* 168:245–251, 1996.
88. MacLeod M, Taylor AD, Baxter G et al: Renal artery stenosis managed by Palmaz stent insertion: technical and clinical outcome, *J Hypertens* 13:1791–1795, 1995.
89. Dorros G, Jaff M, Jain A et al: Follow-up of primary Palmaz-Schatz stent placement for atherosclerotic renal artery stenosis, *Am J Cardiol* 75:1051–1055, 1995.
90. Van de Ven PJ, Beutler JJ, Kaatee R et al: Transluminal vascular stent for ostial atherosclerotic renal artery stenosis, *Lancet* 346:672–674, 1995.
91. Dorros G, Prince C, Mathiak L: Stenting of a renal artery stenosis achieves better relief of the obstructive lesion than balloon angioplasty, *Cathet Cardiovasc Diagn* 29:191–198, 1993.
92. Iannone LA, Underwood PL, Nath A et al: Effect of primary balloon-expandable renal artery stents on long-term patency, renal function, and blood pressure in hypertensive and renal-insufficient patients with renal artery stenosis, *Cathet Cardiovasc Diagn* 37:243–250, 1996.
93. White CJ, Ramee SR, Collins TJ et al: Renal artery stent placement: utility in lesions difficult to treat with balloon angioplasty, *J Am Coll Cardiol* 30:1445–1450, 1997.
94. Taylor A, Sheppard D, Macleod MJ et al: Renal artery stent placement in renal artery stenosis: technical and early clinical results, *Clin Radiol* 52:451–457, 1997.
95. Blum U, Krumme B, Flugel P et al: Treatment of ostial renal artery stenoses with vascular endoprostheses after unsuccessful balloon angioplasty, *N Engl J Med* 336:459–465, 1997.
96. Henry M, Amor M, Henry I et al: Stent placement in the renal artery: three-year experience with the Palmaz stent, *J Vasc Intervent Radiol* 7:343–350, 1996.
97. Graor RA: New techniques for percutaneous renal revascularization: atherectomy and stenting, *Urol Clin North Am* 21:245–253, 1994.
98. Wilms GE, Peene PT, Baert A et al: Renal artery stent placement with use of the Wallstent endoprosthesis, *Radiology* 179:457–462, 1991.
99. Joffre F, Rousseau H, Bernadet P et al: Midterm results of renal artery stenting, *Cardiovasc Intervent Radiol* 15:313–318, 1992.
100. Raynaud AC, Beyssen BM, Turmel-Rodrigues LE et al: Renal artery stent placement: immediate and midterm technical and clinical results, *J Vasc Intervent Radiol* 5:849–858, 1994.
101. Hennequin LM, Joffre FG, Rousseau HP et al: Renal artery stent placement: long-term results with the Wallstent endoprosthesis, *Radiology* 191:713–719, 1994.
102. Kuhn FP, Kutkuhn B, Torsello G et al: Renal artery stenosis: preliminary results of treatment with the Strecker stent, *Radiology* 180:367–372, 1991.
103. Kuhn FP, Malms J, Kutkuhn B: Three-year experience with renal artery stents, *Radiology* 85:209, 1992.
104. Christensen MG, Lorentzen JE, Schroeder TV: Revascularization of atherosclerotic mesenteric arteries: experience in 90 consecutive patients, *Eur J Vasc Surg* 8:297–302, 1994.
105. Lindblad B, Lindh M, Chuter T et al: Superior mesenteric artery occlusion treated with PTA and stent placement, *Eur J Vasc Endovasc Surg* 11:493–495, 1996.
106. Warnock NG, Gaines PA, Beard JD et al: Treatment of intestinal angina by percutaneous transluminal angioplasty of a superior mesenteric artery occlusion, *Clin Radiol* 45:18–19, 1992.
107. Maleux G, Wilms G, Stockx L et al: Percutaneous recanalization and stent placement in chronic proximal superior mesenteric artery occlusion, *Eur Radiol* 7:1228–1230, 1997.

108. Weinberg DJ, Cronin DW, Baker AG Jr: Infected iliac pseudoaneurysm after uncomplicated percutaneous balloon angioplasty and (Palmaz) stent insertion: a case report and literature review, *J Vasc Surg* 23:162–166, 1996.
109. Chalmers N, Eadington DW, Gandanhamo D et al: Case report: infected false aneurysm at the site of an iliac stent, *Br J Radiol* 66:946–948, 1993.
110. Therasse E, Soulez G, Cartier P et al: Infection with fatal outcome after endovascular metallic stent placement. *Radiology* 192:363–365, 1994.
111. Deiparine MK, Ballard JL, Taylor FC et al: Endovascular stent infection, *J Vasc Surg* 23:529–533, 1996.
112. Gordon GI, Vogelzang RL, Curry RH et al: Endovascular infection after renal artery stent placement, *J Vasc Intervent Radiol* 7:669–672, 1996.
113. Glagov S: Intimal hyperplasia, vascular modeling, and the restenosis problem, *Circulation* 89:2888–2891, 1994.
114. Clowes AW, Reidy MA: Prevention of stenosis after vascular reconstruction: pharmacologic control of intimal hyperplasia—a review, *J Vasc Surg* 13:885–891, 1991.
115. Melliere D, Zaouche S, Becquemin JP et al: Antibiotic-impregnated prosthesis: eclectic indications, *J Mal Vasc* 21(suppl A):139–145, 1996.

22
Laser Angioplasty

Warren S. Grundfest

During the early and mid-1980s multiple investigators applied various forms of laser energy in an attempt to recanalize vessels.[1-3] These efforts focused on the use of laser energy to remove atherosclerotic obstructions in an attempt to improve on the limitations of balloon angioplasty. As balloon angioplasty and guidewire techniques improved, and as other devices assisted in recanalization and maintenance of patency, the criteria for measuring the success of laser angioplasty became more stringent. The combination of guidewires, balloons, and stents can now treat most stenoses and short occlusions (less than 3 cm) in peripheral vessels. Highly eccentric lesions can be treated with directional atherectomy catheters, and patency rates can be improved with the use of stents. Thus, as other techniques improved the physician's ability to treat peripheral vascular occlusive disease with percutaneous techniques, the perceived need for laser angioplasty diminished.

Early proponents promulgated the idea that laser angioplasty would replace more conventional techniques.[4,5] These overly optimistic assessments proved dramatically false. The early systems were technologically crude, and their application for vascular recanalization failed to consider the biologic response to thermal injury. These systems applied 10 to 20 watts of light in just a few millimeters, burning the tissue and producing an intense inflammatory response, with subsequent thrombosis and reocclusion.[6,7] Lack of sophistication in delivery systems, a poor understanding of laser–tissue interactions, and the failure to appreciate vascular biology led to disappointing results.[8,9]

At the same time, the magic of the word "laser" and the hype surrounding laser angioplasty resulted in widespread dissemination of the systems before their safety and efficacy had been proved. Comparisons between expensive laser technologies and the simpler, cost-effective balloon- and guidewire-based techniques demonstrated the inadequacy of early laser systems.[10,11] Interventional radiologists, vascular surgeons, and cardiologists became appropriately skeptical of the role of laser recanalization in the treatment of patients with peripheral vascular disease.

Laser Energy Delivery System

At Cedars-Sinai Medical Center in Los Angeles, Frank Litvack, James Forrester, and I attempted to optimize a laser energy delivery system prior to its clinical application.[12] We developed a laser system based on the need to achieve an atraumatic, smoothly recanalized, nonthrombogenic arterial lumen. Implementation of this concept required a thorough understanding of the pathophysiology of atherosclerosis combined with detailed knowledge of the process of ablation. Laser systems that produced high intraarterial temperatures were likely to cause intense thermal damage with high rates of thrombosis and restenosis. We chose instead to apply pulsed ultraviolet energy for arterial recanalization in an effort to minimize thermal damage, maintain precise control of ablation, remove calcified obstructions, and provide a nonthrombogenic arterial lumen.[13]

Laser light achieves tissue removal via one or more of three basic physical processes: photothermal conversion of light to thermal energy, photoacoustic conversion of light to mechanical energy, and photochemical conversion of light to chemical energy. Each of these processes has a different effect on the tissue. *Photothermal* processes produce tissue ablation primarily through the conversion of water to steam and pyrolysis of protein and lipid. As the water vapor and pyrolyzed components expand, hot gases and debris are ejected from the tissue. *Photomechanical* processes generate shock waves in the tissue, rupturing it and causing loss of integrity. As the shock waves expand outward, tissue fragments are blasted away, forming a crater. With *photochemical* ablation, rupture of just a few bonds at relatively low temperature results in ejection of gaseous components of photochemical decomposition. The tissue fragments and gases are ejected rapidly, minimizing energy (heat) transfer to the adjacent tissue.[14,15] Although these processes are not mutually exclusive, infrared wavelengths tend to produce ablation via thermal and mechanical processes.

Ablation Threshold

Pulsed ultraviolet laser energy has a shallow depth of penetration per pulse. Because the volume is small because of the shallow depth of penetration, ablation occurs in thin layers, with minimal thermal damage to adjacent tissue. Ablation occurs only if there are sufficient numbers of photons to energize the entire volume of tissue to be irradiated. This level of energy is called the *ablation threshold*. The ablation threshold is a function of the laser wavelength, pulse duration of the laser light, energy per unit volume, and absorption depth of laser light in the tissue. Below the ablation threshold, the laser energy is converted to heat, but tissue removal does not occur. At energies twice the ablation threshold, photoacoustic phenomena begin to predominate, and tissue ablation is accompanied by intense shock waves that tear the tissue.

Our early studies revealed that pulsed ultraviolet light at 308nm could ablate atherosclerotic tissue with minimal thermal and shock wave damage.[16] Studies were then conducted to understand ablation thresholds for all tissues encountered during vascular recanalization. At 308nm the depth of ablation ranges from 10μm in blood to 30 to 50μm in atherosclerotic tissue to 70 to 80μm in calcified tissue. Studies have shown that corresponding ablation thresholds are $5\,mJ/mm^2$ for blood, 18 to $25\,mJ/mm^2$ for noncalcified atheroma, 35 to $40\,mJ/mm^2$ for moderately calcified atheroma, and in excess of $60\,mJ/mm^2$ for densely calcified atheroma.[17] This variation in energy thresholds sets certain criteria for clinical applications. Ablation in blood or radiography dyes produces significant shock waves and gas bubbles; therefore blood and dyes must be removed from the environment during excimer laser angioplasty. At the same time, an average energy of 40 to $50\,mJ/mm^2$, which ablates most atheromas, is ineffective for removing heavily calcified atheroma.[18]

In vitro and clinical studies have shown the need for adjusting the energy delivery parameters to account for the tissue encountered during recanalization. These adjustments were not implemented during early clinical trials and led to procedure failures.[18] Newer feedback control systems that interpolate tissue type from spectral data and then adjust the laser catheter output energy are under development.

Catheter Design

Studies have shown that catheter design also plays a critical role in procedure success. Early-generation catheters had substantial "deadspace," which refers to the portion of the catheter that does not transmit laser light. As deadspace increases, the ability to ablate a uniform channel decreases. The early catheters did not provide sufficient energy to ablate heavily calcified atheroma, and the systems compensated for deadspace by delivering more intense energy in the fraction of the catheter that transmitted light to the tissue. This solution produced tissue tearing and dissection, as hot spots in the beam exceeded tissue ablation thresholds by a factor of three or four.

Advances in catheter design have reduced this problem. The use of bundles of fibers containing hundreds of small fibers, each 50μm in diameter, and studies that have determined optimal spacing of the fibers, have dramatically improved catheter ablation efficiency. The new generation of catheters should provide a uniform energy output across the face of the catheter while maintaining sufficient flexibility and steerability to negotiate the curves in the peripheral vascular system. Improved catheter performance should translate into improved procedure success and greater tissue debulking. However, correlation with clinical results is required to determine clinical benefit.

Clinical Laser Studies

Initial studies of peripheral excimer laser angioplasty began in August 1987 as part of a US Food and Drug Administration (FDA)-sponsored phase I clinical trial.[19] The goals of these initial studies, sponsored by industrial concerns that made the laser devices, were to demonstrate the feasibility of excimer laser angioplasty, test and modify the techniques and equipment, obtain follow-up data, and develop patient selection criteria. Funding for the trials was limited, and the industry failed to recognize the complexity of the laser and catheter design process. Each new catheter modification required submission to the FDA, thus prolonging development cycles. Limitations in funding also compromised the collection of patient information, and the planned follow-up studies were not completed. The following paragraphs summarize the results of several early excimer-based peripheral laser angioplasty efforts. Follow-up is incomplete, and the data are presented so the reader may understand the potential of laser angioplasty.

Early Trials

Significant changes in delivery system and clinical practice were made based on the experience of the earliest stages of the trials (begun in 1987). The following results reflect two trial phases, described as the first and second groups.

The initial energy source for percutaneous peripheral excimer laser angioplasty was a 308-nm, 140-nanosecond (ns), 20-Hz xenon chloride laser designed and developed by James Laudenslager and Thomas Pacala at the Laser Physics and Materials Science Division of NASA's Jet Propulsion Laboratory (JPL) in Pasadena, CA. Modifications at Advanced Interventional Systems (AIS) in Irvine, CA made the laser appropriate for use in human clinical trials. A variety of early catheter designs were compatible with this laser system. A series of catheters used 400-μm fibers with expanded tips to create a 0.8- to 1.2-mm hole. After several attempts, multifiber concentric catheters with a central lumen for a guidewire were developed. Although primitive by today's standards, these initial catheters were state of the art at the time.

Sixty-two patients were treated in this initial study. The laser catheters permitted successful recanalization in 12 of 14 occlusions of 0 to 5 cm, 17 of 19 occlusions of 5 to 10 cm, 18 of 21 occlusions of 11 to 15 cm, and 5 of 8 occlusions longer than 15 cm. The longest successfully treated occlusion was 33 cm. An overall success rate of more than 84% was achieved. All 10 failures were caused by an inability to maintain the catheters in coaxial alignment within the vessel; 5 of the 10 failures occurred in the first 25 patients treated. Complications included four hematomas; one tip detachment; two distal emboli, which were successfully removed by suction embolectomy; and two early reocclusions, which were successfully treated with urokinase. One episode of transient renal failure was encountered.

Patients with stenoses appeared to have a higher recurrence rate and a lower secondary patency rate. Of the 34 successfully treated occlusions, 26 were available for follow-up, and restenosis occurred in 9 of the 26. Of these nine patients, eight were successfully redilated with balloon angioplasty. While following these patients we noted that long total occlusions recurred as short stenoses. Eight patients with restenosis underwent successful balloon angioplasty, which was patent at 1 year; one declined further treatment and was managed medically. Failure to follow the remaining eight patients is a limitation of this study.

These preliminary efforts demonstrated that excimer laser angioplasty, when combined with balloons, permits effective recanalization for lesions up to 15 cm. Failure to recanalize was primarily due to an inability to guide or steer the catheter into the true lumen. Densely calcified lesions were also a problem if the catheter could not directly engage them. These initial studies demonstrated both the feasibility of the approach and the limitations of the early catheters. They also demonstrated the need for carefully controlled clinical trials and effective database management to facilitate verification of results and ensure follow-up.

Later Studies

After preliminary results were obtained at Cedars-Sinai, the FDA granted permission to expand the trial to 12 centers. This trial, conducted under the auspices of AIS, was closed before its completion date, and many patients were lost to follow-up. Despite these limitations, significant information can be gained from studying the available results.

The initial protocol suggested limiting the procedure to lesions 0 to 15 cm in length, and all patients in the study between 1987 and 1991 had significant symptomatic lower extremity claudication and were candidates for lower extremity revascularization. Delivery systems, developed over the course of the trials, initially consisted of a single core fiber in Teflon catheters and, later, of concentrically arranged multifiber catheters. A fiber inside a balloon catheter that could be inflated to centralize the fiberoptic within the vessel lumen was developed for total occlusions. Finally, systems were developed that consisted of smaller fibers in a densely packed concentric arrangement around the guidewire lumen.

From January 1987 through December 1989, a total of 136 patients were treated at eight institutions. Only 112 of these patients were treated within the established guidelines, however, as some investigators attempted to provide alternative therapy for their patients. Attempts to recanalize 20-cm occlusions or multiple sequential occlusions below the knee with these early systems were successful in only 45% of the procedures. Nevertheless, the overall experience provided a substantial body of knowledge regarding the design of the catheters and the operation of the system. The importance of strict inclusion criteria and careful adherence to defined protocols cannot be overemphasized.

For these studies, acute success is defined as a residual angiographic stenosis of no more than 50% of the original lesion, an ankle-arm index of at least 0.5, and resolution of symptoms. Restenosis was defined as recurrence of symptoms, a change of the ankle-arm index to less than 0.15 improvement, and 50% loss of the luminal diameter originally achieved.

Noninvasive follow-up, such as color flow Doppler or duplex scanning, is preferred because it can demonstrate recurrences before they become symptomatic. As it is much easier to dilate a stenosis than recanalize a column of organized thrombus, we have, in several cases, repeated angioplasty on vessels with stenoses of 70% or more in patients with minimal symptoms.

Patients were followed at 24 to 48 hours, at 1, 2, and 6 months, and at 1 year, noting the following: symptoms, pulses, appearance of stenosis length, ankle-arm indices, and color flow Doppler or duplex scanning. Table 22–1 compares the acute success rates of the first and second groups. In the first group, 112 patients were treated whose mean length of stenosis or occlusion was 8.2 ± 0.1 cm; there were 69 lesions in the superficial femoral artery, 20 in the popliteal artery, and the rest in arteries below the knee. Among these patients, 33% were diabetic and 40% were smokers. Successful recanalization with relief of symptoms and an

TABLE 22–1. Acute Success in Peripheral Excimer Laser Angioplasty

Parameter	First group	Second group
Total lesions	112	106
Technical success	85 (76%)	99 (93%)
Procedural success	88 (79%)	98 (92%)

Note: Procedures performed in lesions longer than 20 cm are not included in these tables ($n = 17$). Several investigators also attempted to treat multiple sequential lesions below the knee with the single-fiber coaxial balloon system ($n = 8$). This system was not designed for vessels less than 4 mm in diameter. For these 25 difficult patients, the acute success rate was 56%. These patients are not included in the analysis.

increase of more than 0.2 in the ankle-arm index was achieved in 79% of the patients whose lesions were treated (a technical success rate of 76%).

In the second group the lesions chosen were significantly shorter but more likely to be calcified. Altogether 106 patients were treated with a mean lesion length of 5.1 ± 5.0 cm; 60 lesions were in the superficial femoral artery, 25 in the popliteal artery, 11 in the peroneal artery, 7 in tibial vessels, and 3 in vein grafts. Among this group, 37% were diabetic and 52% were smokers. Successful recanalization with relief of symptoms and an increase of more than 0.2 in the ankle-arm index was achieved in 93% of the patients treated (a technical success rate of 93%).

Comparison of Early and Subsequent Studies

Changes in patient selection protocols and improvements in the device, procedure, and operator skill improved with experience and significantly affected outcomes in the second group (see comparison in Table 22–2). In the first group, perforation occurred in 17% of cases, a function of attempts to recanalize long and complex lesions with a relatively primitive device. In the second group, the device was revised in response to the need for more accurate placement of the catheter's tip and better control of its motion; moreover, fewer attempts were made to recanalize long, complex lesions (and those that were attempted were limited to lesions crossable by the guidewire). This change reduced the rate of perforation secondary to the device in the second group to 2%. Of note is the relative safety of the device: in the whole series only one patient required urgent bypass, and overall the complications have led to few clinical sequelae. In the second group, primary procedural success was achieved in 98 of the 106 patients treated within the guidelines of the protocol. A combination of devices and laser techniques was responsible for the successful procedures, indicating that excimer laser angioplasty may be a useful adjunct to balloon angioplasty for treatment of peripheral disease, especially in 5- to 10-cm calcified occlusions that can be crossed with the guidewire.

Long-term follow-up (Table 22–3), available in 89 of the patients from the first group and 71 from the second, demonstrates the effect of

TABLE 22–2. Peripheral Excimer Laser Angioplasty: In-Hospital Complications

Complication	First group	Second group
Total patients	112	106
None	70 (62%)	87 (82%)
Bypass	1 (1%)	0
Dissection (device)	3 (3%)	1 (1%)
Dissection (postballoon)	5 (5%)	4 (4%)
Embolus	2 (2%)	0
Fistula	2 (2%)	0
Hematoma	3 (3%)	1 (1%)
Acute occlusion	2 (2%)	1 (1%)
Perforation (device)	17 (17%)	2 (2%)
Perforation (other)	2 (2%)	4 (4%)
Spasm	3 (3%)	4 (4%)
Thrombus	3 (3%)	1 (1%)
Other	0	1 (1%)

Note: Both successful and failed cases are included. Percentages have been rounded off. Angiograms were obtained in most cases before, during, and after each step of the procedure for documentation. Dissections are listed as a result of the laser or of wire passage or balloon angioplasty, and perforations are listed as a result of the device or of wire or balloon manipulation. Data collection forms were designed specifically to record this information. When the cause of a complication was unclear, it was attributed to the laser probe. Complications can be overlapping, so more than one complication may have occurred during the same procedure.

TABLE 22-3. Long-Term Follow-up After Excimer Laser Angioplasty

Follow-up event	First group	Second group
Total patients	83	77
None	43 (52%)	52 (67%)
Reintervention	28 (34%)	12 (16%)
Amputation	4 (5%)	4 (5%)
Bypass	1 (1%)	2 (3%)
Death	4 (5%)	6 (8%)
Lost to follow-up	3 (4%)	1 (1%)

Note: Percentages are rounded to the nearest whole number, so total slightly exceeds 100%. Mean follow-up time for first group is 18 months, with all patients followed for at least 1 year. Mean follow-up for second group is 11 months, with all patients having completed a 6-month follow-up.

patient selection on long-term outcome. The mean lesion length was reduced from 8.2 cm in the first group to 5.1 cm in the second group. In the first group 34% required reintervention, and in the later group only 16% have needed it. Direct comparison is difficult because the second group has not reached the same length of follow-up, but there is a trend toward better long-term patency in this group.

Several patients in the second group were included because of severe concurrent diseases. Note that all six reported deaths resulted from co-morbid diseases, such as cancer and cardiac disease, not from peripheral vascular disease.

The low number of bypass procedures is attributable to several factors. Some patients declined bypass even after repeat balloon angioplasty. Several patients in both groups had at least one bypass prior to attempts at excimer laser angioplasty and declined repeated attempts at bypass. In others, co-morbid illnesses limited the aggressiveness with which they could be treated.

Conclusion

Results of these initial trials indicate that, with appropriate delivery systems, excimer laser angioplasty can expand the role of interventional therapy in the treatment of peripheral vascular disease. However, the initial trials demonstrated that, as then constituted, laser angioplasty did not reduce restenosis rates in peripheral vascular disease. Our experience with 50 patients at Cedars-Sinai proved the procedure to be safe, but the failure to recanalize in 11 patients was due in each instance to the physician's inability to maintain the fiber in a coaxial position. A critical step in the application of laser angioplasty will be the development of a guidance system that maintains the ablation catheter in a coaxial position.

Early clinical trials demonstrated the feasibility of using the technique to treat relatively short occlusions in small-diameter vessels. However, failure to produce catheters that generate holes larger than the diameter of the catheter restricted the application of this technology and is a significant limitation of the technique. To overcome this limitation, several investigators have used "eccentric" catheters. After initial passage of the catheter, multiple passes are made to enlarge the lumen.

One of the pioneers of this technique, Professor Giancarlo Biamino, has reported experience in more than 1800 patients treated in Berlin using excimer laser angioplasty.[20,21] He and his colleagues reported a series of patients treated at one institution with a primary success rate of more than 90%, even in long occlusions of the superficial femoral artery. Biamino has developed a step-by-step laser catheter advancement technique that permits careful advancement of the laser catheter within total occlusions.

To maintain patency after excimer laser angioplasty, Biamino developed an aggressive clinical follow-up strategy. Early reintervention in patients with symptomatic stenoses and in those with asymptomatic stenoses of more than 70% by duplex ultrasonography are standard and have improved the secondary patency rates to 85% at 2 years.

Based on this single-center experience and the American experience, Spectranetics Corp. (Colorado Springs, CO) is initiating an FDA-approved trial of excimer laser angioplasty for treatment of long (more than 10 cm) femoral popliteal occlusions. On August 7, 1998, the FDA approved an investigational device exemption (IDE) for peripheral excimer laser angioplasty (PELA) to use a new series of catheters for percutaneous treatment of peripheral vascular disease. This randomized trial in more than 300 patients should provide information as to the value of this technique in the treatment of patients with occlusions that are difficult to recanalize by guidewire and balloon techniques. Given the rapid progress in the design and implementation of guide catheters, guidewires, balloons, stents, and techniques, defining the role of excimer laser angioplasty for treatment of peripheral vascular disease must await the outcome of this trial.

References

1. Abella GS, Fenech A et al: "Hot tip": another method of laser vascular recanalization, *Lasers Surg Med* 5:327–335, 1985.
2. Geschwind HJ, Boussignac G, Tesseire B et al: Conditions for effective Nd:YAG laser angioplasty, *Br Heart J* 52:484–489, 1984.
3. Ginzberg R, Wechsler L, et al: Percutaneous transluminal laser angioplasty for the treatment of peripheral vascular disease, *Radiology* 156: 619–624, 1985.
4. Lammer J, Pilger E, Karnel F et al: Laser angioplasty: results of a prospective multicenter study at 3-year follow-up, *Radiology* 178:335–337, 1991.
5. Biamino G: Coronary and peripheral laser angioplasty. In Meier B, editor: *Interventional cardiology*, Hogrefe & Huber, 1990, Göttingen, pp 243–260.
6. Katzen BT, Kaplan JO et al: Complication of "hot-tip" laser assisted angioplasty [abstract], *Circulation* 78(suppl II):417, 1988.
7. Isner JM, Donaldson RF, Deckelbaum LI et al: The excimer laser: gross, light microscopic and ultrastructural analysis of potential for use in laser therapy of cardiovascular disease, *J Am Coll Cardiol* 6:1102–1109, 1985.
8. Huppert PE, Duda SH, Helber U et al: Comparison of pulsed laser-assisted angioplasty and balloon angioplasty in femoropopliteal artery occlusions, *Radiology* 184:363–367, 1992.
9. Lammer J, Pilger E, Karnel F et al: Laser angioplasty: results of a prospective multicenter study at 3-year follow-up, *Radiology* 178:335–337, 1991.
10. Biamino G, Dörschel K, Harnoss BM et al: Experience in excimer laser photoablation of arteriosclerotic plaques. In Biamino G, Müller GJ, editors: *Advances in laser medicine. I. First German symposium on laser angioplasty.* Berlin, 1988, Ecomed Verlagsgesellschaft, pp 147–156.
11. Litvack F, Grundfest W et al: Percutaneous excimer-laser and excimer-laser assisted angioplasty of the lower extremities; results of initial clinical trial, *Radiology* 172:331–335, 1989.
12. Cumberland DC, Sanborn TA et al: Percutaneous thermal laser angioplasty: initial clinical results with a laser probe in total peripheral artery occlusions, *Lancet* 1:1457–1459, 1986.
13. Grundfest W, Litvack F, Goldenberg T et al: Pulsed ultraviolet lasers and the potential for safe laser angioplasty, *Am J Surg* 202:394–400, 1985.
14. Grundfest WS, Litvack F, Forrester JS et al: Laser ablation of human atherosclerotic plaque without adjacent tissue injury, *J Am Coll Cardiol* 5:929–933, 1985.
15. Srinivasan R: Ablation of polymers and biological tissue by ultraviolet lasers, *Science* 234:559–565, 1986.
16. Grundfest W, Litvack F et al: Comparison of in vitro and in vivo thermal effects of argon and excimer lasers for laser angioplasty, Circulation 74:8113A, 1986.
17. Grundfest WS, Litvack F et al: Laser ablation and fiber optic damage thresholds for laser angioplasty. In: *International Laser Science—2/American Physical Society/Optical Society of America Conference Technical Digest,* 1986, Paper FE1:66.
18. Adler L, Litvack F, Grundfest W: Excimer laser assisted balloon angioplasty of peripheral vascular stenoses and occlusions, *Semin Intervent Radiol* 8:135–144, 1991.
19. Litvack F, Grundfest W et al: Percutaneous excimer-laser and excimer-laser assisted angioplasty of the lower extremities; results of initial clinical trial, *Radiology* 172:331–335, 1989.
20. Biamino G, Ragg JC, Struk B et al: Long occlusions of the superficial femoral artery:

success rate and 1 year follow-up after excimer laser-assisted angioplasty [abstract], *Eur Heart J* 15(suppl):147, 1994.
21. Biamino G, Skarabis P, Böttcher H et al: Excimer laser assisted angioplasty of peripheral vessels. In Serruys PW et al, editors: *Restenosis after intervention with new medical devices*, Kluwer, 1992, Dordrecht, pp 426–473.

23
Intraluminal Grafts: Historical Perspectives

Marco Scoccianti and Rodney A. White

Abdominal aortic aneurysms (AAAs) are the thirteenth leading cause of death in the United States, and their incidence is increasing.[1] A Mayo Clinic study showed an overall incidence of 36.5 per 100,000 people per year with a sevenfold increase from 1951 to 1980. This increase only partially reflects improved diagnostic capabilities because it is also due to the increased aging of the population.[2] The final endpoint of an untreated AAA is its rupture, but this event is difficult to predict. Although the most important predictor of rupture is size, even small aneurysms rupture. Darling found that the risk of rupture is 9.5% for AAAs less than 4 cm in diameter and 23.4% for those between 4 and 5 cm.[3] It has been calculated that, if hypertension is present, the risk of rupture is 20% for 4-cm AAAs.[4] Even the expansion rate of an aneurysm is difficult to predict because, although the average expansion rate is 0.5 cm per year, great variability has been found in the rate at which individual aneurysms expand.[5] When an aneurysm ruptures, the total mortality is in the order of 78% to 94%, with 27% to 50% of patients dying before reaching the hospital, 24% to 58% dying in the hospital before the operation, and 42% to 80% in the postoperative period.[6] These considerations have suggested that the mere presence of an aneurysm should be regarded as an indication for surgery in low-risk patients. However, although some centers claim a mortality rate of about 2% for elective aneurysm repair, the average operative mortality varies between 4% and 11%, with peaks of 60% in older patients with coronary heart disease, chronic pulmonary insufficiency, or renal failure.[7] In any case, conventional surgical treatment causes significant debility. It requires a large abdominal incision and extensive abdominal dissection, which induce postoperative respiratory impairment and prolonged ileus. The physiologic derangements caused by aortic clamping and declamping may precipitate cardiovascular instability with consequent myocardial ischemia, stroke, or kidney failure. In addition, the need to open the aorta and to suture a graft potentiates intraoperative or postoperative bleeding, which might necessitate giving blood transfusions. This introduces further risks. Dissection of the autonomic plexus around the aortic bifurcation may cause postoperative impotence. Also, the uncomplicated postoperative course requires at least 24 hours in an intensive care unit and averages 10 days in the hospital; high-risk patients clearly require longer hospital stays with considerable increase in the total hospital costs.[8]

It has been therefore logical to look for alternative forms of treatment, especially for those patients with multiple risk factors where the operative mortality is excessive or for those with small AAAs where the risks of correcting the AAA should be minimal.

Evolution in the Treatment of AAA

First Tentatives (Wiring)

The first tentatives of treating AAAs were indeed intravascular and aimed at inducing thrombosis of the aneurysm by insertion of wire into the aneurysmal sac. This technique was first described in 1864 in England by C.H. Moore[9] and modified by Buressi and Corradi in 1879, when they used galvanic current to heat the wire.[10] The first to introduce this concept in the United States was Blackmore, who also developed a special apparatus to induce electrothermic coagulation of the aneurysm lumen and a special needle to cannulate the AAA and introduce the wire.[11] Failures to cause complete thrombosis and late ruptures were common, partially because of inadequate length of wire inserted inside the aneurysm.

Linton was the first to use the wire as a sort of "stent" to induce thrombosis only at the periphery of the aneurysm, thereby increasing its strength. To do so, he used different puncture sites and a mean of 307 feet of wire. In addition to the direct transabdominal approach, he also used an "indirect" posterior approach under local anesthesia to cannulate the aneurysm through a small puncture incision, an approach he reserved for high-risk patients unable to sustain a laparotomy.[12] Even this method was unable to prevent aortic rupture, which occurred in 36% of patients within 18 months; it was therefore abandoned. Hicks and Rob[13] were probably the last to use this method; when they reported their experience (12.5% mortality) in 1976.

Aneurysm Exclusion

The concept of AAA exclusion by proximal and distal ligation and reconstitution of flow by axillobifemoral bypass was introduced by Blaisdell in 1965.[14] Karmody later modified this technique; in an attempt to induce retrograde thrombosis of the aneurysm, he performed bilateral iliac artery ligation and extraanatomic bypass without the proximal aortic ligation. He operated on 60 patients, with an operative mortality of 7% and an incidence of later aortic rupture of 5%.[15] This approach has also been used in collaboration with interventional radiologists to avoid a direct approach to the aneurysm by occluding the iliac arteries with detachable balloons[16] or by inducing thrombosis by transcatheter embolization of bucrylate.[17] A nationwide survey by Lynch showed a hospital mortality of 5.1% for AAA exclusion and 34.0% for distal ligation; the aneurysm rupture rates were 3.3% and 20.0%, respectively.[18] More recently, Pevec reported on 26 patients operated by the Blaisdell technique, with an operative mortality of 7.7% and an incidence of late death resulting from delayed rupture of 11.5%.[19] Both methods have therefore been unable to prevent aneurysmal expansion and rupture, and the operative mortality and the incidence of complications have not been better than those obtained by conventional open repair. It is important to note that, in some cases, persistent aneurysm expansion occurred after complete aneurysm exclusion, presumably because of persistent inflow from patent lumbar or inferior mesenteric arteries. Furthermore, when rupture occurred, it was located at the neck of the aneurysm, suggesting that significant wall stress may persist in this location.

Sutureless Anastomosis

The concept of securing a graft inside the aorta through a rigid ring without the need for sutures was introduced to decrease the total operating time, aortic clamp time, and intraoperative bleeding. Actually, several reports have documented the advantage of using sutureless grafts in the aortic arch, the descending thoracic aorta, and the abdominal aorta.[20-23] Oz described a sutureless endoluminal ring prosthesis made of a Dacron tube graft attached proximally and distally to a rigid metallic stainless steel spool (Figure 23–1). After aortic cross-clamping, an arteriotomy is made in the anterior wall of the aorta, and the proximal and distal spools are inserted through the arteriotomy into the proximal and distal necks. The two spools are then secured by double nylon ties passed around the aorta. In 1989 Oz

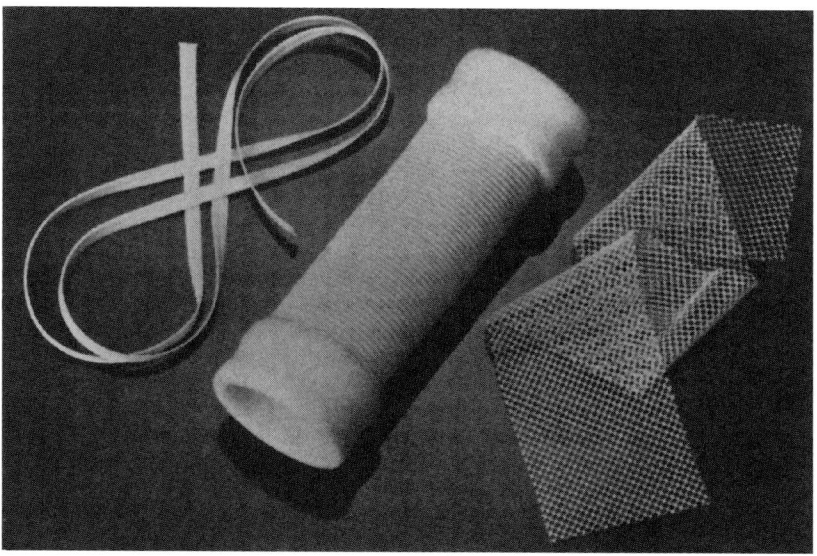

FIGURE 23–1. Intraluminal ring grafts. (From Serra AJ, McNicholas KW, Spagna PM et al: Replacement of the descending thoracic aorta with intraluminal ring graft, *Ann Thorac Surg* 48:689–692, 1989.)

reported that, of 31 patients with AAAs, three were suprarenal and four were ruptured. He had no operative mortality; there were two late deaths resulting from myocardial infarction, but none of the patients with suprarenal or ruptured aneurysms died. Two patients had distal embolization, but there was no kidney failure, postoperative bleeding, pseudoaneurysm formation, graft erosion, or migration.[22]

These reports demonstrated the feasibility of anchoring a graft to the aorta without the need for sutures and provided useful data for intraluminal prosthesis development, including the necessity of having a neck of adequate length and the need to accurately determine (intraoperatively) the length and the diameter of the graft to have a secure fixation and to avoid graft stenosis or aortic erosion. These first prototypes were composed of rigid rings and were therefore difficult to insert; also, securing the spools by ties required circumferential aortic dissection. Elastic rings made either of flat springs[24,25] or of nitinol[26] that could be inserted into a compressed state and remained in position without circumferential aortic ties were then developed and tried in animal studies. These trials demonstrated the feasibility of securing a graft inside the aorta by self-expanding rings and provided important information about the healing response at the site of graft attachment. Histology demonstrated uniform neointima coverage of the graft at the place of insertion into the aorta but also degeneration and reduction in thickness of the media between 40% and 80%. These changes, however, stabilized after 1 month and did not induce aortic perforation or ring migration. These findings are similar to those observed after arterial stent implantation.

First Endoluminal Grafts

Dotter is credited with the development of the first arterial stents for catheter-based insertion through a remote artery. The first stents were made of impervious plastic tubes, and all invariably thrombosed. He then conceived the idea of using tightly wound stainless steel coils; these were deployed into the superficial femoral arteries of three dogs. Although they had a low expansion ratio and were prone to spasm-related migration, two of them remained patent for more than 2 years and at the time of harvesting were well incorporated into the arterial wall and covered by neointima.[27] It was several years later, however, that Cragg overcame the poor expansion ratio of the stain-less steel coiled stent by using nitinol wire. He was able to deploy such a stent in the abdominal aorta of four dogs through a femoral artery cut-down; all grafts remained patent for the 4-week period of the study.[28] He suggested that this method could be used to treat arterial stenosis or aneurysms and venous compressions. One year later, Maas, a Swiss surgeon, reported the successful implantation of 160 double helix spirals made of Mediloy (a high-grade stainless steel) in 65 dogs and 5 calves in the inferior vena cava, thoracic aorta, and abdominal aorta. These spirals could expand up to 32 mm and reach an expansion ratio of 1:5, which is very close to that of current stents. Of note was the absence of migration and perforation 2 years after deployment.[29] However, these devices were too large for peripheral insertion; and, although he predicted their possible use as caval filters, as postangioplasty stents, and to treat aortic dissections, their clinical application was never reported.

The first experiments that focused on exclusion of an artificial AAA using an endoluminal graft were performed by Alexander Balko in 1986. He was also the first to use a Dacron patch model of AAA in sheep. His endoluminal graft was an 8-cm long, 10-mm diameter tube made of polyurethane and totally supported by an S-shaped nitinol frame.[30] The endoluminal graft was compressed in a 15F catheter, inserted into the femoral artery, and manually guided inside the aneurysm; soon after deployment the successful exclusion of the aneurysm was confirmed by the immediate cessation of pulsation in the aneurysm and by the absence of bleeding on opening the aneurysm. Balko not only demonstrated the feasibility of the concept of AAA exclusion but also underscored the potential risks of embolization of thrombotic debris, of prosthesis migration, and of aortic wall erosion. He also predicted that aneurysms not suitable for the technique would be those with renal artery involvement or a short proximal neck, those with a patent inferior mesenteric artery, and those with iliac tortuosity, stenosis, or aneurysms. These concepts are still partially valid today.

Evolution in Endoluminal Graft Design

All of these previously mentioned attempts to develop an endoluminal graft remained substantially isolated because of the lack of a satisfactory anchoring device. Although the increased use of percutaneous balloon angioplasty and improved vascular imaging modalities have produced tremendous advancements in catheter-based technology, the unavailability of stents made AAA exclusion by endoluminal grafts difficult. This problem was eventually solved by the work of two independent teams of investigators led by Julio Palmaz and by Cesare Gianturco, who developed, respectively, a balloon-expandable stent[31] and a self-expanding stent.[32] These stents constituted the basis for the construction of the endoluminal grafts employed in the first animal experiments.

Lawrence and Gianturco initially used a thin-woven Dacron graft attached to a series of Gianturco Zeta stents connected to each other by metallic struts. The leading and the trailing stents had the function to anchor the graft, and the internal stents served to keep the Dacron tube open. The initial device did not have side barbs to help fixation (Figure 23–2). A 12F Teflon sheath housing the device was inserted into the femoral artery, and the endoluminal graft was then deployed under fluoroscopic control into normal canine thoracic and abdominal aortas.[33] The deployment was successful in all dogs, and all the grafts but one remained patent at follow-up. Several important observations were obtained from these experiments. Although collateral branches covered by the Dacron graft occluded, those covered only by the stent remained open. Although a thin neointima covered the stents, a much thicker neointima covered the Dacron; this is similar to that seen in surgically placed grafts. In addition, the importance of correctly sizing the endoluminal graft to the diameter of

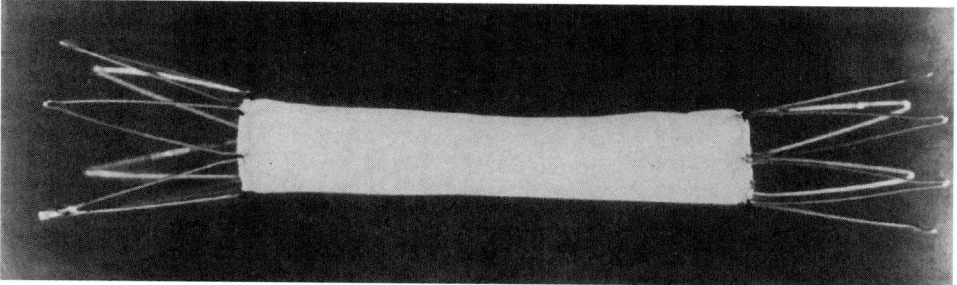

FIGURE 23–2. Woven Dacron graft attached to Gianturco Zeta stents. (From Lawrence DD, Charnsangavej C, Wright KC et al: Percutaneous endovascualr graft: experimental evaluation, *Radiology* 163:357–360, 1987.)

the vessel was demonstrated when an oversized graft caused significant aortic stenosis. The idea of having a totally supported graft is also quite interesting; it has been adopted by other investigators in the development of more recent endoluminal grafts such as the Corvita graft,[34] the tantalum-Dacron co-knit stent,[35] the double-knitted macroporous nitinol stent,[36] and the Cragg stent.[37] The Dacron graft had a tendency to wrinkle and induce excessive fibrous reaction with subsequent arterial narrowing; it also caused thrombosis of the collateral vessels. This observation led Gianturco to modify the device. In subsequent experiments, he used a nylon expandable graft (88% nylon, 12% Lycra spandex; Figure 23–3) and also provided the leading stent with barbs because migration was observed in unanchored devices. The endoluminal graft was then deployed in normal aortas and iliac arteries[38] and in artificially created aortic aneurysms.[39] All well-deployed grafts remained patent, and no migration or stenosis was observed. In addition, the elasticity of nylon allowed for downsizing the graft and obtaining at full expansion a better matching between the diameter of the graft and that of the aorta. This eliminated the longitudinal folds and irregular thickening of the neointima. Although the radial elasticity proved to be an advantage, the longitudinal elasticity of the graft caused some problems during insertion into the loading catheter because nylon had a tendency to bunch up at the distal end. The porosity of nylon was adequate to exclude the aneurysms but insufficient to cause thrombosis of the collateral vessels that remained patent. This property could be useful in endoluminal grafting of vessels affected by athero-

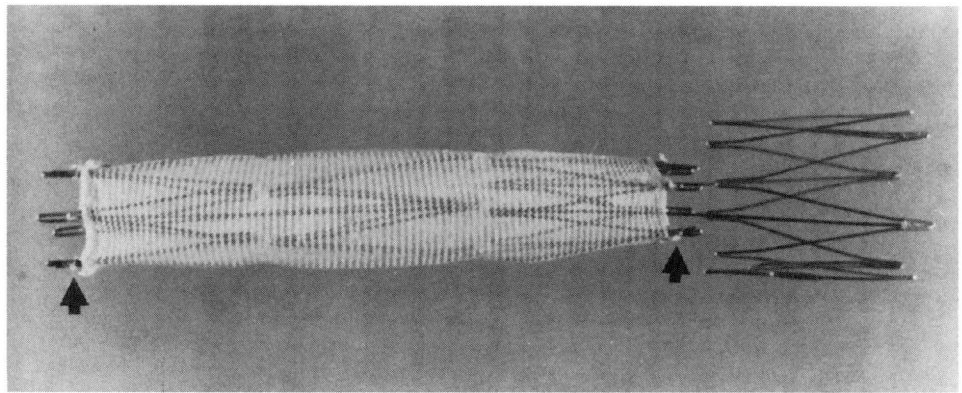

FIGURE 23–3. Nylon expandable graft with barbs (*arrows*) on leading stents. (From Yoshioka T, Wright TC, Wallace S et al: Self-expanding endovascualr graft: an experimental study in dogs, *AJR* 151:673–676, 1988.)

sclerotic occlusive disease, but its value is uncertain in aneurysmal disease. Although these investigators did not proceed to clinical studies, the Gianturco Zeta stent was later incorporated in the endoluminal grafts developed by M.D. Dake at Standford University and by Tim Chuter at the University of Rochester.

At about the same time, Palmaz demonstrated the value of endovascular stenting in the treatment of occlusive arterial disease and showed that, after deployment, a stent gets incorporated into the arterial wall by the formation of a thromboresistant neointima that prevents stent migration. It was logical to use this stent as an anchoring element for endoluminal grafts; and at the 1990 annual meeting of the Radiological Society of North America, Palmaz and Parodi presented the first results of aneurysmal exclusion in a canine model. This device consisted of a thin Dacron tube with two Palmaz stents sutured at each end of the graft by two diametrically opposed 5.0 polypropylene sutures. Two-thirds of each stent was covered by graft, and one-third was exposed. The system was then coaxially mounted over a 10-mm by 10-cm balloon of an angioplasty catheter, preloaded in a 14F Teflon sheath, and inserted into the femoral artery. Under fluoroscopic control the endoluminal graft was positioned at the level of the aneurysm, the sheath was withdrawn, and the balloon inflated, anchoring the graft against the necks of the aneurysm. At follow-up (6 months) all the aneurysms were excluded and the grafts were patent and covered by a thin neointima.[40] In a later and more extensive paper[41] the same authors reported on the exclusion of artificially created aneurysms in eight dogs using a non-crimped, weft-knit Dacron tube connected to two Palmaz stents and coaxially mounted on the same type of balloon angioplasty catheter. All dogs had aneurysm exclusion, but two dogs had torsion of the graft, evident by the presence of spiral folds on angiogram. These folds led to early graft occlusion. In addition, four dogs had evidence of graft kinking (manifested by a decreased interstent distance at follow-up angiogram), but that was ascribed to the shrinkage of the AAA model and was considered an unlikely event in clinical practice. An interesting observation was that in two dogs the graft seemed to collapse soon after deployment; this was corrected by reinflating the balloon for 3 minutes. It is not known if this was due to pressure and flow conditions that produced a Bernoulli effect and predisposed to graft collapse or to the porosity and permeability of the graft itself. Histology of the resected specimens revealed good incorporation of the stents. However, partial and immature endothelialization in the central portion of the grafts was also revealed; these were partially covered by fibrinous thrombus and had an increased number of monocytes compared with the stent, suggesting increased thrombogenicity of the graft surface. These observations suggested that twisting of the graft could possibly be avoided by inflating the stents by two separate balloons and that kinking could be prevented by the use of a crimped graft. It was also pointed out that the choice of the balloon size is critical because oversizing can lead to aortic rupture and undersizing to endoluminal graft migration.

After the successful use of endoluminal grafts in animal studies, the first human application was reported by Parodi in 1991.[42] He successfully treated four high-risk patients with no death; an additional patient was also treated by the same method, but the graft was maldeployed, and he required an open procedure. In these first cases the graft was tailored to the diameter of the aorta and the length of the aneurysm. The device was composed of a large type of Palmaz stent anchored to a thin-walled, crimped, knitted Dacron; to expand the stent to the aortic diameter, a valvuloplasty balloon (3.5 cm long, 23 to 25 mm in diameter) was used. The device was inserted through a femoral arteriotomy, preloaded into a 22F sheath. In three patients the graft was anchored only to a proximal stent, and one of these experienced reflux of blood from the distal graft back into the aneurysm. This event convinced Parodi of the necessity of applying a distal stent, and the subsequent patients were treated accordingly. These first cases stressed the importance of accurate preoperative measurement of the aortic and aneurysm dimensions, the need to have an adequate proximal and distal neck for attachment of the endoluminal graft, and the need to resolve problems related to small or tortuous iliac arteries. Parodi also raised several questions concerning the fate of the aneurysm and the natural history of patent lumbar or inferior mesenteric arteries after exclusion by endoluminal graft and raised concern about the risk of distal embolization of thrombotic material while guiding the endoluminal graft inside the aneurysm. Encouraged by these promising results, Parodi treated eight more patients, one with a subclavian posttraumatic arteriovenous fistula, opening the way to the endoluminal treatment of nonaneurysmatic arterial diseases.[43] Several ingenious maneuvers were employed in some of these cases, for example, the use of a temporary Dacron conduit to insert the endoluminal graft inside an unfavorable iliac artery and the insertion of a second endoluminal graft inside a low-sitting or a too-short previously placed endoluminal graft.

Important and ongoing contributions to the development of endoluminal grafts have also been given by other investigators. Chuter pointed out how only a minority of patients have a distal neck of adequate length to allow deployment of a stent and how often the diameter of the distal neck is different from that of the proximal one precluding the use of a fixed-diameter tube graft.[44] He therefore developed a bifurcated system utilizing barbed Gianturco Zeta stents attached to a polyester graft[45] delivered through a bilateral common femoral artery approach. He successfully deployed this device in both animal studies and human patients with good results (see Chapter 24).

H.M. Lazarus in the mid-1980s experimented with a system consisting of a tube graft incorporating attachment hooks that were then implanted into the aortic wall by balloon expansion. The system was compressed into a flexible capsule, and a pusher rod was used to extrude the device from the capsule.[46] This system was then modified by incorporating a Zeta stent into the graft, which was patented by EndoVascular Technologies (EVT); it is currently undergoing clinical investigation under US Food and Drug Administration (FDA) approval (see Chapter 24).

Currently, many new devices are being developed and evaluated in animal models and are being tested in clinical trials around the world.[34-37,47] Their use has not been confined to the treatment of abdominal or thoracic aneurysms but also to the treatment of pseudoaneurysms, traumatic arteriovenous fistulas, and peripheral occlusive diseases, opening a new and stimulating era in the history of vascular surgery.

References

1. Silverberg E, Lubera J: *Cancer statistics 1983*, New York, 1983, American Cancer Society.
2. Melton LJ, Bickerstaff LK, Hollier LH et al: Changing incidence of abdominal aortic aneurysms: a population based study, *Am J Epidemiol* 120:379–386, 1984.
3. Darling RC, Messina CR, Brewster DC et al: Autopsy study of unoperated abdominal aortic aneurysms. The case for early resection, *Circulation* 56(suppl 2):161, 1977.
4. Cronenwett JL, Murphy TF, Zelenock GN et al: Actuarial analysis of variables associated with rupture of small abdominal aortic aneurysms, *Surgery* 98:472–483, 1985.
5. Sterpetti AV, Schultz RD, Feldhaus RJ et al: Abdominal aortic aneurysm in elderly patients. Selective management based on clinical status and aneurysmal expansion rate, *Am J Surg* 150:772, 1985.
6. Quill DS, Colgan MP, Sumner DS: Ultrasonic screening for the detection of abdominal aortic aneurysms, *Surg Clin North Am* 69(4):713–720, 1989.
7. McCombs RP, Roberts B: Acute renal failure after resection of abdominal aortic aneurysm, *Surg Gynaecol Obstet* 148:175–179, 1979.
8. Breckwoldt WL, Mackey WC, O'Donnell TF: The economic implications of high-risk abdominal aortic aneurysms, *J Vasc Surg* 13:798–804, 1991
9. Moore CH, Murchison C: On a new method of procuring the consolidation of fibrin in certain incurable aneurysms, *Med Chir Trans (London)* 47:129, 1864.
10. Buressi P, Corradi G: *Lo Sperimentale*, 1:445, 1879.
11. Blackmore AH, King BG: Electrothermic coagulation of aortic aneurysms, *JAMA* 111:1821, 1938.

12. Linton RR: Intrasaccular wiring of abdominal arteriosclerotic aortic aneurysms by the "pack" method, *Angiology* 2:485, 1951.
13. Hicks GL, Rob C: Abdominal aortic aneurysm wiring: an alternative method, *Am J Surg* 131(6):664–667, 1976.
14. Blaisdell FW, Hall AD, Thomas AN: Ligation treatment of an abdominal aortic aneurysm, *Am J Surg* 109:560–565, 1965.
15. Karmody AM, Leather RP, Goldman M et al: The current position of non-resective treatment for abdominal aortic aneurysm, *Surgery* 94:591–597, 1983.
16. Leather RP, Shah D, Goldman M et al: Non-resective therapy of abdominal aortic aneurysms, *Arch Surg* 144:1402–1408, 1979.
17. Goldman ML, Sarrafizadeh MS, Philip PK et al: Bucrylate embolization of abdominal aortic aneurysms: an adjunct to nonresective therapy, *AJR* 135:1195–1200, 1980.
18. Lynch K, Kholer TR, Johansen K: Nonresective therapy for aortic aneurysm: results of a survey, *J Vasc Surg* 4:469–472, 1986.
19. Pevec WC, Holcroft JW, Blaisdell FW: Ligation and extraanatomic arterial reconstruction for the treatment of aneurysms of the abdominal aorta, *J Vasc Surg* 20:629–636, 1994.
20. Lemole GM, Strong MD, Spagna PM et al: Improved results for dissecting aneurysms, intraluminal sutureless prosthesis, *J Thorac Cardiovasc Surg* 83:249–255, 1982.
21. Serra AJ, McNicholas KW, Spagna PM et al: Replacement of the descending thoracic aorta with intraluminal ring graft, *Ann Thorac Surg* 48:689–692, 1989.
22. Oz MC, Ashton RC, Oz M et al: Replacement of the abdominal aorta with a sutureless intraluminal ringed prosthesis, *Am J Surg* 158:121–126, 1989.
23. Oz MC, Ashton RC, Lemole GM: Aortic replacement with composite grafts created with a sutureless intraluminal ringed prosthesis, *J Thorac Cardiovasc Surg* 100:781–786, 1990.
24. Matsumae M, Uchida H, Teramoto S: An experimental study of a new sutureless intraluminal graft with an elastic ring that can attach itself to the vessel wall, *J Vasc Surg* 8:33–44, 1988.
25. Matsumae M, Oz MC, Lemole GM: A flexible sutureless intraluminal graft that becomes rigid after placement in the aorta, *J Thorac Cardiovasc Surg* 100:787–792, 1990.
26. Yang C, Sun Y, Dong P et al: Experimental study of a new sutureless intraluminal graft with a shape-memory alloy ring, *J Thorac Cardiovasc Surg* 107:191–195, 1994.
27. Dotter CT: Transluminally-placed coilspring endarterial tube grafts, *Invest Radiol* 4:329–332, 1969.
28. Cragg A, Lund G, Rysavy J et al: Nonsurgical placement of arterial endoprostheses: a new technique using nitinol wire, *Radiology* 147:261–263, 1983.
29. Maas D, Zollikofer CL, Largiader F et al: Radiological follow-up of transluminally inserted vascular endoprostheses: an experimental study using expanding spirals, *Radiology* 152:659–663, 1984.
30. Balko A, Piasecki GJ, Shah DM et al: Transfemoral placement of intraluminal polyurethane prosthesis for abdominal aortic aneurysm, *J Surg Res* 40:305–309, 1986.
31. Palmaz JC, Sibbitt RR, Tio FO et al: Expandable intraluminal vascular graft: a feasibility study, *Surgery* 99(2):199–205, 1986.
32. Wright KC, Wallace S, Charnsangavej C et al: Percutaneous endovascular stents: an experimental evaluation, *Radiology* 156:69–72, 1985.
33. Lawrence DD, Charnsangavej C, Wright KC et al: Percutaneous endovascular graft: experimental evaluation, *Radiology* 163:357–360, 1987.
34. Derume J et al: The Corvita endovascualr graft: device description and early clinical results, personal communication, 1994.
35. Piquet P, Rolland PH, Bartoli JM et al: Tantalum-Dacron coknit stent for endovascular treatment of aortic aneurysms: a preliminary experimental study, *J Vasc Surg* 19:698–706, 1994.
36. Hagen B, Harnoss BM, Trabhardt S et al: Self-expandable macroporous Nitinol stents for transfermoral exclusion of aortic aneurysms in dogs: preliminary results, *Cardiovasc Intervent Radiol* 16:339–342, 1993.
37. Cragg AH, Dake MD: Percutaneous femoropopliteal graft placement, *Radiology* 187:643–648, 1993.
38. Yoshioka T, Wright KC, Wallace S et al: Self-expanding endovascular graft: an experimental study in dogs, *AJR* 151:673–676, 1988.
39. Mirich D, Wright KC, Wallace S et al: Percutaneously placed endovascular grafts for aortic aneurysms: feasibility study, *Radiology* 170:1033–1037, 1989.
40. Palamz JC, Parodi JC, Barone HD et al: Transluminal bypass of experimental abdominal aortic aneurysm, *Radiology* 177(P):202, 1990.
41. Laborde JC, Parodi JC, Clem MF et al: Intraluminal bypass of abdominal aortic aneurysm: feasibility study, *Radiology* 184:185–190, 1992.

42. Parodi JC, Palmaz JC, Barone HD: Transfemoral intraluminal graft implantation for abdominal aortic aneurysms, *Ann Vasc Surg* 5:491–499, 1991.
43. Parodi JC: Endovascular repair of abdominal aortic aneurysms, *Advances in Vascular Surgery* 1:85–106, 1993.
44. Chuter TA et al: Infrarenal aortic structure: implications for transfemoral repair, *J Vasc Surg* 20:44–50, 1994.
45. Chuter TA, Green RM, Ouriel K et al: Transfemoral aortic graft placement, *J Vasc Surg* 18:185–197, 1993.
46. Lazarus HM: Intraluminal graft device: system and method, US Patent No 4,787,799, 1988.
47. May J, White J, Yu W et al: Treatment of complex abdominal aortic aneurysms by a combination of endoluminal and extraluminal aorto-femoral grafts, *J Vasc Surg* 19:924–933, 1994.

24
Endovascular Treatment of Traumatic Arteriovenous Fistulas and Pseudoaneurysms and of Arterial Occlusive Disease

Carlos E. Donayre

Traumatic AV Fistulas and Pseudoaneurysms

The incidence of arterial injuries continues to increase owing either to urban crime and violence or the widespread use of invasive interventional procedures.[1,2] The close proximity of arteries to veins makes them vulnerable to the formation of arteriovenous fistulas and pseudoaneurysms when subjected to penetrating or iatrogenic trauma. Operative management is often complex owing to hemorrhage from an arterialized venous bed or difficult access, which may require morbid surgical exposures. The concept of minimally invasive endovascular techniques to exclude traumatic arteriovenous fistulas or to bypass pseudoaneurysms was realized with the introduction of stented grafts.

The first published report on the use of an intraluminal lined stent to treat an arterial injury appears to be that of Becker and associates.[3] A 43-year-old woman had a large-bore catheter mistakenly placed in her left subclavian artery during attempts at cannulating her subclavian vein. A balloon-expandable, Palmaz iliac stent was completely covered with a thin layer of silicone and percutaneously deployed under fluoroscopic guidance in the patient's left subclavian artery. The covered stent was removed shortly afterward at the time of operative repair. The report on this patient focused on the use of lined stents to obtain vascular control, minimize blood loss, and decrease operative exposure, not as a form of definitive arterial repair.

The endoluminal treatment of arterial injuries by covered stents was a natural progression of Parodi's success with endovascular repair of abdominal aortic aneurysms. Modification of his initial concept led to further clinical applications, such as the endovascular treatment of arterial injuries. A 62-year-old patient initially diagnosed as suffering from a "subclavian aneurysm" was found to have a large subclavian arteriovenous fistula. The fistula developed from a gunshot wound to the right chest suffered by the patient 2 years earlier.[4] A Dacron graft was sutured to a Palmaz stent that could be fully expanded by a 10-mm balloon. In contrast to the Parodi aortic endoluminal grafts, this graft was totally supported by a stent (Figure 24–1). The delivery sheath was introduced through the ipsilateral axillary artery and the stented graft deployed under fluoroscopic guidance. The fistula was immediately eliminated as demonstrated by the completion angiogram (Figure 24–2), and the patient continues to do well 3 years later.

The technical and clinical success in the above case led to its use in six other patients (Table 24–1).[5] One case merits further discussion. It involved a patient suffering from acquired immunodeficiency syndrome (AIDS) and a traumatic common carotid arteriovenous

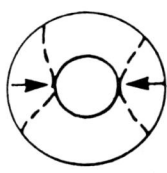
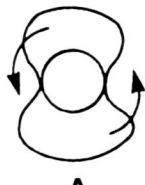
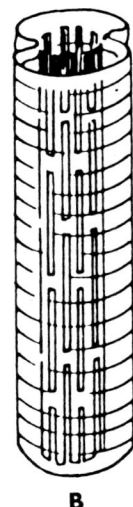
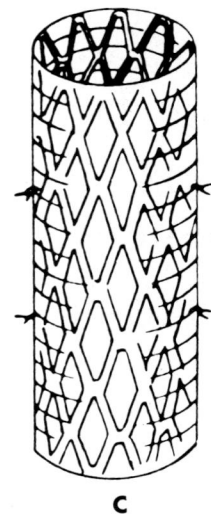

FIGURE 24–1. Covered stent. **A**, Cross-section of collapsed stent with graft attached, showing how graft is wrapped around the stem (*arrows*). **B**, Collapsed stent with Dacron graft attached before folding. **C**, Fully expanded stent with graft fully supported by the stent. (From Parodi JC: Endovascular repair of abdominal aortic aneurysms. In Whitemore et al, editors: *Advances in Vascular Surgery*, vol 1, 1993, p 96.)

fistula secondary to a gunshot wound to the neck. To avoid placing Dacron or polytetrafluoroethylene (PTFE) material in an immunologically compromised patient, and in a freshly contaminated field, a properly selected Palmaz stent was wrapped with autologous, thin-walled vein and deployed in a fashion similar to that described above.

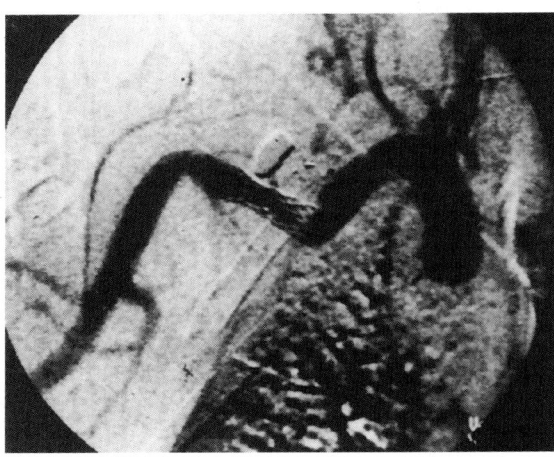

FIGURE 24–2. Right subclavian angiogram 1 month after covered stent deployment demonstrates a patent subclavian artery without stenoses and absence of arteriovenous fistula. (From Parodi JC: Endovascular repair of abdominal aortic aneurysms. In Whitemore et al. editors: *Advances in Vascular Surgery*, vol 1, 1993, p 97.)

The endovascular repair of peripheral arterial injuries lends itself to a percutaneous approach, as a small-caliber carrier can be utilized to house a single stent covered by relatively thin material. Graft strength is no longer a major consideration, as the graft is supported by a stent in its entirety. Furthermore, unlike the endovascular treatment of aortic aneurysms, this stented graft does not have to heal inside thrombus.

Marin, Parodi, and associates were also the first to report percutaneous transfemoral insertion of a stented graft to repair a traumatic arterial injury.[6] An 18-year-old man sustained a gunshot wound to the left thigh and on physical and angiographic examination was found to have a traumatic arteriovenous fistula (Figure 24–3A). Duplex ultrasonography was used to define the size of the arterial defect

TABLE 24–1. Anatomic Location of Traumatic Arteriovenous Fistulas Treated with a Covered Stent

Fistula location	No. ($n = 7$)
Subclavian artery and vein	3
Aorta and IVC	1
Right iliac artery and IVC	1
SFA and femoral vein	1
Common carotid and internal jugular vein[a]	1

[a] Treated with vein-covered stent.
SFA, superior femoral artery; IVC, inferior vena cava.

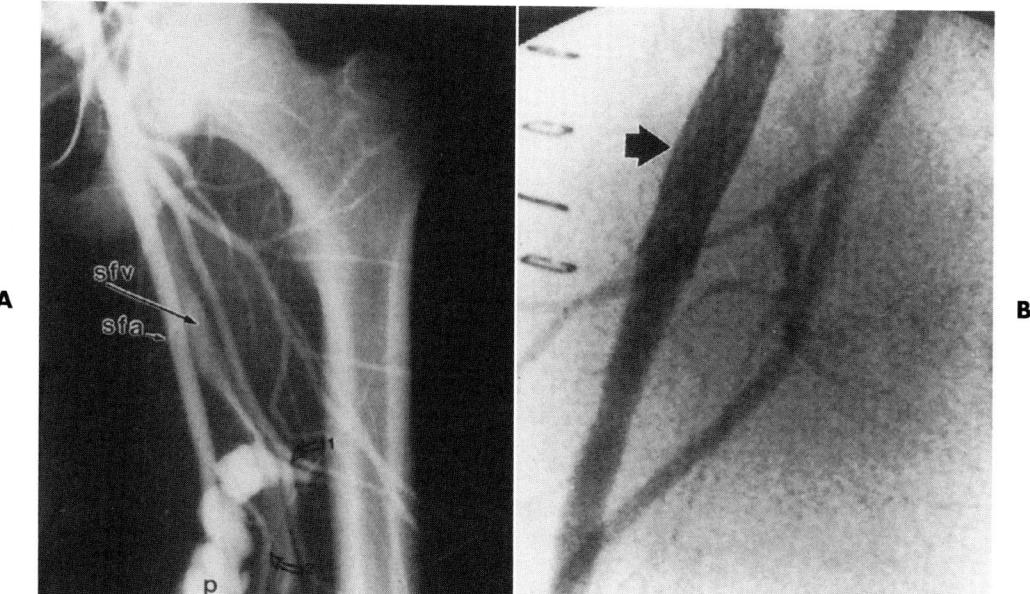

FIGURE 24–3. **A**, Femoral angiogram after a gunshot wound to the left thigh. Arteriovenous fistula is seen between the left superficial femoral artery (*sfa*) and femoral vein (*sfv*). Selective injection of deep femoral arterial branches (*1*) and SFA branch (*2*) showed that these vessels were intact. *p*, pseudoaneurysm. **B**, Completion arteriogram demonstrates patent SFA, proper positioning of stented graft (*arrow*), and no evidence of arteriovenous fistula or contrast extravasation. Metal clips were applied to skin before procedure to facilitate fluoroscopic localization and proper placement of stented graft. (From Marin ML, Veith FJ, Panetta TF et al: Percutaneous transfemoral insertion of a stented graft to repair a traumatic femoral arteriovenous fistula, *J Vasc Surg* 18:299–300, 1993.)

and the diameter of the superficial femoral artery above and below the fistula. A Palmaz stent was covered with a thin-walled PTFE graft and percutaneously deployed utilizing a 12F catheter through an ipsilateral common femoral artery approach. Distal pulses returned immediately following graft deployment. Completion arteriography documented closure of the arteriovenous fistula and patency of the superficial femoral artery (Figure 24–3B).

Parodi and associates have reported their initial experience with the endovascular treatment of traumatic pseudoaneurysms and arteriovenous fistulas, with a follow-up of 2 to 20 months (average 8 months). Their results have been impressive, with 100% patency of the treated vessels, persistent eradication of the fistulas or pseudoaneurysm, and no major complications. Parodi's concept of endovascular repair has also been successfully reproduced or modified by other investigators. May, White, and colleagues reported on the treatment of an iatrogenic subclavian artery pseudoaneurysm utilizing a prosthetic graft-stent device.[7,8] This 78-year-old patient developed a 5 cm subclavian artery pseudoaneurysm following attempts at placement of a central venous catheter. Two PTFE patches (Gore-Tex; W. L. Gore & Associates, Flagstaff, AZ) 0.4 mm in thickness were cut to the appropriate length and sutured together to form a cylinder 1 cm in diameter; they were then secured to an unexpanded 8-mm Palmaz steel stent. The stent-graft was successfully deployed using an open brachial artery approach (Figure 24–4). The patient has not had any complications and continues to have a normal circulation in the right arm 18 months after the endovascular repair.

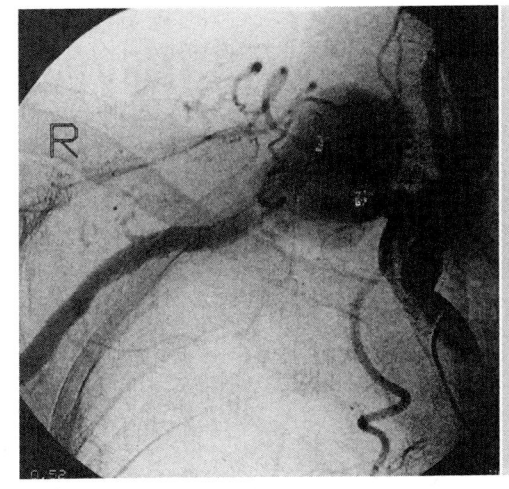 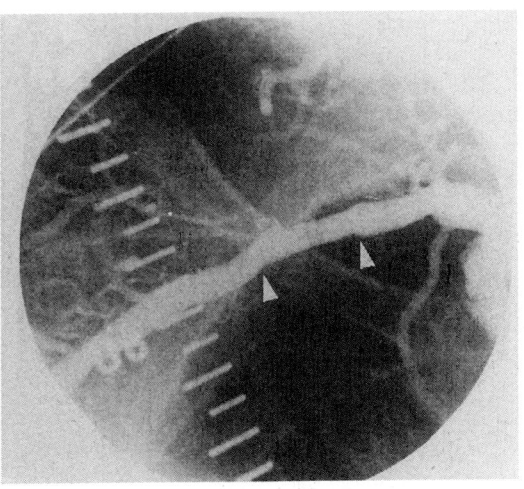

FIGURE 24–4. **A**, Preoperative angiogram showing false aneurysm of the right subclavian artery. Subclavian and axillary arteries distal to the aneurysm are of normal caliber. **B**, Completion arteriogram showing normal flow through the right subclavian artery without leakage of contrast into the aneurysm sac. Proximal and distal ends of the graft-stent device are indicated (*arrows*). (From May J, White G, Waugh R et al: Transluminal placement of a prosthetic graft-stent device for the treatment of a subclavian artery aneurysm, *J Vasc Surg* 18:1057, 1059, 1993.)

Other experimental covered stents have been developed to reduce the diameter of the device and permit percutaneous delivery and deployment. One such prosthesis, which appears suitable for percutaneous use, is the Corvita endovascular graft, first conceived by Jean-Pierre Derume. The stent component of this endovascular graft is comprised of a Didcott braided self-expanding stent constructed of Elgiloy wire and covered with polycarbonate urethane fibers.[9] This endovascular graft is produced in various lengths, with one or both ends of the stent exposed, and can be easily cut to the appropriate length prior to insertion in the operating room.

Implants of an early version of the Corvita endovascular graft began in February 1993 in Europe. Only high-risk patients requiring urgent vascular intervention were initially eligible for enrollment in this study. Altogether 14 patients afflicted with a variety of vascular lesions were enrolled, and successful deployment was achieved in 11 of them. Technical difficulties accounted for failure of device deployment in three of the patients. In one the endovascular prosthesis was cut too short to cover the full length of the lesion, and in the other two iliac artery angulation did not permit passage of the loaded introducer system. This fully stented elastomeric prosthesis is particularly well suited for the percutaneous endovascular repair of traumatic arteriovenous fistulas or pseudoaneurysms, as it can be compressed into a low profile delivery sheet (Table 24–2).[10] With the exception of one patient, who had an

TABLE 24–2. Corvita Endovascular Graft: Clinical Experience in Europe

Indication	No. ($n = 11$)
True aneurysms	3
Aortic arch	
Thoracic aorta	
Iliac artery	
Pseudoaneurysms	3
Subclavian artery	
Iliac artery (2)[a]	
Arteriovenous fistulas	4
Iliocaval (2)	
Axilloaxillary (2)	
Iliac artery stenosis	1

[a] One iliac artery pseudoaneurysm was associated with a dissecting aneurysm.

expanding aneurysm of the aortic arch and died 2 weeks postoperatively from a myocardial infarction, all patients were doing well with a follow-up of 5 weeks to 13 months.[11]

The initial endovascular experience with the repair of traumatic arteriovenous fistulas and pseudoaneurysms utilizing covered stents has met with high technical success and low morbidity. These injuries are usually localized to a small arterial segment, with normal vessel architecture at either end. Even if the vessel is totally transected, bleeding may be contained by muscle and fascial compartments, creating a pulsatile hematoma. The major morbidity associated with an operative repair is directly related to the difficulty encountered achieving adequate exposure and control of the injured vessel.

Endovascular access is achieved from a remote site located distant from the area of injury and occasionally can be gained by percutaneous techniques. Only the affected vessel is manipulated, minimizing injury to the surrounding structures. If successful, the patient benefits by having a shortened hospitalization and quicker return to normal function. The major concern is the long-term function and patency of stented grafts placed in young individuals. Patency of this type of endovascular grafts is favored by the following factors: relatively short length, placement in vessels with relatively large diameter and high flow rates, and entire graft support across normal vessels.

Stent-Graft Revascularization for Arterial Occlusive Disease

The success and durability of aortoiliac reconstructive surgery is currently being challenged by endoluminal therapy. Percutaneous balloon angioplasty (PTA) has gained wide acceptance as an alternative therapy to direct surgical repair of aortoiliac occlusive disease. In 1989 Becker et al. reviewed data from 2697 iliac artery angioplasties reported in the literature.[12] They calculated a 2-year patency rate of 81% and a 5-year patency rate of 72%. Use of more stringent criteria based on both clinical and vascular laboratory assessment lowers these figures. Kalman et al. reviewed data from 667 iliac PTAs utilizing the above criteria and found a *success* rate of 64.9% at 2 years and 53.4% at 5 years.[13] When PTA was limited to the aorta the long-term success rose to 80.1% at 2 years and to 70.1% at 5 years.

Further analysis revealed that intimal dissection and elastic recoil were hindering the technical success of PTA. The development of arterial stents made it possible to overcome the above-mentioned limitations. Stents overcome recoil forces by performing as a scaffold and simultaneously compressing any intimal irregularities against the vessel wall. A prospective, randomized trial of iliac stent placement versus angioplasty utilizing the Palmaz stent proved this to be correct.[14] A 5-year cumulative angiographic patency of 94% was obtained in the stent group versus 65% in the angioplasty group ($p = 0.001$). However, even though stents play a role in improving the early results of failed or inadequate PTAs, they do not appear to prevent restenosis due to intimal hyperplasia and may even be thrombogenic.[15]

The addition of prosthetic grafts to stents became the next logical step to extend the clinical range of transluminal angioplasty. Covered stents were introduced to provide a mechanical barrier to the intraluminal encroachment by intimal hyperplasia seen after endothelial injury following balloon angioplasty. Endovascular prostheses provided an uninterrupted, relatively nonthrombogenic flow surface to reline fractured, dissected, and diseased luminal segments. Their use appears to be of greatest benefit in the management of long aortoiliac occlusive lesions. The aorta and iliac arteries with their large size, paucity of critical side branches, and ease of direct local access makes them highly suitable for endoluminal bypass.

Stented grafts for the treatment of arterial occlusive disease have been championed and mastered by Marin and associates by relying on basic endovascular techniques.[16] Their deployment differs from techniques used for endoluminal exclusion of aortic aneurysms by the addition of an extra step—diffuse vessel dilatation—before endovascular grafting.

Arterial Access

The arterial pathology to be treated with a stent-graft is usually approached from a remote site. Direct access can then be obtained by one of two methods: If the access vessel is patent, it may be approached through a percutaneous puncture technique. However, in many patients with extensive limb-threatening aortoiliac occlusive disease the access arteries are occluded. The presence of an occluded vessel at the site of arterial access does not preclude performance of an endovascular stent-graft procedure. When occluded vessels are present, they can be approached by open surgical exposure of the access artery.

Recanalization of an occluded vessel can be performed in a *prograde* fashion by traversing it with a guidewire inserted from the contralateral limb (Figure 24–5). These recanalization wires (often with hydrophilic coatings) are fed *up and over* the bifurcation and used to develop a prograde arterial wall dissection plane. This technique allows maximal control of arterial inflow, and ensures that the recanilization process begins within the native arterial lumen.

If this approach is not technically feasible, a *retrograde* recanalization can be performed. Here the guidewire is passed through the ipsilateral occluded vessel, often through a dissection plane into the common iliac or aortic

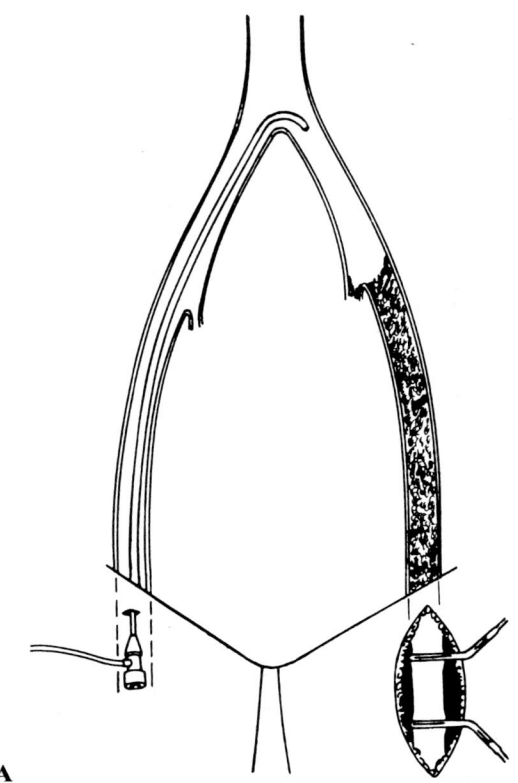 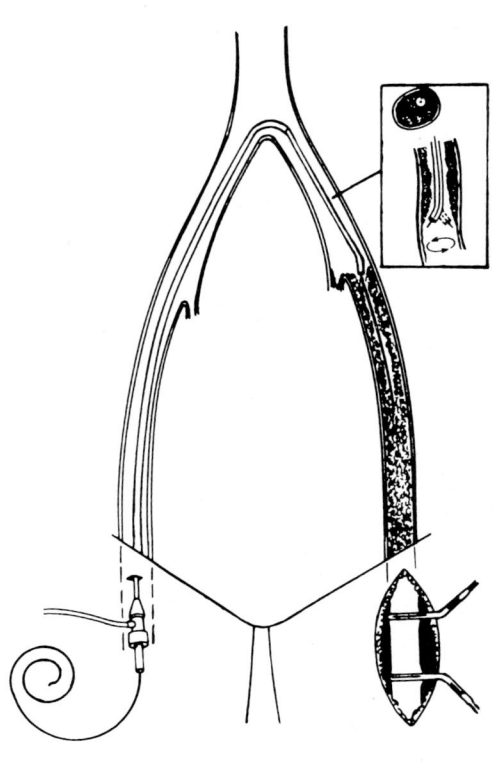

FIGURE 24–5. **A**, Prograde technique demonstrating percutaneous access of a patent ipsilateral femoral artery with introducer catheters in place. It is through these introducer catheters that all subsequent interventions on contralateral occluded vessel are accomplished. **B**, Directional catheter in place with hydrophilic wire working its way through an occluded external iliac artery. The directional catheter provides support to the flexible hydrophilic wires and assist in gaining access to the patent femoral artery (**inset**). (From Marin ML, Veith FJ, Sanchez LA et al: Endovascular aortoiliac grafts in combination with standard infrainguinal arterial bypasses in the management of limb-threatening ischemia: preliminary report, *J Vasc Surg* 22:316–325, 1995.)

24. AV Fistulas/Pseudoaneurysms and Occlusive Disease

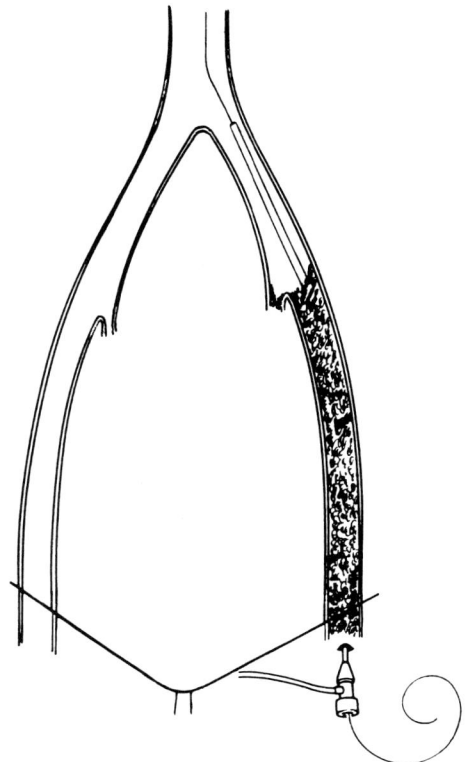

FIGURE 24–6. Retrograde technique with directional and hydrophilic wire across an ipsilateral occluded external iliac into the patent aorta above. (From Marin ML, Veith FJ, Sanchez LA et al: Endovascular aortoiliac grafts in combination with standard infrainguinal arterial bypasses in the management of limb-threatening ischemia: preliminary report, *J Vasc Surg* 22:316–325, 1995.)

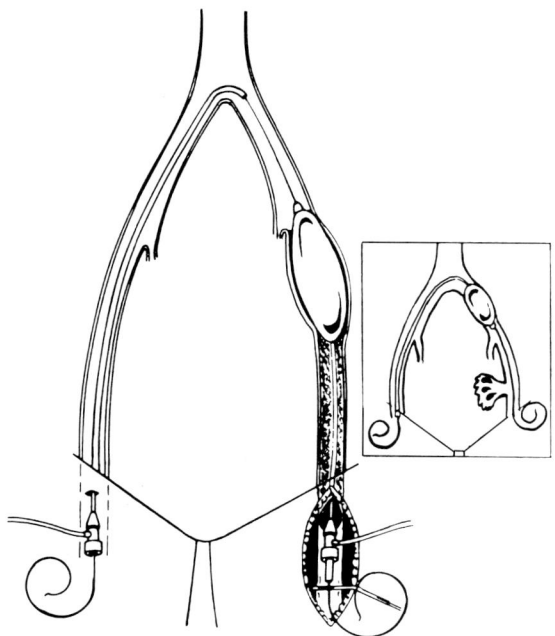

FIGURE 24–7. Following recanalization, balloon dilation is then performed over the wire along the entire length of the occluded or diseased arterial segments. If vessel rupture or perforation occurs, a proximal occlusion balloon can be inflated above the site of injury from the contralateral access vessel (**inset**). Repair can be achieved by deploying a stent-graft across the injured site. (From Marin ML, Veith FJ, Sanchez LA et al: Endovascular aortoiliac grafts in combination with standard infrainguinal arterial bypasses in the management of limb-threatening ischemia: preliminary report, *J Vasc Surg* 22:316–325, 1995.)

lumen (Figure 24–6). Guidewire access into the central axis of the occluded vessel is greatly assisted by the use of directional catheters, which provide support and direction to the flexible hydrophilic guidewire.

Arterial Dilation

Once the recanalization wires have established a connection between the remote access site and the patent segment of the proximal artery, properly selected angioplasty balloons are inserted over a stiff guidewire. Next the diseased segment of artery is submitted to extensive balloon angioplasty. Such dilation permits formation of a widened tract through the atheromatous arterial wall and facilitates insertion of the new endovascular graft within this tract (Figure 24–7).

Stent-Graft Insertion

The device most commonly utilized for endovascular repair of aortoiliac occlusive disease employs PTFE graft material attached to Palmaz stents. This configuration allows the assembly of low profile devices, which can be deployed inside the lumen of narrow vessels. After creation of a neoarterial tract within the wall of the occluded or diseased artery, a carrier system composed of a guiding catheter or sheath containing the endovascular stent-graft is inserted over the previously placed wire and advanced under fluoroscopic control to the patent proximal arterial segment. After the stent-graft is properly positioned, confirmed angiographically, it is secured into position by a stent attachment device (Figure 24–8). The attachment device provides a watertight seal between the proximal end of the graft and the patent portion of the proximal artery. Either direct suture anastomosis or the use of a second stent can be utilized to achieve distal graft fixation. When distal fixation is performed with sutures, it may be accomplished by a standard end-to-side or end-to-end arterial anastomosis.

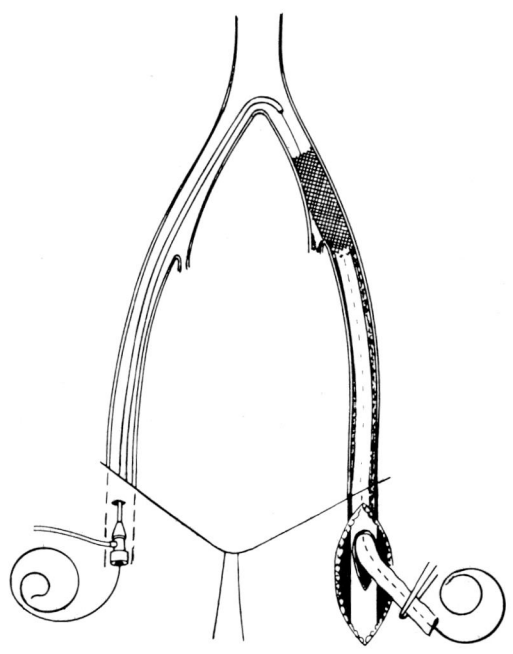

FIGURE 24–8. After creation of a neointimal tract the endovascular stent-graft is deployed at a selected site under fluoroscopic guidance. The distal end of each graft can be endovascularly anastomosed to the common femoral artery utilizing a series of 6-0 Prolene tacking sutures placed within the prosthetic graft. (From Marin ML, Veith FJ, Sanchez LA et al: Endovascular aortoiliac grafts in combination with standard infrainguinal arterial bypasses in the management of limb-threatening ischemia: preliminary report, *J Vasc Surg* 22:316–325, 1995.)

Alternatively, the endovascular stent-graft may be sutured to the patent portion of the outflow artery using an endovascular anastomotic technique.

There are several distinct advantages to use of a suture anastomosis to achieve distal graft fixation. The ability to hand-sew the distal anastomosis allows the graft to cross the inguinal ligament, something that is not recommended with stented anastomoses. Furthermore, the distal graft can be tailored to any length, enabling all aortoiliac grafts to be manufactured at the same length and subsequently modified for each patient. Finally, the endovascular procedure can be combined with standard reconstructive procedures such as femoral endarterectomy or profundaplasty. All procedures are followed by a completion arteriogram to inspect the technical adequacy of the procedure, document patency of the outflow arteries, and look for the presence of distal embolization.

Endovascular prosthetic repair of aortoiliac disease combined with conventional infrainguinal bypass surgery has been reported as a technically feasible, safe option in patients with multilevel lower occlusive disease.[16–18] Marin et al. published data involving 17 patients with multilevel aortoiliofemoral limb-threatening occlusive disease.[19] All patients had an endovascular stent-graft placed proximally using the techniques described above. Distal conventional bypasses were constructed from either PTFE or saphenous vein and extended to the popliteal, tibial, or contralateral femoral artery. One-year primary and secondary patency rates for the endovascular prosthetics were 94% and 100%, respectively. The 1-year primary and secondary cumulative life table patency rates for standard extravascular bypass were 92% and 100%, respectively. Three endovascular grafts required thrombectomy during a 24-month follow-up period. One graft failed owing to progression of distal disease, one because of proximal embolic disease, and one because of a proximal iliac stenosis. All three were successfully revised. Three extraluminal grafts also required revision: One failed while the associated proximal graft maintained normal function, and the other two presented

TABLE 24–3. Aortoiliac Stent-Graft Results

Study	Patients (no.)	Technical success	Primary patency	Secondary patency	Limb salvage (%)	Deaths	Minor complications
Marin (1995)[16]	18	17/18 (94%)	94% at 12 mo	100% at 18 mo	94	0	4/18 (22.2%)
Ohki (1996)[17]	7	7/7 (100%)	100% at 9–28 mo		100	0	1/7 (14.3%)
Marin (1996)[18]	42	39/42 (93%)	89% at 18 mo	100% at 18 mo	94	1/42 (2.3%)	4/42 (9.5%)

in the failing state with outflow vessel lesions. All three grafts were revised, with either distal extension or thrombectomy.

Ohki et al. presented seven patients with bilateral critical ischemia and tissue necrosis in association with severe co-morbid medical illnesses.[17] They underwent implantation of unilateral aortofemoral endovascular stent-grafts followed by standard femorofemoral bypass. In all cases, the symptoms completely resolved, and no graft thromboses occurred during follow-up ranging from 9 to 28 months.

Table 24–3 summarizes the results regarding placement and patency of the aortoiliac segment in the previously cited articles. Technical success refers to the ability to recanalize the occluded vessel with guidewire techniques. Minor complications included wound hematoma, lymphocele, and subendocardial myocardial infarction. Overall technical success was 94%, attesting to the fact that most of the occlusive lesions can be traversed with these methods. Patency rates have been uniformly excellent. The sole death was due to heart failure following an endovascular procedure, for an overall mortality rate of 1.5%. The limb salvage rate overall was 96%.

Endovascular stent-grafts have several theoretic advantages over standard arterial reconstructions.[18] Revascularization procedures are carried out through previously unusable, totally occluded vessels. The occlusion is repaired in an "anatomic" fashion so axillary arteries or the contralateral femoral artery are not jeopardized, as might be the case with an extraanatomic bypass. Devices can be inserted through remote access sites, avoiding the need to expose inflow vessels directly, a point particularly attractive in patients with a history of previous surgical interventions. Because these procedures are generally performed through small superficial incisions, the need for extensive transabdominal or retroperitoneal dissections is obviated. The avoidance of a wide surgical exposure eliminates the potential for prolonged intestinal dysfunction, pulmonary complications, and large fluid shifts, which may be responsible for cardiac and pulmonary failure. Furthermore, this minimally invasive approach allows a wide range of choices for anesthesia. Lastly, preservation of sexual function can be anticipated with the avoidance of aortic and pelvic dissection.

Conversely, there are several potential disadvantages. The biologic behavior of a prosthetic endovascular graft placed in a diffusely dilated, atherosclerotic artery is unknown. Specifically, concern exists regarding the potential of arterial recoil after dilatation, disease progression, and smooth muscle cell proliferation within atheromatous material extrinsic to the endovascular graft. Extrinsic compression can be treated with intragraft balloon dilatation or placement of an additional intragraft stent.[16] Early studies analyzing the plaque extrinsic to the graft in a limited number of recovered specimens have not demonstrated the presence of a significant smooth muscle hyperplastic response.[19] However, animal studies have revealed an exuberant neointimal response between the native vessel and the stent-graft, specifically when the metallic stent lies exposed between the vessel wall and the outside of the prosthetic graft material.[20]

Technical problems may arise specific to this method of repair. Arterial rupture and hemorrhage could result from the long-segment balloon angioplasty of the native vessel performed prior to graft insertion. This complication occurred in 4.7% of patients reported by Marin et al.[18] Local wire perforation during recanalization may also occur.

When these disruptions are significant, they can be managed successfully by placing a proximal occlusion balloon, a technique more easily accomplished when the "up and over" approach is used. As the device is deployed, these injuries are repaired by exclusion.

Endovascular stent-grafts appear to be an important advance in the management of complex aortoiliac occlusive disease and may have particular merit in the treatment of patients with significant co-morbid medical illnesses or those with failed, previous aortoiliac reconstructions. In these situations, stented grafts represent a way to reestablish arterial continuity without extensive operative procedures and their associated complications. Long-term follow-up and careful comparisons with standard operative and endovascular techniques are needed before widespread application of this technique can be advocated.

References

1. Feliciano DV, Bitondo CG, Mattox KL et al: Civilian trauma in the 1980s: a 1 year experience with 456 vascular and cardiac injuries, *Ann Surg* 199:717, 1984.
2. Youkey JR, Clagett GP, Rich NM et al: Vascular trauma secondary to diagnostic and therapeutic procedures: 1974 through 1982, *Am J Surg* 146:788, 1983.
3. Becker GJ, Benenati JF, Zemel G et al: Percutaneous placement of a balloon-expandable intraluminal graft for life-threatening subclavian arterial hemorrhage, *J Vasc Interv Radiol* 2:225–229, 1991.
4. Parodi JC, Barone HD: Transluminal treatment of abdominal aortic aneurysms and peripheral arteriovenous fistulas. Paper presented at the 19th Annual Montefiore Medical Center/Albert Einstein College of Medicine Symposium on Current Critical Problems and New Technologies in Vascular Surgery, New York, November 1992.
5. Parodi JC: Endovascular treatment of abdominal aortic aneurysms. Paper presented at International Congress VII. Endovascular interventions: on the cutting edge, Scottsdale, Ariz, February 1994.
6. Marin ML, Veith FJ, Panetta TF et al: Percutaneous transfemoral insertion of a stented graft to repair a traumatic femoral arteriovenous fistula, *J Vasc Surg* 18:299–302, 1993.
7. May J, White G, Waugh R et al: Transluminal placement of a prosthetic graft-stent device for the treatment of a subclavian artery aneurysm, *J Vasc Surg* 18:1056–1059, 1993.
8. White G, May J: Transluminal placement of a prosthetic graft-stent device for the treatment of a subclavian artery aneurysm, personal communication, 1994.
9. Wilson GJ, Mac Gregor DC, Klement P et al: A complaint Corethane/Dacron composite vascular prosthesis: comparison with 4mm ePTFE grafts in a canine model, *ASAIO J* 39:M526–531, 1993.
10. Donayre CE, Scoccianti M: Applications in peripheral vascular surgery: traumatic arteriovenous fistulas and pseudoaneurysms. In Chuter TA, Donayre CE, White RA, editors: *Endoluminal vascular prostheses*, Boston, 1995, Little, Brown.
11. Derume JP, Mac Gregor DC, Kontges H et al: The Corvita endovascular graft: device description and early clinical results, Department of Vascular Pathology, Free University of Brussels, personal communication.
12. Becker GJ, Katzen BT, Dake MD: Noncoronary angioplasty, *Radiology* 170:403–412, 1989.
13. Kalman PG, Johnston KW, Sniderman KW: Indications and results of balloon angioplasty for arterial occlusive lesions, *World J Surg* 20:630–634, 1996.
14. Richter GM, Roeren T, Brado et al: Further update of the randomized trial: iliac stent placement versus PTA—morphology, clinical success rates, and failure analysis, *J Vasc Intervent Radiol* 4:30, 1993.
15. Ahn SS, Concepcion B: Indications and results of arterial stents for occlusive disease, *World J Surg* 20:644–648, 1996.
16. Marin ML, Veith FJ, Sanchez LA et al: Endovascular aortoiliac grafts in combination with standard infrainguinal arterial bypasses in the management of limb-threatening ischemia: preliminary report, *J Vasc Surg* 22:316–325, 1995.
17. Ohki T, Marin ML, Veith FJ et al: Endovascular aortofemoral grafts and femorofemoral bypass for bilateral limb-threatening ischemia, *J Vasc Surg* 24:984–997, 1996.
18. Marin ML, Veith FJ, Sanchez LA et al: Endovascular repair of aortoiliac occlusive disease, *World J Surg* 20:679–686, 1996.

19. Marin ML, Veith FJ, Cynamon J et al: Human transluminally placed endovascular stented grafts: preliminary histopathological analysis of healing graft in aortoiliac and femoral artery occlusive disease, *J Vasc Surg* 21:595–604, 1995.

20. Dolmatch BL, Tio FO, Li XD et al: Patency and tissue response related to two types of polytetrafluoroethylene-covered stents in the dog, *J Vasc Intervent Radiol* 7:641–646, 1996.

25
Endovascular Repair of Thoracic Aortic Aneurysms

Bradley B. Hill, Christopher K. Zarins, and Thomas J. Fogarty

The detection of thoracic aortic aneurysms has increased since the early 1970s along with the overall increasing prevalence of aneurysmal disease in our aging population. Frequently, patients with thoracic aneurysms have additional serious medical co-morbidities that make them high risk surgical candidates. The results of endovascular repair of abdominal aortic aneurysms indicate that stent-graft techniques, compared to conventional repair, are associated with decreased morbidity and mortality rates, shorter hospitalization, and a more rapid, less painful recovery from the patient's perspective. Thoracotomy for repair of thoracic aortic aneurysms is associated with an even higher risk of serious morbidity and mortality than conventional repair of abdominal aortic aneurysms particularly in patients with significant cardiopulmonary disease. Recognition of this problem has spurred an initiative to develop less invasive approaches to repairing descending thoracic aortic aneurysms. The adaptation of stent-graft technology to the treatment of thoracic aneurysms is limited because most aneurysms that involve the descending thoracic aorta extend into the abdominal viscerorenal aortic segment. In select patients, endovascular repair of thoracic aortic aneurysms offers the possibility of reducing morbidity and mortality by avoiding thoracotomy.

This chapter outlines the indications for endovascular repair of thoracic aneurysms, patient selection and preoperative assessment, device selection, operative approaches, and postoperative considerations. Early results of endovascular repair, current trends, and future perspectives for the treatment of thoracic aneurysms are considered.

Natural History of Descending Thoracic Aortic Aneurysms

Aneurysmal disease of the descending thoracic aorta is typically associated with atherosclerosis and degenerative changes in the aortic wall. These aneurysms are usually fusiform in nature, although, saccular aneurysms can result from penetrating atherosclerotic ulcers or other causes of localized aortic wall compromise. Trauma, infection, dissection of the aortic wall, and autoimmune inflammatory arteritis can cause aneurysmal degeneration of the descending thoracic aorta. Irrespective of the etiology, the natural history of descending thoracic aortic aneurysms is progressive enlargement and rupture, causing death in most cases. Mural thrombus and calcification do not protect against rupture.[1]

Most descending thoracic aortic aneurysms are asymptomatic and are detected incidentally on routine chest radiographs or other diagnostic imaging studies. Occasionally, mechanical compression of adjacent structures or emboli originating from the aneurysm can cause symptoms.[1] Unless elective repair is carried out, the long-term outlook for these patients is grim. The actuarial 5-year survival rate for patients with untreated abdominal aortic aneurysms is 9% to 13%.[2]

Direct Surgical Repair

Operative repair is the treatment of choice in the patient with a descending thoracic aorta measuring 6 cm or more in diameter or twice the diameter of adjacent normal aorta. Complications of operative repair may vary depending on multiple factors, including the extent of aneurysmal disease and patient co-morbidities. The mortality rate for elective repair of descending thoracic aortic aneurysms was 12% in a large single institutional study.[3] The mortality rate for emergent repair of ruptured descending thoracic aortic aneurysms is 50% for patients who survive the acute event and do not die in an emergency room.[4] Other significant complications of direct repair include stroke, paraplegia, and renal, cardiac, and pulmonary failure.

Stent-Graft Repair

Endovascular repair of descending thoracic aortic aneurysms offers the advantages of reduced procedure-related complications and mortality rates, decreased hospital length of stay, and less expensive treatment than conventional operative therapy. The first series of patients was reported by Dake and colleagues in 1994.[2] Thirteen consecutive patients were treated for atherosclerotic, anastomotic, and posttraumatic aneurysms and for aortic dissections. Custom-designed stent-grafts were made from self-expanding stainless steel stents and woven Dacron grafts. Device placement was successful in all 13 patients. No deaths or instances of paraplegia, distal embolization, or infection occurred during a mean follow-up of 12 months.

Stent-grafts have been used successfully to treat acute ruptures of the descending thoracic aorta and posttraumatic aneurysms.[5–9] Eleven patients had acute descending thoracic aortic ruptures treated with endoluminal stent-grafts. Eight patients (73%) had ruptures from aneurysms, and three (27%) had ruptures from trauma. There were no perigraft leaks, stent migrations, paraplegia, or intraoperative deaths. Two deaths occurred during the follow-up period, neither of which was related to the aneurysm or stent-graft procedure.[5]

Mycotic aneurysm of the descending thoracic aorta has also been successfully treated with stent-grafts and antibiotic therapy in high risk surgical patients.[10] An example of a saccular descending thoracic aortic aneurysm treated with an endoluminal stent-graft is illustrated in Figure 25–1.

Patient Selection and Preoperative Assessment

Indications for endoluminal stent-graft repair include aneurysms and penetrating ulcers of the descending thoracic aorta. Patients who have been treated with aortic endografts typically have one or more serious medical co-morbidities, such as severe chronic obstructive pulmonary disease, cardiomyopathy, congestive heart failure, renal disease, or advanced age.[4]

Stent-graft repair of thoracic aortic aneurysms is currently performed at relatively few research centers through institutional review board (IRB)-approved or US Food and Drug Administration (FDA)-approved clinical trials. Patients who have high risk aneurysms but who do not meet the criteria for enrollment in clinical trials, under circumstances that preclude open surgical aneurysm repair, may have approval for compassionate use of devices granted by IRBs, the FDA, and the device industry.

Accurate assessment of aneurysm dimensions and morphology is critical for successful treatment. Measurements needed to select or construct a stent-graft of appropriate dimensions for a given aneurysm include proximal neck length (long and short sides), aneurysm length, distal neck length, and proximal and distal neck diameters. To qualify as a candidate for endoluminal repair, a patient must have

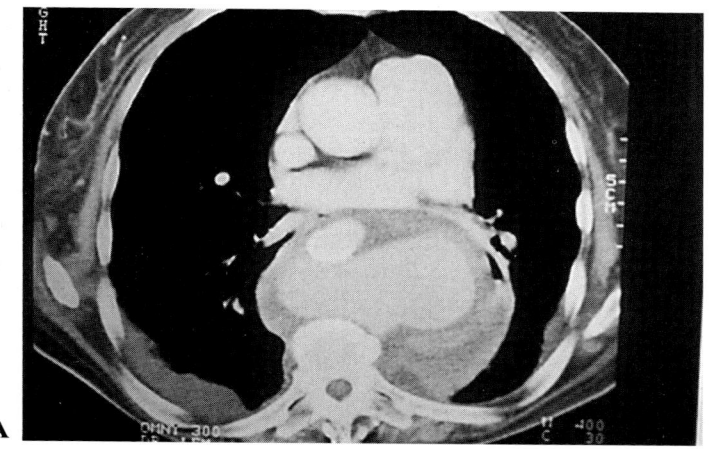

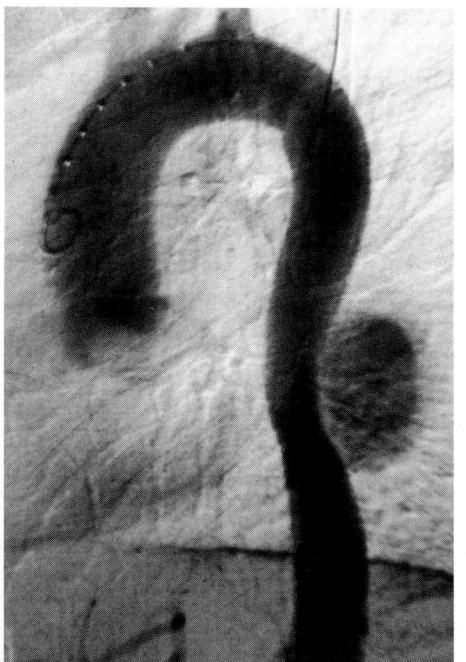

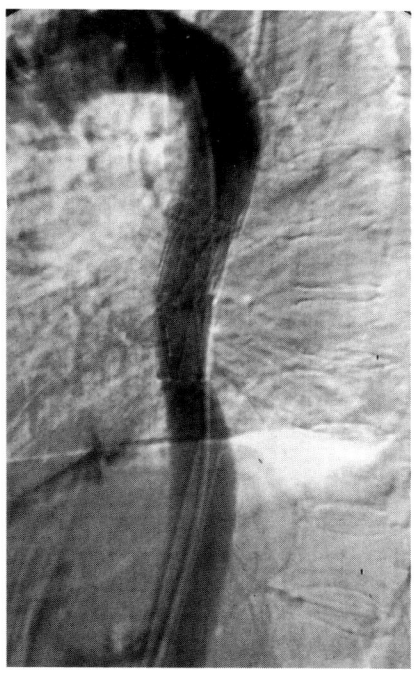

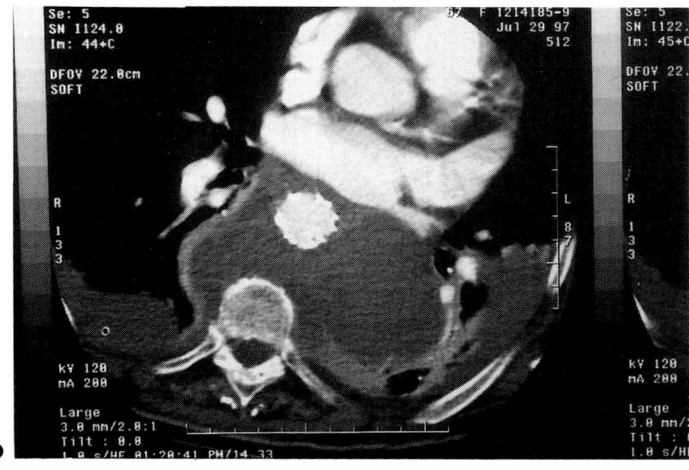

FIGURE 25–1. **A**, Contrast-enhanced thoracic CT scan shows a 10 cm diameter saccular descending thoracic aortic aneurysm with a contained rupture. **B**, Thoracic aortography reveals the saccular aneurysm above the level of the diaphragm. **C**, Aortography shows exclusion of the aneurysm by a 24 mm diameter, 7.5 cm long Gianturco-Dacron stent-graft that was introduced through a 20F delivery sheath inserted into the patient's right femoral artery. **D**, Postoperative CT scan shows successful exclusion of the aneurysm.

adequate proximal and distal aneurysm necks, each at least 15mm long and no more than 40mm in diameter, for device fixation.[4] Imaging the entire aorta and iliac arteries is important to rule out other aneurysms. Twenty to thirty percent of thoracic aortic aneurysms have associated abdominal aortic aneurysms.[11] Associated aortoiliac occlusive disease is also frequently seen with calcification of the terminal aorta and iliac arteries. Severely stenosed or noncompliant iliac arteries may preclude a femoral artery approach to the aorta.

Imaging Studies

Imaging studies helpful for assessing descending thoracic aortic aneurysms include spiral computed tomographic (CT) angiography, magnetic resonance angiography (MRA), standard invasive aortography, transesophageal ultrasonography, and intravascular ultrasonography (IVUS). Volumetric spiral CT and MRA data can be used to study endoluminal surface detail and measure center-of-flow aortic length, accurate cross-sectional diameters of proximal and distal necks, and aneurysm volume and angulation.

Aortography with digital subtraction provides excellent images for evaluating the left subclavian artery position relative to the proximal aneurysm neck. Aortic length measurements are also made using endoluminal measuring catheters. Aortography delineates the contours of the endoluminal aortic surface and is helpful for defining the locations and patency of intercostal arteries. If a dominant intercostal artery is present in the lower thoracic region near the diaphragm, the artery should be spared, if possible, to avoid anterior spinal cord ischemia and paraplegia.

The MRA technique utilizes gadolinium, which is not harmful to the kidneys. Patients who have renal insufficiency with a serum creatinine higher than 1.5mg/dl should have MRA instead of CT angiograms, which require iodinated contrast.

Device Selection

Devices are selected based on their availability, preoperative and intraoperative measurements, and any access limitations imposed by the iliac arteries. A number of graft types have been tested. Basic designs include (1) graft with an internal stent at each end, without columnar support; (2) graft with internal tandem stents; (3) graft with metallic endoskeleton; and (4) graft with metallic exoskeleton. Both polyester and polytetrafluoroethylene (PTFE) graft materials have been utilized extensively. Self-expanding and balloon-expandable stainless steel and nitinol stents have been used. No long-term data have proved the superiority of one device over another.

Device delivery systems vary among the devices. The most common delivery mechanism is the delivery sheath. The larger the device diameter, the larger is the required sheath, up to 28F for a 46mm diameter stent-graft.

Operative Approaches and Technical Considerations

The most appropriate environment for placing aortic endografts is the operating room, where immediate operative intervention can be performed should the aneurysm rupture during device manipulation. A C-arm fluoroscope with digital subtraction capability is the minimum system required for adequate imaging. Transesophageal echocardiography is also used for cardiac monitoring and to confirm proximal and distal aneurysm necks.

The most commonly used approach for placing thoracic aortic endografts is through the femoral artery. It is performed by mobilizing and controlling the common femoral artery through a groin incision. The artery is punctured and a 0.035-inch guidewire is advanced into the thoracic aorta. An introducer is advanced over the guidewire into the iliac system, and an aortogram is obtained to image the proximal aneurysm neck.

Intravascular ultrasonography and endoluminal measuring catheters may be used if additional aortic diameter or length measurements are needed. A device with correct dimensions is selected, and the appropriate-sized delivery sheath is exchanged at the femoral level over a stiff guidewire. The stent-graft device is delivered into the thoracic aorta and positioned utilizing fluoroscopic guidance, road mapping, transesophageal ultrasonography, or bony landmarks for reference. The device is deployed such that the seal between the device and the aorta at the proximal and distal neck is maximized. A completion angiogram is obtained to check device position and patency and to rule out the presence of an endoleak.

If preoperative assessment determines that the iliac or femoral arteries are too small, diseased, or tortuous for a femoral approach, an external iliac or common iliac artery can be used for aortic access. This involves making an incision proximal to the inguinal ligament for mobilization and control of the common, external, and internal iliac arteries. The external iliac is punctured as described above for the femoral approach. If the external iliac artery is too small, the common iliac artery can be used for access in the same fashion, or one end of a 10-mm tube graft of Dacron or PTFE can be sewn to the side of the common iliac artery. This maneuver usually facilitates passage of the delivery sheath. Femoral and iliac artery access sites are generally repaired primarily. Side-limb grafts sewn to a common iliac artery are removed, and the iliac artery is repaired with a patch. If an intimal flap is created during dilation of the femoral or iliac artery, endarterectomy and patch angioplasty may be necessary. In rare instances, significant arterial injury may require arterial reconstruction with an interposition graft. Some patients have a combination of aneurysms involving the descending thoracic and infrarenal aorta. Replacement of the infrarenal aortic segment through a retroperitoneal approach provides access to the thoracic aorta by sewing a side-limb graft onto the infrarenal aortic graft.[11]

The best strategy is to approach the aorta through the smallest artery that can clearly accommodate the device delivery system. If the external iliac is heavily calcified, tortuous, or small, initial exposure of the common iliac artery for access is the wisest approach and may markedly simplify the procedure and avoid unnecessary blood loss.

The proximal aneurysm neck may be problematic if it arises less than 15 mm from the origin of the left subclavian artery. Left subclavian to common carotid artery transposition can be performed to allow the proximal end of the graft to cover the left subclavian orifice for better proximal fixation.[12]

Patients who have aortic endografts placed through the femoral arteries are managed in a monitored setting overnight. An oral diet is usually started the evening of surgery. Patients ambulate on the first postoperative day and are discharged home on the second postoperative day. A chest radiograph and CT angiogram are obtained before hospital discharge to document the position of the device and the presence or absence of endoleaks. Clinic visits and CT angiograms are scheduled at 1, 3, 6, and 12 months after operation to assess patient progress and device function.

Results of Stent-Graft Repair

In 1997 Mitchell et al. reported the cumulative results of 108 patients treated with thoracic aortic stent-grafts at Stanford University Medical Center.[13] The mean aneurysm diameter was 6.3 cm. Vascular access was obtained through the femoral artery in 64 patients (59%). The abdominal aorta, native or graft, an iliac artery, or the ascending aorta was used for access in 44 patients. Twenty-two patients (20%) had stent-grafts placed in conjunction with abdominal aortic aneurysm repair.

Ehrlich and colleagues prospectively studied stent-graft repair versus direct repair of descending thoracic aortic aneurysms at the University of Vienna in Austria and reported their results in 1998.[12] Sixty-eight patients were deemed good candidates for stent-graft repair. Because of limited device availability, only 10 patients (15%) had stent-graft repair, and 58 (85%) had conventional open repair. The mean procedure time was 320 minutes in the conventional group and 150 minutes in the stent-graft group. Five patients (12%) in the open surgical group developed paraplegia, whereas no patient in the stent-graft group developed any neurologic sequelae. The mean hospital length of stay for the surgical group was 26 days versus 10 days for the stent-graft group. Five patients (50%) required transposition of the left subclavian artery onto the left common carotid artery to increase the length of the proximal aneurysm neck. Stent-grafts were placed through a femoral artery in eight cases (80%) and the aorta in two (20%).

In the Stanford series of 108 patients treated with thoracic aortic endografts, 10 patients (9%) died within 30 days from the time of stent-graft placement, and four deaths (4%) were directly attributable to the procedure.[13] In the Austrian comparative study of stent-graft treatment versus conventional surgery, the 30-day mortality was 30% in the conventional group versus 10% in the stent-graft group.[12]

The risk of paraplegia during operative repair increases with the sacrifice of intercostal arteries. In the Stanford series of 108 patients with descending thoracic aortic aneurysms, four patients (4%) had postoperative paraplegia and four patients had perioperative strokes. Paraplegia occurred in two patients who underwent repair of suprarenal abdominal aortic aneurysms immediately followed by thoracic aortic stent-graft placement and in two patients who had thoracic aortic stent-grafts placed across the orifices of intercostal arteries at the T10 level. One of the latter two patients also had undergone a previous abdominal aortic aneurysm repair.[13] In an effort to prevent this devastating complication, Ishimaru et al. described a retrievable stent-graft that can be used in conjunction with somatosensory evoked potentials to "test" for spinal cord ischemia prior to the permanent deployment of a thoracic aortic stent-graft.[14] Seventeen aneurysms were excluded using this technique, and no patient had postoperative paraplegia.

Perigraft leak, or "endoleak," is a condition that exists when some blood flow within an aneurysm is outside the lumen of a previously deployed endograft. Endoleaks have occurred in up to 47% of patients after placement of abdominal and thoracic aortic stent-grafts.[15] In the Stanford series of 108 patients, 5 patients (4.6%) did not have complete aneurysm thrombosis after stent-graft placement. Of five late deaths, occurring more than 30 days after stent-graft placement, one was caused by exsanguination from an aortoesophageal fistula in a patient with a persistent perigraft leak. Two additional late deaths may have resulted from graft failure and aneurysm rupture.[13] In the Austrian comparative study reported by Ehrlich, two of the stent-graft patients (20%) had persistent perigraft leaks that required restenting.[12]

Helical CT scanning has been shown to be more sensitive than angiography for detecting endoleaks following placement of aortic endografts.[15,16] Endoleaks can occur at the proximal and distal fixation sites, through the graft material itself ("transgraft leak"), or through patent intercostal or other patent branch vessels. Most endoleaks seem to involve a combination of leaks, usually a graft fixation site and a patent aortic branch vessel. For instance, in the case of an endoleak following repair of an abdominal aortic aneurysm, a proximal fixation site is the source of blood that flows through a narrow tract into a patent inferior mesenteric artery. Selective embolization of intercostal branches prior to deployment of a thoracic aortic endograft is a strategy to prevent endoleaks. After device deployment, embolization of patent intercostal arteries is not possible. Endoleaks identified at proximal or distal fixation sites can be treated by placing a short extender cuff directly over the source. Kato et al. have described successful coil embolization of perigraft leaks in 10 consecutive patients.[17]

Embolization of mural thrombus and atheromatous material from the aorta may occur during aortic endograft placement. Emboli to the cerebral, visceral, renal, and extremity arteries have been reported.[13] The risk of embolization can be minimized by precise fluoroscopic imaging during the placement of intraluminal guidewires, catheters, and devices, and by working through sheaths whenever possible.

Future Perspectives

Catheter-based technologies have enhanced the surgeon's ability to treat a variety of vascular disease pathologies with less invasive and less morbid approaches. Many challenges lie ahead for evolving aortic endograft technology. The durability of devices beyond a few years and the natural history of small endoleaks remain unknown. Downsizing of devices and their delivery systems may make the femoral approach possible in most if not all patients in the future; however, the likelihood for totally percutaneous thoracic aortic endograft systems is doubtful. Improved preoperative CT and MRA imaging may facilitate more precise preoperative evaluation of spinal cord blood supply without the need for aortography, which in turn could assist in important strategies to decrease the risk of paraplegia in these patients.

References

1. Coselli JS, de Figueiredo LF: Natural history of descending and thoracoabdominal aortic aneurysms, *J Card Surg* 12(suppl):285–289, 1997.
2. Dake MD, Miller DC, Semba CP et al: Transluminal placement of endovascular stent-grafts for the treatment of descending thoracic aortic aneurysms, *N Engl J Med* 331:1729–1734, 1994.
3. Moreno-Cabral CE, Miller DC, Mitchell RS et al: Degenerative and atherosclerotic aneurysms of the thoracic aorta: determinants of early and late surgical outcome, *J Thorac Cardiovasc Surg* 88:1020–1032, 1984.
4. Semba CP, Mitchell RS, Miller DC et al: Thoracic aortic aneurysm repair with endovascular stent-grafts, *Vasc Med* 2:25–30, 1997.
5. Semba CP, Kato N, Kee ST et al: Acute rupture of the descending thoracic aorta: repair with use of endovascular stent-grafts, *J Vasc Intervent Radiol* 8:337–342, 1997.
6. Kato N, Dake MD, Miller DC et al: Traumatic thoracic aortic aneurysm: treatment with endovascular stent-grafts, *Radiology* 205:657–662, 1997.
7. Scharrer-Pamler R, Gorich J, Orend KH et al: Emergent endoluminal repair of delayed abdominal aortic rupture after blunt trauma, *J Endovasc Surg* 5:134–137, 1998.
8. Deshpande A, Mossop P, Gurry J et al: Treatment of traumatic false aneurysm of the thoracic aorta with endoluminal grafts, *J Endovasc Surg* 5:120–125, 1998.
9. Desgranges P, Mialhe C, Cavillon A et al: Endovascular repair of posttraumatic thoracic pseudoaneurysm with a stent graft, *AJR* 169:1743–1745, 1997.
10. Semba CP, Sakai T, Slonim SM et al: Mycotic aneurysms of the thoracic aorta: repair with use of endovascular stent-grafts, *J Vasc Intervent Radiol* 9:33–40, 1998.
11. Moon MR, Mitchell RS, Dake MD et al: Simultaneous abdominal aortic replacement and thoracic stent-graft placement for multilevel aortic disease, *J Vasc Surg* 25:332–340, 1997.
12. Ehrlich M, Grabenwoeger M, Cartes-Zumelzu F et al: Endovascular stent graft repair for aneurysms on the descending thoracic aorta, *Ann Thorac Surg* 66:19–24, 1998.
13. Mitchell RS, Miller DC, Dake MD. Stent-graft repair of thoracic aortic aneurysms, *Semin Vasc Surg* 10:257–271, 1997.
14. Ishimaru S, Kawaguchi S, Koizumi N et al: Preliminary report on prediction of spinal cord ischemia in endovascular stent graft repair of thoracic aortic aneursym by retrievable stent graft, *J Thorac Surg* 115:811–818, 1998.
15. Golzarian J, Dussaussois L, Abada HT et al: Helical CT of aorta after endoluminal stent-graft therapy: value of biphasic acquisition, *AJR* 171:329–331, 1998.
16. Rozenblit A, Marin ML, Veith FJ et al: Endovascular repair of abdominal aortic aneurysm: value of postoperative follow-up with helical CT, *AJR* 165:1473–1479, 1995.
17. Kato N, Semba CP, Dake MD: Embolization of perigraft leaks after endovascular stent-graft treatment of aortic aneurysms, *J Vasc Intervent Radiol* 7:805–811, 1996.

26
Techniques, Case Selection, and Pitfalls Associated with Endovascular Aneurysm Repair

Robert C. Allen and Thomas J. Fogarty

Endovascular repair of abdominal aortic aneurysms (AAAs) is an evolving procedure that allows treatment of one of the most complex forms of vascular pathology in a minimally invasive manner. The survival and future success of AAA stent-grafting is critically dependent on early clinical experience and continued excellence in AAA endovascular repair. Therefore the results must truly reflect the minimally invasive nature of the procedure as reflected in shorter operative times, less blood loss, lower operative morbidity and mortality, shortened length of hospital stay, and a quicker return to normal activities. These goals have been achieved by many investigators, with the patient the primary beneficiary.[1-3] These results also reflect the expertise of the leaders in the field of endovascular AAA stent-graft repair. The factors behind these excellent results are endovascular technical prowess, proper case selection, and experience, which avoids the many possible pitfalls associated with AAA stent-grafting. Technical expertise in the most basic to the most complex catheter/guidewire skills and a thorough knowledge of the stent-graft procedure are essential requirements for successful AAA endovascular repair. Proper case selection is crucial, and important components include patient selection, complete diagnostic evaluation, device sizing, and importantly a realistic knowledge of the skill level of the operator. Endovascular AAA repair is similar to conventional AAA repair in that there is no substitute for experience, and the volume of cases performed directly relates to the avoidance of the many pitfalls along the learning curve of AAA stent-graft repair.[4]

Techniques

Basic Catheter/Guidewire

One of the basic rules of aortic stent-grafting is *not* to start your endovascular experience with AAA endovascular repair. Basic catheter/guidewire skills are an essential tool and the ability to pass all wires and catheters easily and swiftly a strict prerequisite. This should include introducer sheath insertion, abdominal and pelvic angiography, selective catheterization, and brachial/axillary guidewire insertion. These skills must be performed with a high level of expertise by the vascular surgeon or by another member of the group of treating physicians (interventional radiologist or invasive cardiologist). The success of aortic stent-graft repair of AAA is highly dependent on the catheter/guidewire skills of the treating physician(s) and must not be overlooked as a major determinant in the success of the procedure.

Device Access: Femoral Artery

Access of the delivery catheter to the site of stent-graft deployment is an obvious prerequisite to the performance of the procedure. Most stent-graft devices presently in use are loaded in main delivery catheters with an outer diameter of 18F to 27F outside diameter, and may require the use of a delivery sheath with an outside diameter that is larger by 3F to 4F. This size of delivery catheter mandates surgical exposure of the common femoral arteries for device insertion, which is best accomplished by an oblique incision in the groin crease over the common femoral artery pulse (Figure 26–1). A vertical incision is not needed, as the device is optimally inserted in the proximal common femoral artery where it is least diseased and of largest diameter. Device insertion in the more distal common femoral artery is more troublesome, as the vessel is more diseased and smaller with repair following catheter insertion more complicated. In addition, the oblique incision allows subsequent percutaneous access below the entry site at a later date for additional tests or other procedures. The device delivery catheter is always inserted over a superstiff wire in the femoral artery to facilitate passage and tractability. The femoral arteriotomy may be transverse or vertical. The transverse arteriotomy is preferred because of ease of closure, but a vertical arteriotomy is advantageous in small or diseased femoral arteries to facilitate delivery catheter access. The vertical arteriotomy in these cases facilitates femoral artery closure and may require patch angioplasty in select cases.

Device Access: Iliac Arteries

Passage of the main delivery catheter through challenging iliac arteries can be a major impediment to the endovascular repair of AAA. Iliac artery access difficulties can be due to small size (less than 6mm), occlusive disease (especially calcific), angulation, tortuousity, and most frequently a combination of these factors. The worst scenario is dense iliac calcification in combination with either angulation/tortuousity or small/diseased vessels. Endovascular specialists have many techniques and tools at their disposal to help overcome these obstacles such that failed iliac access should be a rare cause of treatment failure. The use of a superstiff wire is essential to facilitate delivery catheter tractability and straighten the iliac artery. External iliac artery angulation or tortuosity is effectively dealt with by mobilization of the common femoral/external iliac artery in the groin incision. An introducer sheath with a long tapered "Coons"-type dilator can be invaluable and helps negotiate even the most challenging iliac arteries. A left brachial-femoral guidewire under tension is a useful technique for facilitating delivery catheter access by straightening the iliac vessels in addition to pulling, rather than pushing, the device through the iliac arteries (Figure 26–2). This aortic "body floss" technique is facilitated by use of an exchange length hydrophilic wire and requires the use of a catheter to protect the origin of the left subclavian artery. A final technique to facilitate delivery catheter passage in the iliac arteries is the use of deep manual hand pressure on the opposite side of the abdomen or pelvis as countertraction. This is performed slowly under

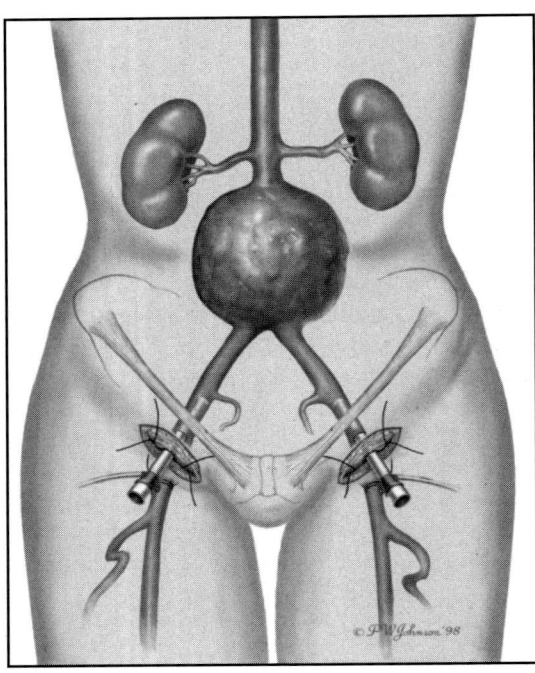

FIGURE 26–1. Small bilateral oblique groin incisions allow easy access to the proximal common femoral arteries and are minimally traumatic. Silastic vessel loops are placed proximally and distally for vascular control with the proximal tape double looped to provide hemostasis around the stent-graft delivery catheter.

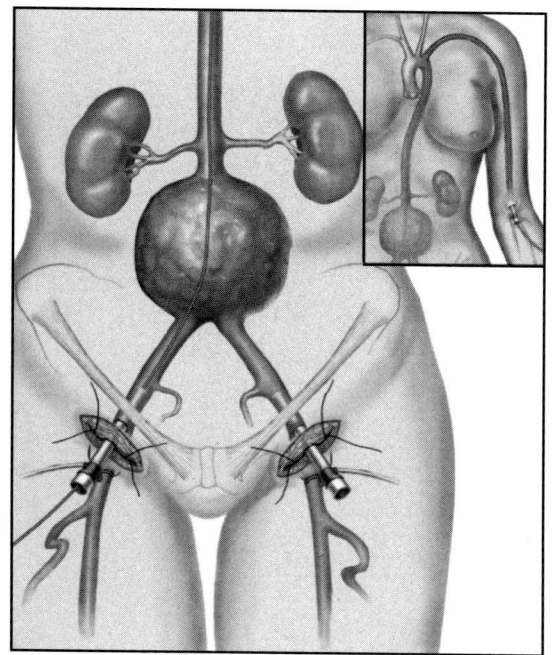

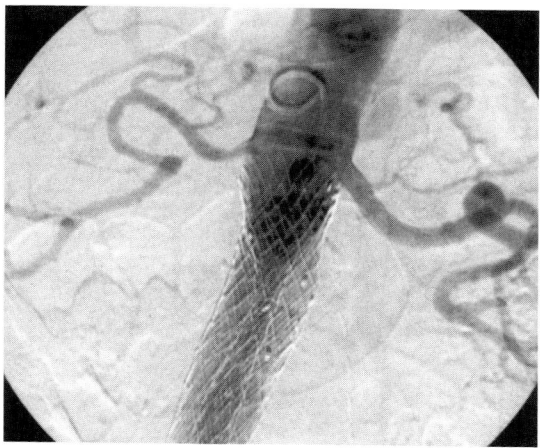

FIGURE 26–3. AneuRx stent-graft perfectly positioned at the lower borders of the orifices to the main renal arteries. This position reduces any possible prosthesis movement during completion of stent-graft insertion and helps minimize the incidence of proximal endoleak.

FIGURE 26–2. Left brachiofemoral guidewire is an important adjunct in select cases. Tension on the guidewire from both ends straightens the iliac access vessels and greatly facilitates delivery catheter insertion. An angiographic catheter should be used to protect the origin of the left subclavian artery.

fluoroscopic guidance and in select cases is highly effective.

Proximal Device Deployment

Accurate deployment of the proximal end of the stent-graft immediately below the lowest major renal artery is the most critical portion of the stent-graft procedure. Deployment of the proximal end of the stent-graft at this level secures a stable base of fixation for the completion of stent-graft insertion (Figure 26–3). The proximal aortic neck just below the renal arteries is the strongest part of the infrarenal aorta and of the best quality. The operator should strive for this position in each case regardless of the length of the proximal length to help ensure a good long-term result. Numerous techniques have been used to mark the position of the renal arteries and avoid parallax errors, including the use of radiopaque rulers, spinal needles in the anterior abdominal wall, bony landmarks, and road mapping techniques. Imaging techniques include keeping the image in the center of the screen and immobilizing the image intensifier following acquisition of the predeployment angiogram. These techniques are helpful but do not totally eliminate parallax errors, as the proximal neck anatomy and position may change when the 18F to 27F main delivery catheter is inserted into its proper position. A superior technique to facilitate excellent proximal positioning in each case is the use of a control or check angiographic catheter to visualize precisely the proximal stent-graft position during deployment. This control or check angiographic catheter can be a straight multi-side-hole catheter inserted from the contralateral femoral artery or a pigtail catheter inserted via the left brachial artery (Figure 26–4). The control or check catheter is positioned several centimeters above the level of the renal arteries. The contralateral straight flush catheter can be pulled down at any time during stent-graft deployment. Several stent-graft devices now utilize uncovered bare stents at the proximal end of the stent-graft to provide added security to the

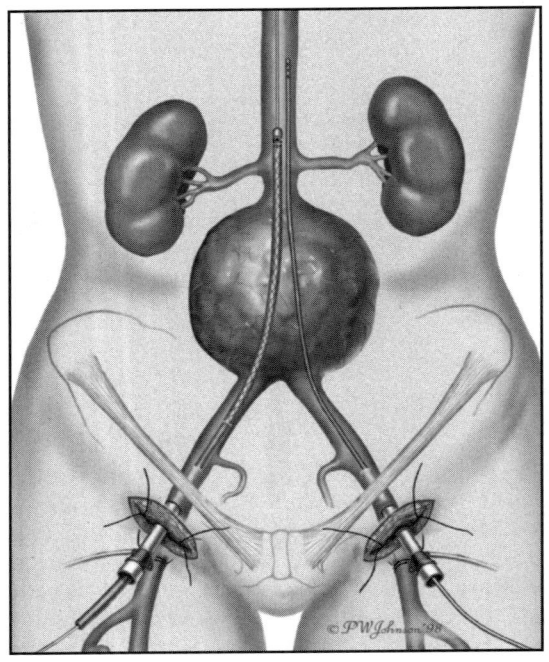 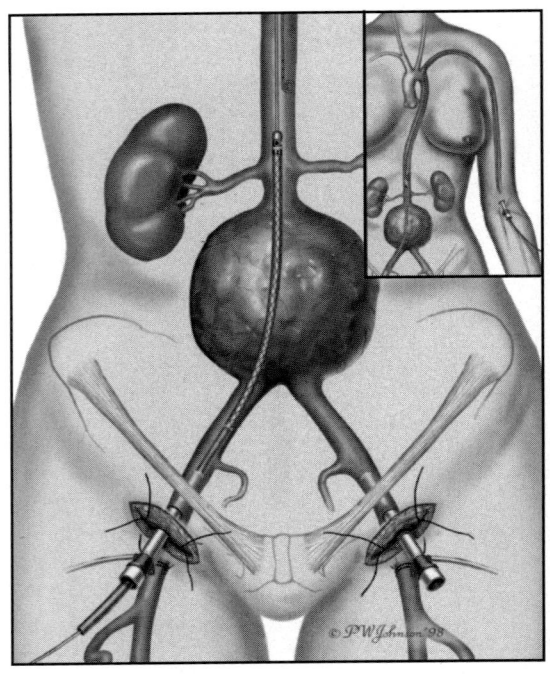

FIGURE 26–4. **A,** Straight multi-side-hole catheter inserted from the contralateral groin allows precise proximal stent-graft positioning at the level of the renal arteries. This catheter allows angiography to confirm proximal stent-graft position and thus eliminates parallax errors. **B,** Pigtail catheter inserted from the left brachial artery approach can serve the same role but, in addition, facilitates cannulation of the contralateral stump of a modular bifurcated stent-graft and can be used for completion angiography.

proximal implantation via suprarenal fixation. Results using this design feature to date have not revealed an increased incidence of renal artery stenosis or thrombosis.[5]

Modular Stent-Graft Contralateral Leg

Modular stent-grafts employ the concept of device construction in vivo with the component parts being put together to exclude the AAA.[6] Most of the modular devices now available utilize a main body with attached ipsilateral iliac limb and an attached short pant leg for insertion of the contralateral iliac limb. The main body with attached ipsilateral limb is deployed first, and then the contralateral short pant leg must be accessed for insertion of the contralateral iliac limb. Access to the contralateral short pant leg can be accomplished by three techniques: (1) retrograde "freestyle" cannulation from the contralateral femoral artery; (2) "up and over" guidewire passage from the ipsilateral to the contralateral side; and (3) antegrade via a left brachial/axillary guidewire (Figure 26–5). Each technique has advantages, and each stent-graft device may be more readily accessed by a specific technique. The method used for short pant leg access is highly variable depending on the institution/operator and specific stent-graft.

Distal Stent-Graft Implantation

Most AAAs (more than 95%) are not amenable to endovascular repair with an aortoaortic stent-graft.[7] The distal aortic neck if present is frequently too short and of poor

26. Endovascular Aneurysm Repair

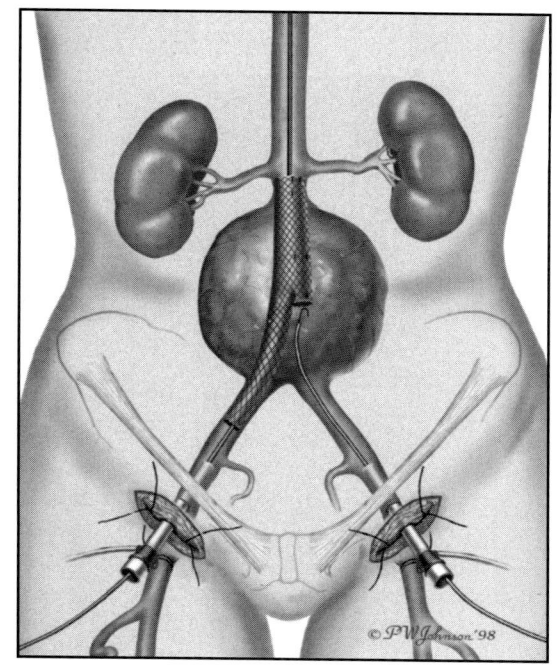

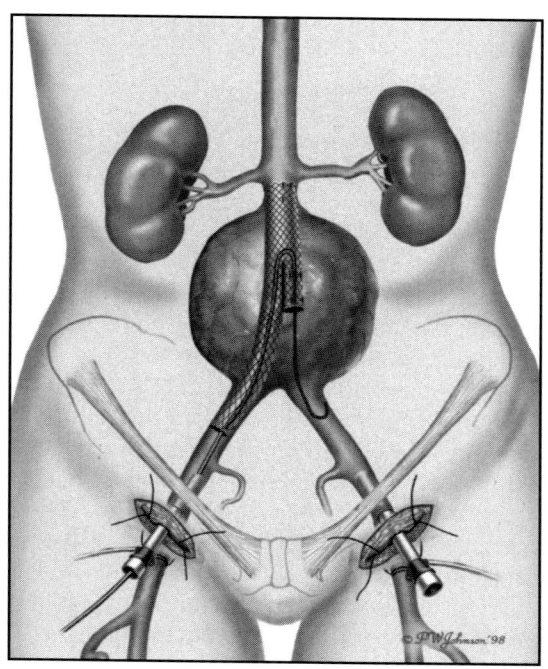

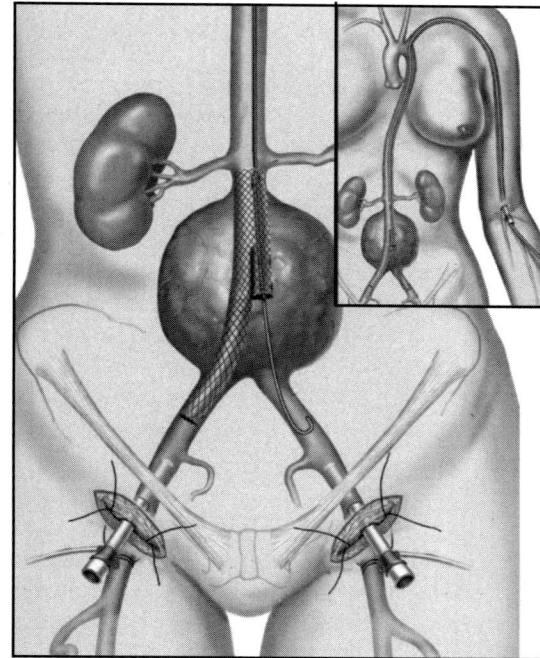

FIGURE 26–5. Access to the contralateral short pant leg or stump of a bifurcated modular stent-graft can be accomplished by three routes or techniques. **A**, "Freestyle" method involves retrograde cannulation from a contralateral groin sheath. This is the fastest (less than 5 minutes) and easiest technique in most (more than 90%) of cases. A variety of angled catheters (e.g., multipurpose, cobra), and a hydrophilic guidewire are the most commonly used equipment. **B**, "Up and over" technique requires passage of a guidewire from the ipsilateral iliac limb over the septum of the stent-graft body and down the contralateral iliac/femoral vessel. The guidewire can be snared in the iliac artery or passed directly into the femoral artery. Curved angiographic catheters or guide catheters (e.g., Simmons, shepherds crook) and a hydrophilic guidewire have proven most useful. **C**, Left brachial approach utilizes a guidewire inserted antegrade from a sheath in the left brachial artery. An exchange length hydrophilic guidewire is essential, as is a curved angiographic catheter to direct the guidewire and protect the left subclavian artery. This technique is especially advantageous for aortic/contralateral iliac angulation and tortuousity.

quality (calcification). Therefore most patients require aortobiiliac stent-graft insertion for AAA exclusion. Accurate stent-graft length determination is imperative to achieve a good seal in the appropriate iliac landing zone. Stent-graft length measurements can be obtained with spiral computed tomography (CT), calibrated catheter angiography, intravascular ultrasonography (IVUS), or any combination of these modalities. Modular extension cuffs as an integral part of the endovascular toolbox can be helpful for optimizing stent-graft position in the ideal iliac implantation site. Oblique pelvic angiography is also helpful for defining the iliac landing zone and internal iliac artery origin. Routine or selective balloon angioplasty of the iliac stent-graft limb following implantation helps achieve a good seal. A select group of AAA patients do not have iliac anatomy suitable for a bifurcated stent-graft and are best treated with an aortouniiliac stent-graft.[8] These patients require placement of the appropriately sized occluding "plug" in the contralateral common iliac artery and a femoro-femoral graft.

Completion Angiography

It is imperative at the end of the procedure to assess for complete AAA exclusion following stent-graft insertion. Completion angiography is performed to document AAA exclusion and detect any possible endoleak. Endoleak is defined by continued contrast extravasation into the AAA sac following stent-graft insertion.[9] The primary concern is a proximal or distal endoleak due to inadequate stent-graft apposition to the proximal aortic neck or distal iliac landing zone. Therefore completion angiography should be performed to assess both proximal and distal implantation sites. A single anteroposterior (AP) view may be possible and helps detect late blush but does not clearly or accurately depict the proximal and distal landing zones. Separate angiograms of the proximal and distal landing sites are far more accurate, and the addition of oblique or lateral views can be helpful in detecting and defining occult endoleaks. Completion angiography should also doc-

ument renal artery and internal iliac artery patency.

Case Selection

Patient Selection

Proper patient selection is the key to good results as with any operation or procedure. The ideal patient to benefit from aortic stent-graft repair for AAA is the high risk patient with multiple co-morbidities that preclude conventional AAA repair. These patients are, however, also at high risk for stent-graft repair.[10] High risk patients with suitable anatomy are good candidates for endovascular repair and greatly benefit from the procedure. The problem group comprises the high risk patients with challenging anatomy who are thought to be candidates for stent-graft repair because it is their last chance for survival. This high risk group may also benefit from endovascular AAA repair, but it should be attempted only at the most experienced and talented centers of excellence. The opposite end of the spectrum, the low risk group, is also a matter of controversy. The low risk group are good candidates for open surgical repair and most also are good anatomic candidates for stent-graft repair. The younger age of this patient population and the unproved long-term durability of stent-graft repair raises the question of the appropriateness of stent-graft insertion in this group. Insertion of an aortic stent-graft for AAA in patients less than 60 years of age is not recommended in many centers at this time.

Anatomic Criteria

The percentage of patients with an AAA who are suitable anatomic candidates for endovascular AAA repair is often discussed but variable. The percentage varies from 10% to 60% and depends on a multitude of factors including the specific stent-graft and the operator.[11-13] Anatomic criteria vary greatly and are merely guides, as each patient/case must be individualized. Standard anatomic criteria are seen in Table 26-1.

TABLE 26–1. AAA Anatomic Inclusion Criteria

Parameter	Criteria
Proximal aortic neck	Diameter ≥ 14mm and ≤ 32mm Length ≥ 10mm
Iliac landing zone	Diameter ≥ 8mm and ≤ 18mm Length ≥ 10mm
Aortic angulation and tortuosity	No set limit Multiple variables Individualize each patient
Iliac angulation and tortuosity	No set limit Multiple variables Individualize each patient

Diagnostic Evaluation

Endoluminal repair of AAA requires a much more detailed evaluation to determine the suitability of endovascular repair and select the appropriate-size stent-graft for endoluminal AAA exclusion.[14,15] Duplex ultrasonography (US) is an appropriate screening tool for AAA, but is not adequate for dimensional assessment prior to endovascular AAA repair. Abdominal spiral CT scan imaging and complete abdominal/pelvic angiography with a marker catheter are essential to obtain all the AAA dimensional and morphologic data prior to endovascular AAA repair.[16,17]

Spiral CT scanning has become an important tool in the evaluation of patients prior to stent-graft insertion. The protocol used for the acquisition of data at the time of the CT scan is crucial for optimizing the amount of information obtained from the study. Frequent errors include improper slice thickness (3mm optimal) and failure to include the entire area from the celiac artery to the femoral arteries in the field of study. The spiral CT scan yields routine transverse axial cuts as well as three-dimensional reconstruction images. Dimensional data (diameter and length) can be evaluated from either image set. The transverse axial images of the proximal and distal landing zones with a magnified field of view are highly accurate. The reconstructed images yield excellent data but are dependent on the computer operator making the measurements. The morphologic data regarding the AAA gained from the reconstructed images are excellent and may assist in case planning.

Angiography of the abdomen and pelvis yields data complementary to those obtained from the spiral CT scan. A complete study with a calibrated angiography catheter may be helpful, especially in complex cases. It should include AP and lateral views of the proximal neck and AP and oblique views of the common and external iliac arteries. Diameter measurements taken with the calibrated catheter are complementary to those obtained from the CT scan, as proper sizing/oversizing is necessary to minimize possible endoleaks. Length measurements (renal arteries to the aortic bifurcation and renal arteries to the internal iliac arteries) obtained with the calibrated catheter are helpful as a guide to stent-graft length in most cases.

Intravascular ultrasonography is a diagnostic modality that may aid in more precise aortic stent-graft sizing and also be of great benefit in evaluating AAA exclusion following deployment.[18,19] IVUS provides precise intraluminal diameter and length measurements to size the prosthesis optimally. IVUS is advantageous in select cases, but the modality is also invasive, expensive, and time-consuming; and it may increase blood loss.

The stent-graft diameter is sized based on the intraluminal diameters of the aortic neck and iliac landing zones. Oversizing by 10% to 20% is essential to obtain a proximal and distal seal for complete exclusion of the AAA. The amount of oversizing varies based on the quality and length of both the proximal and distal landing zones. Stent-graft length is more difficult to determine precisely and may be based on spiral CT scan reconstructions, calibrated marker catheter angiography, or intraluminal IVUS manual pullback.[20]

Case Level Complexity

Case selection must also be predicated on the overall anatomic complexity of the case. This factor is of course intertwined with the experience level of the operator and the risk level of the patient. Level 1 cases are generally easy cases from an anatomic perspective with straight iliac access and long proximal aortic necks (Figure 26–6). They are ideal cases early

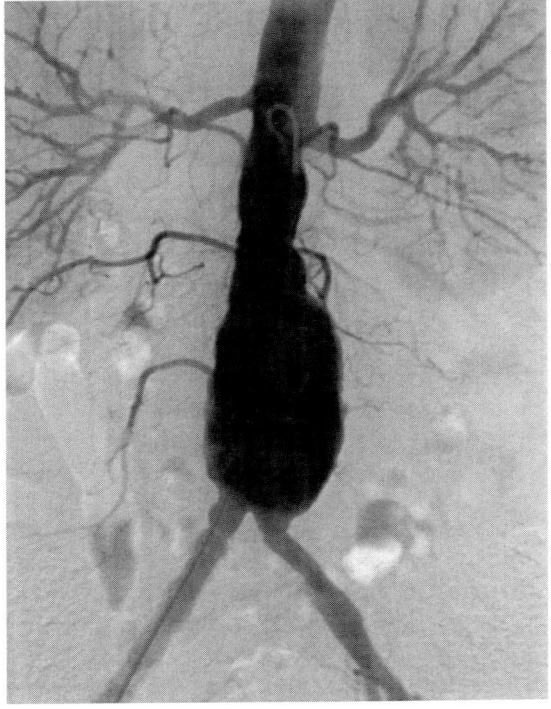

FIGURE 26-6. Classic level 1 case with a long proximal aortic neck below the renal arteries and straight iliac arteries of good caliber. This is an ideal case to start your experience with aortic stent-grafts.

Pitfalls

The following list summarizes the most common problems and errors encountered during the endovascular repair of AAAs and the correct solution (*).

1. Vascular surgeons start their endovascular career with an aortic stent-graft for AAA. *Start an endovascular experience with diagnostic angiography and peripheral interventions.

2. Spiral CT scans and abdominal angiograms are not performed to protocol. *Spiral CT scans of the abdomen and pelvis with 3 mm cuts are obtained, along with calibrated catheter angiograms of the abdomen and pelvis including a lateral aortogram and oblique views of the pelvis.

in an operator/institution's experience, allowing them to learn the stent-graft and implantation techniques. Unfortunately, they comprise only 10% to 15% of cases.

Level 2 cases are the predominant variety (75% to 80%) and feature a main area of anatomic complexity, such as a short or angulated proximal neck, difficult iliac access, or a concomitant iliac artery aneurysm (Figure 26-7). These cases are challenging for a new investigator but routine for the highly experienced stent-graft expert. Level 3 cases have multiple concurrent areas of anatomic complexity and usually occur in high risk patients (Figure 26-8). Level 3 cases (5% to 10% of total) should be avoided if possible, especially early along the learning curve; ideally they are referred to the most experienced center with an excellent record.

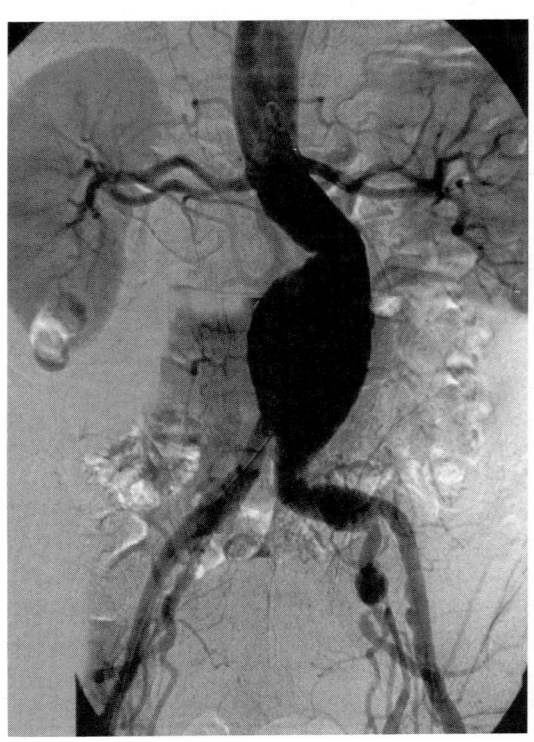

FIGURE 26-7. Level 2 case featuring proximal aortic neck angulation and left common iliac lateral angulation and distal dilatation. Such an anatomic challenge is easily overcome with experience.

26. Endovascular Aneurysm Repair

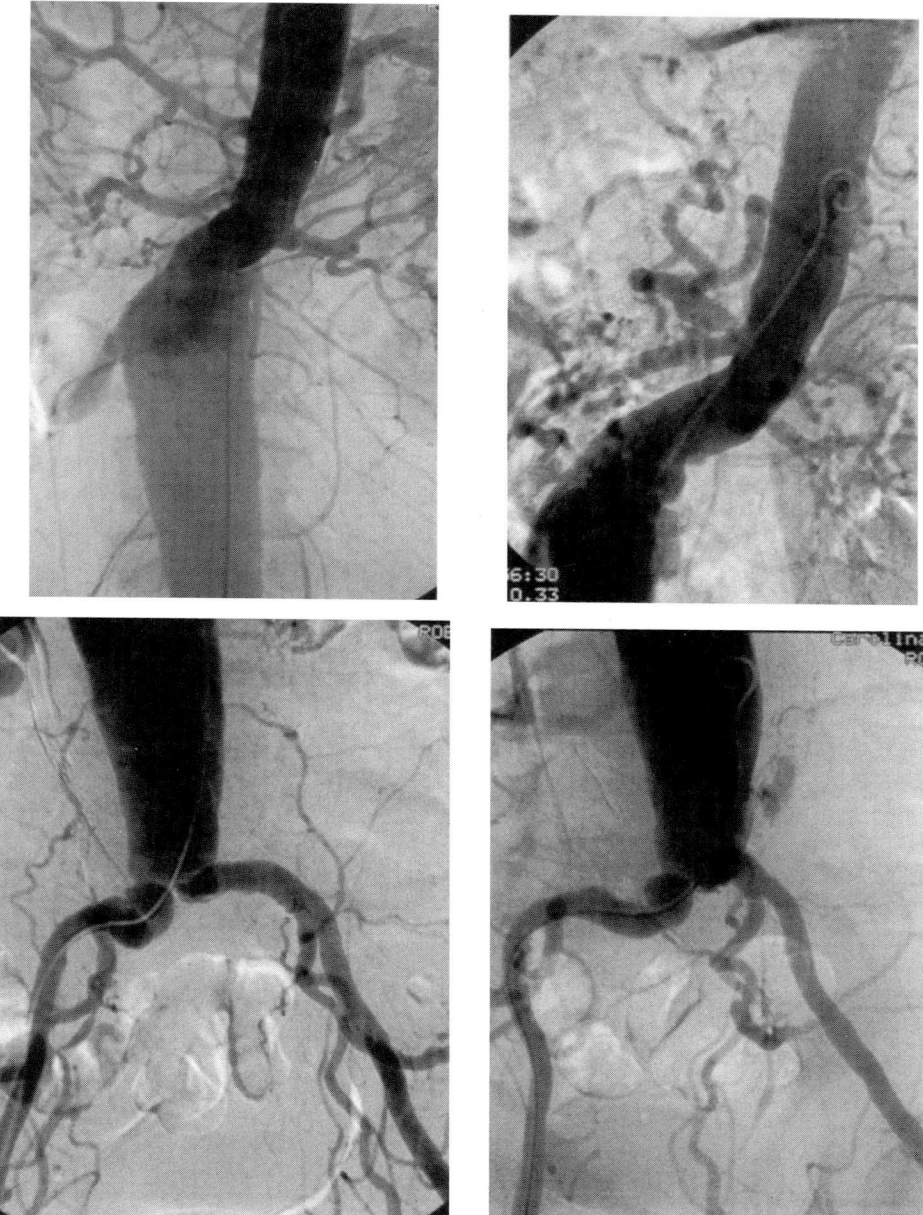

FIGURE 26–8. High risk level 3 patient with coronary disease/chronic obstructive pulmonary disease with a symptomatic 7.0-cm AAA and a hostile abdomen due to diverticular disease. Angiogram reveals a short proximal neck with lateral and anteroposterior angulation. The pelvic angiograms show left iliac lateral angulation and aneurysmal disease of the proximal right common iliac. The patient was discharged home 2 days following stent-graft insertion.

3. A complex case in a high risk patient is submitted as a first case because it is the only chance for patient survival. *Delay the case as long as possible or refer it to another center, Start with straightforward easy cases to learn the device and technique.

4. First case is long with significant blood loss. *The learning curve can be largely elimi-

nated by use of a proctor to scrub in for the first few cases to teach and assist in the procedure.

5. Main delivery catheter refuses to pass through the iliac arteries. *Always use a super-stiff guidewire and apply slow traction on the guidewire during iliac passage. In addition, always lubricate the outside of the delivery catheter.

6. Proximal stent-graft implantation site was lower than expected. *The use of a control or check angiographic catheter to guide proximal deployment precisely is essential.

7. There is difficulty accessing the short pant leg of a modular stent-graft. *Technical expertise with a catheter and guidewire are essential to success. Obtain the requisite experience and skills or make an interventional radiologist/invasive cardiologist an integral part of the team.

8. The length of the iliac limb is too short to reach the iliac landing zone and achieve a seal. *An endovascular toolbox is a must, including iliac extension cuffs because stent-graft length measurements can be highly variable.

9. A single-view completion angiogram reveals a possible endoleak. *Detailed completion angiograms of the proximal and distal landing zones are essential.

10. Patient is febrile postoperatively for several days, requiring prolonged hospitalization. *A febrile reaction following AAA stent-graft repair is not unusual and in most cases is benign. All patients are covered perioperatively with antibiotics, and the fever is treated with nonsteroidal drugs.

References

1. Parodi JC: Endovascular stent graft repair of aortic aneurysms, *Curr Opin Cardiol* 12:396–405, 1997.
2. Allen RC, Fogarty TJ: Aortic stent-grafting for abdominal aortic aneurysms: state of the art, *Intervention* 2:3–10, 1998.
3. Blum U, Voshage G, Lammer J et al: Endoluminal stent-grafts for infrarenal abdominal aortic aneurysms, *N Engl J Med* 336:13–20, 1997.
4. May J, White GH, Yu W et al: Concurrent comparison of endoluminal versus open repair in the treatment of abdominal aortic aneurysms: analsis of 303 patients by life table method, *J Vasc Surg* 27:213–221, 1998.
5. Lawrence-Brown M, Hartley D, MacSweeney STR et al: The Perth endoluminal bifurcated graft system—development and early experience, *Cardiovasc Surg* 4:706–712, 1996.
6. Allen RC, White RA, Fogarty TJ et al: What are the characteristics of the ideal endovascular graft for abdominal aortic aneurysm exclusion, *J Endovasc Surg* 4:195–202, 1997.
7. Armon MP, Yusuf SW, Latief K et al: Anatomical suitability of abdominal aortic aneurysm for endovascular repair, *Br J Surg* 84:178–180, 1997.
8. Yusuf SW, Whitaker SC, Chuter TAM et al: Early results of endovascular aortic aneurysm surgery with aortouniiliac graft, contralateral iliac occlusion, and femorofemoral bypass, *J Vasc Surg* 25:165–172, 1997.
9. White GH, Yu W, May J: "Endoleak"—a proposed new terminology to describe incomplete aneurysm exclusion by an endoluminal graft, *J Endovasc Surg* 3:123–125, 1996.
10. Yusuf W, Wenham PW, Hopkinson BR: The Nottingham experience. In Hopkinson BR, editor: *Endovascular surgery for aortic aneurysms*, Philadelphia, 1997, Saunders, pp 221–229.
11. Brewster DC, Geller SC, Kaufman JA et al: Initial experience with endovascular aneurysm repair: comparison of early results with outcome of conventional open repair, *J Vasc Surg* 27:992–1005, 1998.
12. Ohki T, Veith FJ, Sanchez LA et al: Varying strategies and devices for endovascular repair of abdominal aortic aneurysms, *Semin Vasc Surg* 10:242–256, 1997.
13. Mialhe C, Amicabile C, Becquemin JP et al: Endovascular treatment of infrarenal abdominal aneurysms by the Stentor system: preliminary results of 79 cases, *J Vasc Surg* 26:199–209, 1997.
14. Beebe HG, Jackson T, Pigott JP: Aortic aneurysm morphology for planning endovascular aortic grafts: limitations of conventional imaging methods, *J Endovasc Surg* 2:139–148, 1995.
15. Schumacher H, Eckstein HH, Kallinowski F et al: Morphometry and classification in abdominal aortic aneurysms: patient selection for endovascular and open surgery, *J Endovasc Surg* 4:39–44, 1997.
16. Bayle O, Branchereau A, Rosset E et al: Morphologic assessment of abdominal aortic aneurysms by spiral computed tomographic scanning, *J Vasc Surg* 26:238–246, 1997.

17. Whitaker SC: Preoperative imaging. In Hopkinson BR, editor: *Endovascular surgery for aortic aneurysms*, Philadelphia, 1997, Saunders, pp 17–39.
18. White RA, Donayre CE, Walot I et al: Preliminary clinical outcome and imaging criterion for endovascular prosthesis deployment in high-risk patients who have aortoiliac and traumatic arterial lesions, *J Vasc Surg* 24:556–571, 1996.
19. White RA, Donayre CE, Walot I et al: Modular bifurcation endoprosthesis for treatment of abdominal aortic aneurysms, *Ann Surg* 226:381–391, 1997.
20. Donayre CE, White RA: Application and use of intravascular ultrasound in the placement of endovascular prostheses. In Hopkinson BR, editor: *Endovascular surgery for aortic aneurysms*, Philadelphia, 1997, Saunders, pp 48–56.

27
Inferior Vena Caval Filters: Impact of Endovascular Technology

Mary C. Proctor and Lazar J. Greenfield

Advances in technology often challenge the safe and effective use of established therapies and diagnostic methods. Such new technologies may positively or negatively affect existing treatments or may lead to new indications for their use. This is a well recognized fact in pharmacology, and it is becoming increasingly more evident with medical devices. In light of these considerations, we examine the effects of the newer endovascular interventions on the vena caval filter, one of the original endovascular devices.

Interruption of the vena cava by means of an endovascular device held major advantages over the extracaval clips and suturing grids. Filtering devices were placed transvenously under local anesthesia, eliminating the need for a major abdominal procedure under general anesthesia. Some early devices, such as the Hunter balloon[1] and the Mobin-Uddin umbrella,[2] were withdrawn from the market owing to the high rate of caval thrombosis.[3] In contrast, the cone-shaped Greenfield filter has continued to provide a high degree of efficacy (95% to 98%) coupled with a low long-term rate of occlusion (3% to 5%).[4,5]

Pulmonary Embolectomy

The Greenfield filter was developed to be used in conjunction with another endovascular procedure, suction catheter pulmonary embolectomy.[6] Using a specially designed catheter and control device, the suction cup was advanced into the pulmonary circulation to retrieve emboli causing systemic hemodynamic compromise[7-9] (Figure 27-1). Reviewing the experience with the first 10 patients, it became evident that despite successful embolectomy patients remained at risk for fatal recurrent embolism. In fact, two patients died while awaiting surgical placement of a caval clip.[10] Therefore prevention of recurrent pulmonary embolism (PE) following pulmonary embolectomy became the first indication for filter placement.

Over time, the efficacy and safety of the Greenfield filter became established, and additional indications became commonly accepted, including a major contraindication to anticoagulation or following a serious complication of anticoagulation, forcing it to be discontinued.[11] The appropriate use of vena caval interruption in situations when there is no underlying thromboembolic disease has been an issue since the 1970s. Fullen and Miller first discussed this indication with respect to using the Mobin-Uddin device in patients with hip fractures.[12] Later, Korwin et al. studied the effect of prophylactic caval clips in patients undergoing aortic surgery.[13] In both of these cases there was no underlying thromboembolic disease at the time of placement. However, our initial use of prophylactic placement was as an adjunct in cases in which the patient had acute thromboembolic disease, was concurrently anticoagulated, and had reduced respiratory or cardiac reserve. The added protection was justified by the risk of an embolic event that could prove fatal.[14] Later, the definition was expanded to

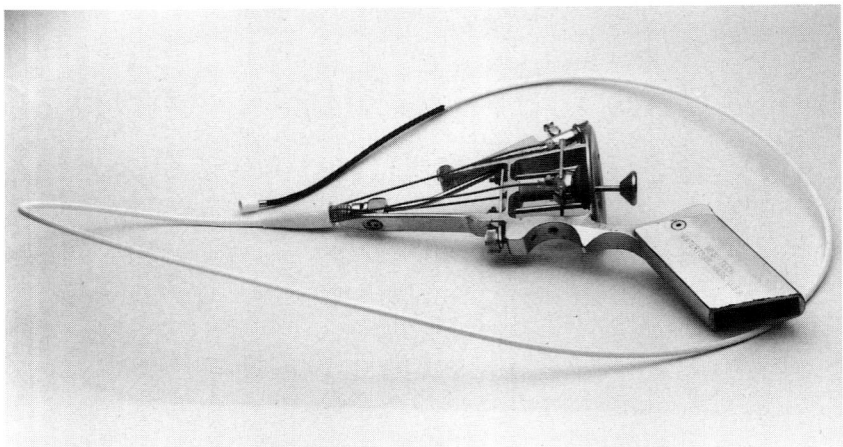

FIGURE 27–1. Greenfield suction embolectomy device is designed to remove emboli from the pulmonary arteries. The steerable end is controlled by the "joy stick" on the distal handle of the device.

include cases in which thromboembolic disease was likely but not yet present.[4]

During the 1980s interventional techniques were adopted by radiologists, which led to major changes with respect to insertion of vena caval filters. Initial reports of percutaneous placement of a filter by Tadavarthy et al.[15] were followed by others including reports by Rose et al.[16] and Pais et al.[17] Hye et al. reported on the first large series of patients (48 surgical, 120 percutaneous) in which outcomes were documented.[18] In this report, the incidences of recurrent PE (1%) and caval occlusion (3%) when filters were placed percutaneously were comparable to surgical outcomes. The incidence of clinically important insertion site thrombosis was only 5%, and the cost of percutaneous placement was 58% lower than for surgical placement. One result of these reports was to open the placement of filters to radiologists as well as to surgeons. However, the relatively large size of the delivery system (28F outer diameter) of the original Greenfield filter was associated with insertion site thrombosis in several reports, with the incidence reaching 41% in one series.[19]

The logical outcome was the development of vena caval filters designed specifically for percutaneous insertion. Lower insertion profiles were achieved either through the use of innovative materials such as the Simon nitinol filter[20,21] or the nontraditional designs such as the Bird's Nest filter (Figure 27–2).

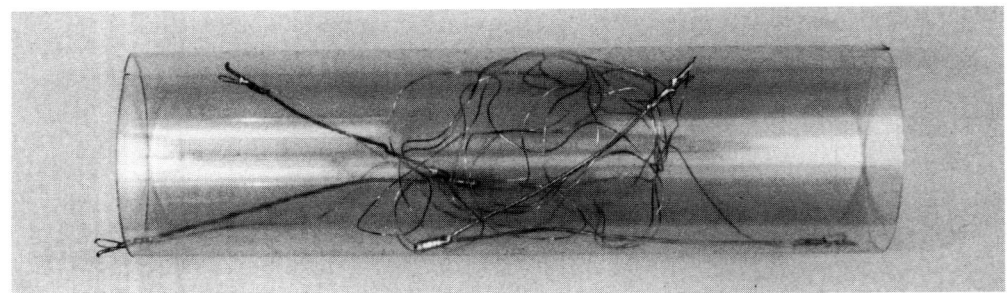

FIGURE 27–2. Bird's Nest filter is composed of four struts and wires delivered into a 6- to 7-cm segment of the vena cava. It is the only marketed filter that does not use the cone shape.

Lytic Treatment

A second technologic advancement that affected the role of vena caval filters was the use of catheter-directed pulse-spray thrombolysis for treatment of deep vein thrombosis (DVT) and pulmonary embolism. Some patients with extensive iliofemoral DVT or phlegmasia cerulea dolens are being aggressively treated with an infusion of lytic agents such as urokinase or t-PA. Initially a wire must be advanced into the thrombus followed by tracking of the infusion catheter. The therapy is associated with an estimated risk of embolism of the thrombus to the pulmonary artery ranging from 1% to 65%.[22] For this reason some authors have recommended placing an inferior vena caval (IVC) filter to trap a potential embolus.[23] Others believe this measure is necessary only if there is a free-floating tail of thrombus, and still others believe that the risk of embolism is so small that a filter is not necessary at all. Finally, there is some interest in having a temporary filter that can be used during the lytic therapy[24] and then removed. This potential indication for the use of IVC filters remains to be evaluated.

Thrombolysis in Lower Extremities and Dialysis Grafts

Innovative thrombectomy devices are also currently being evaluated that remove or destroy lower extremity thrombus or clear hemodialysis grafts. Here again some physicians believe that an IVC filter is necessary, and temporary filters have been tested in Europe for this indication.[25] Further experience is needed to evaluate this approach.

The concept of a temporary filter is not new. In 1968 Eichelter and Schenk described a temporary filter catheter.[26] This device is similar in appearance to the "Protect" infusion catheter. The Eichelter Sieve was withdrawn from the market out of concern for the fate of the trapped or attached thrombi, which could embolize during removal of the catheter. This liability remains unaddressed with many of the current temporary devices.

Several other issues regarding temporary filters remain. The major concerns are efficacy and duration of protection. The decision to place a filter indicates that the patient is at risk for PE. Regardless of the length of time it is in place, the device must be able to trap and hold potentially lethal emboli. In the case of the catheter-infusion device, which has a filter connected to the distal end, the ability of these devices to trap emboli has not been demonstrated in clinical trials as the device has US Food and Drug Administration (FDA) approval as a catheter, not a filter.

A second concern is determining the period at risk. The duration of therapy for thromboembolism remains a disputed question. Our experience and that of others suggests that patients remain at risk well beyond hospitalization.[27] In a pilot study, Trowbridge et al. found a 10% incidence of new DVTs up to 2 months following total hip arthroplasty.[28] In a larger study, Planes et al. found that without prophylaxis there was an 11% incidence of DVT following hospital discharge.[29] Most temporary devices must be removed within 7 to 10 days, leaving the patient unprotected. Only one experimental device, the Tempo filter, has been left for up to 30 days.[30] Clinical trials with this device have currently been put on hold by the FDA because of an unforeseen death from PE.

A third concern is the problem of removing the filter that has effectively trapped an embolus. In a study by Buecker et al. attempts to remove thrombus from temporary filters using a thrombectomy device were technically successful, but there were significant amounts of embolized fragments, making it clinically unsafe.[31] The risk of dislodging or fragmenting a thrombus is of great concern. Finally, most of the temporary devices are not designed for secure attachment to the IVC and depend on an external tethering system. Should the patient become septic, the catheter and the device would have to be removed, resulting in additional costs.

A temporary European device, the Gunther filter, has been investigated by Millward et al.[32] In a study of 17 patients there were no clinically evident PEs, although autopsy did reveal a nonfatal embolism. All filters were successfully removed, but permanent filters were required in two patients with malignancy. Two patients (12%) developed IVC thrombosis; and following filter removal both developed a PE. In addition, two other patients were found to have insertion site thrombosis, and one had a major bleeding complication. The significant incidence of filter-related complications suggest that there may be no advantage to using temporary devices.

The concept of a vena caval filter designed for permanent placement but could be removed if necessary has greater appeal. In vivo animal studies of the original and titanium Greenfield filters have demonstrated that they could be safely removed from the vena cava for at least 14 days using an experimental retrieval system.[33] (Figure 27–3). Cope et al. reported using a Bird's Nest filter as prophylaxis during iliocaval thrombolysis. The filter trapped multiple embolic fragments, which were subsequently lysed; and the device was safely removed 6 hours after treatment.[24]

It is difficult to defend a rationale for temporary devices, as they are subject to the same liabilities as permanent devices. Their use is time-limited, and they require a second interventional procedure to remove them. Until the question of the duration of risk for thromboembolism is resolved, the use of temporary devices is difficult to justify, as is evident from the study by Millward et al.[32]

Subclavian Vein Thrombosis

Experience with subclavian vein thrombosis treated with lytic therapy, angioplasty, and stents suggests that a filter can be a valued adjunct to these procedures, as the risk of embolism of these thrombi is real. Early animal studies by Langham et al. demonstrated the feasibility, efficacy, and safety of superior vena caval placement of the Greenfield filter.[34] Devices were successfully placed in 10 of 11 animals and then challenged with experimental emboli. Pulmonary embolism did not occur, and there was good resolution of thrombus with no caval occlusion. Owen et al.[35] reported one case of superior vena caval (SVC) placement with 1 year follow-up demonstrating efficacy and safety in this location. Lidagoster et al.[36] reported obstructive problems when an SVC filter was placed in a patient with lung cancer and an upper extremity DVT. Ascer et al. reported on patients with SVC filters and reported follow-up in four (4 to 14 months) with no PE or other filter-related complications.[37] The upper extremity veins are an underappreciated source of pulmonary embolism, but the use of a filter in the SVC needs longer follow-up results. The need to insert catheters into the central vessels in patients with filters and the need for long-term anticoagulation are additional issues requiring assessment.

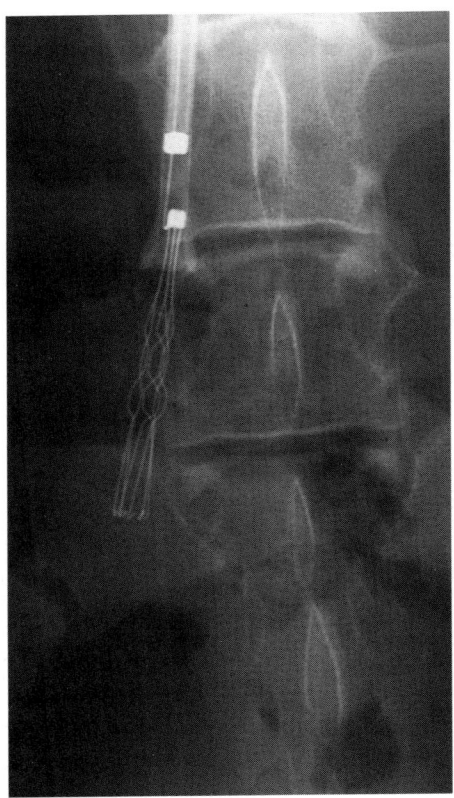

FIGURE 27–3. Percutaneous stainless steel Greenfield filter is being withdrawn into an investigations retrieval system. The retrieval hook can be seen adjacent to the apex of the filter, and the bell-shaped distal end extends over the upper filter limbs.

Use of Central Lines

The use of long-term central lines in patients requiring invasive hemodynamic monitoring or long-term drug or nutritional therapy has increased significantly. Although these devices use materials designed to be nonthrombogenic, they often develop thrombus at the tips or along the catheter. This is especially true for patients with malignancy who are highly thrombogenic or have lines placed via the femoral vein.[38-40] In a study by Dollery et al.[41] the 5-year thrombosis-free rate was only 53%, and the fatal PE 5-year survival rate was 75%. The presence of PEs related to central venous catheters in pediatric intensive care unit cases was reported by Derish et al. In all cases, the PEs were unsuspected prior to death due to masking of symptoms by concomitant respiratory disease.[42] The frequency of this complication in pediatric and cancer patients suggests the need for vigilance and early treatment with lytic therapy and anticoagulation or vena caval filters.

Guidewire Use

Endovascular procedures require the use of various types of guidewires. Following access to the vein with a Seldinger needle, a wire is placed through the needle to maintain access until the procedure is completed. There have been several reports in the literature of these wires becoming entangled in vena caval filters. It occurs when interventionalists fail to scan the IVC using fluoroscopy prior to inserting a wire. Once the wire is trapped, it may cause dislodgement and migration of the filter, with damage to the venous wall. Additional radiologic or surgical intervention to free the wire may be required.[43-46] The wire may also be snared in a filter when it is used to manipulate a misplaced or malpositioned filter.[47-49] A careful history and fluoroscopic scan of the vena cava prior to interventional procedures can prevent these needless complications. Similarly, as new filter designs are introduced to the market, it is important that they be easily identified radiographically and that the materials be compatible with current imaging techniques such as magnetic resonance imaging (MRI). Patients with these or other permanently implanted devices should have some type of identification on their person and in the medical record.

Pediatric Patients

For years, it was thought that children were spared the risk for thromboembolism seen in adults. This belief has been modified as more children are exposed to the risk factors that also affect adults. Major PEs and DVTs have been diagnosed in pediatric patients when they are being treated for various malignancies or when they require central lines for hemodynamic monitoring and resuscitation.[42,50-53] Often these children are at high risk for bleeding complications from anticoagulation,[54,55] making caval interruption the treatment of choice.[56] However, all currently marketed filters are sized for the adult patient. Steinberg et al. reported data on the predicted size of the vena cava based on age, height, weight, and body surface area. They concluded that by the age of 13 the cava has assumed full adult size.[57] Prior to this age, there is little information to guide the physician. An in vivo study in newly weaned lambs to study the effect of Greenfield vena cava filters in the immature vena cava demonstrated that the cava developed to a normal size and shape compared to controls despite the presence of the filter. There was no significant penetration of the cava, and adjacent tissues were not affected. There have also been anecdotal reports to our office supporting the successful use of the filter in patients as young as 4 years of age. The Greenfield titanium filter was selected in these cases owing to its small delivery system and more than 20 years of experience with a cone-shaped device (Figure 27–4). Reed et al.[56] reported outcomes from a small series of eight pediatric patients with vena caval filters demonstrating successful placement in all cases and long-term outcomes similar to those for adult patients. Larger series are necessary to confirm these findings. Whether there is a need for

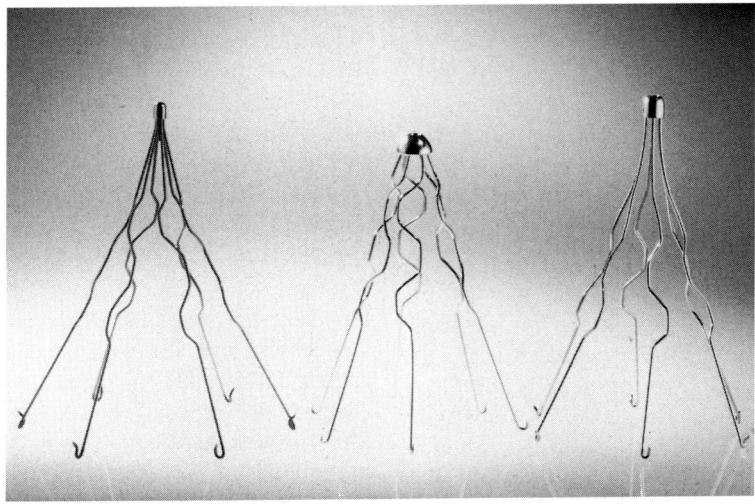

FIGURE 27–4. Narrow apex of the titanium (**left**) and percutaneous (**right**) stainless steel Greenfield filters allow insertion via a 12F delivery system compared to the 24F system required for the original stainless steel filter (**center**).

a filter scaled for pediatric cases remains to be determined.

Conclusion

As less-invasive techniques become the standard of care, it will continue to be necessary to study outcomes for patients who have vena caval filters. Changing indications for filter placement, the use of low-molecular-weight heparins, and the role of temporary filters are just a few of the areas that need to be evaluated. Outcome and cost-effectiveness studies must be done in such a way that data from multiple centers can be combined. One of the problems with the current literature is the lack of reporting standards that require a commonly accepted definition of terms. A consensus conference is currently preparing a set of standards that can be used by radiologists and surgeons to report outcomes in their respective journals. Such efforts have been successful in other areas and should provide a basis for improved communication of clinical results.

References

1. Hunter J, Sessions R, Buenger R: Experimental balloon obstruction of the inferior vena cava, *Ann Surg* 171:315–320, 1970.
2. Mobin-Uddin K, McLean R, Bolooki H: Caval interruption for prevention of pulmonary embolism: long term results of a new method, *Arch Surg* 99:711–715, 1969.
3. Mobin-Uddin K, Callard G, Bolooki H et al: Transvenous caval interruption with umbrella filter, *N Engl J Med* 286:55, 1972.
4. Greenfield LJ, Michna BA: Twelve-year clinical experience with the Greenfield vena caval filter, *Surgery* 104:706–712, 1988.
5. Greenfield LJ, Proctor MC: Twenty-year clinical experience with the Greenfield filter, *Cardiovasc Surg* 3:199–205, 1995.
6. Sherry S: Fifty years of progress with antithrombotic drugs—with much more to come: a perspective, *J Intern Med* 229:113–116, 1991.
7. Greenfield LJ, Pearce H, Nichols R: Recovery of respiratory function and lung mechanics following experimental pulmonary embolectomy, *J Thorac Cardiovasc Surg* 55:160–168, 1968.
8. Greenfield LJ, Bruce T, Nichols N: Transvenous pulmonary embolectomy by catheter device, *Ann Surg* 174:881–886, 1971.

9. Greenfield LJ, Reif M, Guenter C: Hemodynamic and respiratory responses to transvenous pulmonary embolectomy, *J Thorac Cardiovasc Surg* 62:890–897, 1971.
10. Greenfield LJ: Transvenous management of pulmonary thromboembolism, *Surg Rounds* 8(10):86–94, 1985.
11. Greenfield LJ, Peyton R, Crute S, Barnes RW: Greenfield vena caval filter experience: late results in 156 patients, *Arch Surg* 116:1451–1455, 1981.
12. Fullen W, Miller E: Prophylactic vena caval interruption in hip fracture, *J Trauma* 13:403–410, 1973.
13. Korwin SM, Callow AD, Rosenthal D et al: Prophylactic interruption of the inferior vena cava: immediate and long-term hemodynamic effects, *Arch Surg* 114:1037–1040, 1979.
14. Greenfield LJ, Peyton M, Brown P, Elkins R: Transvenous management of pulmonary embolic disease, *Ann Surg* 180:461–468, 1974.
15. Tadavarthy S, Castaneda-Zuniga W, Salamonowitz E: Kimray-Greenfield filter: percutaneous introduction, *Radiology* 151:525–526, 1984.
16. Rose B, Simon D, Hess M, Van Aman M: Percutaneous transfemoral placement of the Kimray-Greenfield vena cava filter, *Radiology* 165:373–376, 1987.
17. Pais O, Mirvis S, De Orchis D: Percutaneous insertion of the Kimray-Greenfield filter: technical considerations and problems, *Radiology* 165:377–381, 1987.
18. Hye R, Mitchell A, Dory C et al: Analysis of the transition to percutaneous placement of Greenfield filters, *Arch Surg* 125:1550–1553, 1990.
19. Kantor A, Glanz S, Gordon DH, Sclafani SJ: Percutaneous insertion of the Kimray-Greenfield filter: incidence of femoral vein thrombosis, *AJR* 149:1065–1066, 1987.
20. Simon M, Athanasoulis C, Kim D et al: Simon nitinol inferior vena cava filter: initial clinical experience, *Radiology* 172:99–103, 1989.
21. Kim D, Grassi CJ, Simon M et al: Simon nitinol filter clinical trial: final results, *RSNA* 1991.
22. Thery C, Bauchart J, Lesenne M et al: Predictive factors of effectiveness of streptokinase in deep venous thrombosis, *Am J Cardiol* 69:117–122, 1992.
23. Tarry WC, Makhoul RG, Tisnado J et al: Catheter-directed thrombolysis following vena cava filtration for severe deep venous thrombosis, *Ann Vasc Surg* 8:583–590, 1994.
24. Cope C, Baum RA, Duszak RA Jr: Temporary use of a Bird's Nest filter during iliocaval thrombolysis, *Radiology* 198:765–767, 1996.
25. Vorwerk D, Schmitz-Rode T, Schurmann K et al: Use of a temporary caval filter to assist percutaneous iliocaval thrombectomy: experimental results, *J Vasc Intervent Radiol* 6:737–740, 1995.
26. Eichelter P, Schenk W: Prophylaxis of pulmonary embolism: a new experimental approach with initial results, *Arch Surg* 97:348, 1968.
27. Kibel AS, Loughlin KR: Pathogenesis and prophylaxis of postoperative thromboembolic disease in urological pelvic surgery, *J Urol* 153:1763–1774, 1995.
28. Trowbridge AA, Boese CK, Woodruff B et al: Incidence of posthospitalization proximal deep venous thrombosis after total hip arthroplasty: a pilot study, *Clin Orthop* 299:203–208, 1994.
29. Planes A, Vochelle N, Darmon JY et al: Risk of deep venous thrombosis after hospital discharge in patients having undergone total hip replacement: double blind randomised comparison of enoxaparin versus placebo, *Lancet* 348:224–228, 1996.
30. Kuszyk BS, Venbrux AC, Samphilipo MA et al: Subcutaneously tethered temporary filter: pathologic effects in swine, *J Vasc Intervent Radiol* 6:895–902, 1995.
31. Buecker A, Neuerburg J, Schmitz-Rode T et al: In vitro evaluation of a rheolytic thrombectomy system for clot removal from five different temporary vena cava filters, *Cardiovasc Intervent Radiol* 20:448–451, 1997.
32. Millward S, Bormanis J, Burbridge BE et al: Preliminary clinical experience with the Gunther temporary inferior vena cava filter, *J Vasc Intervent Radiol* 5:863–868, 1994.
33. Van de Werf F: Thrombolysis for acute myocardial infarction, *Haemostasis* 24:65–68, 1994.
34. Langham M, Etheridge J, Crute S, Greenfield LJ: Experimental superior vena caval placement of the Greenfield filter, *J Vasc Surg* 2:794–798, 1985.
35. Owen E, Schoettle P, Harrington O: Placement of a Greenfield filter in the superior vena cava, *Ann Thorac Surg* 53:896–897, 1992.
36. Lidagoster MI, Widmann WD, Chevinsky AH: Superior vena cava occlusion after filter insertion, *J Vasc Surg* 20:158–159, 1994.
37. Ascer E, Gennaro M, Lorensen E, Pollina RM: Superior vena caval Greenfield filters: indications, techniques, and results, *J Vasc Surg* 23:498–503, 1996.
38. Bolz KD, Aadahl P, Mangersnes J et al: Intravascular ultrasonographic assessment of thrombus

formation on central venous catheters, *Acta Radiol* 34:162–167, 1993.
39. Shefler A, Gillis J, Lam A et al: Inferior vena cava thrombosis as a complication of femoral vein catheterisation, *Arch Dis Child* 72:343–345, 1995.
40. Pollard AJ, Sreeram N, Wright JG et al: ECG and echocardiographic diagnosis of pulmonary thromboembolism associated with central lines, *Arch Dis Child* 73:147–150, 1995.
41. Dollery CM, Sullivan ID, Bauraind O et al: Thrombosis and embolism in long-term central venous access for parenteral nutrition, *Lancet* 344:1043–1045, 1994.
42. Derish MT, Smith DW, Frankel LR: Venous catheter thrombus formation and pulmonary embolism in children, *Pediatr Pulmonol* 20:349–354, 1995.
43. Johnson DR, Harshfield D: Radiological case of the month: inadvertant guidewire entrapment by IVC filter during subclavian line placement, *J Ark Med Soc* 89:517–518, 1993.
44. Urbaneja A, Fontaine AB, Bruckner M, Spigos DG: Evulsion of a vena tech filter during insertion of a central venous catheter, *J Vasc Intervent Radiol* 5:783–785, 1994.
45. Marelich GP, Tharratt RS: Greenfield inferior vena cava filter dislodged during central venous catheter placement, *Chest* 106:957–959, 1994.
46. Granke K, Abraham M, McDowell DE: Vena cava filter disruption and central migration due to accidental guidewire manipulation: a case report, *Ann Vasc Surg* 10:49–53, 1996.
47. Moore B, Vaiji K, Roberts A, Bookstein JJ: Transcatheter manipulation of asymmetrically opened titanium Greenfield filters, *J Vasc Intervent Radiol* 4:687–690, 1993.
48. Sweeney T, Van Aman M: Deployment problems with the titanium Greenfield filter, *J Vasc Intervent Radiol* 4:691–694, 1993.
49. Isaacson S, Gray RR, Pugash RA: Manipulation by catheter of unopened LGM filter. *Can Assoc Radiol J* 44:217–220, 1993.
50. Rohrer MJ, Cutler BS, MacDougall E et al: A prospective study of the incidence of deep venous thrombosis in hospitalized children, *J Vasc Surg* 24:46–50, 1996.
51. Manco-Johnson M: Disorders of hemostasis in childhood: risk factors for venous thromboembolism, *Thromb Haemost* 78:710–714, 1997.
52. McBride WJ, Gadowski GR, Keller MS, Vane DW: Pulmonary embolism in pediatric trauma patients, *J Trauma* 37:913–915, 1994.
53. Uderzo C, Faccini P, Rovelli A et al: Pulmonary thromboembolism in childhood leukemia: 8-years' experience in a pediatric hematology center, *J Clin Oncol* 13:2805–2812, 1995.
54. Andrew M: Indications and drugs for anticoagulation therapy in children, *Thromb Res* 81(suppl):S61–S73, 1996.
55. Massicotte P, Adams M, Marzinotto V et al: Low-molecular-weight heparin in pediatric patients with thrombotic disease: a dose finding study, *J Pediatr* 128:313–318, 1996.
56. Reed RA, Teitelbaum GP, Stanley P et al: The use of inferior vena cava filters in pediatric patients for pulmonary embolus prophylaxis, *Cardiovasc Intervent Radiol* 19:401–405, 1996.
57. Steinberg C, Weinstock D, Gold J, Notterman D: Measurements of central blood vessels in infants and children: normal values, *Cathet Cardiovasc Diagn* 27:197–201, 1992.

Part V
Specialized Endovascular Techniques

28
PTA and Stenting of Subclavian and Innominate Arteries

Amir Motarjeme

Following successful percutaneous transluminal angioplasty (PTA) of the aortoiliac and renal arteries, multiple reports of PTA in the vertebral, carotid, innominate, and subclavian arteries appeared in the radiology literature. The first report of subclavian artery angioplasty in the European literature was by Mathias et al.,[1] and in the United States a single case was reported by Backman et al.,[2] both in 1980. Multiple patient studies of vertebral, carotid, and subclavian artery angioplasty were reported by my group.[3,4] Other notable interventionists such as Sundt et al. and Vitek et al. simultaneously helped advance support for brachiocephalic PTA with strong experimental and clinical research.[5–7]

Today, balloon angioplasty and placement of intravascular stents for proximal arch vessel lesions is considered the treatment of choice by most interventionists.[8] In addition to stenosis, total occlusion of the proximal subclavian arteries in subclavian steal syndrome can be effectively treated in most cases. This is mainly because of having superior balloon catheters and guidewires and, of course, vascular stents.[9]

Indications and Contraindications

Stenosis of the left subclavian artery is one of the most common atherosclerotic occlusive disease of the proximal supraaortic vessels,[10] but few are symptomatic. In a study of 1114 patients with occlusions of the innominate and subclavian arteries, only 168 patients demonstrated signs and symptoms of the subclavian steal syndrome.[11]

The subclavian steal syndrome was first described by Reivich et al. in 1961.[12] Its diagnosis is not difficult. The ipsilateral brachial pressure is considerably lower than the contralateral pressure among patients who complain of a variety of symptoms including vertigo, ataxia, diplopia, paresis, numbness, and arm claudication. Other symptoms of vertebrobasilar insufficiency are nausea, vomiting, vascular headaches, facial numbness, cortical blindness, memory disturbance, and nystagmus.

A Doppler examination of the brachiocephalic arteries usually confirms the diagnosis by showing retrograde flow in the ipsilateral vertebral artery. On rare occasions, on the right side when the vertebral artery is occluded severe stenosis or occlusion of the innominate artery may cause reverse flow in the carotid artery (Figure 28–1).

The diagnosis of subclavian steal syndrome is confirmed by thoracic aortography. Selective injections into the subclavian artery can incorrectly show temporary antegrade flow within the vertebral artery.

On occasion, the patient complains only of intermittent claudication of the arm, which is usually experienced during manual exercise, such as writing, shaving (among men), driving, and housework such as vacuuming and peeling potatoes. We have also seen unusual symptoms such as aching of the suprascapular and shoulder areas.

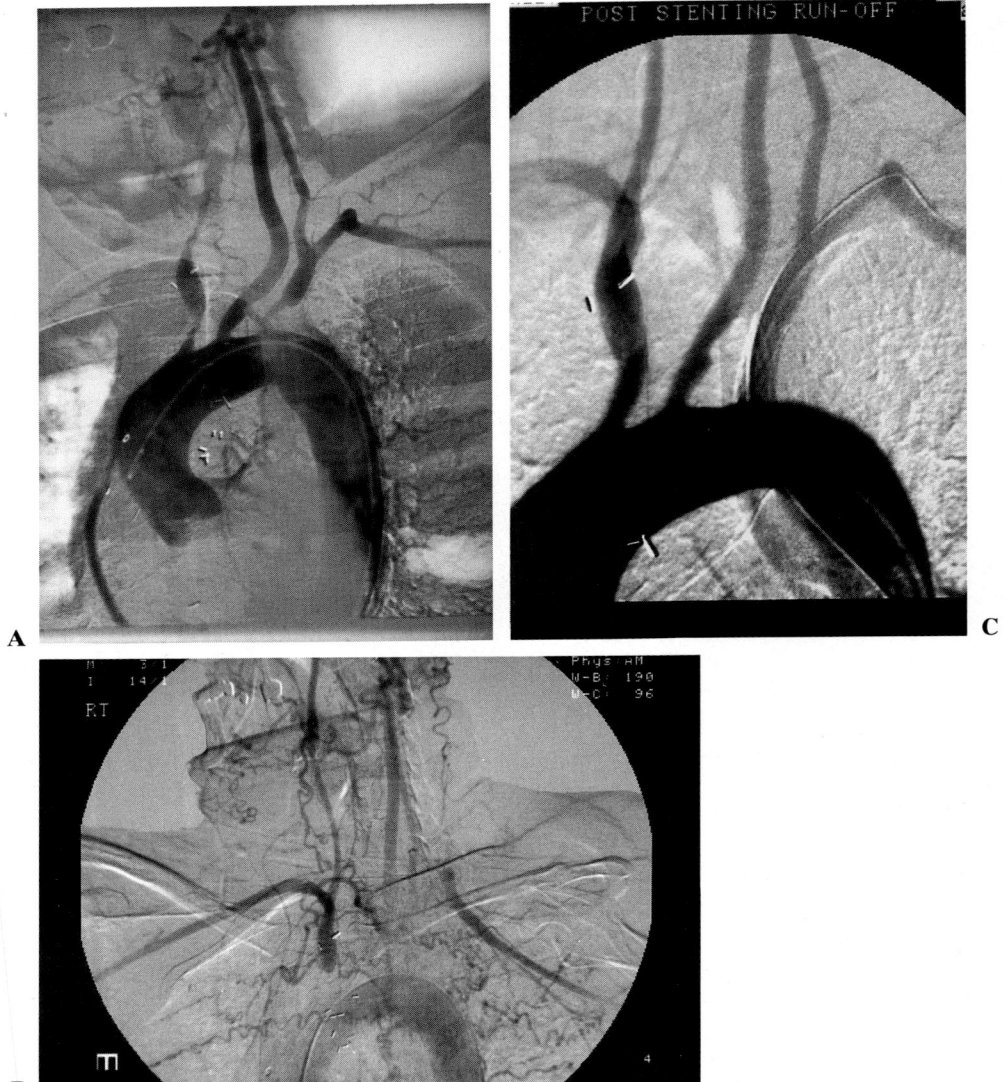

FIGURE 28–1. **A**, Arch aortogram shows stenosis of the left subclavian and more severe stenosis of the innominate arteries. No visualization of the right carotid and subclavian arteries is seen. The left vertebral artery is widely patent. **B**, Late arterial phase shows retrograde flow through the right carotid and good visualization of the subclavian arteries. The right vertebral artery is totally occluded. **C**, Arch aortogram after successful angioplasty of the innominate artery and stenting of the left subclavian artery shows correction of right subclavian steal. There is now antegrade flow in the right carotid and visualization of the right subclavian artery.

Cerebral and arm symptoms are usually exaggerated with arm exercise. Severe stenosis of the innominate artery can duplicate these symptoms. The symptoms could be more severe because of sharing the arterial flow with the right carotid artery. Proximal occlusion of the innominate artery causes retrograde flow down the right vertebral artery to feed both the right subclavian and carotid arteries.

Contraindications to angioplasty and stenting of the subclavian and innominate arteries include allergy to contrast medium, fresh thrombosis, and heavily ulcerated plaques. In the case of thrombosis, thrombolysis is advised

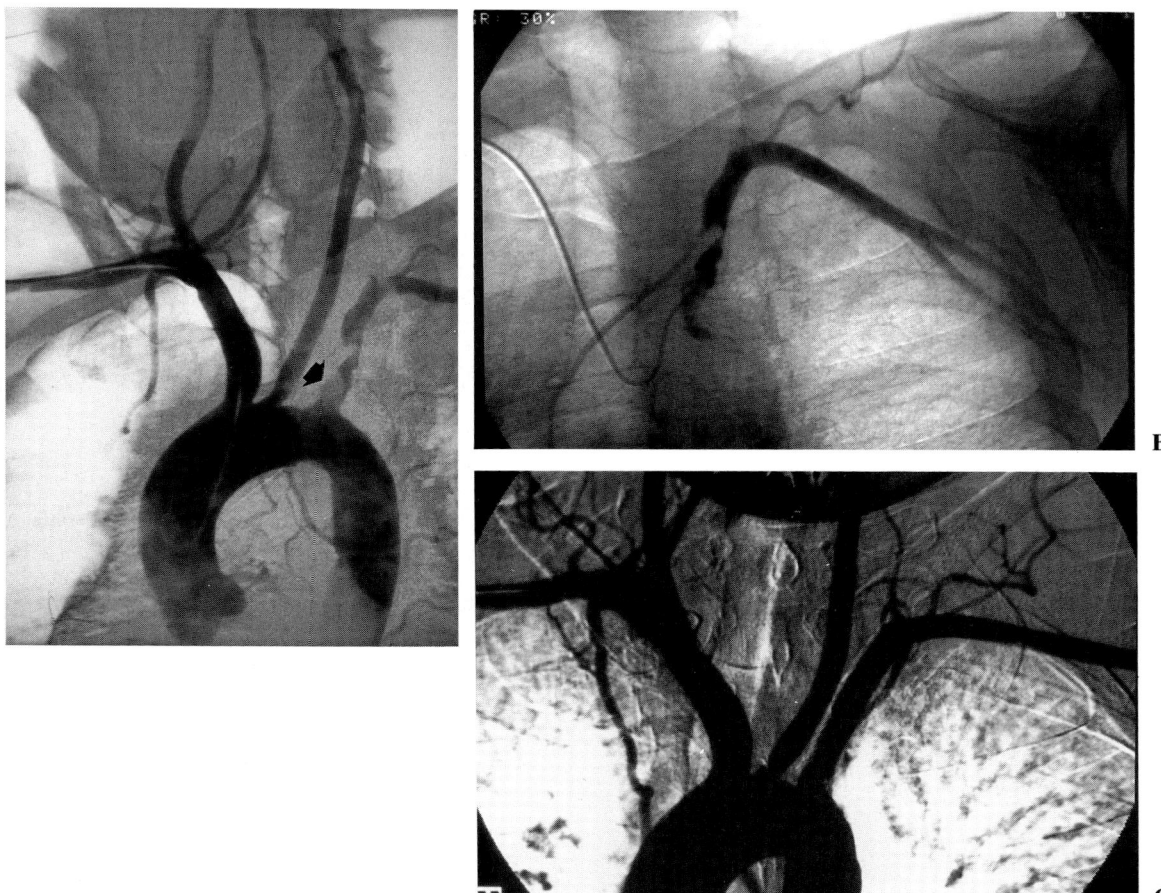

FIGURE 28–2. This 64-year-old man, a double amputee, complained of severe claudication of the left arm, especially while operating his wheelchair. **A**, Arch aortogram performed via the right brachial artery shows severe stenosis of the subclavian artery. Partial thrombosis is seen proximal to the stenosis (*arrow*). **B**, Postthrombolysis left subclavian arteriogram shows complete clot lysis and high-grade eccentric stenosis of the subclavian artery. **C**, After angioplasty and stenting (performed through the left brachial artery) the aortogram now shows total patency of the left subclavian artery. There is also antegrade flow in a small vertebral artery (*arrow*).

prior to angioplasty and stent placement (Figure 28–2). The presence of atherosclerotic plaque adjacent to or involving the vertebral artery is not a contraindication but requires a double balloon angioplasty technique (Figure 28–3).

Methodology

High quality thoracic aortography and an additional selective subclavian arteriogram are needed to study the type and morphology of the lesion. Its extent and location in respect to the origin of the vertebral and internal mammary arteries are especially needed to detect the presence of an associated thrombosis. A transfemoral approach for diagnostic angiography is preferred, although a brachial approach on the contralateral side can also be used. The ipsilateral arm should not be used for diagnostic angiography. The width of the subclavian artery is measured on angiographic film. An anteroposterior (AP) projection on a cut film usually represents 20% magnification, but the actual size of the artery can be measured by

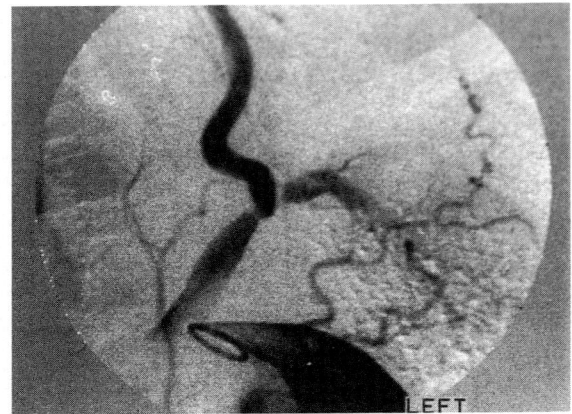
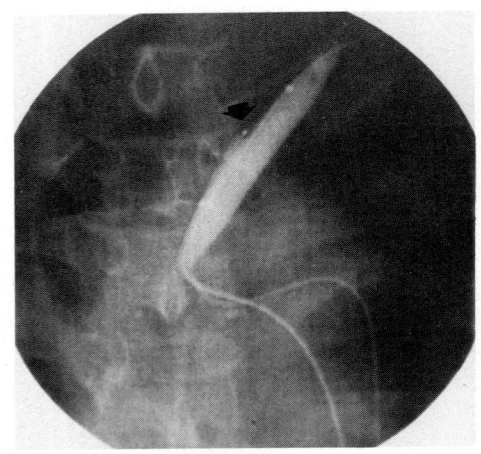
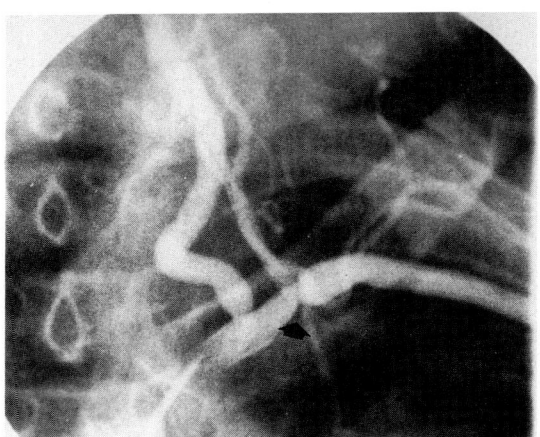

FIGURE 28–3. **A**, This 54-year-old man had severe stenosis of the left subclavian artery adjacent to both sides of the origin of the vertebral artery. **B**, Dilatation of the left subclavian artery with the two-balloon technique. The large balloon is within the subclavian artery, and the smaller balloon (*arrow*) is within the proximal left vertebral artery. The smaller balloon is protecting the integrity of the vertebral artery. **C**, Postangioplasty arteriogram shows dilatation of the subclavian artery on both sides of the vertebral artery. The vertebral artery is widely patent. The distal mild stenosis of the subclavian artery (*arrow*) was purposely not dilated so as to preserve the internal mammary artery.

computerized digital subtraction angiography. An angiogram is usually obtained in the AP and right posterior oblique views for the left side and a left posterior oblique view for the right subclavian arteries. The subclavian artery is then selectively catheterized using preshaped cerebral catheters. We prefer the headhunter no. 1. The stenosis is then negotiated with a steerable wire, usually a 0.035-inch glidewire (Glidewire; Medi-tech, Watertown, MA). The catheter is then advanced over the wire to the axillary artery. The steerable wire is exchanged for a J-shaped stiffer wire. After removal of the angiographic catheter, an 8F guiding catheter, of hockey stick shape, preloaded with an appropriate-size balloon catheter, is inserted over the wire to the subclavian artery. At this time contrast material is injected, and a road map obtained. The balloon is then inserted, and the stenosis is well dilated. The balloon is maintained within the stenosis for one full minute. After deflation the balloon is pulled back to the guiding catheter, and brief angiography is performed to assess the result of angioplasty. If satisfactory, an arch aortogram is obtained for final evaluation. If the lesion is to be stented, the balloon catheter is removed, and a balloon catheter loaded with the stent is inserted. Just before deployment a road map is obtained, and the stent is deployed precisely (Figure 28–4). For eccentric stenosis and residual stenosis with a recoil, a J & J stent is used; and for longer lesions having intimal dissection, a Wallstent is preferred (Figure 28–5, 28–6).

If using a guiding catheter, the smaller J & J stent and a balloon catheter of 5F shaft is used. For Wallstents of any size, a guiding catheter of

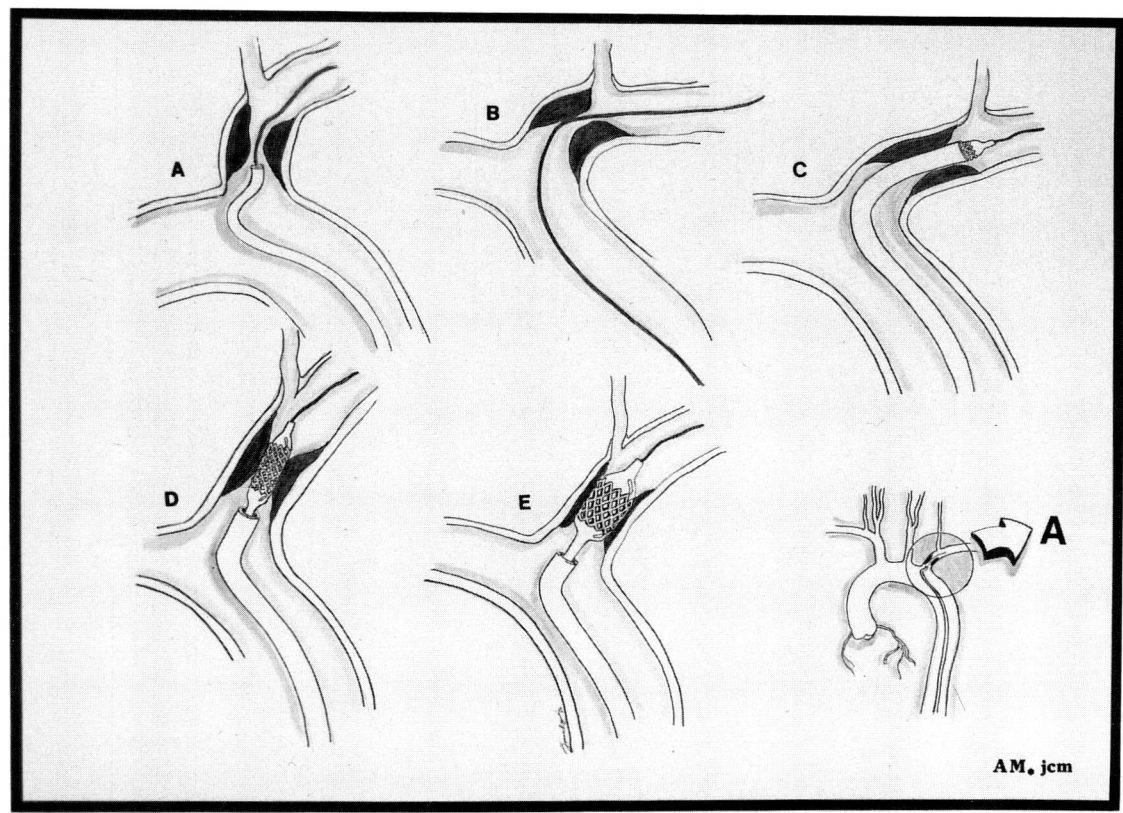

FIGURE 28–4. Stenting a left subclavian stenosis. **A**, Selective catheterization of the left subclavian artery and insertion of a guiding wire across the lesions. **B**, Angiography catheter is removed while the guide wire is kept in place. **C**, Preloaded guiding catheter with stent is inserted within the stenosis. **D**, While the stent is kept within the stenosis, the guiding catheter is pulled back. An angiogram obtained through the guiding catheter can confirm the precise placement of the stent. **E**, Stent is fully deployed. Additional poststent arteriography and intravascular ultrasonography can be performed at this time.

7F or 8F can easily be used (Figure 28–6). After obtaining an initial angiogram, angioplasty and stenting can be performed via the ipsilateral brachial artery. A brachial approach might be preferred for total occlusion, although a transfemoral approach can be tried and is occasionally successful (Figure 28–6).

Preangioplasty and Postangioplasty Management

The patients are treated with aspirin 325 mg daily and dipyridamole (Persantine) 75 mg t.i.d. prior to angioplasty. Heparin 3000 to 5000 units is used during the procedure. The patient's activated clotting time (ACT) is monitored during the procedure; we prefer to keep it around 250 seconds. The heparin dose is adjusted individually to meet this goal.

After the procedure the catheter is removed when the ACT is not more than 30 seconds over baseline. The patient is discharged on aspirin and dipyridamole, as prior to the procedure. Warfarin is not used unless it is required for another pathologic entity, and protamine sulfate is not used for heparin reversal. Hemostasis is obtained manually or with closure devices.

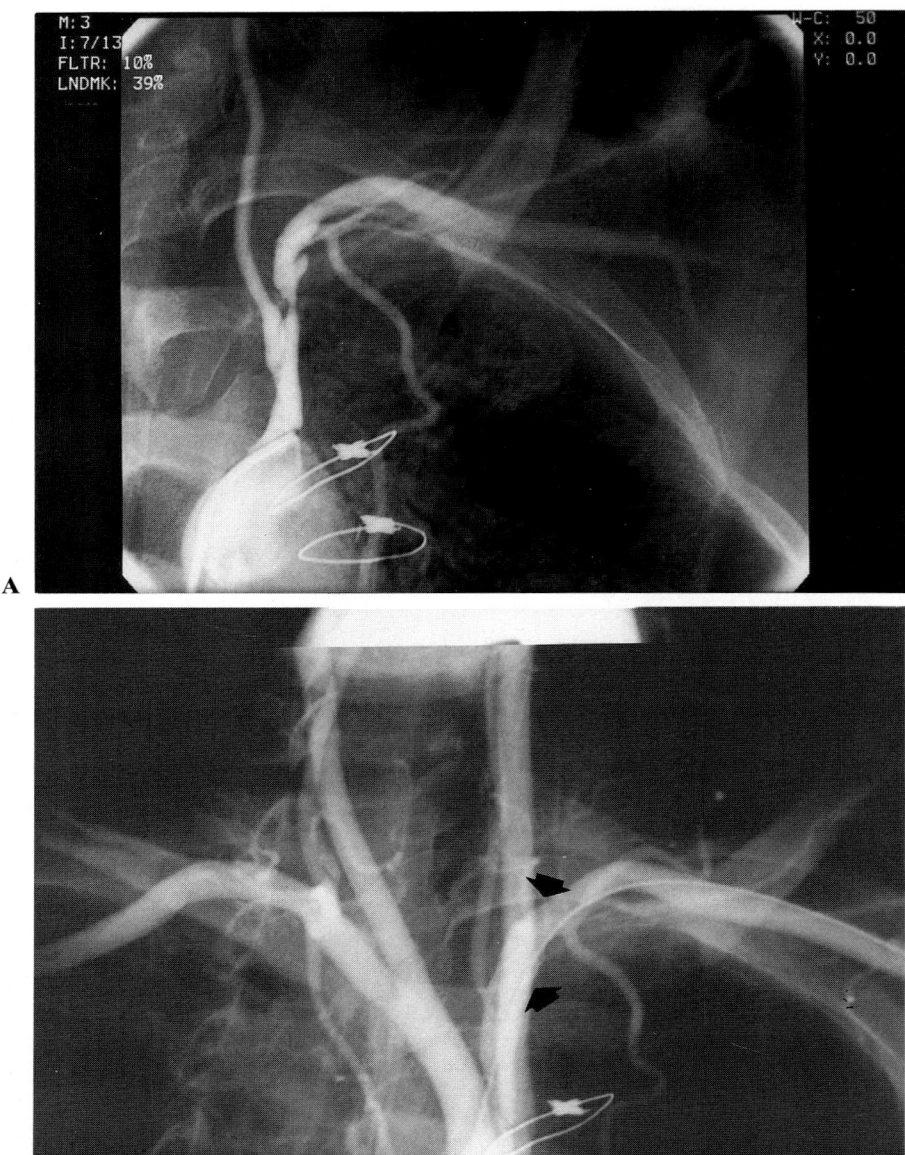

FIGURE 28–5. **A**, Selective left subclavian arteriogram from a 52-year-old woman with chest pain shows a severe eccentric ulcerated stenosis just proximal to the internal mammary artery, which was used to bypass to the anterior descending coronary artery. The stenosis is extended down to the origin of the vertebral artery. **B**, Arch aortogram shows perfect placement of the stent between the origin of the vertebral and internal mammary arteries (between *arrows*). A 154 Palmaz stent was dilated up to 8mm.

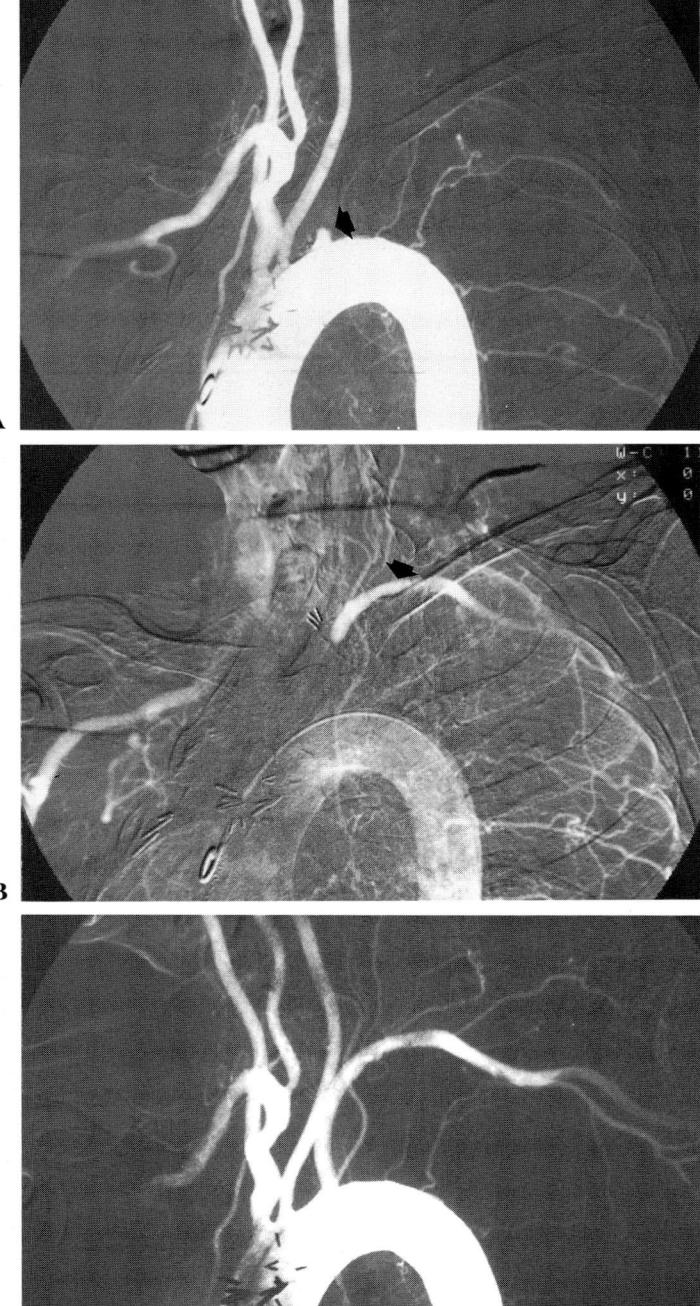

FIGURE 28–6. **A**, A 58-year-old woman with left arm and shoulder pain and occasional dizziness had total occlusion (*arrow*) of the left subclavian artery. Note the prominent intercostal arteries. **B**, Left subclavian steal via the thoracocervical trunk (*arrow*) was also seen. The vertebral artery is occluded. **C**, After recanalization and stenting, the left subclavian artery is widely patent. An 8×20 mm. Wallstent was used.

Results

The primary success of dilatation and stenting of the subclavian and innominate artery stenosis exceeds 90%. All of our 84 patients with stenosis of the subclavian or innominate arteries have been treated successfully. Treatment of total occlusion of the subclavian arteries, however, is not as successful. Occlusion of the subclavian arteries, even a short segment, is difficult to recanalize. We have successfully recanalized only 7 of 14 totally occluded subclavian arteries (Table 28-1). An upgraded pool of 417 patients, which includes those with both stenosis and total occlusion, shows a 95% success rate.[13] The complication rate was 2.6%. In our series, one patient developed thromboembolism of the left brachial artery originating from a totally occluded left subclavian atherosclerotic lesion. This plaque embolus was subsequently removed surgically without untoward effect.

Because of the large number of out-of-area patient referrals and poor patient compliance, long-term follow-up is difficult. The standard protocol is follow-up at 1 month after the procedure and then every 3 months the first year and every 6 months during subsequent years.

The long-patency rate of proximal lesions is superior to that for lesions distal to the vertebral artery. The patency of the stented total occlusion appears to be superior to that after balloon angioplasty. Of seven successfully recanalized occluded left subclavian arteries, four were stented. These have remained patent 1 to 4 years, whereas two of three occlusions treated with angioplasty have reoccluded: one at 6 months and the other at 18 months. One was treated with a left common carotid subclavian bypass, and the other was successfully recanalized and dilated.

Discussion

Over the last 17 years, PTA of the supraaortic vessels, including the subclavian and innominate arteries, has progressed from an experimental procedure to an accepted treatment with an outcome equal or superior to that with surgery in specially defined cases. Among the pathologies that respond particularly well to PTA is stenosis of the subclavian and innominate arteries.[7-9,14,15]

Indications for PTA and stenting of the subclavian arteries are the same as those for surgery.[8] PTA offers the advantage of lower intraoperative morbidity and mortality as well as decreased emotional and financial burden in certain circumstances. Although our long-term follow-up results are by no means complete, there are only a few patients with restenosis/reocclusion of their treated vessel.

The use of PTA as the treatment of choice for subclavian artery stenosis has much support. We have had a 100% (70/70) initial success rate treating these lesions. Pooled data from several studies document a similar outcome (395/417, 94%).[13] In addition, we have seen only three cases of reocclusion over a 5-year period.

The alternative surgical treatment for subclavian and innominate stenosis involved intrathoracic or extrathoracic bypass. Complication rates for these procedures run as high as 23%, with chylothorax, endarterectomy thrombosis, pneumothorax, pleural effusion, neck lymph fistula, phrenic nerve palsy, and Horner syndrome among the most serious.[16]

In contrast, we experienced only one postoperative complication associated with percutaneous treatment of this type of lesion: a thromboembolus to the brachial artery, which was successfully treated by surgical thrombectomy. Pooled data demonstrate a similar inci-

TABLE 28-1. Results of PTA and Stenting in 98 Patients with Subclavian and Innominate Artery Lesions

Pathology	No.
Subclavian artery	77/84 (91.6%)
Stenosis	70/70 (100%)
Occlusion	7/14 (50%)
Innominate artery (stenosis)	14/14 (100%)

dence of complications (2.6% complication rate) with most involving thromboemboli.[13] Fortunately, these thrombi rarely embolized to the brain owing to an apparent delay in the reversal of retrograde flow through vertebral arteries after subclavian angioplasty. This phenomenon was demonstrated by Ringelstein and Zeumer,[17] who used ultrasound monitoring of the ipsilateral vertebral arteries before, during, and after subclavian angioplasty proximal to the vertebral arteries. Despite sufficient recanalization of the proximal subclavian artery, flow within the vertebral artery became antegrade slowly over a period of 20 seconds to several minutes. These authors concluded that the delayed flow reversal served as a protective mechanism against cerebral embolism during and shortly after PTA of the subclavian artery.

For subclavian artery occlusions, PTA has been less successful. We were able to dilate only 50% (7/14) of occluded subclavian arteries. Although thrombolytic therapy was adequate in some of these PTA failures, this approach also was unsuccessful. Moreover, the adequately recanalized occlusions had a 25% restenosis rate at 6 months and a 50% rate at 2 years. Whereas stenotic subclavian lesions may be treated by PTA, surgical intervention is the treatment of choice at the present time for total subclavian occlusions when PTA or stent deployment (or both) failed.

The treatment strategy for subclavian stenoses also holds true in the innominate artery. In our experience, the innominate behaves similarly to the proximal left subclavian artery. When we reviewed the population with subclavian lesions alone, we saw a disparity between the number of diseased left versus right vessels; there was a disproportionately higher number of left subclavian lesions. When we included the innominate vessels with the subclavian vessels, however, the disparity was less evident. In addition, the technical difficulties and pathologic properties of these two vessels are almost identical. We therefore believe innominate artery stenoses should be treated in the same manner as proximal subclavian artery stenoses (Figure 28–1).

References

1. Mathias VK, Schlosser V, Reimke M: Katheterrekanalisation-eines Subklaviaverschlusses, *Rofo Fortschr Geb Rontgenstr Neuen Bildgeb Verfahr* 132:326–347, 1980.
2. Bachman DM, Kim RH: Transluminal dilatation for subclavian steal syndrome, *AJR* 135:995–996, 1980.
3. Motarjeme A, Keifer JW, Zuska AJ: Percutaneous transluminal angioplasty of the brachiocephalic arteries, *AJR* 138:457–462, 1982.
4. Motarjeme A, Keifer JW, Zuska, AJ et al: Percutaneous transluminal angioplasty for treatment of subclavian steal, *Radiology* 155:611–613, 1985.
5. Sundt TM Jr, Smith HC, Campbel JK et al: Transluminal angioplasty for basilar artery stenosis, *Mayo Clin Proc* 55:673–680, 1980.
6. Vitek JJ, Morawetz RB: Percutaneous transluminal angioplasty of external carotid artery: preliminary report, *AJNR* 3:451–456, 1982.
7. Vitek JJ, Raymon BC, Oh SJ: Innominate artery angioplasty, *AJNR* 5:113–114, 1984.
8. Motarjeme A, Gordon GI: Percutaneous transluminal angioplasty of the brachiocephalic vessels: guidelines for therapy, *Int Angiol* 12:260–269, 1993.
9. Motarjeme A: Percutaneous transluminal angioplasty of supra-aortic vessels, *J Endovasc Surg* 3:171–181, 1996.
10. Hass WK et al: Joint study of extracranial arterial occlusion. II. Arteriography, techniques, sites and complications, *JAMA* 203:961, 1968.
11. Fields WS, Lemak NA: Joint study of extracranial arterial occlusion. VII. Subclavian steal: a review of 168 cases, *JAMA* 222:1139–1143, 1972.
12. Reivich M et al: Reversal of blood flow through the vertebral artery and its effect on cerebral circulation, *N Engl J Med* 265:878, 1961.
13. Graor RA, Gray BH: Interventional treatment of peripheral vascular disease. In Young JR, Graor RA, Olin JW, et al, editors: *Peripheral vascular disease*, St Louis, 1991, Mosby Year Book, pp 111–133.
14. Damuth HD, Diamond AB, Rappoport AS et al: Angioplasty of subclavian artery stenosis proximal to the vertebral origin, *AJNR* 4:1239–1242, 1983.
15. Wilms G, Baert A, Dewaele D et al: Percutaneous transluminal angioplasty: early and late

results, *Cardiovasc Intervent Radiol* 10:123–128, 1987.
16. Beebe HG, Stark R, Johnson ML et al: Choices of operation for subclavian-vertebral artery disease, *Am J Surg* 139:616–623, 1980.
17. Ringelstein EB, Zeumer H: Delayed reversal of vertebral artery blood flow following percutaneous transluminal angioplasty for subclavian steal syndrome, *Neuroradiology* 26:189–198, 1984.

29
Role of Angioplasty in Limb Salvage

D.E. Schwarten

Dotter and Judkins[1] included three cases of infrapopliteal angioplasty in their 1964 report on percutaneous transluminal angioplasty. In 1986, eight years after Gruentzig's report of the successful utilization of balloon angioplasty for dilatation of coronary artery stenoses, the use of these more refined systems designed for small-caliber vessels was reported for the management of chronic infrapopliteal atherosclerosis.[2] The development of sophisticated devices for the percutaneous management of infrapopliteal disease has resulted in significantly improved technical and clinical success rates. These improved results have helped broaden the indications for percutaneous intervention for chronic atherosclerotic disease in the distal popliteal artery and infrapopliteal arteries.

Patient Population

Patients undergoing distal angioplasty, as a group, are older, have more extensive vascular disease, and are more frequently diabetic than patients treated by angioplasty at more proximal sites. Angioplasty of the infrapopliteal vessels is associated with higher complication rates and requires enhanced skill levels compared to angioplasty of larger, more proximal vessels. Brown et al.[3] has reported a 17% overall complication rate in a series of patients undergoing infrapopliteal angioplasty without antecedent thrombolysis and a 33% complication rate when the procedure was associated with preangioplasty thrombolysis.

The consequences of complications of infrapopliteal angioplasty are not as easily managed, percutaneously or surgically, as those in more proximal vessels. Therefore most series[4,5] have included primarily patients with ischemic rest pain or more advanced changes. Except in diabetic patients, where limb-threatening disease is not uncommonly confined to the infrapopliteal vessels, multilevel vascular disease is usually present in patients with critical ischemia. These patients have a poor prognosis with an anticipated 5-year mortality rate of nearly 50%.

Management of inflow disease may achieve adequate perfusion to eliminate rest pain or allow healing. The intervening physicians must anticipate, however, that relatively simple inflow procedures may not produce adequate perfusion and that distal and more complex procedures are required. Some publications[6] have suggested that it is acceptable to perform infrapopliteal angioplasty for life style-limiting intermittent claudication. This may be acceptable for patients with disease in the popliteal artery, the tibial-peroneal trunk, or the proximal posterior tibial artery, but in our experience it is distinctly unusual to discover patients presenting with intermittent claudication and isolated proximal infrapopliteal disease. Our decision to include patients with intermittent claudication is made on an individual case-by-case basis and includes multiple variables, not the least of which is the availability of a suitable conduit for distal bypass grafting in the event of a complication.

Angioplasty enjoys the highest clinical success rate and long-term patency rates in all vascular territories when focal atherosclerotic disease is targeted. The infrapopliteal vessels offer no exception to this general rule; therefore ideally angioplasty for limb salvage should be reserved for patients with relatively focal disease. Unfortunately, most patients presenting with threatened limbs do not have focal disease.

We have arbitrarily defined acceptable angiographic anatomy as "focal disease" when there are fewer than four or five focal lesions in a single vessel or when a total occlusion is present that is less than 6cm in length. Even broadening the definition of relatively focal as we have, only a few patients meet these criteria; currently 85% of our patients with infrapopliteal disease undergo distal bypass graft surgery. When there is a compelling reason to avoid operative intervention (high operative risk, lack of suitable conduit) our arbitrary anatomic contraindications are abandoned and angioplasty for limb salvage is attempted.

Technical Aspects

Treatment of a threatened limb by percutaneous techniques is a multidisciplinary approach. Patients are initially worked up by board-certified vascular surgeons who provide clinical and noninvasive data that are helpful when planning the angiographic approach. Usually, diagnostic arteriography is performed from the contralateral approach. This permits completion of the intervention as part of the initial procedure via a contralateral guiding catheter around the aortic bifurcation or via ipsilateral antegrade puncture.

Pharmacologic Adjuncts

Antiplatelet therapy is begun at least 24 hours prior to the anticipated intervention. Intraprocedural systemic anticoagulation is achieved with heparin, with the goal of achieving and maintaining an activated clotting time of more than 200 seconds throughout the procedure. Rarely, systemic heparinization is maintained after the procedure in patients who have resistant vasospasm or subjectively slow runoff. Chronic anticoagulation is rarely necessary.

Guidewire- or catheter-induced vasospasm is almost always easily overcome with 100-μg boluses of nitroglycerin delivered through the catheter directly to the site of spasm. We discourage the routine use of prophylactic calcium antagonists, as they are not necessary and, contrary to widespread opinion, may cause a profound hypotensive response.[7] Persistent mild vasospasm may be managed successfully with transdermal nitroglycerin. If a more aggressive approach is necessary, transcatheter papaverine (60mg) or small doses (1mg) of transcatheter verapamil may be used.

Angioplasty Procedure

Most angioplasty procedures are performed via an ipsilateral antegrade approach through a 5F or 6F sheath. I believe that this approach facilitates better control of guidewire and catheter manipulation than is afforded by the contralateral approach.

In general, in the proximal to mid calf, 0.018-inch guidewire-based systems are employed using catheters in the 4.0F range. More distally, however, catheters based on 0.100- to 0.014-inch guidewires with catheter sizes of 2.5F to 3.3F are employed. These systems are mandatory when performing angioplasty distal to the ankle. Most vendors make catheters designed for below-the-knee angioplasty in 90-cm lengths. Therefore to maintain guidewire position while exchanging angioplasty catheters, a guidewire longer than 145cm is necessary. A 175cm long guidewire permits maintenance of guidewire position across a lesion during catheter exchange. Preservation of branch vessels at bifurcations is easily accomplished by placing "safety" guidewires in any jeopardized branches any performing angioplasty as necessary.

Failure to achieve a technical success with balloon angioplasty because of elastic recoil or an unacceptable dissection may be a good reason to consider stent deployment. There are few published data related to stenting in infrapopliteal vessels. We do know that straight-line outflow to the foot, especially with an intact plantar arch, is associated with a favorable prognosis for PTA. I believe this is essential when stenting. The absence of adequate inflow–outflow predisposes to in-stent thrombosis and potentially catastrophic results.

The stents considered for use in the infrapopliteal vessels is relatively limited. No peripheral stents are approved for use in this anatomic territory. Coronary stents are probably the best choice; although expensive, when viewed in the context of potential limb loss or major operative procedure their use seems appropriate.

Angioplasty of Threatened Grafts

Vein grafts that are threatened by intimal hyperplasia in the vein graft or at the anastomosis or progressive atherosclerosis in the native artery can be treated using percutaneous techniques. Careful ultrasonographic interrogation of grafts frequently allows us to proceed with a planned antegrade puncture, confirmation of the pathologic anatomy with angiography, and percutaneous treatment of the pathology. Progression of atherosclerosis in native vessels is treated the same way it would be in a nongrafted vessel, that is, with balloon angioplasty. Intimal hyperplasia, however, responds poorly to balloon angioplasty;[8] and several authors[9] have suggested that better results may be achieved with directional atherectomy. Our results suggest the same, so lesions thought to be due to intimal hyperplasia are treated with directional atherectomy.

Alternative Techniques

Is there a role for laser or atherectomy in infrapopliteal vessels? No clinical studies have confirmed the efficacy of laser therapy for peripheral vascular disease.

The use of the "subintimal" approach has been advocated, particularly for diffuse disease. Bolia et al.[10] reported an 86% technical success rate with this technique. Long-term follow-up data have not yet been reported.

We have not found directional atherectomy to be of value in the native infrapopliteal vessels, and others have pointed to the dismal 1- and 2-year patency rates when rotational atherectomy has been used for management of infrapopliteal atherosclerotic disease.

A combination of surgical and interventional procedures has been shown to yield good results. Specifically, use of intraoperative angioplasty of outflow vessels may be helpful to maintain an above-knee position for bypass, which is particularly useful in patients who have limited conduit available.[11]

Results

Our personal experience originally reported[12] now includes a series of 194 patients in whom angioplasty was attempted in 248 vessels; technical success was achieved in 243 (98%) of the vessels. We were able to achieve an acceptable anatomic result in 98% of the stenotic lesions and in 88% of total occlusions. At a mean follow-up time of 6.5 years, 115 (84%) of the patients had viable pain-free extremities with average ankle-brachial indices of 0.55. Fifty-eight patients (29%) were either lost to follow-up or had died.

The ability to achieve technical success with currently available technology was illustrated in the series reported by Bakal et al.[13] When using balloon angioplasty catheters designed for small vessels, a technical success rate of 86% was achieved. However, when older methodology was employed in their series, a technical success rate of 29% was reported.

The influence of experience was well illustrated by the initial report of Brown et al.[14] They reported a group of 11 patients for whom a technical success rate of 72% was achieved, but in a follow-up article,[3] with a total of 40 patients, the technical success rate had climbed to 95% with no failures in the latter part of the series.

In addition to our long-term data, Horvath et al.[15] reported a cumulative patency rate by life table analysis of 79.8% at 1 year and 75.3% at 2 years. It is important to note, I believe, that whereas Horvath et al. reported patency rates, our data report limb salvage rates. It is well established that patients undergoing operative intervention for threatened limbs and who subsequently have a healed limb may go on to occlude their graft and not revert to their preoperative clinical status.[16] Multiple factors influence both the initial success and the long-term results of infrapopliteal angioplasty. Bakal et al.[17] emphasized the need to restore straight-line flow to the foot in at least one of the tibial vessels if a clinical benefit is to be realized. Their group reported a 97% early clinical improvement and 80% limb salvage rate at 2 years after successful infrapopliteal angioplasty with restoration of straight-line outflow and reported the absence of significant clinical benefit in patients with obstruction distal to the angioplasty site. Clearly, angioplasty proximal to collaterals is not likely to be a productive endeavor. Diffuse disease has an adverse effect on the results of infrapopliteal angioplasty. Bull and coworkers found a cumulative clinical success rate at 2 years of 83% in patients with a single stenosis and a 57% clinical success rate in patients with multilevel disease. They also noted the adverse effect of associated lytic therapy where the patency rate at 2 years dropped to 55%.[16]

Bull et al. and others have concluded that statistically significant factors in predicting the long-term benefit include (1) a single patent tibial artery; (2) anastomotic stenoses; (3) acute ischemia; and (4) straight-line outflow indirectly supported by posttreatment ankle-branchial indices.

In our series we did not precede angioplasty with lytic therapy in any patient. Brown et al.[14] reported major complications in 6% of their patients and minor complications in 11%; 75% of the complications were associated with lytic therapy. There were complications in 33% of the patients in whom concomitant urokinase was administered. Bakal's group reported three major complications, including one death 5 hours after PTA.[17] Horvath et al. reported an overall major complication rate of 4% and a minor complication rate of 26.4%.[15] These "minor" complications included vessel occlusion and transient renal failure. Bull et al. reported that 3 of their 168 consecutive patients died following periprocedural complications.[16]

Conclusion

Two publications have extensively reviewed infrapopliteal percutaneous angioplasty and have made some interesting comparisons and conclusions. Fraser et al.[18] pointed out that the utilization of infrapopliteal PTA is increasing and called for controlled randomized trials. Bakal et al.[19] concluded that current knowledge regarding infrapopliteal angioplasty supports its role in the management of patients with threatened limbs. Their summary of literature leads to the conclusion that the 2-year benefit of percutaneous angioplasty in properly selected patients is approximately 80%. Bakal et al.[19] agreed with Frasier on the value of randomized trials with angioplasty versus surgery, but such a trial would be difficult to orchestrate.

Infrapopliteal angioplasty has a well defined role in the management of limbs at risk and perhaps in some claudicants. In properly selected patients we agree with Bakal et al. that the results of PTA are equivalent to those achieved with surgical revascularization. PTA is the treatment of choice in the presence of appropriate clinical and anatomic criteria and should be considered for all patients with threatened limbs and an inadequate conduit.

References

1. Dotter CT, Judkins MP: Transluminal treatment of arterial obstruction: description of a new technique and a preliminary report of its application, *Circulation* 30:654, 1964.
2. Schwarten DE: Extracranial uses for the "steerable" coronary balloon angioplasty systems, *Ann Radiol* 299:1209, 1986.
3. Brown KT, Moore ED, Getrajdman GI, Saddeni S: Infrapopliteal angioplasty: long term follow up, *J Vasc Intervent Radiol* 4:139–144, 1993.
4. Schwarten DE, Cutcliff WC: Arterial occlusive disease below the knee: treatment with percuta-

neous transluminal angioplasty performed with low profile catheters and steerable guidewires, *Radiology* 169:71, 1988.
5. Matsi PJ, Manninen MI, Schonnen MT et al: Chronic critical lower limb ischemia: prospective trial of angioplasty with 1–36 months follow up, *Radiology* 188:381–387, 1993.
6. Jagust MB, Sos TA: Infrapopliteal revascularization. In Baum S, Pentecost MJ, editors: *Abrams angiography interventional radiology*, Boston, 1997, Little Brown, pp 284–293.
7. Grossman E, Messerli FM, Gradzicki T, Kowey P: Should a moratorium be placed on sublingual nifedipine capsules given for hypertensive emergencies and pseudoemergencies, *JAMA* 276: 1328–1331, 1996.
8. Perler BA, Osterman FA, Mitchell S: Balloon dilatation versus surgical revision of infrainguinal autogenous vein graft stenosis: long term follow up, *J Cardiovasc Surg* 31:656–661, 1990.
9. Dolmatch BL, Grey RJ, Horton KM: Treatment of anastomotic bypass graft stenosis with directional atherectomy: short-term and intermediate results, *J Vasc Intern Radiol* 6:105–113, 1995.
10. Bolia A, Sayers RD, Thompson MM, Bell PRF: Subintimal and intraluminal treatment of occluded crural arteries by percutaneous transluminal angioplasty, *Eur J Vasc Surg* 8:214–219, 1994.
11. Veith FJ, Gupta SK, Wengester VR et al: Changing arteriosclerotic disease patterns and management strategies in lower limb threatening ischemia, *Ann Surg* 212:402–414, 1990.
12. Schwarten DE: Clinical and anatomic considerations for nonoperative therapy in tibial disease and the results of angioplasty, *Circulation* 83(suppl I):186–190, 1991.
13. Bakal CW, Sprayregen S, Scheinbourn K et al: Percutaneous transluminal angioplasty in infrapopliteal arteries: results in 53 patients, *AJR* 154:171–174, 1990.
14. Brown KT, Schoenberg NY, Moore ED, Saddekni S: Percutaneous angioplasty of infrapopliteal vessels: preliminary results and technical considerations, *Radiology* 69:75–78, 1988.
15. Horvath W, Oertl M, Haidinger D: Percutaneous transluminal angioplasty of crural arteries, *Radiology* 177:565–569, 1990.
16. Bull PG, Mendel M, Hold M et al: Distal popliteal and tibioperoneal angioplasty: long term follow up, *J Vasc Intervent Radiol* 3:45–53, 1992.
17. Bakal CW, Cynamon J, Sprayregen S et al: Infrapopliteal artery angioplasty: followup and factors influencing clinical response in 53 patients. Presented at the 17th annual meeting of the Society of Cardiovascular and Interventional Radiology, Washington, DC, April 1992.
18. Fraser SCA, Al-Kuatoubi MA, Wolfe JHN: Percutaneous transluminal angioplasty of the infrapopliteal vessels: the evidence, *Radiology* 200:33–36, 1996.
19. Bakal CW, Cynamon J, Sprayregen S: Infrapopliteal angioplasty: what we know, *Radiology* 200:36–43, 1996.

30
Carotid Angioplasty and Stenting

Edward B. Diethrich

Carotid stenosis causes disturbing symptomatology in many patients and is known to increase the risk of stroke. Indeed, the cumulative 5-year risk of stroke in those with severe carotid stenosis and transient ischemic attacks (TIAs) is 30% to 35%.[1,2] The gold standard of therapy for carotid artery stenosis is carotid endarterectomy, a surgical technique that has been perfected over more than 40 years.[3] The success of percutaneous endovascular intervention in a variety of anatomic regions has led to the introduction of carotid angioplasty and stenting as a means of treating carotid stenosis. Although those of us evaluating the technology would welcome the opportunity to study carotid endovascular interventions in a large clinical trial, sufficient funding has not yet been made available. In the absence of results from a major trial, there is heated debate about the appropriateness of carotid angioplasty and stenting. It has become clear that some carotid lesions are considerably more amenable to endovascular treatment than others. However, we do not yet have a definitive answer about the equivalency of these less invasive procedures with carotid endarterectomy. The current indications for carotid artery angioplasty and stenting are reviewed in this chapter, as are the techniques and clinical results.

Indications for Carotid Artery Angioplasty and Stenting

At the present time, the indications for cervical carotid artery angioplasty and stenting are unclear. Carotid stenting procedures are being performed in most institutions with investigational review board (IRB) approval, and US Food and Drug Administration (FDA) protocols are in place to ascertain their safety and efficacy.

Patients in a category potentially well suited for carotid angioplasty and stenting are those who have previously undergone one or more endarterectomy procedures and have recurrent disease (Figure 30–1A,B). The reported incidence of restenosis with endarterectomy varies from 1.2% to 36.0%,[4,5] but it is generally agreed that only approximately 10% of the recurrent cases are clinically significant.[6,7] Unless the recurrence is creating a stenosis of 80% or more or a contralateral internal carotid artery (ICA) is occluded, reintervention may not be indicated in the absence of specific symptoms. This latter position may not be universally accepted and may indeed become more liberalized as more experience is gained with stenting.

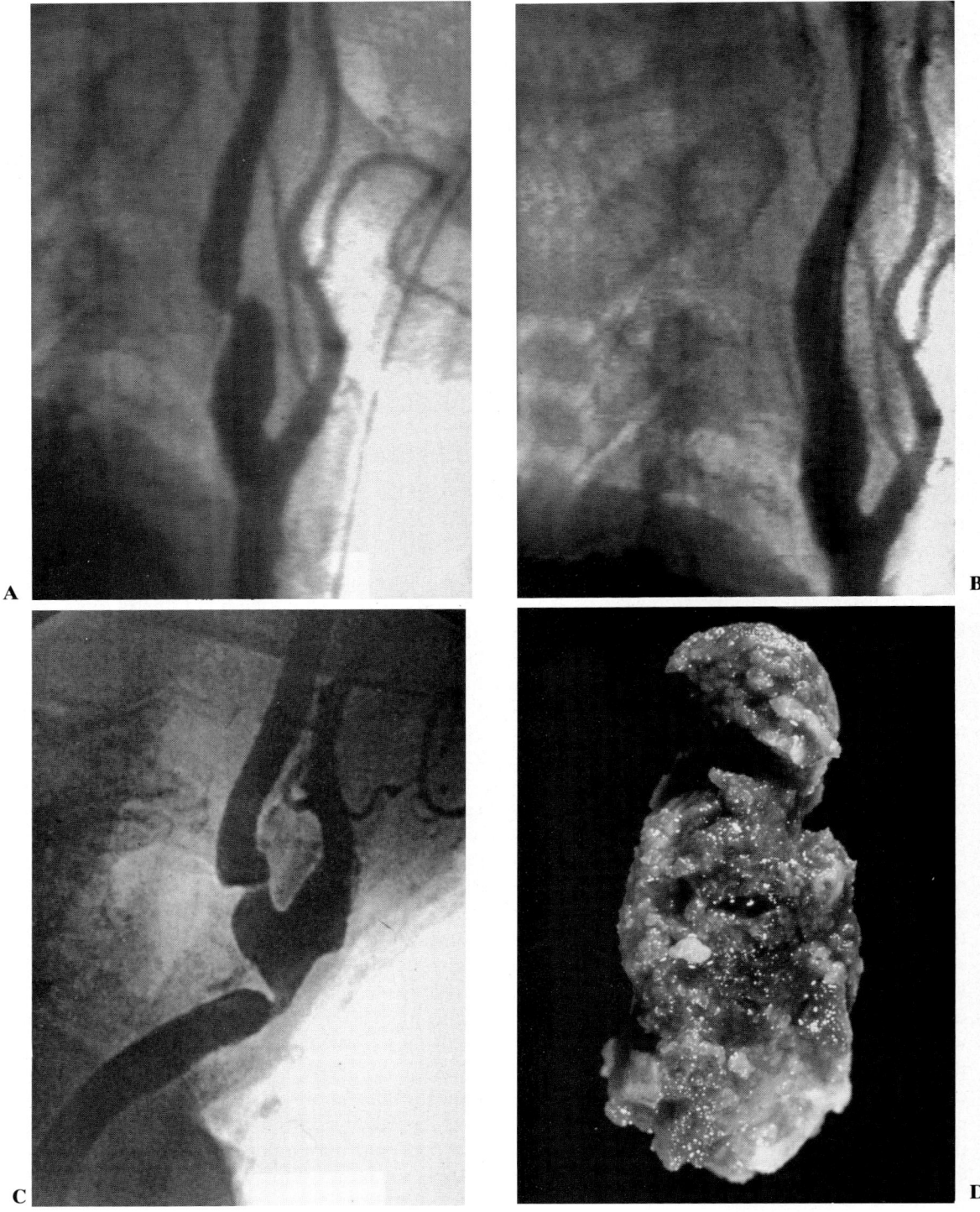

FIGURE 30–1. **A**, Angiogram of the carotid artery in a patient who, only 8 months before, underwent endarterectomy. **B**, Recurrent lesions that develop within the first 12 to 18 months after surgery may be highly suited to endovascular treatment. **C**, After a few years, recurrent lesions may appear suitable for stenting based on angiographic images. **D**, The nature of the plaque in these lesions may result in embolization.

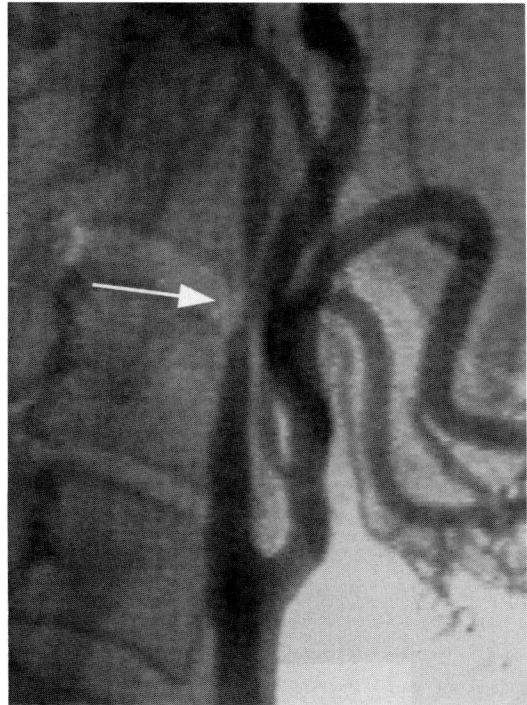 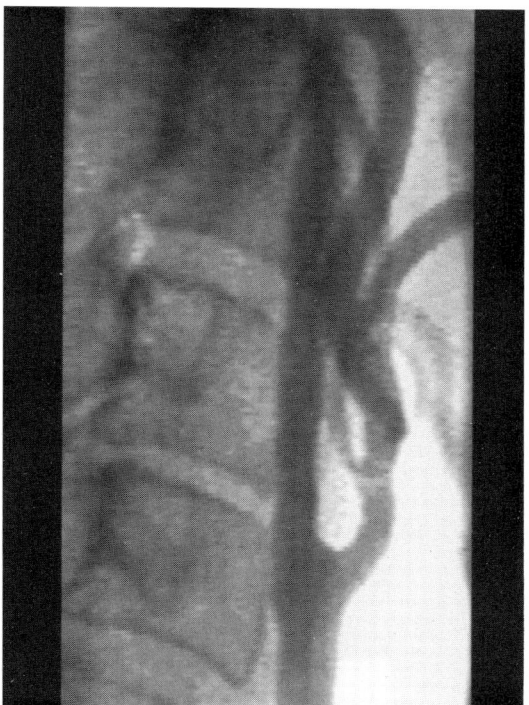

FIGURE 30–2. **A**, Angiogram showing high internal carotid stenosis. **B**, These lesions appear ideal for angioplasty and stenting rather than treatment with classic carotid endarterectomy.

When dealing with recurrent lesions, it is important to recognize that all recurrences are not the same with regard to their potential appropriateness for stenting. Lesions that develop within the first 12 to 18 months following endarterectomy are usually the result of a technical error or a myoproliferative response at the endarterectomized site. They are usually well localized and do not contain the atherosclerotic debris characteristically seen in de novo bifurcation lesions. For these reasons, primary stenting—which is accomplished without ballooning—may be used with a low incidence of neurologic episodes. The pathology of recurrent lesions that develop over a longer period (e.g., several years) is usually different; these lesions are not well localized and frequently contain atherosclerotic material similar to that in the original plaque (Figure 30–1C,D). Duplex scanning often reveals a diffuse lesion with loose material in the lumen. In these cases stenting, with or without prior balloon dilation, may risk embolization of the material within the lesion.

We have sometimes elected to stent patients who present with lesions in the distal ICA at the base of the skull, as these lesions are difficult to access surgically without otolaryngeal and neurologic sequelae. This category of high ICA lesions is almost ideal for stenting (Figure 30–2). The lesions are frequently short and often appear as an "hourglass" configuration located well beyond the bifurcation, where atherosclerotic debris is common. In some cases the midportion of the lesion is narrow, requiring the use of small balloon dilation at low pressure before stent application. The potential complications associated with surgical intervention (i.e., difficulty with adequate surgical exposure of the distal extent of the lesion, the need for subluxation of the mandible and rewiring of the jaw, and the potential for nerve damage) may make this procedure obsolete given the relative simplicity of the endoluminal approach.

Endoluminal treatment is also preferable to the classic surgical approach when extensive scar tissue develops after irradiation and is

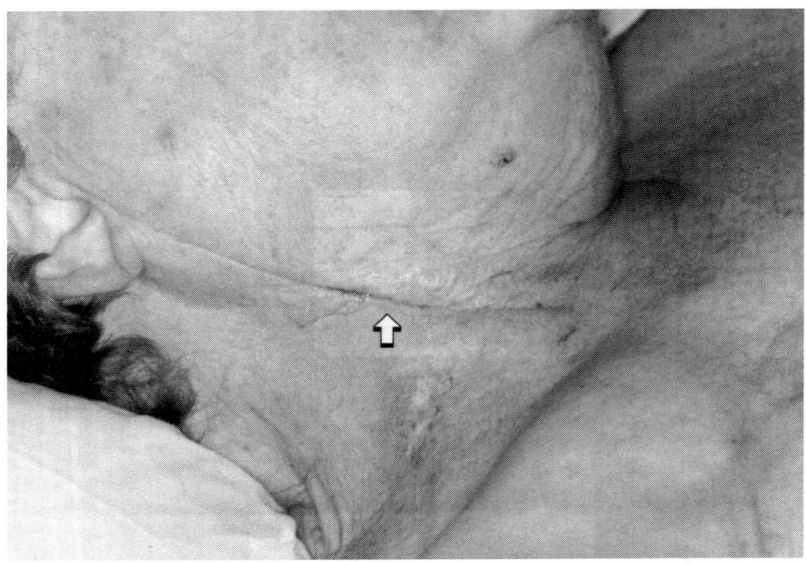

FIGURE 30–3. Patient who underwent radical neck dissection followed by radiation therapy. Surgical exposure of lesions can be difficult in these cases, and stenting may be preferable.

coupled with the aftermath of radical neck dissection (Figure 30–3), creating a veritable "no man's land" for the vascular surgeon. In these cases, even identifying the artery can be a surgical challenge, and the potential for arterial trauma and neurologic damage is considerable. Lesions may be long and diffuse, requiring extensive patching with vein or synthetic materials. Stents are available in a variety of lengths and may be used to cover diffuse lesions with relative ease. Compared to surgical intervention, fewer complications are associated with stenting, making it an attractive alternative to surgical intervention.

Significant changes are underway in the preoperative and postoperative management of patients undergoing carotid endarterectomy, making cost-benefit comparisons with carotid endovascular procedures difficult. Many institutions are eliminating preoperative angiographic studies in most patients. The carotid bifurcation is now frequently assessed via duplex scanning (Figure 30–4), which reduces expenses compared with more invasive imaging techniques. Stent programs may eventually embrace less invasive imaging as well, but currently most protocols mandate extensive preprocedural angiographic analyses.

Current postoperative care of the endarterectomy patient frequently entails direct transfer from the recovery room to the surgical ward, completely eliminating a stay in the intensive care unit (ICU) and its attendant costs. Stent procedures do not require ICU monitoring, but the cost of the device itself is considerable. Given the current similarities in postoperative care, the costs of stenting and endarterectomy may not ultimately be appreciably different.

Techniques for Carotid Artery Angioplasty and Stenting

Anesthesia

Most endovascular procedures do not require the use of a general anesthetic. At the Arizona Heart Institute, we prefer a local anesthesia with mild sedation for percutaneous retrograde femoral interventions. It is possible to use agents that allow the patient to be completely comfortable and conversant during the procedure such that any neurologic change may be immediately assessed.[8–10] In the rare case in which a neurologic deficit arises from ischemia caused by balloon inflation, rapid deflation quickly reverses the symptoms. Balloon inflation at the

30. Carotid Angioplasty and Stenting

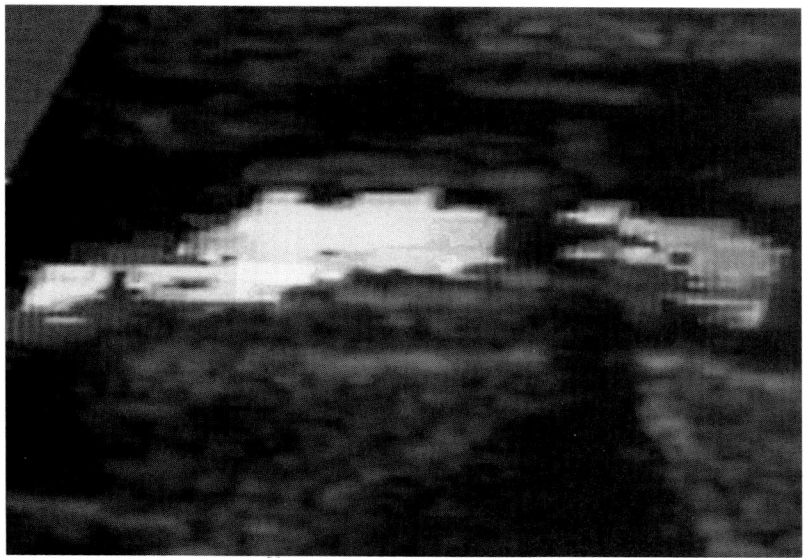

FIGURE 30–4. Duplex scanning of the carotid artery is the most commonly employed noninvasive technique used to evaluate carotid artery disease.

carotid bifurcation commonly yields baroreceptor stimulation, causing bradycardia. Cardiac standstill may result, and momentary sternal compression may be required. Atropine sulfate (1 mg) administered 60 seconds before balloon expansion usually prevents this complication but does not guarantee against it. Thus careful attention should be paid to the electrocardiogram (ECG) monitor during ballooning.

When direct access techniques are used, the positioning of the patient and the need for him or her to remain still during the procedure may dictate a preference for general anesthesia. Short-acting, rapidly reversible drugs should be used so the patient may be awake and extubated in the endovascular suite immediately following the procedure.[8] Although cervical block and local anesthesia have been used successfully for carotid interventions,[9,10] immobilizing the head and neck during the procedure is difficult, particularly if the patient is not intubated, and the anesthesiologist must support a mask over the patient's face.

Access

The carotid region is usually accessed using a retrograde femoral approach, although direct common carotid artery access may also be indicated. For nearly all carotid procedures, a radiopaque ruler (Burkhart Roentgen, Pinellas Park, FL) is placed underneath the patient's shoulder, and its position relative to the target carotid artery is confirmed with fluoroscopy. Because the lesions to be treated reside within the thorax, the fluoroscopy unit is moved over to the field, and radiopaque objects such as tubing and ECG leads are positioned so as not to interfere with imaging during the procedure.

Common Carotid Artery Access

Direct, percutaneous carotid access is associated with a relatively high rate of complications, and we no longer use it at our institution. Our current procedure employs a short, 2- to 3-cm incision just above the clavicle to expose the artery before insertion of the 18-gauge needle (Figure 30–5). The common carotid artery is dissected free from the carotid sheath and held with a heavy silk or vessel loop. This variation in our technique avoids the potential for postprocedural hematoma and prevents the stent compression

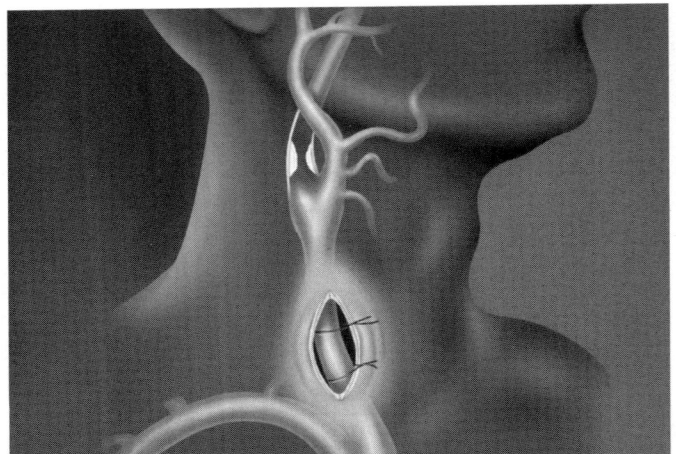
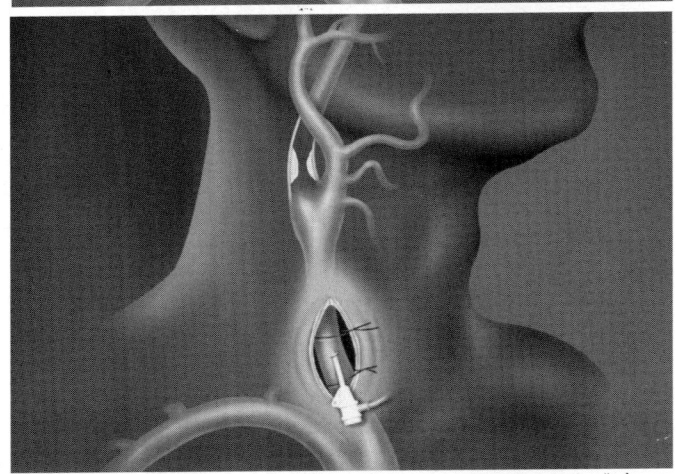
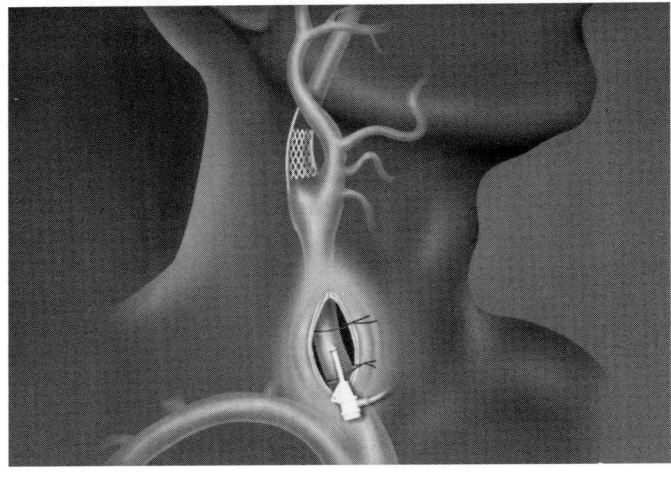

FIGURE 30–5. **A**, Short segment of the common carotid artery is exposed approximately 3 cm above the clavicle. **B**, A 6F or 7F sheath is introduced using a technique similar to that used for percutaneous interventions. **C**, Stent is deployed, and a control angiogram is obtained. **D**, A 4-0 Prolene purse-string suture is placed around the sheath before it is removed. **E**, This technique avoids clamping the artery following stent delivery.

30. Carotid Angioplasty and Stenting

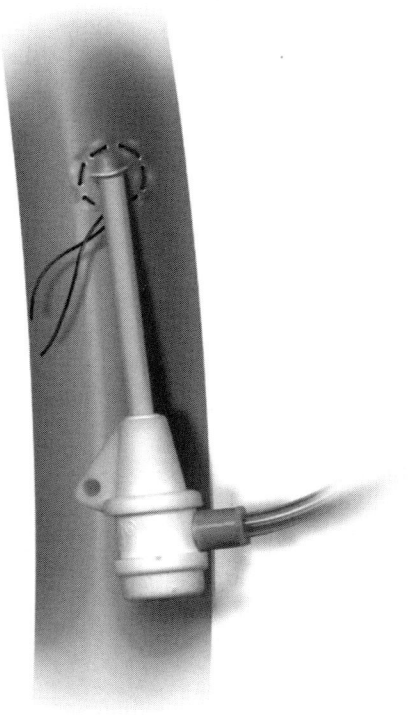
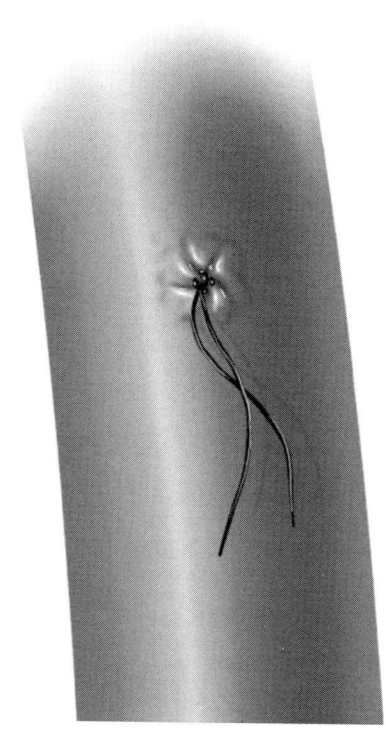

FIGURE 30–5. *Continued.*

seen with the percutaneous approach (Figure 30–6).

The techniques for antegrade and retrograde carotid artery access (Figure 30–7) are identical except for their direction. The antegrade approach to the ICA is documented below.

The entry site into the common carotid artery can be variable distances above the clavicle, depending on the location of the lesion. A short incision (as described above) is made to expose a segment of the common carotid artery, and an 18-gauge, $2\frac{3}{8}$-inch single-wall entry needle (Cook, Bloomington, IN) is used for the puncture.

An angled hydrophilic guidewire (Glidewire; Medi-tech/Boston Scientific, Watertown, MA) is passed cephalad into the external carotid artery. Crossing the ICA is avoided, as it may result in embolic complications. We use a 7F Coons dilator (Cook) to expedite sheath placement and then insert a 7F, 6cm long sheath (Cordis, Warren, NJ), releasing a short bolus of contrast to confirm sheath placement. A fluoroscopic road mapping image is acquired on disk, and the fluoroscopic unit remains stationary for the rest of the procedure. Intravenous heparin sodium (approximately 5000 units) is given to maintain the activated coagulation time (ACT) above 250 seconds, and the sheaths and catheters are irrigated with a heparinized saline solution (10,000 units of heparin in 1000ml normal saline).

Preprocedural duplex scanning is valuable for assessing the nature of the lesion and the degree of narrowing; and, angiographic visualization is used to judge the length and diameter of the lesion and is the basis for deciding whether to predilate. Predilation is frequently necessary before stent deployment in severely stenotic lesions. The balloon diameter is usually one or two sizes smaller than the stent delivery balloon. Preparing the stent delivery balloon at this time shortens the interval between balloon predilation and stent deployment.

Selecting the appropriate stent depends on the diameter and length of the lesion. The most

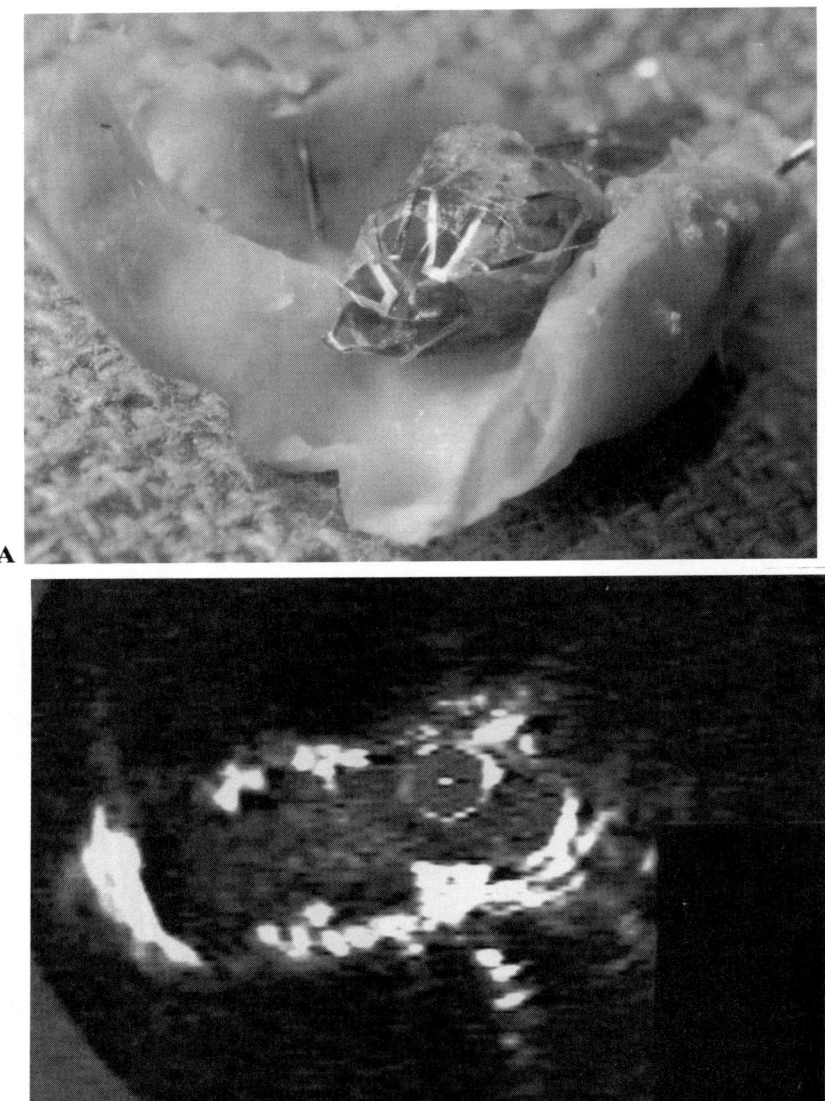

FIGURE 30–6. **A**, Palmaz stent with a severe deformity due to compression on the neck at the time of sheath removal after a percutaneous procedure. **B**, These stent deformities can easily be detected with duplex surveillance. The direct, percutaneous carotid stick has now been abandoned at our institution.

common balloon dilation catheter sizes are 4 mm × 2 cm and 5 mm × 2 cm balloons followed by stent delivery on the same-size or next larger-size balloon. In general, two types of stent are being used today, neither of which has been approved by the FDA for use in the carotid location. Several newer designs are under development, and corporate sponsors are initiating clinical trials of them. Most experience with stents to date has been gained using the rigid, balloon-expandable Palmaz stent (Cordis) or the Wallstent (Schneider, Minneapolis, MN), which is a flexible, self-expanding stent.

After preparation of the balloon and stent, the guidewire is withdrawn from the external carotid artery, and a smaller Roadrunner wire (Cook) is passed across the lesion into the ICA. The wire is kept low in the extracranial ICA to avoid vascular trauma or arterial spasm. The

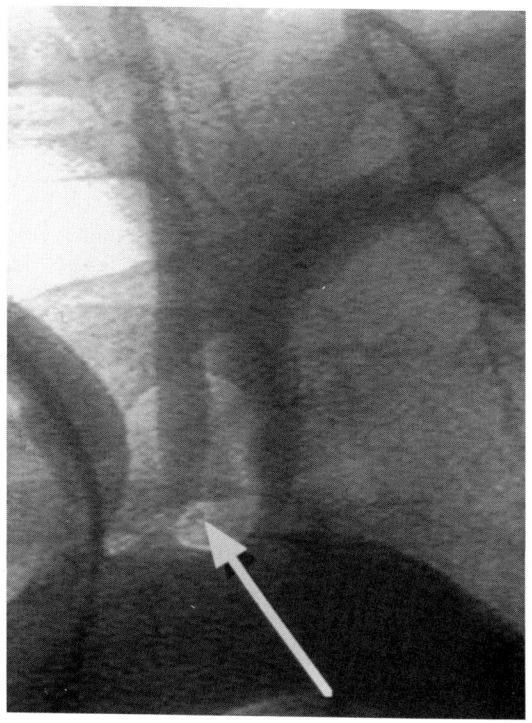 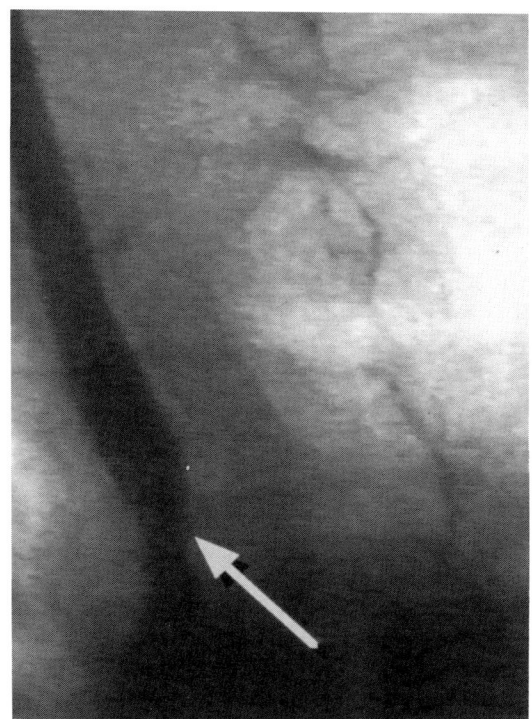

FIGURE 30–7. Angiographic study showing an occlusive lesion at the origin of the left internal carotid artery. This type of lesion can be accessed easily via the retrograde common carotid approach.

anesthesiologist administers atropine (1 mg) to block bradycardia and resulting hypotension during balloon expansion.

The road-mapping image is used to help center the balloon across the lesion, and a short burst of contrast is injected to allow visualization of its final position. The balloon is expanded for a few seconds at 8 to 10 atm. If bradycardia occurs, the balloon should be deflated immediately. When the expansion is complete and the balloon has been deflated, the shaft of the angioplasty catheter is rotated to furl the balloon before it is retracted. Contrast injection confirms the result of balloon dilation and establishment of an adequate passageway for stent deployment.

The balloon catheter with the stent is then advanced into position, and the stent is situated between the dots on the balloon. If the patient moves and the road map is lost, a repeat contrast injection is necessary. When a rigid stent moves on the balloon or is misaligned, it must be repositioned, even if it requires complete removal of the balloon and the stent delivery catheter. After the operator is satisfied with the stent's position, the balloon is expanded to deploy the device or, in the case of a self-expandable stent, is simply released. A short inflation, over 5 seconds, is generally sufficient for balloon expansion. The ECG is carefully monitored for any changes.

Following stent deployment, contrast is injected to confirm patency and assess proper positioning. In all cases, regardless of the approach, a cerebral angiogram is performed at the conclusion of the stent deployment. This step is particularly important to confirm the absence of cerebral embolization, a scenario requiring a neuro-rescue technique such as thrombolytic infusion.

Although it has not been our standard practice to image the intracranial area prior to manipulations across the carotid lesion, it might be advantageous to image at baseline for comparison with the control study. It has become clear that inadequate stent expansion contributes to complications such as stent occlusion and thrombus formation, and we frequently use real-time intravascular ultrasound (IVUS) to determine the adequacy of stent deployment.

Once the procedure is complete and the incision is closed, anesthesia may be discontinued. It is still important that blood pressure be monitored closely at this time as uncontrolled hypertension may result in significant hematoma formation. Before transfer, the patient should be awakened and assessed for any neurologic deficits. After the transfer, we perform a duplex scan of the treatment site within the first hour.

Femoral Access

The retrograde femoral access method is the most familiar, frequently used access technique in endovascular intervention and is often used for both diagnostic and therapeutic modalities. Both iliac arteries are evaluated, and the side with the less tortuous and stenotic artery is chosen to facilitate placement of the sheath and advancement of the guiding catheter into the aortic arch. Occlusion of the abdominal aorta or the femoral/iliac vessels precludes retrograde femoral access.

An 18-gauge $2\frac{3}{8}$-inch needle is inserted in the common femoral artery followed by a 0.035-inch guidewire (Glidewire) and a 7F or 9F sheath (Cordis). Intravenous heparin (approximately 5000 units) is then administered, and a 260-cm, 0.035-inch angled hydrophilic guidewire (Medi-tech) is passed into the aortic arch. A JB2 catheter (Cook) is passed into the high ascending aorta, and the wire is withdrawn to expose the angle of the JB2 catheter. The catheter is then pulled back slowly to engage selectively either the brachiocephalic trunk or the origin of the left common carotid artery. Once the angled guidewire has been passed into the appropriate common carotid artery, the JB2 catheter is advanced over it to the midlevel of the carotid artery. The angled guidewire is then passed into the external carotid artery followed by the JB2 catheter. The guidewire is removed and replaced with a 260-cm Super Stiff Amplatz wire (Cook), which is passed into the external carotid artery. The JB2 catheter is removed, and the fluoroscope is panned in the anteroposterior position from the cervical carotid artery across the arch to allow assessment of the angle and origin of the great vessel (Figure 30–8). The operator should observe the angle of the vessels carefully; an angle that is too acute at the carotid or innominate artery junction may kink the delivery sheath. Conversion to the open approach may be appropriate when vessel angles are deemed too acute.

When the arch anatomy is favorable, a flexible delivery catheter such as the Flexor catheter by Cook (Figure 30–9) is inserted into the midcarotid position, the Amplatz wire is removed, and a 0.014-inch Roadrunner wire is passed across the lesion in the ICA. Contrast is injected for road mapping, and the dimensions of the artery and the nature and length of the lesion are determined. In some cases a stent can be deployed without ballooning. When ballooning is required, a small balloon (usually 4 mm × 2 cm or 5 mm × 2 cm with 120 cm shaft length) is selected and passed to the lesion. When atropine has been administered, the balloon is inflated for a few seconds at 8 to 10 atmospheres. At this point in the procedure, a small bolus of contrast is injected to assess the angioplasty result.

Once a stent has been selected and passed to the lesion, a second contrast bolus is injected to confirm proper location. The stent is deployed using a 5-second balloon inflation in the case of the Palmaz stent. The self-expanding Wallstent is released quickly into the vessel. At this time, we favor imaging with ultrasonography, and the IVUS catheter is passed through the stent. If deployment is adequate, a final control angiogram is obtained. As mentioned previously, it may be advantageous to image at baseline (before any manipulation) for comparison with the control study. When deployment is not adequate, additional dilation of the stent with a larger balloon is performed. After dilation the guiding catheter is withdrawn into the descending thoracic aorta, and a short 9F sheath is substituted in the groin. The patient is then transferred to the ICU for observation and duplex scanning. The groin sheath is removed when the ACT returns to normal. The primary complication associated with femoral access is

30. Carotid Angioplasty and Stenting

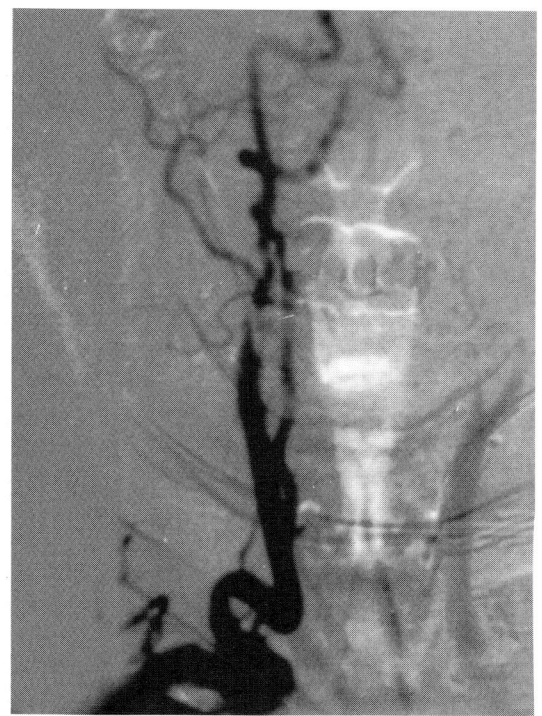 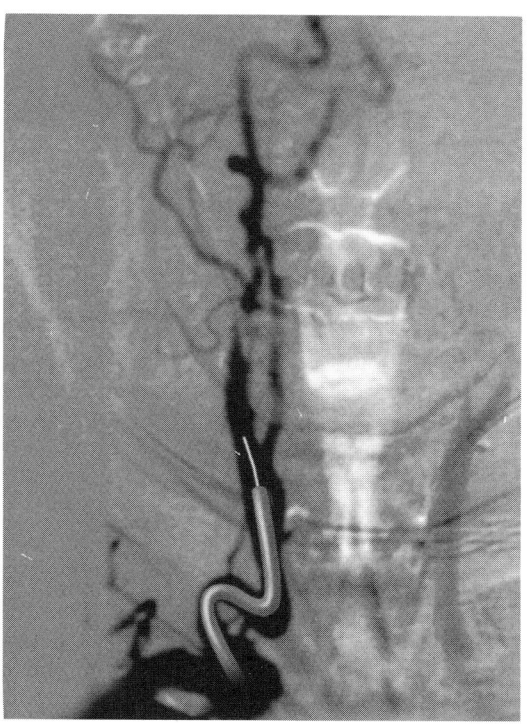

FIGURE 30–8. **A**, Arch angiogram showing marked kinking at the origin of the vessel. Such abnormal vessel takeoff from the arch can make stent passage difficult. **B**, The delivery catheter must traverse the tortuosity.

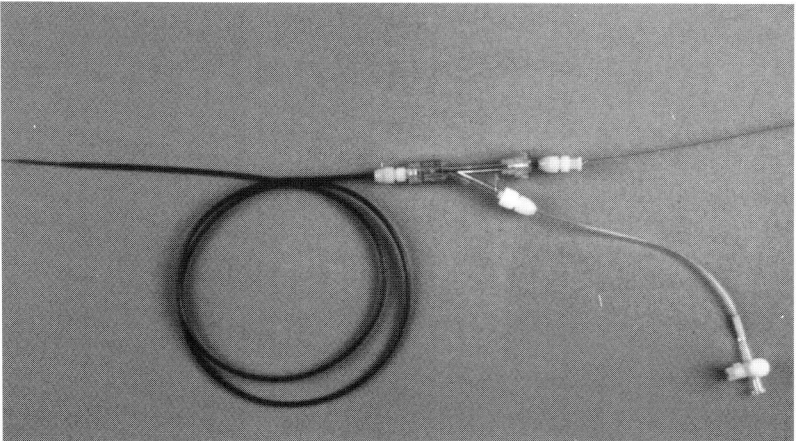

FIGURE 30–9. Flexor guiding sheath. This product has proved helpful for dealing with torturous and kinked arteries in the aortic arch.

groin hematoma; careful sheath removal and attention to the patient's coagulation status are preventive measures. Pseudoaneurysm and arteriovenous fistula are also potential complications but are relatively uncommon.

Clinical Results

The results of carotid angioplasty have been reviewed by several investigators,[11-13] and comprehensive comparison of carotid angioplasty and endarterectomy is forthcoming from the Carotid and Vertebral Artery Transluminal Angioplasty Study (CAVATAS).[14,15] CAVATAS is an international multicenter randomized trial aimed at determining the risks and benefits of carotid and vertebral artery transluminal angioplasty compared to those associated with surgery or medical treatment. Early results from the first 100 patients indicated there was no evidence of any difference in risk between angioplasty and carotid surgery.[14] A single-center update revealed that the procedural TIA rate has improved with experience, and the initial safety data compared favorably with published surgical series.[15] In another evaluation of angioplasty in 774 supraaortic artery lesions, the overall technical success rate was 95.3%; major and minor complication rates were 0.5% and 3.5%, respectively.[11] A more recent study suggested that among more than 500 patients undergoing carotid angioplasty there was zero mortality and 2.1% morbidity.[12] Use of the triple coaxial catheter for protection against embolization was studied in a different series ($n = 259$)[13]; and although dissection (5%) and embolic complications (8%) were seen in those treated without cerebral protection for atherosclerotic bifurcation lesions, no embolic complications were seen in patients in whom the coaxial catheter was used. Despite this published report, I have personal knowledge of complications resulting from the use of that particular protective device.

Our initial series in 110 symptomatic patients with 70% or more arteriographically defined carotid stenoses or ulcerative lesions allowed successful treatment of 109 patients with 129 stents.[16] One percutaneous procedure failed (0.9%) because the stent could not be deployed; the procedure was converted to carotid endarterectomy. The procedures were performed either via direct percutaneous access to the cervical common carotid artery or through a retrograde femoral artery approach. Minor complications included four cases of spasm (successfully treated with papaverine); one flow-limiting dissection (stented); and six access-site problems. There were seven strokes (two major, five reversible) (6.4%) and five minor transient events (4.5%) that resolved within 24 hours. Three procedures were converted to endarterectomy (2.7%) prior to discharge; one stroke patient expired (0.9%), and another patient died of an unrelated cardiac event in the hospital. During the 30-day postprocedural period, two ICA stents occluded (patients were asymptomatic). Clinical success at 30 days (no technical failure, death, endarterectomy, stroke, or occlusion) was 89.1% (98/110). Life-table analysis showed an 89% cumulative primary patency rate at 18 months.

Additional experience in 100 patients who underwent balloon angioplasty and a total of 157 stent placements in 110 extracranial internal/common carotid arteries has also been reported.[17] Following stent deployment, the mean baseline percent stenosis was reduced from $70 \pm 12\%$ to $3 \pm 16\%$. Five external carotid arteries required stenting. Procedures were successful in 97 of 100 patients. Inability to access the carotid artery transfemorally ($n = 2$) and suboptimal coverage of the dissection flap were the cause of the three failures. Complications included TIAs (three), minor strokes (six), major stroke (one), and death (one). The major stroke in this series occurred in a patient with severe mitral regurgitation and atrial fibrillation. The death resulted from a direct retrograde puncture of a carotid artery while the patient was under general anesthesia. There were no late neurologic events. Angiographic follow-up in 38 vessels indicated that there was one restenosis (2.6%). Deformation of a Palmaz stent was seen in eight vessels (21%).

A global view of carotid artery stent placement has been made by Wholey and Wholey in the International Carotid Stent Survey, which evaluated 2591 procedures worldwide. The overall technical success was 98.8%, and at 30 days complications included minor stroke (2.8%), major stroke (1.1%), and death (1.1%). The restenosis rate at 6 months was 2.9%.

Discussion

As the review of clinical results suggests, one of the greatest concerns about carotid angioplasty and stenting is the potential for cerebral embolization and neurologic complications. There are major differences in complication rates and postprocedural results, depending on the exact location of the intervention. For example, a stent placed at the origin of one of the great vessels emanating from the aortic arch, in our experience, is seldom associated with an embolic event. The lesions in this region are characteristically short and concentric and typically absent of loose atherosclerotic debris. The long-term results of stenting in these lesions have been excellent, with low rates of restenosis, intimal hyperplasia, or stent deformity. As with lesions at the level of the aortic arch, lesions in the high internal carotid are often smooth with an "hourglass" appearance and are frequently devoid of rough or fragmented atherosclerotic debris. Treatment of this type of lesion with angioplasty and stenting is unlikely to result in periprocedural embolization.

The potential for periprocedural embolization is greatest in lesions at the level of the carotid bifurcation. Loose atherosclerotic debris is frequently present in lesions at the bifurcation, and passing a wire and balloon and deploying a stent under these circumstances may dislodge it. Use of devices such as umbrellas, sieves, and strainers may allow the interventionist to retrieve and collect loose particulate matter released during the angioplasty procedure, but it seems likely that more sophisticated technology is required to ensure the safety of endoluminal procedures in the carotid bifurcation area.

Preventing complications is clearly preferable, and identification of lesions with potential for embolization via duplex scanning is under study.[18,19] At the Arizona Heart Institute and Heart Hospital, we routinely perform a duplex scan before angioplasty and stenting procedures. We have found that the duplex scan often reveals pathology that predisposes the patient to embolization, and we expect that further refinement of imaging techniques and equipment will continue to aid patient selection for endovascular therapy. Additional modification of stents and new covered stent designs (Figure 30–10) are certain to help limit the potential for embolization.

Other potential complications of carotid angioplasty and stenting include arterial spasm, dissection or occlusion, restenosis, and the inability to dilate a lesion. Indeed, dilation of a tight lesion may be difficult, and it is sometimes difficult even to pass a guidewire or place a balloon under these circumstances. Predilation with a small-diameter balloon with progressive advancement to the desired balloon size is an option in these cases. The internal and external carotid arteries are relatively resistant to spasm, but its consequences can be serious if ischemia results. A vasodilator, such as papaverine, should be used to treat spasm in these vessels. Dilation of the carotid lesion seldom results in dissection, but this is a potentially serious complication. Stenting, rather than angioplasty alone, may decrease the risk of dissection. Occlusion of the external carotid artery with angioplasty in patients in whom it is a significant source of collateral flow may have serious consequences. Simultaneous angioplasty of the ICA and external carotid artery avoids this problem.

At present, we have relatively short-term follow-up of endoluminal therapy that prohibits any definitive projection about the ultimate fate of carotid angioplasty and stenting. Restenosis has proven to be a major limitation of angioplasty and stenting in other vessels, but as yet there are no comprehensive studies of incidence in patients who have undergone carotid procedures. Among our first 100 patients treated with carotid stents at the Arizona Heart Institute, the incidence of restenosis and significant arterial hyperplasia on the stent has been low. The cervical carotid region is an area of high velocity blood flow, which may limit the potential for intimal hyperplasia and restenosis. Clearly, further study is necessary to determine long-term outcomes.

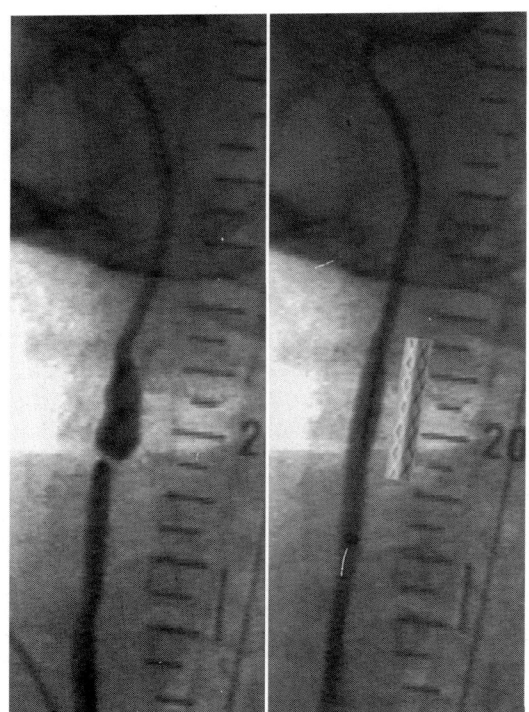
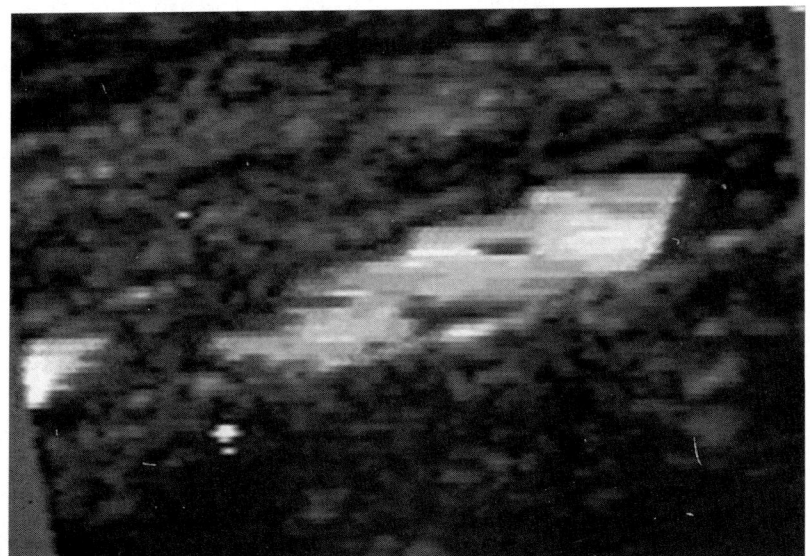

FIGURE 30–10. **A**, Angiogram before and after deployment of a covered stent in the carotid artery. **B**, Duplex scan 4 years later shows patency of the covered stent.

Conclusion

The successful carotid endovascular procedure has the potential to alleviate symptoms and reduce the risk of stroke without a cervical incision or general anesthesia. In addition, the length of hospitalization and recovery required after an endovascular procedure may be less than that associated with endarterectomy, although this has yet to be proven. The technical success of the endovascular procedure depends on careful patient selection, the optimal choice of access, and the skill and experience of the operator. The retrograde femoral approach is generally preferred but may have some limitations due to the configuration of the aortic arch vessels in certain patients. When direct puncture of the carotid artery is required, an open technique may be preferable to reduce periprocedural complications.

Although experience with carotid endovascular intervention is relatively recent, it has already become evident that some anatomic locations within the region are more amenable to endovascular treatment than others. Neurologic event rates may be unacceptably high in endovascular treatment of complicated bifurcation disease. However, the results of stenting in aortic arch lesions, high ICA lesions, and restenotic lesions in patients with damage from radical neck dissection or irradiation indicate that endovascular surgery is likely to advance rapidly as the therapy of choice for these interventions. As improvements in imaging equipment and techniques further our ability to identify lesions that have high and low potential for embolization, we may be able to screen and select patients whose lesions are most suited to endovascular intervention. It seems likely that, in carefully selected patients, these procedures represent a viable treatment alternative to carotid endarterectomy.

References

1. Whisnant JP, Wiebers DO: Clinical epidemiology of transient cerebral ischemic attacks on the anterior and posterior circulation. In: Sundt TM Jr, editor: *Occlusive cerebrovascular disease: diagnosis and surgical management*, Philadelphia, 1987, Saunders, pp 60–65.
2. Dennis M, Bamford J, Sandercock P et al: Prognosis of transient ischemic attacks in the Oxfordshire Community Stroke Project, *Stroke* 21:848–853, 1990.
3. Zarins CK: Carotid endarterectomy: the gold standard, *J Endovasc Surg* 3:10–15, 1996.
4. Gagne PJ, Riles TS, Jacobowitz GR et al: Long-term follow-up of patients undergoing reoperation for recurrent carotid artery disease, *J Vasc Surg* 18:991–1001, 1993.
5. Carbello RE, Towne JB, Seabrook GR et al: An outcome analysis of carotid endarterectomy: the incidence and natural history of recurrent stenosis, *J Vasc Surg* 23:749–754, 1996.
6. Mansour MA, Kang SS, Baker WH et al: Carotid endarterectomy for recurrent stenosis, *J Vasc Surg* 25:877–883, 1997.
7. Raithel D: Recurrent carotid disease: optimum technique for redo surgery, *J Endovasc Surg* 3:69–75, 1996.
8. Kharrazi MR: Anesthesia for carotid stent procedures, *J Endovasc Surg* 3:211–216, 1996.
9. Bergeron P, Chamabran P, Benichou H et al: Recurrent carotid disease: will stents be an alternative to surgery? *J Endovasc Surg* 3:76–79, 1996.
10. Alessandri C, Bergeron P: Local anesthesia in carotid angioplasty, *J Endovasc Surg* 3:31–34, 1996.
11. Kachel R, Basche S, Heerklotz I et al: Percutaneous transluminal angioplasty of supra-aortic arteries, especially the internal carotid artery, *Neuroradiology* 33:191–194, 1991.
12. Kachel R: Results of balloon angioplasty in the carotid arteries, *J Endovasc Surg* 3:22–30, 1996.
13. Theron J: Angioplastie carotidienne protegee et stents carotidiens, *J Mal Vasc* 21(suppl A):113–122, 1996.
14. Gaines P: The European carotid angioplasty trial [abstract], *J Endovasc Surg* 3:107, 1996.
15. Gaines PA: Carotid angioplasty and CAVATAS update [abstract], *J Endovasc Surg* 4(suppl I):12, 1997.
16. Diethrich EB, Ndiaye M, Reid DB: Stenting in the carotid artery: initial experience in 110 patients, *J Endovasc Surg* 3:42–62, 1996.
17. Iyer SS, Roubin G, Yadav S et al: Elective carotid stenting [abstract], *J Endovasc Surg* 3:105–106, 1996.
18. El-Barghouty N, Geroulakos G, Nicolaides A et al: Computer-assisted carotid plaque characterization, *Eur J Vasc Endovasc Surg* 9:389–393, 1995.
19. El-Barghouty N, Nicolaides A, Tegos T et al: The relative effect of carotid plaque heterogeneity and echogenicity on ipsilateral cerebral infarction and symptoms of cerebrovascular disease, *Int Angiol* 15:300–306, 1996.

31
Complications and Troubleshooting

Frank J. Criado, Omran Abul-Khoudoud, and Eric Wellons

Endovascular intervention is fundamentally and unequivocally different from "cut-and-sew" conventional surgery. Conceptually, this difference can be best characterized by recognizing the two hallmarks of percutaneous intraluminal therapy: remote catheter-mediated actions and indirect visualization. From a practical standpoint, this requires an enabling environment (workshop) and special instruments and tools designed for percutaneous transluminal application, as well as a different mindset on the part of the operator. It is, in a word, *nonsurgical* in nature. From conceptualization to bioskills, instrumentation and technical strategies, catheter-based interventional therapy has a distinct personality and an entirely unique set of needs in the three fundamental areas of *workshop*, *instrumentation*, and *operator skills*.[1]

Most complications associated with an endovascular intervention are related to poor case selection or suboptimal technical performance. As such, they are largely *preventable*.[2] Technical complications only are discussed in this chapter, as case selection strategies are covered in other areas of the book.

Surgeons often struggle to contain the impulse to "react surgically" when faced with technical difficulties. This is not helpful and often makes a bad situation worse. Instead of wider exposure, a longer incision, more forceful retraction, or an extra suture, the *endovascular attitude* should focus instead on patience, finesse, thoughtful catheter/wire selection, restrained physical motion, and a better angle of visualization. They represent the most common sources of potential complications: poor conceptualization and inadequate *"endo-habits."*

Complications Related to Inadequate Endo-habits

The following is a list of the most common factors that can negatively affect the results of endovascular interventions.

1. *Failure to visualize.* Losing guidewire access is the most common consequence[3]; others include percutaneous arterial access problems and vessel dissection or perforation. *Prevention/troubleshooting*: Fluoroscopic visualization and guidance are *mandatory* whenever wires, catheters, and other devices are being introduced and advanced transluminally. Instead of the surgical routine of keeping one's eyes on the field, the eyes must focus on the fluoroscopy monitor instead (Figure 31–1).

2. *Inefficient/wasteful use of fluoroscopy.* This leads to unnecessary radiation exposure (patient and team) and overheating of the x-ray unit. *Prevention/troubleshooting*: Use fluoroscopy only when real-time visualization is necessary. *There must be a perfect coordination between the eyes on the monitor and the foot on the pedal.*

3. *Failure to act interventionally.* Surgeons tend to resort to a surgical approach for access difficulty or technical complications without first examining the available options for cor-

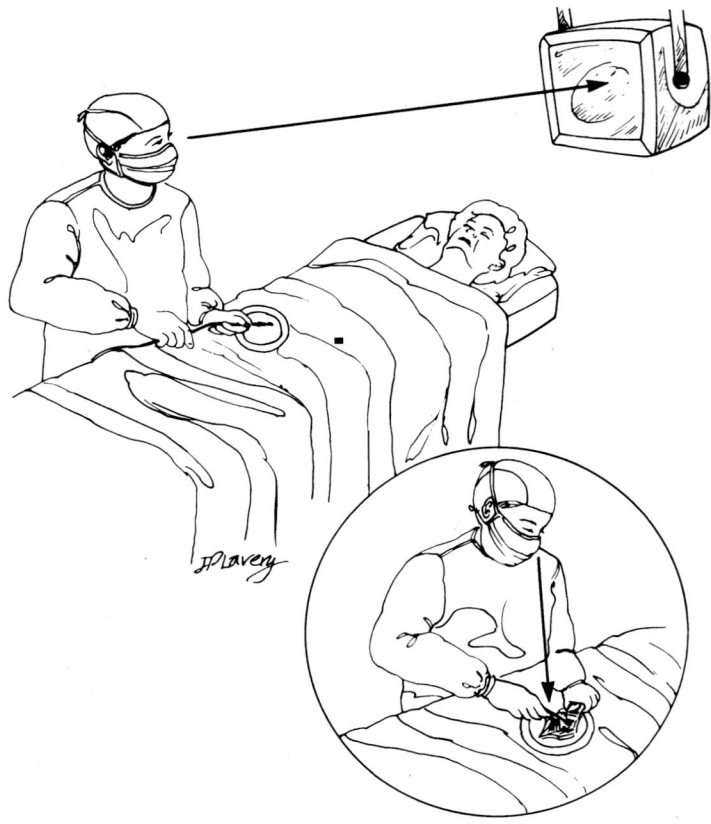

FIGURE 31-1. Unlike conventional surgery (**bottom**), endovascular intervention requires indirect visualization through fluoroscopy. The operator must develop the habit of watching and guiding the catheter and wire motions on the fluoroscopy monitor where real-time visualization is displayed (**top**). Although the concept is clear and simple, this fundamental endo-habit is not an easy one for beginner endovascular surgeons to develop.

rection and troubleshooting. In truth, situations that require open surgical repair are rare. Most difficulties can be resolved through a change in strategy or a different device selection and can almost always be addressed interventionally (nonsurgically).[2,4] *Prevention/troubleshooting*: There is no substitute for adequate training and properly supervised initial endovascular experience. Proctoring in a preceptorship setting may also be helpful to the beginner interventionist who has not yet acquired refined interventional skills and has only partial knowledge of the potential device, imaging, and technical options available.

Access-Related Complications

Percutaneous vascular access and catheterization techniques are the Achilles' heel of endovascular surgeons' learning experience.[5]

Femoral Puncture

1. (a) *High, suprainguinal puncture* should be avoided because it is associated with increased risk of retroperitoneal hemorrhage and pseudoaneurysm formation related to ineffective external compression of the puncture site caused by mechanical interference from the overlying inguinal ligament.[6,7] (b) *Low puncture* (proximal superficial femoral artery, SFA) likewise has been reported to be associated with a higher than expected complication rate.[8] This contradicts, at least in part, the author's experience, which has demonstrated that puncture of the proximal SFA is well tolerated. *Preven-tion/troubleshooting*: The target area defined by Rupp et al.[9] is most useful to ensure infrainguinal puncture of the common femoral artery (Figure 31-2). This information should also prove helpful in the case of diminished or absent femoral pulse. The groin crease is, gen-

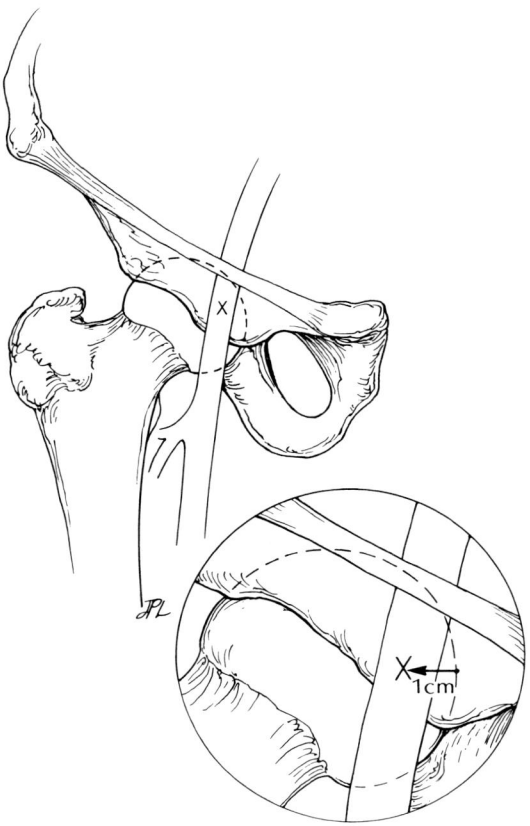

FIGURE 31–2. Infrainguinal puncture of the common femoral artery is facilitated by the recommendation of Rupp et al.[9] The target area is 1 cm lateral to the most medial cortex of the femoral head as seen fluoroscopically. In most individuals it locates the mid common femoral artery approximately 1.5 cm below the inguinal ligament.

erally speaking, a poor marker of the position of the inguinal ligament.

2. *Angle of puncture* should be 30° to 45° (Figure 31–3). Steeper angles may lead to significant bending of the access pathway between the skin and the arterial lumen resulting in angulation of the introducer sheath. Likewise, obese individuals present a significant risk for this type of mechanical mishap as tissue layer shifts results in an S-shaped deformity of the access catheter (Figure 31–4), impeding frictionless passage of rigid devices; balloon-mounted stents are especially prone to motion and dislodgement when passed across severe angulations (Figure 31–4b). *Prevention/ troubleshooting*: Puncture angles of more than 45° must be avoided (Figure 31–3). In case of obesity and excess tissue layer mobility, use of a superstiff guidewire prevents (or corrects) such angulations and permits creation of a smooth, gently curved access pathway (Figure 31–4c). Similarly, densely scarred groins may present the same challenges; here too the routine use of a superstiff guidewire is strongly recommended. Fluoroscopic visualization of the access site should be part of the operator's endo-habit whenever introduction of catheters and devices is met with any degree of resistance.

3. *Femoral bifurcation anatomy* can be easily defined during antegrade puncture by injecting contrast material through the needle prior to the introduction of guidewires and catheters.[2] This simple maneuver (Figure 31–5) immediately reveals whether the artery has been entered at the desired location and may provide the information needed to initiate corrective maneuvers. *Prevention/troubleshooting*: The "test dye injection," described elsewhere,[10] constitutes an excellent endo-habit that effectively facilitates an-tegrade femoral access and prevents sheath misplacement into the profunda femoris artery.[10]

4. *Choice of puncture needle.* (a) The *single-wall needle* is preferred by most; its beveled

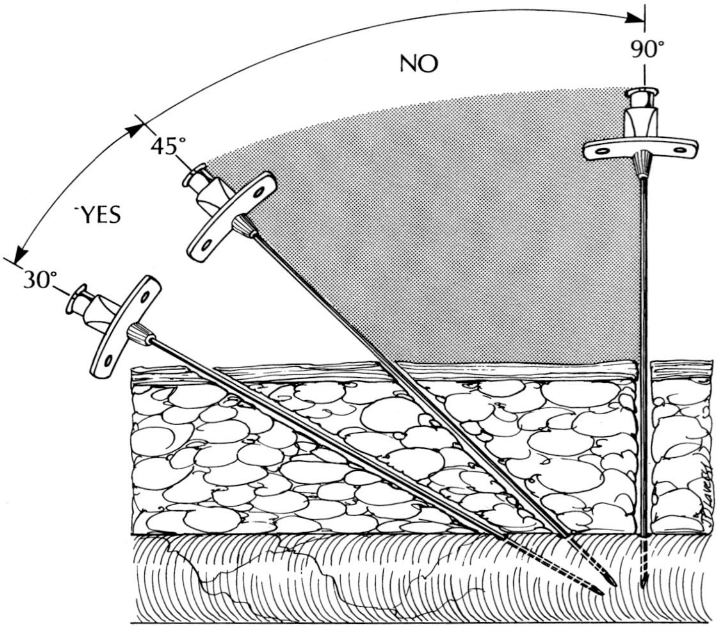

FIGURE 31–3. Proper puncture angle is 30° to 45°.

leading point is advanced toward the vessel, finding the lumen "on the way in" (Figure 31–6a). A 0.035-inch entry guidewire is then passed through the needle after obtaining pulsatile blood return from the hub; once again, a small "puff" of contrast should be injected to ascertain a free intraluminal position if it is in doubt because of the poor quality of blood return or a difficult wire introduction. The latter, in particular, represents the most important potential disadvantage of this type of needle as the long bevel on the end of the needle can be partially within the vessel wall while still obtaining adequate pulsatile blood flow (Figure 31–7). Needless to say, this can lead to subintimal dissection of the punctured vessel. The second potential risk relates to possible peeling off of the wire's plastic or hydrophilic coating by the sharp needle point.[11,12] It is therefore advisable to use coating-free steel guidewires for initial entry after puncture with a single-wall needle. *Prevention/troubleshooting*: Subintimal dissection is suspected whenever smooth and easy introduction of the wire is impaired and, in particular, when the guidewire can be seen (fluoroscopically) curling or stopping a short distance after emerging from the needle (Figure 31–7). Such findings require that the wire be removed and the needle position determined precisely by contrast injection. In all likelihood, a new puncture is then necessary. As described above, a coating-free steel guidewire should be selected for initial access through a single-wall puncture needle. (b) The *double-wall needle* (Figure 31–6b) continues to be used by some interventionists. It has a blunt tip and contains an inner beveled stylet that constitutes the leading point. Transfixing puncture of the vessel is followed by removal of the stylet and then gradual withdrawal of the needle until luminal entry is signaled by pulsatile blood return (Figure 31–6). This needle was designed to secure the intraluminal position with little or no risk of subintimal dissection (see above). Its principal risk is potential bleeding caused by the creation of a small ("unplugged") hole in the back wall of the artery. *Prevention/ troubleshooting*: Bleeding from the hole in the back wall is a potential concern in essentially three situations only: when thrombolysis is anticipated (or considered to be likely), puncture of a synthetic vascular graft, one of polytetrafluoroethylene (PTFE) in particular, and obviously during the course of direct puncturing after cutdown and surgical vessel dissection. All these situations require a single-wall (not double-wall) puncture technique.

5. *Open cutdown approach* is not necessary (or justifiable) for most endovascular inter-

ventions. Contrary to "conventional surgical wisdom," a femoral cutdown is not "totally benign" as it carries a potential for subsequent morbidity in up to 3% to 5% of instances.[5] It is, additionally, poorly accepted by patients and referring physicians alike. *Prevention/ troubleshooting*: Surgical cutdown must be viewed as a valuable but rarely necessary access option. It should be reserved for well defined situations, three in particular: (1) use of high-profile devices larger than 12F to 14F; (2) planned combined endoluminal/reconstructive procedures[10]; and (3) within 4 weeks of surgical exposure/vessel dissection in the same area. Errors in conceptualization and poor catheter/access skills cannot be used as justification for not practicing *percutaneous* intervention in most cases.

6. *Use of an introducer sheath* following arterial puncture and guidewire insertion is a common denominator to all endovascular interventions, both diagnostic and therapeutic. It secures and maintains intraluminal access and establishes a direct pathway to the vascular system for safe, rapid catheter exchanges,

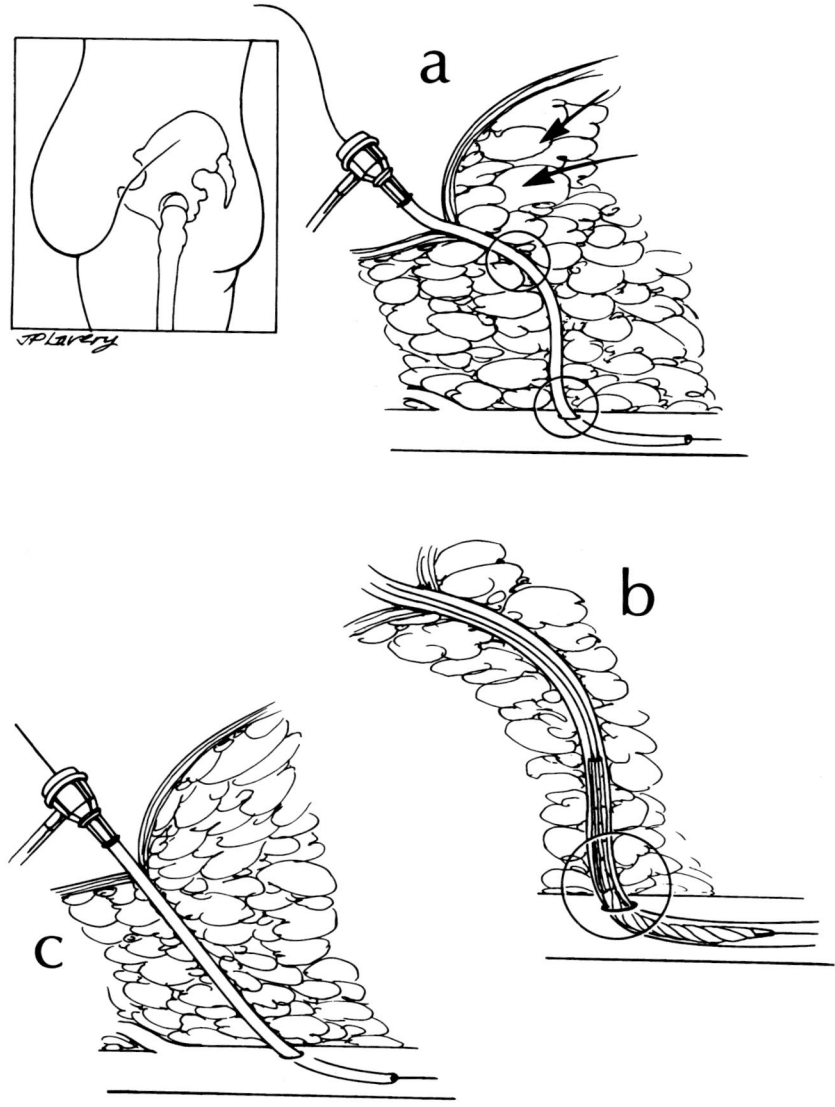

FIGURE 31–4. Potential S-shaped angulation of femoral access pathway in obese patients (**a**). Balloon-mounted stents may be dislodged by passage through deformed access catheters due to excessive friction (**b**). Use of a superstiff guidewire can easily prevent this problem (**c**).

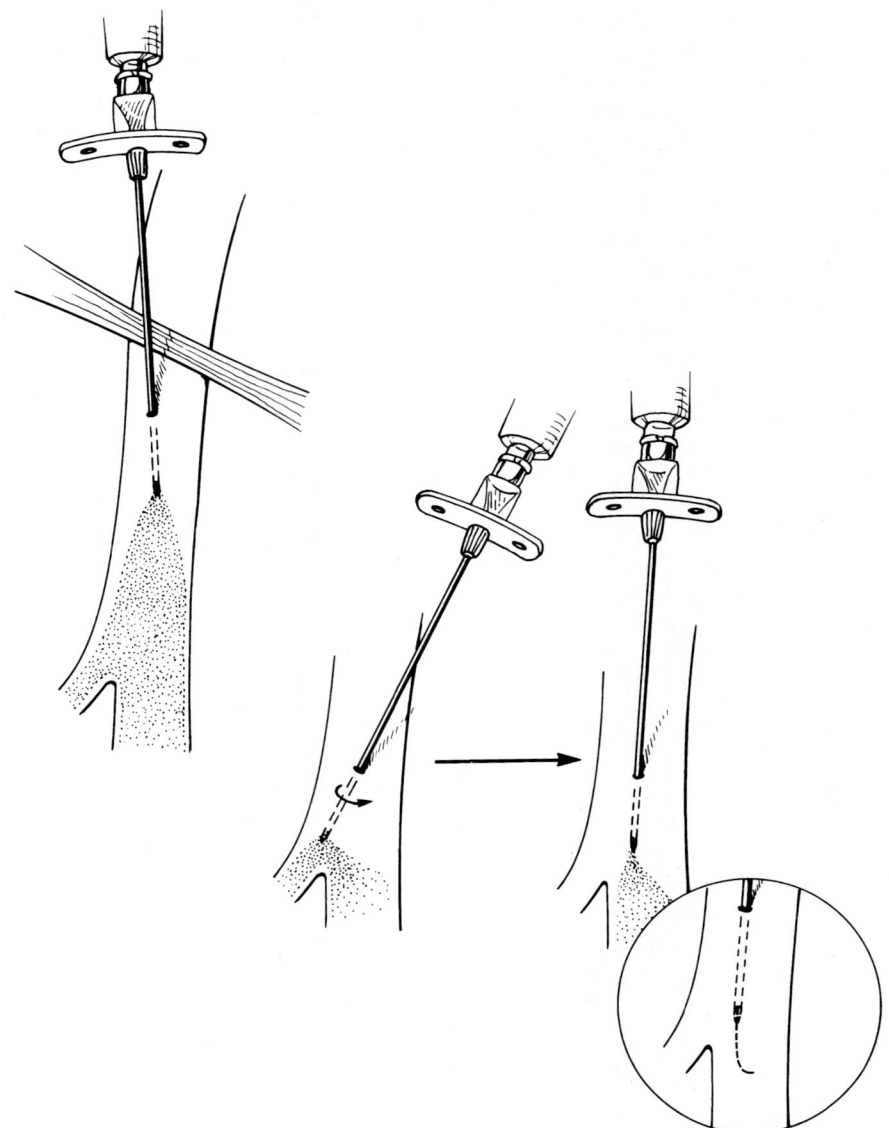

FIGURE 31–5. Injection of contrast by attaching a 10-cc syringe to the hub of the 18-gauge puncture needle clearly reveals the anatomy of the femoral bifurcation and site of puncture during antegrade puncture. At times the needle can be maneuvered, under fluoroscopy, from the profunda to the superficial femoral artery (**middle, right**), and the guidewire can be directed along the desired pathway (**inset**). If, on the other hand, the puncture is in the profunda well beyond the bifurcation, the needle should be removed and a new higher puncture attempted after applying pressure to the puncture site to ensure hemostasis.

contrast injections, and the administration of heparin and other pharmacologic agents. *It has enormous advantages, with only limited disadvantage.*[2] *Prevention/troubleshooting*: A 5F sheath is placed initially during most interventions. It can be later exchanged for a larger introducer depending on the ultimate requirements of the chosen therapeutic strategy and device. (1) *The length of the sheath* is an important consideration; we find ourselves using long 23- to 35-cm radiopaque-tipped sheaths increasingly during transfemoral and trans-

31. Complications and Troubleshooting

FIGURE 31–6. **a**, Arterial puncture with a single-wall needle. **b**, Sequential technique with a double-wall needle.

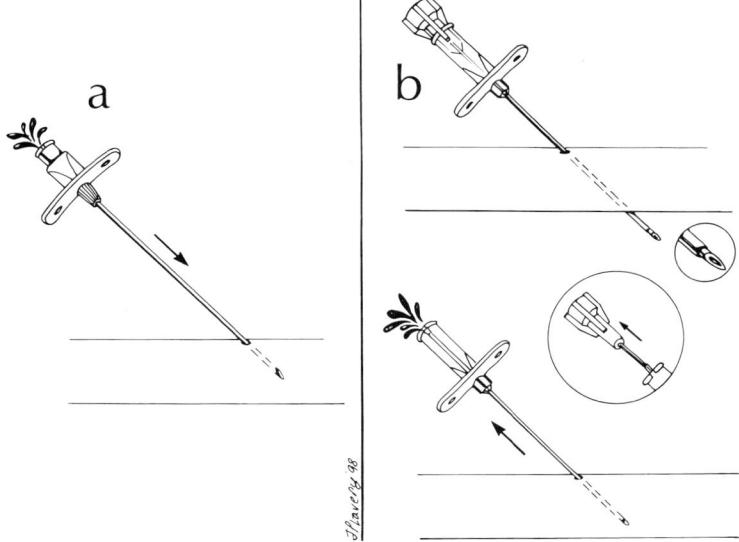

brachial endoarterial procedures (Figure 31–8). They facilitate angiography, guidewire exchanges, deployment of balloon-expandable stents, and contralateral aortoiliac interventions. (2) *Contralateral access* (Figure 31–9) has been optimized by the availability of long, flexible sheaths with radiopaque tips. Important principles include (a) the need for guidewire access first (the wire must be advanced down to the level of the inguinal ligament as a minimum to obtain enough support across the bifurcation; (b) use of, or exchange for, a wire stiff enough to support advancement of the sheath across the aortic bifurcation (without buckling up into the aortic lumen); (c) careful assessment of sheath curvature at the bifurcation: if a tight curve persists, adjustment of device choice (flexible stent or short rigid Palmaz stent) should follow.

7. *Puncture-site complications* are mostly hemorrhagic in nature and largely related to inadequate technique used for initial access and faulty or untimely sheath removal and external compression.[3,13] Haparin utilization and body habitus (obesity) are also influential. *Prevention/troubleshooting*: (1) *Level of puncture* is critical; suprainguinal punctures must be avoided (as previously discussed, Figure 31–2). (2) A smooth angle and access pathway are paramount: proper puncture technique and use of a stiff wire as necessary address these concerns appropriately. (3) The *"difficult groin"* (obesity, scars) requires use of a stiff guidewire (Figure 31–4) and careful fluoroscopic visualization as rigid devices are passed. (4) Heparin utilization should be judicious; only small doses (2000 to 3000 units) are necessary for most

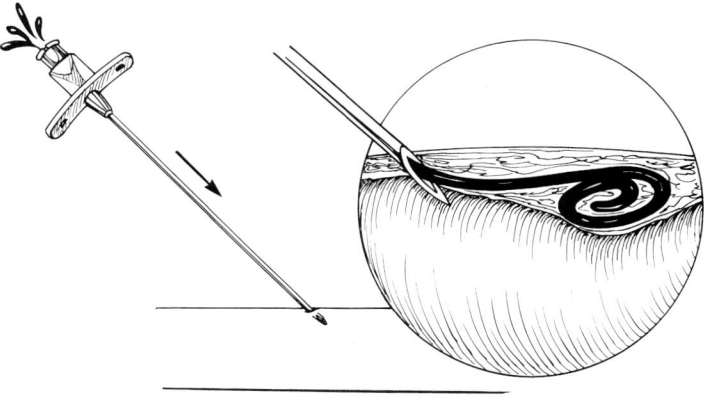

FIGURE 31–7. Mechanism of subintimal dissection as entry guidewire is passed into the arterial wall when the long bevel of the single-wall needle is only partially intraluminal.

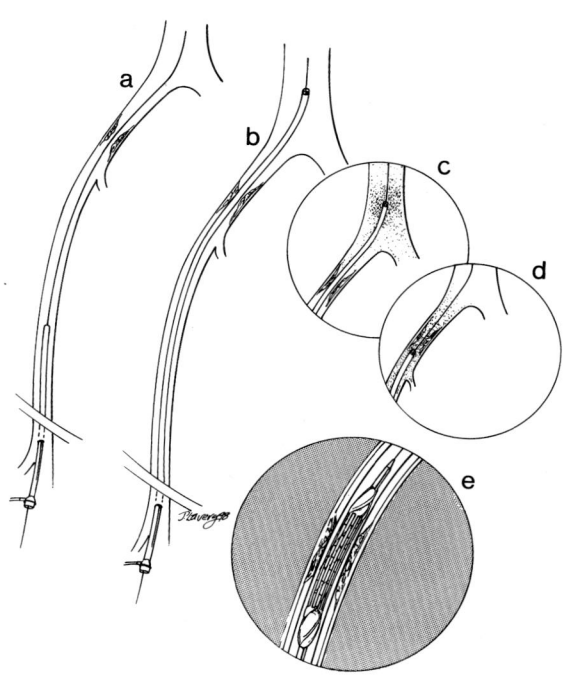

FIGURE 31–8. **a,b,** Use of a long introducer sheath with a radiopaque tip can be helpful, as it facilitates retrograde angiography (**c,d**) and provides a protective conduit for placement of balloon-expandable stents (**e**).

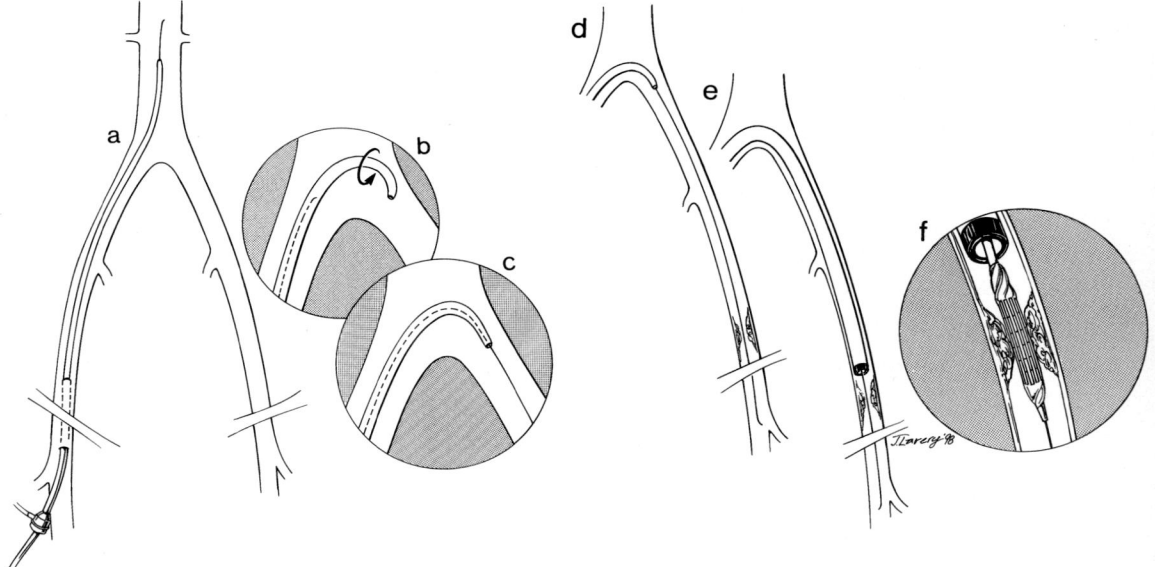

FIGURE 31–9. **a,b,** Crossover contralateral iliac access is achieved with a preshaped curved catheter. The guidewire is then advanced antegrade down the contralateral iliac (**c**) to the level of the inguinal ligament or beyond (**d**) to provide best support for catheter and device tracking across the bifurcation. A bright-tip flexible sheath or similar is then passed over the guidewire to facilitate stent deployment (**f**) and other interventions. Additionally, the sheath provides easy access for contrast injections.

simple interventions.[14] Monitoring the activated clotting time (ACT) is important when full anticoagulation has been induced, with sheath removal performed only after the ACT has decreased to 180 seconds or less. (5) Sheath removal/groin compression is a critical component of every endovascular procedure. It must be performed by a motivated, experienced team member. (6) Percutaneous sealing devices are now available but remain nonstandard.[13] We are favorably impressed by the performance of the Vaso-Seal collagen extravascular plug technique and have adopted it nearly routinely for most outpatient percutaneous endovascular interventions involving retrograde femoral puncture: Patients can usually ambulate and be discharged home within 1 hour.

Axillary-Brachial Access Techniques

These techniques are frequently performed for diagnostic and therapeutic vascular interventions. Significant complications with serious potential can occur.[3,13] Nevertheless, it is a useful vascular access route for a variety of situations involving visceral/renal, brachiocephalic, and lower extremity vascular disease. *Prevention/troubleshooting*: Use of the left arm is preferred whenever possible to minimize the risk of cerebrovascular complications, as it avoids, in most individuals, crossing the vessels and flow path to both carotid arteries and one vertebral artery. We frequently use access "from the top" and have found puncture of the left brachial artery at the upper margin of the antecubital fossa to be technically simple and quite safe. Introducer sheaths 5F to 7F are well tolerated, and hemostasis upon completion is facilitated by the superficial and relatively fixed position of the brachial artery in this area, making it amenable to secure compression against the humerus. A "micropuncture kit" (Cook, Bloomington, IN) is used for brachial artery puncture. As a new technical option, we are now exploring the usefulness and safety of percutaneous catheterization of the radial artery at the wrist for some diagnostic studies. Puncture of the axillary artery is accompanied by a 2% to 3% incidence of axillary sheath hematoma significant enough to cause neurologic compromise.[13] Prompt recognition and surgical decompression offer the only hope of nerve function recovery. Our strong view is that brachial artery puncture (as described) is far safer and technically simpler. We *virtually never* perform percutaneous puncture of the axillary artery on the basis of such considerations.

Imaging-Related Complications

Fluoroscopic imaging and guidance are essential components of endovascular intervention. A complete discussion of radiographic equipment and techniques is well beyond the scope of this chapter, but three relevant aspects, leading potentially to technical error and complication, deserve to be described briefly.

1. *Poor image quality* can derive from a number of factors, including the capabilities and resolution powers of the equipment itself. A few important aspects are under one's control: (a) *Avoidance of motion* is important, particularly when using digital subtraction angiography and road mapping. The anatomic area of visualization and anesthetic technique may have a profound influence on the ability to minimize motion artifacts. (b) *Failure to obtain more than one view* is a significant source of misdiagnosis, especially in areas of arterial bifurcation and those overlying bony structures. One or more oblique views are often revealing during diagnostic studies and interventional procedures. The iliac arteries and femoral and carotid bifurcations are some of the most notorious examples where this principle applies.

2. *Parallax* is a principle that every interventionist would do well to understand. It is conditioned by the fact that x-ray tubes emit cone-shaped radiation (Figure 31–10). Vascular segments can "change position" relative to radiopaque markers that are not in the same plane (i.e., ruler on the table behind the patient). Additionally, only targets that are perfectly centered in the fluoroscopic image can be accurately referenced to such landmarks. Disregard for such potential error can have serious consequences during the course of stenting procedures, particularly endoluminal grafting for abdominal aortic aneurysms.

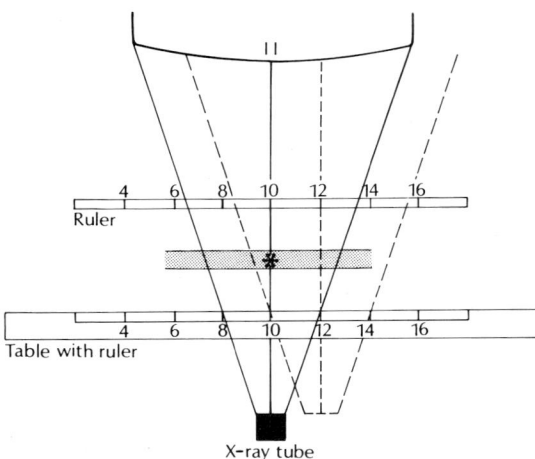

FIGURE 31-10. Parallax concept. It is related to the fact that x-ray tubes emit cone-shaped radiation. Vascular targets can "change position" relative to markers that are not in the same plane (i.e., ruler on the table under the patient or on the patient).

3. *Magnification* of vascular images is partly related to the cone-shaped radiation described above and constitutes another source of potential misadventure. Approximately 20% magnification is consistently seen with cut-film radiography; digital subtraction angiography is far less predictable, as the magnification varies with the choice of image intensifier size and distance from the patient. Unfortunately, radiopaque rulers on or behind the body yield, respectively, reduced or amplified measurements as they are in a different plane from the target structure. Accurate angiographic measurements of vascular length and diameter can only be obtained using an intraluminal reference standard such as a graduated ("measuring") guidewire or catheter.

On balance, it is within the interventionist's purview to minimize the complications of endovascular therapy. Even when they do occur, one still has available devices and techniques ("toolbox") that provide a good opportunity for percutaneous catheter-based troubleshooting and successful correction. Surgical repair is only rarely necessary. Such capability is attainable only through a sound conceptual foundation, hands-on endovascular training, and sufficient ongoing experience.

References

1. Criado FJ: The surgeon as an endovascular interventionist: why and how? *J Cardiovasc Surg* 37(suppl 1):17–25, 1996.
2. Criado FJ, Clark NS, Twena M et al: Common technical complications in endovascular surgery: prevention strategies. In: *SVS/ISCVS handbook on endovascular procedures*, 1997, pp 184–191.
3. Kinney EV, Fogarty TJ, Newman CE: Catheter skills. In White RA, Fogarty TJ, editors: *Peripheral endovascular interventions*, St Louis, 1996, pp 235–247.
4. Criado FJ: On becoming an endovascular surgeon [editorial], *J Endovasc Surg* 3:140–145, 1996.
5. Criado FJ, Twena M, Halsted M et al: Percutaneous femoral puncture for endovascular treatment of occlusive arterial lesions, *Am J Surg* 176:119–121, 1998.
6. Hessel SJ, Adams DS, Avrams HL: Complications of angiography, *Radiology* 138:273–281, 1991.
7. Illescas FF, Baker ME, McCann et al: CT evaluation of retroperitoneal hemorrhage associated with femoral arteriography, *AJR* 146:1289–1292, 1996.
8. Altin RS, Flicker S, Naidech HJ: Pseudoaneurysm and arteriovenous fistula after femoral artery catheterization: association with lower femoral punctures, *AJR* 152:629–631, 1989.
9. Rupp SB, Vogelzang RL, Nemcek AA et al: Relationship of the inguinal ligament to pelvic radiographic landmarks: anatomic correlation and its role in femoral arteriography, *J Vasc Intervent Radiol* 4:409–413, 1993.
10. Criado FJ, Queral LA, Patten P: Transluminal re-canalization, angioplasty and stenting in endovascular surgery: techniques and applications. In Greenhalgh RM, editor: *Vascular and endovascular surgical techniques*, London, 1994, Saunders, pp 49–70.
11. Kim JK, Kang HK: Percutaneous retrieval of the peeled-off plastic coating from a guide wire [letter], *J Vasc Intervent Radiol* 5:657–658, 1994.
12. Reagan K, Matsumoto AH, Teitelbaum GP: Comparison of the hydrophilic guidewire in double-and single-wall entry: potential hazards, *Cathet Cardiovasc Diagn* 24:205–208, 1991.
13. Hodgson KJ, Mattos MA, Sumner DS: Access to the vascular system for endovascular procedures: techniques and indications for percutaneous and open arteriotomy approaches, *Semin Vasc Surg* 10:206–221, 1997.
14. Criado FJ, Twena M, Abul-Khoudoud O et al: Outpatient endovascular intervention: is it safe? *J Endovasc Surg* 5:236–239, 1998.

32
Thrombolysis: Peripheral Arterial Applications

Carlos E. Donayre and Kenneth Ouriel

Vascular surgeons have been able to perform complex revascularization procedures by relying on pharmacologic advances. The discovery of heparin by Jay McLean made this possible. The ability to dissolve occluding thrombus by activating the thrombolytic system with a variety of agents is currently being pursued to reestablish blood flow to an ischemic vascular bed, with the hope of achieving greater long-term clinical success and lower operative mortality.

Catheter-based techniques for thrombus removal remain limited to relatively large vessels. Thrombolytic agents offer the potential of clearing thrombus in small, catheter-inaccessible vessels along with preservation of the vascular endothelium. They are being used as first-line agents for acute thrombotic and embolic occlusions, as well as adjuncts to standard mechanical embolectomy. However, clinical indications, patient selection, and long-term success are still being defined.

Thrombolytic Agents

Streptokinase

Streptokinase is a single-chain nonenzymatic glycoprotein with a molecular weight of 45,000 to 50,000 daltons (D) that is produced by beta-hemolytic streptococci.[1] Discovered by Tillet and Garner in 1933,[2] it was also the first thrombolytic agent to be used clinically, when it was injected by Tillet and Sherry[3] into the pleural space of patients suffering from postpneumonic and chronic empyemas to lyse clotted blood and fibrin.

Its mechanism of action is through an indirect activation of plasminogen via the formation of an equimolar streptokinase-plasminogen activator complex. This complex then converts both free plasminogen and the plasminogen within the activator complex to plasmin, which cleaves fibrin and fibrinogen. Streptokinase is not clot-specific; it causes breakdown of both circulating and clot-bound fibrinogen. Since streptokinase requires plasminogen as a cofactor and a substrate, plasminogen is depleted by this two-stage process more than any other thrombolytic agent. The metabolism and excretion of streptokinase is unclear because its clearance rate depends on a variety of factors. The intricacy of these interactions is manifested in vivo by two half-lives that have been identified for streptokinase. The first is 18 minutes and represents neutralization by circulating antistreptococcal antibodies and inhibitors.[4] The second half-life is approximately 83 minutes, when the remaining drug combines with circulating plasminogen to form the activator complex.

Because streptokinase is not produced by human tissue, it can induce the production of antibodies that can cause fever and both minor and severe anaphylactic reactions. Early clinical experience was hampered by an assortment of these responses, but manufacturers have been able to purify this compound, with febrile and allergic reactions seen now in less than 3%

of treated patients.[5] This incidence can be further lowered by using prophylactic measures such as pretreatment with antihistamines or corticosteroids.

The antigenic property of streptokinase is also responsible for the formation of binding, neutralizing antibodies, which reach peak titers in 7 to 10 days. Streptokinase antibody titers remain elevated for about 3 months before declining to baseline in about 6 months.[6] Large loading doses of streptokinase need to be used to overcome baseline titers of these neutralizing antibodies, and other thrombolytic agents should be considered when dealing with patients recently treated with streptokinase.

Urokinase

The high incidence of allergic reactions to the early streptokinase preparations led to a search for the presence of nonantigenic thrombolytic agents in the human body. MacFarlane and Pilling were the first to describe the presence of fibrinolytic activity in urine in 1947.[7] Williams[8] and Astrup[9] independently identified a plasminogen activator in urine 4 years later; this new agent was named urokinase by Sobel[10] in 1952.

Urokinase is a trypsin-like serine protease composed of two polypeptide chains with a molecular weight of 20,000 and 34,000 D. The light chain contains 158 amino acids and is connected to a 253-amino-acid heavy chain by means of a disulfide bond, which is required for enzymatic activity.[11] Urokinase directly activates plasminogen by cleaving its Arg_{560}-Val_{561} bond. After intravenous administration, urokinase has a half-life of approximately 15 minutes, it undergoes rapid hepatic clearance, and only 3% to 5% is cleared by the kidney.

Normal human urine contains only few micrograms of urokinase; about 1500 liters of urine are required to produce enough agent to treat a single patient.[12] Larger quantities of urokinase can be produced by synthetic methods using fetal kidney cell cultures. Recombinant deoxyribonucleic acid (DNA) techniques with *E. coli* have been used to produce this agent.[13] All of these forms of urokinase are biochemically similar and capable of producing a fibrinolytic state.

Clinical results with urokinase compare well with streptokinase, but the incidence of bleeding complications seems to be lower.[14,15] Urokinase direct plasminogen activation, rather than the formation of an intermediate activator complex seen with streptokinase, results in a lower depletion of plasminogen. Unlike streptokinase, urokinase inhibitors in plasma are relatively constant and allow for the use of fixed therapeutic dosages. Thus the reduced incidence of plasminemia and the ability to induce a more predictable fibrinolytic state may account for the decreased rate of bleeding complications seen with urokinase. Furthermore, urokinase is nonantigenic and nonpyrogenic, and severe anaphylactic reactions are rarely seen after its administration. Urokinase is more expensive to use when compared with streptokinase; but when the cost of complications are factored in, both agents are comparable in price.

Tissue Plasminogen Activator

Natural tissue plasminogen activator (t-PA) is a serine protease composed of a single polypeptide chain of 562 amino acids with a molecular weight of 63,000 to 65,000 D resulting from a heterogeneity of glycosylation patterns.[16] The human t-PA is endogenously synthesized and secreted by vascular endothelial cells under regulation of a gene located on chromosome 8.[17] t-PA can be obtained in large quantities from the Bowes melanoma cell line and by using recombinant DNA technology. The recombinant molecule (rt-PA) is 527 amino acids long and differs from the naturally occurring molecule only with respect to its spatial arrangement.

t-PA, just like urokinase, directly activates plasminogen by cleaving its Arg_{560}-Val_{561} peptide bond and converting it to plasmin. Its main advantage is its high affinity for thrombus-bound fibrin. In addition, when t-PA and plasminogen are both bound to the fibrin surface, the conformation of the two molecules accelerates plasminogen activation 400-fold.[18] t-PA is cleared from plasma by specific uptake and hepatic degradation and exhibits a half-life of approximately 4 minutes.

The expected lower incidence of bleeding complications with the use of t-PA resulting from its higher affinity for thrombus-bound fibrin has not been realized in clinical trials.[19] t-PA binds to platelet receptors, leading to a rapid cleavage of glycoprotein 1b and loss of platelet binding to von Willebrand's factor.[20] Continuous infusion of t-PA leads to accumulation of fibrin fragments, which increase its affinity for plasminogen severalfold. Thus early inhibition of platelet aggregation by t-PA and an increased plasminogen activation in the peripheral circulation may account for the unexpected increased incidence of bleeding complications seen with this agent.

Arterial Applications

Acute Limb Ischemia

Clifton,[21] using a mixture of plasminogen and streptokinase in 1957, was the first to report and document the beneficial effects of direct intraarterial infusions in two patients with peripheral arterial occlusion. However, Dotter is credited with the introduction of low-dose intraarterial thrombolytic therapy, in 1972.[22] He demonstrated that effective local fibrinolysis could be achieved with much lower doses of streptokinase compared with those of standard systemic therapy, along with a reduction of bleeding complications.[23] Twenty years later we are still plagued by controversy as to which therapy, thrombolysis or operative thromboembolectomy, is best in the initial management of acute limb ischemia.

The first obstacle that needs to be overcome for the successful treatment of acute limb ischemia is making an accurate determination of its etiology. Arterial occlusion results from embolism or thrombosis, but their clinical differentiation is not always obvious. Because of the decreased incidence of rheumatic valvular disease and aggressive implementation of anticoagulation therapy in recent years, thrombotic etiologies are observed more frequently (by a ratio of 4:1) in most series of acutely compromised lower extremities.[24] Diagnostic accuracy is important, since it appears to correlate with mortality and amputation rates. Jivegard reported a misdiagnosis rate of 29% in 122 patients undergoing emergency embolectomy with the preoperative diagnosis of acute lower limb embolism.[25] In the 29% of patients who were misdiagnosed, the surgical failure rate was 50%, compared with 13% in the true embolic group. One-half of surgical failures developed gangrene, and most died from septic complications. The thrombotic occlusion group experienced a 50% amputation rate among survivors, as opposed to a 6% amputation rate in those correctly diagnosed as having embolic occlusion.

Balloon catheter thromboembolectomy is able to remove soft thrombus, but it may leave residual thrombus adherent to atherosclerotic plaque. Thrombus in distal arteries and smaller branches is not accessible to the reach of the balloon catheter, and arteriographic follow-up has revealed 30% of residual thrombus in surgically performed thromboembolectomies (Figure 32–1A,B).[26] Direct angioscopic evaluation of the completeness of thromboembolectomy revealed adherent thrombus to the vessel wall of 80% of studied patients.[27]

Blaisdell in 1978 reviewed the published results of 3345 patients who had undergone operative treatment for acute lower extremity ischemia. He found that the average mortality rate exceeded 25% and was accompanied by a 30% amputation rate among survivors.[28] The cause of death in 82% of the cases was either cardiopulmonary or embolic in nature. A more recent review of the literature from 1978 to 1984, which included 2495 patients treated with emergency thromboembolectomy for acute lower extremity ischemia, revealed a 30-day mortality of 18% and a 16% amputation rate in the survivors.[29]

Catheter-directed thromboembolectomy is hampered by its inability to completely clear thrombus and its failure to correct the underlying atherosclerotic lesion responsible for the acute arterial thrombosis. Its use may cause

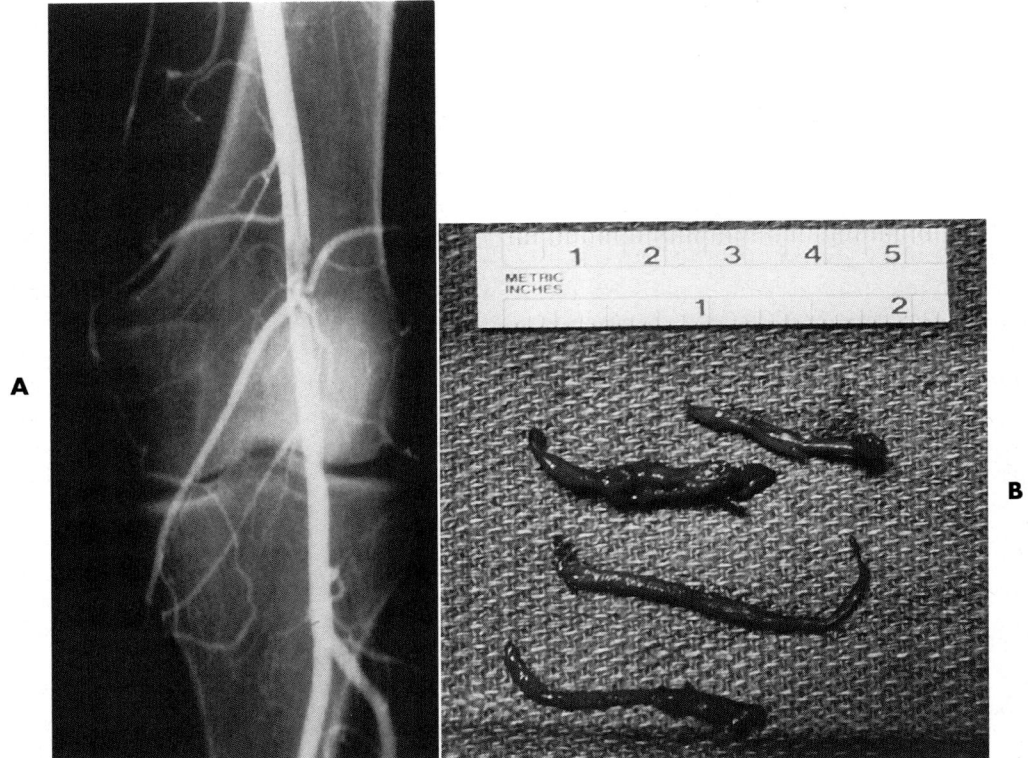

FIGURE 32–1. **A**, Embolus to left popliteal artery of a 42-year-old woman whose presenting symptoms included acute left lower leg ischemia resulting from a cardiac embolus. After an 8-hour infusion of urokinase, she had total resolution of symptoms (ABI = 0.6), but since she required cardioversion for medically uncontrolled atrial fibrillation, the urokinase was stopped at the request of the cardiology service. The angiogram showed only a small filling defect. **B**, Popliteal thrombus. Operative thrombectomy retrieved a larger amount of thrombus than was predicted by the angiogram.

vasospasm, create intimal tears or flaps, and make the vessel more thrombogenic and susceptible to recurrent occlusion. Furthermore, patients with a high incidence of cardiopulmonary co-morbidities are submitted to an emergent operation. It is not surprising that despite technical advances and refinements in anesthetic and postoperative care the mortality for this process has not been significantly lowered.

Direct intraarterial thrombolytic therapy has several potential advantages when it is used for the treatment of acute limb ischemia. Since it requires angiographic evaluation of the ischemic extremity before intervention, it allows for a more accurate preoperative diagnosis and optimum treatment planning. As opposed to catheter thromboembolectomy, thrombolytic therapy can unmask a hemodynamically significant lesion and permits direct corrective interventions. It avoids intimal trauma and can improve outflow resistance by opening small tibial and pedal vessels that are inaccessible to an operative approach. Lastly, patient survival may be improved by restoring arterial flow in a less invasive fashion, and operative interventions may be reduced in complexity or totally avoided (Figures 32–2, 32–3).

The perceived benefits of intraarterial thrombolytic therapy have been difficult to validate. Published reports have offered limited objective data defining the clinical status of the threatened extremity, are retrospective and nonrandomized, have short length of follow-up, and use ill-defined endpoints when making conclusions. Results are also difficult to compare because of wide discrepancies in dosage regimens and interventional techniques used to deliver thrombolytic agents.

One of the best retrospective series of intraarterial thrombolysis as the initial treatment for acute limb ischemia is the one by McNamara and associates.[30] The authors selected 63 patients who had less than a 7-day history of acute limb ischemia manifested by coldness, pain and pallor of the lower extremity, and persistent physical findings of ischemia at the time of admission. They underwent 72 infusions, with a mean time between onset of symptoms and administration of thrombolytic therapy of 30 hours. On entry into the study, all patients were graded as to the degree of ischemia by Society of Vascular Surgery/International Society for Cardiovascular Surgery (SVS/ISCVS) criteria (Table 32-1).[31]

The thrombolytic infusion consisted of an initial transcatheter intrathrombus continuous infusion of urokinase 4000 units/min with serial advancement of the catheter into any remaining occluded segment at 1- to 2-hour intervals until reestablishment of antegrade flow was accomplished. Afterward, the catheter tip was repositioned proximal to any residual clot within the previously occluded segment and the dose decreased to 1000 units/min. This dose was continued for 8 to 12 hours before reexamination. The infusion was continued until complete clot lysis had occurred, unless complications or the patient's degree of ischemia required cessation. Concurrent intravenous heparin therapy was administered in 70 of 72 infusions (97%). After completion thrombolysis, if an arterial stenosis of 50% or more was found, it was referred for either percutaneous transluminal angioplasty (PTA) or elective operative repair. This decision was made after consultation between the interventional radiologist and the vascular surgeon.

A positive thrombolytic outcome (PTO), defined as complete thrombolysis of a previously occluded segment with restoration of antegrade flow, augmented by balloon angioplasty or surgery when necessary, with symptomatic and hemodynamic benefit maintained for at least 30 days, was obtained in 61 of the 72 infusions (85%). There was a strong correlation between the pretreatment degree of ischemia and outcome. All category I (viable) limbs, 13 of 13 (100%), had a PTO; in category II (threatened), 43 of 51 (84%); and in category III (irreversible), 5 of 8 (63%).

PTO was accomplished in 46 of 56 (82%) thrombotic occlusions, 15 of 16 (94%) embolic occlusions, 37 of 42 (88%) native artery occlusions, and 24 of 30 (80%) graft occlusions. The differences, although not statistically significant, showed a trend toward better results with embolic and native artery occlusions. Underlying flow-limiting lesions were demonstrated in 39 of 46 (85%) of successfully treated thrombotic occlusions, with 31 of them undergoing percutaneous balloon angioplasty. Of the remaining eight, three were treated with surgery alone, and five underwent proximal site balloon angioplasty in combination with a distal bypass. Since 7 of the 46 thrombotic occlusions had no underlying lesion demonstrated and none of the 15 successfully treated embolic occlusions required further treatment, thrombolysis was the definitive therapy in 31% (22 of 72) of ischemic limbs. Sixteen surgical procedures were undertaken, eight after successful thrombolysis with a 100% success. Surgical procedures performed after failed thrombolysis were only 50% successful, all of them requiring amputation. Significant bleeding occurred in only 2.8% and distal clot migration in 15%. These results were achieved with an 8.5% amputation rate and with only a single mortality.

Despite having excellent results, this study was criticized for being retrospective in design and lacking a comparable control group.[32] These limitations were addressed by two prospectively randomized trials comparing surgery and thrombolysis for acute limb ischemia.

Rochester Trial

In the Rochester study,[32] patients with limb-threatening ischemia of less than 7 days' duration were randomly assigned to intraarterial

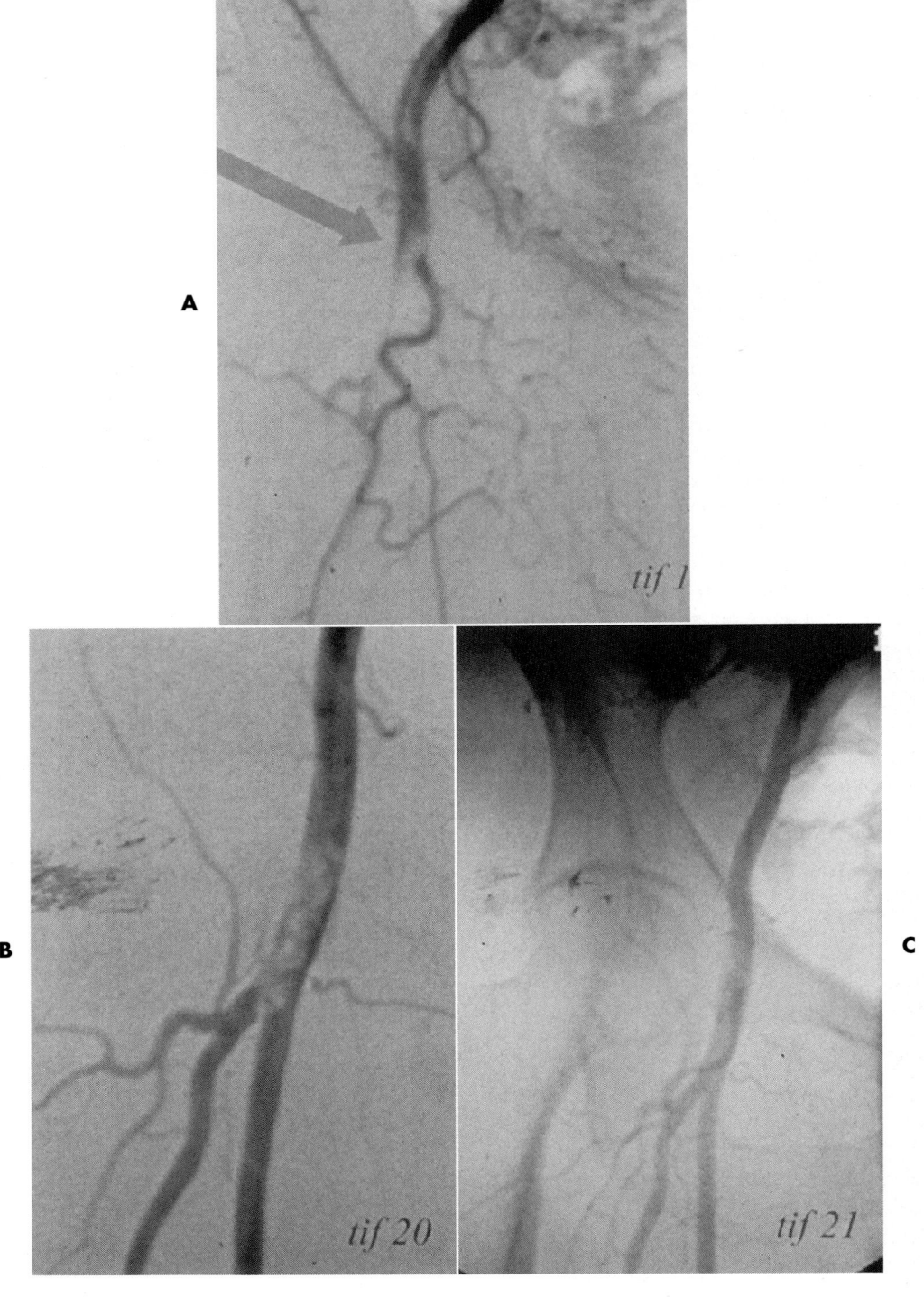

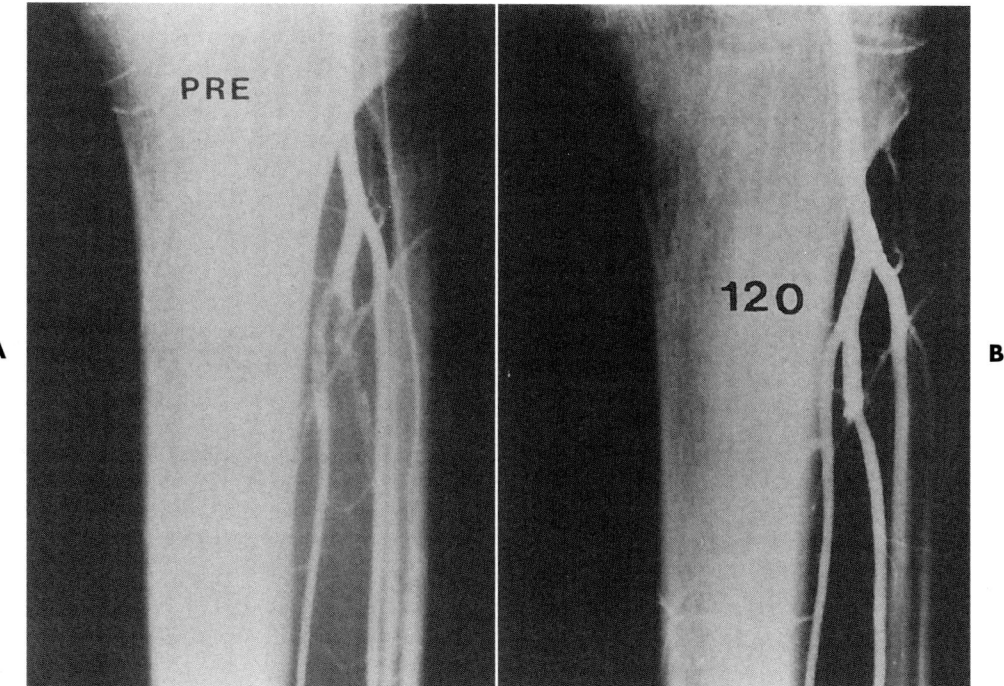

FIGURE 32–3. **A**, All infrapopliteal vessels are occluded in this patient after resuscitation and repair of a gunshot wound of his common femoral artery. The anterior tibial artery was occluded distally. A catheter was placed around the aortic bifurcation, through the repaired femoral artery and into the distal tibioperoneal trunk. **B**, After 2 hours of infusion of streptokinase at 35,000 IU/hr, all infrapopliteal thrombus was lysed (except for a small peroneal branch), with reperfusion of the foot and palpable distal pulses. (From Comerota AJ, White JV: Intraoperative intraarterial thrombolytic therapy as an adjunct to revascularization in patients with residual and distal arterial thrombus, *Semin Vasc Surg* 5:112, 1992.)

catheter-directed urokinase therapy (57 patients) or operative intervention (57 patients). Patients with extremities that were nonfunctional, deemed irreversible (class III), or could not undergo angiography (creatinine > 2.5 mg/dl, dye allergy) were excluded. Acute limb ischemia was due to an embolic occlusion in 21% of the enrolled patients, whereas the remaining 79% of the patients suffered from a thrombotic occlusion (Table 32–2). Native artery occlusions occurred in 46%, and 54% had occluded bypass grafts. Upper extremity occlusions that have a better clinical prognosis because of localized disease, greater collateral

FIGURE 32–2. **A**, 90-year-old woman with a history of atrial fibrillation who had sudden onset of right leg pain. Physical examination revealed a warm contralateral lower extremity with palpable pedal pulses. The right leg was cool and had a diminished femoral pulse. Urokinase infusion rapidly resolved her symptoms. Right femoral angiogram revealed large thrombus with complete occlusion of the common femoral artery (*large arrow*). **B**, Four-hour angiogram revealed distal reconstitution of superficial femoral and profunda arteries, but thrombus was still present. **C**, Twenty-four-hour angiogram showed widely patent femoral system without any evidence of thrombus. Patient was treated with chronic warfarin anticoagulation.

Table 32-1 Clinical Categories of Acute Limb Ischemia

Category	Description	Capillary return	Muscle weakness	Sensory loss	Doppler signals Arterial	Venous
Viable	Not immediately threatened	Intact	None	None	Audible (AP >30 mm Hg)	Audible
Threatened	Salvageable if promptly treated	Inact, slow	Mild, partial	Mild, incomplete	Inaudible	Audible
Irreversible	Major tissue loss, amputation regardless of treatment	Absent (marbling)	Profound, paralysis (rigor)	Profound, anesthetic	Inaudible	Inaudible

From Rutherford RB, Flanigan DP, Gupta SK et al: Suggested standards for reports dealing with lower extremity ischemia, *J Vasc Surg* 4:81, 1986.
AP, ankle pressure.

flow, and lower muscle mass than lower extremities were seen in only 10 patients (9%).

Patients randomized to receive intraarterial thrombolytic therapy were given urokinase through a *single bole catheter* in the following fashion: 4000 IU/min × 2 hours, 2000 IU/min × 2 hours, and 1000 IU/min an hour for up to 44 hours *continuously*. They were also pretreated with 325 mg of aspirin, but systemic heparin anticoagulation was not used. Only two of the patients randomized to thrombolytic therapy could not receive urokinase because of an inability to place the catheter proximal to the occlusive process (96% technical success). Arteriographically successful thrombolysis (>80% clot lysis) was achieved in 70% (40 patients). An anatomic lesion responsible for the native or arterial bypass graft occlusion was uncovered in 21 (37%) patients, and each underwent correction by means of percutaneous balloon angioplasty (two patients) or operation (19 patients). No anatomic lesion was found in 19 (33%) of the patients, and they were treated with long-term warfarin anticoagulation (Figure 32-4). The 17 patients (30%) with unsuccessful thrombolysis underwent either operative revascularization (15 patients) or primary amputation (two patients). Major bleeding complications occurred in five of the patients receiving urokinase and resulted in one mortality resulting from intracranial bleeding with uncal herniation. All other bleeding episodes in this group of patients were related to the site of arterial puncture. Pseudo-

Table 32-2 Etiologic Diagnoses of Acute Peripheral Arterial Occlusion

Diagnosis	Thrombolytic therapy (n = 57)	Operative therapy (n = 57)
Embolic occlusion	11 (19%)	13 (23%)
Thrombotic occlusion	46 (81%)	44 (77%)
Native artery	13 (23%)	14 (25%)
Atherosclerotic stenosis	8 (14%)	10 (17%)
Popliteal aneurysm	3 (5%)	4 (7%)
Antiphospholipid syndrome	2 (4%)	0
Bypass graft	33 (58%)	30 (53%)
Aortofemoral	5 (9%)	5 (9%)
Infrainguinal	26 (46%)	23 (40%)
Axillofemoral	2 (4%)	2 (4%)

From Ouriel K, Shortell CK, DeWeese JA et al: A comparison of thrombolytic therapy with operative revascularization in the initial treatment of acute peripheral ischemia, *J Vasc Surg* 19:1021, 1994.

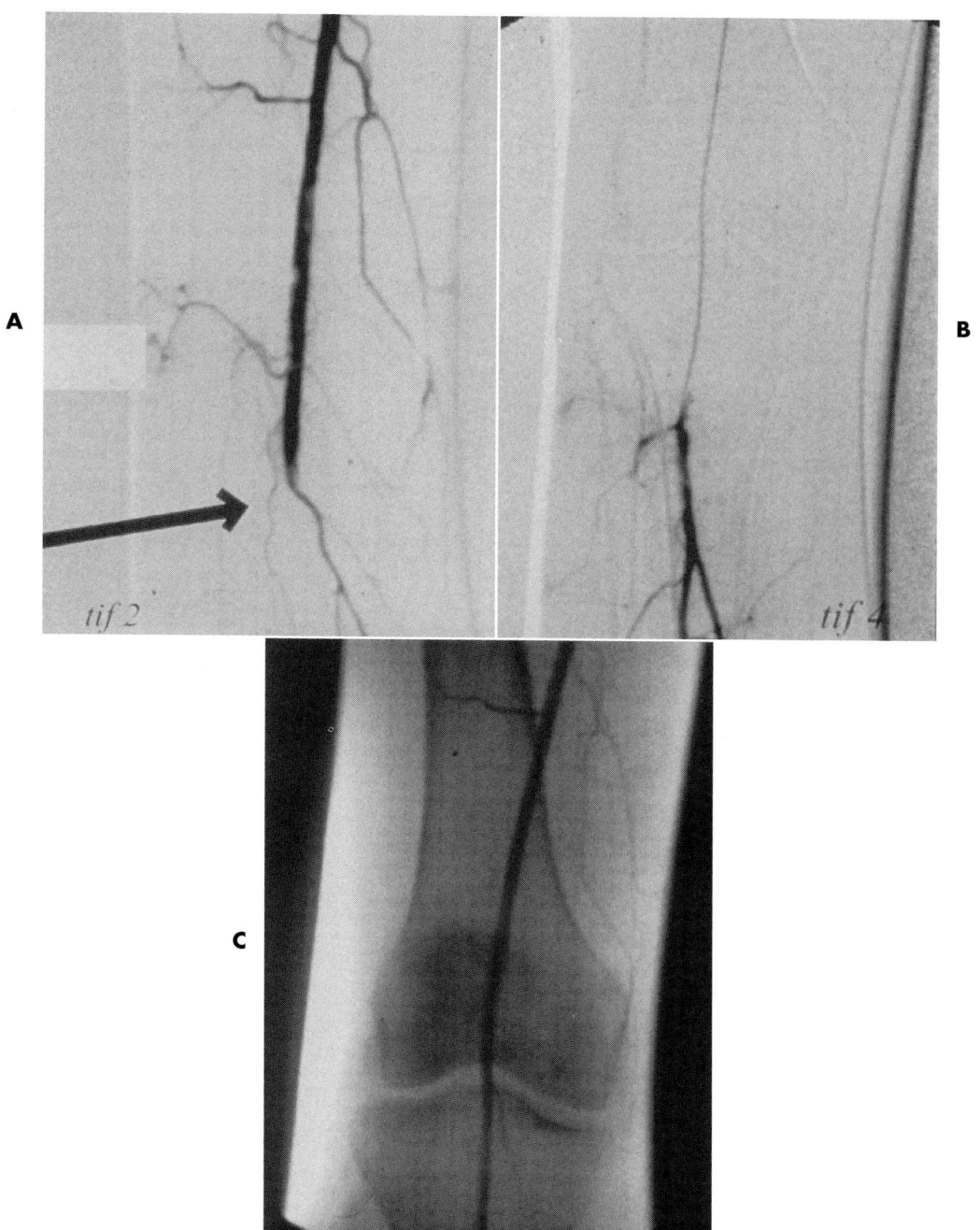

FIGURE 32–4. **A**, Angiogram showing acute occlusion of distal popliteal vessel and runoff vessels (*large arrow*). Patient's foot was cool and mottled, with no Doppler signals. She had a decreased sensory examination but no motor deficits. **B**, Catheter advanced into occluding thrombus and urokinase infusion started with reconstitution of distal vessels. **C**, After 20 hours all thrombus was lysed, no underlying defect was unmasked, and patient was treated with chronic warfarin therapy.

aneurysms developed in three patients and required operative correction.

In-hospital mortality occurred in 8 (14%) of the patients in the thrombolytic arm and 10 (18%) of the patients in the operative arm. There were also no significant differences in the frequency of major amputations during the initial hospitalization (9% versus 12%), and the median length of stay was 11 days for both groups. The event-free survival at 12 months was 75% in the thrombolytic group and 52% in the operated group. This difference was achieved because of a significant decrease in mortality, 16% in the thrombolytic group versus 42% in the operated group, since the limb salvage rate was essentially the same, 18% versus 20%. This benefit was achieved at a cost of approximately $3400 per patient and appears to be directly attributed to the cost of the lytic agent.

STILE Study

The Surgery versus Thrombolysis for Ischemia of the Lower Extremity (STILE) study, a prospective trial, randomized patients with nonembolic lower extremity ischemia with symptomatic progression during the preceding 6 months. Randomization followed angiographic documentation of the obstruction of either native arteries or bypass grafts. Patients were randomized to either rt-PA infusion (0.05 mg/kg/hr) or urokinase infusion (4000 IU/min × 4 hours, followed by 2000 IU/min) versus operative intervention.

Within 14 days of worsening ischemia, 30% of the patients were randomized, 44% of the patients had symptoms for 1 month or more, and 26% of them had symptoms for 2 months or more. Symptoms occurred earlier in patients with bypass graft occlusions than in patients with native artery occlusions, 48% versus 24%, respectively, in the group with worsening ischemia of less than 14 days in duration.

Randomization was terminated after enrolling 393 patients because patients assigned to catheter-directed thrombolysis had significantly greater ongoing/recurrent ischemia, 54.0% versus 25.7% for the surgery group, at the first interim analysis. Technical failure to institute the chosen therapy had a large negative impact, since the ischemic event could not be initially reversed. Failure to properly place delivery catheters occurred in 28% of the patients randomized to lysis, 41% with occluded grafts, and 22% with occluded native arteries (p = NS). The thrombolytic group had also a greater incidence of life-threatening hemorrhages (5.6% versus 0.7%) and more vascular complications (9.7% versus 3.5%) when compared with the surgical patients.

Of the patients randomized to catheter-directed thrombolysis, 55.8% had a major reduction in their planned revascularization procedure, and those patients had a 90.1% amputation-free survival at 6 months, compared with 71.1% for patients without a reduction in their planned procedure. Thrombolysis benefited patients with acute ischemia (<14 days' duration), since this group had a death and amputation rate (15.3%) that was significantly lower (p = 0.01) than the rate seen for the patients undergoing operative repair (37.5%). Major amputations were performed in 30% of the acutely ischemic patients who underwent operations, compared with 11% of patients who underwent thrombolysis (p = 0.02). In patients with more chronic limb ischemia (>14 days), this trend was reversed, with only 3.0% of the surgical patients having major amputations, compared with 12.1% of the thrombolysis patients (p = 0.01). Length of hospitalization was also positively affected by thrombolytic therapy management in patients with acute ischemia; surgical patients had a mean hospital stay of 9.7 days (p = 0.04).

It appears that in the patients with acute reversible limb ischemia (<14 days in duration) angiographic evaluation accompanied by the initiation of thrombolytic therapy is safe and achieves a significant reduction in mortality. Most of these occlusions are due to thrombotic events secondary to an anatomic lesion that when unmasked can be treated either by a properly planned operative procedure of lesser magnitude or an endovascular procedure. In up to one-third of treated patients no anatomic lesion will be found, and those patients benefit from chronic warfarin therapy alone. The ability to embed the delivery catheter within the obstructing clot and pass the guidewire through the occlusion is associated with a high success rate (>85%).[34] Technical advances such as the use of multihole catheters and pulse spray techniques may increase the success rate of recanalization of acute occlusions. These developments await properly controlled trials, but they may nonetheless result in quicker reperfusion periods, shorter indwelling catheter times, and a decrease in the quantities of thrombolytic agents used. These factors may favorably affect the higher incidence of bleeding complications and cost associated with their use.

TOPAS Trial

The Thrombolysis or Peripheral Arterial Surgery (TOPAS) trial was the next randomized, prospective, multicenter study designed to compare the efficacy and safety of catheter-administered urokinase and conventional open surgery as the initial treatment in patients with acute peripheral arterial occlusion threatening leg viability.[35,36] The urokinase used in the trial was a plasminogen activator of 48,000 D produced from genetically engineered mouse hybridoma cell line. This recombinant form of urokinase (r-UK) is similar to the naturally occurring urokinase found in human urine.

To be eligible for the study patients had to have an acute thrombotic or embolic occlusion of a leg (native artery or bypass graft) within 14 days before randomization that met the guidelines for reversible limb-threatening ischemia.[31] Between August 1993 and December 1994 a total of 544 patients underwent randomization in 13 medical centers in North America and Europe. No significant differences were found between the surgery and thrombolytic groups with regard to the duration of symptoms or the nature, location, or length of arterial occlusion (Table 32-3). Thrombotic events were much more frequent than embolic events, and patients with occluded bypass grafts slightly outnumbered those with native arterial occlusions. The occluded bypass grafts were made of polytetrafluoroethylene (PTFE) in 57%, polyester in 11%, autogenous vein in 19%, a composite of PTFE and vein in 4%, and other or

TABLE 32-3. Patient Characteristics in TOPAS Trial ($n = 544$)

Characteristic	Urokinase group ($n = 272$)	Surgery group ($n = 272$)
Age (years)	64.9 ± 0.78	64.5 ± 0.78
Sex (no.)		
Male	192 (71%)	170 (62%)
Female	80 (29%)	102 (38%)
ABI	0.15 ± 0.015	0.18 ± 0.015
Type of occlusion (no./total patients)		
Native artery	122/272 (45%)	120/272 (44%)
Bypass graft	150/272 (55%)	152/272 (56%)
Thrombosis	233/270 (86%)	231/272 (85%)
Embolism	37/270 (14%)	41/272 (15%)
Duration of symptoms before randomization (days)	4.20 ± 0.23 ($n = 272$)	4.00 ± 0.23 ($n = 272$)
Length of occlusion (mm)	32.40 ± 1.42 ($n = 266$)	31.70 ± 1.44 ($n = 259$)
Amputation		
At 6 months	48	41
At 1 year	58	51
Open (major) surgical procedures at 6 months (no.)	102	177
Percutaneous procedures (no.)	128	55
Endovascular procedures (mean)	16.9	2.1
Medical treatment alone (mean)	14.6	3.7
Deaths (no.)		
At 6 months	16.0	12.3
At 1 year	20.0	17.0

ABI, ankle-brachial blood pressure index.

unknown materials in 9%. There were no significant differences between the groups in the frequencies of the planned surgical procedures, as recorded by the patients' physicians before randomization. Thromboembolectomy was the most common planned surgical procedure chosen in 66% of patients, followed by bypass grafting in 32%. Amputation was not selected as a planned procedure for any patient.

Amputation-free survival rates 6 months after randomization were 71.8% in the urokinase group and 74.8% in the surgery group ($p = 0.43$). There were also no significant differences in the rates of amputation-free survival at discharge from the hospital. The mortality rates for the urokinase and surgery groups were 8.5% and 5.9%, respectively, at hospital discharge, 16.0% and 12.3% at 6 months, and 20.0% and 17.0% at 1 year after randomization.

At the end of 6 months Kaplan-Meier analysis showed that 31% of the patients in the urokinase group had had only percutaneous procedures, compared with 5.8% of the surgical patients. The length of hospitalization was similar, with a median of 10 days for both treatment groups.

During the initial hospitalization 54% of the urokinase group and 91% of those in the surgery group required an open surgical procedure, underwent amputation, or died. Twenty-three percent of the patients assigned to initial thrombolysis needed no further interventions before discharge from the hospital. During the first 6 months after treatment patients who were randomly assigned to surgery underwent 551 open surgical procedures, whereas the patients assigned to initial thrombolysis had 315.

The big drawback of this study was that major hemorrhagic complications occurred in 32 patients (12.5%) in the urokinase group compared with 14 patients (5.1%) in the surgery group ($p = 0.005$). Twenty-one of the patients in the urokinase group had major bleeding at the site of vascular access (e.g., sites of catheterization and venipuncture); in four patients bleeding was associated with an open surgical procedure after thrombolysis. In addition, 14 patients in the urokinase group had bleeding in areas other than vascular access sites, compared with 5 patients assigned to surgery ($p = 0.04$). There was a significant association between the co-administration of heparin and the risk of major bleeding. Transfusions of more than 1 unit of packed red blood cells were required in 92 patients in the urokinase group and 69 patients in the surgery group ($p = 0.03$). Intracranial hemorrhage occurred in four patients in the urokinase group. By contrast, there were no incidents of intracranial bleeding in the surgery group.

Distal embolization of partially thrombolyzed material occurred 41 times in 36 patients treated with urokinase. The emboli were disolved in 19 of 26 cases treated only with continued urokinase therapy. Distal emboli did not appear to have a negative impact, as amputation or death during the initial hospitalization occurred in 19% of patients with emboli and in 16% of patients without distal embolization.

These current results differ from those of the single center study performed in Rochester.[24] In the TOPAS study initial thrombolytic therapy was not superior to operative intervention with respect to the major endpoints of survival and limb salvage. Indeed, there was a trend toward higher amputation-free survival rate in the surgical group. The use of 14 days as the measure of ischemia allowed inclusion of patients who were less acutely ill than those in the Rochester study, as manifested by the duration and magnitude of limb ischemia, age differences, and the incidence of coronary artery disease.

Treatment philosophies and patient selection appear to be critical factors requiring further study on identifying candidates suitable for thrombolytic therapy. An initial strategy of thrombolysis compared with immediate surgery appears to reduce the number of open procedures required for the treatment of acute ischemia of the lower leg. For some patients it also allows the avoidance of surgical intervention altogether without a significant increase in mortality, amputation rate, or the duration of hospitalization. In many instances thrombolysis can offer patients definitive treatment with less accompanying trauma than major surgery. Because the ability to embed the delivery catheter within the obstructing clot and pass the guidewire through the occlusion is associated with a high success rate (more than 85%)[36] the use of multihole catheters and pulse spray techniques may increase the success rate of recanalization of acute occlusions. These developments await properly controlled trials, but they may nonetheless result in quicker reperfusion periods shorter indwelling catheter times, and a decrease in the quantity of thrombolytic agents used. These factors may favorably affect the higher incidence of bleeding complications and cost associated with their use.

The concern over the higher incidence of hemorrhagic complications associated with thrombolytic therapy has also led to the search of fibrin-specific plasminogen activators. Human plasma contains at least two physiologic activators of the fibrinolytic system: urinary-type (comprised of urokinase and its parent compound prourokinase) and tissue-type plasminogen activator (t-PA). Both agents catalyze conversion of the proenzyme plasminogen to plasmin, which hydrolyzes fibrin into soluble products. Both prourokinase (Pro-UK) and t-PA have fibrin-dependent modes of action, showing higher activity against fibrin-bound plasminogen and less systemic generation of plasmin compared to urokinase or streptokinase. However, the mechanisms responsible for fibrin-specific fibrinolysis by Pro-UK and t-PA are distinctive. t-PA is activated upon binding to certain polymeric surfaces, including fibrin,[37] specific sites on the platelet membrane,[38] and soluble fibrin degradation products.[39] In contrast, Pro-UK is not activated by direct fibrin binding; rather, it preferentially activates fibrin-bound plasminogen.[40] Plasmin thus formed can locally activate more Pro-UK. This activation is primarily localized to the clot surface where lysis is initiated. The relatively fibrin specificity of these plasminogen activators, with their promise of limited systemic effects compared to urokinase and streptokinase, may usher in safer thrombolytic regimens.

Arterial Bypass Grafts

Noninvasive surveillance of infrainguinal bypass grafts can identify and allow the correction of significant underlying lesions that threaten their long-term patency.[41] Late thrombosis of an arterial graft is largely determined by restenosis at the anastomotic sites, usually the distal site resulting from neointimal hyperplasia, and progression of the underlying atherosclerotic process in the inflow and outflow vessels. Conventional operative thrombectomy, conducted with direct intraoperative or angiographic assessment, and appropriate revision have been disappointing, with 2-year patency rates of less than 40%.[42] As a consequence, thrombolytic therapy has been aggressively pursued to salvage these grafts. It offered the potential benefits of decreasing conduit injury, identifying underlying defects more accurately, improving a compromised distal outflow, and decreasing the magnitude of the planned operative procedure (Figure 32–5).

In the suprainguinal location this concept has worked well. Late occlusion of aortofemoral bypass grafts result from progressive infrainguinal arteriosclerosis. In most of these patients, after the graft limb is recanalized, patency is maintained by extending the graft as a profundaplasty, or a new infrainguinal bypass may be necessary to provide adequate outflow. Preoperative arteriography of the infrainguinal vasculature is needed to plan the proper operative procedure; thrombolytic therapy can be invaluable in providing this information (Figure 32–6).

Most studies of infrainguinal graft thrombolysis report an immediate success rate of greater than 80% for restoration of graft patency, but 50% of these grafts reocclude within 6 months.[43-45] Detection and elimination of uncovered stenoses appear to be crucial to graft survival. Sullivan reported that the patency rates for grafts with corrected lesions was 89% at 1 year and 79% at 2 years, compared with 23% at 1 year and 10% at 2 years for grafts without an underlying correctable lesion.[45] Growing experience suggests that balloon angioplasty may not be adequate in correcting the underlying infrainguinal lesions, and operative correction may yield better long-term results.

There is also a tendency for improved patency when a graft has been functional for

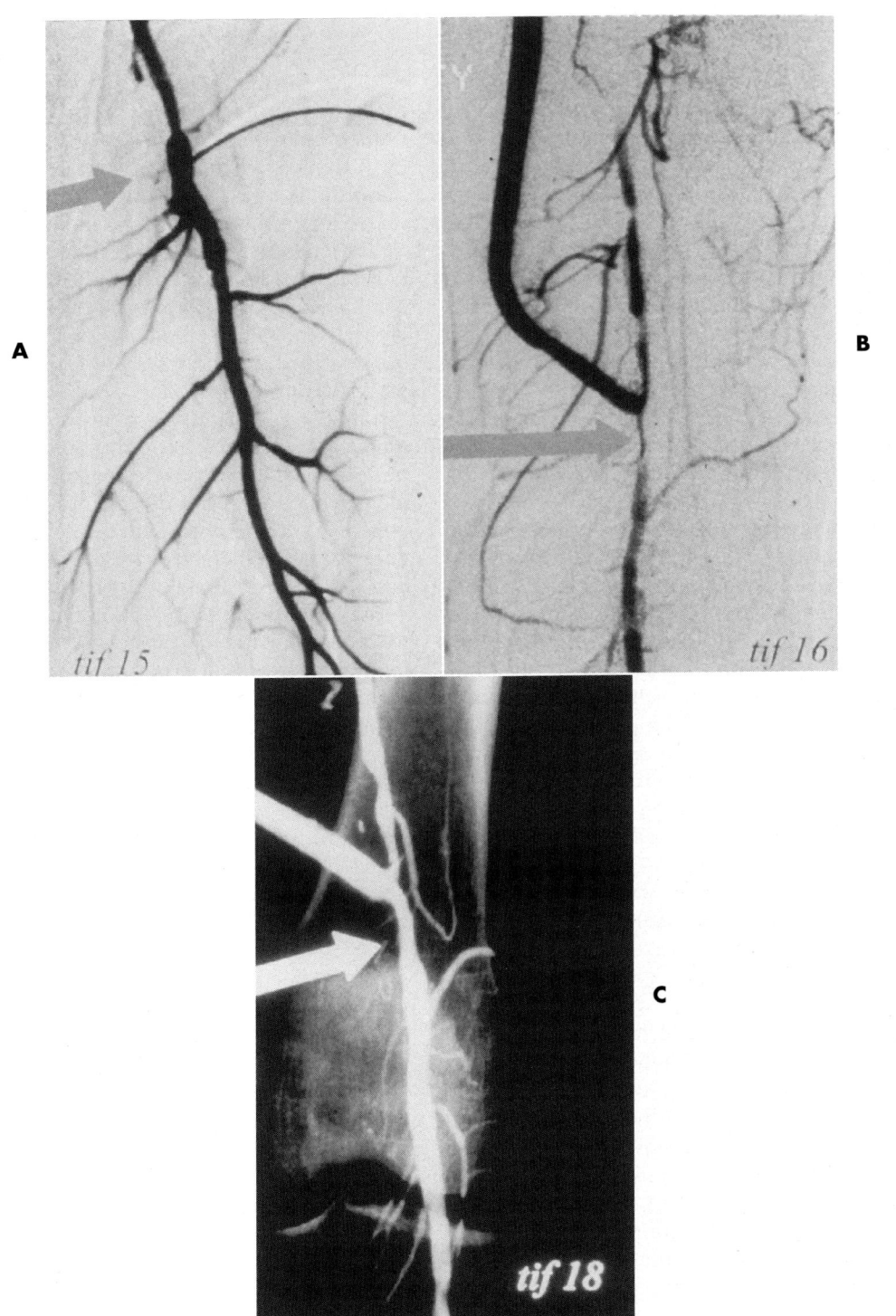

FIGURE 32–5. **A**, A 65-year-old patient after undergoing left femoropopliteal bypass with PTFE for severe disabling claudication had acute limb ischemia. Takeoff thrombosed PTFE graft marked by large arrow. **B**, Urokinase infused into graft with initial reperfusion at 10 hours. Tight stenosis just beyond distal anastomosis was unmasked (*large arrow*). **C**, Balloon angioplasty was performed with salvage of the graft.

a longer period before failing.[46] In the series by Hye, grafts that had been in place and functioning for greater than 1 year fared significantly better than those that had been in place for less than 1 year.[47] Secondary patency in older grafts was 21.5 months, but it was only 7.5 months in grafts less than 1 year old. This may be attributed to a selection factor, with the older grafts having a more favorable anatomy, vein caliber, and coagulability environment, which lead to a greater primary patency. Grafts occluding within 1 year appeared to be smaller in caliber and associated with compromised outflow tracts.

Graft material is another factor that significantly affects long-term patency. Vein grafts have a higher patency rate when compared with prosthetic grafts.[45,46] This may be related to the fact that underlying correctable lesions were present twice as often in vein grafts than in prosthetic grafts.

Thrombolytic therapy should be pursued in patients with a vein graft that has been in place for over a year and has recently occluded. This tends to minimize endothelial injury, allows detection of an underlying lesion in a great percentage of such grafts, and permits their salvage by means of a simple patch angioplasty or vein graft interposition. It should also be pursued in patients with prosthetic grafts with no available vein or with thrombus present in the runoff vessels. Thrombolysis offers both therapeutic and diagnostic advantages when compared with surgical management alone, but long-term results will only be realized with proper patient selection.

Intraoperative Intraarterial Thrombolytic Therapy

The intraoperative use of lytic agents as an adjunct to balloon catheter thromboembolectomy has gained acceptance as an effective method for clearing arterial vessels of residual clot or dealing with persistent ischemia after lower extremity revascularization. The direct intraoperative use of thrombolytics offers several advantages when compared with percutaneous intraarterial administration. Patients with severe ischemia can have flow reestablished without having to wait for diagnostic arteriography and dissolution of a large thrombus load. Since surgical thrombectomy removes most of the thrombus responsible for native artery or graft occlusions, the amount of thrombus that must be lysed is greatly reduced. In addition, occlusion of inflow concentrates the agent to the site with residual thrombus, helping to decrease the amount of thrombolytic agent that is used and shortening the infusion time. All of these factors help to minimize the activation of systemic fibrinolysis, theoretically reducing the incidence of hemorrhagic complications.[48]

Laboratory data confirms the clinical observations that balloon catheter thrombectomy frequently leaves residual thrombus. Quinones-Balrich et al.,[49] in a controlled hind limb perfusion study, showed that intraarterial infusion of 60,000 units of streptokinase after incomplete embolectomy significantly improved the angiographic appearance of the vascular bed compared with embolectomy alone and produced a marked trend toward improved blood flow compared with control limbs. They also pointed out that the criterion of two consecutive clean passes of a balloon catheter after embolectomy is an unreliable sign for establishing the completeness of this form of treatment.

Other studies have suggested that acute muscle ischemia is associated with an inflamed endothelium with increased procoagulant activity,[50] and it impairs endogenous microvascular fibrinolysis.[51] This may promote local thrombosis during acute ischemia and suggests that infusion of exogenous fibrinolytic agents may help to maintain and restore patency by supplementing or replacing endogenous fibrinolysins. Belkin, using an isolated canine gracilis muscle preparation, demonstrated that urokinase infusion significantly decreased muscle infarction, salvaged more ischemic muscle, and lessened the degree of injury as shown by reperfusion edema when compared with the control group.[52] Thus arterial perfusion can be restored with increased tissue salvage and decreased incidence of reperfusion injury with the appropriate use of thrombolytic agents.

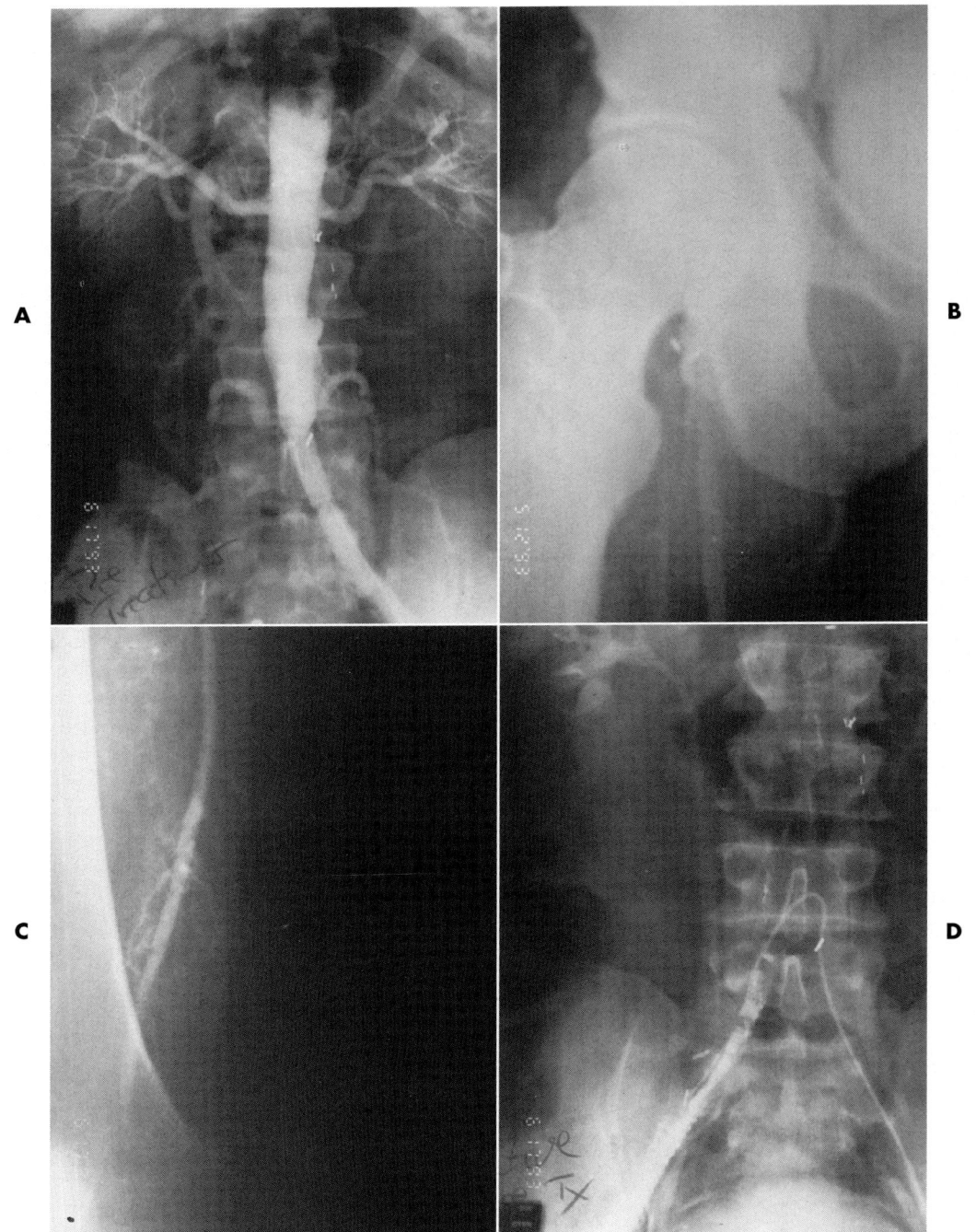

FIGURE 32–6. **A,** A 57-year-old man 4 years after aortobifemoral bypass for thigh claudication had a 7-day history of a painful right leg. Physical examination revealed a cool right leg, decreased foot sensation, absent right femoral pulse, and absent pedal Doppler signals. Angiogram demonstrated an occluded right femoral limb graft. **B,** Reconstitution of right superficial and profunda femoral arteries. **C,** Right superficial femoral artery is occluded at the level of the adductor canal (proximal popliteal artery); distal vessels are not visualized. **D,** Single-hole infusion catheter embedded in soft thrombus achieved rapid clot lysis with symptom improvement.

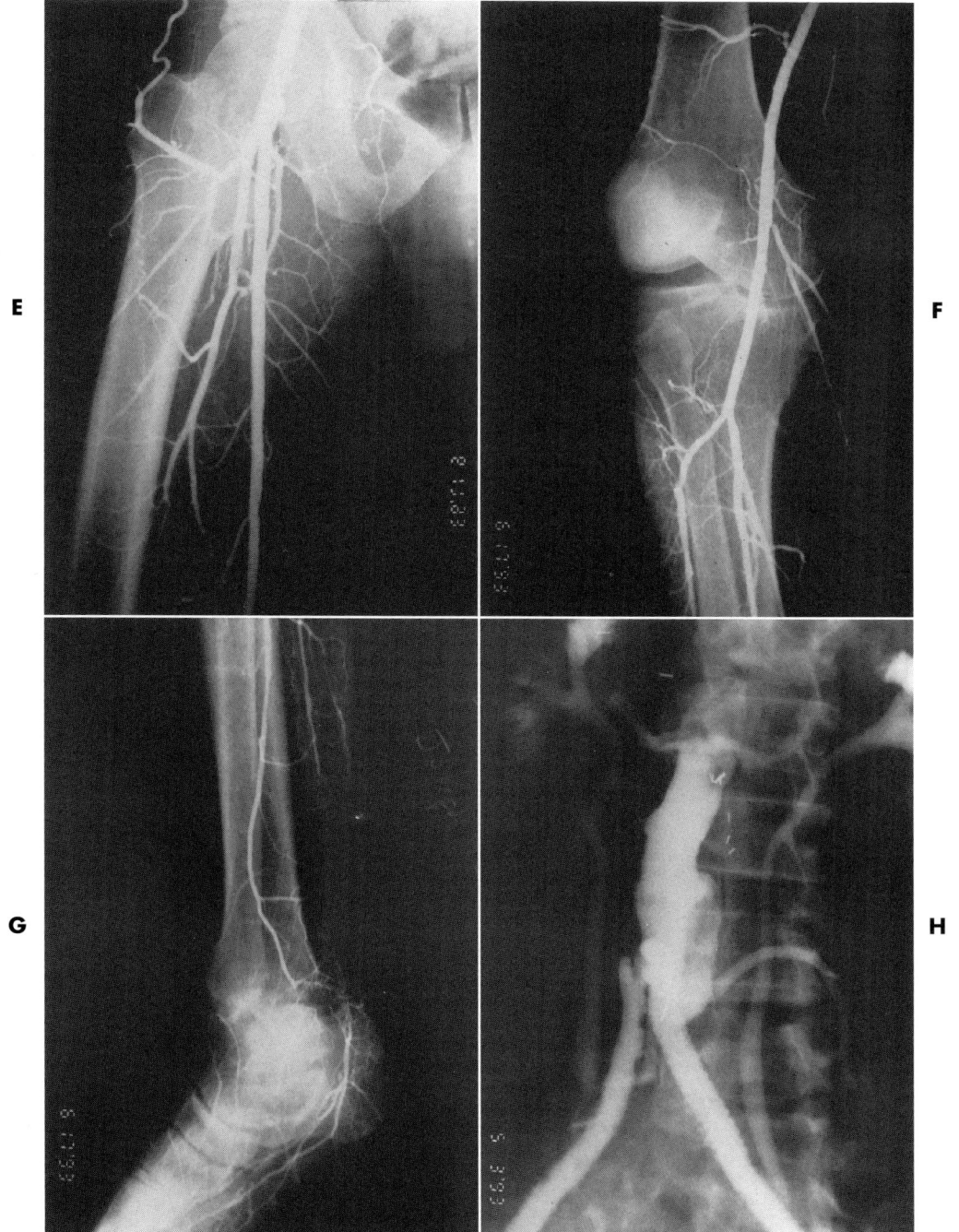

FIGURE 32–6. *Continued.* **E**, By 12 hours, femoral system is completely cleared of any thrombus and catheter is advanced into the popliteal artery. **F**, At 24 hours the popliteal artery is free of thrombus and the origin of the trifurcation vessels is visualized, and catheter advanced distally. Patient was now symptom-free. **G**, At 48 hours, infusion is terminated, peroneal is only vessel patent to ankle level and reconstitutes the posterior tibial artery. **H**, The ischemic cause was not due to a stenosis of the femoral anastomosis causing proximal and distal vessel thrombosis as initially suspected. Angiogram after urokinase infusion revealed a large pseudoaneurysm had formed at the aortic/graft anastomosis and caused distal embolization. The patient underwent aortic reconstruction 5 days after admission; a bifurcated graft was sewn end-to-end just below the renal vessels and anastomosed to the "old" iliac limbs. Since there were no anatomic defects of the femoral anastomoses, groin reconstructions were avoided. Thrombolytic infusion relieved the patient's ischemic symptoms and was instrumental in the planning of the correct operative repair.

Repeated embolectomy after the intraoperative infusion of thrombolytic agents removes additional thrombus that was missed on earlier passes or that was freed or mobilized by intraoperative thrombolysis.[53] Aggressive use of arteriography before and after intraoperative lytic therapy is useful in the evaluation of thrombus removal, and it has a prognostic significance. If no change is seen on arteriography performed after intraoperative lytic therapy, the likelihood of failure for that reconstruction is high and alternatives should be considered during that intervention.[54] If arteriography documents improvement, high likelihood of continued patency is seen.

Comerota has the most extensive experience with the use of intraoperative thrombolytic agents. He treated 53 patients who had impending limb loss and occlusions of their runoff vessels with inflow occlusion and intraoperative dosages of up to 50,000 IU of streptokinase, 250,000 IU of urokinase, or up to 10 mg of rt-PA.[55] Inflow was then restored to the site of infusion by thrombectomy or bypass. Limb salvage was achieved in 70% and was directly attributable to lysis in 47%. Although there was a 9% mortality rate, none of the deaths was thought to be due to the use of lytic agents. A major bleeding complication was seen in only one patient; it occurred on the third postoperative day and was thought to be related to the use of heparin.

In patients with multiple vessel occlusion in whom bolus infusion will not be effective, or in those patients in whom any degree of systemic thrombolysis, however transient, will pose a significant risk, a *high-dose isolated limb perfusion* technique has been advocated.[56] The patient is fully anticoagulated, venous blood is exsanguinated from the limb with a rubber bandage, tourniquet is applied to achieve complete arterial and venous occlusion, and high doses of a lytic agent (1 million IU or more of urokinase/40 mg or more of rt-PA) are directly infused into the affected vessels, followed by drainage of the venous effluent (Figure 32-7). Direct exposure of lytic agents to the thrombus for 45 to 60 minutes has yielded impressive results in a small number of patients suffering from acute multivessel distal thrombi or emboli. If distal vessel occlusion is due to atheromatous emboli or well-formed thrombus, such treatment has not been successful.

A prospective multicenter randomized, blinded, and placebo-controlled study was performed to address the systemic effects on the fibrinolytic system and safety of intraarterial thrombolytic therapy.[57] One-hundred and thirty-four patients were prospectively randomized to receive one of three bolus doses of urokinase (125, 250, 500 units $\times 10^3$) or saline placebo infused into the distal circulation before lower extremity bypass for chronic limb ischemia. Regional (femoral vein) and systemic (vein) blood was sampled before drug infusion, before reperfusion, and after reperfusion. Systemic blood was also sampled 2 hours after reperfusion. Intraoperative bolus of urokinase infusions produced no significant fibrinogen breakdown as compared with placebo. Dose-related plasminogen activation only became significant at a dose of 500,000 units. The change in plasma markers for the breakdown of fibrinogen and fibrin was similar in the regional and systemic circulations. More importantly, there was no increase in operative blood loss, blood replacement, or wound hematoma formation.

Just as in the Rochester Trial, there was also an unexplained survival benefit in patients receiving urokinase (2% mortality) as compared with those receiving placebo (12% mortality). Most of the patients entered into this study did not suffer from acute limb ischemia, only 22% of the patients had rest pain, 54% suffered from tissue necrosis, and the remaining had claudication. The causes of death in the placebo group were either myocardial infarction or progressive cardiopulmonary dysfunction. It is known that increased levels of certain hemostatic factors may play a part in the development of acute coronary syndromes. In patients with angina pectoris, higher levels of fibrinogen, von Willebrand's factor antigen, and t-PA antigen are independent of predictors of subsequent acute coronary events.[58] In addition, low fibrinogen concentrations characterize patients at low risk for coronary events despite

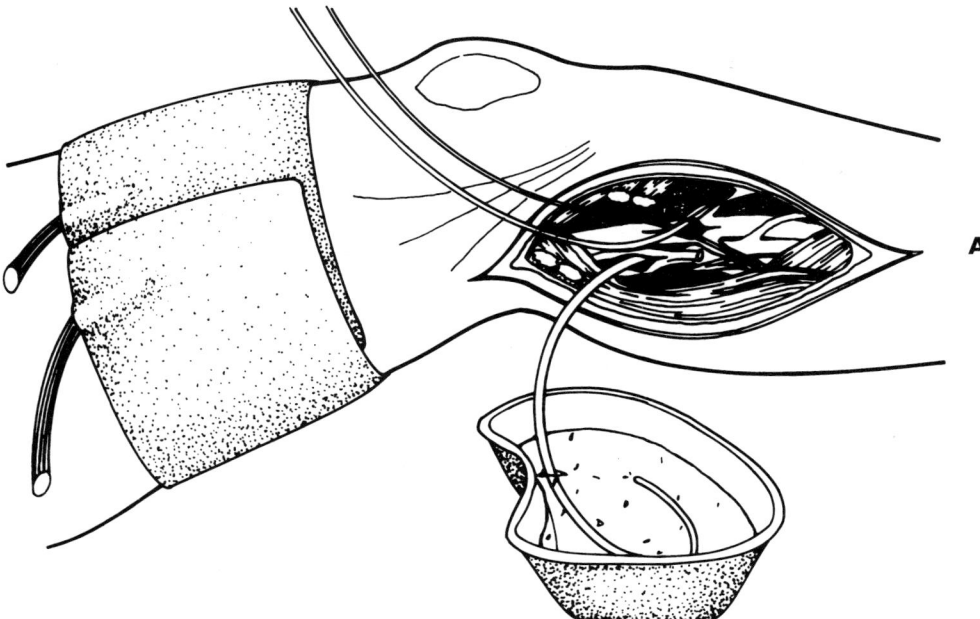

FIGURE 32–7. **A**, High-dose isolated limb perfusion. The patient's limb was elevated and the venous blood exsanguinated with a rubber bandage. A sterile blood-pressure cuff was placed on the distal thigh and inflated to 350 mm Hg. The popliteal vein was cannulated with a red rubber catheter and drained into a basin. One million units of urokinase were dissolved in 1 liter of saline and infused into the lower leg (500,000 IU into each of the anterior and posterior tibial arteries). After completion of the urokinase infusion, the limb was flushed with a heparin-saline solution. The venotomy was closed primarily and the arteriotomy closed with a patch. **B**, Intraoperative angiogram after balloon catheter thrombectomy of the popliteal and tibial vessels after acute embolic/thrombotic occlusion after percutaneous removal of an intraaortic balloon pump (required after emergency coronary artery bypass). Additional thrombus could not be mechanically removed. Catheters were placed into the posterior and anterior tibial arteries, and the arteriogram was obtained with this selective injection technique. There was no evidence of contrast entering the foot. Since no additional thrombus could be retrieved, it was believed that the patient would suffer a major amputation. Patient underwent a high-dose isolated limb perfusion with 1 million units of urokinase as described above. **C**, Postinfusion arteriogram documented significant improvement of perfusion to the foot. The patient had a palpable dorsalis pedis pulse and a pink foot after wound closure. (From Comerota AJ, White JV: Intraoperative intraarterial thrombolytic therapy as an adjunct to revascularization in patients with residual and distal arterial thrombus, *Semin Vasc Surg* 5:116, 1992.)

increased serum cholesterol levels. In the Rochester Trial, plasma fibrinogen concentration decreased during thrombolytic infusion, reaching a nadir of 288 mg/dl (24% below initial concentration) at 24 hours, but it increased in patients randomized to the operative group (Figure 32–8).[33] The patients with acute limb ischemia may be in a procoagulant phase that could be adversely affected by operative intervention, anesthetic use, and wide fluid shifts. In the patients receiving thrombolytic therapy the fibrinogen levels are lowered directly, reperfusion occurs at a slower pace, and the patient may avoid or have a shorter anesthetic exposure resulting from the performance of a less invasive procedure. Patients with higher fibrinogen concentrations may have silent and minor coronary events that manifest as myocar-

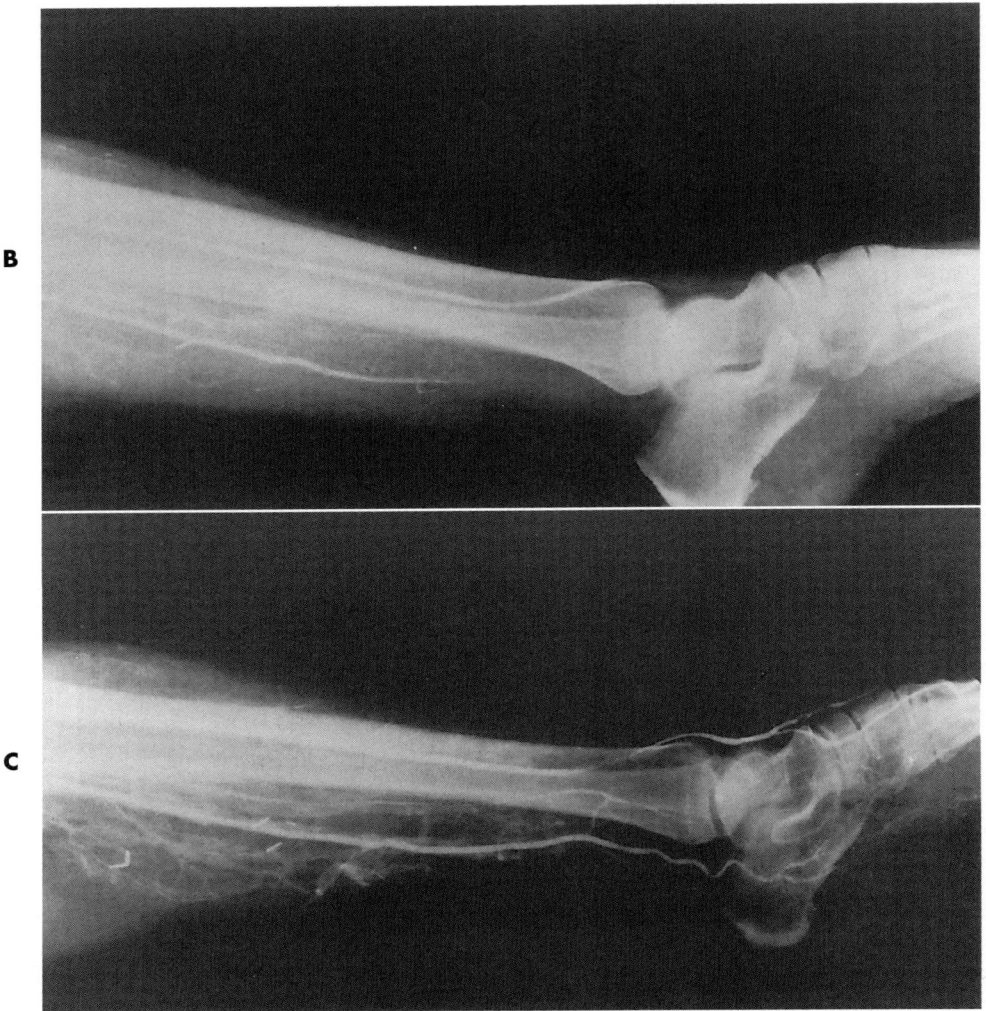

FIGURE 32–7. Continued.

dial infarctions either during their initial hospitalization or as a late event because of the progressive loss of cardiac reserve.

Persistent ischemia of the distal lower extremity despite successful proximal thromboembolectomy has prompted an aggressive use of intraoperative thrombolytic infusions to clear runoff vessels. This technique can be used safely, with bleeding complications associated with the use of heparin anticoagulation in the postoperative period. Despite demanding postoperative management and the need for frequent reoperations required in these patients, the excellent limb salvage rates that can be obtained without an increase in mortality justify the use of this aggressive adjuvant technique.

Popliteal Artery Aneurysms

Although popliteal aneurysm is the most frequently encountered atherosclerotic peripheral artery aneurysm, it is still an uncommon condition. The prevalence is not known, but symptomatic popliteal aneurysms account for 1 in 5000 hospital admissions, with one popliteal aneurysm seen for every 15 abdominal aortic aneurysms.[59] Although rupture is rare, it is asso-

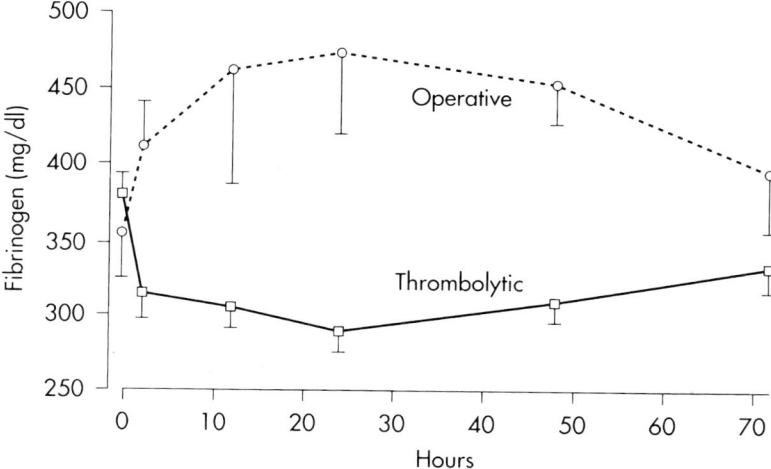

FIGURE 32–8. Patients with acute limb ischemia receiving thrombolytic therapy displayed a gradual decrease in plasma fibrinogen concentration during the period of infusion. This contrasts with the patients on the operative group, who had an increase in their plasma fibrinogen concentration.

ciated with a high incidence of thromboembolic complications and limb loss. Asymptomatic aneurysms when left untreated are associated with a 26% to 50% complication rate, with most occurring within 2 years.[60,61] On the other hand, when reconstruction of popliteal aneurysms is performed, graft patency and limb salvage rates of 64% and 95% at 10 years, respectively, have been achieved.[62]

The role of surgical bypass is accepted for large-diameter (>2 cm) popliteal aneurysms with mural thrombus and for patients who have claudication, digital embolization, and acute limb ischemia. In patients whose symptoms include acute thrombosis, the risk of limb loss depends on the patency status of the tibial vessels.[62] Patients with popliteal aneurysm thrombosis and tibial vessel occlusion were shown to have a 69% amputation rate within 3 years. By contrast, those patients who had patent tibial vessels suffered an amputation rate of only 6% at 6 years. Runoff also affects graft patency; at 3 years extremities with good runoff (> 2 vessels) had an 89% patency.[63] This was significantly better than in extremities with poor runoff (< 2 vessels), which had a patency rate of 40% at 3 years. By 10 years a 64% patency rate was observed in the good runoff group, but no grafts in the poor runoff group were found to be patent.

Not surprisingly, thrombolytic therapy has been used to reopen the outflow tract of acutely thrombosed popliteal aneurysms to improve their clinical outcome. Cotton in 1962 was the first to use streptokinase after a partially successful embolectomy.[64] He used a loading dose of 50,000 units of streptokinase via an intraarterial catheter followed by 56,000 units over the next 5 hours to achieve radiologic clearance to the foot. The first successful use of intraarterial streptokinase for thrombosis of a popliteal artery aneurysm was reported 12 years later by Schwartz, with lysis of the thrombosed aneurysm and outflow tracts being followed by successful grafting the next day.[65] Ferguson treated 10 patients with acute limb ischemia secondary to thrombosed popliteal aneurysms with intraarterial streptokinase. In seven of these patients the correct diagnosis was made only after streptokinase infusion.[66] Limb salvage was achieved in seven patients, five had subsequent bypass procedures, and two were maintained on oral anticoagulation. In another patient, streptokinase initially produced dramatic results with return of the tibial pulse at the ankle, but 24 hours later the pulses disappeared and profound ischemia developed and led to an amputation. Distal embolization resulting from clot and atheroma fragmentation was implicated.

Similar results were achieved by Carpenter in seven patients; in six patients, initial arteriography revealed complete thrombosis of the popliteal artery and runoff vessels.[67] In five of these patients, complete clearing of thrombus from the popliteal artery and runoff vessels was accomplished; and in the sixth patient, popliteal and peroneal artery patency was restored along with reconstitution of the distal posterior and anterior tibial arteries. The last patient had a patent infrageniculate popliteal artery and runoff vessels, but residual intraluminal thrombus was seen in each of these arteries. He was treated with intraoperative thrombolytic therapy with complete clot dissolution. All of these patients underwent successful bypasses without any limb loss or bleeding complications.

The Joint Vascular Research Group reported their experience with thrombolytic therapy in popliteal artery aneurysms in conjunction with acute limb ischemia.[68] Twenty-three patients underwent thrombolysis, with 18 undergoing bypass afterward. Of these bypass patients, 13 were found to be patent at follow-up and five thrombosed, resulting in four amputations. In three recently thrombosed popliteal aneurysms, intraarterial thrombolysis revealed a small aneurysm (<2 cm) with a smooth vessel wall and no residual thrombus. These patients were given long-term anticoagulation and remained well without further intervention. The remaining two patients required above-knee amputation because the runoff could not be cleared by preoperative lysis or by catheter embolectomy.

Approximately 12% of limbs undergoing intraarterial thrombolysis develop distal embolization; these are usually of little clinical consequence and are treated by increasing the rate of administration of the lytic agent or advancing the delivery catheter. However, this complication has been found to be more common during the treatment of thrombosed popliteal aneurysms (13%) than during that of thrombosed arteries (1.5%) or grafts (2.7%).[69] Acute ischemic deterioration of thrombosed popliteal aneurysm undergoing thrombolytic therapy has been treated with emergent catheter thrombectomy supplemented by intraoperative infusion of streptokinase and graft bypass with excellent results in two patients.[70] These investigators also used the same approach in four patients who could not wait for thrombolytic infusion because of severe ischemia. Limb salvage was achieved in all six patients without any bleeding complications or mortalities.

Patients with thrombosed popliteal aneurysms whose presenting symptoms included acute limb ischemia (category II) should undergo diagnostic angiography. If the distal popliteal artery and runoff vessels are thrombosed, a trial infusion of intraarterial urokinase seems prudent. If patency of the popliteal artery and outflow vessels is restored, bypass should be undertaken to the appropriate target vessel (Figure 32-9).

If patency is not restored or ischemia worsens, immediate catheter embolectomy supplemented by intraoperative urokinase therapy and surgical bypass should be performed. In

FIGURE 32-9. **A**, Arteriogram showing thrombus outlined in occluded, large superficial femoral artery proximal to a thrombosed popliteal artery aneurysm. **B**, Arteriogram showing complete lysis of clot and restoration of antegrade flow in the superficial femoral, popliteal, and anterior tibial arteries. These segments had received 4 hours of direct intrathrombus coaxial infusion of urokinase; the still-occluded tibioperoneal trunk had not received intrathrombus infusion. **C**, Arteriogram showing that direct intrathrombus infusion of the tibioperoneal trunk and posterior tibial artery resulted in complete lysis of acute clot. Residual occlusion of distal posterior tibial artery was impenetrable and judged to be due to chronic clot. The anterior tibial artery was demonstrated to be the most suitable vessel for subsequent in situ saphenous vein bypass graft. (From McNamara TD: Thrombolysis as an alternative initial therapy for acutely ischemic lower limb, *Semin Vasc Surg* 5:94, 1992.)

32. Thrombolysis: Peripheral Arterial Applications 477

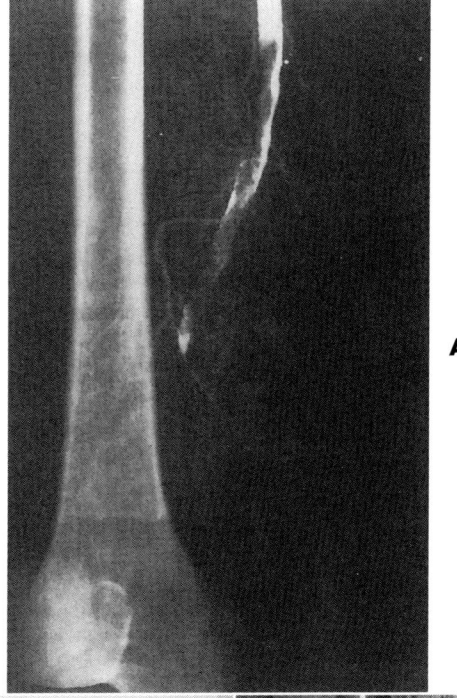

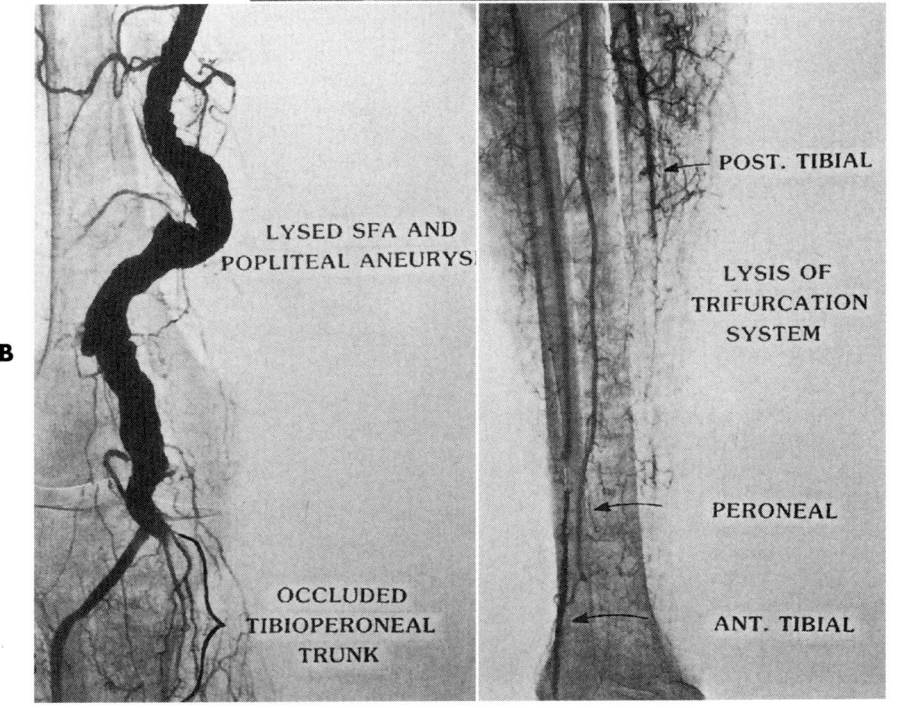

patients with large popliteal aneurysms (>3 cm) and at least one patent runoff vessel, operative thrombectomy along with intraoperative infusion of urokinase is recommended to minimize the risk of distal embolization. Successful thrombolysis of a thrombosed popliteal aneurysm (<2 cm) with a smooth vessel wall and no residual thrombus can be treated with long-term anticoagulation if the patient has underlying co-morbid medical conditions.

Careful patient selection and judicious use of thrombolytic therapy in patients who have thrombosed popliteal aneurysms should be rewarded with a high limb salvage and patency rates.

References

1. Taylor FB Jr, Botts J: Purification and characterization of streptokinase with studies of streptokinase activation of plasminogen, *Biochemistry* 38:1627, 1968.
2. Tillet WS, Garner RL: The fibrinolytic activity of hemolytic streptococci, *J Exp Med* 58:485, 1933.
3. Tillet WS, Sherry S: The effect in patients of streptococcal fibrinolysin (streptokinase) and streptococcal deoxyribonuclease on fibrinous, purulent, and sanguineous pleural exudations, *J Clin Invest* 28:173, 1949.
4. Chesterman CN, Cederholm-Williams SA, Allington MJ: The degradation of streptokinase during the production of plasminogen activator, *Thromb Res* 5:413, 1974.
5. Rubin RN: Choosing a thrombolytic agent in acute myocardial infarction, *Pharmacol Ther* 17:617, 1992.
6. James DC: Antistreptokinase levels in various hospital groups, *Postgrad Med* 49:26, 1973.
7. MacFarlane RG, Pilling J: Fibrinolytic activity in normal urine, *Nature* 159:779, 1947.
8. Williams JRB: The fibrinolytic activity of urine, *Br J Exp Pathol* 32:530–537, 1951.
9. Astrup T, Sterndorff I: An activator of plasminogen in normal urine, *Proc Soc Exp Biol Med* 81:675, 1952.
10. Sobel GW, Mohler SR, Jones NW et al: Urokinase, an activator of profibrinolysin extracted from urine, *Am J Physiol* 171:768–769, 1952.
11. Guenzler WA, Steffens GJ, Oetting F et al: The primary structure of high-molecular-mass urokinase from human urine: the complete amino acid sequence of the A chain, *Hoppe-Seylers Z Physiol Chem* 363:1155, 1982.
12. Verstraete M: Biochemical and clinical aspects of thrombolysis, *Semin Hematol* 15:35, 1978.
13. Ratzkin B, Lee SG, Schrenk WJ et al: Expression in *Escherichia coli* of biologically active enzyme by a DNA sequence coding for the human plasminogen activator urokinase, *Proc Natl Acad Sci USA* 78:3313–3317, 1981.
14. Belkin M, Belkin B, Bucknam CA et al: Intraarterial fibrinolytic therapy: efficacy of streptokinase versus urokinase, *Arch Surg* 121: 769, 1986.
15. Van Breda A, Katzen BT, Deutsch AS: Urokinase versus streptokinase in local thrombolysis, *Radiology* 165:109, 1987.
16. Pennica D, Holmes WE, Kohr WJ et al: Cloning and expression of human tissue-type plasminogen activator cDNA in E. coli, *Nature* 301:214, 1983.
17. Rajput B, Degen SF, Reich et al: Chromosomal locations of human plasminogen activator and urokinase genes, *Science* 230:672, 1985.
18. Hoylaerts M, Rijken DC, Lijnen HR et al: Measurement of human tissue-type plasminogen activator by a two-site immunoradiometric assay, *J Lab Clin Med* 101:274, 1983.
19. TIMI Study Group: The thrombolysis in myocardial infarction (TIMI) trial: phase I findings, *N Engl J Med* 312:932, 1985.
20. Gao S, Morser J, McLean K et al: Differential effect of platelets on plasminogen activation by tissue plasminogen activator, urokinase, and streptokinase, *Thromb Res* 58:421–433, 1990.
21. Clifton EE: The use of plasmin in humans, *Ann NY Acad Sci* 68:209–229, 1957.
22. Dotter CT, Rosch J, Seaman AJ et al: Streptokinase treatment of thromboembolic disease, *Radiology* 102:283–290, 1972.
23. Dotter CT, Rosch J, Seaman AJ: Selective clot lysis with low dose streptokinase, *Radiology* 111:31–37, 1974.
24. Ouriel K, Shortell CK, DeWeese JA et al: A comparison of thrombolytic therapy with operative revascularization in the initial treatment of acute peripheral ischemia, *J Vasc Surg* 19:1021–1030, 1994.
25. Jivegard L, Holm J, Shersten T: The outcome in arterial thrombosis misdiagnosed as arterial embolism, *Acta Chir Scand* 152:251–256, 1986.
26. Plecha FR, Poires WJ: Intraoperative angiography in the immediate assessment of arterial reconstruction, *Arch Surg* 105:902–907, 1972.
27. White GH, White RA, Kopchok GE et al: Angioscopic thromboembolectomy; preliminary obser-

vation with a recent technique, *J Vasc Surg* 7:318–325, 1988.
28. Blaisdell FW, Steele M, Allen RE: Management of acute lower extremity arterial ischemia due to embolism and thrombosis, *Surgery* 84:822–834, 1978.
29. Jivegard L, Holm J, Shersten T: Acute limb ischemia due to arterial embolism or thrombosis, *J Cardiovasc Surg* 29:32–36, 1988.
30. McNamara TO, Bomberger RA, Merchant RF: Intra-arterial urokinase as the initial therapy for acutely ischemic lower limbs, *Circulation* 83(suppl 1):106–119, 1991.
31. Rutherford RB, Flanigan DP, Gupta SK et al: Suggested standards for reports dealing with lower extremity ischemia, *J Vasc Surg* 4:80–94, 1986.
32. Ricotta J: Intra-arterial thrombolysis: a surgical view, *Circulation* 83(suppl 1):120–121, 1991.
33. The STILE Investigators: Results of a prospective randomized trial evaluating surgery versus thrombolysis for ischemia of the lower extremity: the STILE Trial, *Ann Surg* 220:251–268, 1994.
34. Shortell CK, Ouriel K: Thrombolysis in acute peripheral arterial occlusion: predictors of immediate success, *Ann Vasc Surg* 8:59–65, 1994.
35. Ouriel K, Veith FJ, Sasahara AA: Thrombolysis or peripheral arterial surgery: phase I results, *J Vasc Surg* 23:64–73, 1996.
36. Ouriel K, Veith FJ, Sasahara AA et al: A comparison of recombinant urokinase with vascular surgery as the initial treatment for acute arterial occlusion of the legs, *N Engl J Med* 338:1105–1111, 1998.
37. Hoylaerts M, Jijken DC, Lijnen HR, Collen D: Kinetics of the activation of plasminogen by human tissue plasminogen activator: role of fibrin, *J Biol Chem* 257:2912–2919, 1982.
38. Stricker RB, Wong D, Tak Shiu D et al: Activation of plasminogen by tissue plasminogen activator on normal and thrombasthenic platelets: effects on surface proteins and platelet aggregation, *Blood* 68:275–280, 1986.
39. DeMunk GAW, Caspers MPM, Chang GTG et al: Binding of tissue-type plasminogen activator to lysine, lysine analogues, and fibrin fragments, *Biochemistry* 28:7318–7325, 1989.
40. Pannell R, Gurewich V: Pro-urokinase: a study of its stability in plasma and of a mechanism for its selective fibrinolytic effect, *Blood* 67:1215–1223, 1986.
41. Mills JL, Harris EJ, Taylor LM et al: The importance of routine surveillance of distal bypass grafts with duplex scanning: a study of 379 reverse vein grafts, *J Vasc Surg* 12:379–389, 1990.
42. Quinones-Balrich WJ, Prego A, Ucelay-Gomez R et al: Failure of PTFE infrainguinal revascularization: patterns, management, alternatives, and outcome, *Ann Vasc Surg* 5:163–169, 1991.
43. Seabrook DF, Mewissen MW, Schmitt DD et al: Percutaneous intra-arterial thrombolysis in the treatment of thrombosis of lower extremity arterial reconstruction, *J Vasc Surg* 13:646–651, 1991.
44. Gardiner GA, Harrington DP, Koltun W et al: Salvage of occluded arterial bypass grafts by means of thrombolysis, *J Vasc Surg* 13:646–651, 1991.
45. Sullivan KL, Gardiner GA, Kandarpa K et al: Efficacy of thrombolysis in infrainguinal bypass grafts, *Circulation* 83(suppl 1):99–105, 1991.
46. Green RM, Ouriel K, Ricotta JJ et al: Revision of failed infrainguinal bypass grafts: principles of management, *Surgery* 100:646–653, 1986.
47. Hye RJ, Turner C, Valji K et al: Is thrombolysis of occluded popliteal and tibial bypass grafts worthwhile? *J Vasc Surg* 20:588–597, 1994.
48. Garcia R, Saroyan RM, Senkowsky J et al: Intraoperative intra-arterial urokinase infusion as an adjunct to Fogarty catheter embolectomy in acute arterial occlusion, *Surg Gynecol Obstet* 171:971–978, 1990.
49. Quinones-Balrich WJ, Ziomek S, Henderson TC et al: Intraoperative fibrinolytic therapy: experimental evaluation, *J Vasc Surg* 4:229–236, 1986.
50. Bevilacqua MP, Gimbrone: Inducible endothelial functions in inflammation and coagulation, *Semin Thromb Hemost* 13:425–433, 1987.
51. Jacobs GR, Reinisch JF, Puckett C: Microvascular fibrinolysis after ischemia: its relation to vascular patency and tissue survival, *Plast Reconstr Surg* 68:737–741, 1981.
52. Belkin M, Valeri R, Hobson RW: Intraarterial urokinase increases skeletal muscle viability after acute ischemia, *J Vasc Surg* 9:161–168, 1989.
53. Norem RF, Short DH, Kerstein MD: Role of intraoperative fibrinolytic therapy in acute arterial occlusion, *Surg Gynecol Obstet* 167:87–91, 1988.
54. Quinones-Balrich WJ, Baker JD, Busuttil RW et al: Intraoperative infusion of lytic drugs for thrombotic complications of revascularization, *J Vasc Surg* 10:408–417, 1989.
55. Comerota AJ, White JV: Intraoperative, intraarterial thrombolytic therapy as an adjunct to revascularization in patients with residual and

distal arterial thrombus, *Semin Vasc Surg* 5:110–117, 1992.
56. Comerota AJ, White JV, Grosch JD: Intraoperative, intra-arterial thrombolytic therapy for salvage of limbs in patients with distal arterial thrombosis, *Surg Gynecol Obstet* 169:283–289, 1989.
57. Comerota AJ, Rao AK, Throm RC et al: A prospective, randomized, blinded, and placebo-controlled trial of intraoperative intra-arterial urokinase infusion during lower extremity revascularizations: regional and systemic effects, *Ann Surg* 218:534, 1993.
58. Thompson SG, Kienest J, Pyke SDM et al: Hemostatic factors and the risk of myocardial infarction or sudden death in patients with angina pectoris, *New Engl J Med* 332:635–641, 1995.
59. Williams NS: Treatment of asymptomatic popliteal aneurysm: protection at a price, *Br J Surg* 79:731–732, 1992.
60. Gifford RW, Hines EA, James EA: An analysis and follow-up study of 100 popliteal aneurysms, *Surgery* 84:775–783, 1953.
61. Dawson I, van Bockel H, Brand R et al: Popliteal artery aneurysms: long term follow-up of aneurysmal disease and results of surgical management, *J Vasc Surg* 13:398–407, 1991.
62. Bouhoutsos J, Martin P: Popliteal aneurysms: a review of 116 cases, *Br J Surg* 61:469–475, 1974.
63. Shortell CK, DeWeese JA, Ouriel K et al: Popliteal artery aneurysms: a 25 year experience, *J Vasc Surg* 14:771–779, 1991.
64. Cotton LT, Flute PT, Tsapogas MJC: Popliteal artery thrombosis treated with streptokinase, *Lancet* ii:1081–1083, 1962.
65. Schwartz W, Berkowitz H, Taormina V et al: The preoperative use of intra-arterial thrombolysis for a thrombosed popliteal artery aneurysm, *J Cardiovasc Surg* 25:465–468, 1984.
66. Ferguson LJ, Faris I, Robertson A et al: Intra-arterial streptokinase therapy to relieve acute limb ischemia, *J Vasc Surg* 4:205–210, 1986.
67. Carpenter JP, Barker CF, Roberts B et al: Popliteal artery aneurysms: current management and outcome, *J Vasc Surg* 19:65–73, 1994.
68. Varga ZA, Locke-Edmunds JC, Baird RN et al: A multicenter study of popliteal aneurysms, *J Vasc Surg* 20:171–177, 1994.
69. Galland RB, Earnshaw JJ, Baird RN et al: Acute limb deterioration during intra-arterial thrombolysis, *Br J Surg* 80:1118–1120, 1993.
70. Thompson JF, Beard J, Scott DJA et al: Intraoperative thrombolysis in the management of thrombosed popliteal aneurysm, *Br J Surg* 80:858–859, 1993.

33
Combined Surgical and Endovascular Approaches

James May and Geoffrey H. White

Combined surgical and endovascular approaches continue to play an important role in vascular surgery. Despite increasing experience and improvements in technology since the first edition of this book, the combined approach is still required in a significant proportion of endovascular cases. Endovascular procedures are ideally carried out entirely by the intraluminal route. In some situations, however, adjunctive open surgical procedures are required. They may be performed synchronously or sequentially with the endovascular procedure. The areas where this combined surgical and endovascular approach may be used include the treatment of aneurysmal disease, occlusive arterial disease, thrombotic venous disease, and endoscopic techniques. They are summarized in Table 33–1. We present the indications for combined surgical and endovascular approaches and describe how they may best be used.

Combined Surgical and Endovascular Approaches for Aneurysmal Arterial Disease

As of March 1998 we have had experience with 260 clinical cases of endoluminal graft implantation for aneurysm disease.[1–15] The site of the aneurysm was the abdominal aorta ($n = 222$), thoracic aorta ($n = 7$); the iliac ($n = 19$), femoral ($n = 6$), popliteal ($n = 2$), subclavian ($n = 1$), and internal carotid ($n = 1$) arteries; and a vein bypass graft ($n = 2$). Included in this experience are 32 patients who had combined surgical and endovascular approaches in the circumstances listed in the Aneurysmal Disease section of Table 33–1.

Synchronous Approach

Temporary Conduit for Access

The method described by Parodi[16] of using a tubular Dacron graft sutured to the common iliac artery as a temporary conduit to gain access to the aorta is still useful. We have used this technique in 20 of 222 patients undergoing endoluminal repair of abdominal aortic aneurysms (AAAs). The development of more flexible introducing systems of smaller diameter, however, has considerably decreased the need to resort to this maneuver.

Endoluminal Aortoiliac Grafts Combined with Extraluminal Crossover Grafts

A combined extraluminal and endoluminal method of repair (aortoiliac grafts with crossover grafts) remains useful in patients with unilateral iliac artery occlusion or widespread occlusive disease and in patients with extreme iliac tortuosity on one side. We have used this technique in 29 patients, compared with 60 tubular and 133 bifurcated configurations. With the availability of commercially produced,

TABLE 33–1. Summary of Situations in which a Combined Surgical and Endovascular Approach May Be Used

Aneurysmal disease
Synchronous approach
    Dacron tube graft to the common iliac artery used for temporary access to aorta for endoluminal repair of abdominal aortic aneurysms (AAAs) in patients with narrow iliac arteries
    Endoluminal aortoiliac graft combined with an extraluminal crossover graft in complex AAA
    Open AAA repair combined with endoluminal descending thoracic aneurysm repair
    Surgical arteriotomy combined with endoluminal repair of false aneurysms situated in the
        Abdominal aorta
        Internal carotid artery
        Junction of supra- and infrainguinal grafts
    Management of complications of endoluminal repair of AAA by open arterial operations
Sequential approach
    Sequential surgical and endovascular repairs in patients with multiple aneurysmal disease

Occlusive arterial disease
Synchronous approach
    Bypass or endarterectomy combined with
        Angioscopy
        Balloon angioscopy/atherectomy/laser
        Thrombolysis
    In situ bypass with adjunctive endovascular manipulation
    Endoluminal bypass
    Surgical exposure/endarterectomy combined with stent deployment at a remote site
        Common femoral endarterectomy and aortic stent deployment
        Right common carotid arteriotomy and brachiocephalic stent deployment
Sequential approach
    Balloon angioplasty followed by bypass
        Femorofemoral
        Femorodistal

Venous disease
    First rib resection followed by thrombolysis in subclavian vein thrombosis

Endoscopic treatment
    Thoroscopic dorsal sympathectomy
    Endoscopic ligation of incompetent perforating veins

second-generation prostheses it is no longer necessary to use the complicated aortoiliac techniques described in the first edition of this book.

Open AAA Repair Combined with Endoluminal Descending Thoracic Aneurysm Repair

Dake and his colleagues at Stanford now have treated 121 patients by endoluminal repair of their thoracic aneurysms.[17] In 27 of these patients the procedure was combined with open repair of AAA. Sixty-four patients are now 1 year or more from operation and have either a stable or decreasing aneurysm diameter. The incidence of paraplegia was commendably low at 4%. It is important to note that each of the four patients who developed paraplegia had had a prior AAA repair.

Surgical Arteriotomy Combined with Endoluminal Repair of False Aneurysms

False Aneurysm in Abdominal Aorta

An 80-year-old male patient presented with a large anastomotic aneurysm at the superior end of an aortic graft (Figure 33–1A). The patient had had an AAA repaired by open operation using a bifurcated Dacron graft. He was unfit for open repair of the anastomotic aneurysm because of severe respiratory

33. Combined Surgical and Endovasculer Approaches

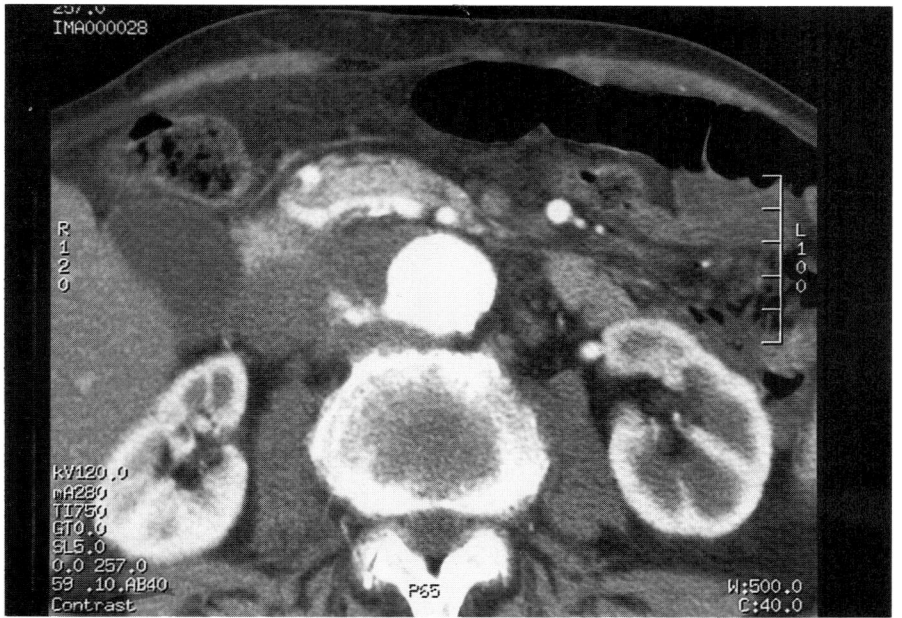

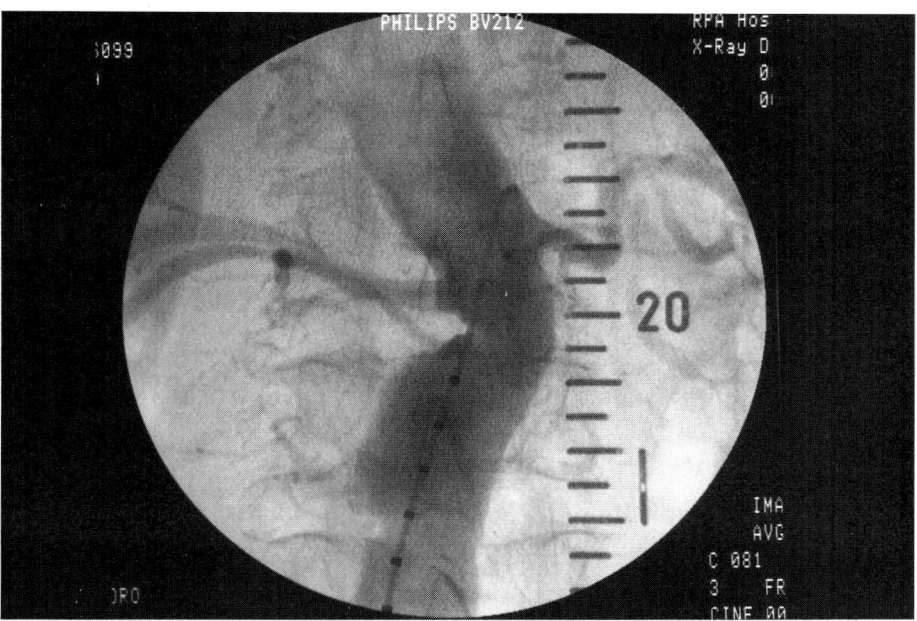

FIGURE 33–1. **A**, Contrast CT demonstrating anastomotic aortic aneurysm between the renal arteries and previous bifurcated aortic graft implanted previously by open operation. **B**, Aortogram demonstrating a short cuff of normal aorta between the renal arteries and anastomotic aneurysm. The aneurysm was successfully excluded from the circulation by deployment of an endoluminal bifurcated graft within the existing bifurcated graft implanted at a previous open operation. (From May J, White G, Waugh R, and Brennan J: Endoluminal repair of internal carotid artery aneurysm: a feasible but hazardous procedure. Journal of Vascular Surgery 1977;26(6):1055–1060.)

impairment. A surgical arteriotomy was used to obtain access for endoluminal repair. Under more favorable circumstances, an endoluminal cuff would have been sufficient to exclude the anastomotic aneurysm. In this case, however, the length of normal aorta between the renal arteries and the anastomotic aneurysm was less than 1 cm (Figure 33–1B). A bifurcated endoluminal prosthesis was chosen to give column strength to the superior end of the device and minimize the chances of migration in the presence of a short proximal neck. The endoluminal bifurcated prosthesis was successfully deployed within the bifurcated graft previously implanted at open operation. Postoperative contrast computed tomography (CT) confirmed exclusion of the anastomotic aneurysm.

False Aneurysm in Internal Carotid Artery

A 70-year-old male patient presented with a golfball-size pulsatile swelling in the right side of his neck 22 years after carotid endarterectomy. Contrast CT demonstrated a 3-cm aneurysm containing a large amount of thrombus in the right internal carotid artery. Because the aneurysm extended to within 2 cm from the base of the skull and manipulation of the aneurysm at open operation was likely to produce distal embolization, the endoluminal method was chosen for repair. Surgical arteriotomy of the common carotid artery immediately above the clavicle was used to provide access for a Passager endograft (Figure 33–2). Successful exclusion of the aneurysm sac from the circulation was achieved (Figure 33–3), but the patient experienced a perioperative embolic stroke, resulting in paralysis of the left arm. Return of movement commenced 1 hour after operation. One month after operation power had returned to normal, but coordination for fine movements was still absent. Duplex scans at 6 months confirmed continued exclusion of the aneurysm sac from the circulation in addition to thrombosis of the endograft. We concluded from this experience that endoluminal repair of aneurysms in the carotid arteries is feasible but hazardous.

False Aneurysm at the Junction of Supraintimal and Infraintimal Grafts

A 78-year-old male patient presented with a large (8 cm diameter) false aneurysm in the

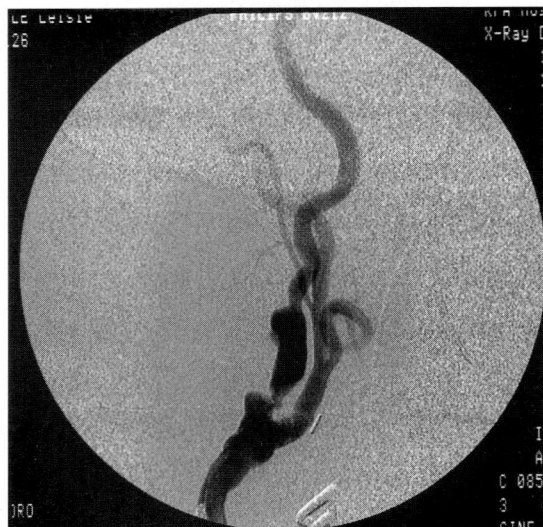

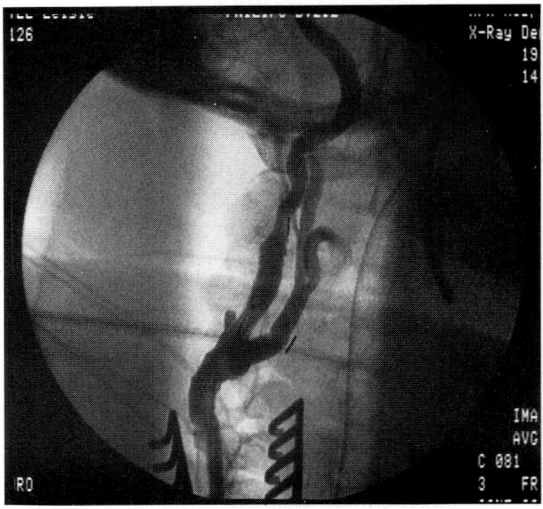

FIGURE 33–2 **A**, On-table preprocedure arteriogram of a 3 cm diameter aneurysm of the right internal carotid artery demonstrating an irregular lumen due to intraluminal thrombus. **B**, On-table postprocedure arteriogram demonstrating exclusion of the aneurysm sac and flow through the endoluminal graft. (From May J, White G, Waugh R, and Brennan J: Endoluminal repair of internal carotid artery aneurysm: a feasible but hazardous procedure. Journal of Vascular Surgery 1977;26(6):1055–1060.)

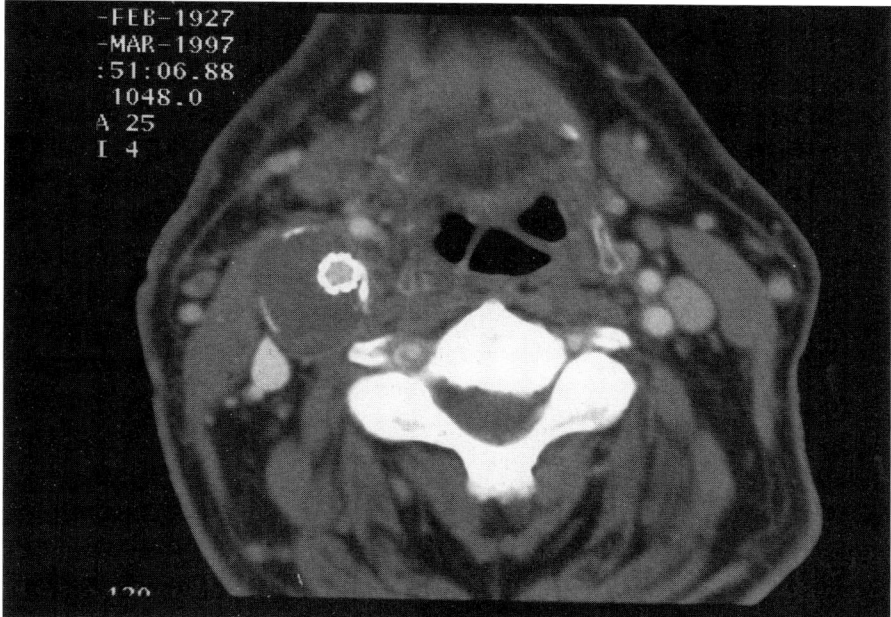

FIGURE 33–3 Postoperative CT demonstrating exclusion of the aneurysm sac from the circulation. Note the calcifications at 3, 8, and 11 o'clock positions, which were also present on the preoperative scans.

right groin. He was experiencing increasing pain from the enlarging aneurysm. Angiography demonstrated that the aneurysm was situated at the junction of the right limb of a previous aortobifemoral graft and a femoral artery bypass graft to the popliteal artery. There was no communication with the underlying common femoral artery. The femoral artery bypass was exposed surgically in the midthigh to obtain access for endoluminal repair. A Passager endograft was used to exclude the aneurysm sac, which resulted in complete relief of the patient's symptoms. Thrombosis occurred in the endograft during the second postoperative week, but the collateral circulation was sufficient to maintain viability of the limb without requiring further intervention.

Management of Complications of Endoluminal Repair of AAA by Open Arterial Operations

Peripheral Embolization

Peripheral embolization has occurred in four patients undergoing endoluminal repair of AAA. Preoperative contrast CT demonstrated thrombus in the proximal neck of the aneurysm, which was considered to be responsible for the peripheral embolization. A surgical embolectomy was required in one patient. Minor skin manifestations in the remainder required no surgical intervention.

Iliac Artery Dissection Requiring Iliofemoral Bypass

In addition to the two patients requiring iliofemoral bypass for perforation of the external iliac arteries reported in the first edition, we have seen dissection of the external iliac artery in four patients. They were treated by iliofemoral bypass, which achieved the dual function of providing access to the aorta for endoluminal AAA repair and revascularization of the ipsilateral limb.

Hand Suturing of the Distal End of an Endoluminal AAA Endograft

Following successful deployment of an aorto-uniiliac endograft, the delivery catheter became incarcerated within the external iliac artery due to a broken steel wire becoming impaled in the arterial wall and acting as an anchor. It was managed via an extraperitoneal incision, which allowed the delivery catheter to be released, and the distal endograft was sutured by hand to the external iliac artery.

Surgical Exposure of the Common Femoral Artery to Enable Endoluminal Repair of Secondary Endoleaks

We have observed secondary endoleaks resulting from distraction of component parts of a modular prosthesis on five occasions (Figure 33–4). They were treated by surgical exposure of the common femoral artery, enabling a further tubular endograft to be positioned between the distracted components of the existing modular endograft (Figure 33–5). It resulted in reexclusion of the aneurysm sac from the circulation.

Sequential Approach

In addition to the four patients who had undergone an aborted attempt at open AAA repair and one patient who had undergone a successful AAA repair with residual large aneurysms of the common iliac arteries reported in the first edition of this book, we have used sequential endoluminal and open surgical approaches in the following situations.

1. Endoluminal AAA repair followed by subsequent open repair for ruptured AAA in four patients. These patients had known endoleaks and were being observed in the hope of spontaneous sealing of the endoleak. All survived open repair.

2. Limb occlusion following endoluminal AAA repair. We have observed occlusion of the limb of an endograft in four patients following endoluminal repair. All were treated by femorofemoral crossover grafts rather than thrombolysis.

3. Operation for sigmoid volvulus following endoluminal AAA repair. One patient

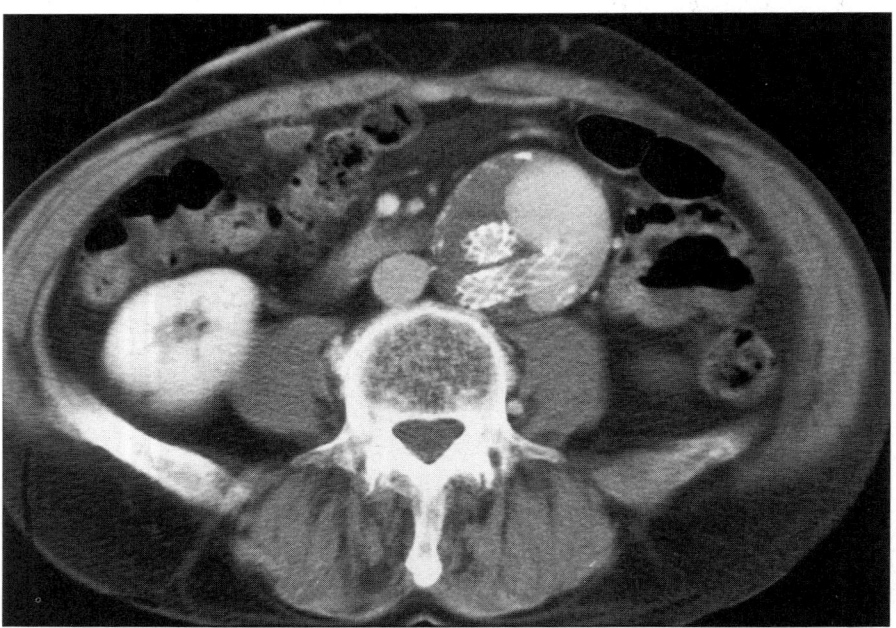

FIGURE 33–4 Contrast CT demonstrating normal vertical right limb of bifurcated graft and horizontal contralateral limb with associated endoleak. (From Whitmore AD, Bandyk D, Cronenwett J, Hertzner N, and White RA, Eds: Endoleak–a complication unique to endovascular grafting. Advances in Vascular Surgery. St. Louis, Mosby (in press).)

33. Combined Surgical and Endovasculer Approaches

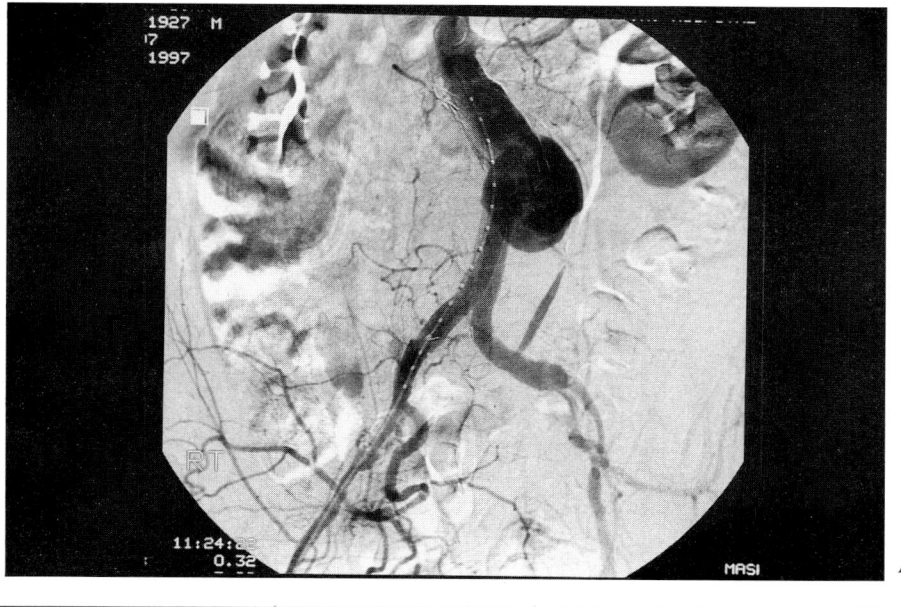

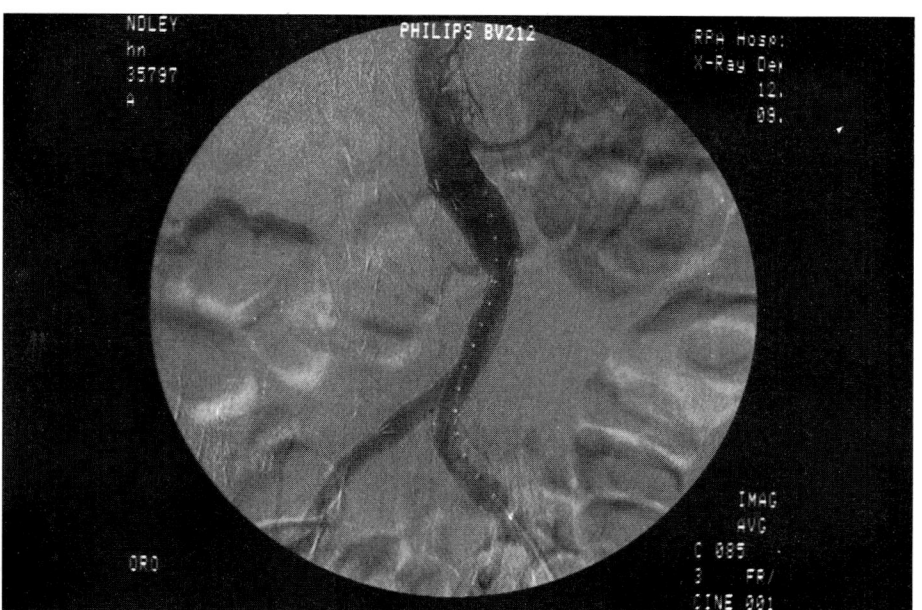

FIGURE 33–5 On-table preprocedure aortogram confirming an endoleak resulting from dislocation of the contralateral limb from the contralateral stump. **B**, On-table postprocedure aortogram demonstrating exclusion of the aneurysm sac following deployment of an intersegmental endograft between the contralateral stump and contralateral limb. (From Whitmore AD, Bandyk D, Cronenwett J, Hertzner N, and White RA, Eds: Endoleak–a complication unique to endovascular grafting. Advances in Vascular Surgery. St. Louis, Mosby (in press).)

re-presented to another hospital 3 weeks after successful endoluminal AAA repair with an acute abdomen. Surgical intervention was undertaken, but the patient died during the perioperative period.

Combined Surgical and Endovascular Approaches for Occlusive Arterial Disease

Synchronous Approach

Bypass procedures or endarterectomy for occlusive arterial disease may be combined with a number of endovascular procedures. Despite the common use of radiologic guidance it has become increasingly obvious that the two-dimensional vessel outline given by this method is limited in its efficacy for accurate representation of intraluminal pathology. Angioscopy may be used to increase the accuracy of characterization of lesions and enhance the selection of treatment options. The ability to make the important distinction between obstruction resulting from embolus, thrombus, or atherosclerotic plaque may be assisted by operative angioscopy. This modality may also be used to monitor the adequacy of the distal anastomosis and runoff at the completion of bypass grafts. It is particularly useful for assessing the adequacy of thrombectomy in thrombosed bypass grafts.

Synchronous percutaneous transluminal angioplasty (PTA) and surgical lower limb revascularization have been recommended for multilevel occlusive disease.[18,19] Various atherectomy devices and laser probes have been used during infrainguinal bypass procedures in an attempt to improve the outcome.[20] The administration of intraarterial thrombolytic agents at operation has also been used successfully for this purpose.[21,22]

A number of adjunctive endovascular procedures have been used in combination with in situ saphenous vein bypass. They have ranged from angioscopy to monitor valve disruption[23–25] to the endoluminal insertion of coil springs to obliterate the tributaries.[26] Miller and coworkers reported that by adopting angioscopic technique for direct visual control of valve division during in situ procedures they were able to reduce the incidence of retained valve leaflets from 18.9% (using the "blind" technique) to 0%. At the same time, the incidence of observed valvulotome injury to the vein wall was decreased from 85.0% during the blind technique to 15.6% by the angioscopic technique.[23]

Angioscopy has also been advocated as a technique for checking the result of extended semiclosed endarterectomy of the aortoiliac and femoral arteries.[27,28] Semiclosed procedures may be performed with the knowledge that lumen irregularities, intimal flaps and dissections, residual atherosclerotic plaque, thrombus, and inadequate or raised endpoints may be detected immediately and corrected while the vessels are still open.[27]

Endoscopic intravascular surgery, such as angioscopically guided intravascular removal of intimal flaps, dissections, and thrombus using flexible grasping forceps and other instruments, may be achieved in selected patients during percutaneous interventions or intraoperatively.[29] The use of vascular endoscopy has introduced the possibility of such intravascular interventions under direct vision, providing immediate assessment of the result. Removal of thrombogenic arterial dissections and flaps of the iliac, femoral, and popliteal arteries by flexible forceps, introduced remotely via the femoral artery under angioscopic control, was reported in a series of patients with traumatic intimal flaps of the femoropopliteal or iliac arteries (either iatrogenic or as a result of external trauma).[29] In addition, tightly adherent arterial thrombi were removed with flexible biopsy forceps in 17 of 154 (11%) patients who had undergone angioscopic monitoring of thromboembolectomy of native arteries or bypass grafts.

Transluminal Insertion of Endoluminal Grafts or Coated Stents in Peripheral Arteries

An emerging alternative technique for treating occlusive disease of peripheral arteries—transluminal insertion of endoluminal grafts or coated stents—blends an operative arteriotomy and remote endovascular intervention, followed by transluminal implantation of a vascular graft, to minimize the extent of surgery. The use of stented grafts or endoluminal prosthetic grafts has been reported for treatment of peripheral artery pseudoaneurysms, popliteal aneurysms, arteriovenous fistulas, and femoropopliteal occlusions.[8,16,30–36]

Endoluminal femoropopliteal or iliofemoral "bypass" may be performed via exposure of the common or superficial femoral artery or by the percutaneous approach.[35] The small incisions required for surgical approach allow use of local anesthesia.[36] The occluded arterial segment is recanalized by guidewire and angioplasty balloon (or alternative endovascular devices), and the lumen is then lined internally by a graft, usually supported at each end or along its entire length by stents. Overdilatation of the treated segment may help accomodate the graft, and self-expanding covered stents or balloon-expandable stent-graft devices may be deployed. This technique is in an early experimental phase. It is not clear whether it is advantageous to remove all atheromatous material from the lumen rather than simply dilating it, and as yet there is no evidence that this technique conveys better long-term patency than simply using a conventional arterial stent.

Surgical Exposure/Endarterectomy Combined with Stent Deployment at a Remote Site

Common Femoral Endarterectomy and Aortic Stent Deployment

Two patients with severe aortic stenosis and advanced occlusive disease in the common femoral arteries were treated by common femoral endarterectomy, which allowed access for balloon dilatation and stent deployment in the aorta at the site of the stenosis (Figure 33–6). A disabling short distance claudication that had been present preoperatively was relieved in both. Care was taken during deployment of the stent in the patient with a large inferior mesenteric artery to avoid stenting over the origin of this artery or interfering with the blood flow through it.

Right Common Carotid Arteriotomy and Brachiocephalic Stent Deployment

A female patient who presented with right arm fatigue and subclavian steal syndrome due to a tight stenosis in the brachiocephalic artery was treated by open arteriotomy of the right common carotid artery and stent deployment in the brachiocephalic artery (Figure 33–7). Despite care being taken to flush out any debris following stent deployment, the patient developed weakness of the contralateral arm on the second postoperative day. Contrast CT confirmed the patency of the stent and the absence of mural thrombus.

Comment

These three cases demonstrate the utility of combining stent deployment with an open surgical approach. In the first two patients a laparotomy was avoided, and in the third patient a thoracotomy was avoided.

Sequential Approach

Symptomatic occlusive disease of the iliac arteries was originally managed by aortoiliac and aortofemoral bypass or endarterectomy. The significant morbidity and mortality of these procedures, particularly for high-risk patients, led to a search for alternative procedures: Extraanatomic crossover bypass and PTA. A patient with symptomatic unilateral iliac artery occlusion with contralateral iliac artery stenosis cannot be managed by PTA or femorofemoral bypass alone. Porter et al.[37] achieved successful limb salvage by combining the procedures and dilating the iliac stenosis before femorofemoral bypass. Kadir and his colleagues[38] reported 12 patients treated by combined iliac PTA and femorofemoral bypass in their experience with PTA as an adjunct to the surgical management of peripheral arterial disease. We have also reported our experience with PTA of contralateral iliac stenosis and extraanatomic bypass of the occluded iliac artery.[39] Thirty-one patients were treated, and a

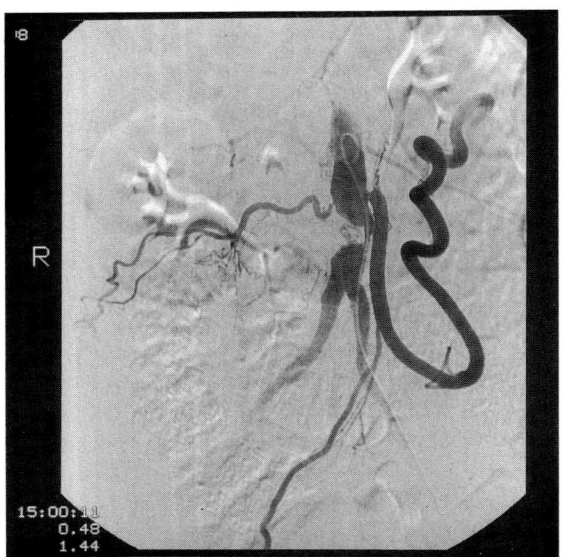

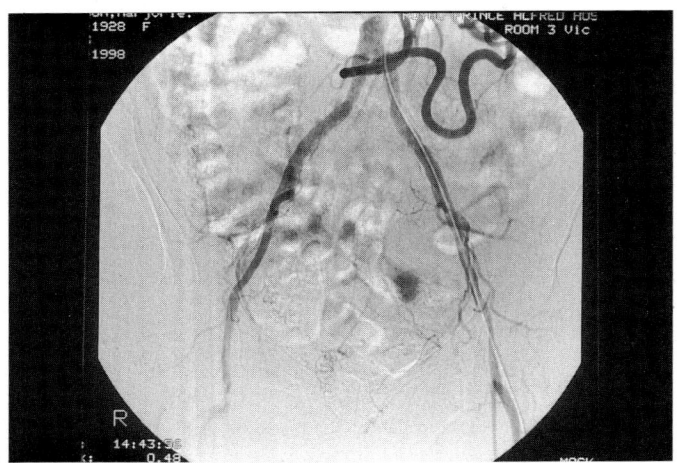

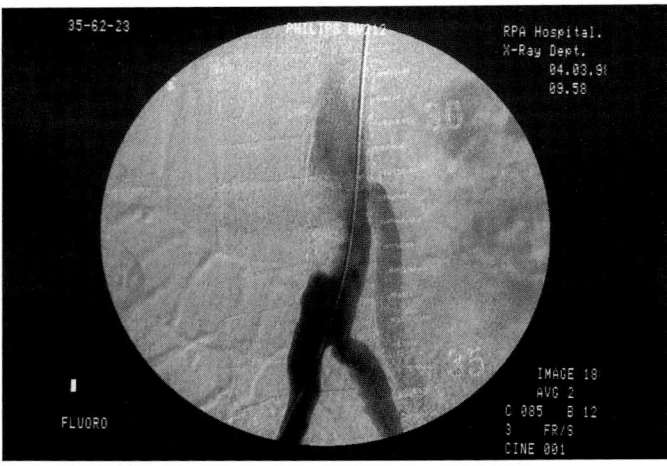

FIGURE 33–6 **A**, Aortogram demonstrating a tight stenosis in the abdominal aorta. Note the enlarged inferior mesenteric artery supplying the marginal artery of the left colon. **B**, Aortogram demonstrating comparatively normal iliac arteries and tubular stenosis in the right common femoral artery. **C**, On-table aortogram following balloon dilatation of aortic stenosis. Access was obtained during open operation on right common femoral artery. **D**, On-table aortogram following deployment of a self-expanding Wallstent in the distal aorta. **E**, Postprocedure aortogram demonstrating restoration of the aortic lumen and maintenance of inflow into the inferior mesenteric artery.

FIGURE 33-6. *Continued.*

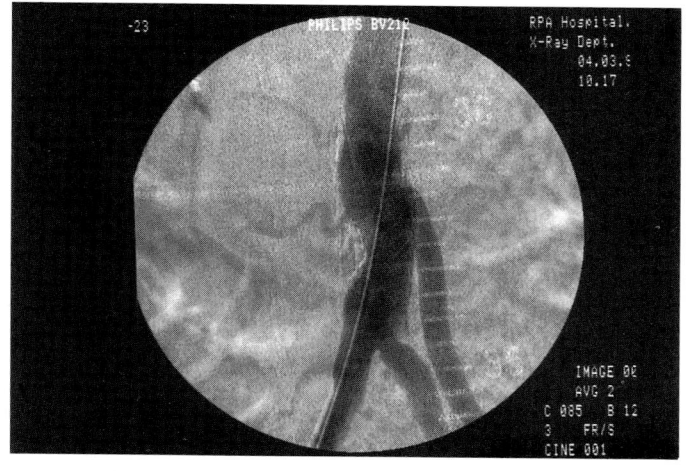

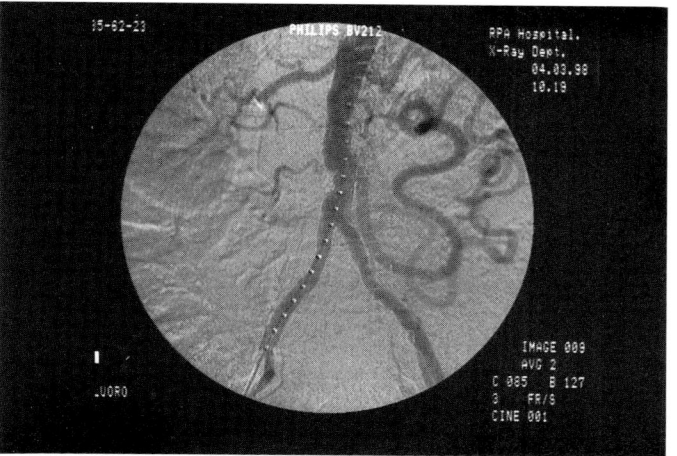

cumulative primary graft patency rate of 89% at 1 year and 81% at 3 years was achieved. The mean resting ankle-brachial systolic pressure index increased significantly on the side of the iliac occlusion from 0.35 ± 0.21 to 0.70 ± 0.20 ($p < 0.05$) after the combined procedure. During the same period (1980 to 1988) 90 patients underwent aortobifemoral or aortobiiliac grafts for occlusive iliac artery disease, and 164 patients had femorofemoral bypass grafts without preceding iliac artery dilatation. The combination of iliac PTA and extraanatomic bypass has several advantages compared with aortobifemoral bypass. The operation can readily be performed under regional anesthesia and takes less time to perform than the aortobifemoral bypass. The hemodynamic changes associated with aortic cross-clamping are avoided. Postoperative ileus and respiratory complications are minimized, and sexual function is not imperiled.

Multisegment arterial occlusive disease involving the iliac arteries and infrainguinal arteries may also be managed by iliac PTA followed by infrainguinal bypass on the ipsilateral limb with the same advantages mentioned previously. This combination has been identified as one of the strategies contributing to the improved limb salvage rate seen with modern vascular surgery.[40] As noted by Brewster and his colleagues,[41] many vascular surgeons remain hesitant to carry out an infrainguinal arterial reconstruction based on inflow established by iliac PTA, especially if the PTA was recent. We

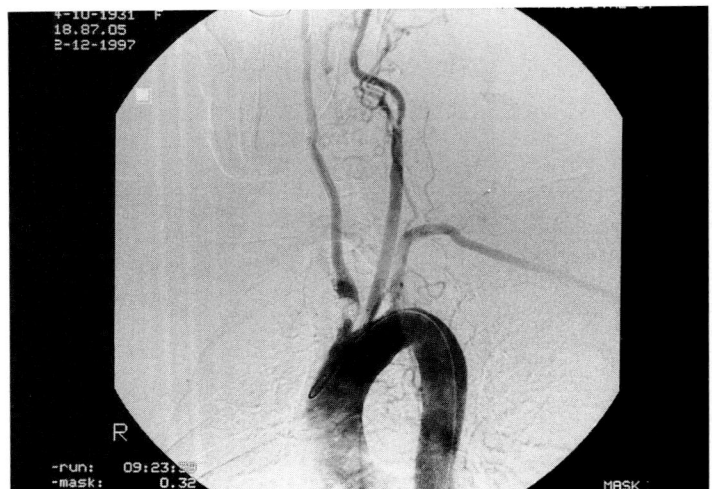

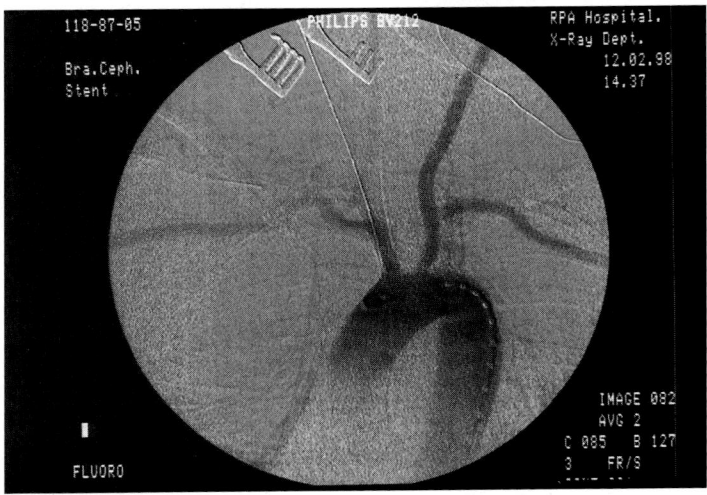

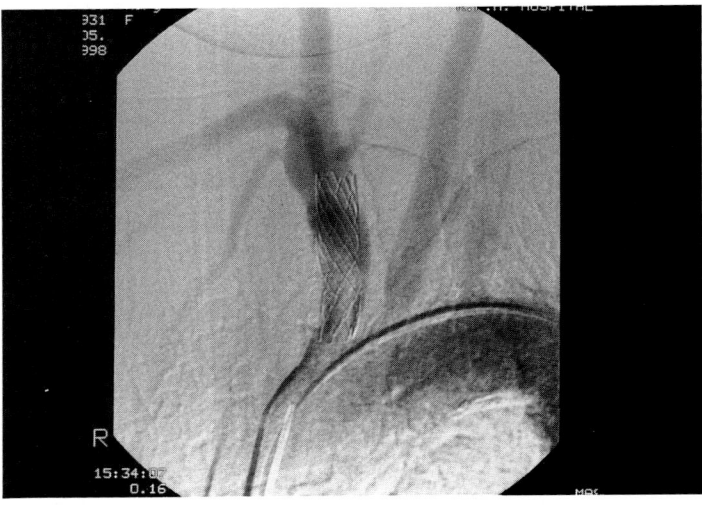

FIGURE 33–7 **A**, Aortogram demonstrating a tight stenosis in the brachiocephalic trunk. **B**, A guidewire has been passed via an arteriotomy in the right common carotid artery through the brachiocephalic stenosis enabling balloon dilatation to be performed. A pigtail catheter from the groin was used to monitor the brachiocephalic interventions. **C**, Aortogram demonstrating restoration of the brachiocephalic lumen by deployment of a self-expanding Wallstent that was introduced through the common carotid arteriotomy.

reviewed our experience over a 10-year period in which 66 patients with iliac artery stenosis and occlusion of the ipsilateral superior femoral artery were treated by iliac PTA and infrainguinal bypass.[42] The 4-year primary and secondary patency of the bypass graft was 65% by life table analysis. The early graft failure rate was significantly higher if the bypass followed PTA within 2 days. We concluded that for selected patients acceptable patency with low morbidity could be obtained with the combined procedures.

Combined Surgical and Endovascular Approaches for Subclavian Vein Thrombosis

Subclavian vein thrombosis following repetitive compression at the thoracic outlet has been recognized for years. Traditionally it has been treated by continuous infusion of heparin for 7 to 10 days with or without oral anticoagulation for the following 3 months. Thrombolytic agents have also been infused into the veins of the arm in an attempt to lyse the clot. Thrombolytic therapy has been combined with surgical excision of the first rib and any associated fibrous band causing compression of the subclavian vein.

The steps in this combined protocol are as follows. Coagulation studies are performed initially followed by a continuous intravenous infusion of heparin to prevent propagation of the thrombus. The diagnosis is confirmed by venogram. This step is followed by intravenous infusion of urokinase with the arm elevated and in a forward position. Sequential venograms are performed until lysis is complete. With completion of lysis, intravenous heparin is given until surgical decompression of the thoracic outlet and subclavian vein is undertaken. Oral anticoagulation is maintained for the following 3 months. We have used this combined mode of treatment with only moderate success in nine patients. Although initial patency of the subclavian vein was achieved in seven patients, long-term patency following thoracic outlet decompression was maintained in three patients.

Because of unsatisfactory results from the above protocol we have modified it in the following way during the past year. Patients are treated initially by continuous infusion of heparin but undergo resection of the first rib and any associated anomalies at the first available operating time. Thrombolysis is commenced 24 to 48 hours later. Any associated intraluminal pathology such as stenosis is dealt with following lysis of the clot. Oral anticoagulation is maintained for 3 months. As yet, the numbers are too small and follow-up is too short to say if this modification is an improvement on the earlier protocol.

Endoscopic Techniques

Endoscopic techniques represent a merging of surgical and endovascular approaches. Thorocoscopic dorsal sympathectomy has represented a major advance in sympathetic denervation of the upper extremity. We have performed this procedure on 187 occasions in 95 patients between 1992 and 1998. Finger sudorometry was used to confirm the completeness of sympathetic denervation.[43] Morbidity was restricted to pneumothorax, requiring chest tube reinsertion in two patients.

We have also subjected endoscopic ligation of perforating veins to trial in patients with the postphlebitic syndrome and leg ulceration. The procedure is feasible and avoids making an incision in skin and subcutaneous tissue with poor healing potential.

References

1. May J, White GH, Yu W et al: Results of endoluminal grafting of abdominal aortic aneurysm are dependent on aneurysm morphology, *Ann Vasc Surg* 10:254–261, 1996.
2. May J, White G, Yu W et al: Treatment of complex abdominal aneurysms by a combination of endoluminal and extraluminal aorto-femoral grafts, *J Vasc Surg* 19:924–933, 1994.
3. May J, White G, Yu W et al: Transluminal placement of aorto-iliac grafts for treatment of large abdominal aortic aneurysms. In Weimann S, editor: *Thoracic and thoracoabdominal aortic aneurysm,* Bologna, 1994, Monduzzi Editore.

4. May J, White G, Yu W et al: Endoluminal stent-grafts for intrathoracic and abdominal aortic aneurysm. In Liermann DD, Kollath J, editors: *Stents—state of the art—proceedings of international stent symposium 3*, Boston, 1994, Boston Scientific.
5. May J, White G, Waugh R et al: Advantages and limitations of intraluminal grafts for thoracic and abdominal aortic aneurysm [abstract], *Angiology* 44(suppl):21, 1993.
6. May J, White G, Waugh R et al: Endoluminal repair of large and small abdominal aortic aneurysm [abstract], *J Intervent Cardiol* 7:109, 1994.
7. May J, White G, Yu W et al: Importance of graft configuration in outcome of endoluminal aortic aneurysm repair: a five year analysis by life table method, *Eur J Vasc Endovasc Surg* (in press).
8. May J, White G, Waugh R et al: Transluminal placement of a prosthetic graft-stent device for treatment of subclavian aneurysm, *J Vasc Surg* 18:1056–1059, 1993.
9. White GH, Yu W, May J: Experimental endoluminal grafts and coated stents [abstract], *Angiology* 4(suppl): 26, 1993.
10. White GH, May J, Yu W: Stented and nonstented grafts for aneurysmal disease: the Sydney experience. In Chuter T, Donayre C, White R, editors: *Endoluminal vascular prostheses*, Boston, 1994, Little, Brown.
11. White GH, Yu W, May J et al: A new non stented endoluminal graft for straight or bifurcated repair of aneurysms, *J Endovasc Surg* 1:16–24, 1994.
12. White GH, May J, McGahan T et al: Historic control comparison of outcome for endoluminal versus open repair of abdominal aortic aneurysms, *J Vasc Surg* 23:201–212, 1996.
13. May J, White GH, Waugh RC et al: Endoluminal repair of abdominal aortic aneurysms, *Med J Aust* 161:541–543, 1994.
14. May J, White GH, Yu W et al: Endoluminal grafting of abdominal aortic aneurysms: causes of failure and their prevention, *J Endovasc Surg* 1:44–52, 1994.
15. May J, White GH, Yu W et al: Concurrent comparison of endoluminal versus open repair in the treatment of abdominal aortic aneurysms: analysis of 303 patients by life table method, *J Vasc Surg* 27:213–222, 1998.
16. Parodi JC: Endovascular repair of abdominal aortic aneurysms. In Whittemore A, editor: *Advances in vascular surgery*, St Louis, 1993, Mosby.
17. Kee S: Stanford experience of endoluminal repair of thoracic aneurysms. Presented at Critical issues in endovascular surgery, Nottingham, January 22–23, 1998.
18. Lowman BG, Queral LA, Holbrook WA et al: Transluminal angioplasty during vascular reconstructive procedures, *Arch Surg* 116:829, 1981.
19. Pfeiffer R Jr, String ST: Adjunctive use of the balloon dilatation catheter during vascular reconstructive procedures, *J Vasc Surg* 3(6):84, 1986.
20. Lorenzi G, Domanin M, Costantini A: PTA and laser assisted PTA combined with simultaneous surgical revascularization, *J Cardiovasc Surg (Torino)* 32:456, 1991.
21. Quinones-Baldrich WJ, Baker D, Busuttil RW et al: Intraoperative infusion of lytic drugs for thrombotic complications of revascularization, *J Vasc Surg* 13:646–651, 1991.
22. Comerota AJ, White JV, Groshe JD: Intraoperative intra-arterial thrombolytic therapy for salvage of limbs in patients with distal arterial thrombosis, *Surg Gynecol Obstet* 169:283–289, 1989.
23. Miller A, Stonebridge PA, Tsoukas AI et al: Angioscopically directed valvulotomy: a new valvulotome and technique, *J Vasc Surg* 13:813–821, 1991.
24. Fleisher HL, Thompson BW, McCowan TC et al: Angioscopically monitored saphenous vein valvulotomy, *J Vasc Surg* 4:360–364, 1986.
25. LaMuraglia GM, Cambria RP, Brewster DC et al: Angioscopy guided semiclosed technique for in situ bypass, *J Vasc Surg* 12:601–604, 1990.
26. Cikrit DF, Dalsing MC, Lalka SG et al: Early results of endovascular assisted in situ saphenous vein bypass grafting, *J Vasc Surg* 19:778–787, 1994.
27. Vollmar JF, Storz LW: Vascular endoscopy possibilities and limits of its clinical application, *Surg Clin North Am* 54:111–122, 1974.
28. Vollmar JF, Loeprecht H, Utschenreiter S: Advances in vascular endoscopy, *Thorac Cardiovasc Surg* 35:334–341, 1987.
29. White GH, White RA, Kopchok GE et al: Endoscopic intravascular surgery removes intraluminal flaps, dissections and thrombus, *J Vasc Surg* 11:280–286, 1990.
30. Parodi JC, Barone HD, Schonholz C: Transfemoral endovascular treatment of aortoiliac aneurysms and arteriovenous fistulas with stented Dacron grafts. In Veith FJ, editor: *Current critical problems in vascular surgery*, St Louis, 1993, Quality Medical Publishing.

31. Parodi JC, Palmaz JC, Barone HD: Transfemoral intraluminal graft implantation for abdominal aortic aneurysms, *Ann Vasc Surg* 5:491–499, 1991.
32. Becker GJ et al: Percutaneous placement of a balloon-expandable intraluminal graft for life-threatening subclavian arterial hemorrhage, *J Vasc Interv Radiol* 2:225–229, 1991.
33. Marin ML, Veith FJ, Panetta TF et al: Percutaneous transfemoral insertion of a stented graft to repair a traumatic femoral arteriovenous fistula, *J Vasc Surg* 18:299–302, 1993.
34. Marin ML, Veith FJ, Panetta TF et al: Transfemoral endoluminal stented graft repair of a popliteal artery aneurysm, *J Vasc Surg* 19:754–757, 1994.
35. Cragg AH, Dake MD: Percutaneous femoropopliteal graft placement, *Radiology* 187:643–648, 1993.
36. Marin ML, Veith FJ, Cynamon J et al: Transfemoral endovascular stented graft treatment of aorto-iliac and femoropopliteal occlusive disease for limb salvage, *Am J Surg* 168:156–162, 1994.
37. Porter JM, Eidemiller LR, Dotter CT et al: Combined arterial dilatation and femorofemoral bypass for limb salvage, *Surg Gynecol Obstet* 137:409–412, 1973.
38. Kadir S, Smith GW, White RJ et al: Percutaneous transluminal angioplasty as an adjunct to the surgical management of peripheral vascular disease, *Ann Surg* 195:768–795, 1982.
39. Walker PJ, Harris JP, May J: Combined percutaneous transluminal angioplasty and extra-anatomic bypass for symptomatic unilateral iliac artery occlusion with contralateral iliac artery stenosis, *Ann Vasc Surg* 5:209–217, 1991.
40. Veith FJ, Gupta SK, Wengerter KR et al: Changing arteriosclerotic disease patterns and management strategies in lower limb threatening ischemia, *Ann Surg* 222:402, 1990.
41. Brewster DC, Cambria RP, Darling RC et al: Long-term results of combined iliac balloon angioplasty and distal surgical revascularisation, *Ann Surg* 210:324, 1989.
42. McGahan TJ, Harris JP, Sachinwalla T et al: Infrainguinal bypass distal to ipsilateral iliac transluminal angioplasty: long term results. Unpublished manuscript, 1995.
43. Satchell P, Ware S, Barron J et al: Finger sudorometry and the sudomotor drive. Unpublished manuscript, 1995.

34
Laparoscopic Aortic Surgery

Carlos R. Gracia and Yves-Marie Dion

The ability to access various body parts remotely through tiny incisions has revolutionized the practice of surgery with minimally invasive surgical (MIS) techniques. The development of superior optics, video imaging equipment, and design of instrumentation to work remotely has grown rapidly. A growing number of surgical disciplines have been applying these advances focusing predominantly on gastrointestinal, gynecologic, urologic, and general thoracic procedures and more recently on coronary bypass surgery. Provided it allows equivalent immediate and long-term results, a less invasive treatment can replace a more invasive one if it improves the patient's well-being and decreases overall cost.

The field of vascular surgery has now begun to unfold the role for new advances in operative procedures. Minimally invasive techniques using scopes and specialized instrumentation have been evolving for saphenous vein harvesting and for subfascial endoscopic perforator vein surgery (SEPS).[1] With the proclaimed advantages of laparoscopic surgery, such as diminished postoperative pain, shorter hospital stay, and earlier return to work, have been documented,[2-5] this often high risk group of patients for vascular surgery would seem to benefit greatly from other techniques for minimally invasive surgery.

Vascular surgeons overall have been slow to apply MIS techniques to aortoiliac disease. This slowness of adoption of operative MIS to aortoiliac disease may in part be due to various items. First is the fact that laparoscopy has grown predominantly within nonvascular circles. This has limited the current laparoscopic experience of vascular surgeons and centered current MIS instrument technology on gastrointestinal laparoscopy. Advances in MIS technology for cardiovascular disease have centered attention on MIS cardiac surgery, not peripheral vascular reconstructions. The application of technology for laparoscopic vascular reconstruction has lagged significantly behind. The fundamentals of vascular surgery (exposure, vascular control, vascular occlusion, anastomosis of vessels and/or grafts, and hemostasis) are significant. They are not readily accomplished without instrumentation dedicated to solving their challenges. Finally, modern-day vascular surgeons have been consumed with primarily pursuing the only other currently available minimally invasive option: endovascular therapies.

In aortoiliac disease, arteriosclerosis is frequently segmental in distribution, making it amenable to effective treatment. A wide range of options for therapeutic management of aortoiliac disease has emerged, yet no one single option for inflow revascularization is ideal or applicable to all cases. In some situations, combinations of interventions may be desirable. Therapeutic options may be categorized as: (1) anatomic (direct reconstructive procedures on the aortoiliac vessels); (2) extraanatomic (indirect bypass grafts that avoid normal anatomic pathways); or (3) nonoperative catheter-based endoluminal therapies that emphasize a minimally invasive approach to treatment of occlusive lesions by a remote, often percutaneous, access site to the arterial system.[6] Ongoing technologic developments and the focus on MIS have revolved around endoluminal therapies by both the industry and surgeons. These modalities have grown owing to an investment in the technology to enable their reproducibility and applicability.

The current minimally invasive vascular techniques for arterial disease are endoluminal and include angioplasty, stent placement, and angioscopy. Experience is also being reported with stent-grafts not only for aneurysmal disease but also aortoiliac occlusive disease.[7] However, confusion exists because of differences in reported early and late results of the various options for the various therapeutic modalities. On the other hand, standard bypass procedures for aortoiliac disease have achieved excellent long-term patency.[8]

For most patients with diffuse aortoiliac occlusive disease, aortobifemoral grafts remain the most durable and functionally effective means of revascularization and should continue to be rightfully regarded as the gold standard (or basis of comparison) with which other options must be properly compared.[6] Although still in its infancy, for aortoiliac occlusive lesions laparoscopy-assisted techniques[9-11] and totally laparoscopic procedures have been offered to humans.[12-15] We review here the experimental and developmental aspects of this field and its current successful application in clinical settings.

Feasibilibty of Laparoscopy in Aortoiliac Surgery

Early work was completed leading to the conclusion that exposure and surgery of the aorta was feasible via laparoscopy. From 1991 through 1992, work was performed to evaluate the possibility of accessing and providing exposure to the aorta. An original abdominal wall-lifting device (Laborie Surgical) was utilized by Dion et al. in Quebec, Canada. A porcine model was selected. Their work represents one of the earliest applications of laparoscopic experience to vascular surgery. Major concerns were addressed by the use of an abdominal wall-lifting device: the lack of ability to suction while working on vascular structures under pneumoperitoneum and of venous air embolism while working near the major venous structures in the retroperitoneum under insufflation. A gasless approach with abdominal wall-lift eliminated these concerns.

This model allowed conventional vascular instrumentation (particularly occlusive clamps and needle drivers) to be utilized, as early instrumentation was nonexistent. Conventionally based vascular instruments could be inserted through blunt ports without concerns for leakage of pneumoperitoneum. Early successes with exposure and surgery on the animal model led to some early instrument design with adaptation of standard vascular instrumentation onto remote handles for laparoscopic application. At the time, the most important were laparoscopic clamps for control of the aorta.

The result of this early work was the first application of laparoscopy to major vascular reconstructive surgery in humans. A surgical team led by Dion of Quebec[10] performed an aortobifemoral bypass (AFB) in March 1993. This early case was followed by four more AFBs.[16] These cases were laparoscopically assisted with all of the dissection, control, insertion, and tunneling of graft completed laparoscopically. Operative details include the use of a transperitoneal approach under pneumoperitoneum. A small minilaparotomy was performed to construct an end-to-side proximal anastomosis, which allowed use of traditional occlusive clamps and needle drivers. All patients demonstrated improved postoperative courses characterized by early ambulation with less pain and need for analgesics.

A small variety of cases, including one AFB, one aortoiliac endarterectomy, and two iliofemoral bypasses, were performed by Berens and Herde.[9] Similarly, a transperitoneal route was used in this experience. The laparoscopic portion was performed with an abdominal wall-lifting device. A minilaparotomy was utilized for vascular suturing and occlusion and for an avenue for insertion of more conventional retractors and packing pads for small bowel retraction. This experience is also more appropriately termed laparoscopy-assisted, as was the experience of Dion et al.[10,16] These patients experienced a faster postoperative recovery with less pain.

These early experiences demonstrated reproduction of the standard operative approach for the aortoiliac arteriosclerotic occlusive disease in each circumstance. The experiences are correctly termed laparoscopy-assisted because of application of the minilaparotomy. The minilaparotomy was thought necessary for several reasons. It was used to perform a continuous sutured vascular anastomosis, a task considered tedious and difficult with current endoscopic instrumentation. The lack of instrumentation was solved as a result of being able to insert conventional occlusive clamps through these small incisions. Finally, they aided the necessary task of retracting abdominal viscera, which was required because of the transperitoneal approach. By combining MIS techniques with minilaparotomy and avoiding xiphopubic incisions, patients experienced improved and shortened postoperative courses.[9,16] It now seemed feasible to apply laparoscopy to vascular reconstructions.

Experimental and Laboratory Background

These pioneering experiences identified important issues. Gasless and traditional gas-insufflation techniques were used. Frustrations were present with both techniques. Were these difficulties the result of problems intrinsic to either of these techniques or to the transperitoneal route common in both experiences? The early human clinical experience of Dion et al.[10] confirmed the difficulty of using the transperitoneal route with respect to bowel retraction. This experience was shared by Berens and Herde.[9] Consequently, aortic dissection and end-to-side aortoprosthetic anastomosis remained tedious. A retroperitoneal approach may provide a solution, as the peritoneal sac would function as an organ "container" and provide improved exposure to the major vessels.

Dion et al.[17] in 1995 reported the first work in an animal series using a retroperitoneal approach. Initially, the anterior approach of Schumaker[18] was used. It was abandoned for a lateral approach to access the retroperitoneum with piglets placed in a right lateral decubitus position. Retroperitoneal dissection to create a retroperitoneal space was facilitated by use of balloon dissectors. After dissection, visualization of the aorta from the left renal artery distally was possible. To address the previous concerns regarding the ability to suction under insufflation, abdominal wall suspension (Laparolift, Origin Medsystems) was utilized. This also allowed the use of instrumentation not designed to work in a sealed gas environment. Totally laparoscopic aortoprosthetic anastomoses were accomplished. However, to complete the aortobifemoral bypass procedure, the animals had to be turned to a supine position for exposure of the femoral vessels and tunneling of the prosthetic graft to the groins. Because of the retroperitoneal approach, bowel retraction became less of a problem.

The success of the previous experience still left major concerns about applying this approach in patients. To translate this model completely to human application would require the undesirable task of having to turn the patient from a lateral position. Turning the patient could allow breaks in sterile technique and would not allow access for proximal control once the patient was repositioned. With the consequences of aortic prosthetic infection and bleeding, it is necessary that the patient remain in a supine rather than a lateral position. Further work would be necessary to modify this approach.

Completely endoscopic anastomoses were accomplished in this experience, in contrast to the need for a laparoscopy-assisted anastomosis thought necessary from the early clinical experiences.[9] This accomplishment went on to identify other limitations of working via a laparoscopy-assisted approach. Variability in the thickness of the abdominal wall of patients of different sizes is problematic. It is difficult to make small incisions in patients with thick or obese abdominal walls. Incisions must increase in size with increasing abdominal wall thickness to obtain and maintain exposure. Eventually, one begins to lose any advantages sought by minimizing trauma from the access. Therefore a completely laparoscopic approach incorporating the anastomosis may ultimately be more reproducible and overcome limitations imposed by small incisions. Further resolution of technical challenges and the development of appropriate instrumentation would be required.

Prior to this last experience, a totally laparoscopic approach to the anastomosis was undertaken by Dion et al. between 1993 and 1994. A canine model was utilized under CO_2 insufflation. A side biting Satinsky style clamp (adapted for laparoscopy) was applied to the infrarenal aorta and a 2-cm aortotomy was performed. A Hemashield (Bard) vascular prosthesis was sutured into this aortotomy as a hemostatic patch. Running monofilament suture was used to accomplish this totally laparoscopically under pneumoperitoneum. This and the prior experience confirmed that standard vascular maneuvers, such as occlusion, opening of the vessel, and its direct suturing, could be successfully performed in a totally laparoscopic environment. A gasless environment was utilized in one, whereas pneumoperitoneum was utilized in the other.

Other investigators were looking at the challenges of applying laparoscopy to vascular surgery. Jones et al.[19] reported in 1996 on an evaluation of transperitoneal and retroperitoneal approaches for aortofemoral bypass. Ten procedures were performed with five animals used for each approach. Retroperitoneal dissection was accomplished by serial balloon dissection to open the retroperitoneum. A transperitoneal approach had been used in the first five animals. An abdominal wall-lift device was used to maintain the working space in both cases. The anastomoses were performed via minilaparotomy with the overall experience demonstrating acceptable clamp times and overall operative times. These investigators reported both approaches to be effective for gasless laparoscopy-assisted exposure of the aorta but noted that the retroperitoneal approach facilitated bowel retraction by using the intact peritoneal sac. The only laparoscopic technique-related complication in this experience pertained to retraction of the small bowel, occurring only in the transperitoneal group. As a result of this work and that of previous investigators, it appeared that a totally endoscopic approach was feasible, as is the case in other laparoscopic procedures. In addition, a retroperitoneal approach appeared to have advantages over a transperitoneal approach.

Pneumoperitoneum Versus Gasless Techniques

The question as to whether a gasless environment or a traditional insufflation approach would be best remained unanswered. A gasless approach seemed promising because of the ability to suction with impunity, as there would be no loss of working space volume due to consumption of the carbon dioxide used to maintain the working space. In addition, the lack of a need for a leakproof seal at the insertion trocar site would allow insertion of a variety of traditional instrumentation. In fact, more than one instrument could be inserted through a given port depending on the relative sizes of the instruments and the port. It was also presumed by many that the ability to insert conventional instrumentation would also improve some of the learning curve issues, as the surgeon would be using familiar tools. All of these factors were considered desirable for approaching vascular surgery remotely by laparoscopy.

Although a gasless technique would represent an alternative to pneumoperitoneum when surgery is performed in localized regions of the abdomen, such as the pelvis or upper abdomen, its application to the peritoneal cavity at large can become problematic. Despite its potential advantages, most laparoscopies were still being performed with insufflation, which is still the case for gastrointestinal and gynecologic procedures. Why is this the case? It was even noted that insufflation with pneumoperitoneum could compromise cardiac output and renal flow.

Variation in body size and morphology of pateints could make working under a gasless environment more difficult. Making small incisions to facilitate retraction or to insert multiple conventional instruments creates conflicts. The limitations noted earlier with varying thickness of the abdominal wall is important. Despite the heartiest intention to start with small incisions, common sense and experience dictate that the incisions must increase in size with increasing abdominal wall thickness to obtain and maintain exposure. Eventually, you begin to lose any advantages sought by minimizing trauma from the access.

On the other hand, a standard-size trocar placed in an insufflated space standardizes that space. The same-size puncture site is present based on the diameter of the trocar, 3 to 12 mm, inserted into the body cavity despite the thickness of the abdominal wall. Common sense also dictates that large patients have more intracavitary fat and bulk. In these cases, the pneumoperitoneum does not make the retraction process any simpler, particularly with a transperitoneal route. Yet the overall compressing effect of carbon dioxide under normal working pressures (12 to 15 mmHg) is not present under a gasless environment. Therefore the small bowel tends to occupy more space in the abdominal cavity. The three-dimensional compressing effect of working with gas insufflation was known, workable, and potentially desirable. The safety of its use would require further investigation.

Carbon dioxide embolization during laparoscopy is a recognized, potentially lethal complication.[20,21] The potential for pulmonary embolization following major venous laceration while under laparoscopic conditions was evaluated by Dion and coworkers.[22] A model to evaluate gas embolization under carbon dioxide pneumoperitoneum was constructed. Anesthetized dogs with hemodynamic monitoring via an arterial line and Swan-Ganz catheter were used. The status and amount of embolism within the heart chambers was evaluated by transesophageal echocardiography. Euvolemic dogs were submitted to a 1-cm longitudinal incision made in the vena cava while maintaining a carbon dioxide pneumoperitoneum with pressures between 12 and 15 mmHg. No gas embolism was seen in 82% of the cases after exposure of the venotomies to the pneumoperitoneum. Only 18% had gas bubbles visible in the right heart cavities by transesophageal echocardiography. In contrast, direct intravenous bolus injection of only 15 ml carbon dioxide led to visualization of many more gas bubbles in the right heart cavities. Massive intravenous injections of carbon dioxide (> 300 cc) led to the appearance of gas bubbles in the left heart cavities and death.

These experiments also identified transesophageal echocardiography as more precise than relying on elevation of pulmonary artery pressure for detecting gas embolism. A bolus of 15 cc carbon dioxide was easily visualized by the transesophageal echocardiography probe without concomitant elevation of pulmonary artery pressure. The routine use of transesophageal echocardiography has not been clinically encouraged because in clinical practice few episodes of gas embolism have been reported. In three studies the incidence of gas embolism was, respectively, 1 in 63,845 patients, 15 in 113,253 pateints, and 8 in 50,247 patients.[23] Because of these studies, it was thought that it would be safe to proceed in this area under routine pneumoperitoneum if it were determined necessary or helpful.

Further Laboratory Development

The advantages of a retroperitoneal approach were beginning to be appreciated. It would be desirous to allow simultaneous access to proximal aortic control and to the groins. A standard supine position is required to provide access to the groins for exposure of the femoral arteries and to tunnel the limbs of the vascular graft. An anterolateral laparoscopic approach with the subject supine was subsequently performed and reported by Dion and Gracia[24] (Figure 34–1, see color plate). The goal was to reproduce the exposure and control obtained by the lateral approach for the distal aorta, iliac arteries, and inferior mesenteric artery. As significant bleeding could occur from the lumbar vessels at the time of incision or division of the aorta, their exposure and control was also necessary. This

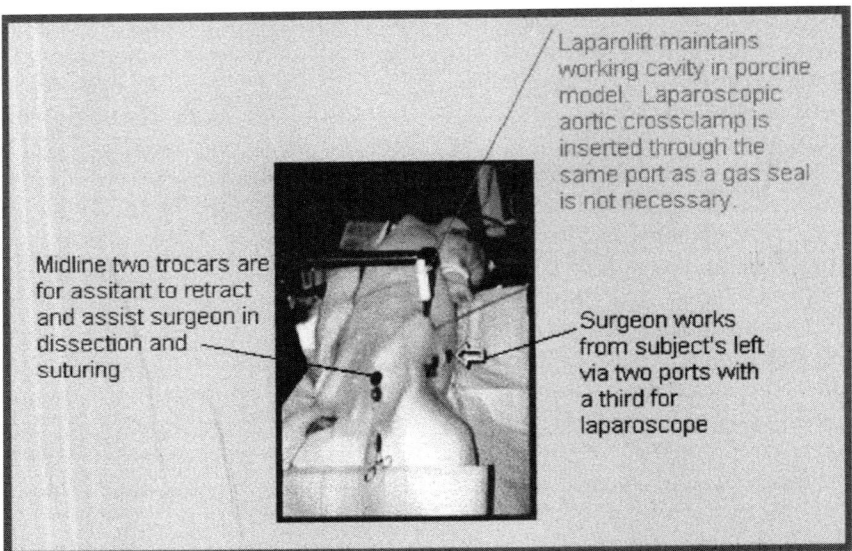

FIGURE 34-1. Porcine model as described by Dion and Gracia[24] depicting the ability to work in the retroperitoneum with the subject supine. This is in contrast to previous reported models of retroperitoneal exposure requiring the subject to be lateral. The latter is not ideal for vascular bypass, as it does not allow simultaneous access to groins and proximal aortic control. (See color plate).

point would also be important for a successful laparoscopic approach to abdominal aortic aneurysms.

Dion and Gracia paid attention to approaching the aorta in models for occlusive disease as well as aneurysmal disease. After proximal occlusion and oversewing the distal aorta, the aorta was transected and an end-to-end aorto-prosthetic anastomosis performed for an occlusive model. In the aneurysmal model the aorta was opened longitudinally, with the lumbar arteries controlled not only from outside the aorta but oversewn intraluminally while bleeding, as with an open repair. Similar to the open technique of endoaneurysmorrhaphy, the anastomosis was constructed in end-to-end fashion by suturing from within the aorta and incorporating an intact posterior wall. All anastomoses were constructed with standard running monofilament 4-0 Prolene suture with curved vascular needles.

Piglets were selected as the model of choice because of several similarities to the human. However, some differences from human anatomy were present, particularly when comparing the porcine and human aortas and iliac arteries. The large size of this animal model (Yorkshire piglets, 75 to 80 kg) makes comparison with human surgery more realistic. It allows performance of an aortobifemoral bypass under conditions similar to those in humans, with the surgeon and assistant working in the same fashion as if the abdomen were opened. Despite the enormous size of the torso of the Yorkshire-cross piglet (75 to 80 kg), reproducing that of the human torso well, it has an aorta that typically measures 7 to 8 mm in diameter. The vascular graft must be custom-made from 6 mm diameter grafts sewn in end-to-side fashion to form an appropriate bifurcated prosthesis for aortobifemoral bypass. In addition, the porcine aorta contains no atheromas. The abdominal wall of the piglet is composed of the same muscles as that of humans.[17] Also, the porcine anatomy in the retroperitoneal aorta and surrounding structures is comparable to that in humans. In the case of aneurysms, however, an aneurysmal mass and the resultant difficulties it would generate are obviously absent. The commonplace destruction of the posterior wall of the aorta in aneurysmal disease is not available in the nonatheromatous porcine aorta.

Construction of an AFB was consistently performed in less than 4 hours with blood loss never exceeding 550 ml. Bleeding most commonly occurred at the time the aorta was opened and flushed. On occasion bleeding came from the oversewn aortoiliac stump after the limbs of the gafts were opened; this was corrected with additional sutures as necessary. The totally laparoscopic aortic anastomosis did not take more than 60 minutes to perform. No operative mortality was encountered in this or the previous series, which together account for 34 consecutive totally laparoscopic AFBs.

The anterolateral retroperitoneal approach has numerous advantages over a lateral approach and is better than the transabdominal technique. Once a consistent exposure and the anastomosis could be constructed in the laboratory animal model without excessive blood loss, excessive surgery times, or operative mortality, it seemed appropriate to begin to offer patients the option of laparoscopic AFB. Based on the completed animal experiments where a retroperitoneal approach solved many of the exposure and retraction difficulties, it was thought to be the approach for clinical application. It was believed it would solve the troublesome problem of small bowel retraction, which had proved problematic in the first human transperitoneal work. A totally endoscopic approach was also selected based on laboratory successes.

Early Clinical Experience

The first human aortic vascular experience was completed in 1993 by Dion et al.,[10] as previously noted. A 63-year-old man with a history of myocardial infarction underwent laparoscopy-assisted AFB grafting performed for ischemic rest pain due to aortoiliac occlusive inflow disease. Four additional procedures were performed and reported[16] with the same technique. The only intraoperative complication was a small bowel perforation due to retraction difficulties in this transperitoneal route. Postoperatively, there were no complications, and the patients felt less pain, being able to cough better and walk more easily.

A second series was reported in 1995 by Berens and Herde.[9] Their experience included one left iliofemoral bypass, one AFB, one right iliofemoral bypass, and one aortoiliac endarterectomy. The two iliac patients were ambulating early and taking a diet within 24 hours, with discharge in 24 hours. The aortic procedure patients were taking a diet at 48 hours postoperatively and discharged on the third postoperative day. There were no complications.

Details of both Dion's experience and Berens and Herde's work were previously noted. Whereas both approaches used a transperitoneal route, Dion et al. utilized gas insufflation for maintenance of the working space and Berens and Herde used an abdominal wall lift device (Origin Medsystems). The difficulty retracting intraabdominal organs, rendering aortic dissection and end-to-side aortoprosthetic anastomosis tedious, was noted by both groups. Despite the inspirational improvements observed in the postoperative recoveries of their patients, improvement in various areas, alone or in combination, would be necessary. Multihour operative procedures are not destined to be highly reproducible or enjoy widespread adoption. Refinements to the approach would be beneficial to avoid spending so much time and effort battling the intraabdominal organs in retraction. Improvements in instrumentation would be critical to begin to establish some form of reproducibility that would drive the operative process more in line with traditional approaches.

A third experience with a laparoscopy-assisted technique was reported by Fabiani et al.[25] in 1997. A combination of procedures and access were used. A transperitoneal approach was used for AFB completed in three patients. Unilateral aortofemoral bypass was performed by a retroperitoneal approach in four patients. Conversions to open laparotomy in two other patients were due to inadequate aortic exposure in one and extensive aortic calcification in the other. Dissection, vascular control, tunneling, and placement of graft were accomplished under laparoscopic view. The authors termed the technique video-assisted when they made a small 3-cm median minilaparotomy incision. This allowed insertion of a Satinsky clamp, at which time the aortotomy and anastomosis were performed through this route with visibility and video guidance provided by the laparoscope in place. Patient experience was again favorable. Short postoperative ileus was noted, with enteral diets started 48 hours postoperatively. Lengths of stay in the hospital ranged from 4 to 7 days. This experience very much reproduced the original laparoscopy-assisted experience reported by Dion et al. but with decreasing operative times.

As a result of our own laboratory experiences[24,26-29] we began to evaluate the retroperitoneal approach for a completely laparoscopic AFB in human cadavers. Evaluation in the human cadaver laboratory is appropriate before embarking on further clinical work. A series of experiences were collected by recreating the retroperitoneal working space in human cadavers. Application of balloon technology (General Surgical Innovations) allowed rapid, reproducible dissection of the retroperitoneum from a virtual space to actual space. This space was maintained with carbon dioxide insufflation, pneumoretroperitoneum, with pressures of 12 to 14 mm Hg.

Our clinical experience began in March 1995. Four patients underwent successful AFB ($n = 2$) and iliofemoral graft ($n = 2$) using a completely endoscopic and retroperitoneal approach. All four were men with ages ranging from 62 to 71 years. The indications for surgery were rest pain in one (ABI less than 0.20) and severe claudication in three (ABI less than 0.60). All had aortoiliac occlusive disease and were not considered ideal candidates for endoluminal procedures based on the extent and distribution of the arteriosclerotic disease on arteriography. All were given the option of endoluminal interventions. All patients were candidates for standard open surgery based on routine preoperative cardiopulmonary evaluation.

The first clinical case in which a completely retroperitoneal approach was used was a right iliofemoral bypass graft for a completely occluded right external iliac artery (Figure 34-2, see color plate). Retroperitoneal dissection established a satisfactory working space. Gas insufflation was utilized to maintain a working space that was sufficient. There was concern that pneumoretroperitoneum would not be successful for exposing the infrarenal aorta. As we did not need to extend past the aortic bifurcation, it was thought that insufflation would be adequate. The approach was also from the iliac fossa superiorly. The typical abdominal wall suspension was carried out from the umbilicus, and there did not seem to be an ideal location for an abdominal

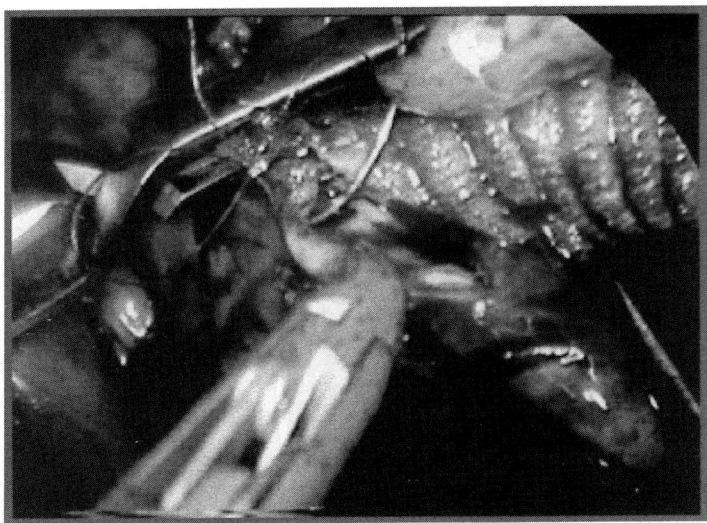

FIGURE 34-2. Laparoscopic view of intracorporeal suturing to anastomose the right common iliac artery to a prosthetic Dacron graft for a right iliofemoral bypass graft. This type of bypass could be performed via an entirely retroperitoneal dissection and space. When applied to the infrarenal aorta, this approach becomes more problematic without a peritoneal "apron". (See color plate).

wall-lift. The space was adequate, and an end-to-end anastomosis was constructed completely endoscopically without difficulty. This patient required minimal analgesics and was discharged from the hospital in 48 hours. A second right iliofemoral bypass with end-to-side anastomosis also proceeded well with the same technique.

Encouraged by this, we moved on to the first patient for AFB. Based on our extensive laboratory work we used the gasless space with abdominal wall suspension with which we were familiar. At the time and for the reasons previously outlined, it seemed to hold promise to complete a completely endoscopic retroperitoneal procedure. However, there were difficulties maintaining the working space and exposure for dissection and proximal anastomosis, resulting in a lengthy operation of about 12 hours. The crossclamp time approached 240 minutes. Most of the operation dealt with efforts to maintain adequate exposure. Although lengthy, steady progress was made throughout the procedure, and the patient developed no intraoperative difficulties. However, he did develop a compartment syndrome, which was immediately identified and treated. A lengthier hospital stay was also experienced due to myoglobinuria before the patient was ready for discharge.

Valuable experience had been gained from these first two cases. The iliofemoral bypass proceeded smoothly with insufflation. Instrumentation appeared to be the largest obstacle, requiring adaptation of some endoscopic bulldogs as occlusive devices. With the AFB the gasless environment was significantly more difficult to maintain in the human torso than the porcine model, despite their similarities. The advantages of working under insufflation were not easily dismissed, and we began to work with insufflation on the next aorta and all subsequent cases. If exposure could be performed consistently and maintained better with insufflation, adaptation of basic vascular instrumentation for laparoscopy should allow vascular anastomosis to be constructed in this totally laparoscopic environment.

The second AFB was performed under insufflation. Surgical time remained long at about 10 hours but improved overall, with the aortic crossclamp time decreased to 70 minutes. The improved exposure and visibility under insufflation was notable, with most of the operative time spent in orientation and careful dissection in the retroperitoneum. Intraoperatively, minute ventilation was adjusted to cope with rising end-tidal carbon dioxide. There were no major pH shifts and no postoperative problems with subcutaneous emphysema. The patient ambulated, started a diet within 48 hours of surgery, and required minimal analgesics postoperatively. Although he could have been discharged in 72 hours, he was observed for an additional 24 hours. This was now more in line with the recovery expected for MIS procedures.

The lengthy surgical time should be evaluated in light of learning curve issues. Many of the early applications of laparoscopy to gastrointestinal procedures were commonly several hours. The operating time for early attempts at colectomy, for example, were 6 to 8 hours. With flat learning curves and appropriate instrumentation, many laparoscopic operations are now within the normal open operating times of many laparoscopic surgeons. Technology and experience improved the reproducibility and ability to do laborious tasks in shorter times. However, patient disease and morphology affect overall operating times for both the experienced surgeon and the neophyte. Consequently, operating times are difficult to compare overall because of many variables and lack of documentation in the literature. For laparoscopy to be successful in ABF or iliofemoral bypass grafting, further improvement and evolution of what has been learned would be necessary. Surgical times would need to continue to improve. Attention must be applied to the technology and instrumentation that would not only improve operating times but contribute to the reproducibility of the procedure.

Difficulties were identified that were significant, and dealing with them accounted for a large part of the operating time in the first cases. Review of these first cases demonstrated that the more isolated procedures, such as iliofemoral bypass, lend themselves to rapid extraperitoneal dissection under insufflation. With a larger space needed for aortic exposure and control, insufflation appeared to work better. However, pneumoretroperitoneum created three problems. First, with a larger space there is more peritoneum that can be violated, allowing intraperitoneal leak and collapse of the retroperitoneal working space. Second, it was noted that over time there would be competitive insufflation of the peritoneal cavity across thinned out areas of the peritoneum. The most susceptible area was the anterior portion of the peritoneum. Even without violation of the peritoneal lining, we experienced a gradual decrease in the retroperitoneal working space. The third problem was that the volume of the retroperitoneal working cavity was small and highly sensitive to suctioning. There would need to be solutions to these challenges to improve on time, reproducibility, and patient safety.

On the other hand, some potential problems did not materialize. The human iliac artery was more accurately approximated by the porcine aorta, allowing adequate re-creation of operating on the actual iliac vessel. The larger human aorta (16mm diameter prosthesis being utilized) had proved technically easier to work with. Its size facilitates many of the maneuvers utilized for laparoscopic suturing in a confined space (e.g., the retroperitoneum). The tactile feedback critical to a surgeon working with instruments was just as palpable with the laparoscopic tools as would be experienced with open tools. Assessment of the calcified plaque with the needle tip to determine how and where to place it was comparable between open and laparoscopic needle drivers.

These overall experiences were taken back to the laboratory to evaluate how the difficulties may be solved. A solution was found when working with the vulnerable area of anterior peritoneum. Much time had been spent to develop the retroperitoneal space without violating the susceptible anterior peritoneum for fear the space would collapse. Rather than avoiding it, Dion and Gracia[13] described construction of a peritoneal "apron" by incising this area anteriorly under the left rectus sheath. This could be suspended with transabdominal sutures toward the right of the abdomen. It succeeded in terms of the primary reason for the retroperitoneal approach—containment of abdominal viscera—while solving other problems as well. There was no longer a concern regarding creation of a leak in the peritoneal lining. It eliminated problems between the two compartments. In essence, by connecting the two it avoided competitive insufflation and collapse of the retroperitoneum. We could now use the entire peritoneal cavity with its larger volume of insufflation, which stabilized the operating field despite aggressive suctioning with the use of modern insufflators of 20 to 30 l/min.

This "apron" modification of the retroperitoneal approach would prove to be one of our most significant developments in moving forward with AFB. Its application in the subsequent three cases was reported[13]: two men and one woman with ages similar to those of previous patients, all with severe claudication (ABI less than 0.60). All three had aortoiliac occlusive disease and were either not ideal candidates for interventional procedures or were failures of previous interventions (Figure 34–3, see color plate). Improvement in overall surgical times continued with performance of these next three AFBs (5 to 6 hours). Considerably decreased time and effort were spent maintaining adequate exposure. All aortic anastomoses were accomplished in end-to-end fashion with intracorporeal laparoscopic suturing using continuous running monofilament suture in all cases (Figure 34–4, see color plate). These cases were done completely endoscopically. Crossclamp times would also vary depending on whether additional reconstruction was required at the femoral or profunda femoris vessels. Operative times had now been decreased by 50% with a relatively brief clinical experience. Hospital stays averaged 4 to 5 days, with one patient staying 6 days. All patients could have been discharged sooner, but they were kept for observation of their progress. There were no further postoperative complications after the first case, as noted earlier.

This operative experience continued with the next seven cases, reported by Dion, Gracia, and coworkers,[26] all with an end-to-end anastomoses. In a review of these cases, the operating

34. Laparoscopic Aortic Surgery

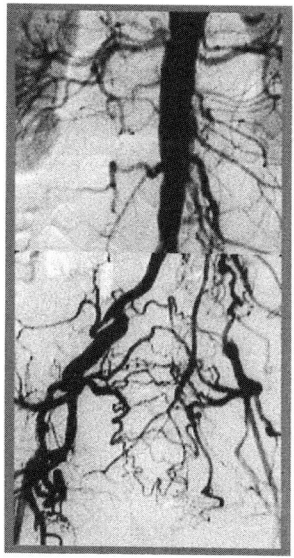
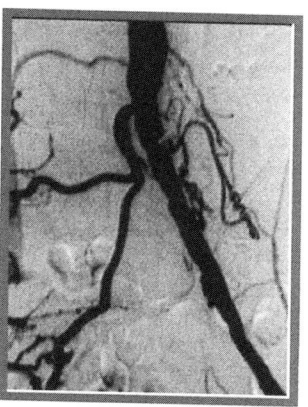
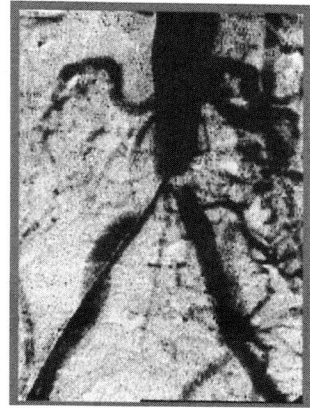
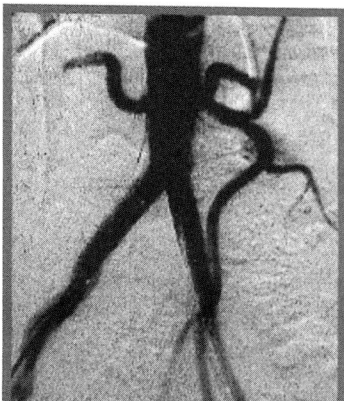
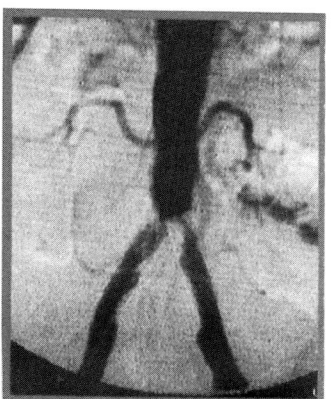

FIGURE 34–3. Preoperative arteriograms of patients with aortoiliac occlusive disease. **A**, A 61-year-old woman had diffuse bilateral iliac disease of both external and internal iliac arteries. **B**, A 57-year-old male patient had an occluded right iliac system and contralateral disease. **C-1**, A 61-year-old man had bilateral common iliac artery stenosis. **C-2**, Same patient after successful placement of bilateral common iliac artery stents following angioplasty. **C-3**, Same patient about 14 months after stent placement with recurrent disease and symptoms. He elected to not have any further endoluminal procedures but to have aortobifemoral bypass. A laparoscopic approach was then discussed with the patient. (See color plate).

times were decreased from 510 minutes to 245 minutes. The mean total aortic clamping time was 121 minutes with the time required to perform the aortic anastomosis 66 minutes. The last two cases of this experience were performed in just over 4 hours with aortic anastomotic times of 34 and 28 minutes, respectively. The mean blood loss was 820 ml, and the average amount of fluids administered was 6975 ml (4500 to 8500 ml). Only one patient was transfused with homologous packed red blood cells, donated by the patient preoperatively. Cell saver for autotransfusion was used in two other patiens.

There were three conversions from the totally laparoscopic approach to a laparoscopy-

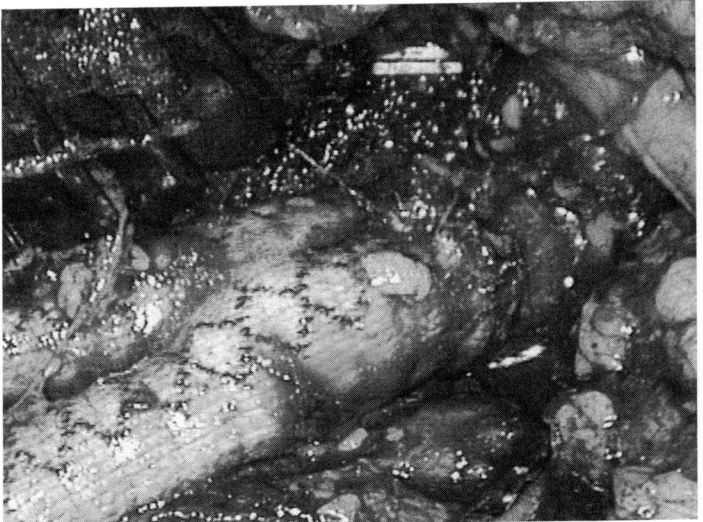

FIGURE 34–4. Laparoscopic view of the aortoprosthetic anastomosis completed in end-to-end fashion. (See color plate).

assisted procedure by minilaparotomy. Conversions never required performance emergently. All three were for proximal aortic difficulties associated with calcifications of the aorta. Two patients required revision at the time of conversion, with one patient having developed immediate graft occlusion after unclamping by disruption of a calcified plaque by the aortic clamp. A minilaparotomy of 4 to 5 cm was performed to explore the anastomosis and endarterectomize the site of crossclamping in these two patients. The utilization of the retroperitoneal approach via the "apron" allowed excellent ecposure for the conversions. Small renal vein retractors could be inserted behind the retroperitoneal "apron" to readily expose the infrarenal anastomotic area without interference or difficulties in bowel retraction (Figure 34–5, see color plate). During the third conversion there was no need for further inter-

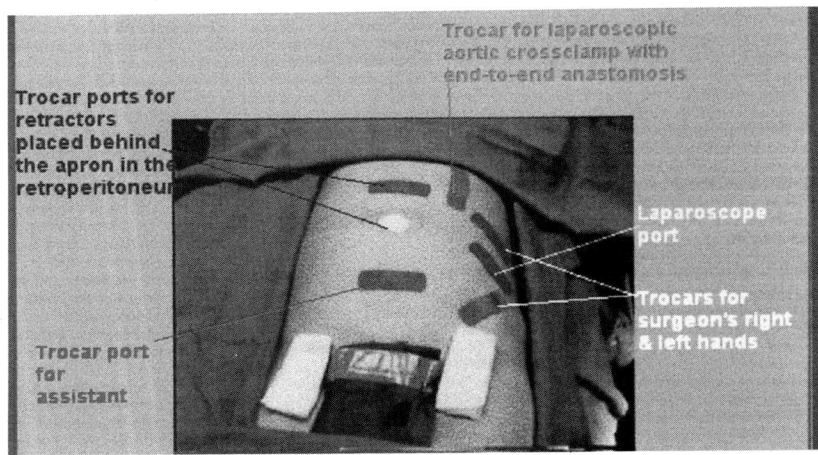

FIGURE 34–5. Patient position with identification of trocar sites for totally laparoscopic aortobifemoral bypass, not requiring minilaparotomy. If minilaparotomy were necessary, connecting the two superior midline trocars (in blue) would provide ready access to the retroperitoneum with the use of renal vein retractors. They are placed behind the retroperitoneal "apron" facilitating exposure of the infrarenal aorta up to the renal vein without difficulty from the small intestine. (See color plate).

vention at the time of conversion. What was learned in these three cases was valuable. As all conversions were for calcific arteriosclerotic plaque, we have advocated being more aggressive with endarterectomy of the proximal cuff at the time of anastomosis. In addition, the retroperitoneal approach and "apron" provide exposure in cases where a conversion to laparoscopy-assisted by minilaparotomy is required.

The key to successful completion of the bypass was in the careful creation of the retroperitoneal cavity, aided by the "apron." It allowed the necessary exposure for the surgeons to work. Most of the operating time involved in these cases was spent on the careful creation of the retroperitoneal cavity. In contrast, the aortic anastomosis were generally completed within 50 to 60 minutes. All of the reported cases for totally endoscopic completion were with an end-to-end anastomosis. Five more cases have now been completed with similar results, with modifications allowing end-to-side anastomosis (Figure 34–6, see color plate).

The continued improvement in decreasing surgical time was due in part to overall increased familiarity with the retroperitoneal anatomy as seen laparoscopically. Moreover, dedicated instrumentation (Karl Storz Endoscopy America) had been provided that has contributed greatly to decreased operating times. The time now required to establish a retroperitoneal work space and complete the dissection has decreased from more than 4 to 5 hours to less than 1.5 hours. With continued improvement in technique and instrumentation, the operating time for laparoscopic operations for occlusive aortoiliac surgery should rivel those of open surgery. This would impart to the modern vascular surgeon a new tool to add to the arsenal for treatment of arteriosclerotic occlusive disease. The ability to provide the long-term known advantages and patency rate of standard bypass graft techniques in minimally invasive fashion is beneficial to the patients. It should combine to work with the interventional technologies and techniques to provide the best long-term and cost-effective solution for our patients.

Abdominal Aortic Aneurysms

The surgical approach to infrarenal aortic aneurysm requires a lengthy xiphopubic incision, which is associated with considerable postoperative pain. The surgical treatment for abdominal aortic aneurysm involves placement of a prosthetic graft in the involved area. The gold standard for aortic aneurysm repair was

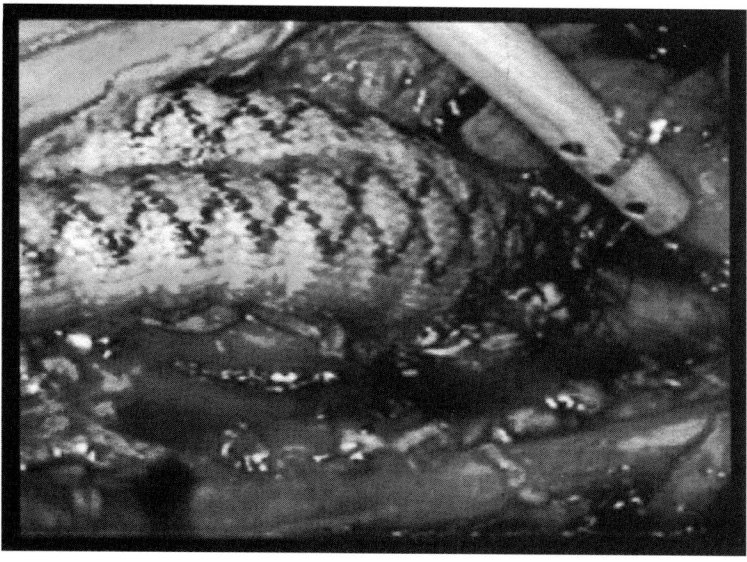

FIGURE 34–6. Laparoscopic view of the aortoprosthetic anastomosis completed in end-to-side fashion. (See color plate).

described by Creech in 1966 with the technique of endoaneurysmorrhaphy.[27] Until this time, mortality rates had remained high. Continued improvements in modern anesthetic techniques and critical care have contributed to the decreased mortality rates of 2% to 4%.[28] Postoperative care requires a critical care stay, which typically causes hospital stays to be 5 to 10 days and so increases the cost.

The MIS techniques used with other abdominal laparoscopic procedures may give similar advantages to patients if applied to aortic aneurysm repair. The challenges for the successful application of MIS techniques to aneurysms are significant. Despite these challenges, there have been efforts to pursue this goal. The earliest work on laparoscopic aortic aneurysm repair was reported by Chen et al.[29] In their experiments there were 15 successful graft insertions in 21 pigs undergoing transabdominal dissection of the aorta. Six were unsuccessful because of technical, anatomic, or bleeding difficulties. The retroperitoneal approach was attempted in two cases with only one being successful: Tears in the peritoneum occurred in the other. Other complications were noted, including injuries to bladder, ureter, renal vein, inferior vena cava, aorta, and lumbar vessels. The operating time decreased from 6 hours to less than 2 hours with a concomitant decrease in estimated blood loss from 1000ml to less than 150ml with experience. Chen and coworkers secured endoluminal grafts with extraluminal umbilical tapes after insertion by aortotomy. This is in contrast to our experience,[24] where the endoaneurysmhorrhaphy technique of suturing the graft in place with an intact back wall was used. Lumbar vessels could also be controlled intraluminally as well as extraluminally.

In these attempts to develop MIS techniques to approach an aneurysm, one must recognize the limitation of the animal models (i.e., the lack of an aneurysmal mass or calcification in the wall). Without this mass the dissection is simpler; and without the calcification there is no risk of distal embolization. We have subsequently undertaken a series of laboratory experiments to create and work with an aneurysmal mass in animals laparoscopically.[30]

Twelve experiments were performed on 12 female piglets (70 to 75kg) by submitting them to two procedures. First, via laparotomy an aortic aneurysm was created according to the technique described by White.[31] After a period of 4 to 15 days, the laparoscopic resection was performed. A peritoneal apron was constructed according to the method previously described.[13] The laparoscopic repair was performed with aortobifemoral graft with proximal end-to-end anastomosis. Lumbar arteries could be successfully controlled from within the lumen at the time the aneurysmal mass was open using laparoscopic clip appliers. Laparoscopic repairs were completed in all 12 cases with an average duration of surgery of 210 minutes (150 to 300 minutes), aortic crossclamping 55 minutes (38 to 72 minutes), and blood loss 150ml (80 to 250ml).

The result of the work of Chen and colleagues[32] has been the successful completion of laparoscopy-assisted repair of infrarenal abdominal aortic aneurysm in humans. An asymptomatic 6-cm aortic abdominal aneurysm in a 62-year-old man was successfully repaired. This first case was performed with 10 trocars and a 10-cm minilaparotomy. The approach was transabdominal, and bowel retraction was facilitated by a modified "fish" retractor for the special task. Total operating time was 4 hours, and estimated blood loss was 1000ml. Decreased operative fluid requirement with early mobilization of fluids was observed. A more rapid return of bowel function with an earlier discharge on postoperative day 6 was reported. Chen and coworkers have since simplified the approach, reducing the number of trocars to six (personal communication). This work contributes to determining the feasibility of performing laparoscopic aortic surgery, whether totally laparoscopic or laparoscopy-assisted.

Percutaneous placement of endoluminal stent-grafts is directed at avoiding any of the morbidity and mortality associated with major abdominal surgery. Despite the technical success achieved in most cases, endovascular grafts require high skill for implantation[33] and are subject to complications themselves. In a phase I trial May et al. reported a vascular complication rate of 10% for a tube graft, which rose to 43% for a bifurcated endovascular graft.[34] In another phase I trial with 46 patients, Moore and Rutherford[35] reported contrast enhancement outside the graft but within the aneurysmal sac in 17 grafts (44%), of which 9 (51%) resolved spontaneously. The hospital stay varied between 1 and 14 days.[33,34] Uncontrolled lumbar vessels and endoleaks have raised concern over continued aneurysmal growth and risk of rupture.[36-38] Updated results of ongoing trials should allow further assessment of the role of endoprosthesis for treatment of abdominal aortic aneurysm. An interesting approach to the treatment of abdominal aortic aneurysm is to combine laparoscopic and endovascular techniques, which may help solve many of the challenging problems encountered during the performance of one of these two described techniques. We have initiated work in the laboratory to explore this possibility.

Conclusions

The development of minimal access vascular aortoiliac surgery must follow accepted rules.[39] In the opinion of the authors, laparoscopic aortic surgery is feasible. It has been developed in the laboratory,[16,17,19,24,29,30] and performed on a few well selected patients.[9-13,25,26,32] A totally laparoscopic approach to the aortoiliac segment in our experience and evaluation appears to be more appealing than a laparoscopy-assisted method utilizing an 8- to 10-cm incision or a purely minilaparotomy approach.[40] This is similar to the experience with laparoscopic cholecystectomy, but it has demonstrated wider acceptance and higher adoption than the minilaparotomy approach to cholecystectomy.

To promote the further development, safety, efficacy, reproducibility, and ability to teach the procedures, many areas require improvement. Thus far, the procedure has been safely performed with current "off the shelf" instrumentation, including conventional open and laparoscopic instrumentation. As previously mentioned, dedicated and purposely built laparoscopic vascular instrumentation (Karl Storz Endoscopy) has been available to the authors and has greatly aided the safe completion of the most recent procedures, enabling shorter surgery times. Not only must standard vascular instruments be adapted to work laparoscopically, but new technology and concepts are required. Improvements in occlusive devices such that they can function extracorporeally or intracorporeally are necessary. Instrumentation that allows consistent construction of safe and durable anastomosis is also required. A number of technologies are under evaluation for this express purpose. As stapling technology has revolutionized the fashion in which gastrointestinal anastomoses are performed, one can envision an automated anastomotic device. This instrumentation would contribute to the safety and reproducibility of these procedures and broaden their appeal.

On cannot ignore the improved clinical advantages and potential for patients as a result of these minimally invasive procedures. Vascular surgeons have a wide variety of exposure and experience in laparoscopy, from none to extensive (those who also do laparoscopic gastrointestinal surgery). Over the next several years experience should be more uniform as many of tomorrow's vascular surgeons come from training programs where they had laparoscopic training and experience. Other procedures, as in venous disease, are exposing more vascular surgeons to nonendoluminal minimally invasive techniques, skills, and instrumentation. With an understanding of the importance of increased skills and experience in laparoscopy, the ability to perform laparoscopic suturing will become more prevalent.

Laparoscopic vascular surgery of the infrarenal aortoiliac segment has the potential to benefit the patient. For use in patients with occlusive disease, it differs only by the approach (laparoscopic versus open). Therefore the long-term results are expected to be similar. Performing laparoscopic surgery for occlusive disease is presently easier than attempting to treat abdominal aortic aneurysms completely laparoscopically. The role of laparoscopy in the ultimate treatment of aortic aneurysm requires definition and investigation, which depends on the continued interest in and fate of endoluminal stent-grafts. Ongoing experience supports the continued investigation and development of these techniques, with laparoscopic aortoiliac surgery clearly in the feasibility stage.

References

1. Bergan J, Murray J, Greason K: Subfascial endoscopic perforator vein surgery: a preliminary report, *Ann Vasc Surg* 10:211–219, 1996.
2. Périssat J, Collet D, Belliard R: Traitement laparoscopique par lithotripsie intra-corporelle suivi de cholécystostomie ou de cholécystectomie, *Chirurgie* 116:243–247, 1990.
3. Peters JH, Ortega A, Lehnerd SL et al: The physiology of laparoscopic surgery: pulmonary function after laparoscopic cholecystectomy, *Surg Laparosc Endosc* 3:370–374, 1993.
4. Poulin EC, Mamazza J, Breton G et al: Evaluation of pulmonary function in laparoscopic cholecystectomy, *Surg Laparosc Endosc* 2:292–296, 1993.
5. Svenberg T: Pathophysiology of pneumoperitoneum. In Ballantyne GH, Leahy PF, Modlin IM, editors: *Laparoscopic surgery*, Montreal, 1994, Saunders, pp 61–68.
6. Brewster DC: Current controversies in the management of aortoiliac occlusive disease, *J Vasc Surg* 25:365–379, 1997.
7. Marin M, Veith F, Cynamon J: Transfemoral endovascular stented graft treatment of aortoiliac and femoropopliteal occlusive disease for limb salvage, *Am J Surg* 168:16–62, 1994.
8. Veith F, Gupta S, Wengerter K et al: Changing arteriosclerotic disease patterns and management strategies in lower-limb-threatening ischemia, *Ann Surg* 212:402–414, 1990.
9. Berens ES, Herde JR: Laparoscopic vascular surgery: four case reports, *J Vasc Surg* 22:73–79, 1995.
10. Dion YM, Katkhouda N, Rouleau C, Aucoin A: Laparoscopy-assisted aortobifemoral bypass, *Surg Laparosc Endosc* 3:425–429, 1993.
11. Fabiani JN, Mercier F, Carpentier A et al: Video-assisted aortofemoral bypass, *Ann Vasc Surg* 11:273–277, 1997.
12. Ahn SS, Hiyama DT, Rudkin GH et al: Laparoscopic aortobifemoral bypass, *J Vasc Surg* 26:218–232, 1997.
13. Dion YM, Gracia CR: A new technique for laparoscopic aortobifemoral grafting in occlusive aortoiliac disease, *J Vasc Surg* 26:685–692, 1997.
14. Dion YM, Gracia CR, Demalcy JC: Laparoscopic aortic surgery [letter], *J Vasc Surg* 23:539, 1995.
15. Said S, Muller JM: Introduction to video endoscopic vascular surgery of the pelvic area, *Zentralbl Chir* 122:757–761, 1997.
16. Dion YM, Rouleau C, Aucoin A: Laparoscopy-assisted aortobifemoral bypass, *Surg Endosc* 8:438, 1994.
17. Dion YM, Chin AK, Thompson TA: Experimental laparoscopic aortobifemoral bypass. *Surg Endosc* 9:894–897, 1995.
18. Schumaker HB: Midline extraperitoneal exposure of the abdominal aorta and the iliac arteries, *Surg Gynecol Obstet* 135:791–792, 1972.
19. Jones DB, Thompson RW, Soper NJ et al: Development and comparison of transperitoneal and retroperitoneal approaches to laparoscopic-assisted aortofemoral bypass in a porcine model, *J Vasc Surg* 23:466–471, 1996.
20. Chui PT, Gin T, Oh TE: Anaesthesia for laparoscopic general surgery, *Anaesth Intensive Care* 21:163–171, 1993.
21. McQuaide JR: Air embolism during peritoneoscopy, *S Afr Med J* 46:422–423, 1972.
22. Dion YM, Levesque C, Doillon CJ: Experimental carbon dioxide pulmonary embolization after vena cava laceration under pneumoperitoneum, *Surg Endosc* 9:1065–1069, 1995.
23. De Plaizer RMH, Jones ISC: Non-fatal carbon dioxide embolism during laparoscopy, *Anaesth Intensive Care* 17:359–361, 1989.
24. Dion YM, Gracia CR: Experimental laparoscopic aortic aneurysm resection and aortobifemoral bypass, *Surg Laparosc Endosc* 6:184–90, 1996.
25. Fabiani JN, Mercier F, Carpentier A et al: Video-assisted aortofemoral bypass: results in seven cases, *Ann Vasc Surg* 11:273–277, 1997.
26. Dion YM, Gracia CR, Estakhri ME et al: Totally laparoscopic aortobifemoral bypass: a review of 10 patients, *Surg Laparosc Endosc* (in press).
27. Creech O Jr: Endo-aneurysmorrhaphy and treatment of aortic aneurysm, *Ann Surg* 164:936–946, 1966.
28. Cambria RP, Brewster DC, Abbott WM et al: Transperitoneal vs. retroperitoneal approach for aortic reconstruction: a randomized prospective study, *J Vasc Surg* 11:314–325, 1990.
29. Chen HM, Murphy EA, Levison J, Cohen JR: Laparoscopic aortic replacement in the porcine model: a feasibility study in preparation for laparoscopically assisted abdominal aortic

aneurysm repair in humans, *J Am Coll Surg* 183:126–132, 1996.
30. Dion YM, Cardon A, Gracia C, Doillon C: A model for laparoscopic aortic aneurysm resection. Unpublished, May 1998.
31. Verbin C, Donayre C, Kopchok G et al: Anterior patch aortic aneurysm model for the study of endoluminal grafts, *J Invest Surg* 8:381–388, 1995.
32. Chen HM, Murphy EA, Halpern V et al: Laparoscopic-assisted abdominal aortic aneurysm repair, *Surg Endosc* 9:905–907, 1995.
33. Veith FJ, Marin ML: Endovascular surgery and its effect on the relationship between vascular surgery and radiology, *J Endovasc Surg* 2:1–7, 1995.
34. May J, White JH, Yu W et al: Results of endoluminal grafting of abdominal aortic aneurysms are dependent on aneurysm morphology, *Ann Vasc Surg* 10:254–261, 1996.
35. Moore WS, Rutherford RB: Transfemoral endovascular repair of abdominal aortic aneurysm: results of the North American EVT phase 1 trial, *J Vasc Surg* 23:543–552, 1996.
36. Marty B, Sanchez LA, Ohki T et al: Endoleak after endovascular graft repair of experimental aortic aneurysms: does coil embolization with angiographic "seal" lower intraaneurysmal pressure? *J Vasc Surg* 27:454–461, 1998.
37. Matsumura JS, Moore WS: Clinical consequences of periprosthetic leak after endovascular repair of abdominal aortic aneurysm, *J Vasc Surg* 27:606–613, 1998.
38. Wain RA, Marin ML, Ohki T et al: Endoleaks after endovascular graft treatment of aortic aneurysms: classification, risk factors, and outcome, *J Vasc Surg* 27:69–78, 1998.
39. Schrock TR: The endosurgery evolution: no place for sacred cows, *Surg Endosc* 6:163–168, 1992.
40. Weber G, Jako GJ: Retroperitoneal "mini" approach for aortoiliac reconstructive surgery, *Vasc Surg* 29:387–392, 1995.

35
Endovenous Surgery

John J. Bergan and Patricia E. Thorpe

Surgery of the veins was dominant in the early days of the modern era of vascular surgery. Now it has languished in performance and in progress. One of the many reasons for this is that arterial reconstruction is so spectacular and appealing to both patient and surgeon that performance of its procedures has crowded out teaching of venous disorders to students and surgical residents. Consequently, several generations of surgeons have learned little about venous pathophysiology and treatment. For them, endoluminal techniques of sclerotherapy and internal vein stripping have become an anathema. Therefore treatment of vein problems has lagged behind progress made on the other side of the circulation, in the arteries.

However, there is a sense of change in the surgical field. A new generation of surgeons is beginning to see the importance of venous surgery. They realize that diagnostic tools such as magnetic resonance phlebography and color duplex ultrasonography can unravel mysteries of venous pathophysiology. They see that minimally invasive interventions, so important to the patient's perception of success of operations, can be applied to veins. Therefore the future looks bright for endoluminal venous surgery. It is certainly appropriate to include a summary of its present status and future promise in this book.

At this time a variety of techniques have joined sclerotherapy and stripper introduction as endoluminal manipulations in the veins. Included in this armamentarium are angioscopy and several endoluminal endovenous ablative techniques. In addition, endoluminal, catheter-directed thrombolysis can be supplemented by percutaneous transluminal angioplasty (PTA) and stent placement. Also, subfascial video-endoscopy, although not truly endoluminal, must be considered in the same category because it provides outpatient, minimally invasive treatment to achieve the objectives of more traditional, older operations. This chapter considers the status of these advances in exploration of the venous system.

Current Status: Diagnosis

Progress in developing endoluminal venous surgery can proceed only after there is knowledge of the current status of venous interventions and the pathophysiology that they are designed to correct. Currently, in diagnosis, clinical examination provides a subjective categorization of venous dysfunction. This is then corroborated by instrumental objectivity. The hand-held, continuous-wave Doppler instrument lends such objectivity and has become an integral part of the venous examination.[1] It performs the same function as the Brodie-Trendelenburg test.

Commonly, the physical examination is supplemented by duplex examination. This is conducted in the supine patient when acute or chronic venous obstruction is suspected and in the erect patient when reflux is assessed.[2] Additional imaging to search for venous obstruction can be achieved by magnetic resonance or contrast phlebography.[3] Physiologic importance of chronic venous occlusions remains elusive to evaluate. Among the methods that are being employed are impedance plethysmography (IPG), mercury strain gauge (MSG), and air plethysmography (APG).

Global information about whole-limb reflux is obtained by venous pressure recovery time (VRT), photoplethysmography (PPG) recovery time, or LRR or APG examination. The venous pressure, PPG, and LRR recovery times are rendered imprecise by the vagaries of tourniquet application[1] but remain in common use. It is easily appreciated that precisely targeted therapy requires specific venous segment information regarding venous obstruction or reflux rather than the whole-limb data obtained by PPG, LRR, and APG, which may not even accurately assess grades of venous insufficiency.

After detection of venous reflux by continuous-wave Doppler sonography, duplex study identifies precisely the refluxing segment. This information is directly useful clinically. Duplex software can also give information about volume and velocity of reflux, as well as diameter and cross-sectional area of interrogated veins, but the utility of that information is questioned.[4]

Accumulated information derived from imaging techniques and physiologic studies has led to better terminology in the diagnosis of venous disorders. For example, the term *postphlebitic state* has been replaced by *chronic venous insufficiency* (CVI). The former, easily traced to the pioneering observations of Homans,[5] carried the connotation of an irreversible condition. CVI, in contrast, includes the entire cutaneous spectrum of findings of the postphlebitic state with the understanding that these may be caused by primary venous insufficiency, which can be treated for palliation and even cured.[6] This fact is of great importance to the development of endovenous surgery. Repair of venous valves, for example, can be done in primary venous dysfunction but not in the secondary, postthrombotic state. The patient with the most advanced stigmata of CVI may profit from the manipulations of endovascular repair. The limb may not have to be relegated only to treatment with elastic support.

Despite the spate of new tools to measure venous physiology and pathophysiology, the ascending[7] and descending[8] phlebograms remain the standard against which all other tests are measured. Often in practice, these are left to be performed after an advanced surgical procedure is chosen.

Current practice holds that venous problems in their simplest form, the telangiectasias, and perhaps even reticular varicosities, need only physical examination and study by hand-held, continuous-wave Doppler. Varicose veins, the next step up the hierarchical ladder of severity, require physical examination supplemented by the hand-held, continuous-wave Doppler and, if surgery is contemplated, corroboration by duplex scanning. Economic constraints of managed care limit the use of duplex scanning, although it is held to be the gold standard in detection of reflux in superficial and deep veins. If duplex examination or clinical assessment suggests the presence of obstruction either in the iliofemoral segment or in the femoropopliteal segment, imaging techniques need to be performed, such as ascending phlebography or magnetic resonance phlebography. If surgical reconstruction is thought to be necessary, or if subfascial perforator vein interruption is contemplated, ascending phlebography supplemented by descending phlebography for valve repair is usually done. Physiologic studies including APG are performed primarily as research tools rather than in selecting therapy.

Current Status: Treatment

Sclerotherapy and surgery are no longer considered to be competitive. Detection of axial reflux in the saphenous systems usually indicates surgical intervention rather than sclerotherapy. Size and location of varicosities also affect this judgment. Small varices, especially below the knee where compression therapy is most effective, may suggest treatment by sclerotherapy, whereas large varices, especially those arising in the medial thigh, may dictate treatment by surgery.

Reluctance to remove the saphenous vein led to a resurgence of interest in proximal saphenous vein ligation for correction of the gravitational reflux component of venous stasis after 1980. However, repeated comparisons of proximal ligation and stripping of the saphenous vein to the knee continue to show long-term superiority of the latter procedure when used in combination with varicectomy, perforator interruption, or sclerotherapy.[9] Saphenous ligation has the ability to return the operated patient back to work or military duty immediately. In situations where this is requisite, the lesser procedure may be justified.

Thus, after the various options have been explored, the one that produces the best long-term results has proven to be selective greater saphenous vein stripping to the knee combined with multiple stab avulsions of varices.[10]

Because reflux is the dominant pathologic finding in nearly all cases of venous dysfunction, the first step in surgical treatment is usually directed toward correction of this abnormality. Superficial reflux, rather than deep insufficiency, has proven to be an important component of the total problem in well over 50% of legs with the most severe manifestations of CVI.[11] Therefore removal of the refluxing superficial veins by the endoluminal techniques to be described is a logical first step in surgical therapy. If this is inadequate treatment, surgical venous reconstruction should be considered.

Options in venous reconstruction, which are part of the current armamentarium, include bypass of physiologically important obstruction, repair or transplantation of venous valves, or redirection of the venous stream through competent proximal valves. All of these have acceptable late results[12] but are not endoluminal.

Endoluminal Venous Stripping

The actual technique of saphenous removal (stripping) became endoluminal after Van Der Stricht[13] revived the technique first proposed by Babcock at the turn of the century.[14] In brief, the method includes selection of patients by Doppler or duplex ultrasound to ensure that saphenofemoral reflux is present, introducing the disposable plastic stripper through an open venotomy in a distal direction after transecting the vein and ligating the stump proximally (Figure 35–1). After the stripper is exposed distally at or just below the knee, a heavy ligature is tied around the vein and the stripper at its proximal end. The vein wall is grasped so that distal traction on the stripper will invert the vein into itself. Further traction allows it to exit through the lower incision. This technique minimizes tissue trauma because the relatively large stripper heads formerly used in saphenous stripping are not used. Thus the procedure accomplishes the objectives and needs of proximal saphenous vein removal and does so, incidentally, in an endovenous fashion.[15]

Although saphenous vein removal has received criticism, it has been tested against the other vein-sparing techniques and remains convincingly the best method of preventing persistent distal reflux and recurrent varicosities. Proximal saphenofemoral junction ligation with or without excision of clusters of varicosities is the other surgical option. Duplex scanning has determined the natural history of proximal saphenous vein ligation in treatment of greater saphenous reflux.[16] In 52 of 54 limbs in which actual proximal ligation was achieved, there were 24 in which reflux persisted. Similarly, Rutherford found that 70% of limbs undergoing proximal ligation for venous insufficiency showed persisting reflux,[17] and others have documented a similar experience.[18] Even when proximal ligation is supplemented by distal sclerotherapy, phlebographically controlled perforator ligation, or even surgical stab avulsion, the results are not as satisfactory as when the same maneuvers are added to saphenous vein removal to knee level.[9]

Endoluminal Sclerotherapy

Treatment of venous dysfunction by purely endoluminal sclerotherapy has a time-honored history that dates back to the invention of the syringe over 150 years ago. Modern studies have clarified indications for this form of venous ablation.[19,20] Sclerotherapy is used for the treatment of telangiectasias, reticular varicosities, postoperative persistence of varicosi-

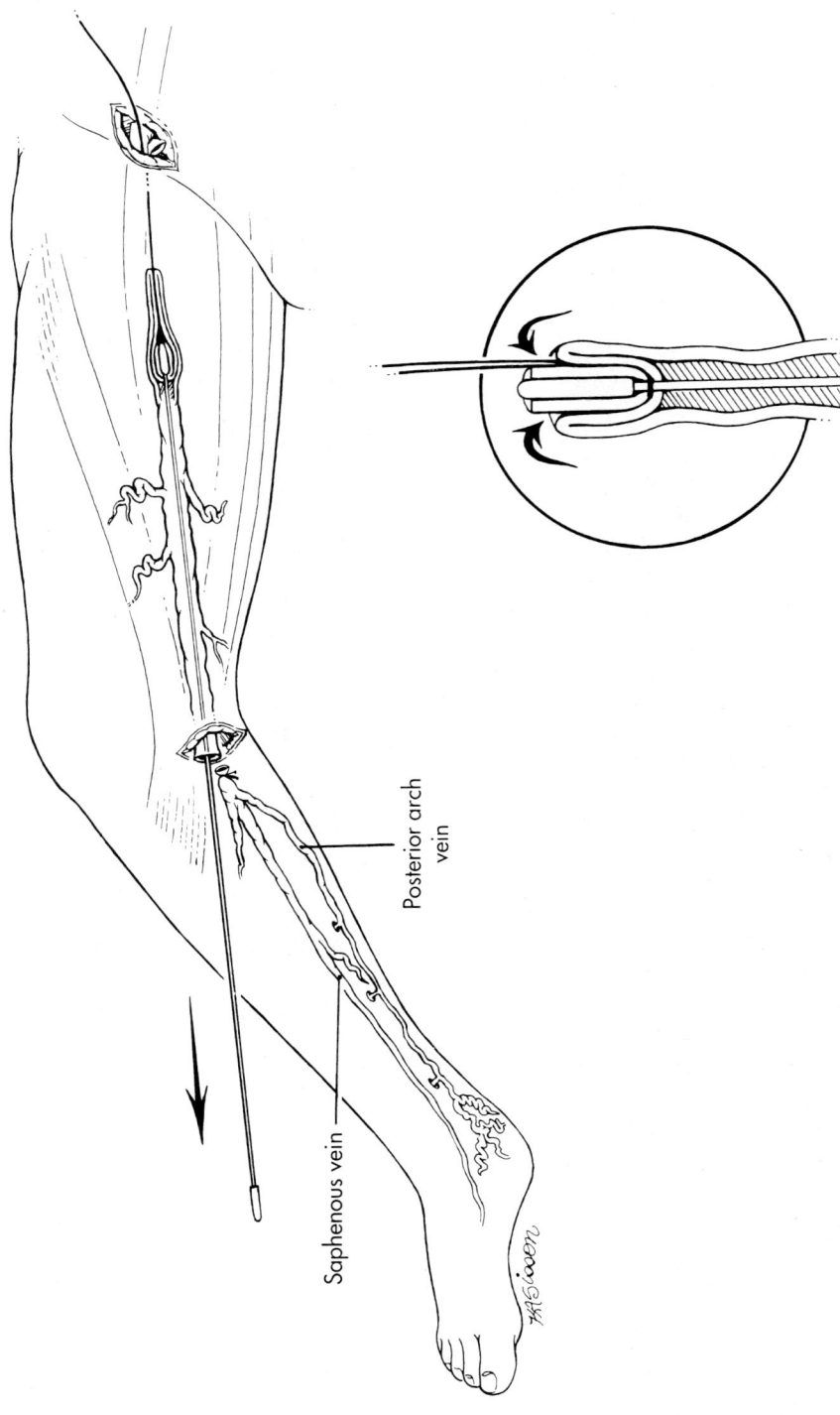

FIGURE 35–1. Removal of the thigh portion of the saphenous vein is the mainstay in surgical treatment of primary venous insufficiency. The endoluminal device, commonly a disposable plastic stripper, can be introduced from above downward and the vein ligated around the stripper proximally. As distal traction is applied, the vein is inverted into itself and removed distally in the region of the knee. This minimizes tissue trauma but accomplishes the desired result of detaching the superficial venous system from perforating veins that are transmitting intercompartmental pressure to unsupported subcutaneous venous networks.

ties, or when treatment is requisite in the aged or infirm.[21]

When patients are found with no saphenofemoral or saphenopopliteal reflux, sclerotherapy can be considered. Such sclerotherapy must be planned so as to deal with the source of venous hypertension and the distribution of the various varicose clusters. No universally accepted single sclerotherapy technique has emerged. An important contribution of the French school of sclerotherapy was emphasis on proximal-to-distal treatment.[22] A completely opposite point of view held that the largest-diameter vessels must be treated first, since these are most likely to be transmitting pressure to smaller vessels. This is especially true when the source of venous hypertension is a perforating vein such as the anteromedial-calf-perforating vein named for Boyd. This method could result in distal-to-proximal treatment. Despite this and other controversies, some guiding principles remain in sclerotherapy: (1) empty veins should be treated rather than full veins; (2) the most dilute solution that will accomplish sclerosis should be used; (3) small amounts of sclerosant should be instilled at each injection site; (4) duration of compression will vary directly with the size of the vessel being treated: telangiectasias may need no compression or require only 12 to 24 hours of compression, whereas large varicosities (4 to 6 mm in diameter) may require as much as 7 to 14 days; and (5) ambulation is believed to cause rapid dilution of sclerosing solution, which prevents high concentrations of this solution from affecting deep veins.

Risks of deep venous thrombosis are lessened by adhering to the principle of injecting no more than 0.5 to 1.0 ml per injection site.[23] The greatest success is obtained when treating the smallest vessels. Subdermal reticular veins that are in intimate contact with telangiectasias are in this category. This technique requires 30-gauge needles, and the volume injected is 0.1 to 0.5 ml per injection site. Treatment of the reticular veins before treatment of the telangiectasias greatly reduces the recurrence rate and minimizes side effects.[24]

Endoluminal Endoscopy

Although venous thrombectomy is little used in the United States, the angioscope has been found to be invaluable in controlling completeness of thrombectomy in those situations where it has been requisite. Venous thrombectomy of the left iliofemoral system in particular lends itself to intravenous angioscopy. When this shows proximal thrombus clearance to be incomplete, the procedure can be terminated by a cross-femoral bypass from the left femoral vein to the right external iliac vein with or without an arteriovenous fistula. Since venous thrombectomy is used only in situations of great need, having the option of intraoperatively monitoring clearance of thrombus is a valuable adjunct.

Miniaturization of endoscopic equipment allows exploration of the superficial venous system with visualization of the inside of the veins in situ and in vivo. Video recording of the morphology, dynamics, and kinetics of the valves is possible. Although this technique is currently in a stage of exploration, clearly the future holds hope for endovenous therapy, as is indicated below. Just as duplex ultrasound permits observation of the movements of valve leaflets, endoscopy provides a direct view of these valves. These are not seen in a physiologic state as the patient is supine, and the valves are subject to irrigating fluid. However, many observations have been made that are of some value.

The classification of venous valves into three types has been made by Van Cleef.[25] Further, when passed from below, the angioscope with its internal illuminating system is able to transilluminate the veins from within, allowing very accurate location of the saphenofemoral junction and thus minimizing the external incision to control this point. This can be a very important adjunct when operations are done for varicose recurrence after proximal ligation. After failed proximal ligation of the saphenous vein, the angioscope passed from below minimizes the proximal dissection by identifying the exact point of ligature so that this can be exposed and dealt with properly.

Endoscopic evaluation of the saphenous vein has revealed it to have a preferential flattening

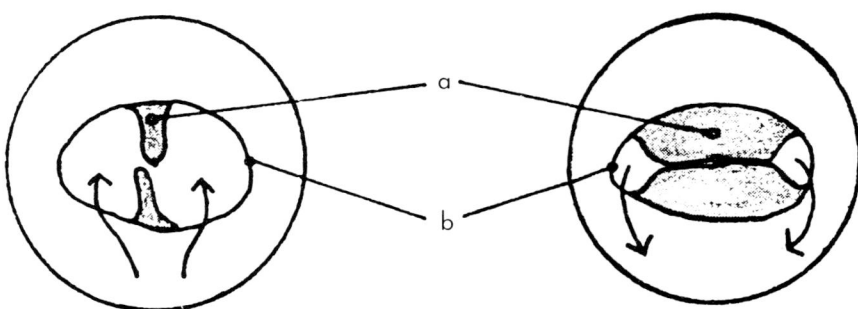

FIGURE 35-2. Angioscopic observation of valve function has clarified origin of venous reflux. This occurs at the valve commissure (a) and initiates reflux, which then proceeds along the margin of the valve (b). (From Van Cleef JF, Hugentobler JP, Desvaux P et al: Etude endoscopique des reflux vavulaires sapheniens, *J Mal Vasc* 17:113–116, 1992.)

that acts parallel to the outside of the skin. This gives a vein two walls, one internal and the other external, and two borders. The valves are inserted on each of the vein walls. The valve commissures are located on the borders; thus the free margins of the valves are parallel with the surface of the skin. Observation of valve function has revealed that transitory functional incompetence does occur in the valves (Figure 35-2). This results from inertia of the valve leaflets and adherent flattening of the valve leaflet against the vein wall with resultant loss of coaptation.

The intercorunal or commissural space allows reflux along the margin of the valve. This important observation, made by Van Cleef, implies that external suture of the commissural space may restore competency to a refluxing valve. This observation supports the work of Kistner in performing external valve plasty successfully. Finally, endoscopic observation has identified actual valve lesions such as stretching, splitting, and tearing that are de novo lesions clearly distinct from thickening, retraction, and adhesion of valves typically caused by previous phlebitis.[26]

Angioscopy of the saphenous vein in particular has therapeutic implications. The frequent finding of long segments of apparently valveless greater saphenous veins suggests that total obliteration of the valve cusps has occurred.[27] Although chronic venous hypertension is a possibility in producing this type of valve destruction, a more likely possibility is leukocyte trapping, collagenase activation, and destruction of the supporting structure of the valve. Angioscopic observation of long, valveless segments of saphenous vein confirms the earlier work of Leonard Cotton. He reported long segments of avalvular greater saphenous vein in his dissections of veins removed from varicose vein patients.[28]

Of further therapeutic importance are our observations that the greater saphenous vein is valveless or has no hemodynamically functional valves from the groin to the upper calf. These competent valves are frequently found near the anteromedial-calf–perforating vein (vein of Boyd). This observation confirms the advantage of greater saphenous stripping only to the upper calf.[10]

Since veins draining clusters of varicosities can readily be identified through the angioscope, it is logical to assume that endoscopically controlled obliteration of such veins might be of great therapeutic advantage in treating varicose clusters. Several groups have tried endovascular obliteration of tributary veins to the saphenous trunk in performance of in situ saphenous vein arterial bypass. Occlusion coils have been used. However, the technique is technically challenging, is sometimes ineffective, and causes intimal damage.

Endovenous Obliteration

More relevant to venous surgery, Gradman used venoscopically controlled endovascular obliteration of tributary veins in treatment of varicose clusters.[29] Monopolar electrocautery, available in most operating rooms, was used, and the electric current was delivered through a long, 0.4-mm steel alloy electrode insulated for most of its length with Teflon (Figure 35–3). The 1-cm exposed electrode was directed into tributary veins where a 1-second burst was delivered with the energy system set for delivery of 10 to 15 W of power. Postoperatively, the appearance of varices thrombosed using endovascular coagulation was comparable with similar varices treated with sclerotherapy. The most effective treatment was in patients with a cluster of varices arising from a single tributary from the saphenous vein. Varices with long variceal tributaries did not fare well, since the electrode usually advanced only a short distance into the tributary and the varices were seen to fill from alternate sources. There is no doubt that these initial explorations will be supplanted by improvements in all phases of the procedure in the future.

Another endovenous approach to therapy has been explored by the VNUS Medical Technologies Company of Sunnyvale, California. Their two projects have included endovenous occlusion and endovenous shrinking. The former is to obliterate grossly refluxing valve segments such as the saphenous vein, and the latter is to restore valve competence in axial veins when shrinkage could be applied

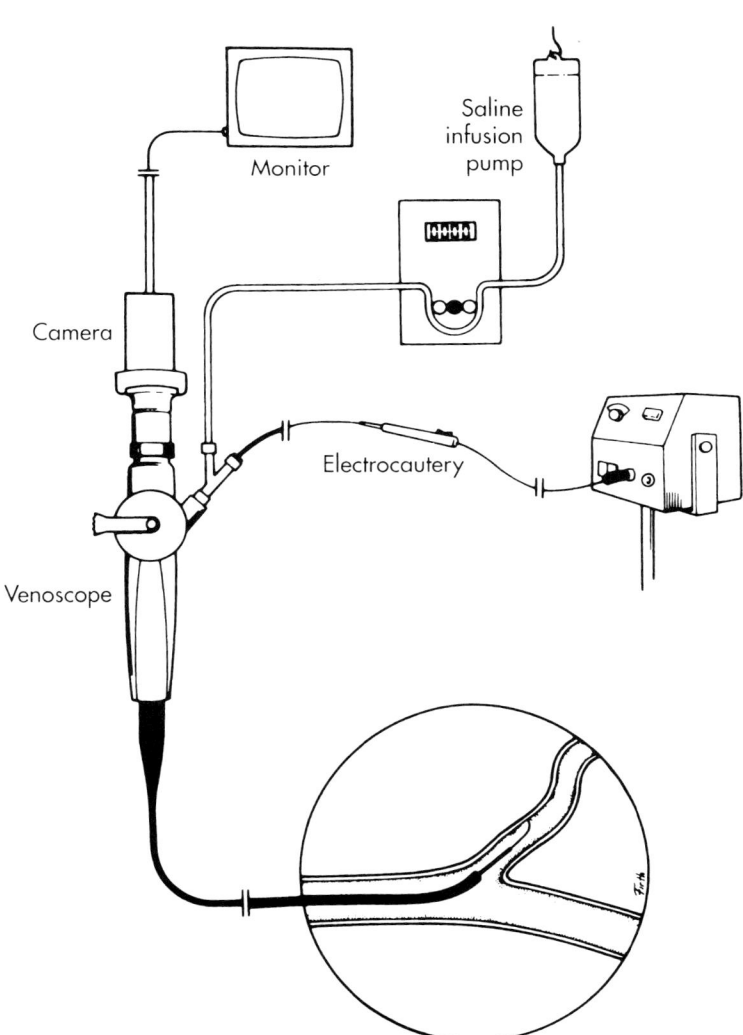

FIGURE 35–3. Monopolar electrocautery delivered to the orifice of veins draining varicose clusters can obliterate those tributaries and the control points for the cluster itself. (From Gradman WS, Segalowitz J, Grundfest W: Venoscopy in varicose vein surgery: initial experience, *Br J Surg* 48:589–598, 1961.)

(e.g., a refluxing but small-diameter saphenous vein).

The VNUS system consists of a radiofrequency generator that displays power, impedance, temperature, and the time elapsed during which the pulse is delivered. There is a temperature control, and the system delivers the minimum power necessary to maintain a preset electrode temperature. Messages to the operator are supplied. The closure catheter consists of four collapsible electrodes surrounding a microthermacouple, which measures and delivers information about vein temperature. It is designed to be used in 2- to 6-mm veins through a 5F (1.7 mm) catheter. In practice, the closure catheter is inserted into the desired segment of vein; once in position, the electrodes are deployed, and a radiofrequency energy is initiated. The vein wall contracts owing to the increased temperature initiated by the electrodes, and the catheter is slowly withdrawn, closing vein segments as it moves.

The system in practice is designed to close segments of the greater saphenous vein or lesser saphenous vein. It theoretically could be inserted into major tributaries to the greater saphenous vein at the groin such as the anterolateral vein or the posteromedial vein with its connections to the vein of Giacomini. Whether the system could be used for recurrent varices depends on the potential accessibility of those varices and the ability to thread the catheter through them. If a given limb has an established posterior arch vein with its connections to perforating veins, theoretically the obliterating catheter could perform a great service in closing the perforating veins at their connection with the posterior arch vein, thereby reducing perforating vein reflux.

Because of the ability of the intravenous electrode to measure temperature precisely and deliver this information to the operator, the system may be used to restore valve competence. It is known that the collagen in the vein wall components does shrink in response to heat. Heat is delivered to the vein wall by the expandable electrodes, which are activated by radiofrequency energy. The physician then can control the extent of shrinkage of the vein diameter, and temperature can be controlled by the system to maintain heat in the therapeutic range. Identification of refluxing valves would be done by duplex ultrasonography. Restoring valve competence to the saphenous vein could reduce the diameter of the vein and maintain its patency should it be necessary for coronary or peripheral bypass procedures. Vein wall shrinkage is apparently caused by acute contraction of myocytes and fixation by fibroblasts due to thermal denaturation. The acute constriction and folding of intracellular matrix and collagen bundles allows the valve competence to be restored in a vein of lesser diameter. Chronic studies on veins treated in this manner has shown abundant new collagen and intracellular matrix formation with the thickened vein wall and a constricted luminal diameter.[29]

Another use for the angioscope in venous surgery has been found in direct femoral vein valve repair. As that type of repair has progressed from the open technique[31] to the external suture method,[32] it has been found to be advantageous to monitor such external repair by angioscopy.[33] This method combines the advantages of external repair with avoidance of venotomy yet with accurate suture placement to ensure that the needle passes through the vein lumen and captures the edges of the elongated valve cusps. The angioscope allows discovery of hypoplastic or absent valve leaflets, which would preclude valve repair. Further, the angioscope allows final direct assessment of the repair so that valve competence is assured before surgical closure of the incision. With external vein plasty, multiple vein valves can be repaired at one operative sitting. Even greater saphenous vein valvular incompetence can be corrected if the angioscope is passed through one of the tributary veins near the saphenofemoral junction. A disadvantage of the technique is angioscope-induced trauma to venous intima or valve leaflets. Further, intraluminal pressures must be controlled very accurately to avoid disruption of the delicate valve repair.

Advocates of sclerotherapy would herald the development of the small-caliber angioscope as a possible way of obliterating greater saphenous reflux without open operation. Biegeleisen explored this possibility.[34] In 16 patients, attempts were made to obliterate 18 veins by angioscopic sclerotherapy. The angioscope was successfully passed to the saphenofemoral junction in 14 patients, and there was short-term success in 12 of them. In nine veins followed for up to 12 months, all nine recanalized in that time period. Biegeleisen's conclusion was that the magnitude of reflux through the saphenofemoral junction was much greater than had been imagined previously. This finding of complete recanalization was disparate from the patient's observations. Patients were generally satisfied with the results, but it was "evident however, that we had not obtained durable obliteration of greater saphenous varicosities with this method." Because some believe that greater saphenous ablation can be done with purely endoluminal, sclerotherapeutic techniques, the subject is not closed.[35] The future holds that this technique may receive selective application.

Clearly, angioscopy will find a place in direct venous surgery in the near future.

Endovenous Thrombolysis

Though thrombolyic therapy offers the potential of removing acute thrombus and preserving valvular integrity, concern for patient safety (based on bleeding complications associated with early trials of systemic infusions) has prevented its widespread use.[36] In addition to bleeding complications, systemic thrombolytic therapy is ineffective for treating lower extremity venous occlusion, as flow is shunted to collaterals and the superficial veins, away from the thrombosed segments.

The introduction of catheter-directed thrombolysis, unlike systemic thrombolysis, which has limited benefit in lower extremity deep venous thrombosis (DVT) due to preferential flow into collateral veins, offers a alternative method for treating DVT. Catheter-directed thrombolysis with urokinase has shown promise in treating both arterial and venous peripheral vascular disease.[37-40] Evidence reveals that 75% to 79% of patients treated for DVT with this technique demonstrated complete or partial lysis of thrombus, improved vessel patency, and alleviation of symptoms.[41,42] Although some investigators have stated that the estimated age of the thrombus is inversely correlated with technical success, we have shown clinical benefits from improved venous flow after treating chronic thrombosis as well.[41,43] Urokinase has been recommended as the agent of choice for treating DVT because of its margin of safety and low complication rate.[44,45]

With its varying degrees of severity, DVT is a complex disease to treat. Experience suggests that thrombolysis offers advantages over anticoagulation alone, particularly for maintaining valvular competence. We have concluded that thrombolysis with urokinase is a safe, effective alternative to heparin anticoagulation for treating DVT. Furthermore, when comparing patients treated for a first known episode of DVT, urokinase patients experienced significantly less postthrombotic pain. This observation endured throughout the 10-year follow-up and suggests that removal of thrombus mitigates, if not prevents, valvular damage that leads to venous hypertension. Although most patients with chronic venous insufficiency have reflux without thrombosis, 10% to 15% of this population are afflicted by residual obstruction. This represents a large number of patients who suffer from apparently preventable postthrombotic sequelae.

Patient selection for thrombolysis remains a challenge and appears to include active patients with extensive, multisegmental obstructing thrombosis. Our unreported data suggest that thrombolysis versus standard therapy provides a clinical challenge to this group. This advantage could result in less venous disease over a lifetime and might represent a significant decrease in health care costs to society.

Venous Stenting

Intravascular stents have been designed for use in arteries; experience with stents in the venous system is more limited. Further, the longest reported clinical follow-up of arterial stenting is in the 5- to 10-year range. Therefore there is no conclusive evidence that long-term results will be satisfactory in the venous system. At present, venous stenting, a truly endoluminal technique, is restricted to a highly selected group of individuals who are poor surgical can-

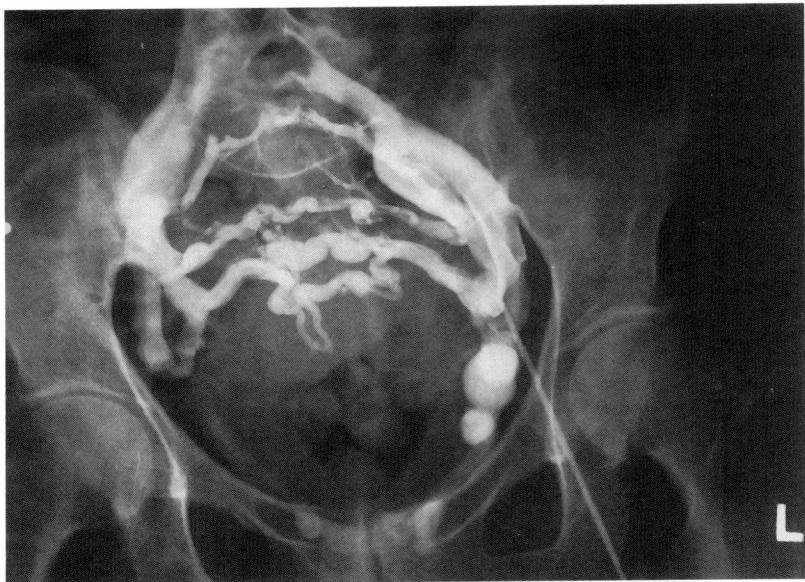

FIGURE 35–4. This left iliac phlebogram shows the characteristic appearance of the May-Thurner syndrome with right iliac artery compression of the left common iliac vein. The patient is a 27-year-old woman with refractory venous stasis ulceration who demonstrated superficial reflux in the greater saphenous system distal to this lesion. Ablation of such reflux did not result in ulcer healing, and therefore the procedure of left iliac venous dilation and stenting was planned.

didates but who have venoocclusive disease caused by thrombosis, prior surgery, and even angioplasty. Despite this, it has become increasingly apparent that percutaneous procedures are useful in opening venous conduits that are closed, compressed, or stenotic.

Endoluminal stents are fully described elsewhere in this book. Stents currently in use include stainless steel, tantalum, and nickel-titanium alloy. These have been fashioned into rigid tubes, flexible wire cylinders, woven meshes, and other designs that have been created to enhance desirable characteristics. The future holds that complex polysaccharide matrixes may be employed in an effort to obtain bioresorptive lattice works. The stents may be balloon expandable, such as the Palmaz stent, or self-expanding such as the Wallstent or the Gianturco Z stent. The latter are stainless steel, but their designs and methods of deployment are quite different.

The largest experience of venous stenting reported to date is that of the Stanford group.[46] Their experience includes treatment of the vena cava, the innominate, the subclavian, thoracic outlet venous compression, and iliofemoral veins (Figures 35–4, 35–5). Nearly half of their patients have had regional thrombolysis. In those without thrombus, a significant pressure gradient and/or residual stenosis was observed after percutaneous transluminal dilatation. They averaged placement of 2.8 stents per patient, with a resolution of venous obstructive symptoms in 97% of treated patients. Late follow-up revealed a 10% occlusion rate, but secondary patency was achieved in 95% of these. The Stanford group, with its vast experience, favors placement of stents in malignant obstructions. However, they have addressed the problem of failing hemodialysis access conduits in which the results are usually palliative but safe. In treating venous thrombosis, results with acute thromboses have been dramatic, and even chronic deep venous thrombosis has been benefited by treatment with catheter-directed thrombolysis and stent placement.

When lytic agents are used before stent placement, access can be gained through prox-

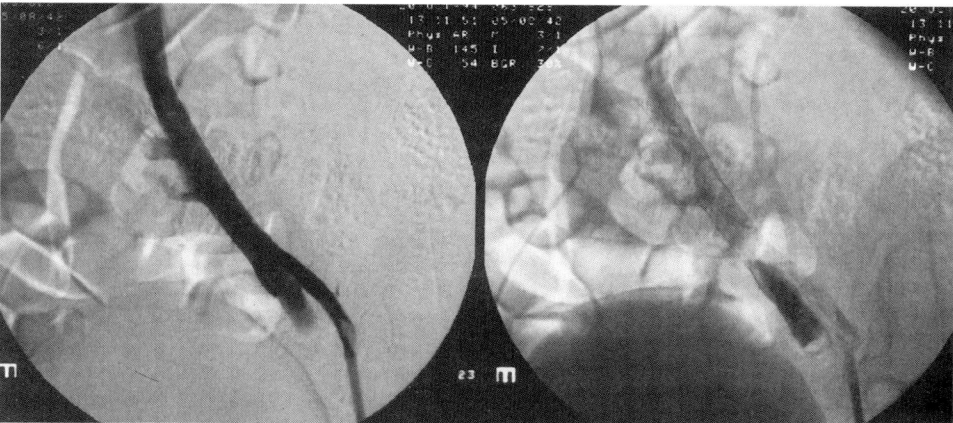

FIGURE 35-5. These photographs taken during venous stenting in Figure 35-4 demonstrate placement of the self-expanding Wallstent and the smooth venous channel that results after its insertion. Note the absence of crossover venous collateral vessels. This indicates that the physiologic obstruction present with they May-Thurner syndrome has been totally relieved.

imal arterial infusion or retrograde installation into foot veins with external compression. Ultrasound-directed popliteal puncture or even ipsilateral or contralateral femoral vein access are also possibilities. The transjugular placement of an infusion catheter directly into the thrombus has been found to be a favorable alternative because this provides easy access, prevention of further deep venous thrombosis from catheter placement, and sparing of the femoral vein from catheter-related trauma.

Advantages of the thrombolysis stent placement technique are obvious. No surgical procedure is required; no arteriovenous fistula is constructed.[47] However, as with any new treatment modality, long-term careful observation is mandatory. These techniques may be only of short-term benefit.

Subfascial Endoscopy

Although technically not endovenous, subfascial operations using endoscopy should be included in this review because they fulfill the requirements of achieving therapeutic objectives in a minimally invasive fashion that allows outpatient, economically advantageous procedures to be accomplished. Perforator vein interruptions have been performed for decades in the treatment of severe chronic venous insufficiency. However, long hospitalization time required by slow secondary healing of long incisions from knee to ankle have discouraged wide application of these procedures.

Introduction of laparoscopic general surgery spurred investigation of minimally invasive approaches to venous surgery. Accumulating experience suggested that video-assisted techniques might be applicable to subfascial perforator interruption because 90% of incompetent perforating veins occur in the lower leg in the posterior arch vein distribution.[48]

Clinically significant perforators include the gastrocnemius point, soleal point, and perforating veins identified at varying distances from the heel pad.[49] All of these are accessible by endoscopic coagulation or clipping. Such interruption occludes the perforating vein proximal to its branchings, and this approach allows transsection of all perforators that are thought to be clinically significant. An appealing aspect of the procedure is that it can be performed on an outpatient basis. Furthermore, the surgical incision is made proximal to affected skin even in patients with far-advanced changes of lipodermatosclerosis and healed ulceration.

We have chosen to modify the open technique of Reinhard Fischer of St. Gallen, Switzerland.[50] The incision is made on the

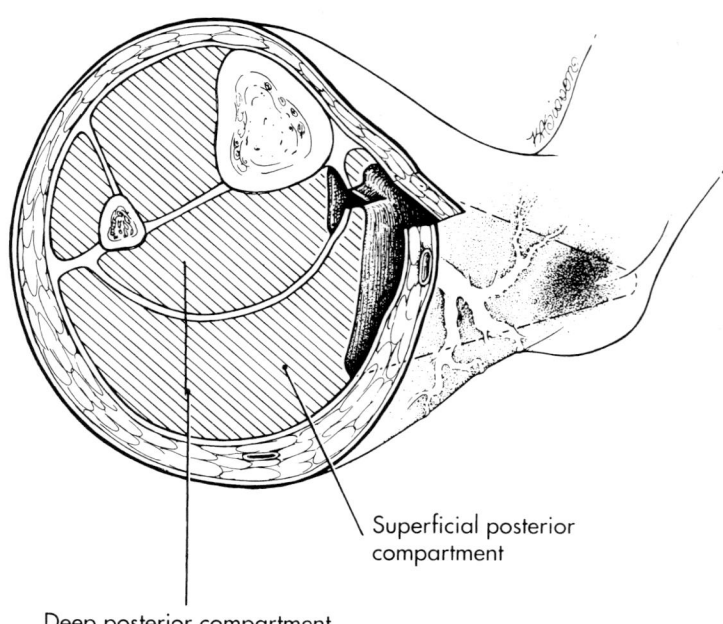

FIGURE 35–6. Proximal incision and space that can be treated by subfascial endoscope. Perforator veins emanating from the superficial posterior compartment can be clipped and divided or electrocoagulated and divided using endoscope and video visualization. Paratibial perforating veins emanating from the deep posterior compartment can be identified after incision into fascia of the deep posterior compartment and exposure of those very important paratibial perforating veins.

anteromedial leg posterior to the tibia. The 3-cm skin and subcutaneous incision is retracted to expose the fascia that is incised. A subfascial space is created by inserting the endoscope and manipulating it anteriorly as far as is feasible and then posteriorly as far as needed.

It is relatively easy to distinguish a normal perforating vein that is competent from one that is incompetent. The normal perforator exhibits one or more veins with parallel walls that are not tortuous or dilated. The accompanying artery is often seen. In contrast, the incompetent perforating vein is often thick, passes transversely, is apparently white, and looks bloodless if a tourniquet is used and exsanguination of the limb has preceded the exploration. Without the tourniquet the incompetent perforating vein looks like any other varicose vein. Frequently the incompetent perforating vein is seen to branch into one or more tributaries before penetrating the fascia. Recognition of perforating veins is much more accurate by the subfascial approach than by phlebography or preoperative Doppler or duplex techniques.

Limitations of subfascial video endoscopic perforator interruption are found in the most distal aspect of the leg. This is a dangerous area anatomically. Here there is reduced maneuverability of the instrumentation. The most serious distal consequences of the procedure include damage to the posterior tibial nerve. Complications may be avoided by keeping strictly to the fascia in every step throughout the endoscopy. Also, no structure should be divided unless one is absolutely sure it is a perforating vein. Before applying the cautery, extreme care must be taken that the structure being clamped, cauterized, or clipped is a perforating vein and not the accompanying artery or posterior tibial nerve.[51]

Division of the crural fascia in patients with the most severe forms of chronic venous insufficiency has been advocated by many.[52,53] The subfascial endoscopic perforator interruption technique lends itself to such fasciotomy. After division of the perforating veins and thorough exploration of the available space, the procedure is terminated by passing a fasciotomy knife through the scope and incising the fascia from above downward or from below upward (Figure 35–6). The pathophysiologic indication for this is the severe fascia fibrosis and elevated compartment pressures found in the fascia in severe chronic venous insufficiency.[54] Thickening, induration, and elevated pressures are thought to limit transfascial blood flow. Transcutaneous partial pressure of oxygen ($TCPO_2$) levels have been measured in patients before and after fasciotomy. In all instances the measurements were made 2 cm proximal to the ulceration and 2, 5, and 10 days afterward. An increase in $TCPO_2$ was observed immediately postoperatively, and by the 10th postoperative day all patients showed $TCPO_2$ levels that were at least 100% higher than before surgery. The impressive increase in $TCPO_2$ was confirmed at 8 weeks after the procedure.[53]

Von Langer measured compartment pressures in 12 patients with varicose veins, 18 with severe chronic venous insufficiency, and 6 with the postthrombotic syndrome. Compartment pressures were lowest in those patients with primary venous insufficiency, intermediate in patients with severe chronic venous insufficiency, and highest in those with the postthrombotic syndrome. In all instances in these 36 patients a laser fasciotomy decreased the postoperative compartment pressures to one-half of the preoperative level. Since the broad fasciotomy split has been observed to remain open at least 6 months after the procedure, it appears that fasciotomy in situations of most severe chronic venous insufficiency is clearly an important addition to the minimally invasive armamentarium.

Conclusion

Endovenous surgery is clearly in its infancy. However, standard endoluminal techniques of saphenous ablation and sclerotherapy have now been joined by endoluminal thrombolysis and stenting in selected cases. Furthermore, explorations and angioscopy, electrodesiccation of selected venous tributaries, and monitoring by intravenous ultrasound are clearly within the capabilities of surgeons today. Finally, subfascial endoscopic techniques, although not precisely endoluminal, show promise in offering treatments that formerly required hospitalization to afflicted individuals on an outpatient basis.

References

1. Van Bemmelen JS, Bergan JJ: *Quantitative measurement of venous incompetence*, Austin, 1992, RG Landes.
2. Van Bemmelen PS, Bedford G, Beach K et al: Quantitative segmental evaluation of venous valvular reflux with ultrasound scanning, *J Vasc Surg* 10:425–431, 1989.
3. Bergan JJ: New developments in the surgical treatment of venous disease, *J Cardiovasc Surg (Torino)* 1:624–631, 1993.
4. Moulton S, Bergan JJ, Beeman S et al: Gravitational reflux does not correlate with clinical status of venous stasis, *Phlebology* 8:2–6, 1993.
5. Homans J: Thrombophlebitis of the lower extremities, *Ann Surg* 87:641–651, 1928.
6. Walsh JC, Bergan JJ, Beeman S et al: Femoral venous reflux is abolished by greater saphenous vein stripping, *Ann Vasc Surg* 8:566–570, 1994.
7. Lea Thomas M et al: A simplified technique of phlebography for the localization of incompetent perforating veins of the legs, *Clin Radiol* 23:486, 1972.
8. Kamida CB, Kistner RL: Descending phlebography: the Straub technique. In Bergan JJ, Kistner RL, editors: *Atlas of venous surgery*, Philadelphia, 1992, WB Saunders.
9. Neglen P, Einarsson E, Eklof B: The functional long-term value of different types of treatment for saphenous vein incompetence, *J Cardiovasc Surg (Torino)* 34:295–301, 1993.
10. Sarin S, Scurr JH, Coleridge-Smith PD: Assessment of stripping the long saphenous vein in the treatment of primary varicose veins, *Br J Surg* 79:889–893, 1992.
11. Shami SK, Sarin S, Cheatle TR et al: Venous ulcers and the superficial venous system, *J Vasc Surg* 17:487, 1993.
12. Bergan JJ: Reconstruction of deep veins. In Negus D, editor: *Leg ulcers: a practical approach to management*, ed 2, London, 1994, Butterworth-Heinemann.
13. Van Der Stricht J: La crossectomie. Quant et Pourquoi? *Extrait de Phlebologie* 39(1):47, 1986.
14. Babcock WW: A new operation for extirpation of varicose veins, *NY Med J* 86:1553, 1907.
15. Bergan JJ: Ambulatory surgery of varicose veins. In Bergan JJ, Goldman MP, editors: *Ambulatory treatment of venous disease: an illustrative guide*, St Louis, 1995, Mosby.
16. McMullin GM, Coleridge-Smith PD, Scurr JH: Objective assessment of high ligation without stripping the long saphenous vein, *Br J Surg* 78:1139–1142, 1991.

17. Rutherford RB, Sawyer JD, Jones DN: The fate of residual saphenous vein after partial removal or ligation, *J Vasc Surg* 12:422–428, 1990.
18. Friedell ML, Samson RH, Cohen MJ et al: High ligation of the greater saphenous vein for treatment of lower extremity varicosities. The fate of the vein and therapeutic results, *Ann Vasc Surg* 6:5–8, 1992.
19. Hobbs JT: A random trial of the treatment of varicose veins by surgery and sclerotherapy. In Hobbs JT, editor: *The treatment of venous disorders*, Phildelphia, 1977, JB Lippincott.
20. Jakobsen BH: The value of different forms of treatment for varicose veins, *Br J Surg* 66:182–184, 1979.
21. Goldman MP, Weiss RA, Bergan JJ: Diagnosis and treatment of varicose veins: a review, *J Am Acad Dermatol* 3:393–414, 1994.
22. Tournay R, Caille JP, Chatard H et al: *La Sclerose des Varices*, Paris, 1980, Expansion Scientifique.
23. Weiss RA, Weiss MA: Sclerotherapy. In Wheeland RG, editor: *Cutaneous surgery*, Philadelphia, 1994, WB Saunders.
24. Weiss RA, Weiss MA: Painful telangiectasias: diagnosis and treatment. In Bergan JJ, Goldman MP, editors: *Varicose veins and telangiectasias: diagnosis and treatment*, St Louis, 1993, Quality Medical Publishers.
25. Van Cleef JF, Desvaux P, Hugentobler JP et al: Endoscopie Veneuse, *J Mal Vasc* 16:184–187, 1991.
26. Van Cleef JF, Hugentobler JP, Desvaux P et al: Etude endoscopique des reflux valvulaires sapheniens, *J Mal Vasc* 17:113–116, 1992.
27. Gradman WS, Segalowitz J, Grundfest W: Venoscopy in varicose vein surgery: initial experience, *Phlebology* 8:145–150, 1993.
28. Cotton LT: Varicose veins: gross anatomy and development, *Br J Surg* 48:589–598, 1961.
29. Gradman WS: Venoscopic obliteration of variceal tributaries using monopolar electrocautery: preliminary report, *J Dermatol Surg Oncol* 20:482–485, 1994.
30. VNUS Medical Technologies Presentation, North American Society of Phlebology, Nov 7, 1997.
31. Kistner RL: Surgical repair of the incompetent femoral valve, *Arch Surg* 110:1336–1342, 1975.
32. Kistner RL: Valve reconstruction for primary valve insufficiency. In Bergan JJ, Kistner RL, editors: *Atlas of Venous Surgery*, Philadelphia, 1992, WB Saunders.
33. Gloviczki P, Merrell SW, Bower TC: Femoral vein valve repair under direct vision without venotomy: a modified technique with use of angioscopy, *J Vasc Surg* 14:645–648, 1991.
34. Biegeleisen K: Failure of angioscopically guided sclerotherapy to permanently obliterate greater saphenous varicosity, *Phlebology* 9:21–24, 1994.
35. Raymond-Martimbeau P: Two different techniques for sclerosing the incompetent saphenofemoral junction: a comparative study, *J Dermatol Surg Oncol* 16:626–631, 1990.
36. Ricotta JJ, Dalsing MC, Ouriel K et al: Research and clinical issues in chronic venous disease, *Cardiovasc Surg* 5:343–349, 1997.
37. Graor RA, Young JR, Rusius B, Ruschhaupt WF: Comparison of cost-effectiveness of streptokinase and urokinase in the treatment of deep venous thrombosis, *Ann Vasc Surg* 1:524–528, 1987.
38. Ouriel K, Shortell CK, DeWeese JA et al: A comparison of thrombolytic therapy with operative revascularization in the initial treatment of acute peripheral arterial ischemia, *J Vasc Surg* 19:1021–1030, 1994.
39. Janosik JE, Bettmann MA, Kaul AF, Souney PF: Therapeutic alternatives for subacute peripheral arterial occlusion: comparison by outcome, length of stay, and hospital charges, *Invest Radiol* 26:921–925, 1991.
40. Van Breda A, Graor RA, Katzen BT et al: Relative cost-effectiveness of urokinase versus streptokinase in the treatment of peripheral vascular disease, *J Vasc Interv Radiol* 2:77–87, 1991.
41. Bjarnason H, Kruse JR, Asinger DA et al: Iliofemoral deep venous thrombosis: safety and efficacy outcome during five years of catheter-directed thrombolytic therapy, *J Vasc Interv Radiol* 8:405–418, 1997.
42. Comerota AJ, Katz ML, White JV: Thrombolytic therapy for acute deep venous thrombosis: how much is enough? *Cardiovasc Surg* 4:101–104, 1996.
43. Thorpe PE, Zhan XX, Sides SN: Endovascular therapy for chronic venous disease [abstract], *J Vasc Interv Radiol* 9:175, 1998.
44. Semba CP, Dake MD: Venous thrombosis. In: Ouriel K, editor: *Lower extremity vascular disease*, Philadelphia, 1995, Saunders, pp 312–330.
45. Tomera JF, Kaul AF: Regional thrombolytic infusion for peripheral arterial occlusion and deep venous thrombosis: tried and true, *Am J Health Syst Pharm* 54:1988–1991, 1997.

46. Semba CP, Dake MD: Iliofemoral deep venous thrombosis: aggressive therapy with catheter-directed thrombolysis, *Radiology* 191:487–494, 1994.
47. Janssen HJ, Antonucci F, Stuckman G et al: Behandlung von venenstenosen und verschlussen benigner Atiologie mit vaskularen endoprothesen: ein neues, nichtoperatives therapiekonzept, *Vasa* 23:66–73, 1994.
48. Jugenheimer M, Junginger T: Endoscopic subfascial sectioning of incompetent perforating veins in treatment of primary varicosis, *World J Surg* 16:971–975, 1992.
49. Sherman RS: Varicose veins: anatomy, reevaluation of Trendelenburg tests, and operating procedure, *Surg Clin North Am* 44:1369, 1964.
50. Fischer R: Erfahrungen mit der endoskopischen Perforantensanierung, *Phebologie* 21:224–229, 1992.
51. Fischer R, Sattler G, Vanderpuye R: Le traitement endoscopique des perforantes (TEP) situation actuelle, *Phlebologie* 46:701–707, 1993.
52. Hauer G et al: Endoskopische subfasziale diszision der perforansven. In Bruner H, editor: *Der Unterschenkel. Aktuelle Probleme in der angiologie*, Stuttgart, 1988, Huber.
53. Vanscheidt W, Peschen M, Kreitinger J et al: Paratibial fasciotomy, *Phlebology* 23:45–48, 1994.
54. Von Langer C, Vorpahl U, Atamer C, Schück R: Die endoskopische laserfasciotomie. In Schütz R, Bruch H-P, Weiss H-d, editors: *Neue Trends in Diagnostik und Therapie von Venenleiden*, Lübeck, 1993, Norddeutsche Angiologentage.

36
Thoracic Outlet Syndrome: Endoscopic Transaxillary First Rib Resection and Thoracodorsal Sympathectomy for Causalgia

Bernardo D. Martinez

Thoracic outlet syndrome is a condition related to compression of the subclavian axillary vein, artery, and brachial plexus due to significant congenital anomalies of the scalenus muscle insertion at the first rib. In situations associated with trauma or occupational demand on the upper extremity, the functional relationship between these neurovascular structures, scalenus muscles, and the first rib appear to be altered.

Surgical Decisions

The surgical procedure elected depends on the patient's clinical presentation. Most importantly, the decision for surgical intervention is based on worsening of the clinical symptoms of the patient, confirmation of the abnormal physical examination findings, the degree of disability, and failure of a conservative home exercise program to relieve neurogenic symptoms of compression. When symptoms of arterial and veins compression manifest, a thoracic outlet home exercise program is contraindicated.

Transaxillary Surgical Decompression

A transaxillary approach for first rib resection was first described by Roos in 1966,[1] offering an alternative to the anterior or supraclavicular approach[2], or the posterior approach.[3] The concept of adjunctive endoscopic video was adopted in 1983 because of the relative inaccessibility of the anatomic surgical area during the transaxillary approach.[4] This technique demonstrated the benefits of magnifying the anatomic surgical area, which ensures a greater measure of safety during the transaxillary approach.[5,6] In 1982 the safety of transaxillary first rib resection was widely reported.[7] In addition, intraoperative endoscopic video during the transaxillary approach offers direct visualization of the congenital anomalies of the scalenus muscles and their compression of vital structures, greatly enhancing the likelihood of preserving functional integrity of the nerve, artery, and vein.

Congenital cervical band anomalies were first described in 1976[8] and provided the key to the problem of thoracic outlet syndrome.

Endoscopic Transaxillary First Rib Resection

To understand the biomechanics of this surgical procedure, it is essentially important to review the basic anatomic landmarks of the first rib and its muscular insertions. Figure 36–1 (see color plate), shows the left first rib from a superior view, indicating that the most anterior muscular structure insertion is the subclavius muscle. This muscle orientation and hypertrophy are important in the development of venous compression in association with the costoclavicular ligament and the most anterior fibers of the scalenus anterior muscle, which inserts behind the vein. These three elements are key to the pathogenesis of extrinsic venous compression by a type 7 band,[6,8] particularly in

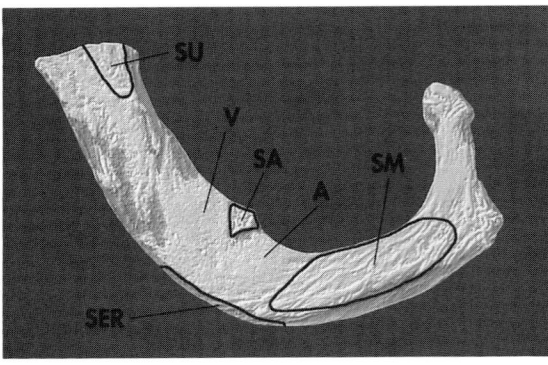

FIGURE 36-1. The left first rib shows its muscular insertions. *SU*, subclavius; *V*, venous space; *SA*, scalenus anterior; *A*, arterial space; *SER*, serratus anterior; *SM*, scalenus medius. (See color plate).

athletic muscular individuals. It is important to appreciate that the length of rib that lies underneath the clavicle remains anterior to the vein (Figure 36-1), joining the sternum to create a relatively large surface area.

On traversing the rib, venous and arterial rib notching is noted (Figure 36-1) as well as the scalenus tubercle, the site of insertion of the scalenus anterior. This muscle usually has a wide variation of anatomic insertion. Obviously, a wide insertion narrows the thoracic outlet space, producing neurovascular compression.

The scalenus medius is an important muscle and a key factor in neurogenic compression. Its broad insertion can be seen in Figure 36-2. Type 3 band, which is a derivative of the most medial fibers of the scalenus medius in the inner border of the first rib, is the most common of all the congenital bands. Type 3 band is a critical factor in the compression of C8-T1 branches of the brachial plexus (Figures 36-2, 36-3, 36-4, see color plate). The second most common band is type 5, scalenus minimus (Figures 36-5, 36-6, see color plate), which may have its lower insertion in the first rib or the Sibson fascia, between the artery and the nerve.

Type 4 band, although seen less frequently, is a powerful band, capable of compressing the nerve and the artery. This band, like a sling under the artery and the nerve, is composed of the most posterior fibers of the scalenus anterior and the most medial fibers of the scalenus medius. Figure 36-7 (see color plate) shows severe neurovascular compression from type 4 band with practically no outlet. Figure 36-8 (see color plate) shows the posterior stump of the first rib with attachments of the scalenus medius muscle and the "arcuate" ligament, or type 4 band, still around the nerve and the artery. Figure 36-9 (see color plate) shows complete resection of the first rib and partial resection of the scalenus medius. When completely resected, decompression of the nerve and artery is achieved. The area of indentation resulting from the previous compression can be easily recognized.

Figure 36-1 also indicates a significant length of the first rib behind the scalenus medius insertion, including its tubercle. Complete excision of the first rib at the articular surface of the transverse process of T1 vertebrae is seen in Figure 36-4.

Position and Incisions

The patient is placed under general anesthesia using the bibronchial Univent endotracheal tube technique. The patient is positioned in a modified lateral decubitus attitude, at approximately 35° to 40°.

Two incisions are made. A 4-cm instrumental working incision is made transversally at the axillary hairline level. This is done at the third rib level between the pectoralis major and latissimus dorsi muscles. An endoscopic incision to accommodate a 10-mm trocar (Ethicon, Cincinnati, OH) is made more inferiorly and anteriorly at the fourth rib level.[5,6]

It is recommended that a 10 mm (W) × 20 cm (L) rigid endoscope, with a 0° lens (0°, Wolf, 8960.40, Germany) attached to a microvideo camera, be utilized for visualization. The trocar-endoscope system serves as a support over the second and third ribs to facilitate access to the first rib and the thoracic outlet anatomy.

Creation of the Surgical Space

Sharp and blunt instrumental dissection is used to gain access to the intercostal muscle plane. Advancing superiorly in this landmark facilitates creation of a surgical working space.

36. Thoracic Outlet Syndrome

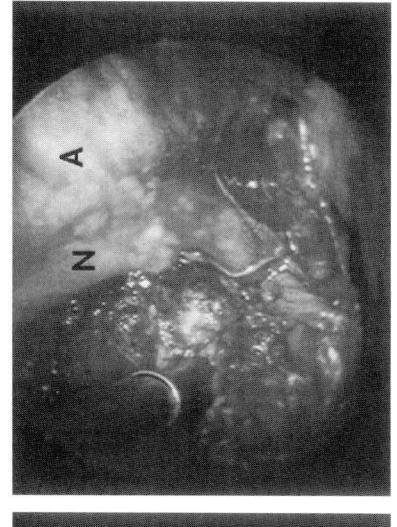

FIGURE 36–2. Right transaxillary approach. *Arrow* shows area of the compression of the nerve by a type 3 band. *SM*, scalenus medius; *N*, nerve; *A*, artery; *R*, rib; *SA*, scalenus anterior; *V*, vein. (See color plate).

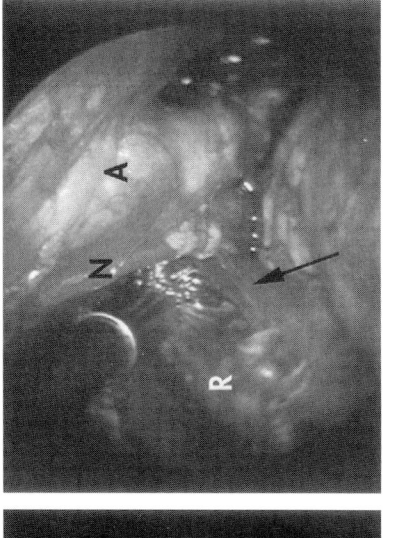

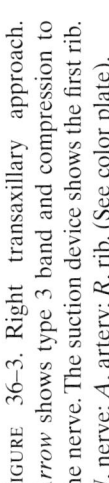

FIGURE 36–3. Right transaxillary approach. *Arrow* shows type 3 band and compression to the nerve. The suction device shows the first rib. *N*, nerve; *A*, artery; *R*, rib. (See color plate).

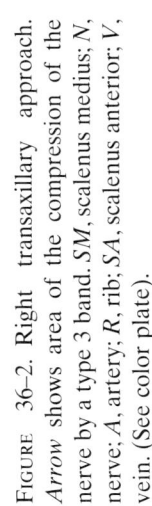

FIGURE 36–4. Completion of the transaxillary first rib resection. Suction device shows cartilaginous surface of the transverse process of thoracic I vertebra. *N*, nerve; *A*, artery. (See color plate).

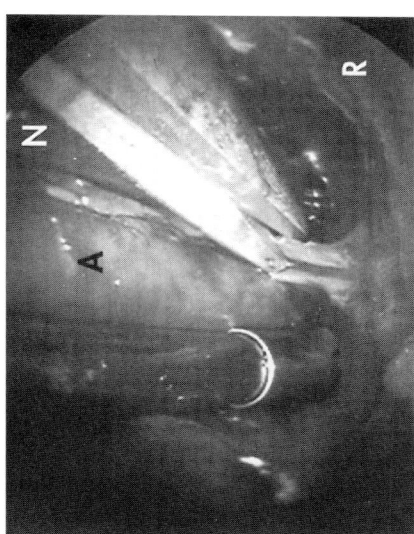

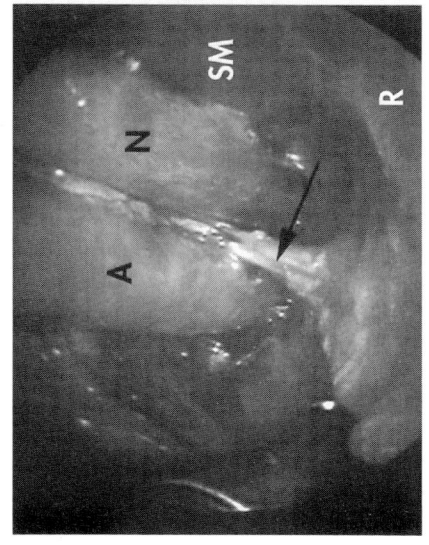

FIGURE 36–5. Left transaxillary approach. *Arrow* shows type 5 band between the artery and the nerve. *A*, artery; *N*, nerve; *SM*, scalenus medius; *R*, rib. (See color plate).

FIGURE 36–6. Left transaxillary approach. Scissor is cutting a type 5 band. *A*, artery; *N*, nerve; *R*, rib. (See color plate).

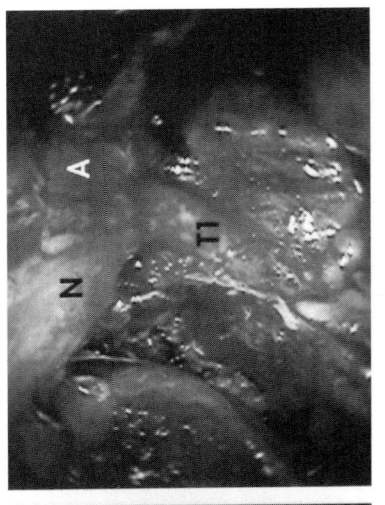
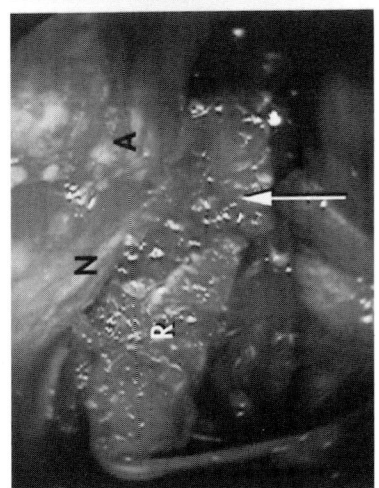
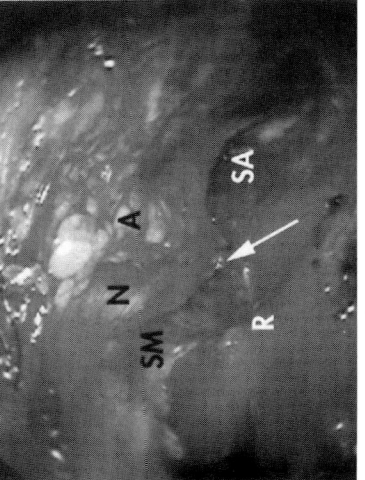

FIGURE 36–7. Right transaxillary approach. *Arrow* shows critical compression of the nerve and the artery by a type 4 band. *N*, nerve; *A*, artery; *SM*, scalenus medius; *SA*, scalenus anterior; *R*, rib. (See color plate).

FIGURE 36–8. Right transaxillary approach. Anterior and middle third of the first rib is already excised. *Arrow* shows that abundant muscle fibers (type 4) are still compressing the nerve and artery. *R*, rib; *N*, nerve; *A*, artery. (See color plate).

FIGURE 36–9. Completed right first rib resection. The nerve and the artery are decompressed. *N*, nerve; *T1*, lower branch of brachial plexus; *A*, artery. (See color plate).

Venous and arterial branches encountered in the subcutaneous tissue layer and near the vicinity of the first rib and axillary artery are usually controlled by ligation techniques.

A second intercostal brachial cutaneous nerve branch is frequently encountered. As pushing and stretching the nerve may produce undesirable paresthesias in the area, it is recommended that this branch be sacrificed even though it provokes regional numbness in the posteromedial aspect of the arm.

Maintenance of the Surgical Space

An important concept in endoscopic surgery is that the surgery is greatly enhanced when a thoroughly complete dissection of the space is achieved, as described in our previous step. This surgical space is maintained using a controlled biomechanical traction device comprised of a pneumatic air-filled arm support (Jobst, Charlotte, NC). The system is suspended by orthopedic bars and ropes attached to the operating table. Minimal weights and manual surgical assistant control provides the traction delivered throughout the procedure. The surgical working space is also maintained by an Omni retractor, applying a single blade in the subpectoral space just anterior to the axillary vein. A lateral narrowed Deaver retractor is placed to control the latissimus dorsi, taking care not to exert any pressure on the long thoracic nerve.

Identification of Soft Tissue Muscular Anomalies, Brachial Plexus, Subclavian Axillary Artery and Vein

The endoscopic technique described ensures a great measure of safety by offering direct, continuous visualization of the vital structures indicated in Figure 36–10 (see color plate). Complete evaluation of the neurovascular compression by these soft tissue bands is essential to the surgical strategy during surgical decompression.

Disengagement of Scalenus Muscles

Proper instrumentation is required to disengage the scalenus muscle with precision and safety (Figure 36–11). The straight Urschel,

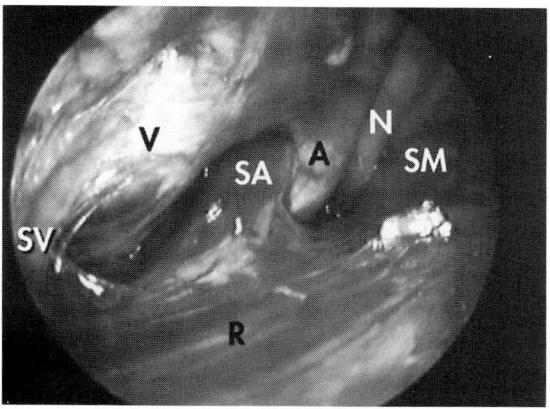

FIGURE 36–10. Left transaxillary approach, overall view. *SV*, subclavius; *V*, vein; *SA*, scalenus anterior; *A*, artery; *N*, nerve; *SM*, scalenus medius; *R*, rib. (See color plate).

single action rongeur and the angled Urschel modified by Martinez are used to excise the fibers of these muscles by small bites under direct endoscopic visualization (Figure 36–12, see color plate). The muscle resection usually starts at the scalenus medius, followed by the scalenus anterior, and is finalized by resecting the intercostal muscle and some digitation fibers of the serratus anterior. It is important to excise as much muscle tissue as possible under direct endoscopic control to facilitate mobilization of the first rib.[6]

Resection of the First Rib

The periosteal rib elevator is used to mobilize the anterior and middle thirds of the first rib. The rib cutter (Figure 36–13, see color plate) is placed under endoscopic control at three levels: (1) posterior to the nerve; (2) anterior to the vein; and (3) wedge diagonal cut to ensure a safe margin toward the vein, which lies immediately behind the rib.

Approximately 50% of the first rib resection has been accomplished at this stage, and a larger working space has been obtained. Further space can be gained, if needed, by collapsing the ipsilateral lung field using the Univent endotracheal intubation technique. Bleeding is controlled by use of bipolar electrocautery.

The first rib resection anterior to the vein is completed to the sternal cartilage junction.

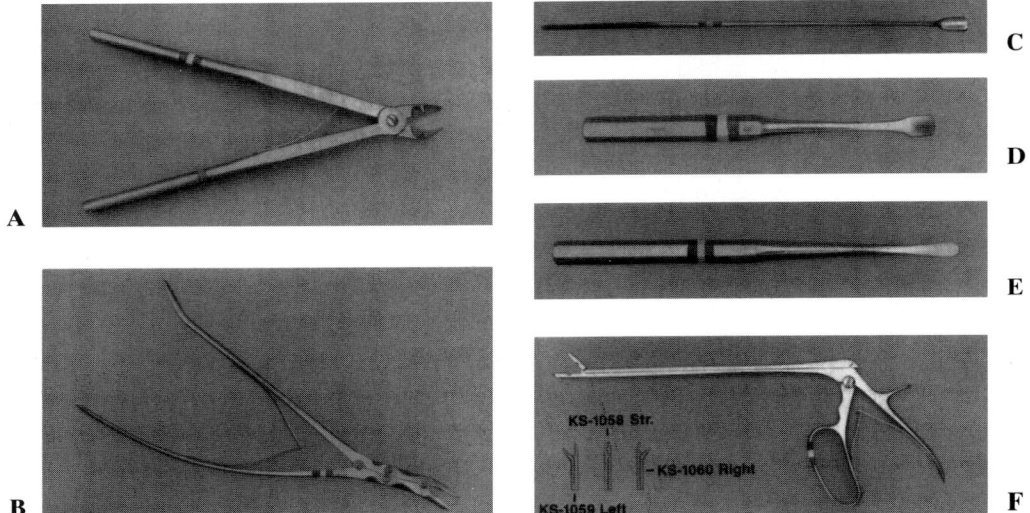

FIGURE 36–11. Instruments. **A**, Rib cutter. **B**, Dale rongeur. **C**, Roos nerve retractor. **D**, **E**, Rib elevators. **F**, Urschel rongeur (angled by Martinez).

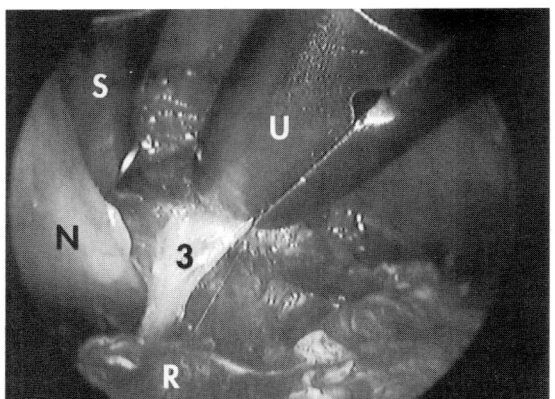

FIGURE 36–12. Left transaxillary approach. Urschel instrument is excising residual muscular fibers of a type 3 band in close proximity to the nerve. *N*, nerve; *U*, Urschel rongeur; *3*, type 3 residual fibers; *S*, suction device; *R*, rib. (See color plate).

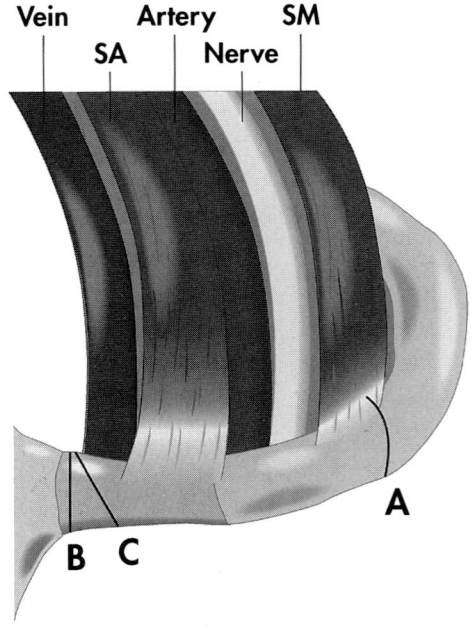

FIGURE 36–13. Left transaxillary first rib resection. Placement of the rib cutter instrument: *A*, posterior to the nerve; *B*, anterior to the vein; *C*, wedge diagonal cut to ensure a safe margin toward the vein. *SA*, scalenus anterior; *SM*, scalenus medius. (See color plate).

Approximately 4 cm of the posterior segment of the first rib is easily mobilized, as the scalenus medius, serratus, and intercostal muscles have already been excised. The posterior rib is best removed by small fragments, "crushing" bites, under direct endoscopic control using the Dale double rongeur, the Urschel single action rongeur, and the angled Urschel rongeur modified by Martinez. It is at this point that relaxation of the arm is beneficial to carefully dissect around the C8–T1 branches of the brachial plexus (as indicated in Figure 36–12). Visualization of the bright, smooth surface of the T1 vertebra transverse process cartilage (lying posterior to the first rib) indicates that the first rib has been completely resected (Figure 36–4).

Final Review of Surgical Decompression, Closure, and Drainage

Video and hard copy photographic documentation is processed at this final stage to compare with the previous compression findings. This step ensures that the three vital structures are fully decompressed, and all the soft tissue bands have been properly taken care of, as shown in Figures 36–4 and 36–9.

The functional integrity of the pleura is investigated. In cases where incidental violation of the pleura has occurred, a soft red rubber catheter is placed in the intrapleural space. If the pleura is intact, a similar drainage catheter need be placed only in the extrapleural space. Approximately 70 to 120 ml of serosanguineous fluid may be expected to drain during the first 24 hours. Closure of the wounds is accomplished using absorbable subcutaneous material and subcuticular skin closure. Chest radiography is routinely done in the operating room to check the expansion of the lung and completion of the first rib resection.

Limitations of Transaxillary First Rib Resection

The limitations of transaxillary first rib resection have been previously described.[5,9–11] The high incidence of interdigitations of the scalenus anterior and medius muscles and associated anomalies are the main reason for recurrent symptoms; therefore concomitant scalenectomy as a combined procedure with the first rib resection is done in approximately two-thirds of patients.

Transaxillary first rib resection alone is probably indicated only for patients with isolated venous symptoms and those with neurogenic compression syndrome, predominantly of the lower brachial plexus distribution with a type 3 band. On the other hand, if an associated type 5 band is present, it implies the need for further scalenectomy.

Complications

In my clinical series 96% of the patients were free of complications. Only 2% had complications related to the transaxillary endoscopic approach. An inflammatory reaction is manifested by slight engorgement of the mammary gland. This reaction did not appear to be of infectious origin, but perhaps an alteration of lymphatic drainage; it responded empirically to antibiotic and supportive therapy. The remaining complications (2%) were related to supraclavicular scalenectomy.

Results

No nerve, artery, or vein injury was seen. Incidental violation of the parietal pleura was experienced in 23%. All patients responded favorably to a soft rubber closed-drainage system therapy.

Thoracodorsal Sympathectomy

Thoracodorsal sympathectomy is performed in association with surgical thoracic outlet decompression whenever thoracic outlet and causalgia syndromes are present concomitantly. In a clinical situation of isolated causalgia or reflex sympathetic dystrophy, thoracodorsal sympathectomy can be done with or without first rib resection. A similar technique is followed in the former situation, as already described. The apical pleural layer can be dissected downward to the level of the third and fourth posterior ribs. The sympathetic chain and ganglia can be easily recognized against the head of the ribs. The third and second thoracic ganglia are removed, followed by the lowest portion of the first thoracic ganglion (which is fused to the inferior cervical ganglion, comprising the stellate ganglia) is removed. The apex of the lower portion of the first thoracic ganglion is removed, taking care to preserve the anterior and superior branches to avoid potential damage to the ocular branches (Horner syndrome).

If the transaxillary approach for sympathectomy is not elected, endoscopic thoracodorsal sympathectomy can be accomplished by three 10-mm port incisions. The endoscopic port should be placed at the midaxillary line in the fourth intercostal space. The left and right working instrument ports are best placed in the anterior and posterior axillary lines at a lower level. The posterior axillary line port is best placed under direct vision to avoid injury to the long thoracic nerve. The Univent endotracheal intubation technique is recommended to create and maintain a working space.

Figure 36–14 (see color plate) demonstrates the opening of the pleura and dissection of the thoracic ganglia. Resection of the third, second, and lowest portion of the first ganglia are carried out as previously described. After placing intrapleural tube drainage and closing the wound, chest radiographs are obtained to confirm lung expansion.

Acknowledgments. I thank Christine Newman for her valuable help in the writing of this chapter, and John Salazar and Jeff Coomer from St.Vincent Hospital, Toledo, Ohio, for helping me in the development of the endoscopic video technique.

References

1. Roos DB: *Transaxillary approach for first rib resection to relieve thoracic oustlet syndrome,* Ann Surg 163:354–358, 1966.
2. Falconer MA, Li FWP: *Resection of first rib in costoclavicular compression of the brachial plexus,* Lancet 1:59–63, 1962.
3. Clagett OT: *Presidential address: research and pro-search,* J Thorac Cardiovasc Surg 44: 153–166, 1962.
4. Martinez BD: *Thoracic outlet syndrome, intraoperative endoscopic video recording evaluation,* American College of Surgeons Library, October 1985, Catalog ACS-1397.
5. Martinez BD: *Thoracic outlet syndrome.* In Cameron J, editor: *Current surgical therapy,* ed 4, 1992, pp 753–757.
6. Martinez BD: *Adjunctive endoscopic video technique in transaxillary first rib resection for thoracic outlet syndrome: ten years experience,* American College of Surgeons Library, October 1996, Catalog ACS-2008:8.
7. Dale WA: *Thoracic outlet compression syndrome: critique in 1982,* Arch Surg 117:1437–1445, 1982.
8. Roos DB: *Congenital anomalies associated with thoracic outlet syndrome, anatomy, symptoms, diagnosis and treatment,* Am J Surg 132:771–778, 1976.
9. Sanders RJ, Monsour JW, Gerber FG et al: *Scalenectomy versus first rib resection for treatment of the thoracic outlet syndrome,* Surgery 85:109–121, 1979.
10. Roos DB: *The place for scalenectomy and first rib resection in thoracic outlet syndrome,* Surgery 92:1077–1085, 1982.
11. Sanders RJ, Pearce WH: *The treatment of thoracic outlet syndrome: a comparison of different operations,* J Vasc Surg 10:626–634, 1989.

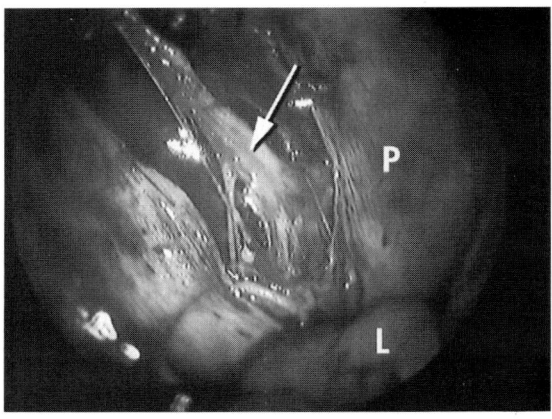

FIGURE 36–14. Left endoscopic thoracodorsal sympathectomy view. *Arrow* indicates thoracic ganglia (T2). *P,* pleura; *L,* lung. (See color plate).

37
Prevention of Lesion Recurrence in Endovascular Devices

Ted R. Kohler and Alexander W. Clowes

Synthetic prosthetic grafts developed over the last 40 years have permitted vascular surgeons to undertake reconstructions of extensively diseased vessels in situations where other forms of repair were not likely to work. The structure and function of these grafts differ from that of normal native vessels in that they lack an endothelial covering at the luminal surface and are prone to sudden thrombosis; they are rigid and do not possess vasomotor activity; and they induce a wound healing response that under some circumstances causes luminal narrowing and reduction in blood flow. In general, these deficiencies are not of major concern if the graft is used to replace a large vessel in a high flow system, but they do become limiting when the graft is used to replace a vessel of small diameter with relatively low blood flow.

Do these general conclusions apply to grafts, stent-grafts, or stents placed intraluminally? Should we expect healing of these conduits to be the same as for regular grafts, or is the healing different because of the intraluminal site? The answers to these questions will come from studies ongoing in humans and animal models. In the meantime, certain predictions can be made based on what we already know of the reparative response of injured vessels and vascular grafts sutured to native vessels but placed in the extravascular space. This chapter provides an overview of this subject.

Arterial Repair in Response to Balloon Injury

Study of the normal vascular response to injury forms the basis for understanding healing in diseased and synthetic blood vessels. Experiments performed over the last two decades provide us with the outline of a mechanism in animals and to a certain extent in humans. Much of the work has been done in rats, although it has been extended to other species.

When the rat carotid artery is damaged by passage of a balloon embolectomy catheter, a series of reproducible events ensue.[1] The endothelial layer is stripped away, and in its place platelets attach and spread on the denuded surface. Fibrin does not accumulate, although it does in other situations, such as deep injury of the media, disruption of atherosclerotic plaque, and repeat injury of an established intima. Ballooning of the vessel also causes a medial injury; 20% to 30% of the smooth muscle cells are destroyed by a combination of stretch and direct trauma. One of the important lessons we have learned from these studies is that there is a correlation between the extent of medial injury and the subsequent wall thickening response. This correlation also holds true in human arteries subjected to trauma during surgical reconstruction. Deep injury causes cell proliferation in the adventitia and the media. Proliferating fibroblasts migrate into the vessel wall where they may contribute substantially to intimal hyperplasia.[2] During this process these cells differentiate into myofibroblasts (positive for α-actin).[3]

A cohort of medial smooth muscle cells start synthesizing DNA beginning 24 hours after injury.[4] This proliferative response depends largely on the extent of the damage. Between 0 and 24 hours genes critical for cell cycle progression out of the resting state (G_0) are induced in the smooth muscle cells. The first few cycles of smooth muscle cell replication allow repletion of the damaged media with cells. At 4 days smooth muscle cells begin to move from the media to the intima. Migration between these two tissue compartments is easily detected, as smooth muscle cells are not normally present in the intima of the rat carotid artery. Migration might occur within the media, but we have no way to identify it. The intimal smooth muscle cells continue to divide for several rounds and then stop spontaneously at 4 weeks regardless of whether endothelial cells have covered the surface. Smooth muscle cell proliferation ceases earlier in regions exhibiting endothelial recovery.[5] The intimal thickening caused by smooth muscle cell proliferation is further enlarged by the accumulation of large amounts of matrix (Figure 37–1). In fact, the intima in its final form is mostly matrix (80%). The general conclusion derived from these studies is that the response to injury is vigorous and immediate but subsides within weeks. The available evidence from studies of coronary arteries subjected to angioplasty, vein grafts, and endarterectomized carotid arteries confirm that the injury response in humans is also immediate and short-lived. Changes that occur after 6 months are likely to be caused by stimuli other than the initial injury.

The endothelial layer is regenerated from sources of nontraumatized cells adjacent to the zone of injury. In all species studied including humans, endothelial ingrowth, the sum of migration and cell replication, is limited to 1 to 3 cm. In the denuded rat carotid artery, an endothelial layer is reestablished at the ends but not in the central portion of the artery.[6] Smooth muscle cells can adapt to this situation and create a pseudoendothelium that substitutes to some extent for normal endothelium. If the sources of endothelium (e.g., microvascular orifices, ends of the zone of trauma) are closely spaced, endothelial repair goes to completion.

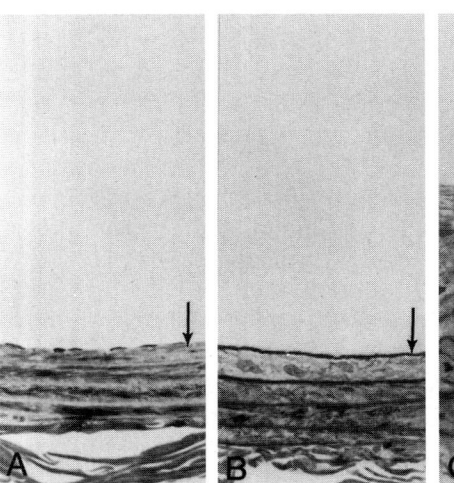
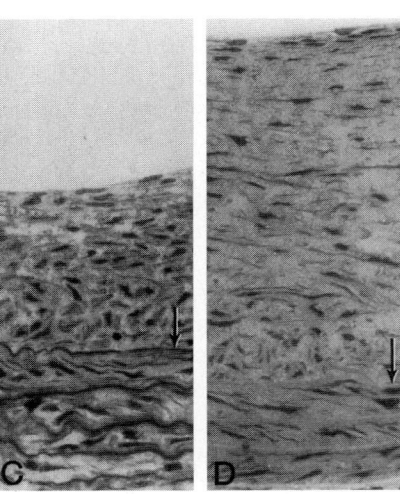

FIGURE 37–1. Histologic cross sections of injured carotid arteries in the region lacking endothelium. **A**, Normal vessel. Note the single layer of endothelium in the intima. **B**, Denuded vessel at 2 days. Note the loss of endothelium. **C**, Denuded vessel at 2 weeks. Intima is now markedly thickened owing to smooth muscle proliferation. **D**, Denuded vessel at 11 weeks. Further intimal thickening has occurred. Internal elastic lamina is indicated by the *arrow*. Lumen is at the top. ×360. (From Clowes AW, Reidy MA, Clowes MM: Mechanisms of stenosis after arterial injury, *Lab Invest* 49:208–215, 1983.)

Many reconstructive procedures (e.g., endarterectomy) delaminate the vessel wall and thereby transect the vasa vasorum. These transected microvessels can then serve as sources of new endothelium. Microvessels derived from the surrounding granulation tissue can also invade synthetic vascular grafts and, as with the transected vasa vasorum, provide new sources of endothelial cells to cover the luminal surface.[7] There has been a suggestion that at times endothelial cells can embolize from remote sites and repopulate the surface of denuded vessels. The data supporting this mechanism of vascular repair come from studies of grafts placed in dogs and humans.[8-10] Islands of endothelium have been identified that have no obvious source other than blood. In summary, there are various salvage mechanisms by which injured vessels or vascular grafts can be covered with endothelium. If possible, endothelial cells cover a luminal surface unless the sources of new cells are separated by more than a few centimeters or their reparative capacity is impaired or blocked.

The blood vessel lumen may or may not be narrowed during the healing phase. In the injured rat carotid artery, intimal thickening and vasospasm contribute to a decrease in luminal area during the early phase. At late times the vessel adapts, and little luminal narrowing is detected regardless of the size of the intima. This set of observations coupled with the seminal findings of Glagov et al.[11] showing that human blood vessels adapt to progressive wall thickening by dilating reinforces the concept that there may be a great discordance between stenosis and intimal hyperplasia except when the vessel is rigid. This is supported by the finding that lumen narrowing following balloon injury in monkeys does not correlate with the extent of intimal hyperplasia.[12] In this model, reduction in vessel caliber was caused by remodeling of the wall.

Molecular Mechanisms Controlling Wall Mass and Lumen Diameter

Over the last decade, we have begun to understand the factors regulating the response of the normal blood vessel to injury, although little is known about the injury response in atherosclerotic vessels and in venous or synthetic substitutes. The first wave of medial smooth muscle cell proliferation is largely controlled by basic fibroblast growth factor (bFGF), a growth factor found and stored in the cytoplasm of most cells and released from damaged endothelium and smooth muscle cells.[13,14] Other molecules, such as thrombin, might also be cofactors for stimulating smooth muscle cell growth. In addition, the loss of inhibitory factors generated by the endothelium, such as nitric oxide, might permit the growth factors to exert their stimulating activity on the smooth muscle cells. bFGF, for example, does not stimulate smooth muscle cell growth unless the endothelium has been removed first. Smooth muscle cell migration from the media to the intima is regulated by molecules transported in platelets. Elimination of platelets from the vasculature has no effect on the first wave of proliferation but still is able to inhibit intimal thickening because migration is blocked.[15] One of the platelet molecules, platelet-derived growth factor (PDGF), stimulates migration and has only a weak effect on smooth muscle cell replication.[16] It should be pointed out that PDGF is a family of molecules and is synthesized and secreted by vascular cells as well as being transported in platelets. Transforming growth factor (TGF) and angiotensin II from the blood or generated in the wall may also regulate intimal mass.

Reparative Mechanisms in Atherosclerotic Arteries

The repair of damaged atherosclerotic vessels is considerably more complex than for normal arteries, and the cellular mechanisms are not as well defined. For example, balloon injury (embolectomy or angioplasty catheter) damages the surface and induces a substantial thrombotic response of platelets, fibrin, and leukocytes. Although the intima does thicken, the source of the smooth muscle cells is unknown. Unlike the normal rat carotid artery, atherosclerotic arteries in animals and humans already have a population of intimal smooth muscle cells. Whether these cells contribute to further intimal thickening is not known. In atherectomy specimens obtained from coronary arteries at various times after angioplasty, smooth muscle cell proliferation is low.17 This observation raises the possibility that smooth muscle cell proliferation is not the mechanism for controlling the cellular mass in the intima; we must now consider the possibility that smooth muscle cell's migrate in from the media or derive from pericytes that accompany the microvascular endothelium. In support of the latter hypothesis is evidence that most of the proliferation seen in human atherosclerotic lesions can be localized to the vasa vasorum!18 Lipid and matrix accumulate in these lesions. The factors controlling these events have not been defined.

The relationship between restenosis of a diseased vessel and changes in intimal mass is far from clear and is being intensively investigated. Recoil and chronic vasospasm, sometimes termed vascular remodeling, contribute to luminal narrowing, or renarrowing, and might be more important than intimal hyperplasia.[12,19]

Intimal Hyperplasia and Luminal Narrowing in Stented Arteries and Synthetic Vascular Grafts

Intimal thickening in stented arteries and synthetic grafts resembles the intimal thickening of the balloon-injured rat carotid artery with some important differences. First, the vascular structure is artificially made rigid and therefore cannot contract or dilate in response to normal stimuli. Second, the endothelial cells and smooth muscle cells are derived from the artery adjacent to the device or, in the case of porous synthetic grafts, from transmural microvessels. Third, the synthetic material induces a chronic inflammatory response. Fourth, so long as the stent or graft remains without an endothelial covering it is thrombogenic. In dogs and swine, stents endothelialize within 2 weeks. These devices become embedded in the vessel wall as neointima grows through the interstices and covers the wires (Figure 37–2).[20] Significant

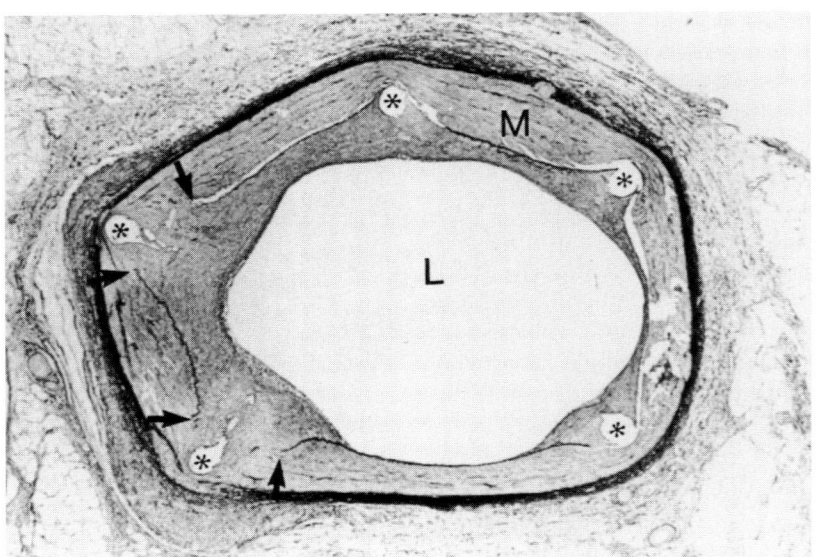

FIGURE 37–2. Photomicrograph of a section of swine coronary artery in which a metallic coil was placed with a balloon catheter. The internal elastic lamina has been broken in several locations (*arrows*). Neointimal thickening is evident and appears greatest where the wires have penetrated deeply into the media. *L*, lumen; *M*, media; *, holes from coil wires. ×30. Elastic-van Gieson stain. (From Schwartz RS, Murphy JG, Edwards WD et al: Restenosis after balloon angioplasty: a practical proliferative model in porcine coronary arteries, *Circulation* 82:2190–2200, 1990.)

restenosis may result from ingrowth of tissue through the open mesh structure. In human iliac arteries, stents that are partially covered with PTFE have been observed by angiography to have much less narrowing in the covered segments than the uncovered segments, possibly due to inhibition of this tissue ingrowth.[21]

Endothelialization of stent-grafts resembles that of similar grafts used for arterial bypass. Endothelium grows onto the graft surface from the adjacent vessel, but this process is limited to a few centimeters. This endothelial growth is sufficient to cover completely open-structure stents and short lengths of graft material (approximately 6 cm). For example, short stent grafts consisting of PTFE and Palmaz stents heal along their entire length by 3 months in dogs.[22] The central portion of longer grafts usually lacks endothelium. In animal models of conventional (not endoluminal) bypasses, even long Dacron and polytetrafluoroethylene (PTFE) grafts can develop a complete endothelial covering if they are porous enough to allow ingrowth of capillaries from the surrounding granulation tissue (Figure 37–3).[7] This endothelialized neointima breaks down over time in Dacron grafts possibly due to chronic inflammation associated with the graft material[23] and in PTFE grafts when the material is too porous (internodal distances of more than 60 μm).[24] Evidence for similar healing by capillary ingrowth in humans is lacking.[25] The reasons for the failure of porous human grafts to generate an endothelial surface is not known but could relate to toxic substances from the graft, a chronic inflammatory reaction, poor growth capacity of human microvascular endothelium, or the lack of sufficient stimulatory substances around the graft.

The local environment is an important factor that influences the healing of endoluminal devices. Subcutaneously placed carotid-femoral Dacron grafts in dogs heal less rapidly than those implanted in the descending thoracic aorta.[26] Porous PTFE grafts heal more rapidly when wrapped with vein or omentum.[27,28] Similarly, wrapping with vein enhances endothelialization of Dacron grafts.[29] It is not surprising to find that endovascular placement of standard-porosity PTFE grafts promotes more

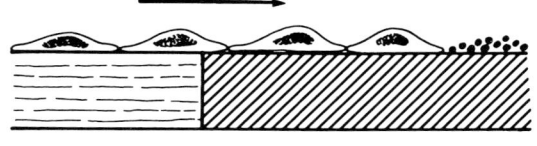

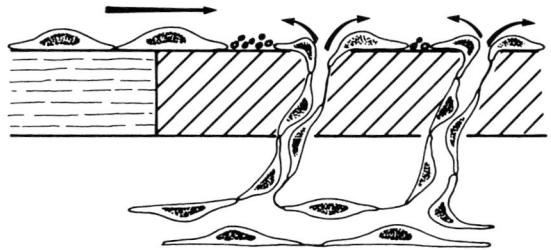

FIGURE 37–3. Healing by endothelium (and smooth muscle cells) of low-porosity (***top***) and high-porosity (***bottom***) PTFE grafts. In low-porosity grafts endothelium is derived from the cut edges of adjacent artery and grows as a continuous monolayer toward the center of the graft. In high-porosity grafts, capillaries derived from surrounding granulation tissue penetrate the graft matrix and provide multiple sources of endothelium at the luminal surface. (From Clowes AW, Clowes MM, Reidy MA: Kinetics of cellular proliferation after arterial injury. III. Endothelial and smooth muscle growth in chronically denuded vessels, *Lab Invest* 54: 295–303, 1986.)

rapid endothelialization.[30–32] This was also observed when grafts were placed in arterial segments denuded of endothelium by a balloon catheter.[33] In these experiments, endothelium grew in from the adjacent vessel for a distance of 2 to 3 cm from the anastomosis. Endovascular grafts also had reduced intimal hyperplasia at the anastomoses. In another study using dog iliac artery, endovascular PTFE grafts endothelialized more completely than conventional bypass grafts but had significantly more narrowing at the distal anastomosis.[34] Dacron endovascular aortic grafts in sheep heal along their entire length and by 3 months develop a neointima composed of cells that appear to be myofibroblasts with a lining of endothelial-like cells.[35,36] In a dog aneurysm model, a thick collagen-rich, elastin-poor neointima formed along the entire length of endoluminal Dacron grafts.[37] There was a monolayer of squamous cells on the luminal surface, which may have been endothelium (positive factor VIII staining in one animal). Grafts appeared to be fully incorporated in the wall. Another study of a sheep model of abdominal aneurysm reported good incorporation of a polyester endovascular device into the arterial wall with development of a cellular pseudointima.

There are some observations from endovascular devices removed from humans. Explants of PTFE grafts have demonstrated endothelium as far as 8 cm from the anastomosis.[38] The origin of these cells is not clear. There was no sign of capillary ingrowth in the graft to suggest transmural healing. These cells could have migrated from the anastomoses or may have derived from a blood-borne source, as has been observed in the canine model.[9,10] Autopsy 7 months after placement of an endovascular graft for abdominal aortic aneurysm in a human revealed good incorporation of the proximal graft with typical pannus ingrowth consisting of endothelium and underlying smooth muscle cells.[39] Pannus at the distal anastomosis was poorly formed and fibrinous.

The traumatized artery should be a good source of microvessels and factors that stimulate microvascular growth such as bFGF. Although the graft might eventually become incorporated by vascular cells, initially it should exhibit the same tendency to develop spontaneous thrombosis as standard extraanatomically located grafts. In contrast to aneurysmal arteries it may be possible to use grafts made of thinner, more porous material in atherosclerotic arteries, as the surrounding wall has adequate strength to resist arterial pressure. These intraluminal grafts may reduce the recurrence of wall thickening in their investing arteries by preventing thrombus from forming on the injured surface. Intimal thickening is reduced by hydrogel barriers that prevent blood from contacting the luminal surface of injured arteries.[40] The extent to which endoluminal grafts are affected by thrombosis, intimal hyperplasia, luminal stenosis, and infection depends on how well they are incorporated into vascular tissue. Furthermore, the formation of thick intima and new atheroma is probably dependent on the properties of the cells lining the luminal surface. If the cells have a normal phenotype and behave as normal, uninjured vascular cells, it is likely that the endoluminal graft is a durable form of reconstruction.

In summary, there is evidence that endovascular stents endothelialize rapidly, but intimal hyperplasia is not prevented by these devices, whose open structure allows ingrowth of vascular tissue. Endovascular grafts incorporate into the surrounding vessel. There is evidence that these devices may have better endothelialization and less intimal hyperplasia at the graft-vessel junction than do grafts placed with sutured anastomoses. Further work will determine if endovascular grafts have improved patency and whether their attachment to the native vessel is durable over many years.

Prevention of Lesion Recurrence

Wall thickening following endovascular grafting may result from organization of thrombus that accumulates on the surface of the graft or injured vessel, vasospasm, or intimal hyperplasia. Lower recurrence rates may result from changing the mechanical properties of endovascular devices to reduce injury to the wall, biologic control using genetic engineering, and drug intervention to reduce thrombosis, smooth muscle cell proliferation, or vessel spasm. Alteration of local, hemodynamic factors, such as wall shear, may also reduce restenosis.

Mechanical Considerations

Because the amount of wall thickening that occurs following arterial injury is proportional to the extent of injury, devices that limit arterial injury may be expected to incite less wall thickening. Proliferation is greatest when the internal elastic lamina is disrupted and deep medial injury occurs. In general, stenting causes more arterial injury than does balloon dilatation. Such injury has been documented in rabbit and swine models[20,41,42] and may result from the inflammatory response to the foreign body or chronic mechanical injury caused by the stent. Lesions found in stented pig coronary arteries resemble those found in human lesions following percutaneous transluminal coronary artery angioplasty (PTCA).[42] Unlike lesions of intimal hyperplasia found in rat arteries following angioplasty, thrombosis is a prominent component of the response, and these lesions produce luminal narrowing. In the swine model the degree of intimal thickening associated with stenting is proportional to the depth of injury.[20,43,44] Wall thickening is increased by oversized stents and is reduced when the stent diameter matches that of the native vessel.[20] Similarly, in human coronary arteries, oversized stents are associated with an increased risk of restenosis.[45] There may be other, fundamental differences between the lesions caused by balloon angioplasty and those caused by stents. In the rabbit, heparin has less effect on stented than on nonstented lesions.[41]

Hemodynamic Factors

Intimal hyperplasia is affected by hemodynamic factors. Shear forces have a profound influence on wall structure in developing, mature, atherosclerotic, and injured vessels. Mature vessels change diameter in response to flow. Acute changes in diameter result from alteration of vasomotor tone. If the flow change persists, wall structure is modified to maintain the new diameter with normal vasomotor tone.[46] In part, this may be due to trophic effects of vasoactive factors, such as nitric oxide. This molecule is the endothelium-derived relaxation factor that causes vasodilatation and decreased proliferation of vascular smooth muscle cells. Endothelial production of nitric oxide increases in response to increased shear. Atherogenesis is enhanced in areas of decreased shear, and intimal hyperplasia is greater when flow is decreased in vein grafts, PTFE grafts, and following experimental balloon injury.[47-57] In high-porosity PTFE grafts, increased blood flow causes regression of the neointima in association with increased expression of endothelial nitric oxide synthase.[58] It is likely that endovascular grafts and stents perform best when runoff is adequate to provide normal or increased flow. A better understanding of the mechanism by which flow reduces intimal thickening may allow us to devise treatment that mimics this action. For example, it may be possible to introduce genes for nitric oxide synthase or drugs that mimic the effect of this or other vasodilators.

Pharmacologic Agents

Drugs may be delivered systemically or locally. Because many of the drugs are directed against cell proliferation, they may have potent, undesirable side effects. Therefore local delivery via a catheter, stent, or micro beads is an attractive alternative. Infusion catheters have been developed to inject pharmacologic agents directly into the vessel wall. The therapeutic benefit of these systems is offset by the fact that they induce endothelial injury and damage to the internal elastic lamina.[59] Technology is being developed to place therapeutic agents on microbeads that are taken up by the vascular cells, where they slowly release the drug into the cytosol.

Many agents have shown potential for reducing intimal hyperplasia in animal models, but none has had convincing therapeutic benefit in large, clinical trials. An extensive review of the literature and a meta-analysis of the available data performed by Herrman and coauthors are summarized in Figure 37–4.[59,60]

Antithrombotic Agents

Antiplatelet therapy may be effective in reducing acute thrombosis following stenting, but its role in preventing restenosis is not yet known. Acute thrombosis is a frequent complication following endovascular stenting. Aspirin and heparin both reduce platelet uptake on experimental stents in an ex vivo shunt model.[61] In clinical studies, antithrombotic therapy using aspirin, with or without dipyridamole, increases early patency rates but is ineffective in reducing later restenosis due to intimal hyperplasia. This is consistent with the finding that in animal models smooth muscle cell proliferation following injury is unaffected by thrombocytopenia. Antiplatelet drugs such as aspirin, dipyridamole, and ticlopidine given during the perioperative period improve the early patency

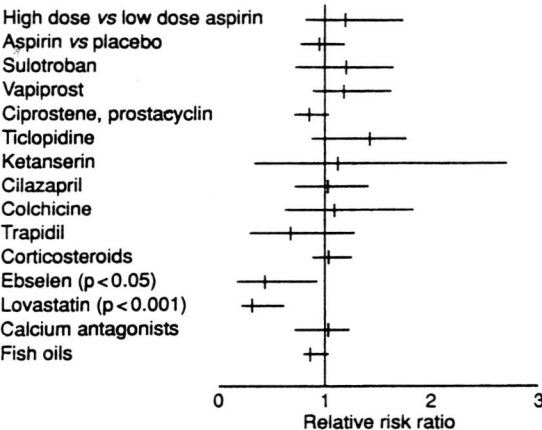

FIGURE 37-4. Relative risk ratio of various drugs compared to controls for prevention of restenosis following PTCA in clinical studies. Bars indicate the 95% confidence intervals. Statistical significance ($p < 0.05$) occurs when the bars do not cross the relative risk of 1. A risk ratio < 1 indicates lower restenosis in the test group. (From Herrman JP, Hermans WR, Vos J, Serruys PW: Pharmacological approaches to the prevention of restenosis following angioplasty: the search for the Holy Grail? Part I, *Drugs* 46:18–52, 1993.)

of coronary artery bypass grafts.[62] Ticlopidine can improve the 2-year patency rate of vein grafts used in lower extremity bypass operations.[63] This finding suggests that antiplatelet therapy may be able to reduce intimal hyperplasia. In further support, a large, prospective clinical trial found that ischemic complications of coronary angioplasty and atherectomy were reduced by a monoclonal antibody directed against the platelet IIb/IIIa glycoprotein receptor.[64,65] A single infusion of this agent improved outcome for as long as 3 years after the procedure.[66] The mechanism of this effect is not fully understood. Currently, there are no data to show that this therapy reduces intimal hyperplasia.

Heparin inhibits intimal hyperplasia in balloon-injured rabbit and rat carotid arteries due to inhibition of smooth muscle cell migration and proliferation.[67] Endothelial regeneration is not affected. In animal models of acute arterial injury, heparin administration can be delayed for several hours after the mitogenic stimulus and has little further effect if continued beyond 72 hours. The mechanism of this action may be inhibition of the induction of metalloproteinases by injured smooth muscle cells.[68] These enzymes are necessary for the cells to degrade surrounding matrix, enabling cell migration and proliferation. To date, clinical trials with heparin have not reduced restenosis following PTCA.[69]

Work by Rogers and coworkers suggested that ineffective drug delivery might explain the failure of clinical trials using drugs such as heparin that are effective antiproliferative agents in animal models.[41] They studied various modes of heparin delivery following balloon injury or stenting of rabbit iliac arteries. Stenting caused more exuberant intimal hyperplasia than simple balloon injury. Occlusive thrombus was common following stenting and was reduced by heparin whether it was administered by continuous infusion or locally with drug-releasing stents or perivascular polymeric, controlled-release matrices. Heparin reduced intimal hyperplasia after balloon injury but was less effective in controlling intimal hyperplasia following stenting. Local delivery was even less effective than intravenous drug administration. This study suggests that the antiproliferative and antithrombotic effects of heparin differ depending on the type of injury. Different therapies may be needed for different types of arterial injury. Both the dose and mode of delivery of the agent are important.

Low-molecular-weight fractions of heparin (LMWH) also have antiproliferative effects but have fewer side effects because of less inhibition of platelet aggregation and thrombin generation. Furthermore, unlike standard heparin, LMWH can be administered by a single, daily, subcutaneous injection. It reduced intimal hyperplasia following coronary stent implantation in hypercholesterolemic miniswine.[70] In a randomized clinical study, LMWH (2500 IU daily) improved graft patency more than aspirin and dipyridamole in patients receiving femoropopliteal grafts for limb salvage.[71] There was no difference in patients who were being treated for claudication only. LMWH can reduce intimal hyperplasia in animal models. However, clinical trials using LMWH following coronary angioplasty have shown no reduction in restenosis.[72]

Hirudin is the anticoagulant of the European leech. It is a peptide that binds thrombin, blocking its ability to activate platelets.[73] Because of its small size, this molecule can penetrate thrombus and inhibit thrombin bound to fibrin. Hirudin reduces fibrin deposition in animal models of deep arterial injury. In high doses it can totally eliminate mural thrombosis and nearly eliminate platelet deposition.[73] Clinical trials are underway testing hirudin in patients undergoing coronary angioplasty.

Antiproliferative Agents

The vessel wall has angiotensin-converting enzyme (ACE) activity that is separate from the plasma renin-angiotensin system. Angiotensin II derived from this enzyme acts as both a vasopressor and a growth factor for smooth muscle cells. This provides a mechanism for local regulation of wall structure by angiotensin.[74] ACE inhibitors can decrease intimal hyperplasia following arterial injury in some but not all animal models.[75,76] This effect is enhanced by the addition of heparin. Clinical studies have been disappointing. Cilazapril failed to reduce the incidence of restenosis following coronary angioplasty in two large, multicenter prospective, randomized clinical trials (MERCATOR in Europe and MARCATOR in North America). Failure to reduce restenosis may be due to the fact that much higher doses of drug are required to inhibit tissue ACE activity than are required to suppress circulating activity and to lower blood pressure.[77] Alternatively, restenosis may have occurred despite reduction of neointimal hyperplasia.[78] In this case, vessel remodeling rather than intimal thickening may determine the luminal area.

Vessel spasm following arterial injury may enhance wall thickening by promoting the formation of thrombus at the site of injury. Calcium channel blockers may block this process. In animal models, these agents can reduce intimal hyperplasia following balloon injury and atherogenesis.[79-82] These effects may result from inhibition of early smooth muscle cell proliferation. Although nifedipine may reduce the formation of new atherosclerotic lesions,[81] clinical trials with a variety of calcium channel blockers have failed to prevent restenosis in coronary arteries.

Cytostatic drugs can prevent smooth muscle cell growth. Because they have potent systemic effects, local delivery is preferred and has been studied using catheter infusion or coated stents. As yet, no benefit has been found in studies using a variety of agents such as doxorubicin, vincristine, methotrexate, and dactinomycin.[59]

Trapidil (triazolopyrimidine) is a pyrimidine derivative that can inhibit cellular proliferation induced by PDGF in cell culture and can limit intimal thickening in animal models.[59] Monoclonal antibodies against PDGF also inhibit intimal thickening in animal models.[83] The primary effect of this treatment appears to be reduction of migration rather than proliferation of smooth muscle cells. Clinical trials have suggested a role for this agent in preventing restenosis.[59,84] It is hoped that large-scale studies will be undertaken soon.

Steroids may reduce restenosis through their antiinflammatory effect and their ability to inhibit smooth muscle cell proliferation and collagen production by fibroblasts. Steroids can reduce intimal hyperplasia in animal models when delivered systemically or by silicone drug-eluting polymers.[85,86] Clinical studies, including one large, multicenter trial of 850 patients, failed to show any benefit of treatment following PTCA.[87] Nonsteroidal antiinflammatory drugs can effectively reduce platelet deposition at the site of arterial injury and in arterial grafts. Their possible clinical role is as yet unknown. One small trial with ebselen, a new selenium-containing antiinflammatory agent, had promising results 3 months following angioplasty.[59]

Fish oils reduce triglycerides, inhibit platelet aggregation, and promote vasodilatation and fibrinolysis. They inhibit atherogenesis and vein graft intimal hyperplasia. Some clinical trials have shown a benefit of fish oils in reducing restenosis following PTCA, but others have not; moreover, side effects leading to discontinuation of the medication were common (approximately 10%). Similarly, lovastatin can reduce intimal hyperplasia in animal models, possibly as a result of inhibition of smooth muscle cell proliferation.[59] Clinical results so far have been conflicting.

Biologic Control

In theory, restenosis can be reduced if the vessel wall at the site of intervention can return to a normal, quiescent, nonthrombogenic state. One of the main components of the normal vessel wall is an intact endothelial lining that inhibits thrombosis and smooth muscle cell proliferation. This has been the goal of cell seeding efforts for artificial grafts and denuded arteries following endarterectomy. Injured or recently regrown endothelium may function abnormally[88] and conceivably may be thrombogenic or stimulatory for smooth muscle cell growth and matrix production. If this were the case, providing such an endothelial lining for a vascular graft may impair rather than improve its long-term function.

It is now possible to introduce foreign genes for various growth factors or other enzymes into endothelial cells or smooth muscle cells.[89–91] Cells may be modified in vitro and then reintroduced into the vasculature, or genes may be introduced directly into the cells of the vessel wall using replication-defective retroviral vectors or liposomes. Antisense oligodeoxynucleotides have been used to block messenger RNA from genes involved with smooth muscle cell proliferation. In one study, transcatheter delivery of an antisense oligomer to the c-*myc* proto-oncogene, which plays a role in smooth muscle cell proliferation, significantly reduced intimal hyperplasia following balloon injury of porcine coronary arteries.[92] Similarly, antisense oligonucleotides directed against the oncogene c-*myb* can inhibit intimal smooth muscle cell proliferation in vitro and intimal smooth muscle cell accumulation in vivo.[93,94]

This approach has enormous therapeutic potential. For example, fibronectin-coated metal stents have been seeded with genetically modified endothelial cells that produce tissue plasminogen activator.[95,96] Transduced smooth muscle cells seeded onto injured rat carotid arteries can produce adenosine deaminase for up to 6 months and erythropoietin for up to 11 weeks.[97,98] It should be possible to add combinations of genes for other antiproliferative or antithrombotic products to inhibit local thrombosis and intimal hyperplasia. This technique may allow biologic control of thrombosis on the surface of these artificial devices. It may also be possible to control intimal hyperplasia following endarterectomy, angioplasty, or bypass by introducing specific growth promoters or inhibitors into cells that are seeded onto the surface of these vessels or into cells within the vessel wall. Another approach is to infect cells with a virus bearing a gene that catalyzes the formation of a cytotoxic drug locally in response to systemic therapy. One group has used this approach to reduce intimal hyperplasia following balloon injury in swine.[99] They used an adenovirus to insert the gene for herpesvirus thymidine kinase into smooth muscle cells in the injured artery. This treatment made the cells sensitive to the nucleoside analog ganciclovir. Intimal hyperplasia decreased after treatment with ganciclovir, and there were no significant systemic effects.

Brachytherapy

There is currently a great deal of enthusiasm for the use of radiation therapy (brachytherapy) to reduce restenosis following coronary artery angioplasty. This therapy treats the intimal lesion like a cancer, with uncontrolled proliferation of smooth muscle cells as the primary cause for wall thickening. Brachytherapy inhibits intimal hyperplasia in animal models of balloon injury.[100] Intracoronary gamma radiation reduces restenosis following coronary balloon angioplasty and stenting of coronary arteries of patients who have previously had an episode of restenosis.[101] One of the main problems with this technique is the difficulty of delivering the precise dose that prevents lesion formation without causing excessive scarring of the local tissue. Also, the logistics of delivering this highly toxic treatment can be challenging. It is conceivable that catheter delivery of a measured dose of radiation to the site of the stent-graft improves long-term patency, particularly for small vessels sensitive to even minor degrees of wall thickening.

Conclusion

Restenosis occurs in up to 30% of cases following all forms of revascularization, including endovascular procedures such as percutaneous angioplasty, atherectomy, and stenting. It is likely that similar rates of restenosis will occur when grafting is added to endovascular techniques. The process of restenosis involves early thrombosis and vasospasm at the site of intervention followed by organization of thrombus, smooth muscle cell proliferation, and production of matrix components by the smooth muscle cells. Restenosis may be minimized by methods that reduce injury to the vessel wall, inhibit thrombosis, minimize vasospasm, or prevent smooth muscle cell proliferation. Although many agents have been successful in reducing intimal hyperplasia in animal models, few have had a convincing, significant effect in clinical trials. This may be due to fundamental differences between animal models of intimal hyperplasia and restenosis in human atherosclerotic arteries. In most animal models thrombosis is a much less prominent component than it is in clinical lesions, and lesions of intimal hyperplasia do not reduce the lumen diameter significantly. Furthermore, human lesions have significant amounts of fibrosis, calcification, and intramural hemorrhage that is not found in most animal models. Early studies with the porcine model of atherosclerosis and restenosis suggest that it may more closely mimic the human lesions. Another potential cause for failure of drug treatment in humans is a discrepancy between the standard therapeutic dose of the agent and the increased dose needed to suppress intimal proliferation. Biologic control using genetically altered vascular cells offers a new and exciting approach to the problem of restenosis. Delivery of these cells directly into the injured wall or as coating on stents or grafts may allow control of wall structure and could provide a route for treatment of systemic disease with specific gene products.

References

1. Clowes AW, Reidy MA, Clowes MM: Mechanisms of stenosis after arterial injury, *Lab Invest* 49:208–215, 1983.
2. Wilcox JN, Waksman R, King SB, Scott NA: The role of the adventitia in the arterial response to angioplasty: the effect of intravascular radiation, *Int J Radiat Oncol Biol Phys* 36:789–796, 1996.
3. Zalewski A, Shi Y: Vascular myofibroblasts: lessons from coronary repair and remodeling, *Arterioscler Thromb Vasc Biol* 17:417–422, 1997.
4. Majesky MW, Schwartz SM, Clowes MM, Clowes AW: Heparin regulates smooth muscle S phase entry in the injured rat carotid artery, *Circ Res* 61:296–300, 1987.
5. Clowes AW, Reidy MA, Clowes MM: Kinetics of cellular proliferation after arterial injury. I. Smooth muscle growth in the absence of endothelium, *Lab Invest* 49:327–333, 1983.
6. Clowes AW, Clowes MM, Reidy MA: Kinetics of cellular proliferation after arterial injury. III. Endothelial and smooth muscle growth in chronically denuded vessels, *Lab Invest* 54:295–303, 1986.
7. Clowes AW, Kirkman TR, Reidy MA: Mechanisms of arterial graft healing. III. Rapid transmural capillary ingrowth provides a source of intimal endothelium and smooth muscle in porous PTFE prostheses, *Am J Pathol* 123:220–230, 1986.
8. Shi Q, Wu HD, Hayashida N et al: Proof of fallout endothelialization of impervious Dacron grafts in the aorta and inferior vena cava of the dog, *J Vasc Surg* 20:546–557, 1994.
9. Kouchi Y, Onuki Y, Wu MH et al: Apparent blood stream origin of endothelial and smooth muscle cells in the neointima of long, impervious carotid-femoral grafts in the dog, *Ann Vasc Surg* 12:46–54, 1998.
10. Shi Q, Wu MH, Hayashida N et al: Proof of fallout endothelialization of impervious Dacron grafts in the aorta and inferior vena cava of the dog, *J Vasc Surg* 20:546–556, 1994.
11. Glagov S, Weisenberg E, Zarins CK, Stankunavicius R: Compensatory enlargement of human atherosclerotic coronary arteries, *N Engl J Med* 316:1371–1375, 1987.
12. Mondy JS, Williams JK, Adams MR et al: Structural determinants of lumen narrowing after angioplasty in atherosclerotic nonhuman primates, *J Vasc Surg* 26:875–883, 1997.
13. Lindner V, Lappi DA, Baird A et al: Role of basic fibroblast growth factor in vascular lesion formation, *Circ Res* 68:106–113, 1991.
14. Lindner V, Reidy MA: Proliferation of smooth muscle cells after vascular injury is inhibited by an antibody against basic fibroblast growth

factor, *Proc Natl Acad Sci USA* 88:3739–3743, 1991.
15. Fingerle J, Johnson R, Clowes AW et al: Role of platelets in smooth muscle cell proliferation and migration after vascular injury in rat carotid artery, *Proc Natl Acad Sci USA* 86:8412–8416, 1989.
16. Jawien A, Bowen-Pope DF, Lindner V et al: Platelet-derived growth factor promotes smooth muscle migration and intimal thickening in a rat model of balloon angioplasty, *J Clin Invest* 89:507–511, 1992.
17. O'Brien ER, Alpers CE, Stewart DK et al: Proliferation in primary and restenotic coronary atherectomy tissue: implications for antiproliferative therapy, *Circ Res* 73:223–231, 1993.
18. O'Brien ER, Garvin MR, Dev R et al: Angiogenesis in human coronary atherosclerotic plaques, *Am J Pathol* 145:883–894, 1994.
19. Geary RL, Williams JK, Golden D et al: Time course of cellular proliferation, intimal hyperplasia, and remodeling following angioplasty in monkeys with established atherosclerosis: a nonhuman primate model of restenosis, *Arterioscler Thromb Vasc Biol* 16:34–43, 1996.
20. Schwartz RS, Murphy JG, Edwards WD et al: Restenosis after balloon angioplasty: a practical proliferative model in porcine coronary arteries, *Circulation* 82:2190–2200, 1990.
21. Marin ML, Veith FJ, Cynamon J et al: Effect of polytetrafluoroethylene covering of Palmaz stents on the development of intimal hyperplasia in human iliac arteries, *J Vasc Interv Radiol* 7:651–656, 1996.
22. Dolmatch BL, Tio FO, Li XD, Dong YH: Patency and tissue response related to two types of polytetrafluoroethylene-covered stents in the dog, *J Vasc Interv Radiol* 7:641–649, 1996.
23. Greisler HP, Schwarcz TH, Ellinger J, Kim DU: Dacron inhibition of arterial regenerative activities, *J Vasc Surg* 3:747–756, 1986.
24. Golden MA, Hanson SR, Kirkman TR et al: Healing of polytetrafluoroethylene arterial grafts is influenced by graft porosity, *J Vasc Surg* 11:838–845, 1990.
25. Kohler TR, Stratton JR, Kirkman TR et al: Conventional versus high-porosity polytetrafluoroethylene grafts: clinical evaluation, *Surgery* 112:901–907, 1992.
26. Durante KR, Wu HD, Sauvage LR et al: Implant site: a determinant of completeness of arterial prosthesis healing in the dog and possibly in humans, *Ann Vasc Surg* 4:171–178, 1990.
27. Bull DA, Hunter GC, Holubec H et al: Cellular origin and rate of endothelial cell coverage of PTFE grafts, *J Surg Res* 58:58–68, 1995.
28. Sterpetti AV, Hunter WJ, Schultz RD, Farina C: Healing of high-porosity polytetrafluoroethylene arterial grafts is influenced by the nature of the surrounding tissue, *Surgery* 111:677–682, 1992.
29. Graham LM, Harrell KA, Sell RL et al: Enhanced endothelialization of Dacron grafts by external vein wrapping, *J Surg Res* 38:537–545, 1985.
30. Ombrellaro MP, Stevens SL, Sciarrotta J et al: Effect of intra-arterial environment on endothelialization and basement membrane organization in polytetrafluoroethylene grafts, *Am J Surg* 174:29–32, 1997.
31. Ombrellaro MP, Stevens SL, Kerstetter K et al: Healing characteristics of intraarterial stented grafts: effect of intraluminal position on prosthetic graft healing, *Surgery* 120:60–70, 1996.
32. Ombrellaro MP, Stevens SL, Sciarrotta J et al: Effect of balloon-expandable and self-expanding stent fixation on endoluminal polytetrafluoroethylene graft healing, *Am J Surg* 173:461–466, 1997.
33. Weatherford DA, Ombrellaro MP, Schaeffer DO et al: Healing characteristics of intraarterial stent grafts in an injured artery model, *Ann Vasc Surg* 11:54–61, 1997.
34. Ohki T, Marin ML, Veith FJ et al: Anastomotic intimal hyperplasia: a comparison between conventional and endovascular stent graft techniques, *J Surg Res* 69:255–267, 1997.
35. Harris EJJ, Harris EJ, Berry GJ, Mitchell RS: Endoluminal aortic grafting: a preliminary animal study of graft-healing, *J Surg Res* 61:404–412, 1996.
36. White JG, Mulligan NJ, Gorin DR et al: Response of normal aorta to endovascular grafting: a serial histopathological study, *Arch Surg* 133:246–249, 1998.
37. Eton D, Warner DL, Owens C et al: Histological response to stent graft therapy, *Circulation* 94(suppl II):182–187, 1996.
38. Marin ML, Veith FJ, Cynamon J et al: Human transluminally placed endovascular stented grafts: preliminary histopathologic analysis of healing grafts in aortoiliac and femoral artery occlusive disease, *J Vasc Surg* 21:595–603, 1995.
39. McGahan TJ, Berry GA, McGahan SL et al: Results of autopsy 7 months after successful endoluminal treatment of an infrarenal abdom-

inal aortic aneurysm, *J Endovasc Surg* 2:348–355, 1995.
40. Hill-West JL, Chowdhury SM, Slepian MJ, Hubbell JA: Inhibition of thrombosis and intimal thickening by in situ photopolymerization of thin hydrogel barriers, *Proc Natl Acad Sci USA* 91:5967–5971, 1994.
41. Rogers C, Karnovsky MJ, Edelman ER: Inhibition of experimental neointimal hyperplasia and thrombosis depends on the type of vascular injury and the site of drug administration, *Circulation* 88:1215–1221, 1993.
42. Karas SP, Gravanis MB, Santoian EC et al: Coronary intimal proliferation after balloon injury and stenting in swine: an animal model of restenosis, *J Am Coll Cardiol* 20:467–474, 1992.
43. Schwartz RS, Edwards WD, Huber KC et al: Coronary restenosis: prospects for solution and new perspectives from a porcine model [see comments], *Mayo Clin Proc* 68:54–62, 1993.
44. Schwartz RS, Huber KC, Murphy JG et al: Restenosis and the proportional neointimal response to coronary artery injury: results in a porcine model, *J Am Coll Cardiol* 19:267–274, 1992.
45. Strauss BH, Serruys PW, de Scheerder IK et al: Relative risk analysis of angiographic predictors of restenosis within the coronary Wallstent, *Circulation* 84:1636–1643, 1991.
46. Langille BL, O'Donnell F: Reductions in arterial diameter produced by chronic decreases in blood flow are endothelium-dependent, *Science* 231:405–407, 1986.
47. Kohler TR, Kirkman TR, Kraiss LW et al: Increased blood flow inhibits neointimal hyperplasia in endothelialized vascular grafts, *Circ Res* 69:1557–1565, 1991.
48. Berguer R, Higgins RF, Reddy DJ: Intimal hyperplasia, *Arch Surg* 115:332–335, 1980.
49. Rittgers SE, Karayannacos PE, Guy JF: Velocity distribution and intimal proliferation in autologous vein grafts in dogs, *Circ Res* 42:792–801, 1978.
50. Morinaga K, Okadome K, Kuroki M et al: Effect of wall shear stress on intimal thickening of arterially transplanted autogenous veins in dogs, *J Vasc Surg* 2:430–433, 1985.
51. Mii S, Okadome K, Onohara T et al: Intimal thickening and permeability of arterial autogenous vein graft in a canine poor-runoff model: transmission electron microscopic evidence, *Surgery* 108:81–89, 1990.
52. Kohler TR, Jawien A: Flow affects development of intimal hyperplasia following arterial injury in rats, *Arterioscler Thromb* 12:963–971, 1992.
53. Kamiya A, Togawa T: Adaptive regulation of wall shear stress to flow change in the canine carotid artery, *Am J Physiol* 239:14–21, 1980.
54. Zarins CK, Zatina MA, Giddens DP et al: Shear stress regulation of artery lumen diameter in experimental atherogenesis, *J Vasc Surg* 5:413–420, 1987.
55. Kohler TR, Jawien A: Flow affects development of intimal hyperplasia following arterial injury in rats, *Atheroscler Thromb* 12:963–971, 1992.
56. Glagov S, Weisenberg G, Kolletis R, Stankunavicius R: Compensatory enlargement of human atherosclerotic coronary arteries prevents narrowing of the lumen, *FASEB J* 45:583, 1986.
57. Zarins CK, Weisenberg E, Kolettis G, Stankunavicius R: Differential enlargement of artery segments in response to enlarging atherosclerotic plaques, *J Vasc Surg* 7:386–394, 1988.
58. Mattsson EJ, Kohler TR, Vergel SM, Clowes AW: Increased blood flow induces regression of intimal hyperplasia, *Arterioscler Thromb Vasc Biol* 17:2245–2249, 1997.
59. Herrman JP, Hermans WR, Vos J, Serruys PW: Pharmacological approaches to the prevention of restenosis following angioplasty: the search for the Holy Grail? (Part II), *Drugs* 46:249–262, 1993.
60. Herrman JP, Hermans WR, Vos J, Serruys PW: Pharmacological approaches to the prevention of restenosis following angioplasty: the search for the Holy Grail? (Part I), *Drugs* 46:18–52, 1993.
61. Breckwoldt WL, Belkin M, Gould K et al: Modification of the thrombogenicity of a self-expanding vascular stent, *J Invest Surg* 4:269–278, 1991.
62. Goldman S, Copeland J, Moritz T et al: Saphenous vein graft patency 1 year after coronary artery bypass surgery and effects of antiplatelet therapy: results of a Veterans Administration Cooperative Study, *Circulation* 80:1190–1197, 1989.
63. Schomig A, Neumann FJ, Kastrati A et al: A randomized comparison of antiplatelet and anticoagulant therapy after the placement of coronary-artery stents [see comments], *N Engl J Med* 334:1084–1089, 1996.
64. Anonymous: Use of a monoclonal antibody directed against the platelet glycoprotein IIb/IIIa receptor in high-risk coronary angio-

plasty: the EPIC investigation, *N Engl J Med* 330:956–961, 1994.
65. Coller BS, Anderson K, Weisman HF: New antiplatelet agents: platelet GPIIb/IIIa antagonists, *Thromb Haemost* 74:302–308, 1995.
66. Topol EJ, Ferguson JJ, Weisman HF et al: Long-term protection from myocardial ischemic events in a randomized trial of brief integrin beta3 blockade with percutaneous coronary intervention: EPIC investigator group: evaluation of platelet IIb/IIIa inhibition for prevention of ischemic complication [see comments], *JAMA* 278:479–484, 1997.
67. Kohler TR, Kirkman TR, Clowes AW: Effect of heparin on adaptation of vein grafts to arterial circulation, *Arteriosclerosis* 9:523–528, 1989.
68. Kenagy RD, Nikkari ST, Welgus HG, Clowes AW: Heparin inhibits the induction of three matrix metalloproteinases (stromelysin, 92-kD gelatinase, and collagenase) in primate arterial smooth muscle cells, *J Clin Invest* 93:1987–1993, 1994.
69. Klein LW: Restenosis after successful percutaneous transluminal coronary angioplasty, *Prog Cardiovasc Dis* 32:365–382, 1990.
70. Buchwald AB, Unterberg C, Nebendahl K et al: Low-molecular-weight heparin reduces neointimal proliferation after coronary stent implantation in hypercholesterolemic minipigs, *Circulation* 86:531–537, 1992.
71. Edmondson RA, Cohen AT, Das SK et al: Low-molecular weight heparin versus aspirin and dipyridamole after femoropopliteal bypass grafting, *Lancet* 344:914–917, 1994.
72. Faxon DP, Minor S, Cot'e G et al: Low molecular weight heparin in prevention of restenosis after angioplasty: results of enoxaparin restenosis (ERA) trial, *Circulation* 90:908–914, 1994.
73. Chesebro JH, Webster MW, Zoldhelyi P et al: Antithrombotic therapy and progression of coronary artery disease: antiplatelet versus antithrombins, *Circulation* 86(suppl III):100–110, 1992.
74. Pipili E, Manolopoulos VG, Catravas JD, Maragoudakis ME: Angiotensin converting enzyme activity is present in the endothelium-denuded aorta, *Br J Pharmacol* 98:333–335, 1989.
75. Powell JS, Clozel JP, Muler RKM et al: Inhibitors of angiotensin-converting enzyme prevent myointimal proliferation after vascular injury, *Science* 245:186–188, 1989.
76. Hanson SR, Powell JS, Dodson T et al: Effects of angiotensin converting enzyme inhibition with cilazapril on intimal hyperplasia in injured arteries and vascular grafts in the baboon, *Hypertension* 18(suppl II):70–76, 1991.
77. Rakugi H, Wang DS, Dzau VJ, Pratt RE: Potential importance of tissue angiotensin-converting enzyme inhibition in preventing neointima formation, *Circulation* 90:449–455, 1994.
78. Cook NS, Zerwes HG, Pally C et al: Decreased lumen size after balloon injury despite inhibition of neointimal thickening and antivasospastic treatment, *Cardiovasc Res* 28:215–220, 1994.
79. Jackson CL, Bush RC, Bowyer DE: Mechanism of antiatherogenic action of calcium antagonists, *Atherosclerosis* 80:17–26, 1989.
80. Jackson CL, Bush RC, Bowyer DE: Inhibitory effect of calcium antagonists on balloon catheter-induced arterial smooth muscle cell proliferation and lesion size, *Atherosclerosis* 69:115–122, 1988.
81. Lichtlen PR, Hugenholtz PG, Rafflenbeul W et al: Nifedipine trial, *Lancet* 335:1109–1113, 1990.
82. El-Sanadiki MN, Cross KS, Murray JJ et al: Reduction of intimal hyperplasia and enhanced reactivity of experimental vein bypass grafts with verapamil treatment, *Ann Surg* 212:87–96, 1990.
83. Ferns GAA, Raines EW, Sprugel KH et al: Inhibition of neointimal smooth muscle accumulation after angioplasty by an antibody to PDGF, *Science* 253:1129–1132, 1991.
84. Maresta A, Balducelli M, Cantini L et al: Trapidil (triazolopyrimidine), a platelet derived growth factor antagonist, reduces restenosis after percutaneous transluminal coronary angioplasty, *Circulation* 90:2710–2715, 1994.
85. Chervu A, Moore WS, Quiñones-Baldrich WJ, Henderson T: Efficacy of corticosteroids in suppression of intimal hyperplasia, *J Vasc Surg* 10:129–134, 1989.
86. Villa AE, Guzman LA, Chen W et al: Local delivery of dexamethasone for prevention of neointimal proliferation in a rat model of balloon angioplasty, *J Clin Invest* 93:1243–1249, 1994.
87. Pepine CJ, Hirshfeld JW, Macdonald RG et al: A controlled trial of corticosteroids to prevent restenosis after coronary angioplasty: M-HEART group, *Circulation* 81:1753–1761, 1990.
88. Azuma H, Funayama N, Kubota T, Ishikawa M: Regeneration of endothelial cells after balloon

denudation of the rabbit carotid artery and changes in responsiveness, *Jpn J Pharmacol* 52:541–552, 1990.
89. Wilson JM, Birinyi LK, Salomon RN et al: Implantation of vascular grafts lined with genetically modified endothelial cells, *Science* 244:1344–1346, 1989.
90. Nabel EG, Plautz G, Nabel GJ: Gene transfer into vascular cells, *J Am Coll Cardiol* 17:189B–194B, 1991.
91. Nabel EG, Plautz B, Boyce FM et al: Recombinant gene expression in vivo within endothelial cells of the arterial wall, *Science* 244:1342–1344, 1989.
92. Shi Y, Fard A, Galeo A et al: Transcatheter delivery of c-myc antisense oligomers reduces neointimal formation in a porcine model of coronary artery balloon injury, *Circulation* 90:944–951, 1994.
93. Simons M, Rosenberg RD: Antisense nonmuscle myosin heavy chain and c-myb oligonucleotides suppress smooth muscle cell proliferation in vitro, *Circ Res* 70:837–843, 1992.
94. Simons M, Edelman ER, DeKeyser JL et al: Antisense c-myb oligonucleotides inhibit intimal arterial smooth muscle cell accumulation in vivo, *Nature* 359:67–70, 1992.
95. Dichek DA, Neville RF, Zwiebel JA et al: Seeding of intravascular stents with genetically engineered endothelial cells, *Circulation* 80:1347–1353, 1989.
96. Flugelman MY, Virmani R, Leon MB et al: Genetically engineered endothelial cells remain adherent and viable after stent deployment and exposure to flow in vitro, *Circ Res* 70:348–354, 1992.
97. Lynch CM, Clowes MM, Osborne WRA et al: Long-term expression of human adenosine deaminase in vascular smooth muscle cells of rats: a model for gene therapy, *Proc Natl Acad Sci USA* 89:1138–1142, 1992.
98. Osborne WR, Ramesh N, Lau S et al: Gene therapy for long-term expression of erythropoietin in rats, *Proc Nat Acad Sci USA* 92:8055–8058, 1995.
99. Ohno T, Gordon D, San H et al: Gene therapy for vascular smooth muscle cell proliferation after arterial injury [see comments], *Science* 265:781–784, 1994.
100. Wiedermann JG, Marboe C, Amols H et al: Intracoronary irradiation markedly reduces neointimal proliferation after balloon angioplasty in swine: persistent benefit at 6-month follow-up, *J Am Coll Cardiol* 25:1451–1456, 1995.
101. Teirstein PS, Massullo V, Jani S et al: Catheter-based radiotherapy to inhibit restenosis after coronary stenting [see comments], *N Engl J Med* 336:1697–1703, 1997.

38
Endoluminal Radiation Therapy

Rudolf P. Tutein Nolthenius and Frans L. Moll

Percutaneous transluminal angioplasty (PTA) and percutaneous transluminal coronary angioplasty (PTCA) are generally accepted and used as a minimal invasive therapeutic intervention for treatment of symptomatic stenoses of the central, peripheral, and coronary arteries. Clinical success and vessel patencies after PTCA are dependent on the pathology and type of lesion and the anatomic location.[1-3] Several mechanisms are responsible for the success after PTA. Recoil, remodeling, and restenosis are factors responsible for reocclusions, but it is not known which factor is most influential. Recoil and remodeling might be prevented or reduced by the use of stents. Many attempts to prevent restenosis have failed.[4-12] An important factor in restenosis is neointimal hyperplasia (NIH). As with other vascular interventions the vessel wall becomes traumatized after PTA. This trauma initiates a cascade of reactions in the vessel wall, the mechanism of which is not completely understood. In addition to smooth muscle cell proliferation with migration of cells from media across the internal elastic lamina and formation of an intimal mass of actively proliferating cells,[13-18] there seems to be an important role for adventitial responses as well.[19-27] Radiation therapy has been used successfully in several benign hyperproliferative diseases to prevent a proliferative response,[28-34] so it was conjectured to be beneficial in reducing NIH as well.

Radiation Therapy

Several methods are available to deliver radiation: external beam radiation, brachytherapy, and radioactive stents or liquids. With *external beam radiotherapy* a beam of radiation from a source outside the patient is aimed at a target of interest within the patient. Usually treatments are given with certain time intervals from several angles to achieve a homogeneous dose at the target while sparing the surrounding tissue. With this technique it is difficult to treat small volumes or targets that need a higher dose than the surrounding tissue allows.

Brachytherapy is a technique for delivering radiation to a target by placing a radioactive source close to or even in the target. In this way it is possible to deliver a high dose of radiation to a target without damaging the surrounding tissues because the intensity of the radiation dose rapidly decreases with increasing distance from the radiation source, thus sparing the tissues farther away from the source. It is possible to calculate exactly the dose volume at a certain target; and by placing several sources around the target it is possible to create complex configurations of dose distributions.[35]

Radioactive stents have the same ability to deliver the radiation close to the target, but exact dose distributions are not yet available. *Radioactive liquids* are still experimental.

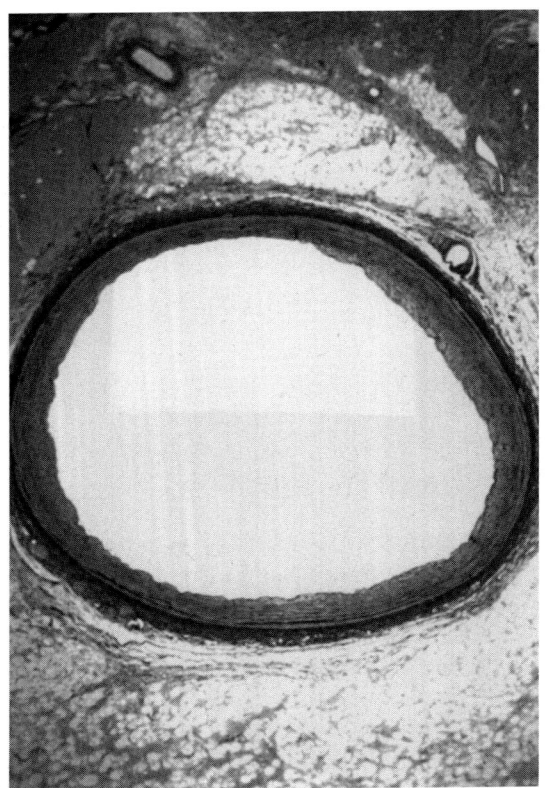 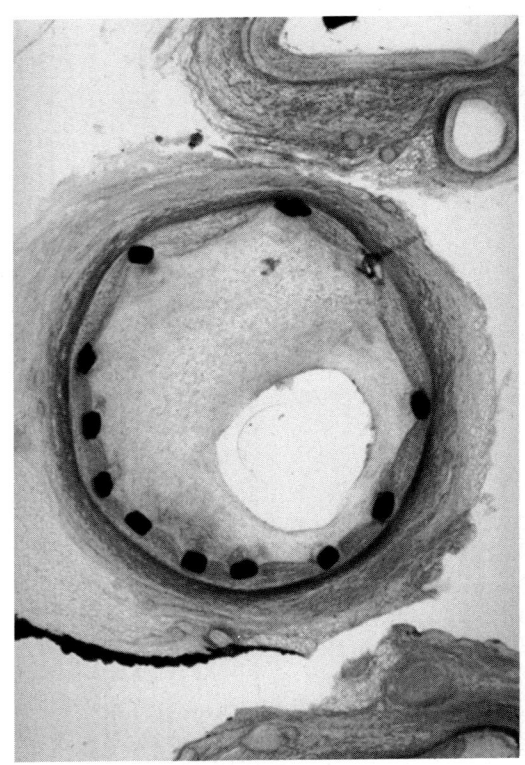

FIGURE 38–1. Light microscopy of normal pig coronary artery (**A**), control, stented but nonirradiated pig coronary artery (**B**), and stented and irradiated pig coronary artery (**C**) 1 month after treatment.

Many animal and human studies have been performed to examine the effect of the various types of radiation on the formation of NIH: External beam radiation, brachytherapy, and radioactive stents have been investigated in (intimal hyperplasia-inducing) animal models. Shimotakahara and Mayberg[36] and Mayberg et al.[37] demonstrated the effect of external beam radiation on NIH in a rat model after overstretching the carotid artery. Schwartz et al.[38] investigated the effect of external beam radiation in coronary arteries. Waksman et al.[39–41] performed a study in swine using brachytherapy and demonstrated a reduction in NIH in a dose-response relationship. This effect was still noted after 6 months of follow-up. Similar results were seen by Wiedermann et al.[42–44] Both Waksman and Wiedermann used low dose rate (LDR) iridium 192 (^{192}Ir). The optimal dose for inhibiting NIH seems to be between 1500 and 2000 cGy. Mazur et al.[45] used a high dose rate (HDR) afterloader with a computerized ^{192}Ir source. Verin et al.[46] used yttrium 90 as an endovascular source in rabbits with similar results. All these studies with different types of radiation in different models and different animals were unequivocal in their results. Figure 38–1 shows a reduced intimal response after irradiation and stenting compared to stenting alone in a pig coronary artery model. The effect on reducing NIH has been demonstrated using both gamma and beta radiation. The advantage of the latter is safety for both personnel and the patient, as beta sources have only short penetration. This trait, however, makes the source valuable only for treatment of small vessels, such as coronary arteries. In large arteries, such as the superficial femoral artery (SFA) and popliteal artery (PA), use of a gamma source seems mandatory to deliver sufficient radiation to the vessel wall.

The first clinical studies were performed by

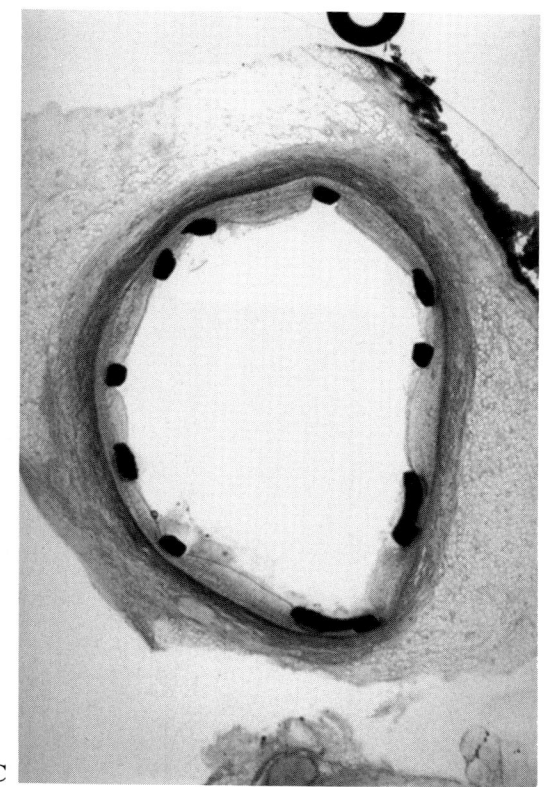

FIGURE 38–1. *Continued.*

Böttcher et al.[47,48] and later Liermann and colleagues.[49-51] They used ^{192}Ir with an HDR afterloader following recanalization and dilatation of a reocclusion in the SFA. Irradiation was performed using a ReKa-catheter to optimize the centering of the radiation source in the vessel, but true centering was not possible owing to the lack of a real (or true) centering catheter. Thirteen patients were described by Böttcher et al. with follow-up of 3 to 27 months. Liermann et al. described four patients with follow-up of 23 to 30 months. In neither study were signs of reocclusion seen, and there were no complications. After these encouraging reports prospective studies were started in the United States and Europe.

An important aspect of endovascular irradiation is the dose distribution. Because there is a dose-effect relationship it is important to obtain an equal dose distribution at the target site. For this reason various companies developed special "centering" balloons (Figures 38-2, [see color plate]; 38-3).

In addition to the new catheters and afterloaders, other endovascular radiation applications are being developed and investigated. In 1994 Fischell et al.[52] reported inhibition of

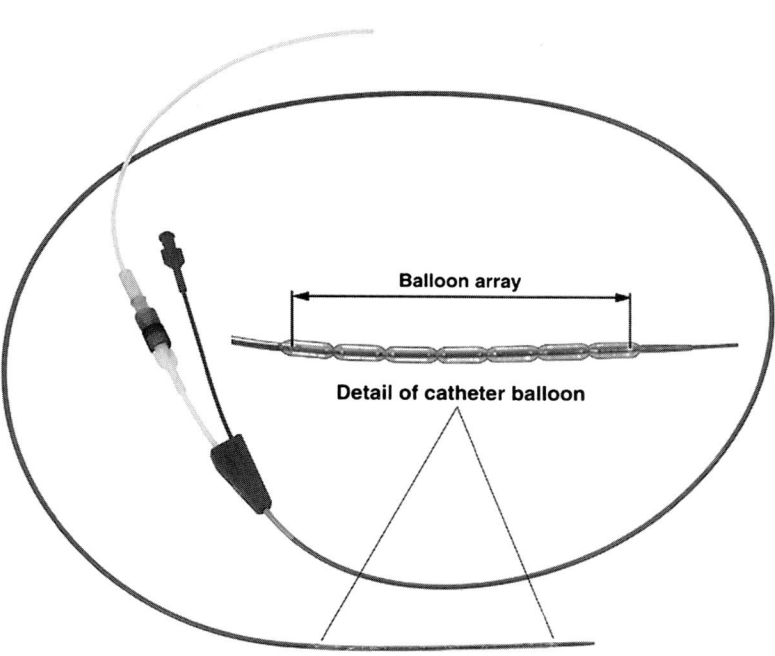

FIGURE 38–2. Centering balloon catheter from Nucletron. (See color plate).

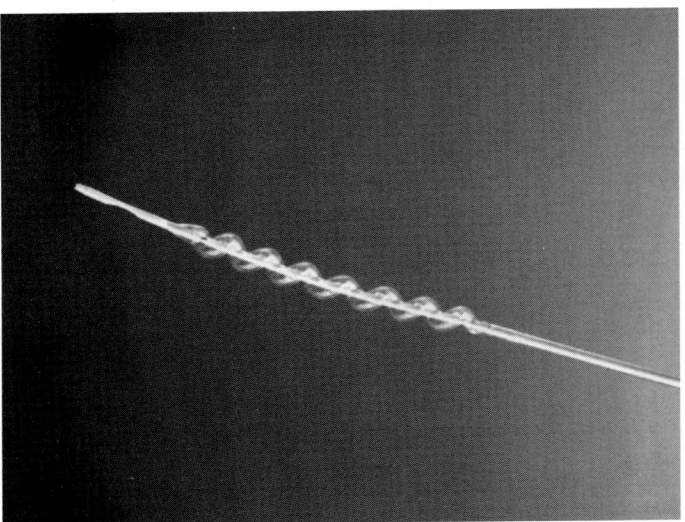

FIGURE 38–3. Centering balloon catheter from NeoCardia/Guidant.

smooth muscle cell proliferation using phosphorus 32 (^{32}P)-impregnated titanium wires in vitro. These positive findings resulted in in vivo studies. Hehrlein et al.[53-55] demonstrated NIH reduction using radioactive Palmaz *stents* in femoral rabbit arteries compared to that achieved with nonradioactive stents. Laird et al.[56] had similar results in a porcine coronary and iliac artery model. These first experiences are promising, but clinical results are not yet available.

Technical Considerations of Endovascular Irradiation

Brachytherapy is readily available in most medical centers with a radiation department. This technique, which delivers a radioactive source on a wire to various sites in the human body, is mostly used for treatment of malignancies of the biliary tract, lesions in the gynecologic system, and head and neck tumors. With this technique it is also possible to irradiate an angioplasty site endovascularly. Special consideration must be taken concerning the radiation source (beta or gamma), how to deliver the source (computerized afterloader or manually), where to deliver it (radiation department or cardiovascular suite), and at what time (before, immediately after, or several days after PTCA or PTA).

Radiation Source

The advantage of beta-emitting sources, such as strontium 90/yttrium 90 (^{90}Sr/^{90}Y) or ^{90}Y, compared to gamma sources such as ^{192}Ir is the reduced dose delivered to normal tissues, which also calls for fewer precautions concerning radiation hygiene safety for the medical staff and patient. Furthermore, it is possible to achieve high doses with sources of only modest activity because they are directly ionizing. The disadvantage of beta sources is the rapid falloff in radial dose distribution, which makes it difficult to create isodosimetric dose distributions several millimeters distant from the radiation source and therefore to treat large arteries. This probably restricts the use of beta-emitting sources to coronary arteries. Beta emitters such as ^{90}Sr/^{90}Y or ^{90}Y are easily handled and can be incorporated in a standard catheterization laboratory. Developments such as the HDR afterloader with an encapsulated ^{32}P beta-emitting source (Neocardia, Houston, Tx) and an "over-the-wire" passive centering ready-to-use intracoronary radiation system (Novoste Corporation, Norcross, GA) with ^{90}Sr are

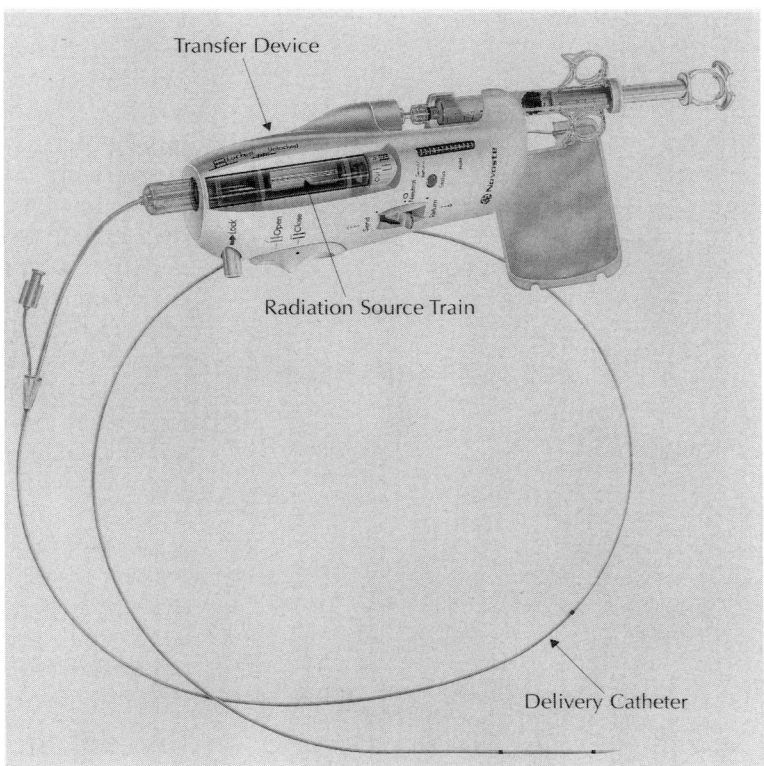

FIGURE 38-4. Novoste Beta-Cath System. This system is under clinical investigation and is not commercially available.

currently being investigated (Figure 38-4). For peripheral arteries the HDR afterloader is the most valuable and precise delivery system at the moment (Figures 38-5 [see color plate]; 38-6).

Mechanism of Delivery

When using gamma radiation manual delivery causes problems regarding the safety of personnel. Moreover, it is difficult to deliver the calculated dose precisely to the target volume. It is therefore more accurate and reliable to use a computer-controlled remote HDR afterloader [Nucletron, Veenendaal, The Netherlands or Columbia, MDY. USA (Figure 38-5) or Neocardia/Guidant (Figure 38-6)].

Site of Delivery

Gamma irradiation requires a special suite, available at all irradiation centers, to protect personnel. Usually these special protection requirements are not available in a standard vascular intervention suite. The patient must be transported from the intervention suite to the radiation department. Alternatively, a specially designed protective shield could be installed around the patient in the conventional angiography suite. This arrangement is currently a matter of investigation and might become commercially available.

Timing of Delivery

It is still unclear if there is optimal timing for radiation therapy in relation to angioplasty. Animal studies[38,39] have suggested a better effect if radiation is started several days after PTA, but the results were not conclusive as little difference was demonstrated. It therefore seems most reasonable to treat patients directly after angioplasty.

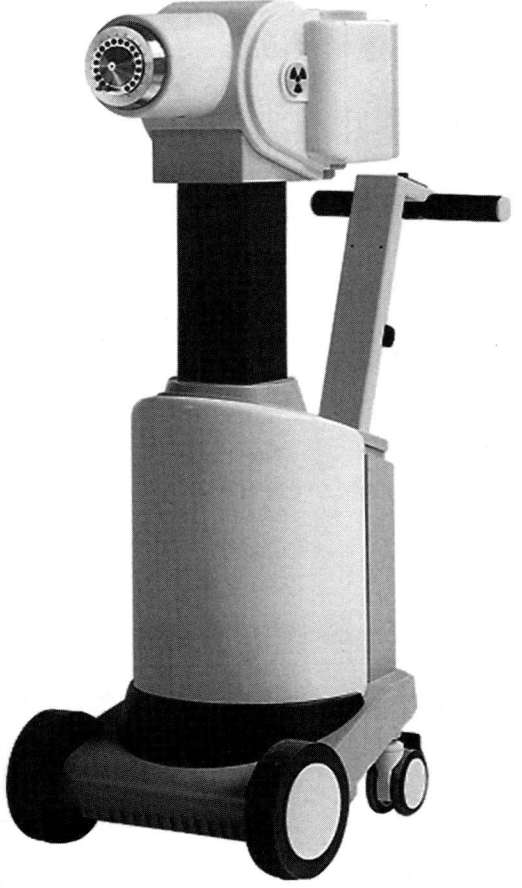

FIGURE 38-5. Nucletron HDR afterloader. (See color plate).

guidewire is kept in situ and the angioplasty balloon is exchanged for a centering balloon. This balloon consists of an open lumen in which a closed 5F source guiding catheter (SGC) can be placed. A dummy source wire is allowed to move freely in the lumen of this SGC. After positioning the centering balloon with the SGC the patient is transported to the radiation department with a deflated balloon. Dosimetric calculations are made based on vessel diameter, length of treated segment, and target volume. The dummy source wire is connected to the HDR, and a test or dummy run is performed. If no resistance is encountered, the dummy wire is exchanged for the ^{192}Ir radioactive wire, which is delivered by the microSelectron HDR afterloader. To optimize the central position of the radioactive source the centering balloon is inflated during this procedure. Irradiation itself takes about 3 to 5 minutes. The wires and sheath are removed immediately after irradiation.

Present Status and Near Future

Based on many experimental and some clinical studies there is evidence that radiation therapy reduces neointimal hyperplasia in arteries. Whether it will result in improved clinical outcome with improved patency is yet

Considering the pros and cons of beta and gamma radiation, the best option seems to use beta radiation in small vessels such as coronary arteries and gamma radiation in larger arteries such as peripheral vessels. In certain situations, such as an arteriovenous fistula where the problem area is superficial, it might even be easier to use external beam irradiation as the primary treatment option.

Technique in Peripheral Vessels

So long as there is no protective shield commercially available to place around the patient, irradiation should be performed in a specially designed suite in the radiation department. After PTA is successfully performed the

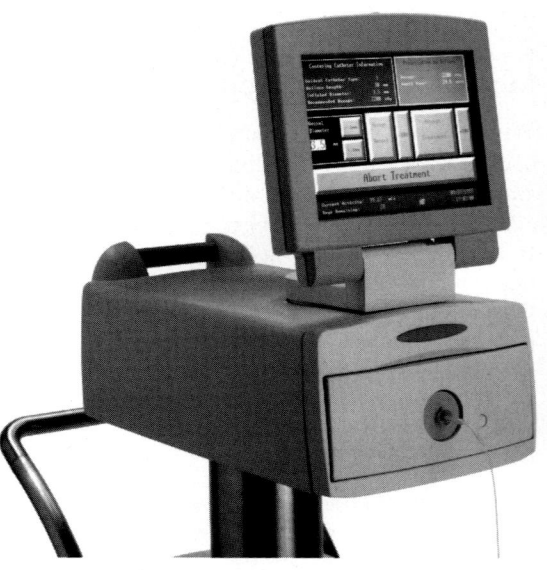

FIGURE 38-6. NeoCardia/Guidant's afterloader.

unknown. Many questions must still be answered. Several clinical studies have been started. The Beta Energy Restenosis Trial (BERT) is a US Food and Drug Administration (FDA)-approved feasibility study limited to 23 patients in two centers. Verins' group[57,58] in Geneva performed a clinical study of 15 patients with intracoronary beta irradiation after PTCA, and early results in the randomized SCRIPPS study seem encouraging.[59,60] In this latter study patients with restenosis underwent coronary stenting and balloon dilatation and were randomly assigned to undergo catheter-based irradiation with ^{192}Ir or placebo. Currently more randomized studies are being started. A prospective randomized study was initiated in 1997 in The Netherlands. The effect of gamma radiation after PTA of the superficial femoral artery is being examined in this study. The study was designed to enroll 226 patients. A double-blind randomized study on peripheral arteries is under investigation in the United States. In this study the effect of gamma radiation after PTA in the SFA is being investigated in a double-blind way. Only the radiotherapist (not the treating physician) knows if only a dummy run or actual irradiation takes place.

On theoretical grounds irradiation might be even more effective if prior to the irradiation debulking of the atheromatous plaque is performed instead of angioplasty. After debulking by means of atherectomy or remote endarterectomy, the lesion is more likely to receive equal dose distribution to the adventitia of the artery because centering of the source seems more accurate. This concept has not yet been investigated. So far, the preliminary results justify further study to determine whether irradiation will find a permanent place in the ongoing battle to reduce restenosis after successful interventional treatment of peripheral arterial occlusive disease.

References

1. Hunink MG, Donaldson MC, Meyerovitz MF et al: Risks and benefits of femoropopliteal percutaneous balloon angioplasty, *J Vasc Surg* 17:183–192, 1993.
2. Johnston KW: Femoral and popliteal arteries: reanalysis of results of balloon angioplasty, *Radiology* 183:767–771, 1992.
3. Murray RRJ, Hewes RC, White RIJ et al: Long-segment femoropopliteal stenoses: is angioplasty a boon or a bust? *Radiology* 162:473–476, 1987.
4. Chesebro JH, Webster MWI, Reeder GS et al: Coronary angioplasty antiplatelet therapy induces acute complications but not restenosis [abstract], *Circulation* 80(suppl 2):64, 1989.
5. Corcos T, David PR, Val PG et al: Failure of diltiazem to prevent restenosis after PTCA, *Am Heart J* 109:926–931, 1985.
6. Dehmer GJ, Popma JJ, Egerton K et al: Reduction in the rate of early restenosis after coronary angioplasty by a diet supplemented with w-3 fatty acids, *N Engl J Med* 319:733–740, 1988.
7. Ellis SG, Roubin GS, Wilentz IJ et al: Effect of 18 to 24 hour heparin administered for prevention of restenosis after uncomplicated coronary angioplasty, *Am Heart J* 117:777–782, 1989.
8. Raizner AE, Hollman J, Abukhalil J et al: Ciprostene for restenosis revisited: quantitative analysis of angiograms [abstract], *J Am Coll Cardiol* 21:321A, 1993.
9. Reis GJ, Boucher TM, Slipperly ME et al: Randomized trial of fish oil for the prevention of restenosis after coronary angioplasty, *Lancet* 2:177–181, 1989.
10. Schwartz L, Bourassa MG, Lesperance J et al: Aspirin and dipyridamole in the prevention of restenosis after PTCA, *N Engl J Med* 318:1714–1719, 1988.
11. Thornton MA, Gruentzig AR, Hollman J et al: Coumadin and aspirin in the prevention of recurrence after transluminal coronary angioplasty: a randomized study, *Circulation* 69:721–727, 1984.
12. Whitworth HB, Roubin GS, Hollman J et al: Effects of nifedipine on recurrent stenosis after PTCA, *Am Coll Cardiol* 8:1271–1276, 1986.
13. Clowes AW, Reidy MA, Clowes MM: Kinetics of cellular proliferation after arterial injury: smooth muscle growth in the absence of endothelium, *Lab Invest* 49:327–333, 1983.
14. Reidy MA, Fingerele J, Lindner V: Factors controlling the development of arterial lesion after injury, *Circulation* 86:1143–1146, 1992.
15. Schwartz RS, Murphy JG, Edwards WD et al: Restenosis after balloon angioplasty: a practical proliferative model in porcine coronary arteries, *Circulation* 82:2190–2200, 1990.
16. Schwartz RS, Huber KC, Murphy JG et al: Restenosis and the proportional neointimal response to coronary artery injury: results in a porcine model, *J Am Coll Cardiol* 19:267–274, 1992.

17. Karas SP, Gravanis MB, Santoian EC et al: Coronary intimal proliferation after balloon injury and stenting in swine: an animal model of restenosis, *J Am Coll Cardiol* 20:467–474, 1992.
18. Schneider JE, Berk BC, Gravanis MB et al: Probucol decreases neointimal formation in a swine model of coronary artery balloon injury: a possible role for antioxidants in restenosis, *Circulation* 88:628–637, 1993.
19. Scott NA, Ross C, Subramanian R et al: Characterization of the cellular response to coronary injury [abstract], *Circulation* 90:1392, 1994.
20. Scott NA, Martin F, Simonet L et al: Contribution of adventitial myofibroblasts to vascular remodelling and lesion formation after experimental angioplasty in pig coronary arteries [abstract], *FASEB J* 9:A845, 1995.
21. Wilcox JN, Waksman R, King SB: The role of the adventitia in the arterial response to angioplasty: the effect of intravascular radiation, *Int J Radiat Oncol Biol Phys* 36:789–796, 1996.
22. Scott NA, Cipolla GD, Ross CE et al: Identification of a potential role for the adventitia in vascular lesion formation after balloon overstretch injury of porcine coronary arteries, *Circulation* 93:2178–2187, 1996.
23. Booth RF, Martin JF, Honey AC et al: Rapid development of atherosclerotic lesions in the rabbit carotid artery induced by perivascular manipulation, *Atherosclerosis* 76: 257–268, 1989.
24. Barker SG, Tilling LC, Miller GC et al: The adventitia and atherogenesis: removal initiates intimal proliferation in the rabbit which regresses on generation of a "neoadventitia," *Atherosclerosis* 105:131–144, 1994.
25. Chignier E, Eloy R, Huc A et al: Adventitial resection of small artery provokes endothelial loss and intimal hyperplasia, *Surg Gynecol Obstet* 163:327–334, 1986.
26. Marmur JD, Rossikhina M, Guha A et al: Tissue factor is rapidly induced in arterial smooth muscle after balloon injury, *J Clin Invest* 91:2253–2259, 1993.
27. Rakugi H, Jacob HJ, Krieger JE et al: Vascular injury induces angiotensinogen gene expression in the media and neointima, *Circulation* 87:283–290, 1993.
28. Van den Brenk HA, Minty CC: Radiation in the management of keloids and hypertrofic scar, *Br J Surg* 47:595–605, 1961.
29. Van den Brenk HA: Results of profylactic postoperative irradiation in 1300 cases of pterygium, *AJR* 103:723, 1968.
30. Finger PT, Berson A, Sherr D et al: Radiation therapy for subretinal neovascularization, *Ophthalmology* 103:878–889, 1996.
31. Grillo HC, Potsaid MS: Studies in wound healing, *Ann of Surg* 154:741–750, 1961.
32. Inalsingh CHA: An experience in treating five hundred and one patients with keloids, *Johns Hopkins Med J* 134:284–290, 1974.
33. MacLennan I, Keys HM, Evarts CM et al: Usefulness of postoperative hip irradiation in the prevention of heterotopic bone formation in a high risk group of patients, *Int J Radiat Oncol Biol Phys* 10:49–53, 1984.
34. Nickson JJ, Lawrence W, Rachwalsky L: Röentgen rays and wound healing: fractionated irradiation: experimental study, *Surgery* 34:859–862, 1953.
35. Levendag PC, Schmitz PI, Jansen PP et al: Fractionated high dose rate and pulsed dose rate brachytherapy—first clinical experience in squamous cell carcinoma of the tonsillar fossa and soft palate, *Int J Radiat Oncol Biol Phys* 38:497–506, 1997.
36. Shimotakahara S, Mayberg MR: Gamma irradiation inhibits neointimal hyperplasia in rats after arterial injury, *Stroke* 25:424–428, 1994.
37. Mayberg MR, Luo Z, London S et al: Radiation inhibition of intimal hyperplasia after arterial injury, *Radiat Res* 142:212–220, 1995.
38. Schwartz RS, Koval TM, Edwards WD et al: Effect of external beam irradiation on neointimal hyperplasia after experimental coronary artery injury, *J Am Coll Cardiol* 19:1106–1113, 1992.
39. Waksman R, Robinson KA, Crocker IR et al: Endovascualr low-dose irradiation inhibits neointima formation after coronary artery balloon injury in swine: a possible role for radiation therapy in restenosis prevention, *Circulation* 91:1533–1539, 1995.
40. Waksman R, Robinson KA, Crocker IR et al: Intracoronary radiation before stent implantaion inhibits neointima formation in stented porcine coronary arteries, *Circulation* 92:1383–1386, 1995.
41. Waksman R, Robinson KA, Crocker IR et al: Intracoronary low-dose beta-irradiation inhibits neointima formation after coronary artery balloon injury in the swine restenosis model, *Circulation* 92:3025–3031, 1995
42. Wiedermann JG, Leavy JA, Amols H et al: Effects of high-dose intracoronary irradiation on vasomotor function and smooth muscle

histopathology, *Am J Physiol* 267:H 125–132, 1994.
43. Wiedermann JG, Marboe C, Amols H et al: Intracoronary irradiation markedly reduces restenosis after balloon angioplasty in a porcine model, *J Am Coll Cardiol* 23:1491–1498, 1994.
44. Wiedermann JG, Marboe C, Amols H et al: Intracoronary irradiation markedly reduces neointimal proliferation after balloon angioplasty in swine: persistent benefit at 6-month follow-up, *J Am Coll Cardiol* 25:1451–1456, 1995.
45. Mazur W, Ali MN, Dabhagi SF et al: High dose rate intracoronary radiation suppresses neointimal proliferation in the stented and balloon model of porcine restenosis [abstract], *Circulation* 90:652, 1994.
46. Verin V, Popowski Y, Urban P et al: Intraarterial beta irradiation prevents neointimal hyperplasia in a hypercholoesterolemic rabbit restenosis model, *Circulation* 92:2284–2290, 1995.
47. Böttcher HD: Endovascular radioprevention of intimal hyperplasia after percutaneous transluminal angioplasty of peripheral blood vessels, *Radiologe* 34:519–524, 1994.
48. Böttcher HD, Schopohl B, Liermann D et al: Endovascular irradiation—a new method to avoid recurrent stenosis after stent implantation in peripheral arteries: technique and preliminary results, *Int J Radiat Oncol Biol Phys* 29:183–186, 1994.
49. Liermann D, Berkefeld J, Herrmann G et al: Intervention and clinical aspects combined with endovascular irradiation of intimal hyperplasia of the vascular system, *Radiologe* 34:524–533, 1994.
50. Liermann D, Böttcher HD: Use of low dose local radiation for treatment of restenosis Presented at the Sixth annnual international symposium on vascular diagnosis and intervention, January 1994, pp 69–71.
51. Liermann D, Böttcher HD, Kollath J et al: Prophylactic endovascular radiotherapy to prevent intimal hyperplasia after stent implantation in femoropopliteal arteries, *Cardiovasc Intervent Radiol* 17:12–16, 1994.
52. Fischell TA, Bassam KK, Fischell DR et al: Low-dose beta particle emission from "stent" wire results in complete, localized inhibition of smooth muscle cell proliferation, *Circulation* 90:2956–2963, 1994.
53. Hehrlein C, Zimmermann M, Metz J et al: Radioactive stent implantation inhibits neointimal proliferation in non-atherosclerotic rabbits, *Circulation* 88(suppl I):65, 1993.
54. Hehrlein C, Gollan C, Donges K et al: Low-dose radioactive endovascular tents prevent smooth muscle cell proliferation and neointimal hyperplasia in rabbits, *Circulation* 92:1570–1575, 1995.
55. Hehrlein C, Stintz M, Kinscherf R et al: Pure beta-particle emitting stents inhibit neointima formation in rabbits, *Circulation* 93:641–645, 1996.
56. Laird JR, Carter AJ, Kufs WM et al: Inhibition of neointimal proliferation with low-dose irradiation from a beta-particle-emitting stent, *Circulation* 93:529–536, 1996.
57. Popowski Y, Verin V, Papirov I et al: Intraarterial 90-yttrium brachytherapy: preliminary dosimetric study using a specially modified angioplasty balloon, *Int J Radiat Oncol Biol Phys* 33:713–717, 1995.
58. Popowski Y, Verin V, Urban P: Endovascular beta-irradiation following percutaneous transluminal coronary balloon angioplasty, *Int J Radiat Oncol Biol Phys* 36:841–845, 1996.
59. Teirstein PS, Massullo V, Jani S et al: Catheter-based radiotherapy to inhibit restenosis after coronary stenting, *N Engl J Med* 336:1697–1703, 1997.
60. Massullo V, Teirstein PS, Jani S et al: Endovascular brachytherapy to inhibit coronary artery restenosis: an introduction to the SCRIPPS Coronary Radiation to Inhibit Proliferation Post Stenting trial, *Int J Radiat Oncol Biol Phys* 36:973–975, 1996.

39
Local Drug Delivery: New Approaches in Endovascular Therapies

Aaron V. Kaplan

The ability to deliver agent directly into the arterial wall holds great promise for the treatment of coronary arterial and peripheral vascular disorders. The initial focus of catheter-based drug delivery has been the delivery of classic pharmaceutical agents in the setting of angioplasty to prevent acute complications and late restenosis. More recently preclinical studies have focused on the delivery of novel agents (e.g., adenoviral vectors) to prevent restenosis and to promote angiogenesis.[1]

The practice of angioplasty has undergone fundamental changes with the incorporation of stents into the clinical armamentarium. It is estimated that stents were used in approximately two-thirds of patients treated in the United States in 1997. Stents have been shown to reduce both acute complications and late restenosis.[2,3] They have provided the interventionist with a means to treat large dissections, leading to a dramatic reduction in acute abrupt closure and the rate of emergency surgery. The mechanical scaffold provided by stents is also responsible for the prevention of arterial recoil and negative geometric remodeling, which make up a significant component of restenosis. The benefit of stent placement within the coronary vasculature has been demonstrated primarily in discrete lesions in large vessels. As more trackable stents become available, allowing treatment of lesions in small vessels, the benefit of stent placement may be reduced. Multiple studies have demonstrated that stent placement increases late lumen loss.[2,3] Furthermore, the treatment of restenosis within a stented artery (i.e., "in-stent" restenosis) presents the interventionist with a far more difficult problem than "old-fashioned" restenosis. Therefore the benefit of a local delivery strategy may be greatest for prevention of in-stent restenosis. Despite encouraging results in animal models, pharmacologic therapies to reduce restenosis have been disappointing. This may be due in part to the inability to achieve sufficient tissue concentration of agent at the site of interest.[4] Another approach to the treatment of restenosis is local therapy, that is, the delivery of agent directly into the arterial wall at the site of angioplasty.

The purpose of this chapter is to review the basic concepts associated with local therapy and to provide an overview of devices presently in use and under development. The scope is limited to systems that deliver agent(s) in an aqueous vehicle. Although the delivery of agent in a bioeluting matrix, in particulate or stent form, holds much promise, a thorough review is beyond the scope of this chapter.

Local Drug Delivery: Definition and Premise

A local therapeutic strategy is most compelling when applied to focal processes, for example, coronary artery disease and peripheral vascular disease. The limitations of systemic therapy for focal processes are illustrated by the current approach to the treatment of acute myocardial infarction. During the past decade several large-scale multicenter trials have demonstrated the benefits of thrombolytic agents. As a result, systemic thrombolytics have become the standard treatment for patients with acute myocardial infarction. Thrombolytic agents are routinely administered systemically via an intravenous route. Dosing regimens have been developed to obtain rapidly and then sustain plasma concentrations within the therapeutic range throughout the systemic circulation. This approach requires dosing regimens to achieve therapeutic levels of agent throughout its volume of distribution even though the site that requires therapy (i.e., occlusive thrombus) has a volume of approximately 500μL. As a result, the entire circulation is exposed to lytic agent at therapeutic concentrations. The major drawback to this approach is that fibrin at distant sites is exposed to fibrinolysis, leading to hemostatic complications. The most dramatic of these complications is intracranial bleeding. Less dramatic bleeding complications are routinely encountered within the gastrointestinal and genitourinary tracts, the retroperitoneal space, and arterial access sites, leading to blood transfusion, prolonged hospitalization, and surgical intervention. The risk of these complications limits the dosing and effectiveness of these agents. Excessive bleeding observed during clinical trials has led to reduction of the doses of thrombolytic agent and anticoagulant.[5,6] A local delivery strategy circumvents these problems. If the agent is delivered only to the site of obstructive thrombus without significant systemic overflow, agent dosing would no longer be limited by these complications.

A local strategy also allows reduction of the amount of agent required, which could significantly reduce the cost of therapy. For agents not stable in the systemic circulation, local therapy allows a means to obtain adequate tissue concentrations. To achieve these goals, we and others have developed approaches to deliver agent directly into the arterial wall at the site of angioplasty.

For a local delivery device to be effective, it must deliver an efficacious agent and attain adequate target tissue concentrations for a sufficient duration without significant injury to the arterial wall. The device must be easy to use and have an acceptable safety profile. Furthermore, the combined cost of the device and drug must be justifiable.

The benefit of a local delivery strategy is based on the efficacy of both the agent and the device. Agent characteristics, including mechanism of action, molecular weight, and partition coefficient, affect the residence time within the arterial wall. Therefore studies of drug delivery systems must be reviewed in the context of the agent delivered.

Drug delivery devices have been reported to have a delivery efficiency in the range of 0.1% to 10.0%. The initial tissue concentration of agent is determined primarily by the characteristics of the drug delivery system and the arterial wall. The therapeutic potential for a delivery efficiency of 1% is formidable. For example, an agent with a volume of distribution of 5 liters delivered into a coronary arterial segment (length 20mm, diameter 3.0mm, estimated mural volume 0.5ml) with a transfer efficiency of approximately 1% has an initial mural concentration approximately 10^4 more than that in plasma. The advantages of starting with such a high tissue level allows a depot to sustain concentrations within therapeutic concentrations.

In the context of a drug delivery device, injury can be divided into two categories: acute (e.g., dissection and perforation) and chronic (e.g., restenosis). Issues surrounding an injury leading to acute complications are common to all new interventional devices and are straightforward to study.[7] A drug delivery catheter must have an acceptable complication rate for it to be accepted into routine clinical practice.

More difficult to study is the injury. Though initially subclinical, it may increase intimal hyperplasia, leading to an increase in clinical restenosis. This type of injury can be further classified as mechanical or chemical. The most commonly discussed mechanical injury is the high-pressure "jet injury" associated with perforated balloons (see below). Another type of injury is the foreign body reaction associated with delivery of bioerodable elements.[8] With well designed animal studies, the acute and chronic effects of drug delivery on the arterial wall can be ascertained. These observations are limited by the animal models in which they are performed. Because it is difficult to randomize patients to a control group in which a vehicle without drug is delivered into the arterial wall, it is difficult to define the effect of delivery on clinical restenosis. In reality, clinical studies can evaluate the efficacy of a drug–device combination. It will be difficult to dissociate the effect of drug from that associated with delivery. The benefit (or lack thereof) of a locally delivered drug is the net effect of both the agent and the mechanism of delivery. Theoretically, the delivery of agent may inflict subtle injury on the arterial wall, which may lead to an increased response to the injury, resulting in an increased restenosis rate (see below). This effect, if present, must be outweighed by the benefits of the drug being delivered.

Specific Devices

Wolinsky Perforated Balloon Catheter

Most local delivery catheters devised to date are modified angioplasty balloon catheters. The simplest angioplasty balloon-based system is the perforated balloon first described by Wolinsky and Thung (USCI/Bard, Bellerica, MA).[9] The Wolinsky catheter is a standard angioplasty catheter with laser-drilled perforations in the balloon membrane. The catheter described in the initial publication has a total of 300 holes with diameters of 25 µm. These holes are arranged in six longitudinal rows of 50 holes each over a span of 12 mm.[9] The catheter is filled with therapeutic solution and positioned at the site of interest using standard technique. When the balloon is pressurized, agent exits the balloon via the perforations. The condition under which agent exits the balloon is determined by the proximal inflation pressure, the size and number of perforations, and the fit with respect to the arterial wall (Table 39–1; Figure 39–1).

The Wolinsky balloon has been evaluated by many investigators in a variety of experimental settings. We have studied the effect of locally delivered antithrombins via the Wolinsky balloon on platelet thrombus formation. In a whole-artery preparation, intramural delivery of D-phenylalanyl-prolyl-arginine-chloromethyl ketone (PPACK), a direct thrombin inhibitor, resulted in a 53% reduction of

TABLE 39–1. Local Drug Delivery Systems

Catheter name and manufacturer	Description	Time required[a]	Clinical testing	Regulatory approval
Wolinsky Balloon, USCI/Bard	Perforated balloon	1 minute	Yes; abandoned	None
LocalMed InfusaSleeve, LocalMed	Sleeve loaded on standard PTCA catheter	< 30 seconds	Yes	US, Europe
Dispatch Catheter, Scimed Life Systems	Helical balloon with perfusion for prolonged bathing of arterial wall	30 minutes	Yes	US, Europe, Japan
Transport Catheter, Cardiovascular Dynamics	Balloon-in-a-balloon	Variable	Yes	Europe, Japan
Hydrogel Balloon, Boston Scientific	Standard PTCA balloon with special coating from which drug is passively dispersed	5 minutes	Yes	Approved for other uses
Channel Balloon, Boston Scientific	Balloon surrounded by array of 24 channels each with a 250-µm hole	Variable	No	None
MIC Catheter, Cordis	Perforated balloon covered with a permeable membrane	Variable	No	None
Iontophoresis Balloon, CorTrak Medical	System in which small electric field is between delivery balloon and skin	5 minutes	No	None

PTCA, percutaneous transluminal coronary angioplasty.
[a] As determined by published protocols.

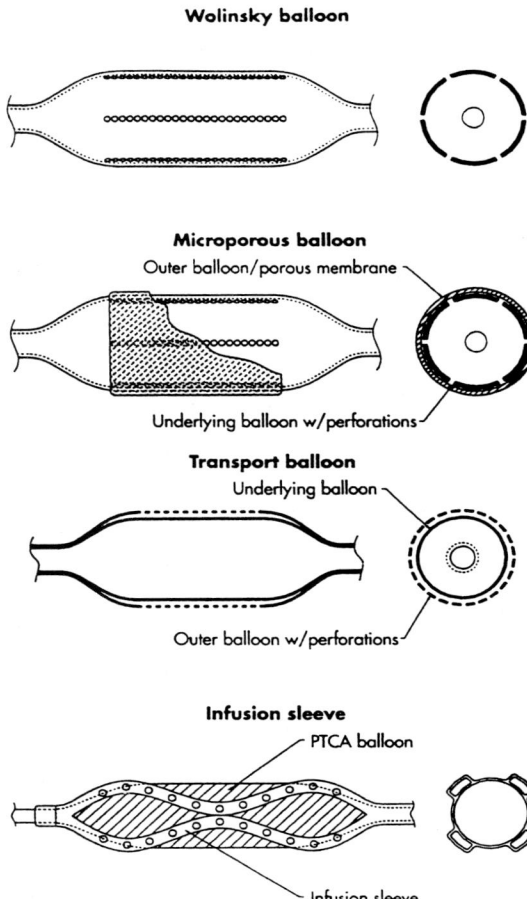

FIGURE 39–1. Local drug delivery systems currently under development: Wolinsky balloon, microporous balloon, transport balloon, and infusion sleeve. See text for descriptions of the construction and use of each device. For other devices under development, see Figure 39–2.

platelet thrombus formation.[10,11] In a porcine model of restenosis, Shi and colleagues studied the effect of c-*myc* phosphothioate antisense delivered intramurally. A significant reduction in myointimal proliferation was observed.[12] In these systems, delivery of a potent agent via a perforated balloon demonstrated beneficial effect on antithrombotic and antirestenotic endpoints.

Not all the evaluations with the Wolinsky type of balloons have resulted in beneficial effects on the endpoint being examined. Muller and colleagues studied the effect of methotrexate on restenosis in a porcine carotid model of restenosis. Using the radiolabeled technique, medial methotrexate levels reached 1000 μM immediately after delivery and remained above 100 μM for 7 days (peak serum concentration for treatment of large cell adenocarcinoma is 100 μM). Despite sustaining "adequate" tissue levels of the agent, no effect was observed on neointimal thickening at 30 days.[13] Gimple et al. examined the effect of local delivery of heparin on intimal proliferation in a double-injury cholesterol-fed rabbit model. No effect on neointimal hyperplasia was observed.[14] The lack of efficacy observed in these studies may be due to ineffectiveness of agent, inadequate drug delivery, or the specifics of the animal model used. It is difficult to compare directly the studies demonstrating a positive effect with those showing a lack of efficacy.

Acceptance of the perforated balloon catheters has been hampered by early reports characterizing jet injury and initial clinical tests that apparently had a high dissection rate.[15,16] Plante and colleagues reported on the effect of delivering saline solution via a perforated balloon catheter on acute and chronic markers of arterial injury in a rabbit iliac model. When compared with controls, no differences in endpoints were observed in the initial angiographic results, ^{3}H-thymidine uptake at 4 days, or neointimal hyperplasia.[17] These findings are consistent with what other groups reported in similar models.[16,18] Still others reported a high degree of injury.[15,19] Review of this literature is made difficult by the fact that design changes in the catheter (i.e., hole size and array) differ from study to study, as do the specific delivery parameters (i.e., proximal infusion study.)[20] Furthermore, different animal models were used. This confusion underlines the main difficulty with the design of this catheter: coupling balloon inflation with drug delivery. This difficulty led us and others to investigate designs that allow more precise control of the fit independent of drug delivery.

Microporous Balloon

The microporous infusion catheter (MIC), under development by the Cordis Corporation

(Miami, FL), is a modified perforated balloon catheter. The MIC balloon was developed to overcome the initial problems associated with the Wolinsky balloon. To limit the energy of the jets, the perforated balloon is covered by a porous membrane (pore size less than 1 μm). When the balloon is inflated, agent "oozes" through the porous membrane (Table 39–1, Figure 39–1).

Lincoff and colleagues, at The Cleveland Clinic, evaluated the ability of this catheter to deliver marker agent (horseradish peroxidase) in vivo into normal porcine coronary arteries after overstretch injury. An overall transfer efficiency of approximately 1% was reported, with most of the agent delivered to the lumen.[21]

The MIC catheter has been used in the phase I evaluation of cytoclasin b sponsored by NeoRx Corporation. Cytoclasin b inhibits actin polymerization and has been evaluated in a porcine restenosis model. It is thought to prevent restenosis primarily by inhibiting vascular remodeling. A phase I study evaluating the safety of locally delivered cytoclasin b has now been completed. In this study a total of 43 patients were randomized to one of five groups (saline control and four concentrations of cytoclasin b) in which the agent was delivered at a constant infusion pressure for 90 seconds. Patients in each group received varying volumes (18.0 ± 6.6 ml) and therefore varying amounts of the agent. Review of angiograms following agent delivery demonstrated a new dissection or worsening of preexisting dissections in 30% (10/33) of patients. Early complications included two deaths. A phase II study is presently in the planning stages.[22]

A more recent generation of the MIC catheter, the MIC-3, marketed as the Crescendo catheter, has received 510k clearance from the US Food and Drug Administration (FDA). This catheter is being evaluated in the Impress Trial, a prospective randomized trial studying the impact of low-molecular-weight heparin (LMWH) on restenosis in patients electively undergoing stent placement.[23] Altogether 245 patients who underwent percutaneous transluminal coronary angioplasty (PTCA)/placement of a Palmaz Schatz stent were randomized to LMWH or control groups. Patients assigned to the LMWH group received 5000 IU of nadroparin (Sanofi, Gentilly, France) in a volume of 2 ml at 3 atm. Patients assigned to the control group received no further treatment. Patient recruitment in this study was completed during the fall of 1997. Technical failure (i.e., failure to deliver the MIC catheter to the index lesion) was reported in 4.1% (5/122) of patients. At six months follow-up there was no difference in the incidence of major adverse events or target lesion revascularizations. Similarly, core angiographic analysis showed no difference in angiographic restenosis or late loss.

Transport/Balloon in a Balloon

The Transport Catheter (SciMed Lifes Systems, Maple Grove, MN) is a dual-purpose angioplasty/drug delivery catheter. The catheter consists of two concentric balloons mounted on the distal end. The inner balloon acts as a traditional angioplasty balloon. The outer balloon membrane contains 36 to 45 holes 250 μm in diameter. Drug is infused via a proximal infusion port into the space between the balloons and exits via the perforations in the outer balloon membrane. Agent can be delivered with the inner balloon inflated or deflated.[25] The effect of inner balloon inflation on the egress of the agent and preclinical data on agent transfer have not been reported (Table 39–1, Figure 39–1).

The initial use of the the Transport Catheter was for the delivery of lytic agents in patients with unstable coronary syndromes.[24,25] Cumberland and colleagues[26] at the Northern General Hospital in Sheffield, England, reported their experience in nine patients primarily with class IV angina. This series demonstrated the ability to use the transport as a primary dilatory catheter. In patients with angiographic thrombus, recombinant tissue plasminogen activator (rt-PA) was administered before (three patients) and after (three patients) angioplasty. Acute closure occurred in one patient and was easily treated by repeat PTCA.

Local delivery of LMWH (enoxaparin) via the Transport Catheter has been evaluated in patients electively undergoing stent placement. A 20-patient pilot series has been performed in Poland in which predilatation patients received 10mg of enoxaparin delivered with a mean pressure of 68 ± 3 psi over 72 ± 4 seconds with a balloon support pressure of 3 atm. The investigators have reported a good safety profile and a low 6-month angiographic restenosis rate. An open-label prospective randomized control study evaluating enoxaparin delivered locally to PTCA patients alone is presently in the recruitment phase.[26]

Local delivery of c-*myc* antisense is also being evaluated with the Transport Catheter in the ITALICS trial. This study is a single-center blinded randomized control study in which patients are randomized to received c-*myc* antisense or saline following placement of a Wallstent. Results presented at the European Society of Cardiology Meeting (August 1998) indicated that there was no significant impact of locally delivered c-myc antisense on angiographic parameters of restenosis detected at 6 months.[27]

Dissociation of Apposition from Drug Delivery

Delivery of agent in an aqueous vehicle requires two distinct steps: (1) apposition of drug delivery elements against the arterial wall; and (2) delivery of agent to the arterial wall. The Wolinsky balloon and the MIC balloon couple apposition with drug delivery conditions. This protocol has some major disadvantages.

In these systems the balloon–artery fit and drug delivery conditions are determined by the inflation/infusion pressure. If the delivery balloon selected is found to be undersized then increased inflation/infusion pressure will be required to ensure adequate apposition commiting to drug delivery at a pressure that may inflict unacceptable arterial wall injury. Santolan et al. reported injury associated with high pressure delivery in connection with the Wolinsky balloon catheter.[16] The impact of this injury in animal models of restenosis remains unclear (see below). Conversely, using a slightly oversized drug delivery catheter engenders a similar conundrum. If agent is infused at optimal conditions for drug delivery, there is a risk of unwanted arterial overstretch, leading to arterial dissection. If the agent inflation/infusion pressure is reduced to avoid excessive arterial overstretch, drug transfer efficiency is reduced because of inadequate drug delivery pressure. Because a precise fit is required for optimal drug delivery, a system that links balloon inflation (i.e., apposition) with drug infusion has limitations.

The coupling of inflation and drug delivery also limits the size and configuration of perforations within the balloon. Large perforations require a high flow rate to achieve significant inflation pressure. Perforated balloons are not well suited for lesion dilatations for the same reason. Furthermore, perforated balloons cannot be used multiple times because during balloon deflation blood elements are entrained into the balloon; additional inflations would deliver a mixture of blood elements and agent into the arterial wall. The difficulties encountered with the perforated balloon have led investigators to evaluate different designs.

The optimal conditions for drug delivery are not yet defined. Investigators studying the basic pharmacokinetics of intramural drug delivery require a system that decouples apposition from drug delivery conditions. These needs have led us and others to design drug delivery catheters that allow independent control of apposition and drug delivery.

Infusion Sleeve

To define the optimal conditions for drug delivery, we have developed a system that dissociates apposition from drug delivery.[28] The Infusion Sleeve (LocalMed, Palo Alto, CA) is a multilumen catheter consisting of a proximal infusion port, a proximal hub, a main catheter shaft, and a distal infusion region with multiple side holes. The catheter has a central lumen for a dilatation catheter and guidewire access, as well as four separate outer lumens for drug delivery. Side holes in each of the drug delivery lumens are located within the infusion region near the distal tip of the Infusion Sleeve. Radiopaque markers are also located in each drug delivery lumen within the infusion region. The agent travels through the proximal infusion port and the outer infusion lumens and exits via side holes (nine 40μm diameter holes per drug delivery lumen). The Infusion Sleeve is designed to track over standard dilatation balloon catheters. During drug delivery the Infusion Sleeve is aligned with the underlying balloon. The Infusion Sleeve has been designed to provide independent control of the apposition of the drug delivery elements against the arterial wall (determined by the inflation pressure of the underlying PTCA balloon) and delivery of agent into the arterial wall (determined by the infusion pressure of the drug delivery elements) (Table 39–1, Figure 39–1).

The Infusion Sleeve is used clinically in the following manner. Before the procedure it is loaded onto a standard balloon dilatation catheter of the operator's choice. PTCA is performed in the usual fashion with the Infusion Sleeve in the guide. After angioplasty the Infusion Sleeve is advanced over the dilatation catheter, aligning the infusion region of the Infusion Sleeve with the balloon of the PTCA catheter. Drug delivery is then performed under specific apposition and infusion conditions. After drug delivery the Infusion Sleeve can be retracted, allowing the unsheathed PTCA balloon to perform additional angioplasty, or the Infusion Sleeve/PTCA balloon catheter assembly can simply be removed.

The Infusion Sleeve has been evaluated in various preclinical, in vitro, and in vivo models. The ability to deliver marker agent (horseradish peroxidase) via the Infusion Sleeve was evaluated in a porcine explanted heart model. Agent transfer was found to be a function of delivery pressure and apposition conditions. At optimal conditions (proximal pressure 100psi, delivery time less than 30 seconds), transmural and adventitial staining was demonstrated without disruption of the arterial architecture.[29] The effect of locally delivered heparin via the Infusion Sleeve on platelet thrombus formation was evaluated in an in vivo porcine carotid overstretch model. Local delivery of heparin (50 or 100 units/kg) reduced platelet thrombus formation by 57%, an effect that was sustained for at least 12 hours.

Clinical evaluation of the Infusion Sleeve was begun in the spring of 1994 at the Red Cross Hospital in Frankfurt.[30] The initial safety of the catheter was demonstrated in a series ($n = 95$) performed at Red Cross Hospital in Frankfurt and the Instituto di Cardiologico in Milan. Bartorelli and colleagues evaluated local delivery of heparin prior to stent placement in elective patients with a 6-month angiographic follow-up.[31] The InfusaSleeve was successfully tracked, and heparin was delivered in 94% of patients. Stent placement was successful in all cases. Ten dissections were observed after PTCA and prior to heparin delivery. Of these, seven remained unchanged, two worsened, and one improved with local heparin infusion. A 6-month clinical follow-up was available for all 33 patients; 30 patients had no symptoms and a negative exercise treadmill test. Angiographic restenosis (at least 50% stenosis) was observed in 4 of the 32 patients who underwent follow-up angiography. The impact of local heparin delivery prior to stent placement is being evaluated in an open labeled multicenter prospective randomized trial (Heparin Infusion Prior to Stenting, HIPS). One hundred seventy nine elective patients were randomized to receive Heparin (5000 U) via the infusion sleeve (5000 units Heparin delivered at 100psi with 2atm balloon support pressure) or by intracoronary infusion prior to placement of a Palmasz-Schatz Stent. Six month angiographic and intravascular ultrasound (IVUS) follow-up failed to demonstrate a significant impact on restenosis. Restenosis is to be measured by intravascular ultrasonography performed at approximately 6 months. The recruitment phase ($n = 179$) of this study was completed during the summer of 1997.[32]

The local PAMI study evaluated local heparin delivery during acute infarct angioplasty in a prospective multicenter 120-patient series.[33] Angioplasty was performed using standard techniques after which heparin (4000 units) was delivered; 25% of patients received stents. Procedural success was reported in 98% of patients; 6.7% of patients suffered death, reinfarction, recurrrent ischemia, or stroke during the index hospitalization. The 6-month target vessel revascularization rate was 12.5%. Local heparin therapy with provisional stenting is thus feasible, may eliminate the need for systemic heparin, and is associated with a low rate of infarct artery revascularization at 6 months.

Channel Balloon Catheter

The Channel Balloon Catheter (Boston Scientific, Boston, MA) is a dual-purpose angioplasty/drug delivery catheter composed of a standard angioplasty balloon surrounded by 24 drug delivery channels, each with a single 250-μm hole. Angioplasty can be performed by inflating the inner balloon without inflating the drug delivery channels. When drug delivery is desired, the drug delivery channels are pressurized while the inner balloon is inflated (Figure 39–2, Table 39–1).[34]

Delivery of horseradish peroxidase via the Channel Balloon Catheter demonstrated areas of full-thickness delivery without disruption of the media in an acute in vivo rabbit iliac model. Quantitative assessment of agent delivery via the Channel Balloon Catheter was evaluated with iodine 125 (^{125}I)-insulin in the same model, demonstrating a 40-fold increase in agent at 30 minutes compared with that in control vessels.[35] Functional evaluation of the Channel Balloon Catheter was performed in a porcine model measuring platelet deposition on Dacron graft material. Conditioning of Dacron graft material with heparin (500 units) via the Channel Balloon Catheter before perfusion reduced platelet deposition by approximately 70%, an effect that was sustained for 100 minutes.[34] The Channel Balloon Catheter has been used to evaluate the delivery of adenoviral vectors in rabbits and other models.[1]

Dispatch Catheter Coiled Balloon

The Dispatch Catheter (Scimed Life Systems, Maple Grove, MN) was designed to provide prolonged bathing of an isolated arterial segment simultaneously with perfusion. This system is an over-the-wire nondilatory system with a helical balloon that spirals around a urethane sheath. Inflation brings the helical

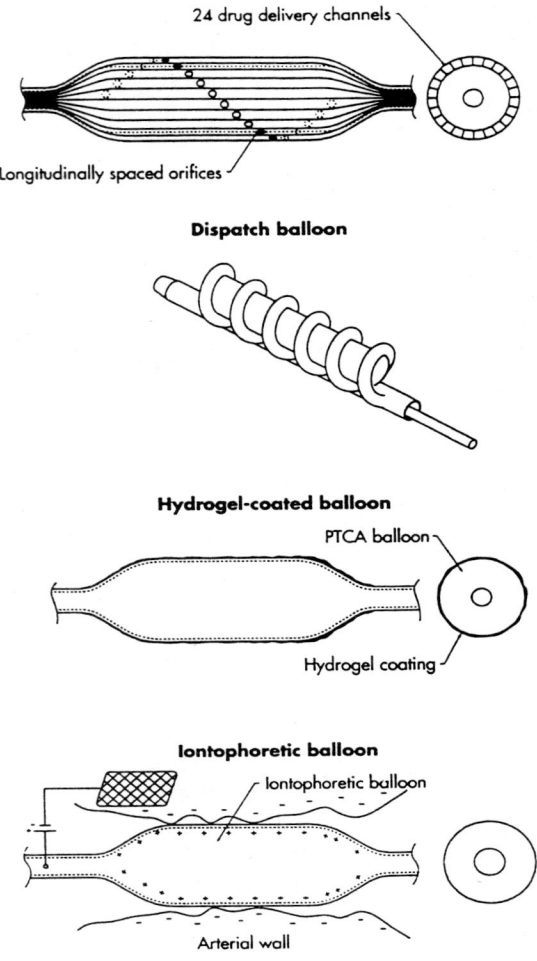

FIGURE 39–2. Local drug delivery systems currently under development: channel balloon, dispatch balloon, hydrogel-coated balloon, and iontophoretic balloon. See text for descriptions of the construction and use of each device.

balloon against the arterial wall while expanding the central urethane sheath, allowing perfusion. Agent is infused through the spaces between the coils (Table 39–1, Figure 39–2).

Using a radiolabeling technique, the kinetics of heparin delivery were studied in a porcine model. In this model, immediate heparin transfer was modest, with an efficiency of 0.04% to 0.08%. Most of the agent delivered to the arterial wall was washed out at 30 minutes (67% to 88%) with 7% to 8% of agent still in the arterial segment at 24 hours. The effect of heparin transfer to the arterial wall via the Dispatch Catheter on thrombus formation was evaluated using radiolabeled platelets. No reduction in platelet deposition was observed at 1 hour.[36] Urokinase transfer via the Dispatch Catheter was studied in a similar model by the same group. The efficiency of transfer was increased (about 1.2%), with 99% washout by 5 hours. The effect of the delivery in an in vitro clot lysis model demonstrated a beneficial effect of urokinase delivery when compared with appropriate controls.[37]

Initial clinical evaluation of the Dispatch Catheter has focused primarily on feasibility. The Hartford group reported on their initial clinical experience in patients with angiographic thrombus ($n = 14$). Patients were treated with 150,000 units of urokinase administered over 30 minutes. The procedure was well tolerated, with angiographic evidence of improvement.[37,38] These investigators pointed out the limitations of the Dispatch Catheter, which included significant ischemia resulting from side-branch obstruction and inadequate distention of the urethane sheath in arteries of small diameter and partially dilated large arteries. Finally, the 30 minutes required for delivery may be too cumbersome in a busy catheterization laboratory. Evaluation of the clinical benefit of treatment is ongoing.

Hydrogel-Coated Balloon Catheter

Hydrogels are interlaced crosslinked polyacrylic acid (PAA) chains that were developed initially as lubricious coatings. When exposed to an aqueous environment, the PAA swells to approximately three times its initial volume in a stable complex. Investigators have taken advantage of this property for the purpose of drug delivery.[39,40] Hydrogel-coated balloons are dipped into solution containing agent. As the hydrogel expands, water along with agent enters the interstices created by the PAA chains. The balloons are then dried, removing the water while leaving agent within the PAA material. When these balloons are subsequently exposed to an aqueous environment (i.e., blood), the hydrogel swells and agent leaves the balloon by diffusion. Drug delivery is performed by simply positioning the agent-coated balloon at the site of interest. As the balloon is inflated, agent is transferred to the arterial wall via "pressure-augmented" diffusion[41] (Table 39–1, Figure 39–2).

This approach has been evaluated in a variety of animal models and attempted in a small number of patients. Fram and colleagues[39] demonstrated the ability to transfer marker agent and fluorescinated heparin in vivo. They demonstrated agent transfer without gross disruption of the arterial wall. When marker agent (horseradish peroxidase) was delivered using this technique, delivery was relatively superficial and remained for only 90 minutes.

The ability of hydrogel balloon technology to deliver direct thrombin inhibitor PPACK was evaluated in a porcine shunt model. When Dacron grafts were treated with PPACK-loaded hydrogel-coated balloons, a significant reduction in platelet deposition was observed, which was sustained for at least 2 hours.[42] Rasheed and colleagues evaluated this method to perform gene transfer in a rabbit iliac model.[16] The Hartford group demonstrated the feasibility of using urokinase-impregnated hydrogel-coated balloons clinically in the setting of ischemic coronary syndromes.[43]

The ability to perform drug delivery by simply performing angioplasty with a specially coated balloon has tremendous appeal, but the technique has several important limitations. The amount of agent that can be loaded onto a balloon is limited to microgram quantities. Moreover, the agent is rapidly washed off the balloon, with more than 95% of it (heparin) removed within 7 seconds.[44] This has forced investigators to cover balloons with sheaths during the initial positioning of the device. When the remaining agent is delivered to the wall, only superficial portions of the artery receive agent. These limitations must be circumvented by advances in hydrogel technologies for this technology to gain acceptance.

Iontophoretic Balloon

The iontophoretic balloon (Cor Track Medical, Minneapolis, MN) employs low-level electric current to drive agent into the arterial wall.[45] The CorTrack catheter is a standard angioplasty balloon with a porous membrane containing an Ag-AgCl electrode. The 7F catheter shaft contains intake and output ports, a wire for the electrode, and a guidewire lumen. The catheter is positioned using standard over-the-wire technique and inflated to a low pressure (0.1 to 0.2 atm) to bring the porous membrane in contact with the arterial wall. Balloon inflation is maintained by recirculating infusate at a rate of 1 to 2 ml/min. During balloon inflation an electric field is generated between the balloon (cathode) and a skin patch (anode) (Table 39–1, Figure 39–2).

Fernando-Ortiz and colleagues reported their experience with the CorTrak catheter in delivering hirudin 125 in a porcine carotid model.[46] Drug was delivered via a small electric field (constant-current density of about 4 mA/cm^2) for 5 minutes. Arteries were harvested at different time points over a 2-hour period. Initial hirudin levels were approximately 80 times higher than in the controls. Tissue concentrations returned to background levels within 2 hours. Qualitative analysis by autoradiography demonstrated transmural delivery of agent.

The iontophoretic balloon is an interesting technology in the earliest stages of development. The appeal of the technology is that the underlying mechanism, iontophoresis, may be a "kinder and gentler" mechanism to deliver drug when compared with pressure-based delivery. Although this conclusion is intuitive, many questions remain. Because agent transfer is charge-dependent, specific drugs have different transfer efficiencies and may require manipulation to enhance their iontophoretic transfer. Also unknown is how atherosclerotic changes within the arterial wall affect agent transfer. Finally, if a transfer time of 5 minutes or more is required, perfusion capability must be added to the catheter. We look forward to the development of this technology.

Infiltrator Catheter

The infiltrator catheter (Interventional Technologies, San Diego, CA) is a novel drug-delivery catheter based on the Barath cutting balloon.[47] The cutting balloon consists of a noncompliant PTCA balloon, with three of four cutting blades arranged longitudinally along the surface of the balloon. When inflated, each blade protrudes about 0.010 inch. The purpose of these blades in the cutting balloon is to incise the arterial wall mechanically in an effort to perform PTCA in a more controlled manner. In a large randomized trial the cutting balloon was shown to be safe, though no benefit in regard to restenosis was observed.[48] The infiltrator balloon resembles the cutting balloon in that there are holes in the blades (injector ports). The injector ports are protected from the arterial wall during tracking by the folding pattern of the balloon. When the balloon is inflated, the injector ports are exposed and engage the arterial wall. Agent is then injected.

The infiltrator catheter has been used to evaluate the impact of locally delivered methylprednisolone acetate on restenosis in patients electively undergoing stent placement. Drug delivery was attempted in 24 patients in a total of 40 lesions. The drug delivery system was unsuccessful in tracking to the lesion site in 10% of cases. After drug delivery 46 stents were implanted (1.2 stents/lesion). Angiographic follow-up was obtained for all lesions in which drug delivery was performed. The angiographic restenosis rate (50% or more diameter stenosis) was observed in 40% of lesions; 44% of the lesions underwent repeat intervention.

Conclusion

The field of site-specific drug delivery is in its infancy. As new catheters become available, the challenge is to determine how to use them effectively for delivering agents, new and old, to address the clinical problems of restenosis and abrupt closure after angioplasty.

References

1. Van Belle E, et al: Successful percutaneous adenovirus-mediated gene transfer performed during stent implantation, *Circulation* 94(suppl 1):259, 1996.

2. Serruys PW, et al: A comparison of balloon-expandable-stent implantation with balloon angioplasty in patients with coronary artery disease, *N Engl J Med* 331:489–495, 1994.
3. Fischman DL, et al: A randomized comparison of coronary-stent placement and balloon angioplasty in the treatment of coronary artery disease, *N Engl J Med* 331:496–501, 1994.
4. Edelman ER, Karnovsky MJ: Contrasting effects of intermittent and continuous administration of heparin in experimental restenosis, *Circulation* 89:770–776, 1994.
5. TIMI Study Group: Comparison of invasive and conservative strategies after treatment with intravenous tissue plasminogen activator in acute myocardial infarction: results of the Thrombolysis in Myocardial Infarction (TIMI) trial, *N Engl J Med* 320:618–627, 1989.
6. Global Use of Strategies to Open Occluded Coronary Arteries (GUSTO) IIa Investigators: randomized trial of intravenous heparin versus recombinant hirudin for acute coronary syndromes, *Circulation* 90:1631–1637, 1994.
7. Ellis SG, et al: Coronary morphologic and clinical determinants of procedural outcome with angioplasty for multivessel coronary disease, *Circulation* 82:1193–1202, 1990.
8. Lincoff AM, et al: Sustained local drug delivery by a novel intravascular eluting stent to prevent restenosis in the porcine coronary artery [abstract], *J Am Coll Cardiol* 23:18A, 1994.
9. Wolinsky H, Thung SN: Use of a perforated balloon catheter to deliver concentrated heparin into the wall of the normal canine artery, *J Am Coll Cardiol* 15:475–481, 1990.
10. Leung W-H, et al: Local delivery of an antithrombin agent by an infusion balloon catheter reduces platelet deposition at the site of balloon angioplasty, *Coronary Artery Dis* 2:699–706, 1991.
11. Kaplan AV, et al: Local infusion of the thrombin inhibitor Argatroban reduces platelet thrombus formation at the site of angioplasty [abstract], *Circulation* 84(suppl II):727, 1991.
12. Shi Y, et al: Transcatheter delivery of c-myc antisense oligomers reduces neointimal formation in porcine model of coronary artery balloon injury, *Circulation* 90:944–951, 1994.
13. Muller DWM, et al: Intramural methotrexate therapy for the prevention of neointimal thickening after balloon angioplasty, *J Am Coll Cardiol* 20:460–466, 1992.
14. Gimple LW, et al: Effect of "in situ" heparin delivery by a porous balloon catheter on restenosis following balloon angioplasty [abstract], *J Am Coll Cardiol* 19:169A, 1992.
15. Santolan EC, et al: Use of a porous infusion balloon in swine coronary arteries: low pressure minimizes arterial damage [abstract], *Circulation* 84(suppl II):591, 1991.
16. Rasheed Q, et al: Local intramural drug delivery using an infusion balloon following angioplasty in normal and atherosclerotic vessels, *Cathet Cardiovasc Diagn* 31:240–245, 1994.
17. Plante S, et al: Porous balloon catheters for local delivery: assessment of vascular damage in a rabbit iliac angioplasty model, *J Am Coll Cardiol* 24:820–824, 1994.
18. Stadius ML, Collins C, Kernoff R: Local infusion balloon angioplasty to obviate restenosis compared with conventional balloon angioplasty in an experimental model of atherosclerosis, *Am Heart J* 126:47–56, 1993.
19. Gellman J, et al: Evaluation of a local infusion catheter for simultaneous balloon angioplasty and vessel wall infusion [abstract], *Circ Res* 38:492A, 1990.
20. Wolinsky H: Local delivery: let's keep our eyes on the wall, *J Am Coll Cardiol* 24:825–827, 1994.
21. Lincoff AM, et al: Efficiency of solute transfer by a microporous balloon catheter in the porcine coronary model of arterial injury [abstract], *J Am Coll Cardiol* 23:18A, 1994.
22. Wilensky RL, et al: The biostent trial: a randomized, double-blind, prospective, multi-center trial evaluating the safety and tolerability of locally delivered cytochlasin B in prophylaxis of angioplasty restenosis, *Circulation* 96(suppl I):650, 1997.
23. Bassand JP, et al: Update: interim results of the IMPRESS randomized trial. In: *Proceedings of the local drug delivery meeting and cardiovascular course on radiation and molecular strategies*, February 1998, p 58.
24. Hong MK, et al: A dual-purpose angioplasty-drug infusion catheter for the treatment of intragraft thrombus, *Cathet Cardiovasc Diagn* 32:193–195, 1994.
25. Cumberland DC, et al: Initial clinical experience of local drug delivery via a porous balloon during percutaneous coronary angioplasty [abstract], *J Am Coll Cardiol* 23:891A, 1994.
26. Deutsch E, et al: Favorable impact of intramural low molecular weight heparin delivered at the time of coronary stent deployment on late loss in de novo lesions, *Circulation* 96(suppl I):650, 1997.

27. Kutryk MJB, et al: Feasibility of the local delivery of antisense oligonucleotide against c-myc for the prevention of in-stent restenosis: acute results of the Thoraxcentra ITALICS trial, *Eur Heart J* 18:507, 1997.
28. Kaplan AV: Infusion sleeve catheter, *Semin Intervent Cardiol* 1:36–38, 1996.
29. Kaplan AV, et al: Intramural delivery of marker agent in ex vivo and in vivo models using a novel drug delivery sleeve [abstract], *J Am Coll Cardiol* 23:187A, 1994.
30. Kaplan AV, et al: Heparin delivery at the site of angioplasty with a novel drug delivery sleeve: initial clinical series [abstract], *J Am Coll Cardiol* 25:286a, 1995.
31. Bartorelli AL, et al: Local heparin delivery prior to coronary stent implantation: acute and six-month clinical and angiographic results, *Cathet Cardiovasc Diagn* 42:1–8, 1997.
32. Wilensky R, et al: The heparin infusion prior to stenting trial (HIPS): safety data and initial results of a randomized, prospective trial evaluating the efficacy of locally delivered heparin in reducing in-stent restenosis [abstract], *Circulation* 96(suppl I):710, 1997.
33. Esente P, et al: Acute and subactue stent thrombosis treated with local heparin therapy, Submitted.
34. Thomas CN, et al: Local delivery of heparin with a PTCA infusion balloon inhibits platelet-dependent thrombosis [abstract], *J Am Coll Cardiol* 23:4A, 1994.
35. Hong MK, et al: A new PTCA balloon catheter, with intramural channels for local delivery of drugs at low pressure [abstract], *Circulation* 86(suppl I):380, 1992.
36. Fram DB, et al: Local heparin delivery in porcine coronary arteries with the Dispatch Catheter: delivery, washout and effect on platelet deposition following balloon angioplasty [abstract], *Circulation* 90(suppl I):493, 1994.
37. Mitchell JF, et al: Enhanced intracoronary thrombolysis using the Dispatch Catheter [abstract], *Circulation* 90(suppl I):493, 1994.
38. McKay RG, et al: Treatment of intracoronary thrombus with local urokinase infusion using a new site-specific drug delivery system: the Dispatch Catheter, *Cathet Cardiovasc Diagn* 33:181–188, 1994.
39. Fram DB, et al: Localized intramural drug delivery during balloon angioplasty using hydrogel-coated balloons and pressure-augmented diffusion, *J Am Coll Cardiol* 23:1570–1577, 1994.
40. Riessen R, et al: Arterial gene transfer using pure DNA applied directly to a hydrogel-coated angioplasty balloon, *Hum Gene Ther* 4:749–758, 1993.
41. Riessen R, Isner JM: Prospects for site-specific delivery of pharmacologic and molecular therapies, *J Am Coll Cardiol* 23:1234–1244, 1994.
42. Nunes GL, et al: Local delivery of a synthetic antithrombin with a hydrogel-coated angioplasty balloon catheter inhibits platelet-dependent thrombosis, *J Am Coll Cardiol* 23:1578–1583, 1994.
43. Mitchell JF, et al: Local, intracoronary thrombolysis using urokinase-coated hydrogel balloons [abstract], *Circulation* 90(suppl I):493, 1994.
44. Azrin MA, et al: Local delivery of heparin on hydrogel-coated balloons decreases vessel wall cellular proliferation following balloon angioplasty [abstract], *Circulation* 88(suppl I):310, 1993.
45. Welsh RG, et al: Iontophoretic drug delivery system, *Semin Intervent Cardiol* 1:40–42, 1996.
46. Fernando-Ortiz A, et al: A new approach for local intravascular drug delivery: iontophoretic balloon, *Circulation* 89:1518–1522, 1994.
47. Barath P, et al: Nipple balloon catheter, *Semin Intervent Cardiol* 1:43, 1996.
48. Reimers B, et al: Persistent high restenosis after local delivery of long acting steroids prior to coronary stent implantation, *Circulation* 96(suppl I):710, 1997.

40
Management of the Percutaneous Access Site

James W. Vetter

In the first edition of this textbook, I discussed overall management of the percutaneous access site. Since that chapter was written, a great deal has changed in endovascular procedures. Rather than restate aspects that have remained the same (e.g., the importance of care and precision when accomplishing a correctly placed sheath), it is more useful to provide an update on the advances in devices, techniques, and strategies that have been developed. It is also useful to resummarize some of the most important principles and techniques that remain unchanged. Because most of the advances involve the Perclose procedure and the ways in which it can be used to permit new diagnostic and interventional strategies, more space is devoted to these devices. There is an obvious bias toward the Perclose devices because their use allows the widest choice of interventional strategies, and they offer the most secure method of access site management. The use of Perclose devices is growing rapidly worldwide, so there is also a section in this chapter dedicated to the practical use of the devices. In particular, the discussion is directed toward new strategies for endovascular procedures.

Introduction

For any procedure, including surgical endovascular intervention and invasive diagnostic procedures, the most important aspect is to minimize patient risk by securely controlling all phases of the procedure, including the site of access and the method for its management. Being able to provide predictably secure surgical closure percutaneously should be the goal of any vascular access site management device or method.

At this point, it is important to make a distinction between the various methods available for this purpose, as it is apparent that confusion exists with respect to the various closure devices. The Perclose device is, at this juncture, the only percutaneous suture-based device among those available. It mechanically draws the edges of the puncture together for secure surgical closure. Thus it achieves its goal using only needles and sutures, without excess material such as collagen or other anchoring devices, thereby requiring no additional follow-up procedures once correctly accomplished. Unfortunately, the closure devices are often mistakenly lumped together as being one and the same. This may lead to erroneous conclusions with regard to the various devices' relative efficacy, capabilities, and potential complications, all of which are different depending on the mechanism utilized by each device. The collagen devices differ in that they do not close the puncture hole per se; rather, they promote local thrombus formation at the site by leaving behind collagen on the outside and, with one of the devices, an absorbable anchor inside the vessel.

Goals of Access Site Management

Ideally, the peripheral interventionist can gain direct, straightforward access to a target lesion no matter where it is located (without having to circumnavigate the aortoiliac junction, for example). It would be ideal to be able to use any sheath size, any level of anticoagulation, or indeed any pharmacologic regimen desired to treat target lesions optimally. It would also be desirable to allow unimpeded outflow and inflow immediately after the procedure. Further more, it would be of additional benefit to allow immediate ambulation regardless of the above factors and to avoid the need for general anesthesia. Finally, immediate reaccess to the same site should be permissible. The only two methods that permit all of the above while providing secure closure are the Perclose device repair method and direct open surgical vascular repair. Other currently available methods, including various fibrin glues, balloons, manual pressure, compression clamps, flexible sheaths, and collagen devices, fall short in one or more of these areas as summarized in Table 40–1.

Alternatives

Perclose Device

The Perclose procedure, in contrast to all other closure procedures including collagen devices, can be thought of as percutaneous surgical repair—possible at the bedside and with only a small skin incision. Proper use of the Perclose devices permits complete control over the arterial (and venous) access sites. Having immediate and secure control over these cannulation sites, regardless of sheath size, level of anticoagulation, or desire for immediate ambulation, allows broader thinking. In fact, the peripheral interventionist is limited only by biases based perhaps on experience with less secure ways of closing the access site. Endovascular diagnostic and interventional procedure strategies can in fact be changed in several ways.

The interventionist can, for example, use retrograde cannulation or antegrade cannulation, or both, in the same groin and at the same sitting if desired. In another example, the patient may have a diagnostic procedure in the morning and then an intervention through the same site at any time thereafter, whether that day or at a later time. Additional specific

TABLE 40–1. Advantages and Disadvantages of Various Management Methods

	Easy to use?	Approved for use by nonphysicians?	Will work for all sheath sizes?	Allow immediate ambulation?	Allow early repuncture?	Can be used at any level of anticoagulation?	Save cost?
Compression (manual or device)	No	Yes	Yes	No	No	Yes	No
Open surgical repair	No	No	Yes	Variable	No	Yes	No
Perclose	Yes	Yes	Yes	Yes	Yes	Yes	probably[†]
Collagen Devices	Yes	Yes	No	No	No	possibly[†]	probably[†]
Balloons, glues, and others	Possibly[*]	No	No	No	No	No	Possibly[†]

[*] Not fully tested
[†] Data is incomplete, but appears favorable.

examples of new or improved approaches made possible by use of the Perclose devices are outlined in a later section. However, several general statements can be made. Anticoagulation need not be interrupted or withheld. Flow through the vein or artery controlled using the Perclose device is not impeded, which is obviously an important advantage for maintaining brisk inflow and outflow. Immediate assessment of the site after the procedure is possible, after which ambulation is allowable. These and other advantages are made possible because Perclose is a percutaneous procedure that, once properly mastered, offers the same security as a direct *open* surgical repair. It can be performed by surgeons, surgical assistants, physician assistants, or specialized teams. It can be performed anywhere from the outpatient environment to the procedure laboratory in the hospital, or even at the bedside on the ward.

Other Devices and Methods

The currently available means to control bleeding at the access site include manual compression, collagen plugs, direct surgical closure, and percutaneous closure (the Perclose procedure discussed above). Only the last two result in mechanical closure by tissue edge apposition, and only these two (surgery and Perclose) reduce the caliber of the puncture site to result in secure, durable control of bleeding. Possible advantages of the collagen-based methods include a less expensive cost for materials and that they may be easier to learn to use initially. Their use in terms of overall patient management, however, is more complex—similar to simple manual compression—because of the initial restrictions they impose for endovascular intervention strategies and because of the reduced security during the postprocedure period. They also carry added restrictions against immediate or even early repuncture at the site,[1] which precludes any possibility of some of the more useful strategies recently developed that are discussed later in the chapter. Although the collagen devices may be simpler to learn to use initially and, thus may be appealing for some cases, such as simple diagnostic or limited interventional cases, their use imposes stricter limitations compared to use of the Perclose devices. Although the initial training for the Perclose devices may be more involved, once mastered the devices are easy to use quickly and routinely. The major advantage of the Perclose method over the collagen devices lies in the patient benefits of the more secure suture-based closure, ease and simplicity of pre- and postprocedure management, and the associated cost savings benefits made possible by the predictability of the result. The most interesting aspect of Perclose device use is in the strategic changes its use allows. Same-day discharge, same-hour discharge, multiple access procedures, popliteal artery closure, venous access closure, immediate recannulation and immediate ambulation, regardless of type of intervention, are some of the advantages for the interventionist. Of the currently available alternatives, the two fastest procedures are those that use the collagen devices and those with the Perclose devices. The difference between the two appears to be relatively insignificant with perhaps a slight advantage for one or the other based on sheath size, level of anticoagulation, and other factors. Both approaches are learnable by nonphysician personnel. There are few data with respect to some of the newer methods for closure, although there are ample data with respect to direct open surgical repair and manual compression. The surgical repair and compression methods are well known. Their limitations are also relatively obvious and familiar to interventionists. Therefore use of these methods is not discussed in detail.

Other less well known but emerging techniques and devices include thrombus accelerators, tissue glues of various kinds, clips, physical barrier applicators, and balloons, with or without energy sources for thrombus formation. The results with some of these methods are encouraging.

When considering the devices already available and those that are emerging, the interventionist should be careful to distinguish the devices that augment or are adjuncts to thrombus formation from those that durably, mechanically reduce or obliterate the vascular puncture or tear.

Nursing Care Considerations

Wound care monitoring for bleeding or loss of distal pulses and the time to ambulation and discharge are the major skilled nursing concerns. The alternative methods for management of the percutaneous access site vary with respect to no or minimal follow-up required with the Perclose devices to many hours of skilled nursing follow-through for manual compression. Follow-up for direct open surgical repair requires mainly wound care, as inflow and outflow are generally unimpeded for all practical purposes. The other methods fall somewhere between Perclose and manual compression. The collagen devices, for example, require less bed rest than compression; but because more late bleeds are likely, particularly when these devices are used after interventions with full anticoagulation, more skilled nursing observation is required for longer periods compared to that needed with the Perclose device.

Cost of Access Site Management

For a complete discussion on the economics of interventions, the reader is referred to Cohen et al.[2] Briefly, it is important to note that major cost savings can be realized by limiting access site complications and permitting optimum target site medications. These medications include not only antiplatelet drugs but also full, continuous anticoagulation and even thrombolytic therapy when necessary. Additionally, whenever conventional (large) sheaths can be used along with conventional femoral equipment, costs can be more easily controlled. The most controllable aspect for reducing health care costs for endovascular procedures is probably related to the length of the hospital stay. In this respect, any device, whether collagen plug or surgical closure, that reduces time to ambulation is likely to provide some benefit in reducing hospital costs. Overall, the Perclose device is the ideal method for potentially reducing costs more effectively than the other approaches given its advantages in security and predictability over the collagen devices and the lack of need for the operating room in the case of direct open surgical repair. The reduction in bed rest and skilled nursing time compared to manual compression is substantial and should lead to overall reduced health care costs.

Specific Endovascular Procedure Approaches

Popliteal Approach

In our experience, the popliteal approach (combined with Perclose closure of the popliteal access site) offers the best chance for successful treatment of superficial femoral artery chronic total occlusions as well as osteo/proximal superficial femoral artery lesions. It is simpler than the contralateral approach; and in the case of a long chronic total occlusion, it is more likely to be successful with less chance of perforation. The popliteal vessel can generally easily accommodate a sheath of 6F, 7F, or 8F and often even 9F for the larger arteries. Compression to close the access site is acceptable but much trickier to manage than with Perclose; and temporarily, at least, it impedes outflow. In contrast, using the Perclose device allows immediate restoration of full outflow; it also permits immediate ambulation.

Combined approaches including the antegrade, retrograde, bilateral groin approach, and combinations of the groin and popliteal approaches are likewise made possible using the Perclose device. In fact, using the Perclose devices the operator may combine two or more sites or the same location in two different directions (antegrade/retrograde cannulation). This is an advantage when treating an iliac and femoral lesion on the same side during the same procedure, for example. The technique obviates the need for the contralateral approach and thus permits more direct access to lesions that are often difficult to cross. The contralateral approach may likewise be awkward when using stiff or bulky equipment such as stents. The contralateral approach also generally necessitates the use of long equipment and the need for awkward exchanges over long lengths.

New strategies and specific case examples follow.

Case 1

Problem: Right iliac occlusion, right superficial femoral artery (SFA) stenosis.

Conventional approach: *Strategy A*: Dilate and then stent the iliac vessel and SFA from the contralateral side. *Strategy B*: Dilate and then stent the iliac vessel via the ipsilateral side, pull the sheath, then compress. Bring the patient back for antegrade cannulation for the SFA at a later date. DISADVANTAGES: *Strategy A*: The iliac lesion may be difficult to recanalize from the contralateral side because it is a total occlusion. *Strategy B*: It necessitates a staged procedure. Inflow is addressed, but the outflow problem remains until later. This may compromise the long-term result.

Perclose approach: *Strategy A*: Dilate/stent the iliac vessel using the preferred ipsilateral (retrograde) approach. Use Perclose to close the retrograde puncture; then, using an antegrade puncture, treat the SFA followed by Perclose of the antegrade puncture site. *Strategy B*: Popliteal approach. Treat both lesions. Use Perclose to close the popliteal access site, immediately restoring outflow.

Case 2

Problem: The patient enters the hospital having a mechanical mitral valve for which warfarin (Coumadin) is used. The patient or the referring physician neglected to stop the warfarin therapy. The patient is now in need of intervention.

Conventional approach: *Strategy A*: Reschedule the case for a time when the international normalized ratio (INR) is nearly normal or normal, at which time the patient can be started on heparin. The procedure can then be performed after which the heparin would be allowed to wear off, the sheath pulled, compression (or use of a collagen device to accelerate local thrombus) could be used followed by reinstitution of heparin and simultaneous reintroduction of warfarin. The heparin then can be discontinued when the INR is therapeutic. *Strategy B*: Use fresh frozen plasma or vitamin K, or a combination of these drugs; heparinize the patient; and repeat the steps above. DISADVANTAGES: Complicated and potentially treacherous patient management process.

Perclose approach: Congratulate the patient (referring physician) on a well managed INR and then perform the intended interventional procedure using the Perclose method to close the access site. Discharge the patient while still on warfarin, which has continued uninterrupted.

Case 3

Problem: The patient is transferred to the hospital after an acute myocardial infarction with sheaths already in place. He is fully anticoagulated, probably on a nitroglycerin or heparin (or both) drip.

Conventional approach: Give antibiotics. Change sheaths. Perform intervention. Stop the heparin; and when the activated clotting time is at an acceptable level, withdraw the sheath and apply compression or use one of the collagen devices. Continue antiplatelet medications and allow resumption of ambulation only after a long period of bed rest to ensure stability at the access site (this period maybe shortened by use of collagen devices). The patient may then be discharged when the coronary and the access site are stable.

Perclose approach: Give antibiotics and change the sheath. Perform the intervention and immediately close the access site with Perclose. Heparin may be continued, antiplatelet regimens begun, and some of the other newer pharmacologic regimens continued indefinitely or gradually tapered off as desired. The patient may be discharged as soon as the coronary situation (or peripheral target lesion) is stable.

Case 4

Problem: The patient comes to the hospital from a referring physician's office in the middle of the afternoon with a diagnosis of possible coronary artery or peripheral vascular disease.

Conventional approach: Proceed with cardiac or peripheral diagnostic studies that day but discharge late at night. *Alternative*: Keep the patient in the hospital until the next day or use one of the other approaches such as the radial approach. The patient may then be discharged later or on the second day.

Perclose approach: Proceed immediately with the diagnostic procedure using a conventional femoral approach, which can then be securely closed with the Perclose device. Allow the patient to return to the referring physician's office with the diagnostic studies, a full report, and recommendations in hand.

Summary

Cases such as those described above are perhaps overly dramatized. They do, however, appear frequently at busy interventional centers. Though every patient may not present the challenges outlined above, all patients, even those with simple and straightforward problems, can benefit from the Perclose approach. Perclose closure allows immediate restoration of downstream flow, the choice of any sheath size, and the choice of any pharmacologic regimen. Perhaps even more importantly, cases like the ones described above are often more difficult, and perhaps even impossible, to treat without the use of the Perclose devices. Retrograde recanalization attempts for opening totally occluded vessels are, in many cases, more likely to be successful than attempts using the antegrade approach (with the flow). This point may be particularly important in the case of the superficial femoral artery, common femoral artery, and iliac vessels. In these cases, use of a popliteal approach followed by Perclose of the site should be considered.

Ways to Take Advantage of the New Devices

Some of the revised thinking made possible by use of new devices is outlined in this section. The Perclose devices are used as examples because they allow the most flexibility with regard to patient management.

1. Consider ways in which the scheduling of cases may be affected by the ability to ambulate immediately and the same-day discharge of patients, both diagnostic and interventional.
2. Plan most cases, both diagnostic and interventional, as outpatient procedures.
3. Consider preanticoagulation/antiplatelet regimens.
4. Work with nursing and administrative personnel to maximize efficiency by changing clinical pathways.
5. Work with billing consultants/insurance carriers/HCFA (Medicare) to obtain advice on how to bill for these new procedures.
6. Consider simple single staging for procedures that in the past may have required a multistaged strategy.
7. Consider other, more efficient strategies made possible by immediate secure access site stabilization.

Using the Perclose system as an example, interventional cases may be performed at any time during the day; and in many cases patients may be discharged during that same day. Use of these devices allows patients to be returned to a short stay or ambulatory unit rather than a specialized area for intense nursing monitoring. Patients may be started on warfarin or simply continued on it if it was begun prior to the procedures. The endovascular procedure may be performed without interruption of anticoagulation.

Specific Aspects of the Perclose Devices

An alternative to direct vascular surgical repair in the operating room is percutaneous surgical closure using the Perclose devices. These devices have been developed in various sizes to close puncture sites ranging from 4F to 12F in size under any pharmacologic regimen. The device is exchanged for the interventional or diagnostic sheath. The Perclose device itself provides intraprocedure hemostasis by occluding the puncture orifice during its use by the operator. This obviates the need for external

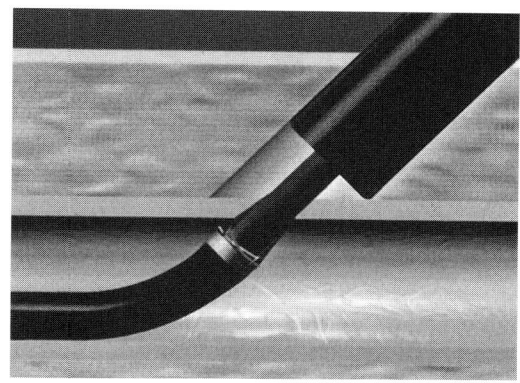

FIGURE 40–1. Correct position of the device prevents bleeding by occlusion of the puncture orifice. (See color plate)

compression during the closure procedure. It also eliminates the need for proximal and distal control of the vessel as would be required during open direct surgery. This feature allows the entire procedure to be performed by a single operator. The device is correctly positioned when indicated by marker tubes that signal when the needle tips are within the vessel lumen (Figure 40–1, see color plate). The needles then are withdrawn through the vessel wall (Figure 40–2, see color plate), puncturing it from the inside (Figure 40–3, see color plate). The device uses a pair of needles, or two pairs of needles, depending on the size of the device. Each pair of needles is attached to each end of a strand of a standard vascular suture. The needles are spaced to penetrate the vessel wall a precise distance from the edges of the puncture orifice; and as they are pushed through the vessel wall from the inside by the push rod mechanism, they draw the ends of the sutures with them (Figure 40–4, see color plate). They present the suture ends above the skin surface to the operator. The operator ties the ends of the sutures after removing the needles and slides the knot (of choice) to the vessel wall surface. If the device has two pairs of sutures, the process is repeated for the second suture. The device is then removed. While removing the device, the knots are further tightened, which results in complete obliteration of the puncture orifice by mechanical edge apposition (Figure 40–5, see color plate). The resulting hemostasis from orifice closure by mechanical approximation is obviously the same mechanism used by the vascular surgeon. The guidewire may be left in place until hemostasis is confirmed, after which the operator may remove it. This safety feature is important and allows access to the orifice if desired. The knots then may be further tightened before placing additional locking throws (in the case of the standard square knot but not required for other types of knots, such as the improved clinch knot).

Safety features and benefits of the Perclose device are several. Allowing the operator to maintain guidewire access until hemostasis is

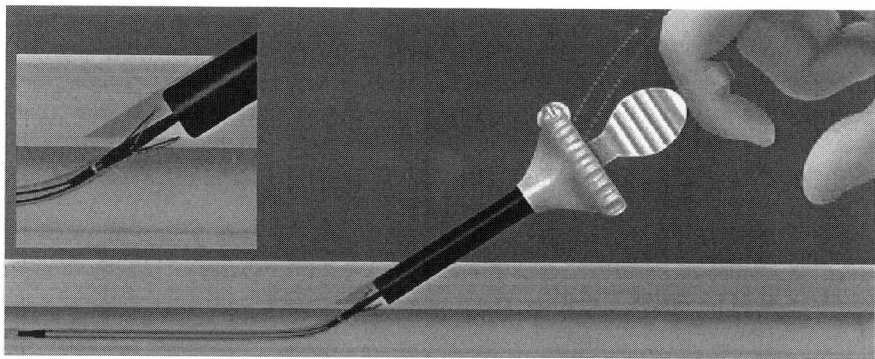

FIGURE 40–2. Confirm that the Interlocks are reengaged and correctly aligned with the locking indents in the hub. Then, unlock the pull handle (90° counterclockwise) and pull the needles fully back. Pull the first few millimeters very slowly. (See color plate)

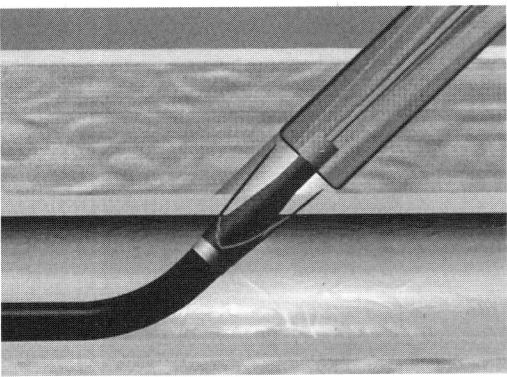 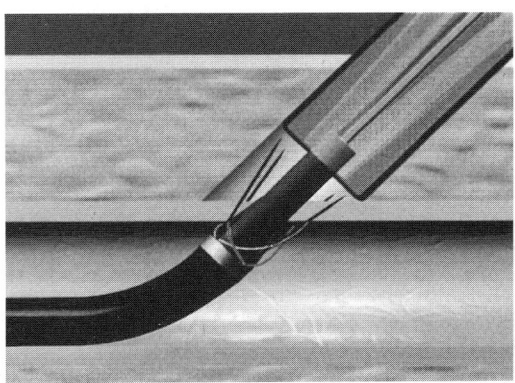

FIGURE 40–3. Backbleeding via the marker port confirms that needle tips will correctly puncture the arterial wall from within. (See color plate)

FIGURE 40–4. Needle tips carry sutures through the vascular wall. They also puncture the wall at a precisely controlled distance from the of orifice edge. (See color plate)

confirmed is an important safety advantage of the Perclose system over other methods, including external compression and the collagen devices. Once the interventional sheath is removed, the collagen devices, for example, provide no reliable means for reaccess to the puncture orifice. As with open surgery, the Perclose device may allow uninterrupted, full systemic anticoagulation. The amount of material left in place by direct surgical repair and by the Perclose devices is minimal (Figure 40–6, see color plate), and with both techniques repeat cannulation of the vessel is immediately possible. Again, this is an important advantage in the case of the potentially unstable patient. Immediate ambulation is allowable, and early hospital discharge is possible with the percutaneous surgical approach (Perclose). Patients have ambulated immediately while fully anticoagulated and can be allowed to stand to void in the catheterization laboratory immediately after an intervention.

Complications associated with use of the Perclose devices have been relatively few—similar or fewer than those associated with conventional methods. The device takes advantage of the long track record of favorable results with direct surgical vascular repair. The suture

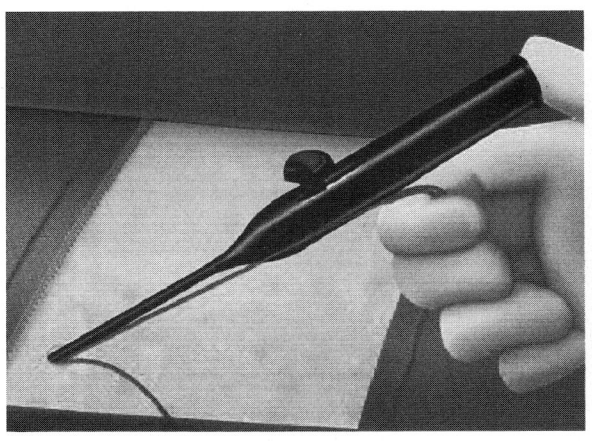 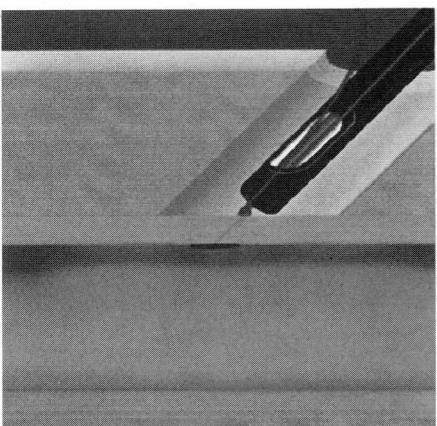

FIGURE 40–5. (A) To avoid an "air knot," apply tension to the suture while advancing the knot. (B) Tension must be applied to remove slack in the suture while advancing the knot. (See color plate)

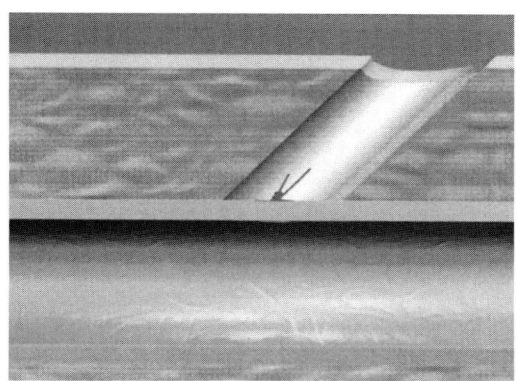

FIGURE 40–6. Completed knot resulting in secure closure of the vascular puncture orifice. The suture ends are trimmed close to the knot allowing minimal, residual material. (See color plate)

patterns and knots used for securing the sutures and the sutures themselves are familiar to vascular surgeons.

Of the alternatives, the Perclose devices appear to offer the most secure and useful management of the puncture site. These devices not only use the proven principles of needle/suture closure, they are also practical because they basically constitute a surgical repair that does not require a large skin incision. Whenever it is desirable to mechanically close the arteriotomy positively without regard to the level of anticoagulation,[3] sheath size, potential need for immediate repuncture of the artery, or hemodynamic considerations (hypertension), the Perclose method should be the method of choice.

Complications

Incidence and Etiology

Femoral artery access site complications, in order of frequency, have been hematoma, rebleeding, pseudoaneurysm, arteriovenous fistula (AVF), local and systemic infection, thrombosis of the access vessel, distal embolization, and neural palsy, as well as anemia from blood loss requiring transfusion. The most common direct cause of AVF formation is probably unintended cannulation of the profunda femoral artery or superficial femoral artery at a point where the vein and artery are more likely to overlap.[4] The most common causes of pseudoaneurysm formation are aggressive anticoagulation, inadequate compression, the use of large sheaths, and uncontrolled hypertension.[4] Access site bleeding complications may result from improper location of the initial puncture. This may lead to an inability to achieve hemostasis with manual external compression because of the lack of sufficient back support usually provided by the surrounding structures and femoral head, or by the enclosing common femoral artery and venous sheath.[4] When the site of cannulation is proximal to the inguinal ligament, effective compression is not possible and bleeding into the peritoneal cavity or retroperitoneal space may result. On the other hand, if the site is distal to the femoral head, again effective compression is generally not possible and the result may be a pseudoaneurysm or a bleed into the thigh. A too distal cannulation may also lead to formation of an AVF because the femoral vein and femoral artery overlie one another more commonly in this area. Other, newer methods to achieve hemostasis may not be as dependent on the site of cannulation, as they may achieve the results without the need for external compression. Common causes of complications also include uncontrolled hypertension, which may lead to insufficient compression, leaking or rebleeding after compression, aortic insufficiency with associated wide pulse pressure, insufficient length of compression time and limb immobilization time, excessive anticoagulation, antiplatelet or thrombolytic therapy, uncontrolled patient coughing, or straining for voiding or evacuation.

Ways to Avoid Complications

Proper placement of the cannulation puncture is an important way to avoid femoral complications such as hematoma and pseudoaneurysm. Use of external landmarks alone can be insufficient, particularly in the obese patient because of the imprecision inherent in deep punctures and the variability in the relationship between the femoral crease and the inguinal ligament.[4] Variability also exists in the relationship between the femoral crease and the femoral head as well as the common femoral artery bifurcation. The use of fluoroscopic landmarks has proved useful in this regard. The method advocated by Kim et al.[2] locates the distal (inferior) border of the femoral head[4] using fluoroscopy, marking it with a Kelly clamp or other radiopaque object; the next step is to penetrate the skin with the needle at that level, which generally results in the tip of the needle entering the common femoral artery (above the bifurcation in 95% of cases) in an area where the femoral head supporting structures provides sufficient backing forces to allow effective external compression.[4] Puncture of the femoral vessel off-center medially or laterally can also result in difficulty achieving effective hemostasis with external compression. Use of the "smart needle" Doppler-guided thin wall device may not only help avoid off-center punctures, it may help avoid the "double wall" or "back wall" puncture, another potential source of AVF hematoma, retroperitoneal bleed, or pseudoaneurysm formation. Knowledge of femoral artery anatomy and meticulous care by the operator is likely to result in fewer lateral or medial punctures and punctures of the "back wall." Efforts to limit complications by decreasing the size of catheters has been of either minimal benefit or no benefit thus far, despite earlier reports of increased complications with the use of large catheters, perhaps because of concomitant use of more aggressive anticoagulation regimens. Current methods of anticoagulation are evolving. It is generally agreed that levels of anticoagulation during interventions vary depending on the site and size of the target vessel. Large femoral or iliac intervention sites generally do not require aggressive anticoagulation during or after interventions, whereas in general coronary interventions are performed under aggressive anticoagulation using an activated clotting time (ACT) of 300 to 400 seconds. Greater ACT levels and use of thrombolytics in the acute myocardial infarction/percutaneous transluminal coronary angioplasty (PTCA) patient have been associated with a high degree of initial success (PAMI study). In an effort to decrease access site bleeding complications, postintervention anticoagulation regimens have been evolving, particularly after coronary stenting. Recently investigators have decreased ACT level requirements, particularly when using antiplatelet regimens such as Reapro. The results of attempts to rely on antiplatelet agents more and heparin less during the period after stenting to limit thrombosis appear favorable in terms of decreasing femoral access site bleeding complications. Determination of which lesions and vessels are candidates for such regimens is in the evolutionary phase. Concurrently, there is a trend among leading coronary intervention centers for more aggressive use of local delivery catheters, such as the Kaplan-Simpson Infusisleeve, and new, even more powerful antiplatelet agents in an effort to decrease thrombosis during the acute and subacute periods. Currently, in general, when the ACT has dropped to acceptable levels, the arterial and venous access sheaths are removed and external compression is applied for a variable time. The patient is then immobilized for several hours (on occasion, up to several days) depending on the level of anticoagulation and whether postprocedure anticoagulation is restarted. In the usual clinical scenario of the unstable patient or the patient with a less than ideal target vessel result, further anticoagulation is necessary. It is generally started approximately 4 hours after the sheaths are removed to permit time for local thrombus formation at the access site. Efforts to decrease the need for aggressive anticoagulation seem to help limit the complications associated with bleeding at the access site, although in some cases they have been associated with worse short-term results at the target artery treatment site, including sudden "subacute" thrombosis (target lesion site) and perhaps worse long-term results.[5]

Patients with acute myocardial infarction, unstable angina, hypercoagulable state, or suboptimal intervention site results, and those for whom certain procedures have been performed (e.g., rotablader, bail-out stent, bail-out directional atherectomy, and recanalization of total occlusions) are not candidates for reduced anticoagulation. Unfortunately, the optimal anticoagulation or antiplatelet regimens for the interventional site generally increases the likelihood of access site complications when manual compression or collagen devices are used for hemostasis. In this regard, direct open surgical access site repair or use of the percutaneous Perclose device has not been associated with increased complications despite high levels of anticoagulation.[3] These methods are the only two so far shown to be able to control access site bleeding during ideal anticoagulation and antiplatelet regimen treatment for the interventional site. Perhaps ongoing trials with the newer stents or use of local catheters such as the Kaplan-Simpson Infusisleeve (Local Med, Palo Alto, CA) to deposit high local heparin concentrations or concentrations of other more effective medications will prove to be useful in this regard.

Treatment of Access Site Complications

Surgical repair of femoral artery access site complications has a long established record of safety and efficacy but obviously is more invasive than other procedures. Other methods to treat pseudoaneurysms and AVFs have been used, including reclamping with one of the compression devices described previously.[6] This method has been gratifyingly effective for selected patients. The major impediment for this method includes the time and expertise required and local discomfort, which is often substantial, frequently exceeding the pain associated with the original compression. There is also the requisite period of further or repeat bed rest, making outpatient treatment less feasible. To be successful, the patient's discomfort must be aggressively managed with local anesthesia and usually some systemic analgesia as well. However, relief of discomfort associated with pseudoaneurysms after noninvasive treatment is highly welcomed by patients and may be an important marker for successful treatment. Hypertension must be controlled, and any coagulation abnormalities should be corrected if possible. Pseudoaneurysms in general are easier to treat successfully than AVF using this method.

Collagen devices have also been used alone, or with external compression, to treat pseudoaneurysms under two-dimensional ultrasound guidance. Ultrasonography is used to identify the abnormality and for correct placement of the collagen plugs to cause obliteration of flow between the artery and the pseudoaneurysm. It is also useful for guiding placement of external compression devices and to document success or failure with this method. Ultrasonography can be used as a screening tool to predict whether external compression or use of collagen plugs is likely to be successful by revealing the location, number, and size of the connecting passageway or passageways.[6,7]

Conclusion

Management of the access site has become recognized as a major challenge for the interventionist. Estimates place the number of interventional procedures alone to be well over one million worldwide, further placing in perspective the importance of successful access site management. Often interventional catheters and medications that are ideal for optimal interventional target site results cause more difficulty for management of the access site. Complications at the access site have been increasing, in contrast to the decrease in complications at the interventional target site. Reversal of the complication trend seems most promising with either direct open vascular surgical repair or percutaneous vascular surgical puncture site closure devices (Perclose). Likewise, complications may be reduced by using devices such as the newer stents and local delivery catheters, which may lessen the need for systemic anticoagulation regimens. Devices such as the Smart Needle (Doppler needle) and use of improved puncture techniques should also lessen complications. Once present, certain selected complications may be treated by less invasive techniques, such as recompression or insertion of collagen plugs. Finally, in the present political climate with attention focused on containment of health care costs, the use of devices such as the Perclose device should permit better utilization of hospital resources, increase patient comfort, and lower overall health care costs. These devices have been used to permit "preanticoagulation" or continuous anticoagulation with warfarin. The device may also make practical the aggressive use of antiplatelet regimens, such as ticlopidine, clopidogrel, abciximab, and others. These approaches could result in significant savings for the in-hospital costs associated with these beneficial procedures. The newer approaches to management of the access site should allow freer choices for both peripheral and coronary interventional procedures. At the same time the trend toward increasing access site complications should be reversible.

When making the decision about which device or method is to be used to assist in access site management, several properties of the method or device should be carefully considered. The device or method must have a high initial success rate for access site closure among the typical interventional or coronary patient population. If, on occasion, it fails to result in closure of a puncture, as an important safety feature it should have a means to provide reaccess to the puncture orifice. Complications related to the device should be rare; that is, the device should not introduce a new set of complications unique to its use. Even after successful puncture site closure, reaccess should be immediately allowable because of the need to reintroduce catheters quickly in cases where target vessel flow is compromised after an initially successful intervention. It must allow multiple reaccess using the same vessel over time; that is, it should not induce excessive scarring, which would make reaccess difficult. It should be secure enough to allow an aggressive anticoagulation and antiplatelet regimen so established and new regimens may be used freely to optimize the results, both short and long term, at the target lesion. It should be useful for a broad range of sheath sizes to accommodate imaging and therapeutic endovascular devices of many guiding catheter size requirements. Therapeutic equipment may then be based on choices ideal for treatment of the target lesion and optimal visualization with contrast. At this time, many compromises from the target vessel standpoint are reluctantly accepted to minimize groin complications by choosing smaller and smaller guiding catheters or inconvenient approaches such as the radial artery approach. Another characteristic of a new device should be the need for less or no groin monitoring by skilled nursing or physician-assistant personnel. The device should also permit early ambulation and hospital discharge. These benefits should together result in lowering hospital costs directly and should also lead to lower indirect costs by allowing more efficient use of resources and more efficient flow of patients through the interventional laboratory and post-laboratory units, resulting from greater flexibility in scheduling of cases, both diagnostic and therapeutic.

Finally, the device should be more comfortable for the patient than standard external compression devices. Patients often complain that the compression and associated required bed rest are the worst part of their treatment experience. In contrast, they often liken their experience with the Perclose device to "flying in first class." This improvement in patient comfort may reduce the need for narcotics and the use of vagolytic medications, which carry their own potential complications and undesirable side effects and result in the need for expert monitoring by professional staff.

When access site complications occur, they must be recognized early to permit appropriate therapy consisting of a period of close observation when spontaneous resolution seems likely, surgical repair when necessary, or use of compression with or without ultrasound guidance when appropriate.

References

1. Kensey KR: Puncture site hemostasis, *J Inv Cardiol* 6(8):273-276, 1994.
2. Cohen DJ, Breall JA, Ho KKL et al: Economics of elective coronary revascularization. Comparison of costs and charges for conventional angioplasty, directional atherectomy, stenting and bypass surgery, *J Am Coll Cardiol* 22(4):1052-1059, 1993.
3. Vetter JW, Ribero EE, Hinohara T et al: Suture-medicated percutaneous closure of femoral artery access sites in fully anticoagulated patients following coronary interventions, *Circulation* 90(4):901-921, 1994.

4. Kim D, Orron D et al: Role of superficial femoral artery puncture in the development of pseudoaneurysm and arteriovenous fistula complicating percutaneous transfemoral cardiac catheterization, *Cath Cardiovasc Diagn* 25:91–97.
5. Foley JB, Brown RI, Penn IM: Thrombosis and restenosis after stenting in failed angioplasty comparison with elective stenting, *Am Heart J* 128(1):12–20, 1994.
6. Felmeth BD, Roberts AC et al: Postangiographic femoral artery injuries: nonsurgical repair with US-guided compression, *Radiology* 178:671–675, 1991.
7. Cohen GI, Chan KL: Physical examination and echo Doppler study in the assessment of femoral arterial complications following cardiac catheterization, *Cath Cardiovasc Diagn* 21(3): 137–143, 1990.

Suggested Readings

Fischman DL, Leon MB, Baim DS et al: Stent restenosis study investigators, *N Engl J Med* 331(8):496–501, 1994.

George BS, Voorhees WD III, Roubin GS et al: Multicenter investigation of coronary stenting to treat acute or threatened closure after percutaneous transluminal coronary angioplasty: clinical and angiographic outcomes, *J Am Coll Cardiol* 22(1):135–143, 1993.

Grossman W, Baim D: Cardiac catheterization, angiography, and intervention, Lea & Febiger Fourth Edition, 1991.

Khoury M, Batra S, Berg R et al: Influence of arterial access sites and interventional procedures on vascular complications after cardiac catheterization, *Am J Surg* 164(3):205–209, 1992.

Kresowik TF, Khoury MD, Miller BV et al: A prospective study of the incidence and natural history of femoral vascular complications after percutaneous transluminal coronary angiography, *J Vasc Surg* 13:328–336, 1991.

Mackenzie DJ, Wagner WH, Kulber DA et al: Vascular complications of the intra-aortic balloon pump, *Am J Surg* 164(3):517–521, 1992.

McCann RL, Schwartz LB, Pieper KS: Vascular complications of cardiac catheterization, *J Vasc Surg* 14:375–381, 1991.

Muller DW, Shamir KJ, Ellis SG et al: Peripheral vascular complications after conventional and complex percutaneous coronary interventional procedures, *J Cardiol* 69:63–68, 1992.

Oweida SW, Roubin GS et al: Post catheterization vascular complications associated with percutaneous transluminal coronary angioplasty, *J Vasc Surg* 12:310–315, 1990.

Popma JJ, Satler LF, Pitchard AD et al: Vascular complications after balloon and new device angioplasty, *Circulation* 88:1569–1578, 1993.

Schatz RA, Baim DS, Leon M et al: Clinical experience with the Palmaz-Schatz coronary stent: initial results of a multicenter study, *Circulation* 83:148–161, 1991.

Semler HJ: Transfemoral catheterization: mechanical vs. manual control of bleeding, *Radiology* 154:234–235, 1985.

Serruys PW, de Jaegere P, Kiemeneij F et al: Benestent study group, *N Engl J Med* 331(8):489–495, 1994.

Skillman JJ, Kim D, Baim DS: Vascular complications of percutaneous femoral cardiac interventions: incidence and operative repair, *Arch Surg* 123: 1207–1212, 1988.

Sridhar et al: Reduction in peripheral vascular complications after coronary stenting by the use of a pneumatic vascular compression device, *Circulation* 90(4), 1994 (abstract).

Vetter JW, Hinohara T, Ribeiro EE et al: Percutaneous vascular surgery: suture-mediated percutaneous closure of femoral artery access site following coronary intervention, *J Am Coll Cardiol* Special Issue: 10A, 1005.

41
Endovascular Chemotherapy Delivery

Dat Nguyen and Stanley R. Klein

The earliest account of a substance used as an antineoplastic agent in humans was by Adair and Bagg in 1931.[1] This first substance was dichloroethylsulfide, a sulfur mustard. It was locally applied as a vesicant to eradicate malignant tumors. Both sulfur and nitrogen mustard were heavily investigated under military secrecy during World War II as potential chemical-warfare agents.[2] One of the most important observations by Gilman and Phillips was the destruction or shrinkage of lymphoid tissues shortly after administration of a "toxic dose of nitrogen mustard."[2] With wide availability of nitrogen mustards to civilian investigators in 1946, many physicians found them to be therapeutically useful in palliative treatment of lymphomas and leukemia but with significant local and systemic toxic effects.[3] Administration of nitrogen mustard into peripheral veins was noted to produce an intense local inflammatory reaction, causing pain and frequently resulting in thrombosis and occlusion. Significant systemic toxic effects, particularly on the gastrointestinal tract and hemopoietic system, were also noted.

Subsequent to the early experiences with chemotherapy, many ingenious ways have been devised to reduce local or systemic adverse effects of antineoplastic drugs. These usually involve one or both of the following general principles: (1) reducing regional venous exposure to high concentrations of a caustic drug by administration into a high-flow region of the venous system and (2) reducing systemic exposure by direct delivery of the drug to the target organ. The history and description of each technique is discussed in the following sections.

Central venous delivery of chemotherapeutic agents obviates many delivery system-related adverse sequela, but a suitable catheter, technique of insertion, and methodology were not known until the early 1950s. Since Sir Christopher Wren accessed a peripheral vein with a pointed-end cannula made from a goose quill in 1656,[4] many investigators had tried to cannulate the central venous system of animals and humans.[5] The most notable attempt was in 1929 by Forssmann, a urologist who introduced a ureteric catheter via his right antecubital vein, advanced into the right side of his heart, and climbed several stairs to the x-ray department to document his achievement. He proposed this route as the most rapid and effective way to deliver cardiac drugs to patients in sudden cardiac arrest and as good access to sample central venous blood. However, there was little interest in central venous cannulation until 1936, when in situ cardiac research blossomed. Furthermore, blood-compatible plastics were discovered in 1932,[6] and most of the catheterization for cardiovascular study was accomplished by insertion of the cannula via direct peripheral vein or arterial exposure. After the availability of plastic catheters, techniques of percutaneous insertion over a guidewire were described by Seldinger in 1952.[7] Later the same year, Aubainac introduced the approach for insertion of a catheter into the subclavian vein.[8] Four years later, Keeri-Szántó advocated this technique further by describing in detail the constant anatomic landmarks for the infraclavicular subclavian puncture.[9] Because the risk for pneumothorax was substantial with the initial application of this technique, the supraclavicular approach for insertion of a subclavian venous catheter was introduced by Yoffa in 1965.[10] The objective of eliminating the risk of pneumothorax was not accomplished. In 1966, percutaneous insertion of a central venous catheter via an internal jugular vein was described by Hermosura, again to avoid pneumothorax.[11]

Indar demonstrated that the complication of venous thrombosis was related in part to the material used for catheter manufacture (polyethylene).[12] After the discovery by Scribner that silicone rubber was relatively inert and could be used for temporary renovascular access with reduction of vascular thrombosis,[13] Steward took advantage of the inert property of silicone rubber and used it for catheter manufacture in 1961.[14] Although improvements were made in the technique of insertion and catheter biomaterial availability, the safety of long-term central venous catheterization was not known until 1968, when Dudrick reported his result of chronic hyperalimentation via central venous catheter.[15] Of note was the significant incidence of catheter-related infection and thrombosis, resulting in the recommendation that central venous catheterization be used only on an inpatient basis. In 1973, Broviac introduced a silicone rubber catheter with a felt cuff and reported a reduction of catheter-related infection and venous thrombosis.[16] Because of its narrow lumen, however, there was a significant incidence of occlusion. In 1979, Hickman modified the implantable catheter by enlarging the inner diameter.[17] Neiderhuber introduced a totally implantable injection port attached to a silicone catheter in 1982 with the objectives of further reducing the incidence of catheter-related infection, improved cosmesis, and patient inconvenience.[18] Currently, adjuvant steps (e.g., heparin and antibiotic binding) in catheter construction and refinement in placement technique (e.g., peripherally introduced central venous access) have made the durability of outpatient long-term central venous cannulation, a necessity for chemotherapy delivery, a reality.

An alternative vascular access with high flow is that created by arteriovenous shunt via a fistula or synthetic graft. Before the wide availability of the Silastic central venous catheter, long-term indirect or direct central venous access was not feasible for chemotherapy. Repeated intermittent peripheral catheterization, especially for chemotherapy, usually resulted in occlusion and eventuated in open methods for continued access. In contrast, with a peripheral arteriovenous fistula (AVF), drug concentration is reduced and thus sclerotic injury is minimized. The enlarged vein, resulting from the creation of the AVF, facilitates repeat venous accesses with ease. In 1974, Steckler reported the use of an AVF for chemotherapy treatment of leukemia patients.[19] Few others subsequently reported such uses.[20,21] The enthusiasm for this form of vascular access waned as the catheter-based technology improved and multiple caveats associated with fistula creation were appreciated.[20,21]

Arterial infusion of regional chemotherapy for cancer treatment was intially introduced in 1950 by Klopp after an accidental administration of nitrogen mustard into the brachial artery of a patient with Hodgkin's disease.[22] Klopp subsequently treated 10 patients with a variety of tumors by arterial infusion of chemotherapy. His results demonstrated significant tumor shrinkage with local arterial chemotherapy infusion in contrast to historical controls treated with systemic infusion. Kinetics of infusion (constant vs. bolus, multiple vs. single agent) became increasingly important.[23] As more drugs were added to the antineoplastic arsenal, prolonged arterial infusion techniques were extended to tumors in many regions of the body including primary and metastatic liver tumor, pelvic tumor, and extremity tumor.[23–26] The infusion was initially accomplished using a portable external pump, and the patient usually required hospitalization. The inconveniences associated with an external pump were eliminated by the introduction of the implantable infusion port developed in the early 1980s.[18,27]

Regional perfusion was designed to further reduce the systemic toxicity of chemotherapy associated with arterial infusion. With vascular isolation of the involved anatomic region, the venous outflow is shunted from systemic circulation to an extracorporeal circuit, where it is oxygenated and returned to the arterial supply of the tumor. This vascular exclusion permits the usage of high-dose chemotherapeutic agents without significant systemic toxic effects. This approach, however, was not possible until the availability of a mechanical heart-lung apparatus in 1953.[28] The first isolation perfusion of chemotherapy, reported by Creech in 1958, was used for treatment of a variety of extremity tumors.[29] Additionally, there have been occasional reports of complete remission of various tumors in patients who had high fever resulting from infection after attempted surgical extirpation. The effect of heat in combination with chemotherapy was investigated and found to significantly increase the cytotoxic effect of chemotherapeutic drugs.[30] Subsequently, isolation perfusion was modified to include sustained regional hyperthermia by extracorporeal circulation.[30,31] With the development of better catheters and a slight modification of the technique, the pelvic circulation can be excluded, and thus unresectable pelvic cancer can be treated with hyperthermic regional perfusion.[32,33]

Arterial ligation was originally conceived by Markowitz in 1952 to eradicate isolated hepatic neoplasms without the need for chemotherapy or surgical resection.[34] With the advance of catheterization techniques, the arterial supplies of various organs can be reached, and embolization of specific branches has been used since 1973 to destroy malignant masses.[35–39] Embolization and arterial occlusion are most frequently applied in the treatment of hepatic tumors, especially unresectable ones.[37–39] Initially, embolic materials were made of autologous clot, subcutaneous tissue, muscle, or Gelfoam. However, more recently, emboli often contain antineoplastic agents and are found to be more effective on hepatic tumor than emboli alone.[38,39] The combination of chemoembolization and radiation has been proposed for preoperative elimination of cancer cells before liver transplantation as a method for treatment of unresectable hepatic cancers.[40]

Vascular access devices and techniques have evolved rapidly since the discovery of the first antineoplastic agent. Whether the access is venous or arterial, the main objective of the evolution has been to increase the efficiency of drug delivery to the tumor, to increase the toxicity of the drug specifically to its target tumor cells, and to reduce the unwanted systemic effects of chemotherapy. The last two goals may be further improved by careful timing of drug administration with circadian rhythm, since there has been evidence that cancer cell proliferation, deoxyribonucleic acid (DNA) synthesis, bone marrow, and white blood cell activities are more affected at certain stages of the rhythm.[41–45] The drug delivery to targeted cancer cells may also be enhanced by tagging chemotherapeutic agents to tumor-specific antigen antibodies. Ultimately, cancer treatment may improve from further understanding of the genetic basis of cellular growth regulation.

Central Venous Catheter

Broviac introduced the first silicone rubber central venous catheter with a felt cuff, facilitating a zone of autogenous incorporation for chronic venous access.[46] Subsequently, there have been an increasing number of indwelling catheters of different sizes and types using the same principles. Variables to be considered include external hub or implantable port, number of lumens, catheter internal and external diameter, and biomaterial thrombogenicity. Furthermore, choosing a catheter must take into account the indication for catheter placement, patient-related variables such as available anatomic sites, and potential adverse cosmetic sequela or procedure-related complications. Placement of a catheter is associated with inherent complications such as pneumothorax or injury of the recipient vein or artery. The relative risk depends on the patient's body habitus, anatomic site, the approach or technique of insertion, and the surgeon's experience. An appropriately selected catheter in conjunction with an appropriately planned strategy of insertion should be formulated for each patient to minimize acute and long-term morbidity.

Catheter Selection

It is important that an appropriately sized catheter be chosen. Disturbance of laminar blood flow results from the placement of any intravascular device. An inappropriately large catheter may increase the risk of venous thrombosis by occluding the majority of the cross-sectional area of the recipient vessel.[47] The specifications of the catheter usually indicate the outer diameter in French gauge and the length in millimeters. Each millimeter is equivalent to 3.1416 (pi) Frech gauge (F). Single-lumen catheter sizes range from 2.7F to 9.6F. Double-lumen catheters are available from 7.0F to 12F. The largest catheter available is a 12.5F triple-lumen catheter. The selection of catheter size depends on the number of lumens required and the size of the vein used for insertion. Because there has been a good correlation between the incidence of catheter-related infection and the lumen number,[48,49] a single-lumen catheter should be the catheter of choice for long-term chemotherapy unless an extra lumen is needed for frequent blood drawing or simultaneous administration of medications.

In pediatric patients, special considerations are necessary. A 4F catheter can be safely placed into the subclavian vein or an internal jugular vein of an infant with a weight of 2 kg or more.[49] For an infant weighing less than 2 kg, a 3F Silastic catheter may be inserted via external jugular or great saphenous vein (GSV) cutdown.[50] Another way of estimating the size of an appropriate catheter is to reduce the French gauge in proportion to the length of the patient, assuming that the vein diameter is linearly correlated with the growth of the patient.[51] For example, an infant with the weight of 3.2 kg and length of 50 cm would need a catheter approximately three times smaller than that of an adult of 70 kg and 175 cm.

Catheter composition is also an important factor in minimizing postplacement thrombosis. Since the discovery of polyethylene in 1933,[52] many other biomaterials have been developed to reduce thrombogenicity and to provide more durability and flexibility to the catheter. The thrombogenicity of each catheter is related to inherent manufacturing material and the presence of any bonded compounds.[53-55] The relative thrombogenicity of commonly used composition materials, ranked from most to least problematic, include polyethylene, polyvinylchloride, polypropylene, fluorocarbons (tetrafluoroethylene or fluoroethylenepolypropylene), polyurethane, and silicone rubber.[53,56-59] Most of the commonly available catheters (e.g., Broviac, Hickman, Leonard, or Groshong) are made of silicone rubber. The risk of venous thrombosis associated with these were reported to be from 1.0% to 3.6%.[60,61] Raad et al. reported that there is a good correlation between the incidence of thrombosis and infectious complications.[62] Thus selection of the least thrombogenic catheter can also minimize risk of catheter-related infection.

Catheters of different designs and sizes are associated with different relative degrees of risk for morbidity. For example, as mentioned previously, a multilumen catheter is at higher risk for infectious complications than a single-lumen catheter.[48,49] The multilumen catheter is also more prone to accidental removal than a single-lumen catheter.[63] Similarly, catheters with external hubs (i.e., transcutaneous catheters) are associated with a higher rate of infection in pediatric patients than those with a subcutaneous implanted port.[64,65]

Acceptability by the patient is another important consideration in selecting a type of catheter. In contrast to external or transcutaneous catheters, subcutaneous implantation of a catheter port avoids an open skin wound and thus eliminates the need for frequent and vigilant dressing changes. Appropriate placement of the access under the skin must incorporate a low-profile design in conjunction with positions in skin crease or at the site of a binding garment. Finally, positioning the access device under skin in commonly exposed areas (e.g., neckline) should be avoided regardless of placement site. Because of the subcutaneous position, accessing the implantable port with a needle is typically associated with some degree of pain and anxiety.[64] Despite this fact, young patients tend to favor a catheter with a subcutaneous port over an unsightly external catheter.[66]

Cost of the catheter and its insertion must also be considered. A catheter with an implantable port is significantly more expensive than an external catheter.[67] However, routine care for external catheters, such as dressing change, frequent heparin flush, and nursing assistance, as well as treatment for catheter-related infection, may offset this initial cost difference. A prospective study found that the cost per day of use with an external catheter will exceed that of a catheter with an implanted port after 6 months.[67]

Approaches for Inserting Central Venous Catheters

A central venous catheter can be inserted into a number of named veins in different regions of the body. Common and less frequently considered options are depicted in Figure 41–1. The insertion procedure involves either a percutaneous Seldinger type of technique or a direct surgical exposure of the vein. In general, insertion through a large, central vein can be done percutaneously in adult patients. In contrast, insertion in pediatric patients most often will require a cutdown to expose the vein. The vein is generally chosen depending on its ease of accessibility, compatibility with catheter size, whether it may interfere with the patient's functional status, and the surgeon's familiarity with the proposed method of vascular access.

Specific approaches are associated with a higher risk for morbidity than others, depending on the vein, method of access (e.g., percutaneous vs. surgical exposure), and the surgeon's experience. Percutaneous catheterization via the subclavian vein is associated with 0% to 4.7% incidence of pneumothorax, which is approximately 20 times that associated with placement via the internal jugular vein.[68,69] However, the incidence of arterial puncture with the subclavian approach is about two to three times lower than with the internal jugular route (1.0% to 2.2%).[70–73] Although hemostasis is usually obtained after arterial puncture with

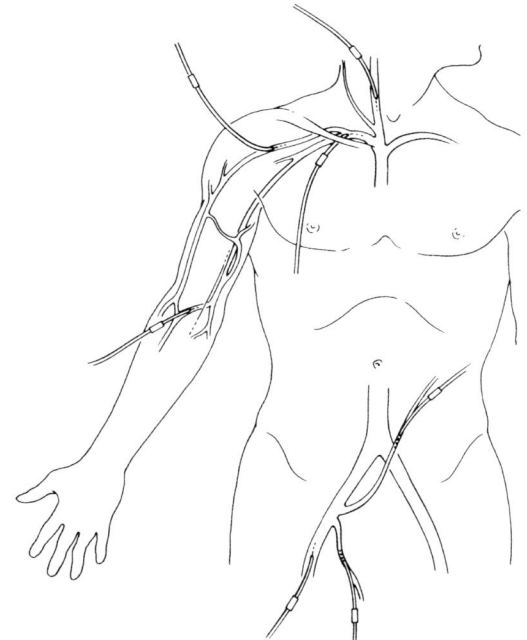

FIGURE 41–1. Sites for placement of a central venous catheter. Subclavian (SV), internal (IJV), and external jugular (EJV) veins are common access routes. Other less frequently used routes include cephalic (CV), femoral (CFV), great saphenous (GSV), and inferior epigastric (IEV) veins.

short periods of compression, complications may result from plaque embolization.[74] These problems associated with catheterization of the subclavian and internal jugular veins may be nearly obviated by inserting the catheter percutaneously or with open access of the external jugular or cephalic vein.[75,76]

Because of the presence of the large lymphatic channels in the thoracic outlet, injury may result from percutaneous catheterization of the right or left subclavian and internal jugular veins. Such injury is rare but may lead to a significant chylous collection.[77–80]

Placement of a chronic catheter into the femoral vein or GSV should be avoided if possible because it will interfere with ambulation. In addition, the potential risk of catheter-related thrombosis or infections may be greater in this difficult-to-manage area.

Percutaneous Techniques

As mentioned previously, percutaneous insertion of a central venous catheter is usually used for placement into large veins of large pediatric or adult patients. Frequently, these percutaneous techniques can be done safely under light sedation with local anesthetic in an outpatient procedure suite or an operating room and are facilitated with fluoroscopy. Subsequent to the catheter insertion and position verification followed by a brief period of postplacement observation, the device can be used for the intended purpose. It is important to provide the patient or party responsible for care of the catheter with appropriate instructions regarding management.

Infraclavicular Insertion into Subclavian Vein

The patient is placed in the supine position on the operating table, and light intravenous sedation is administered (Figure 41–2). The patient's shoulders are slightly hyperextended with a rolled towel positioned between the scapulas directly under the vertebral column. The hyperextended shoulders facilitate access into the subclavian vein. It is recommended that the ipsilateral jugular area also be included in the surgical field in case access into the subclavian vein is difficult.

Before beginning the procedure, the operator should verify that all necessary equipment is present and working. Appropriate patient monitoring should be maintained throughout the entire procedure. The sophistication of the monitoring that is required will depend on the status of the patient.

To begin the procedure, 1% lidocaine is infiltrated into the skin approximately 2 to 3 cm below the junction of the medial and middle third of the clavicle using a 25-gauge needle. Additional lidocaine is used to infiltrate the proposed subcutaneous tissue along the tract of the catheter toward the clavicle and the periosteum just below the clavicle. After the patient is placed in Trendelenburg's position to distend the subclavian vein, a 16-gauge needle connected to a 10-ml syringe is then inserted into the anesthetized skin at the junction of the medial and middle third of the clavicle. The needle is advanced horizontally toward the clavicle with the needle bevel directed upward to a point 1 to 2 cm cephalad to the sternal notch. It is essential that the operator advance the needle in a nearly horizontal plane when attempting to penetrate the vein so that inadvertent puncture of the pleura is reduced. When the clavicle is encountered by the tip of needle, the needle is withdrawn slightly and then readvanced until the tip of the needle is below the clavicle. Again, it is essential to maintain the needle parallel to the horizontal plane during this part of the procedure. At this point the needle should be advanced slowly with constant aspiration on the barrel of the syringe. The subclavian vein is usually entered within 5 to 6 cm. In the obese patient this distance might be greater. The bevel of the needle is then rotated 90° to maximize blood flow. The syringe is disconnected from the needle. It is important to cover the end of the needle when the syringe is disconnected to prevent air embolism. A flexible-tipped guidewire is then advanced into the vein via the needle. Approximately 15 cm of the guidewire can be advanced safely into the subclavian vein. If the wire is advanced too far (i.e., into the heart), cardiac arrhythmias may occur. The incidence of adverse cardiac events can be minimized by noting the wire position using fluoroscopy. Once the wire is in the appropriate position, the needle is removed from the vein. The puncture in the skin is widened with an 11 blade to facilitate catheter placement. At this point, the patient should be taken out of Trendelenburg's position for the remainder of the procedure.

A 1.0- to 1.5-cm skin incision is now made over a flat area of the chest that is best suited to help conceal the catheter beneath clothing (such as just above the nipple line at the lateral sternal border). Be sure to consider and avoid the neckline and breast in the female patient. Anesthetize the proposed tract with 1% lidocaine, and create a subcutaneous tunnel between two incisions using a tunneler. The catheter is then passed from the precordial incision to the infraclavicular incision by tying the end of the catheter to the end of the tunneler. The catheter is positioned such that the fabric cuff that helps to seal the catheter tract from

41. Endovascular Chemotherapy Delivery

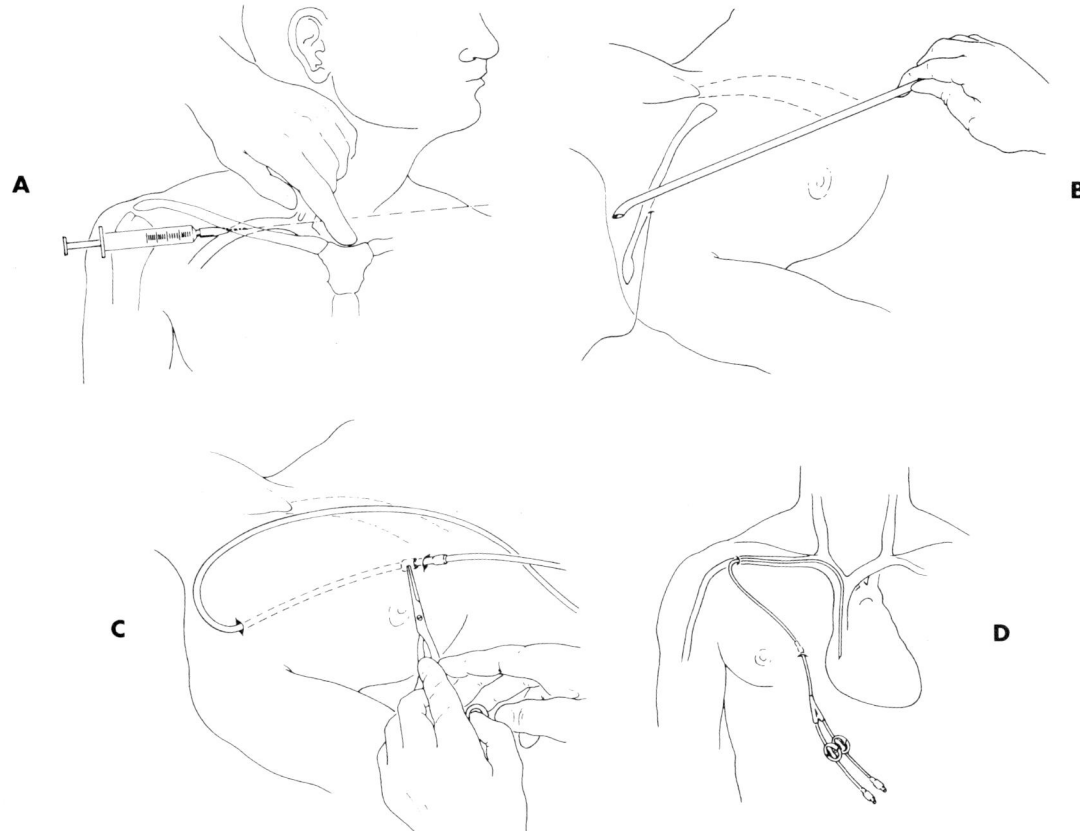

FIGURE 41–2. Infraclavicular technique of subclavian vein catheterization. Advancement of access needle is directed and should be horizontal and toward the opposite shoulder. After entering the vein, a guidewire is threaded into the vein. An appropriate-length catheter is selected and tunneled subcutaneously over the wire. Immediately after placement of the dilator and introducer sheath complex, the dilator is removed, and the catheter is inserted and advanced to the superior vena cava (SVC). The sheath is removed, and a chest x-ray is obtained to confirm position of catheter tip. The procedure is completed by tunneling a length of the proximal catheter beneath the subcutaneous tissues to allow incorporation of the catheter in a desirable position.

outside contamination is approximately 4 to 5 cm inside the subcutaneous tunnel.

The proximal end of the catheter is then tailored to length by placing it along a course that estimates the path of the subclavian and innominate veins and the superior vena cava (SVC). The catheter is cut at the right third costosternal junction. This point is usually correlated with the position of proximal SVC. The lumen(s) of the catheter is (are) then flushed with heparinized saline solution (10 IU/ml). An introducer sheath covering the tract dilator is inserted into the subclavian vein over the guidewire using cinefluoroscopy. If the dilator is inserted too far, perforation of the great veins is a possibility. For this reason, only insert the sheath-dilator complex into the subclavian vein and avoid more proximal advancement. The wire must be straightened by slowly and slightly withdrawing it to facilitate the insertion. This is done to prevent shearing of the dilator and the sheath by a kinked wire and to avoid subsequent laceration of the vein by a damaged dilator. After dilator and sheath placement the wire and the dilator are removed. The open end of the sheath should be covered with a finger to avoid air embolism. The tip of the catheter is inserted into the sheath, and the catheter is advanced through the vein. The sheath is then removed. The catheter may need to be held in place during the removal of the sheath.

The position of the catheter tip is documented with cinefluoroscopy. It should be at the junction of the SVC and right atrium. Blood is withdrawn from the catheter lumen, and the lumen is flushed with heparinized saline solution. If the tip's position is not appropriate, or if difficulty aspirating blood or flushing the catheter is encountered, the position must be adjusted. Examine the system carefully for inadvertent kinds using fluoroscopy with dye injection.

The infraclavicular incision is closed by 4-0 absorbable subcuticular stitches. The precordial skin incision is narrowed around the catheter using 4-0 nonabsorbable sutures before skin approximation. The catheter is temporarily anchored externally to the chest with a nylon suture until adequate incorporation of the subcutaneous fabric cuff has occurred. After both incisions are dressed, the patient is transferred to the recovery room. An upright chest x-ray is taken in the recovery room to exclude a pneumothorax or a hemothorax and to confirm the position of the catheter tip.

Insertion into Internal Jugular Vein

The patient is placed in supine position with the head rotated to the contralateral side (Figure 41–3). The heads of the sternocleidomastoid muscle are noted as the patient is instructed to turn the head toward the neutral position against light resistance. The neck and chest are prepped and draped as described for subclavian vein placement. The patient is then placed in Trendelenburg's position.

Lidocaine 1% is used to infiltrate the skin and subcutaneous tissue at the apex of the triangle where the two heads of sternocleidomastoid muscles converge. A 22-gauge needle connected to a syringe is inserted into the skin at this location. With a finger palpating the carotid artery, the needle attached to the syringe is advanced just lateral to the artery at 30° with respect to the horizontal plane. The caudal advancement of the needle should be parallel the sagittal plane. Constant aspiration of the barrel of the syringe should be performed throughout advancement of the needle. The internal jugular vein is usually entered within 2 to 3 cm of the skin. Once the needle is in the vein, the syringe is removed, leaving the needle in the lumen as a guide for insertion of the access needle. If pulsatile blood flow is noted, the carotid artery may have been entered instead of the jugular vein. The guide needle should be removed and pressure applied. The 22-gauge needle is then advanced in a more lateral position to identify the jugular vein. Once the vein is encountered with the 22-gauge needle, a 16-gauge access needle connected to a syringe is inserted and advanced in parallel to the 22-gauge needle. The position of the needle is secured with one finger covering the hub of the needle to prevent air embolism. A guidewire is threaded into the vein with its tip followed and positioned at the junction of the SVC and right atrium using cinefluoroscopy. Both needles are removed. The Trendelenburg's position is reversed. The puncture site of the access needle is enlarged to accommodate sheath and catheter insertion.

Insertion into Femoral Vein

The patient is placed in the supine position, and the groin and the lower abdominal wall are prepared in a sterile fashion (Figure 41–4). The skin and subcutaneous tissue just medial to the femoral artery pulse and 3 to 4 cm caudal to the inguinal ligament is infiltrated with 1% lidocaine. A 16-gauge access needle attached to a syringe is inserted into the anesthetized skin and advanced cephalad at 30° to 45° with respect to the horizontal plane. The femoral vein is usually entered 3 to 4 cm below the skin. The syringe is removed, and one finger is used to cover the hub of the needle. If no pulsatile blood flow is encountered, a guidewire is inserted into the vein through the needle. The needle is then removed from the vein, leaving the wire in place. The skin puncture is enlarged, and another 1.0- to 1.5-cm skin incision is made

41. Endovascular Chemotherapy Delivery

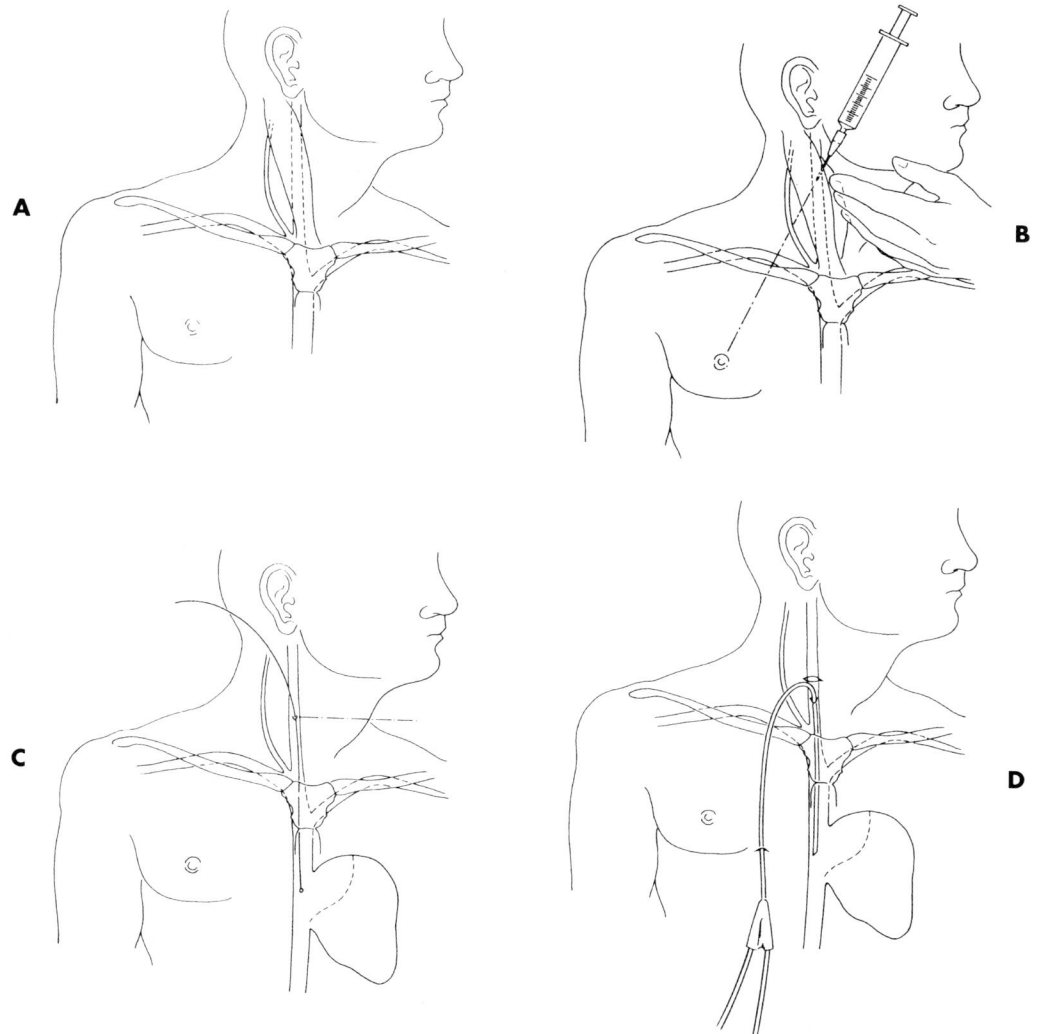

FIGURE 41-3. Internal jugular vein catheterization. With the patient's head turned to the contralateral side and the junction of the heads of the sternocleidomastoid muscle (SCM) are identified, a needle is inserted into the vein at a vertical angle of 30° to 45°. Once the vein is encountered, the remainder of the procedure is similar to that described for subclavian vein catheterization.

in the ipsilateral abdominal wall. This incision is usually created more lateral than the first incision so that a gentle curve can be created between the subcutaneous tunnel and the vein. The remaining portion of the procedure is similar to that described for the placement of catheters in thoracic veins. The catheter length is measured so that its tip will be in the inferior vena cava near the renal vein when it is fully inserted. Careful inspection of the insertion site must be maintained after catheter placement to avoid the risks of catheter displacement, bleeding, and infection in the groin.

Open Surgical ("Cutdown") Techniques

Open surgical exposure is primarily used for small-diameter vascular access. However, the approach is sometimes also used for catheterization of the internal jugular vein. The catheter

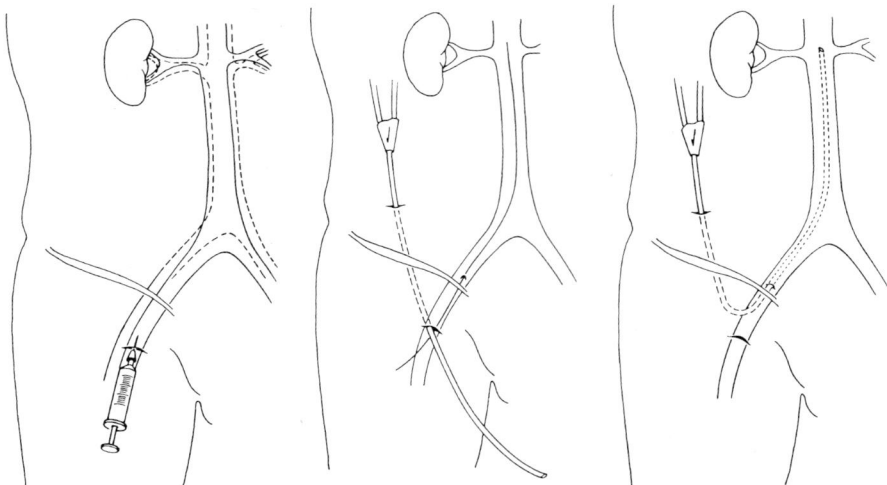

FIGURE 41-4. Femoral catheterization. With the patient in a supine position, the femoral vein is intubated approximately 3 to 4 cm inferior to the inguinal ligament and just medial to the femoral pulse. The catheter can be tunneled from a lower abdominal incision to be inserted into the femoral vein.

is inserted via a venotomy into smaller tributary veins without the need for a dilator or an introducing sheath. With the exception of the internal jugular vein, isolation of these veins from subcutaneous tissue can be performed easily when the cutaneous incision is appropriately placed. The length of the catheter is premeasured by matching the catheter along the course of the vein to the junction of the SVC and right atrium for superior venous system or to the junction of the inferior vena cava (IVC) and renal vein for inferior venous access. An x-ray is always taken after the procedure to confirm the position of the catheter tip. The advantage of the open technique is a lower risk of accidental injury to adjacent structures. This is particularly true for vascular access in pediatric patients. However, pediatric patients often require general anesthesia to obtain adequate sedation.

Open Internal Jugular Vein Access

Similar to percutaneous catheterization of the internal jugular vein, the junction of the two heads of sternocleidomastoid muscle are identified. The patient is placed in the supine position, and the head is turned to the side contralateral to the proposed catheter placement (Figure 41-5). The neck and chest areas are prepared in a sterile field. A 2.0-cm transverse skin incision is placed over the heads of the sternocleidomastoid muscle. The platysma is divided, and the two heads of the sternocleidomastoid are bluntly separated. The jugular vein is freed from the surrounding structures, and vascular tapes are placed around the vessel for proximal and distal control. Before making a venotomy, the catheter is tunneled subcutaneously from a precordial incision to the neck incision. The catheter is tailored to the appropriate length and passed into the vein through a small venotomy in the center of a 5-0 or 6-0 Prolene pursestring suture. After insertion, the catheter is advanced to the SVC. Fluoroscopy is used to confirm the position of the catheter tip. Lumen function is then checked by aspirating blood and flushing the catheter with heparinized solution (2 to 3 ml per lumen). The catheter may be advanced or withdrawn slightly to improve the position or to enhance flow through the lumen. The pursestring suture is tied, and the vascular tapes are then removed from the vein. The platysma is reapproximated, and the neck incision is closed in two layers. The precordial incision is narrowed around the

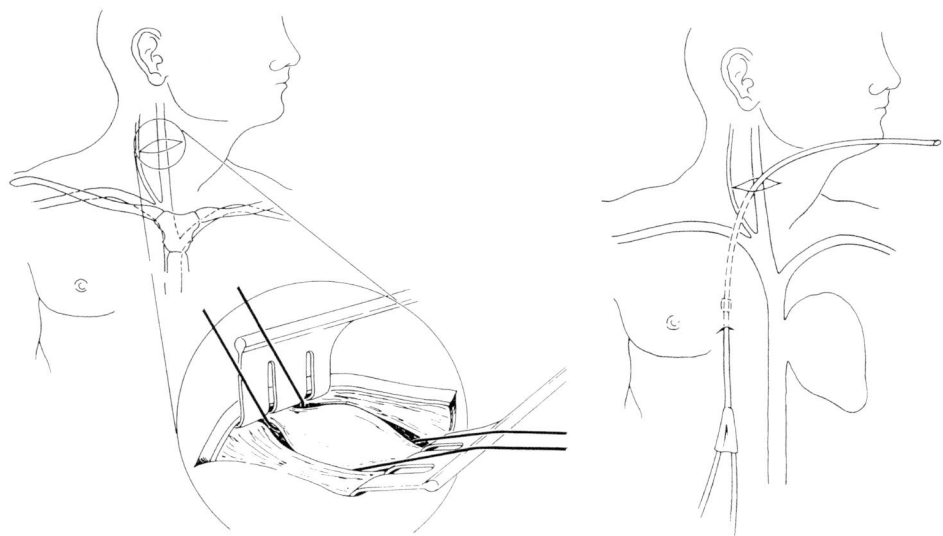

FIGURE 41-5. Direct surgical placement of an internal jugular vein catheter. Through a 2-cm transverse skin incision over the heads of the sternocleidomastoid muscle (SCM), the internal jugular vein (IJV) may be exposed after the platysma is divided and blunt dissection. After a venotomy is created in the middle of a 6-0 Prolene pursestring suture, the catheter is inserted and advanced into the SVC.

catheter with a single nylon suture. The catheter itself is anchored to the skin. After dressing the incisions, the catheter is also anchored to the chest with tape or an Op-Site plastic drape. An upright chest x-ray is taken in the recovery room to document the position of the catheter tip.

Open External Jugular Vein Access

The insertion of a catheter into the external jugular vein is very similar to the approach described for the internal jugular vein access (Figure 41-6). However, the superficial location of the external jugular vein permits a much easier and safer isolation than that of the internal jugular vein. Exposure of the external jugular vein is performed through a 1.0- to 1.5-cm transverse neck incision over the lateral head of the sternocleidomastoid muscle. After dividing the platysma, the vein is dissected free from the surrounding tissue and ligated distally. An appropriate-length catheter that has been tunneled subcutaneously is inserted into the vein through a venotomy. After confirming the position of the catheter tip in the proximal SVC using cinefluoroscopy, the proximal suture is snugly tied to coarctate the vein around the

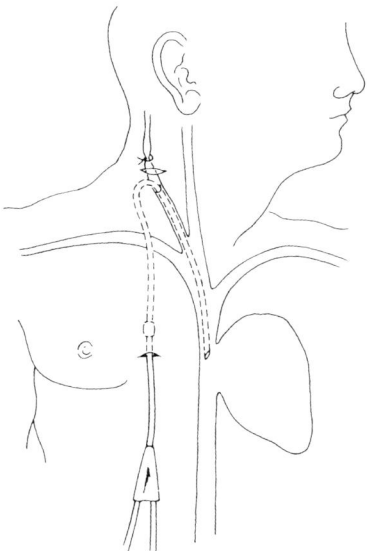

FIGURE 41-6. Open catheterization of the external jugular vein. The vein is exposed through a 1.5- to 2.0-cm skin incision approximately over the lateral head of the sternocleidomastoid. After ligation of the distal limb of the vein, venotomy is created and the catheter is subsequently advanced into the SVC.

catheter. The catheter lumen function is then tested by aspiration of blood and by flushing with heparin solution. The incisions are closed, and postplacement care is initiated as described for the internal jugular vein access.

Open Cephalic Vein Access

The ease of catheterization of the cephalic vein is similar to that of the external jugular vein (Figure 41–7). The cephalic vein can be readily isolated through a 1.0- to 1.5-cm diagonal skin incision across the deltopectoral groove. Careful blunt dissection of the subcutaneous fatty tissue will expose the vein. The distal limb of the exposed vein is then ligated with nonabsorbable suture, and the proximal vein is temporarily controlled with vascular loops. A venotomy is created in the isolated segment, and an appropriate length of catheter that has been turned subcutaneously is inserted into the cephalic vein and advanced to the proximal SVC. Because the cephalic vein joins the subclavian vein at an almost 90° angle, the catheter may persistently turn toward the peripheral vein during catheter advancement. Twisting the catheter while inserting under fluoroscopy may help to guide the tip toward the central venous system. Once the catheter is in place, function of the catheter lumen is assured and the catheter is secured in the vein by a proximal suture.

Open Saphenous Vein Access

In pediatric patients, occlusion of catheters frequently occurs because of the small diameter of access veins and devices. Although a potentially higher risk of infection is associated with catheters placed in the inguinal region, the GSV sometimes provides an alternative route for vascular access (Figure 41–8). The GSV can be readily exposed through a 2.0- to 2.5 cm transverse skin incision approximately 2.0 to 2.5 cm caudal to the inguinal ligament and 1 cm medial to the femoral artery. A combination of sharp and blunt dissection is used to expose the vein. Before catheter insertion, it should be tunneled subcutaneously from an ipsilateral lower

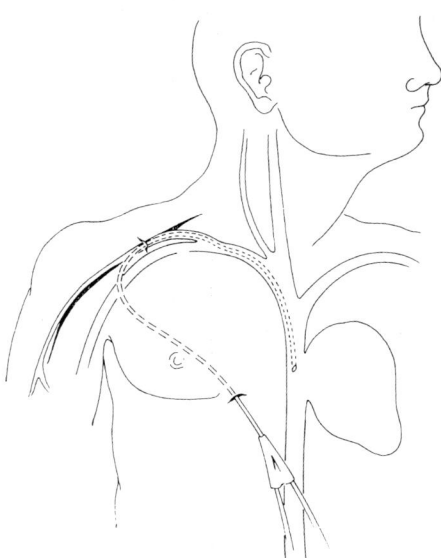

FIGURE 41–7. Direct catheterization of the cephalic vein. The vein is exposed through a 1.5- to 2.0-cm vertical skin incision over the deltopectoral groove. After creation of the venotomy, the catheter is inserted and advanced into the subclavian vein and subsequently into the SVC. Fluoroscopy may be used during catheter advancement to assist in directing the catheter at the junction of cephalic and subclavian veins.

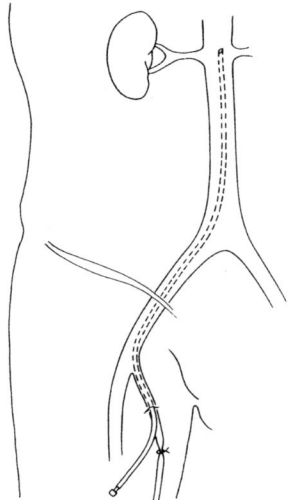

FIGURE 41–8. Catheterization of the great saphenous vein (GSV). In pediatric patients, exposure of the GSV is readily achieved through a small infrainguinal incision just medial to femoral pulse.

abdominal incision. After the vein is isolated, catheterization proceeds as described for other open access rates. Using cinefluoroscopy, the catheter tip should be positioned near the junction of the IVC and renal veins when completely inserted.

Infusion Port

An infusion port can be attached to any catheter system. To accommodate the port, a subcutaneous pocket is constructed in the plane between the subcutaneous fat and the muscle fascia at the precordial or abdominal incision for the thoracic outlet or inguinal approach, respectively. After attaching the catheter to the port, the entire system is flushed with heparin solution. Anchoring sutures are placed in the fascia and threaded through the base of the port. A subcutaneous tunnel is then created between the pocket and the skin incision where the vein is isolated. After pulling the catheter through the tunnel, the port is positioned into the pocket. The catheter is tailored to an appropriate length and inserted into the vein as previously described. The position of the catheter tip should be confirmed with fluoroscopy. A noncoring Huber needle connected to a syringe filled with heparinized saline is inserted into the port. The patency of the catheter-port system is verified by aspiration of blood and subsequent flushing of the system with heparinized saline. Once the patency of the system is confirmed, anchoring sutures are tied to secure the port to the base of the pocket. After the closing of skin incisions, the Huber needle is reinserted into the port to permit immediate chemotherapy treatment and to avoid difficulty in needle insertion at a later time resulting from postoperative edema. At the completion of the procedure, a postoperative upright chest x-ray is require to confirm the catheter tip position and to document the location of the port.

Peripheral Insertion of Central Venous Catheter

The concept of placing a central venous catheter via an antecubital vein began with Forssmann nearly 70 years ago.[5] Because of the relatively high incidence of catheter-related peripheral thrombophlebitis,[53-55] the concept never gained the popularity associated with a centrally placed catheter. With the recent development of less thrombogenic biomaterials, peripheral insertion of a central venous catheter (PICC) has been shown to be safe for long-term hyperalimentation and chemotherapy.[81-83] Its inherent freedom from dangerous acute complications such as pneumothorax and major vascular injury permits minimally trained health professionals to insert a PICC without the need for special equipment or facilities. Therefore PICCs can be readily inserted by trained nurses or primary care physicians with considerably less cost. The current emphasis on cost containment in health care has made PICC an attractive alternative to centrally placed catheters.

Despite the advantages of a PICC, it is not suitable for all patients requiring chronic vascular access. The peripheral veins of patients selected for PICC placement must be in satisfactory condition. However, many patients already have significantly narrowed or occluded veins as a consequence of prior multiple venous punctures and sclerotic reaction from intravenous infusion of chemotherapy. For these patients, a more central venous catheterization is more appropriate. Unfavorable venous anatomy occasionally misdirects the insertion of a PICC and consequently results in failure of a PICC placement. Using fluoroscopy in this situation provides guidance for catheter advancement and enhances successful placement. The reported incidence of insertion failure is approximately 3.8% to 24.0%.[83-90] With fluoroscopic guidance, the failure rate is reduced more than tenfold.[88] In general, PICC catheter placement is most suitable for patients with well-preserved peripheral veins and can be accomplished at the bedside in the hospital, in the clinic, or at home. However, the success rate of insertion is significantly augmented if the insertion is accomplished using cinefluoroscopic guidance.

PICC catheters are typically small catheters designed for small-diameter peripheral veins. Their sizes range from 1.2F to 5.0F. Typically, 2.6F or smaller catheters are used in pediatric patients. Most of the PICC catheters are single-lumen tubes, but double-lumen configurations are available. The small diameter of PICC lumens, especially in double-lumen catheters, significantly limits the rate of infusion. For this reason, a PICC catheter is more prone to occlusion than are central catheters.[15,91] PICC catheters have a reported occlusion frequency of 8.2% to 22.4%.[83,85,86,90,92-94] The higher rates of occlusion occur when a catheter is coupled to an implantable port. PICC catheters coupled to implantable ports are typically used for longer duration than those with external access ports. If occlusion rates are reported as the number of occlusions per day of use, the rate of occlusion for catheters with external and implantable ports is equivalent.

The incidence of catheter-related infection for PICC lines is reported at less than 5%.[92,95] This rate is typical for 2- to 3-week durations of catheter use. With longer use, infection rates may approach 16% (for use up to 12 weeks).[96] With implantable ports, Morris et al. and Winter et al. reported that the infection rate associated with long duration of catheter use is reduced.[85,86] They reported a 3% to 5% infection rate with 4 to 5 months' use.

Although PICC catheters may function up to 430 days,[86] the duration of use should be limited to shorter periods to avoid thrombophlebitis and infectious complications. With an implantable port, the frequency of infection is minimized by frequent heparin flushes by diminishing the likelihood of catheter thrombosis.

The technique of PICC catheter insertion/port implantation is as follows.

With the patients in the supine position, the nondominant arm is abducted to a position almost almost perpendicular to the trunk (Figure 41-9). After placing a deflated pressure cuff around the arm, the volar aspect of the forearm is exposed and the antecubital area and forearm are prepared in a sterile fashion. With the pressure cuff inflated to distend the peripheral veins, either the cephalic or the basilic vein can be catheterized using the Seldinger technique. Without a pressure cuff, an open surgical exposure under local anesthesia provides direct catheterization of the chosen vein. The catheter is tailored to the appropriate length using the third sternocostal junction as a landmark for the junction of the SVC and the right atrium. A subcutaneous pocket over the brachioradialis muscle may be created under local anesthesia if an implantable port is desired. The port should be attached to the catheter, positioned in the pocket, and anchored to the muscle fascia before cutting the catheter to the appropriate length. The catheter-port system should be flushed with heparinized saline before insertion. Although PICC catheter insertion may be accomplished without fluoroscopy, its utilization allows the operator to guide the catheter advancement in the appropriate direction and to confirm the position of the catheter tip on full insertion. After catheter insertion, the lumen function is then checked and the incision is closed. After completion of the insertion, an upright chest x-ray should be obtained to document the catheter tip position.

Arterial Perfusion

After a half-century of experience with systemic chemotherapy, it is now known that many malignancies such as leukemia, Hodgkin's lymphoma, choriocarcinoma, germ cell cancer, Wilms' tumor, and a few other types of cancer are curable.[97] However, the ultimate fate of the vast majority of patients with malignancy remains unchanged despite more sophisticated chemotherapeutic agents. One hypothesis for this limited scope of cure is that significant toxic effects of systemic chemotherapy may prohibit the administration of higher doses of antineoplastic agents to achieve the required therapeutic drug levels to destroy all cancer cells in the target organ. Although the absolute cytotoxic levels of many antineoplastic drugs in vivo are undetermined, the strategy used to achieve the goal of tumor eradication has been to modify the delivery process so as to increase local drug concentration within the tumor environment or to combine the chemotherapy with a second modality (e.g., radiation therapy).

Discovery of alternative modalities for chemotherapy delivery was serendipitous. With

41. Endovascular Chemotherapy Delivery

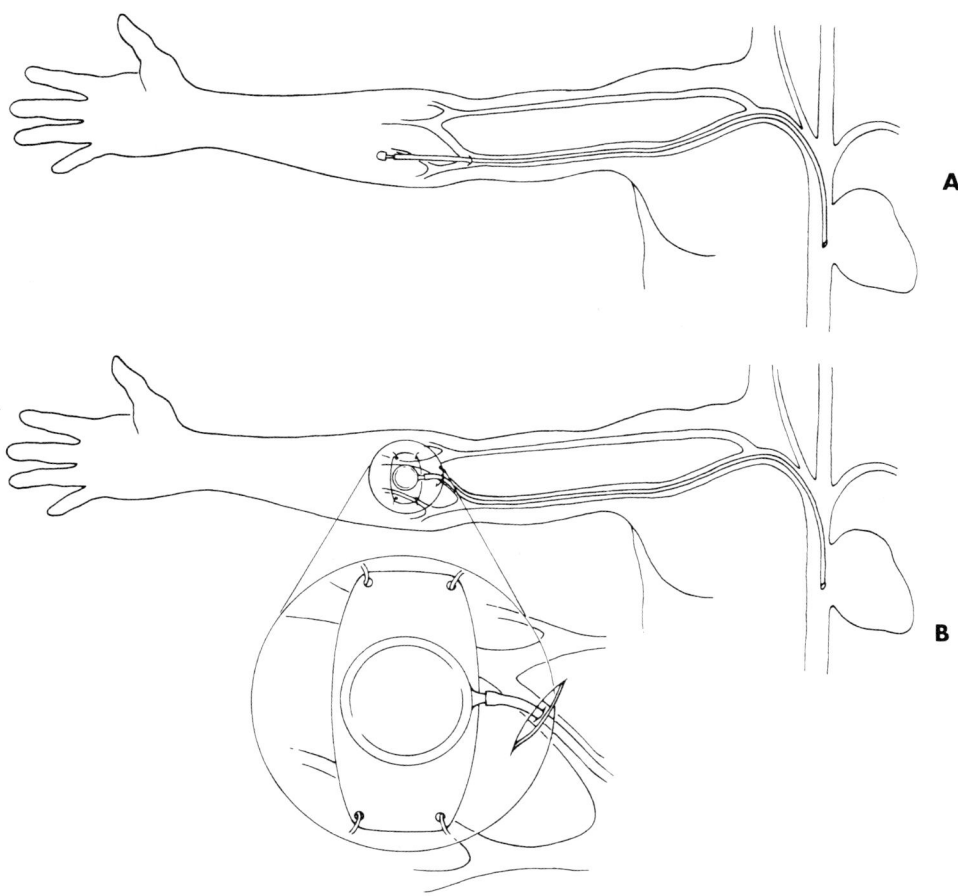

FIGURE 41–9. Peripherally inserted central venous catheter (PICC). **A**, Under local anesthesia, the antecubital vein can be easily accessed and used as a route for placement of a PICC catheter. **B**, A subcutaneous port may also be placed along with the PICC catheter.

very little knowledge of pharmacokinetic properties of antineoplastic agents and the cellular biology of tumor growth, Klopp et al. in 1950 observed the complete resolution of an intense local reaction in normal tissue of a patient's hand and forearm after an accidental brachial artery injection of nitrogen mustard.[22] He subsequently proposed that injection of nitrogen mustard into an artery supplying a tumor might serve as a technique for the treatment of primary head and neck cancers, brain tumors, and a variety of metastatic tumors. Klopp's results were variable, but in several instances there was complete disappearance of the tumor. In addition, less systemic toxicity was noted in conjunction with this technique than with systemic chemotherapy.

Subsequent to Klopp's first report, various techniques of arterial access and delivery have been developed to allow a wider application of intraarterial chemotherapy, to further enhance the therapeutic effect of chemotherapy, and to minimize systemic effects. Initially, intraarterial chemotherapy was possible only through a direct surgical catheterization of the artery supplying the target organ.[22] After the introduction of the Seldinger technique and the availability of improved angiographic capabilities in the mid-1950s, arterial accesses to many organs and regions were more accessible percutaneously via the groin or axilla.[98] The application of intraarterial chemotherapy has since been extended to cancer treatment in almost every region of the body. A variety of tumors have been treated using this mode of therapy. The list includes malignant gliomas, brain metastases, head and neck cancers, bronchogenic carcinoma, primary liver cancer, metastatic liver tumors, prostate cancer, extremity sarcomas, and recurrent malignant melanoma.[99–106]

After a wide clinical application of intraarterial chemotherapy, bolus injection of some antineoplastic agents such as methotrexate and 5-FU over a short duration was noted to be less effective than longer continuous administration in reducing the tumor mass.[23–26] Subsequently, intraarterial chemotherapy was continuously delivered using a large and fixed external pump, and thus patients often required prolonged hospitalization, up to 2 months.[23,24] After the development of a portable external pump, outpatient intraarterial chemotherapy became possible.[25,107] With the availability of an implantable infusion pump since 1979, this mode of delivery provides an attractive option for those requiring a long course of regional chemotherapy.[108]

Despite the local delivery of antineoplastic agents, significant systemic toxic effects are still reported with intraarterial chemotherapy. Bone marrow suppression occurred in 40% of the patients during the course of their treatment. In some cases, the patients' early demises were attributed directly to leukopenia or thrombocytopenia caused by intraarterial chemotherapy.[22] Consequently, the total amount and the concentration of antineoplastic agents delivered through intraarterial infusion are restricted. Theoretically, the toxic systemic effects could be reduced by concurrent administration of an antineoplastic agent and its antidote (such as methotrexate and citrovorum). However, Sullivan and Watkins showed that this combination technique was not significantly effective in reducing systemic toxic effects.[23,24] There was still an 11% to 60% incidence of hematologic toxic effect.

Along with the development of new anticancer agents, modifications have been added to the intraarterial technique to increase tumor exposure to agents and to minimize undesired side effects of chemotherapy. The first modification, isolation perfusion, was initially thought to be so radical that it has been designated a separate entity. In 1958, Creech et al. used a heart-lung pump with an oxygenator to completely isolate an extremity with a cancerous lesion for chemotherapy.[29] The goals of this technique were to allow treatment with "super" high concentrations of antineoplastic drugs in the target organ and to avoid the severe systemic toxic consequence. The details of the isolated perfusion technique are further discussed in the Isolated Perfusion section.

A continuous delivery of very concentrated anticancer drugs for a long period without such sophisticated isolation may exceed the allowable total body dosage and increases the risk for severe toxic effects and death. The therapeutic effect of bolus intraarterial infusion, on the other hand, is limited by the dilution of the agents resulting from high blood flow and consequently by the short exposure of the tumor bed to the agents. In 1979, Karakousis reported the application of a tourniquet around an extermity to occlude venous outflow and to reduce arterial inflow while the extremity was receiving arterial chemotherapy.[100] Through animal experimentation, he demonstrated much higher tissue drug levels with this technique than that achieved by arterial infusion alone. Clinically, he was able to reduce the total dosage of the antineoplastic agent but still obtained good response in treating cancer. Catheters with a balloon have been used experimentally and clinically to occlude the arterial blood flow while administering intraarterial chemotherapy to increase drug level in the target tissues.[109,110]

Another modification was the use of hemodialysis to remove anticancer drugs from venous blood. In 1987, Oldfield et al. described the use of hemodialysis in combination with intraarterial infusion of cisplatin into the carotid artery of a patient with a glioblastoma multiforme.[111] They reported a 50% reduction of venous cisplatin levels in patients treated by this combination technique compared with those treated with intraarterial infusion alone. Moreover, there was no hematologic or renal toxicity in the former group of patients.

Of course, there are other complications associated with intraarterial infusion therapy besides the systemic toxicity of the chemotherapy. In general, these are related to placement of the catheter or the catheter itself. Specific problems include infection, bleeding, arterial thrombosis, stenosis, or erosion of catheter into nearby structures. The incidence of such complications varies and depends on the target organ and the location of vascular access. Further details on complications are discussed along with the description of intraarterial infusion for each target organ.

Primary and Metastatic Liver Tumors

Arterial access to liver tumors can be achieved by either a percutaneous or a direct surgical catheterization. However, before proceeding with the catheterization of the liver tumor bed, an arteriogram should be obtained to ascertain if any anatomic anomaly of hepatic artery exists. An appropriate strategy of catheter placement is then proposed for the circumstance found. Approximately 65% to 70% of the population has the most common vascular anatomy of the common hepatic artery branching into the gastroduodenal and proper hepatic artery, which is subsequently divided into the right and left hepatic arteries.[101,112] In the remaining population a variety of vascular anomalies may be present, including a left hepatic artery branching from the left gastric artery, the right gastric or the gastroduodenal artery arising from the superior mesenteric artery (SMA), or the common hepatic artery as a division of the SMA.[101]

Through a laparotomy, open surgical catheterization of the arterial supply of a liver tumor is typically accomplished by placing a catheter into a ligated gastroduodenal artery with its tip at the bifurcation of the common hepatic artery.[101,103] Alternatively, the catheter can be placed in a ligated branch of a major hepatic artery supplying the liver tumor.[101,112] Occasionally, vascular anomalies obligate a reconstruction such that an infusion into all hepatic tumor beds is feasible with only one catheter.[113] In contrast, percutaneous catheterization of the liver bed is accomplished via the axillary or femoral artery using the Seldinger technique.[114,115] Although the minimal morbidity of the percutaneous approach is desirable, the success rate of percutaneous catheterization is reported at only 85%.[114] Because of anatomic anomalies or vascular atherosclerotic disease, hepatic catheter placement is occasionally achievable only through an open surgical technique.

Similar to the external central venous catheter, long-term use of the external arterial catheter is plagued with a relatively high rate of catheter-related infection and catheter displacement. With a mean life of 8 months, the external arterial catheters have infection and displacement rates reported at 9.8% to 25.0% and 17.6% to 30.0%, respectively.[114-116] Consequently, intraarterial infusion chemotherapy for liver tumors is preferably performed via an implantable infusion pump.

Although the delivery route of chemotherapy is an important factor in increasing drug concentration in the tumor bed, the rate of administration also affects the pattern of drug distribution to the liver.[114] Kaplan et al. discovered that a slow infusion resulted in delivering the majority of the drug to the right hepatic lobe, but a more rapid infusion rate resulted in an equal distribution of the drug to both lobes.[117] However, the higher infusion rate may result in more severe systemic toxic effects and thus defeats one of the goals of arterial chemotherapy. It is interesting that the lack of uniformity of distribution at slow infusion rates may be improved by reducing blood flow with a proximal balloon occlusion of the common hepatic artery.[118,119] Reducing blood flow consequently increases the time of drug exposure to the tumor.[128] However, with a large tumor burden, occlusion of hepatic arterial flow must be done with caution and initially for a short duration only.[120] Massive liver necrosis as a result of prolonged occlusion and arterial thrombosis is a major potential risk of balloon occlusion of the common hepatic artery. Obviously, balloon occlusion of the hepatic artery may not be applicable for those patients with an implantable pump. Because of the relative unresponsiveness of the immature or primitive tumor vasculature to vasoactive agents, blood flow may be shunted toward the tumor bed, and thus drug delivery to the tumor is improved with the concomitant infusion of a vasoactive agent.[121] Since chronic infusion of a vasoactive agent may result in significant deleterious systemic effects, a continuous chemically induced shunt may not be achievable without significant risk to the patients, especially those with cardiovascular diseases.

The concentrations of chemoagents in hepatic tumor beds at or near the liver surface may be significantly lower than expected because of dilution produced by a number of potential collaterals arising from the diaphragm, omentum, or adhesion. The development of such collaterals may partially explain the ineffectiveness of intraarterial chemotherapy for hepatic tumors near the surface.[122] Dividing these collaterals by detaching the liver surface from nearby structures and wrapping the liver with a plastic or rubber sheath may improve the efficacy of hepatic arterial chemotherapy.[122] Besides the development of collaterals, progressive changes of arterial perfusion in the liver often occur during the course of chemotherapy. These changes may occur secondarily to the tumor shrinkage and a decrease in vascularity of the tumor. Consequently, the distribution of anticancer agent may be altered, and ultimately the effectiveness of arterial chemotherapy may be diminished.[123]

There are potential complications associated with intrahepatic arterial chemotherapy of which the surgeon should be aware. Gastrointestinal complications include cholecystitis (20%), hepatitis, gastritis, duodenitis, and gastroduodenal ulceration.[101,116] The incidence of catheter-related complications is dependent on whether an implantable infusion pump is used. For the external hepatic artery catheters, a high incidence of infection (9.8% to 25.0%), catheter displacement (17.6% to 30.0%), and arterial thrombosis (33%) are noted.[115-117] In contrast, for hepatic artery catheters used with implantable infusion pumps, the incidence of catheter-related and pocket infection is lower and in the range of 2.5% to 7.6%.[101,116] Similarly, the incidence of catheter displacement/pump malfunction and incidence of arterial thrombosis are significantly reduced to 2.5% to 3.8% and to 2.5% to 17.3%, respectively.[101,116]

Percutaneous Placement of Hepatic Artery Catheter

As previously mentioned, the external intraarterial hepatic catheter is typically deployed through the axillary or femoral artery (Figure 41–10). After anesthetizing the area around the chosen artery, a small-gauge access needle is inserted into the lumen. A guidewire is then threaded into the artery via the access needle and advanced using fluoroscopy. After removing the access needle, a dilator and an introducer sheath are placed into the artery. After the withdrawal of the dilator, an angiocatheter is inserted into the artery and advanced over the guidewire. An angiogram of the celiac trunk is obtained to provide a road map of the

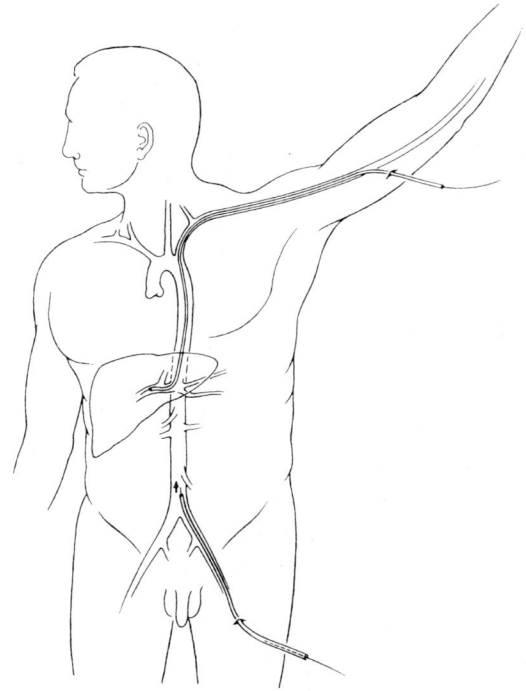

FIGURE 41–10. Percutaneous placement of a hepatic artery catheter. The catheter may be inserted into either the axillary or the femoral artery and advanced over a guidewire into the common hepatic artery.

hepatic vasculature for appropriate catheter placement. If no anatomic anomaly is found, the guidewire is advanced further into the proper hepatic artery and the angiocatheter is completely withdrawn. A properly tunneled, tailored, and flushed 5F catheter (see Central Venous Catheter) is subsequently inserted and advanced over the wire into the proper hepatic artery. The wire is withdrawn, and the catheter lumen function is checked. If no adjustment is needed, the introducer sheath is removed from the artery and pressure is applied over the access site for homostasis. Finally, the skin incision is reapproximated and dressed.

Direct Surgical Placement via Laparotomy

After a careful preoperative evaluation, a laparotomy via a right upper quadrant incision is performed under general anesthesia (Figure 41–11). After an exploration to determine the extent of the liver cancer, the gallbladder is excised. Dissection of the porta hepatis is then required to expose the common bile duct and the proper hepatic artery (PHA). Further proximal dissection of the PHA is necessary to identify the gastroduodenal artery (GDA) and the right gastric artery (RGA). Proximal small branches of the GDA and the RGA itself are ligated and divided. A left hepatic artery arising from the left gastric artery or any arterial branch supplying the liver that is not preceded by a proximal gastroduodenal branch should also be ligated. At this point the common hepatic artery (CHA) should be exposed and compared with the GDA. The catheter should be placed into the smaller of the two arteries. If the GDA is chosen, it is ligated approximately 1.5 to 2.0cm from the origin on the CHA. A noncrushing curved clamp is placed on the CHA before its bifurcation. An arteriotomy is made, and a 5F or 7F beaded catheter is introduced and advanced into the GDA until its tip is positioned at the bifurcation. Ligature is subsequently placed around the GDA on both sides of the catheter bead for anchoring. Additional ligatures are placed along the length of the GDA between the bead and arteriotomy as needed. After catheter placement, a subcutaneous pocket is created for the pump in the right abdominal wall and the free end of the catheter is then brought through the wall into the upper area of the pocket. After lumen function is verified, the catheter is attached to the pump, which is prefilled with heparin solution. The clamp on the common hepatic artery should be released as soon as this attachment is accomplished. The pump is then positioned and anchored firmly into the pocket. Using a Wood's light, the pattern of perfusion is determined by injecting 10% fluorescein into the pump. If the liver is the only organ that is perfused, the laparotomy and pocket incision are closed.

Extremity Malignant Tumors

Intraarterial infusion chemotherapy for soft tissue extremity tumors frequently constitutes one component of multimodality therapy.[102,103,109,110] A catheter is placed for temporary vascular access using a percutaneous technique via the axillary or femoral artery (Figure 41–12). A 4F to 7F Silastic catheter is typically employed. As previously mentioned,

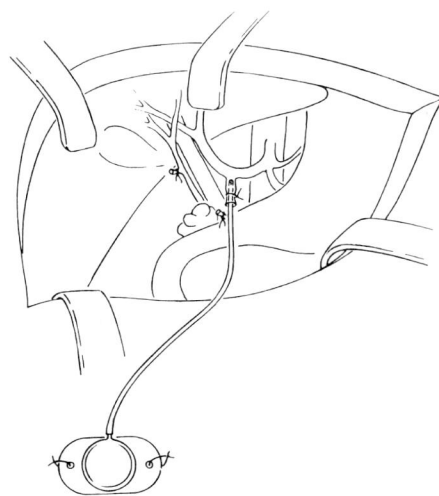

FIGURE 41–11. Open surgical placement of a hepatic artery catheter. The gastroduodenal artery is exposed via a right subcostal laparotomy. After the artery is ligated, the catheter is inserted until its tip just reaches the common hepatic artery. The catheter is then connected to a pump in the right abdominal wall.

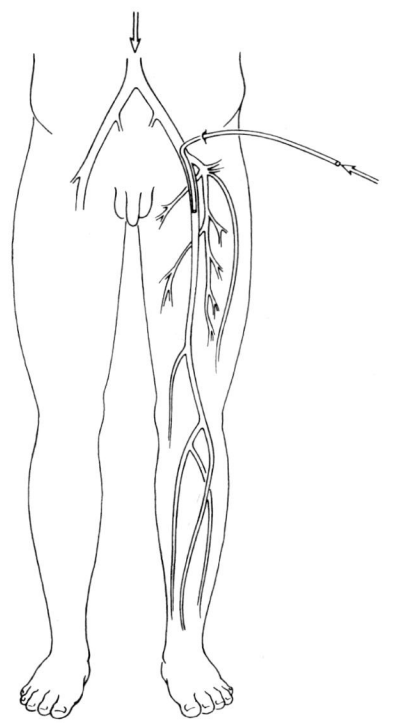

FIGURE 41–12. Catheter placement for arterial infusion of chemotherapy for lower extremity malignancy. Percutaneous insertion technique is commonly used for placement of the catheter into the lower extremities. The catheter can be guided into the main artery supplying the tumor.

antineoplastic drug concentration in the target tissue can be increased significantly with each administration by temporarily occluding the arterial inflow using a balloon catheter with or without concomitant temporary venous outflow obstruction.[102,109,110] Complications associated with arterial chemotherapy for extremity soft tissue tumors include infection (3.6%), arterial thrombosis (17.8%), and systemic toxic effects.[102,103] To date, chemotherapy delivered intraarterially has facilitated limb-sparing surgery and has definitely prolonged ultimate survival.[124–126]

Brain, Head, and Neck Cancer

Glioblastoma multiforme and metastatic brain tumors were described in the first series of intraarterial infusion chemotherapy by Klopp.[22] Originally, either the internal or common carotid artery was the route for chemotherapy administration. However, ophthalmic toxicity is a potential complication associated with the infusion of certain antineoplastic agents such as cisplatin using these routes.[106,127] With the availability of a better catheter, advancement of the catheter tip above the ophthalmic artery permits the completion of the entire course of intraarterial chemotherapy without any adverse ophthalmic-related consequence[106,127] (Figure 41–13).

Head and neck malignant tumors may be treated via a catheter placed retrograde from the superficial temporal artery to the level of the external carotid branch supplying the tumors (Figure 41–14).[24,128] The catheter for this approach is usually a 4F Silastic or polyethylene catheter, which may be left in place up to 45 days.[24] Similarly, catheter placement via the superior thyroid artery may also be accom-

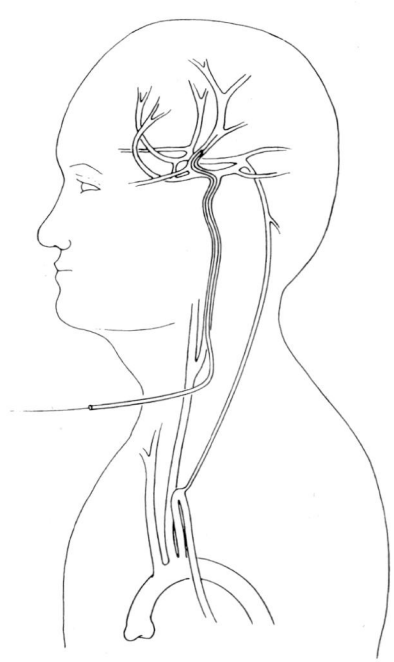

FIGURE 41–13. Technique of catheter placement for arterial infusion of chemotherapy for brain tumor. Catheter tip is advanced superior to the ophthalmic artery to prevent toxicity to the ipsilateral eye.

41. Endovascular Chemotherapy Delivery

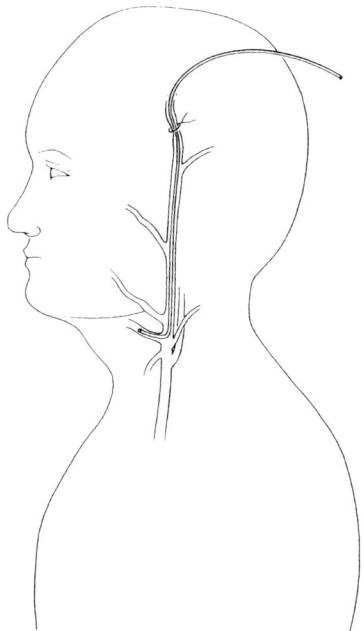

FIGURE 41-14. Catheter placement for arterial chemotherapy of head and neck tumor. The superficial temporal artery can be catheterized directly via surgical exposure of the artery. The catheter is guided into the arterial branch supplying the tumor.

plished.[22] Carotid artery thrombosis is a potential and dreadful complication of placing these catheters. To minimize this complication, superficial transposition of the external carotid artery into the subcutaneous tissue for intermittent repeat accesses for chemotherapy administration has been reported with great success (Figure 41-15).[129]

Others: Bladder and Prostate Cancers

Intraarterial chemotherapy has been used as a neoadjuvant (preoperative) therapy before surgical excision of bladder cancer.[100] The objectives are to facilitate tumor resection and, hopefully, increase cure or the interval to recurrence. Again, the chemotherapy is administered via a percutaneously placed catheter via the groin, with the tip of the catheter positioned at the bifurcation of the aorta. Likewise, prostate cancer has been subjected to neoadjuvant therapy via a catheter placed in the iliac artery.[104] In the pelvis, an area with numerous collateral arterial supplies, the effect of intra-arterial infusion chemotherapy is diluted and brief. Permanent occlusion of collateral branches into the pelvis has been reported to increase antineoplastic drug concentration in pelvic tissue and exposure of the tumor to the drug.[104] Again, the technique of "stop-flow" perfusion using balloon occlusive techniques may be used to improve chemotherapy pharmacokinetics with impressive results for palliative therapy.[120]

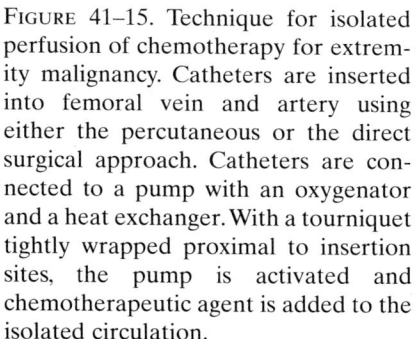
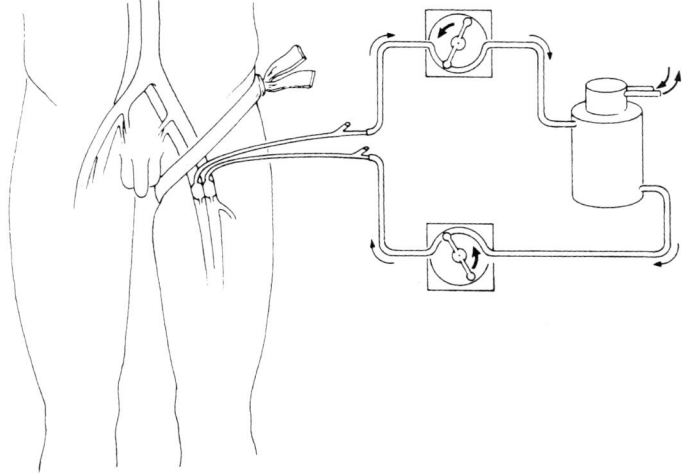

FIGURE 41-15. Technique for isolated perfusion of chemotherapy for extremity malignancy. Catheters are inserted into femoral vein and artery using either the percutaneous or the direct surgical approach. Catheters are connected to a pump with an oxygenator and a heat exchanger. With a tourniquet tightly wrapped proximal to insertion sites, the pump is activated and chemotherapeutic agent is added to the isolated circulation.

Arterial Embolization and Chemoembolization

Arterial embolization of localized but unresectable tumors is accomplished via a temporarily placed percutaneous catheter from either the axillary or femoral artery. The technique for placement of the catheter is similar to that described in previous sections. A wide variety of materials including Gelfoam, coils, Gelfoam and microcrystalline collagen permeated drugs, and solid pellets of antineoplastic agents have been injected into advanced local tumors.[130–134] The local drug reservoir augments agent delivery and produces local ischemia. Care must be taken so as not to induce ischemia too rapidly with aggressive embolization.

Isolated Perfusion

Isolated perfusion, initially used exclusively for tumors of the extremity, now has found application for liver, pelvic, and lung cancers.[32,33,135] In general, the involved organ or region with the tumor has its blood circulation isolated from the rest of the body while administering chemotherapy. The reported duration of the isolated perfusion for the extremity and pelvis in human subjects ranges between 25 to 45 minutes.[29,31–33] The largest investigation using hyperthermic isolated perfusion of the extremities with melanoma was by Stehlin in 1975.[31] In this study, mortality attributable to the perfusion was reported at 1.1% (2 of 165 patients). One patient died of renal failure and the other from a pulmonary embolus. Of all the patients, 1.6% required amputation resulting from excessive necrosis, but little other morbidity occurred. Other reported complications of isolated perfusion of extremity and pelvic cancers include deep vein thrombosis, nerve palsy, pancreatitis, and pelvic abscess. Several human trials of isolated perfusion for liver tumors have been reported and the results are encouraging, but further investigation is needed.[136–138] The perfusion is typically accomplished for 1 to 4 hours, depending on whether antineoplastic agent is administered along with hyperthermic perfusion. Like arterial infusion chemotherapy, massive liver necrosis and excessive bleeding (as a result of coagulopathy) are major potential complications of isolated liver perfusion. Further research to improve the technique of isolated liver perfusion is ongoing using a variety of animal models.[139,140]

Extremity Cancers

As part of the management strategy, sarcoma and melanoma of the extremity are sometimes treated with isolation perfusion (Figure 41–15). In different settings, indications include limb-sparing surgery (sarcoma) or the attempted control of metastatic disease (melanoma). In general, the isolation of extremity circulation involved control of the iliac artery or vein or the common femoral artery and vein. Under general anesthesia, the lower abdomen, groin, and extremity containing the tumor is included in the sterile field. A kidney bump or rolled towel is placed behind the ipsilateral gluteal area. An incision 2 cm cephalad and parallel to the inguinal ligament is used to gain control of the iliac vessels, and a standard vertical incision is preferred for the femoral vessels. The catheters, with or without balloons, are then inserted via arteriotomy and venotomy after appropriate proximal and distal vascular control. Vascular occlusion is obtained by inflating the balloons or by placing noncrushing clamps across the vessels. Before occluding the vessels, the pump/oxygenator is primed with colloid or autologous blood and is warmed to 40° to 42°C. The patient should be administered 5000 to 10,000 units of heparin. An Esmarch bandage is tightly wrapped around the thigh proximal to the catheters. Temperature thermistors are placed in the deep tissues at several loci in the extremity for on-line monitoring. Immediately after vascular occlusion is obtained, the pump/oxygenator is connected to the catheters and the perfusion is commenced with the rate set between 600 to 1000 ml/min. A heating blanket is also wrapped around the extremity to raise its temperature. If deep temperatures reach 40°C, antineoplastic agents are administered and the perfusion is continued for approximately 45 to 60 minutes. Blood is kept

41. Endovascular Chemotherapy Delivery

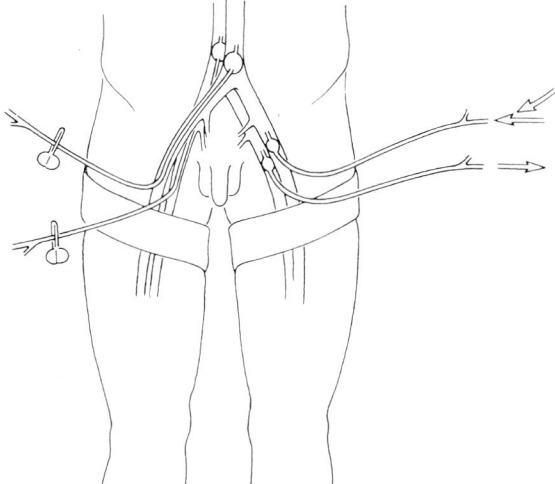

FIGURE 41–16. Isolated perfusion technique for pelvic tumors. A pair of balloon catheters in inserted into the femoral artery and veins and advanced to just above the bifurcations of the aorta and the IVC. Inflation of these catheters is required to exclude the systemic circulation. In the contralateral groin, another pair of catheters is inserted and advanced into the iliac artery and vein. The latter catheters are connected to the pump. The circulation of lower extremities is excluded using tourniquets. After isolation of the pelvic region, pumping is initiated and the antineoplastic agent is administered.

well oxygenated throughout the perfusion. At the conclusion of the perfusion, the pump is stopped and the outflow limb of the pump is disconnected from the arterial catheter. Low-molecular-weight dextran solution is then infused into the arterial catheter to wash out the entire extremity. After completing the washout, the tourniquet is released and major vessels are opened. The catheters are subsequently removed, and pressure is applied to obtain hemostasis. Repair of arteriotomy and venotomy is then accomplished before closing the skin incision.

Pelvic Tumors

For pelvic tumors, except for inserting the catheters proximally to just above the bifurcation of the vena cava and abdominal aorta, and perhaps for exposure of these segments of the vena cava and aorta retroperitoneally, the previous description is to be followed verbatim (Figure 41–16). In addition, proximal occlusions may be obtained on the vena cava or aorta by balloon dilatation with distal vascular control.

Liver Tumors

Isolated perfusion of the liver is accomplished by either open or percutaneous occlusive techniques (Figure 41–17). In general, isolation of the hepatic circulation is obtained by first isolating and draining the hepatic venous blood into the inflow of the heart-lung pump (HLP) and secondly infusing the outflow limb of the HLP into the hepatic artery or portal vein. Because of the interruption of the IVC and portal vein created as the result of this

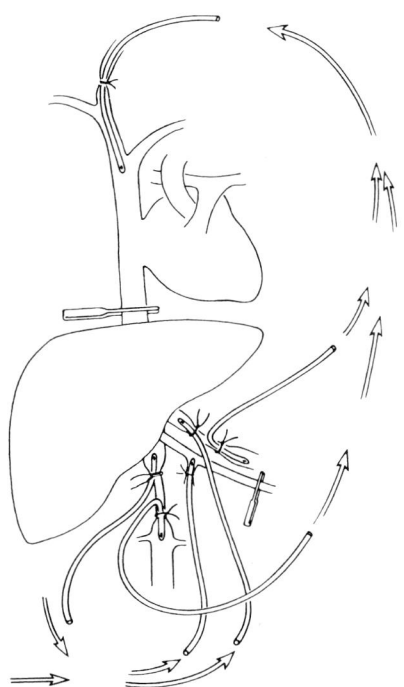

FIGURE 41–17. Isolated perfusion for liver tumor. Complete isolation of the liver requires draining all of hepatic venous blood into a pump and returning to portal vein and/or hepatic artery. As a result of the isolation, the IVC and portal vein are temporarily interrupted. Shunts must be created to return blood from the infrahepatic IVC and mesenteric/splenic vein to the SVC.

isolation, shunts from the infrahepatic IVC and the distal portal vein to the SVC are required.

Under general anesthesia a subcostal abdominal incision is made to provide wide hepatic exposure. The porta hepatis is dissected to isolate the gastroduodenal and common hepatic arteries. Further dissection provides isolation of the portal vein. A Kocher maneuver is performed to expose the infrahepatic IVC. The suprahepatic IVC is exposed at the hiatus through the diaphragm. No attempt is made to encircle the vessel. The axillary vein may be isolated if a venovenous shunt is desired. The shunt is assisted by blood pump and heparin-bonded tubing. A catheter is placed into the gastroduodenal artery. The portal vein and IVC would be cannulated in instances when a veno-veno shunt is desired. A catheter with a single balloon is inserted into the infrahepatic IVC. The suprahepatic IVC is directly clamped after supraceliac aortic cross-clamping. The balloon catheter is used to control the infrahepatic IVC. Before connection to the hepatic circulation, the pump is primed with the patient's blood or colloid. The perfusion circulation is heated to 40° to 42°C, and anticancer agents are added to the gastroduodenal catheter. Perfusion is performed for approximately 1 hour. After removal of all catheters, the gastroduodenal artery is ligated, but other vessels are repaired. The gallbladder is removed. Laparotomy and neck incisions are then closed.

Conclusion

Administration of chemotherapeutic agents can be accomplished through a variety of techniques. Advantages, disadvantages, and theoretic benefits are slightly or completely different for the techniques. Despite these differences, the goals of chemotherapy should include (1) a potential cure for the malignancy, (2) an effective and specific delivery to the target lesion, and (3) minimal adverse systemic effects. These goals may soon be realized with better understanding of tumor molecular biology and with development of target-specific antineoplastic agents.

References

1. Adair FE, Bagg HJ: Experimental and clinical studies on treatment of cancer by dichloroethylsulphide (mustard gas), *Ann Surg* 93:190, 1931.
2. Gilman A, Phillips FS: Biological actions and therapeutic application of the B-chloroethyl amines and sulfides, *Science* 103:499–415, 1946.
3. Carver LF: The nitrogen mustards: clinical use, *Radiology* 50:486–493, 1948.
4. Lower R: Tractatus de Corde, 1669. In *Early science in Oxford*, vol IX, London, 1932, Oxford University Press (translated by KJ Fraklin).
5. Peters JL: Historical review. In Peters JL, editor: *A manual of central venous catheterization and parenteral nutrition*, Boston, Mass, 1983, Wright PSG.
6. Farquhar JW, Lewis IC: Some medical uses of polyethylene with special reference to venoclysis in infants, *Lancet* 2:244–246, 1948.
7. Seldinger SI: Catheter replacement of the needle in percutaneous arteriography: a new technique, *Acta Radiol* 39:368–376, 1953.
8. Aubainac R: L'injection intraveineuse sous-claviculaire, *Presse Med* 60:1456, 1952.
9. Keeri-Szántó M: The subclavian vein, a constant and convenient intravenous injection site, *Arch Surg* 72:179–181, 1956.
10. Yoffa D: Supraclavicular subclavian venepuncture and catheterization, *Lancet* 2:614–617, 1965.
11. Hermosura B, Vanagas L, Dickey MW: Measurement of pressure during intravenous therapy, *JAMA* 195:321, 1966.
12. Indar R: The dangers of indwelling polyethylene catheters in deep veins, *Lancet* 1:284–286, 1959.
13. Quinton W, Dillard D, Scribner BH: Cannulation of blood vessels for prolonged hemodialysis, *Trans Am Soc Artif Intern Organs* 6:104, 1960.
14. Steward RD, Sanislow CA: Silastic intravenous catheter, *N Engl J Med* 265:1283–1285, 1961.
15. Dudrick SJ, Wilmore DW, Vars HM: Long-term total parenteral nutrition with growth, development and positive nitrogen balance, *Surgery* 64:134–142, 1968.
16. Broviac JW, Cole JJ, Scribner BH: A silicone rubber atrial catheter for prolonged parenteral alimentation, *Surg Gynecol Obstet* 136:602–606, 1973.
17. Hickman RO, Buckner CD, Clife RA et al: A modified right atrial catheter for access to the

17. venous system in marrow transplant recipients, *Surg Gynecol Obstet* 148:871–875, 1979.
18. Niederhuber JE, Esminger W, Gyves JW et al: Totally implanted venous and arterial access system to replace external catheters in cancer treatment, *Surgery* 92:706–712, 1982.
19. Steckler RM, Martin RG, Speer JF et al: Vascular access by means of surgically created arteriovenous fistulas in chemotherapy of acute leukemia. A preliminary report, *South Med J* 67:821, 1974.
20. Buckley CJ, Manning LG, Page CP: Experience with central high flow arteriovenous fistulas in patients requiring chronic parenteral chemotherapy or hemodialysis, *Am J Surg* 136:730–734, 1978.
21. Lempert N, MacDowell RT, Karmody A et al: Vascular access for cancer chemotherapy, *Cancer* 43:1943–1946, 1979.
22. Klopp CT, Alford C, Bateman J et al: Fractionated intra-arterial cancer chemotherapy with methyl bis amine hydrochloride: a preliminary report, *Ann Surg* 132:811–832, 1959.
23. Sullivan RD, Miller E, Sikes MP: Antimetabolites-metabolite combination cancer chemotherapy: effects of intraarterial methotrexate-intramuscular citrovorum factor therapy in human cancer, *Cancer* 12:1248–1262, 1959.
24. Watkins E, Sullivan RD: Cancer chemotherapy by prolonged arterial infusion, *Surg Gynecol Obstet* 118:3–19, 1964.
25. Sullivan RD, Norcross JW, Watkins E: Chemotherapy of metastatic liver cancer by prolonged hepatic-artery infusion, *N Eng J Med* 270:321–327, 1964.
26. Cady B, Oberfield RA: Arterial infusion chemotherapy of hepatoma, *Surg Gynecol Obstet* 138:381–384, 1974.
27. Blackshear PJ, Rohde TD, Buchwald H: The implantable infusion pump: a new concept in drug delivery, *Med Prog Technol* 6:149–161, 1979.
28. Gibbon JH: Application of a mechanical heart-lung apparatus to cardiac surgery, *Minn Med* 37:171, 1984.
29. Creech O, Krementz ET, Ryan RF et al: Chemotherapy of cancer: regional perfusion utilizing an extracorporeal circuit, *Ann Surg* 148:616–632, 1958.
30. Cavaliere R, Ciogatto EC, Giovanella BC et al: Selective heat sensitivity of cancer cells. Biochemical and clinical studies, *Cancer* 20:1351–1381, 1967.
31. Stehlin JS, Giovannella BC, de Ipolyi PD et al: Results of hyperthermic perfusion for melanoma of the extremities, *Surg Gynecol Obstet* 140:339–348, 1975.
32. Wile A, Smolin M: Hyperthermic pelvic isolation-perfusion in the treatment of refactory pelvic cancer, *Arch Surg* 122:1321–1325, 1987.
33. Turk PS, Belliveau JF, Darnowski JW et al: Isolated pelvic perfusion for unresectable cancer using a balloon occlusion technique, *Arch Surg* 128:533–539, 1993.
34. Markowitz J: The hepatic artery, *Surg Gynecol Obstet* 95:644, 1952.
35. Almgard LE, Ferstrom I, Haverling M et al: Treatment of renal adenocarcinoma by embolic occlusion of renal circulation, *Br J Urol* 45:474–479, 1973.
36. Feldman F, Casarella WJ, Dick HM et al: Selective intraarterial embolization of bone tumors. A useful adjunct in the management of selected lesions, *AJR Am J Roentgenol* 123:130–139, 1975.
37. Goldstein HM, Wallace S, Anderson JH et al: Transcatheter occlusion of abdominal tumors, *Radiology* 120:539–545, 1976.
38. Yamada R, Sato M, Kawabata M et al: Hepatic artery embolization in 120 patients with unresectable hepatoma, *Radiology* 148:397–401, 1983.
39. Bismuth H, Morino M, Sherlock D et al: Primary treatment of hepatocellular carcinoma by arterial chemoembolization, *Am J Surg* 163:387–394, 1992.
40. Cherqui D, Piedbois, P, Pierga JY et al: Multimodal adjuvant treatment and liver transplantation for advanced hepatocellular carcinoma. A pilot study, *Cancer* 73:2721–2726, 1994.
41. Focan C, Barbason H, Betz EH: Use of synchronization induced by cyclophosphamide in a methylcholanthrene sarcoma with circadian proliferation to rational sequential chemotherapy, *Biomed* 23:230–235, 1975.
42. Focan C: Sequential chemotherapy and circadian rhythm in human solid tumors. A randomised trial, *Cancer Chemother Pharmcol* 3:197–202, 1979.
43. Scheving LE, Burns ER, Pauly JE et al: Circadian variation in cell division of the mouse alimentary tract, bone marrow and corneal epithelium, *Anat Rec* 191:479–486, 1978.
44. Bellamy WT, Alberts DS, Dorr RT: Daily variation in non-protein sulfhydryl levels of human

bone marrow, *Eur J Cancer Clin Oncol* 24: 1759–1762, 1988.
45. Smaaland R, Laerum OD, Lote K et al: DNA synthesis in human bone marrow is circadian stage dependent, *Blood* 77: 2603–2611, 1991.
46. Broviac JW, Cole JJ, Scribner BH: A silicone rubber atrial catheter for prolonged parenteral alimentation, *Surg Gynecol Obstet* 136:602–606, 1973.
47. Virchow R: *Gesammelte Adhandlungen zur Wissenschaftlichen Medicin*, Frankfurt, Germany, 1856, Verlag Von Medindinger Sohn and Comp.
48. Early TF, Gregory RT, Wheeler JR et al: Increased infection rate in double-lumen versus single-lumen Hickman catheters in cancer patients, *South Med J* 83:34–36, 1990.
49. Henriques HF, III, Karmy-Jones R, Knoll SM et al: Avoiding complication of long-term venous access, *Am Surg* 59:555–558, 1993.
50. Matlak ME: Vascular access in pediatric patient. In Wilson ES, editor: *Vascular access surgery*, ed 2, St Louis, 1988, Mosby.
51. Rosen M, Latto IP, Ng WS: Paediatric procedures: choosing the equiment. In Rosen M, Latto IP, Ng WS, editors: *Handbook of percutaneous central venous catheterization*, ed 2, Philadelphia, 1992, WB Saunders.
52. Farquhar JW, Lewis IC: Some medical uses of polyethylene with special reference to venoclysis in infants, *Lancet* 2:244–246, 1948.
53. Borrow M, Crowley JG: Evaluation of central venous catheter thrombogenicity, *Acta Anaesthesiol Scand* Suppl 81:59–64, 1985.
54. Hanfield-Jones RPC, Lewis HBM: Rubber tubing as a cause of infusion thrombophlebitis, *Lancet* 1:585–588, 1952.
55. Hoshal VL, Ause RG, Hoskins PA: Fibrin sleeve formation on indwelling subclavian central venous catheters, *Arch Surg* 102:353–358, 1971.
56. Indar R: The dangers of indwelling polyethylene catheters in deep veins, *Lancet* 1:284–286, 1959.
57. Nejad MS: Clotting on the outer surface of vascular catheters, *Radiology* 91:248, 1968.
58. Jones MV, Craig DB: Venous reaction to plastic intravenous cannulae: influence of cannula composition, *Can Anaesth Soc J* 19:491, 1972.
59. Welch GW, McKeel DW, Silvestein P et al: The role of the catheter composition in the development of thrombophlebitis, *Surg Gynecol Obstet* 138:421–424, 1974.
60. Simmons JR, Buzdar AU, Ota DM et al: Complications associated with indwelling catheters. *Med Pediatr Oncol* 20:22–25, 1992.
61. Dejong PCM, VonMeyenfeldt MR, Rouflart M et al: Complications of central venous catheterization of the subclavian vein: the influence of a parenteral nutrition team, *Acta Anaesthesiol Scan* Suppl 81:48–52, 1985.
62. Raad II, Luna M, Khalil SM et al: The relationship between the thrombotic and infectious complications of central venous catheters, *JAMA* 271:1014–1016, 1994.
63. Hayward SR, Leherwood AM, Lucas CE: The fate of prolonged venous access devices, *Am Surg* 56:515–519, 1990.
64. Ingram J, Weitzman S, Greenberg ML et al: Complications of indwelling venous access lines in the pediatric hematology patient: a prospective comparison of external venous catheters and subcutaneous ports, *Am J Pediatr Hematol Oncol* 13:130–136, 1991.
65. Severien C, Nelson JD: Frequency of infections associated with implanted systems and cuffed, tunneled Silastic venous catheters in patients with acute leukemia, *Am J Dis Child* 145: 1433–1438, 1991.
66. Borst CG, de Kruif AT, van Dam FS et al: Totally implantable venous access ports—the patient's point of view: a quality control study, *Cancer Nurs* 15:378–381, 1992.
67. McCready D, Broadwater R, Ross M et al: A case-control comparison of durability and cost between implanted reservoir and percutaneous catheters in cancer patients, *J Surg Res* 51:377–381, 1991.
68. Sterner S, Plummer DW, Clinton J et al: A comparison of the supraclavicular approach and the infraclavicular approach for subclavian vein catheterization, *Ann Emerg Med* 15:421–424, 1986.
69. English ICW, Frew RM, Pigott JF et al: Percutaneous catheterization of the internal jugular vein, *Anaesthesia* 24:51, 1969.
70. Ryan JA, Abel RM, Abbott WM et al: Catheter complications in total parenteral nutrition, *N Eng J Med* 290:757, 1974.
71. Brachos GJ: Central venous catheterization via the supraclavicular approach, *J Trauma* 17: 872–877, 1977.
72. Mostert JW, Kenny GM, Murphy GP: Safe placement of central venous catheter into internal jugular vein, *Arch Surg* 101:431, 1970.
73. Brinkman AJ, Costley DO: Internal jugular venipuncture, *JAMA* 223:182, 1973.

74. McGoon MD, Benedetto PW, Greene BM: Complications of percutaneous central venous catheterization: a report of two cases and review of the literature, *Johns Hopkins Med J* 145:1–5, 1979.
75. Berthelsen P, Hansen B, Howard-Hansen P et al: Central venous access via the external jugular vein in cardiovascular surgery, *Acta Anaesthesiol Scand* 30:470–472, 1986.
76. Dailey RH: External jugular vein cannulation and its use for CVP monitoring, *J Emerg Med* 6:133–135, 1988.
77. Hinkley ME: Thoracic duct thrombosis with fatal chylothorax caused by a long venous catheter, *N Eng J Med* 280:25, 1969.
78. Khalil KG: Thoracic duct injury: a complication of jugular vein catheterization, *JAMA* 221:908–909, 1972.
79. Ruggiero RP, Caruso G: Chylothorax a complication of subclavian vein catheterization, *J Parenter Enteral Nutr* 9:750–753, 1985.
80. Campistrol JM, Cases A, Lopez-Pedretz J et al: Thoracic duct injury: an unusual complication following subclavian catheterization for hemodialysis, *Nephron* 46:390–391, 1987.
81. Hoshal VL: Total intravenous nutrition with peripherally inserted silicone elastomer central venous catheters, *Arch Surg* 110:644–646, 1975.
82. MacDonald AS, Master SKP, Moffitt EA: A comparative study of peripheral inserted silicone catheters for parenteral nutrition, *Can Anaesth Soc J* 24:263–269, 1977.
83. Bottino J, McCredie KB, Groschel DH et al: Long-term intravenous therapy with peripherally inserted silicone elastomer central venous catheters in patients with malignant diseases, *Cancer* 43:1937–1943, 1979.
84. Starkhammar H, Bengtsson M, Gain T et al: A new injection portal for brachially inserted central venous catheter: a multiple center study, *Med Oncol Tumor Pharmacother* 7:281–285, 1990.
85. Winters V, Peters B, Coila S et al: A trial with a new peripheral implanted vascular access device, *Oncol Nurs Forum* 17:891–896, 1990.
86. Morris P, Buller R, Kendall S et al: A peripherally implanted permanent central venous access device, *Obstet Gynecol* 78:1138–1142, 1991.
87. Adi-Nader JA: Peripherally inserted central venous catheters in critical care patients, *Heart Lung* 22:428–434, 1993.
88. Cardella JF, Fox PS, Lawler JB: Interventional radiologic placement of peripherally inserted central catheters, *J Vasc Interv Radiol* 4:653–660, 1993.
89. Carre MC et al: Central venous brachial catheter (P.A.S. Port TM) and catheter scanning system (Cath-Finder TM), *J Surg Oncol* 55:190–193, 1994.
90. Merell SW, Peatross BG, Grossman MD et al: Peripherally inserted central venous catheters. Low-risk alternatives for ongoing venous access, *West J Med* 160:25–30, 1994.
91. Lam S, Scannell R, Roessler D et al: Peripherally inserted central catheters in an acute-care hospital, *Arch Intern Med* 154:1833–1837, 1994.
92. Markel S, Reynen K: Impact on patient care. 2652 PIC catheter days in the alternative setting, *J Intraven Nurs* 13:347–351, 1990.
93. Graham DR, Keldermans MM, Klemm LW et al: Infectious complications among patients receiving home intravenous therapy with peripheral, central, or peripherally placed central venous catheters, *Am J Med* 91:95s–100s, 1991.
94. Andersen KM, Holland JS: Maintaining the patency of peripherally inserted central catheters with 10 units/cc heparin, *J Intraven Nurs* 15:84–88, 1992.
95. James L, Bledsoe L, Hadaway LC: A retrospective look at tip location and complications of peripherally inserted central catheter lines, *J Intraven Nurs* 16:104–109, 1993.
96. Raad I, Davis S, Becker M et al: Low rate of infection and long durability of nontunneled Silastic catheters, *Arch Intern Med* 153:1791–1796, 1993.
97. Yarbro JW: The scientific basis of cancer chemotherapy. In Perry M, editor: *The chemotherapy source book*, Baltimore, 1992, Williams & Wilkins.
98. Sullivan RD, Jones R Jr, Schnabel TG Jr et al: Treatment of human cancer with intra-arterial nitrogen mustard (methyl-bis(2-chloroethyl)amine hydrochloride) utilizing simplified catheter technique, *Cancer* 6:121–134, 1953.
99. Hellekant C: Bronchial angiography and intra-arterial chemotherapy with mitomycin-C in bronchogenic carcinoma. Anatomy, technique, complications, *Acta Radiol Diag* 20:478–496, 1979.
100. Nakazonono M, Iwata S: Preoperative intraarterial chemotherapy for bladder cancer, *Urol Res* 9:289–295, 1981.

101. Daly JM, Kemeny N, Oderman P et al: Long-term hepatic arterial infusion chemotherapy, *Arch Surg* 119:936–941, 1984.
102. Ingvar C, Eskborg S, Stingson L et al: Tourniquet infusion chemotherapy of lower extremities: clinical and pharmacokinetic results, *Eur J Surg Oncol* 15:375–379, 1989.
103. Kashdan BJ, Sullivan KL, Lackman RD et al: Extremity osteosarcomas: intra-arterial chemotherapy and limb-sparing resection with 2-year follow up, *Radiology* 177:95–99, 1990.
104. Nakamura K, Takashima S, Nakatsuka H et al: Prostate cancer: arterial infusion chemotherapy and alteration of intrapelvic blood flow, *Radiology* 185:885–889, 1992.
105. Simunek A, Krajina A, Hlava A: Selective intra-arterial chemotherapy of tumors in the lingual artery territory by a new approach, *Cardiovasc Interv Radiol* 16:392–395, 1993.
106. Nakagawa H, Fujita T, Kudo S et al: Selective intra-arterial chemotherapy with a combination of etoposide and cisplastin for malignant gliomas: preliminary report, *Surg Neurol* 41:19–27, 1994.
107. Watkins E Jr: Chronometric infusor: apparatus for protracted ambulatory infusion therapy, *New Engl J Med* 269:850, 1963.
108. Blachshear PJ, Rohde TD, Prosl F et al: The implantable infusion pump: a new concept in drug delivery, *Med Prog Technol* 6:149–161, 1979.
109. Karakousis CP, Rao U, Holterman OA et al: Tourniquet infusion chemotherapy in extremities with malignant lesions, *Surg Gynecol Obstet* 149:481–490, 1979.
110. Kudo S, Wright KC, Chuang VP et al: Experimental evaluation of intraarterial occlusion-infusion chemotherapy, *AJR* 143:1069–1073, 1984.
111. Oldfield EH, Clark WC, Dedrick RL et al: Reduced systemic drug exposure by combining intraarterial cis-diaminedichroloplatinum(II) with hemodialysis of regional venous drainage, *Cancer Res* 47:1962–1967, 1987.
112. Curley SA, Chase JL, Roh MS et al: Technical considerations and complications associated with the placement of 180 implantable hepatic arterial infusion devices, *Surgery* 144:928–935, 1993.
113. Eckhauser FE, Knol JA, Strodel WE et al: Complicated access for regional infusion chemotherapy, *Arch Surg* 119:1195–1197, 1984.
114. Petrek JA, Minton JP: Treatment of hepatic metastases by percutaneous hepatic arterial infusion, *Cancer* 43:2183–2188, 1979.
115. Oberfield RA, McCaffrey JA, Polio J et al: Prolonged and continuous percutaneous intraarterial hepatic infusion chemotherapy in advanced metastatic liver adenocarcinoma from colorectal primary, *Cancer* 44:414–423, 1979.
116. Huk I, Entscheff P, Prager M et al: Patency rate of implantable devices during long-term intraarterial chemotherapy, *Angiology* 41:936–941, 1990.
117. Kaplan WD, D'Orsi CJ, Ensminger WE et al: Intra-arterial radionuclide infusion: a new technique to assess chemotherapy perfusion patterns, *Cancer Treatment Reports* 62:699–703, 1978.
118. Barth KH, Lutz RJ, Kremers PW et al: Mixing problem of low flow hepatic artery infusion. Improvement with small caliber double-lumen balloon catheters, *Invest Radiol* 23:519–523, 1988.
119. Kawabata M, Takashima S, Mitsuzane K et al: Balloon occluded arterial infusion therapy for malignant hepatic tumors, *Gan To Kagaku Ryoho* 11:806–813, 1984.
120. El-Domeiri AA: A method of intermittent occlusion and chemotherapy infusion of the hepatic artery, *Surg Gynecol Obstet* 143:107–109, 1976.
121. Golberg JA, Murray T, Kerr DJ et al: The use of angiotensin II as a potential method of targeting cytotoxic microspheres in patients with intra-hepatic tumor, *Br J Cancer* 63:308–310, 1991.
122. Sasaki Y, Imaoka S, Shibata T et al: Decollateralization with silicone rubber sheeting for advanced hepatocellular carcinoma: a preliminary report, *Surgery* 108:840–846, 1990.
123. Roth J, Wallner B, Safi F: Arterial perfusion abnormalities of the liver after hepatic arterial infusion chemotherapy and their correlation with the changes in metastases: evaluation with CT and angiography, *AJR* 153:751–754, 1989.
124. Eilber FR, Mirra JJ, Grant TT et al: Is amputation necessary for sarcomas? A seven-year experience with limb salvage, *Ann Surg* 192:431–437, 1980.
125. Eilber FR, Morton DL, Eckardt J et al: Limb salvage for skeletal and soft tissue sarcomas. Multidiscipline preoperative therapy, *Cancer* 53:2579–2584, 1984.
126. Eilber FR, Eckardt J, Rosen G et al: Neoadjuvant chemotherapy and radiotherapy in the multidisciplinary management of soft tissue sarcomas of the extremity, *Surg Oncol Clin N Am* 2:611–620, 1993.

127. Kapp JP, Parker JL, Tucker EM: Supraophthalmic carotid infusion for brain chemotherapy. Experience with a new single-lumen catheter and maneuverable tip, *J Neurosurg* 823–825, 1985.
128. Simunek A, Krajina A, Hlava A: Selective intraarterial chemotherapy of tumors in the lingual artery territory by a new approach, *Cardiovasc Interv Radiol* 16:392–395, 1993.
129. Claudio F, Cacace F, Comella G et al: Intraarterial chemotherapy through carotid transposition in advanced head and neck cancer, *Cancer* 65:1465–1471, 1990.
130. Wanabe S, Nishioka M, Ohta Y et al: Prospective and randomized controlled study of chemoembolization therapy in patients with advanced hepatocellular carcinoma. Cooperative Study Group for Liver Cancer Treatment in Shikoku area, *Cancer Chemother Pharmacol* 33(suppl):S93–96, 1994.
131. Uchida H, Matsuo N, Sakaguchi H et al: Segmental embolotherapy for hepatic cancer: keys to success, *Cardiovasc Interv Radiol* 16:67–71, 1993.
132. Kyotani S, Nishioka Y, Okamura M et al: A study of embolizing materials for chemoembolization therapy of hepatocellular carcinomas: antitumor effects of cis-diaminedichloroplatinum (II) albumin microspheres, containing chitin and treated with chitosan on rabbits with VX2 hepatic tumors, *Chem Pharm Bull (Tokyo)* 40:2814–2816, 1992.
133. Wang Y, Wu MC, Zhang XH: Hepatic arterial chemoembolization with CDDP microcapsules. Experimental studies, *Chinese Med J (Engl)* 105:120–125, 1992.
134. Kawai S, Okamura J, Ogawa M et al: Prospective and randomized clinical trial for the treatment of hepatocellular carcinoma—a comparison of Lipiodol-transcatheter arterial embolization with and without adriamycin (first cooperative study). The Cooperative Study Group for Liver Cancer Treatment of Japan, *Cancer Chemother Pharmacol* 31(suppl):S1–S6, 1992.
135. Baciewicz FA, Arredondo M, Chaudhuri B et al: Pharmokinetics and toxicity of isolated perfusion of lung with doxorubicin, *J Surg Res* 50:124–128, 1991.
136. Quebbeman EJ, Skibba JL, Petroff RJ: A technique for isolated hyperthermic liver perfusion, *J Surg Oncol* 27:141–145, 1984.
137. Ausman RK, Aust JB: Isolated perfusion of liver with HN_2, *Surg Forum* 10:77, 1960.
138. Aigner KR, Walther H, Link KH: Isolated liver perfusion with MMC/5-FU—surgical technique, pharmacokinetics, clinical results, *Contr Oncol* 29:229–246, 1988.
139. Stone RT, Jabour A, Wilson SE et al: Uptake of 5-fluoracil during isolated perfusion of the canine liver, *J Surg Oncol* 13:347–353, 1980.
140. VanDeVelde CJH, Kothuis BJL, Barenbrug HWM et al: A successful technique of in vivo isolated liver perfusion in pigs, *J Surg Res* 41:539–599, 1986.
141. Bauer GM, Porter JM, Fletcher WS: Human umbilical cord vein allograft arteriovenous fistula for chemotherapy access, *Am J Surg* 138:238–240, 1979.

Suggested Reading

Bauer GM, Porter JM, Fletcher WS: Human umbilical cord vein allograft arteriovenous fistula for chemotherapy access, *Am J Surg* 138:238–240, 1979.

Index

AAA. *See* Abdominal aortic aneurysm(s)
Abdominal aorta
  development of atherosclerosis and, 22
  evaluation of, with ultrasound, 150
Abdominal aortic aneurysm(s) (AAA)
  access to, 481
  artificial, 364
  endoluminal grafts and, 362–363
  evolution in treatment of, 36–364
  grafts for, 481–482
  hypertension and, 361
  incidence of, 361
  intraluminal grafts and, 371–380
  repair, combined with endoluminal descending thoracic aneurysm repair, 482
  surveillance protocols for endo-grafted, 109–115
  sutureless anastomosis and, 362–363
  See also Aortic aneurysm
Abdominal aortic aneurysm(s), endovascular repair of, 391–401
  patient selection, 396
    anatomic criteria, 396–397
    complexity of case, 397–398, 399
    diagnostic evaluation, 397
    pitfalls, 398, 399

  techniques, 391–396
    angiography, 396
    catheter/guidewire, 391
    device access, femoral artery, 391–392
    device access, iliac arteries, 392–393
    distal stent-graft implantation, 394, 396
    modular stent-graft contralateral leg, 394, 395
    proximal device deployment, 393–394
Abdominal procedures, anesthesia for, 81–85
ABI. *See* Ankle-brachial index
Ablation threshold, 354
Absorbed radiation dose, 121–122
Access site
  in abdominal aortic aneurysm(s), endovascular repair of, 391–393
  bleeding, control of, 579–580
  to carotid artery, 433–438
  complications, 585–587
  direct surgical repair of, 580–582
  endovascular approaches, 580–582
  femoral, 438–440
    complications, 585–587
    management of, 578–580
    cost of, 580
  See also Perclose devices
Accreditation Council for (Graduate Medical Education, 33

Acenocoumarol, 340
Acquired immunodeficiency syndrome, stents and, 371–372
Acute limb ischemia, 457–467
  amputation and, 292
Adherent clot catheter, 295–296, 298
β-adrenergic antagonists, 66–67
AIDS. *See* Acquired immunodeficiency syndrome
Air plethysmography, 516
Ai-Nafiis, Ibn, 3
Alfentanil, 61, 72–73, 74
Aluminum, corrosion resistance and, 228
Amides, 65–66
Amiodarone, 68
Amputation, acute ischemia and, 292
Analgesia
  for endovascular procedures, 59–68
  epidural, 78
Analgesic agents and adjuvants, 59–55
Analgesics, for endovascular procedures, 60–62
Anaphylactoid reactions, to contrast media, 147
Anastomoses
  intravascular ultrasound and, 137
  sutureless, 362–363
Anatomic evaluation, intraoperative monitoring and, 94–95

621

Anesthesia
  in cardiac catheterization suite, 74–76
  for carotid procedures, 70–74
  for endovascular procedures, 59–91
  epidural, 78
  for intracranial procedures, 70–74
  local, for percutaneous puncture, 260
  physiologic response to, 69–70
  See also General anesthesia
Anesthesia survey, 83–84
Anesthesiologist, role of, 75–76
Anesthesiology service, endovascular, 79–85
Anesthesiology service chief, role of, 79–80
Anesthetic agents and adjuvants, 59–66
  drug interactions and, 67–68
Anesthetic risk, management of, 81–84
Anesthetics, local, 65–66
AneuRx, 240, 393
Aneurysms
  aortic. See Aortic aneurysm
  Blaisdell technique of exclusion of, 362
  computed tomography and, 46–48
  degeneration of, atherosclerotic, 24
  of femoral artery, 45
  intravascular ultrasound and, 208
  Karmody technique of exclusion of, 362
  of popliteal artery, 474–478
  rupture of, computed tomography and, 153–154
  thoracic aortic, 383–389
  See also Abdominal sortie aneurysm(s); Pseudoaneurysm
Aneurysm exclusion, 362
Aneurysm formation, 23–25
Aneurysmal arterial disease, 481–488
  endovascular reporting standards for, 107, 109
Aneurysmosis, 45
Angina pectoris, anesthetic risk and, 82

Angiogram(s)
  earliest, 3
  intraoperative, 94
  number of, required for credentialing, 34
Angiographic catheters, 250–255
Angiography, 143–149
  anatomic evaluation of, 94–96, 97–98, 99
  catheters for, 250–255
  compared with intravascular ultrasound, 205, 207
  computed tomography, 152–153
  digital subtraction, 144
  endovascular training and, 35
  film screen, 143–144
  techniques of, 143–146
  versus intravascular ultrasound, 201, 204
Angioplasty
  aortic, 278
  balloon, 269–287
  and bypass graft stenosis, 282
  amd carptod arteru. 429–443
  of femoral artery, 279–280
  of iliac artery, 278–279
  infrapopliteal, 280
  laser, 93, 139, 353–360
  and limb salvage, 423–427
  number of, needed for credentialing, 34
  peripheral excimer laser, 353–359
  peripheral laser, 353–360
  of popliteal artery, 279–280
  of subclavian and innominate artery(ies), 417
  See also Carotid angioplasty and stenting; Percutaneous transluminal angioplasty
Angioplasty balloons, 272–274
  biomaterials considerations for, 222–227
Angioplasty catheters, biomaterials considerations of, 225–227
Angiopump, 181
Angioscopes, 177–179
Angioscopic sclerotherapy, 520
Angioscopy
  basic techniques of, 179–183

  for carotid endarterectomy, 187
  clinical applications of, 183–193
  completion, 185, 187
  equipment for, 177–179
  to evaluate operative procedure for arterial occlusion, 299–300
  general principles of, 181–183
  history of, 6
  indications for, 183–184
  infrainguinal bypass grafting and, 184
  instrumentation, techniques, and applications of, 177–194
  interpretation of, 183
  percutaneous applications of, 192–193
  for procedural assessment, 136–137
  of saphenous vein, 520, 522
  thromboembolectomy and, 192
  vascular access surgery and, 187, 189–191
  for vein preparation for bypass grafting, 187
  venous thrombectomy and, 192
Angiotensin II, 547
Angiotensin-converting enzyme inhibitors, 547
Ankle brachial index (ABI)
  to assess ischemia, 43–44
  after bypass surgery, 104
  as gauge of hemodynamic success, 93
  patient selection and, 51
Antegrade femoral artery puncture, 264
Antiarrhythmic agents
  arterial occlusion and, 292
  drug interactions and, 67–68
Anticholinergics, as premedicants, 60
Anticoagulation
  with early operative embolectomy, 292
  percutaneous access site complications and, 585–587
  postintervention regimens of, 586
  surgical incisions and, 266

Index

Antihistamines
  contrast reactions and, 147
  as tranquilizers, 60
Antihypertensive agents,
    common, drug
    interactions and, 67–68
Antiinflammatory agents,
    547–548
Antineoplastic drugs, delivery of,
    591–593
Antiplatelet agents, 545–546
  percutaneous access site
    complications and, 586
Antiproliferative agents, 547–548
Antisense oligodeoxynucleotides,
    548
Antithrombotic agents, 545–546
Aorta
  abdominal, evaluation of with
    ultrasound, 15
  atherosclerosis and, 23–25
  computed tomography and,
    46–48, 152–155
  descending thoracic, 383–389
  dissection of. *See* Aortic
    dissection
  enlargement of, 22
  incidence of occlusion and,
    290–291
  infrarenal abdominal, 21
  magnetic resonance imaging
    and, 48–49, 155–157
  occlusion of, 296, 299–300
  prosthesis for, 289–290
  thoracic, 21
  traumatic rupture of, 154
  See also Abdominal aortic
    aneurysm(s); Aortic
    aneurysm(s)
Aortic aneurysm(s)
  aortograms of, 47
  arterial emboli and, 289–290
  atherosclerosis and, 23–25
  computed tomography and,
    153–154
  computed tomography
    angiography and, 155
  intravascular ultrasound and,
    205, 207
  ultrasound and, 150
Aortic angioplasty, 278
Aortic arch, fluoroscopy and, 136
Aortic branch catheterization,
    femoral approach to,
    253–255
Aortic dissection
  computed tomography and,
    153
  computed tomography
    angiography and, 155
  intravascular ultrasound and,
    204–205
  ultrasound and, 151
Aortic occlusion, operative
    procedure for, 296,
    299–300
Aortic prostheses, arterial emboli
    and, 289–290
Aortic rupture, traumatic, 154
Aortic surgery, laparoscopic. *See*
    Laparoscopic aortic
    surgery
Aortoaortic EVT, 240
Aortobifemoral bypass grafting,
    279–280
Aortofemoral grafts, 486
Aortography
  of aortic aneurysm, 47
  in aortic branch
    catheterization, 251, 253
  in crossiliac catheter
    placement, 170
  development of, 4
Aortoiliac disease, 41–42
Aortoiliac grafts, 377–380, 485
Aortoiliac procedures,
    fluoroscopy and, 136
Aortouniiliac enograft, 485–486
Aprons, radiation protection
    provided by, 122
Argon laser eyewear needed
    with, 127
Arrhythmias, cardiac, 289
  anesthetic risk and, 82
Arterial bypass grafting,
    advantages of
    endarterectomy over,
    310–311, 313
Arterial bypass grafts, 467–471
Arterial access, 376–377
  prograde, 376
  retrograde, 376–377
  up and overp, 376
Arterial dilation, 377
Arterial disease
  aneurysmal, 481–488
  occlusive combined surgical
    and endovascular
    approaches to, 488–493
  stented graft revascularization
    for, 375–380
Arterial dissection, arterial
    puncture and, 248–249
Arterial embolectomy, 289
Arterial emboli, systemic,
    279–281
Arterial embolization and
    chemoembolization, 612
Arterial enlargement, in
    response to
    atherosclerosis, 22
Arterial infusion, of regional
    chemotherapy, 591–593
Arterial injury
  during catheterization, 248–249
  after balloon angioplasty, 283
  covered stents and, 371–372
  wall thickening after, 544–548
Arterial insufficiency, 41–42
Arterial lacerations, during
    catheterization, 248–249
Arterial ligation, 593
Arterial occlusion
  acute adjunctive procedures
    and, 301
  clinical presentation of,
    291–292
  evaluation of, 292–293
  preoperative management
    of, 292–293
  workup of, 292–293
  anatomic distribution of,
    290–291
  angioscopy to evaluate, 300
  antiarrhythmics and 279
  after balloon angioplasty,
    283–284
  of brachial artery, 290–291
  after catheterization or
    dilatation, 249
  digitalis and, 292
  diuretics and, 292
  embolic, 42
  etiologic diagnoses of, 462
  heart disease and, 292
  heparin and, 292
  of iliac artery, 278–279
  of mesenteric artery, 300
  operative procedure for, 296,
    299–300
  pathophysiology of, 289–291
  of popliteal artery, 300

Arterial occlusion (cont.)
   thrombotic, 42
   of visceral arteries, 290–291
Arterial occlusive disease
   endarterectomy for, 488
   stent graft revascularization for, 375–380
Arterial perforation, 283
Arterial perfusion, 604–611
Arterial puncture
   arterial dissection and, 248–249
   double-wall, 261, 262–263
   percutaneous, 261
   single-wall, 261, 264
Arterial repair, in response to balloon injury, 539–541
Arterial revascularization, 301, 375–380
   intraprocedural monitoring and, 93
Arterial rupture, as complication of balloon angioplasty, 283–284
Arterial thrombus, as complication of catheterization, 249
Arteriography, 3–4
Arteriotomy, 266
   carotid, and brachiocephalic stent deployment, 489
   combined with endoluminal repair of false aneurysms, 482–484
Arteriovenous fistula, 585
   chemotherapy treatment and, 592
   traumatic, 371–375
   treatment of, 585
Artery(ies)
   atherosclerotic
     occluded, 14
     reparative mechanisms in, 541–542
     response of wall in, 13–14
     well-adapted, 13
   axillary, percutaneous puncture of, 264
   brachial
     arterial occlusion and, 290–291
     percutaneous puncture of, 264
   carotid
     balloon angioplasty of, 282
     flow field changes at bifurcation of, 18
     occlusion of, 300
     plaque localization and, 21–23
   common iliac, balloon angioplasty of, 278–279
   coronary, plaque localization and, 21
   hepatic, 607–609
   infrapopliteal, angioplasty of, 280
   injury to
     balloon dilatation and, 544
     during catheterization, 248–249
     covered stents and, 371–372
     wall thickening after, 544–548
   innominate, balloon angioplasty of, 281
   intercostal, plaque localization and, 21
   mammary, plaque localization and, 21
   mesenteric
     balloon angioplasty of, 280–281
     evaluation of by ultrasound, 152
     occlusions of, 300
     plaque localization and, 21–23
     repair of, after balloon injury, 539–541
     response of wall of to plaque formation, 13–14
     stented, intimal hyperplasia in, 542–544
   subclavian
     balloon angioplasty and, 281
     percutaneous puncture of, 264, 265
   vertebral, balloon angioplasty and, 281–282
   visceral, occlusion of, 290–291
   wall shear stress in, 17–18
   See also Aorta; Femoral artery; Iliac artery; Popliteal artery; Renal artery
Artificial abdominal aortic aneurysm, 364
Aspirin, 545–546
Asthma, contrast reactions and, 147
Atherectomy
   as adjunct to thromboembolectomy, 302
   directional, 75, 309–310
   disobliteration techniques, 309–310
   dissections and, 309–310
   effect of high-speed rotational, 211–212
   evaluation of by intravascular ultrasound, 210–212
   history of, 7–8
   restenosis and, 310
   success of, 93
Atherectomy catheters, 309–310
AtheroCath, 309–310, 311
Atherogenesis, 545
Atherosclerosis
   abdominal aorta and, 22
   aneurysms and, 23–25
   in animal models, 14–15, 25
   arterial enlargement in response to, 22
   balloon angioplasty and, 278
   cigarette smoking and, 11, 23
   coronary, 20
   diabetes mellitus and, 11
   hemodynamic influences in, 17–21
   hyperlipidemia and, 11
   hypertension and, 11, 20–21
   intravascular ultrasound and, 204–205
   process of, 11–17
Atherosclerotic heart disease, 289. *See also* Atherosclerosis
Atracurium, 65, 74
Auth Rotablator, 309–310, 312
Axial imaging applications, 153–154
Axillary artery, percutaneous puncture of, 264

Backbleeding, 300
Balloon angioplasty
   aortic, 278
   atherosclerosis and, 278
   of brachiocephalic vessels, 281–282
   of carotid artery, 282

Index

catheters used during, 225–227, 272–274
of common iliac artery, 278–279
compared with Wallstent, 340
complications of, 282–284
equipment for, 270–274
history of, 6–7, 269
indications for, 269–270
of infrapopliteal vessels, 280
of innominate arteries, 281
lesions best suited for, 270
mechanism of, 269
of mesenteric arteries, 280–281
psuedoaneurysm and, 283
of renal arteries, 280–281
of subclavian arteries, 281
technique of, 278
vasodilators in, 275, 276
of vertebral artery, 281–282
versus stent graft revascularization, 375–380
Balloon catheter thromboembolectomy, 457
Balloon catheters
hydrogel-coated, 567, 572, 573–574
for local drug delivery, 567–570
Wolinsky, 567–570
See also Catheters
Balloon dilatation
arterial injury and, 544–545
Balloon dilation catheter, ultra-thin polyethelene terephthalate, 274
Balloon expansion
to deploy intraluminal graft, 366
to deploy stems, 366
Balloon materials, 223–224
Balloon mechanics, 222–223
Balloon sizes, typical, 276
Balloon ultrasound imaging catheter, 209
Balloon-centering technique, popliteal puncture and, 258
Balloon-in-a-balloon, 569–570
Balloons
angioplasty, 272–274
biomaterials considerations for, 222–227
microporous, 568
transport, 568

Basic fibroblast growth factor, 541
Bentson wire, 250, 251, 253
Berenstein catheter, 250, 251
Beuhler, William J., 232
Bicitra, 60
Biocompatibility, of endovascular devices, 227–230
Biomaterials considerations for endovascular devices, 219–246
Bird's Nest filter, 404
Bladder cancer, 611
Blaisdell technique of aneurysm exclusion, 362
Blood exposure, 128
Bone marrow suppression, 606
Brachial artery
arterial occlusion and, 290–291
catheterization of, fluoroscopy and, 130
percutaneous puncture of, 264
Brachiocephalic vessels, balloon angioplasty and, 281–282
Brachytherapy, 548, 555
Brain tumors, 610–611
Bretylium, 68
Brodie-Trendelenburg test, 515
Buerger's sign, 42
Bupivacaine, 65
Butorphanol, 61–62
Bypass
femoropopliteal, 488
iliofemoral, 488
postintervention surveillance and, 103–118
venous, 314
Bypass graft(s)
arterial, 467–471
versus endarterectomy, 310–311, 312
versus PTA of subclavian and innominate ateries(ies), 420–421
Bypass graft stenosis, angioplasty and, 282
Bypass grafting
aortobifemoral, 279–280
infrainguinal, 184–187
vein preparation for, 187
Bypass procedures
ankle-brachial index after, 104
for occlusive arterial disease, 488

C-arm fluoroscopy, 35, 135, 266
c-myc phosphothioate antisense, 568
Calcium antagonists, 546
Calcium channel blockers, 547
Calcium entry blockers, drug interactions and, 67
Cancer
of bladder, 611
of head, neck, and brain, 610–611
history of chemotherapy for, 505–593
of liver, 607–609, 612, 613–614
pelvic, 611, 614
prostate, 611
Carbon, 231
Carbon dioxide contrast, 148–149
Cardiac arrhythmias, arterial emboli and, 289
Cardiac catheterization
adult, anesthesia and, 75–76
history of, 4–5, 577
Cardiac disease, contrast reaction and, 147
Cardiac catheterization suite, anesthesia in, 74–76
Cardiac procedures associated with thromboembolectomy, 302, 303
Cardiomyopathy, arterial emboli and, 289
Carotid and Vertebral Artery Translunimal Angioplasty Study, 440
Carotid angioplasty and stenting
balloon angioplasty of, 282, 435–437, 440
clinical results, 440–441
indications for, 429–432, 433
techniques for, 432–440
access, 433–440
anesthesia, 432–433
Carotid artery
flow field changes at bifurcation of, 18
magnetic resonance imaging and, 48–49, 155–157
occlusions of, 300
plaque localization at bifurcation of, 21–23
See also Carotid angioplasty and stenting

Carotid duplex scanning, 151, 435
Carotid endarterectomy, 187
  ultrasound and, 151
Carotid procedures, anesthesia for, 70–85
Carotid sinus
  flow field changes and, 18
  oscillation of flow and, 19–20
Catheter(s)
  adherent clot, 295–296, 298
  angiographic, 250–255
  for atherectomy, 309–310
  balloon angioplasty, 272–274
  balloon dilation, 274
  balloon ultrasound imaging, 209
  biomaterials considerations for, 222–227
  central balloon, 557, 558
  Channel Balloon, 567, 572
  crossiliac placement of, 255–258
  Dispatch, 567, 572–573
  for embolectomy, 293–296
  Fogarty balloon embolectomy, 293–295
  graft thrombectomy, 296, 298–299
  Groshong, 35
  history of, 591–593
  hockey stick, 251, 253
  imager, 251
  in intravascular ultrasound, 195, 196
  laser angioplasty, 354–355
  Microporous Infusion, 567, 568–569
  pigtail, 251, 253, 272, 273
  preformed, 251
  selection of
    for chemotherapy, 593–595
    in pediatric patients, 594
  Simmons, 251, 253
  Simpson, 309–310, 311
  Straight, 251
  TEGwire, 274, 275
  tennis racquet, 272, 273
  thru-lumen, 293–294
  transluminal extraction, 8
  transport, 567, 569–570
  types of for balloon angioplasty, 225–227, 272–274
  Wolinsky, 567–570

See also Central venous catheter
Catheter skills, 247–255
Catheter thromboembolectomy, 289–308
Catheterization
  of aortic branch, 253–255
  arterial lacerations during, 248–249
  arterial occlusion after, 249
  central venous, 600–601
  of cephalic vein, 595
  contrast injection and, 252
  crossiliac, 255–258
  of external jugular vein, 595
  of femoral vein, 600, 601
  of internal jugular vein, 595, 598
  principles and axioms of, 249–250
  pseudoaneurysm and, 248
  of subclavian vein, 595, 596–598
  superficial femoral artery occlusion and, 255, 258
Cathscanner, 137
Caval filters, biomaterials considerations and, 227–230
Celiac axis, evaluation of, 152
Centering balloon catheter, 557, 558
Central venous catheter(s)
  approaches for inserting, 595–603
  chemotherapy and, 593–604
  peripheral insertion of, 603–604
  Silastic, 592
  sites for placement of, 595
Central venous monitoring, intraoperatively, 138
Cephalic vein
  open access to, 602
  percutaneous catheterization via, 595
Certified registerd nurse anesthetists (CRNAs), 81
Cervical plexus block, 72
Channel Balloon Catheter, 567, 572
Chemoembolization, 593, 612
Chemotherapy
  central venous catheter and, 593–604
  endovascular delivery of, 591–619
  history of, for cancer, 591–593
  intraarterial, 604–611
  isolation perfusion of, 592–593
  regional, arterial infusion of, 592–593
  selection of catheter for, 593–595
Chemotoxic reactions to contrast media, 147
Children
  anesthesia management and, 75
  catheter selection in, 594
  open saphenous vein access in, 602–603
2-Chloroprocaine, 65
Choriocarcinoma, 604
Chromium, 231
  corrosion resistance and, 228
  toxicity of, 228–229
Chronic arterial insufficiency, 41–42
Chronic venous insufficiency, 516
Cigarette smoking
  atherosclerosis and, 11, 23
  patient selection and, 51
Cilazapril, 546, 547
Cineradiography, 146
Cisplatin, 610
Citrovorum, 606
Cladding, 177–178
Claudication, 41–42
Clonidine, 68
Clothesline effect, dilating force and, 223
CO_2, laser, eyewear needed with, 127
Cobalt, toxicity of, 229
Cobalt-chromium alloys, 231, 233
Cobra-head catheter, 251, 253
Cocaine, 65
Coherency, of laser light, 124–125
Colchicine, 546
Collagen devices, to manage percutaneous puncture site, 578, 579–580
Collagenase, 23
Collimation, 122
Color-flow imaging, 45, 152
Commissural space, 520
Compartment pressures, venous dysfunction and, 526–527

Completion angioscopy, 185, 187, 191–191
Compression devices, external, 578, 586
Computed tomography (CT), 152–155
 in assessment of aortic aneurysm, 46–48, 152–153
 metallic implants and, 233
 peripheral vascular disease and, 154
 three-dimensional, 154–155
 ultrafast, 48
 vascular applications of, 6
 See also Spiral computed tomography
Computed tomography angiography (CTA)
 aortic aneurysm and dissection and, 152–153
 spiral, 48–49, 109, 111, 114
 See also Spiral computed tomography
Computerized image reconstruction, and intravascular ultrasound, 200–201
Congestive heart failure
 anesthetic risk and, 82
 after balloon angioplasty, 284
Continuous quality improvement (CQI), 85
Continuous-pulse amplitude monitor, 292, 293
Continuous-wave Doppler, 43
Contrast injection, catheterization and, 252
Contrast media
 and digital subtraction angiography, 150
 endovascular training and, 35–36
 to evaluate balloon angioplasty results, 278
 and film screen angiography, 143–144
 iodinated, angiography and, 146–148
 risks associated with, 94
 systemic adverse reactions to, 146–148
Contrast phlebography, of veins, 516

Copper, toxicity of, 229
Coronary artery(ies)
 atherosclerosis and, 21–23
 use of stents in, 209–210
Coronary artery disease, postoperative ischemia and, 82
Corrosion fatigue, 229
Corrosion resistance, 228
Corticosteroids, 546
 contrast reactions and, 147–148
Corvita endovascular graft, 365, 374–375
Coumadin, 313, 317
Cournand, Andre, 4–5
CQI. See Continuous quality improvement
Cragg nitinol spiral IVC filter, 232
Cragg stent
 characteristics of, 234
 endoluminal grafts and, 365
 radiologic considerations and, 233
 spiral, 234, 234
Cragg Thrombolytic Brush, 305, 306
Credentialing, in endovascular surgery, 33–39
Crevice corrosion, 228
CRNAs. See Certified registerd nurse anesthetists
Crookes' tube, 119
Crossability, as catheter characteristic, 225–226
Crossiliac catheter placement, 255–258
Crossover grafts, extraluminal, 481–482
CT. See Computed tomography
CTA. See Computed tomography angiography
Cutdown techniques, for central venous catheter insertion, 599–600
Cytostatic drugs, 547

da Vinci, Leonardo, 3
Dacron, for endovascular grafts, 236–242
Dacron graft, 364–365
 as temporary conduit, 481
Dactinomycin, 547
De Weese, M.S., 8

DeBakey standard knit vascular graft, 238–239
DeBakey woven Dacron vascular graft, 238–239
Deep venous thrombosis
 duplex ultrasonography and, 45–46
 iliofemoral, 493
 lytic treatment, 405
 magnetic resonance imaging and, 157
 vascular ultrasound and, 152
Derume, Jean-Pierre, 374
Desflurane, 64, 74
Diabetes mellitus
 anesthetic risk and, 82
 atherosclerosis and, 11, 23
 contrast reaction and, 147
 patient selection and, 51
 postoperative ischemia and, 82
Dialysis fistulas, ultrasound and, 152
Diastole, shear stress and, 19–20
Diazepam, 60, 62–63, 68, 71, 73
Digital pressures, 43–44
Digital subtraction angiography, 144, 145, 150, 266
Digitalis, 292
Digoxin, 82
Dilator-sheath mismatch, 248–249
Diltiazem, 67
Dipyridamole thallium scintigraphy, 82
Direct current procedures, 76
Directional atherectomy, 75, 309–310
 role of anesthesiologist in, 75
Directionality, of laser light, 124–125
Disobliteration techniques, 309–319
Dispatch Catheter, 567, 572–573
Dissection
 arterial, 249
 atherectomy and, 309–301
 of descending thoracic aorta, 383–389
 iliac, 284
 subintimal, 283–284
Dissociation of apposition from drug delivery, 570–574
Distal stent-graft implantation, 394, 396

Diuretics
　arterial occlusion and, 292
　drug interactions and, 67
Doppler, continuous wave, 43
Doppler flowmetry, 98–99
Doppler spectral analysis, 149–152
Doppler ultrasound, to localize occlusion, 292
Doppler wave recordings, 149–150, 152
Dos Santos, Cid, 309
Dos Santos, Raynaldo, 3, 4, 5
Dotter, Charles, 6–8
Double-wall arterial puncture, 261, 262–263
Doxacurium, 65, 74
Doxorubicin, 547
Droperidol, 60, 68
Drug delivery
　dissociation of apposition from, 570–574
　local, 565–576
Drug interactions, 66–68
Duplex ultrasound, 149
　carotid, 151
　after endarterectomy, 314, 316–317
　to evaluate limb ischemia, 44–46
　intraoperatively, 97–98
　of veins, 516
Dypridamole, 545
Dypyridamole thallium imaging, 51

Ebselen, 547–548
Echocardiography, transesophageal, 156
Edema, after revascularization, 302
Edison, Thomas A., 120
EDRF. *See* Endothelial-derived relaxing factor
Eichelter Sieve, withdrawal from market, 405
Einstein, Albert, 123
Elastase, 23
Elastic modulus, of metals used in endovascular implants, 231
Elastic recoil, 321
Elderly patients
　anesthetic risk and, 82

atherosclerosis and, 12
thrombectomy and reconstruction and, 301
Electromagnetic flowmetry, 99
Elgiloy, 231
Elongation, of metal used in endovascular implants, 231
Embolectomy
　anticoagulation and, 292
　arterial, 289
　history of, 6
　instrumentation for, 293–296
　pulmonary. 403–405
　See also Thromboembolectomy
Embolectomy catheters, 293–296
Emboli
　definition of, 289
　"paradoxical," 277
　removal of with catheter, 293, 295
　See also Thromboembolus
Embolization and chemoembolization, 612
Endarterectomy
　advantages of, 310–311, 312
　femoral, 302, 489, 490, 491
　Mollring Cutter remote, 314–316
　for occlusive arterial disease, 488
　proximal, 302
　results of, 313–314
　semiclosed, 310, 311, 313
　surveillance and medication after, 316–318
　technique of, 313
　transluminal 137, 309–314
　versus venous bypass, 314
Endocarditis, infectious, 289–290
Endoluminal endoscopy, 517, 519–520
Endoluminal grafts, 141–142
　abdominal aortic aneurysms and, 362
　aortofemoral, 485
　aortoiliac, 485
　designs of, 241
　evolution in design of, 364–367
　first, 363–364
　healing characteristics of, 239–240
　transluminal insertion of, 488–489

See also Grafts
Endoluminal radiation therapy, 555–563
　delivery
　　mechanism of, 559
　　site of, 559
　　timing of, 559
　and peripheral vessels, 560
　radiation source, 558, 559, 560
Endoluminal sclerotherapy, 517, 519–520
Endoluminal stent-graft(s), 371
Endoluminal venous stripping, 517, 518
Endoluminal venous surgery, 515–529
Endoscopic transaxillary first rib resection, 531–538
　complications of, 537–538
　incisions, 532
　limitations of, 537
　positions, 532
　scalenus muscles, disengagement of, 534
　surgical space
　　creation of, 532, 533
　　maintenance of, 534
Endoscopy
　endoluminal, 517, 519–520
　subfascial, 525–527
Endothelial ingrowth, 540
Endothelial injury, plaque initiation and, 11–12
Endothelial layer, regeneration of, 540–541
Endothelial-derived relaxing factor (EDRF), 17
Endothelium, sources of, 540–541
Endovascular and surgical approaches, combined, 481–495
Endovascular chemotherapy delivery, 591–619
Endovascular devices
　biomaterials considerations for, 219–256
　design characteristics of, 233–236, 240–242
　healing characteristics of, 229–230
　intraoperative applications of, 266
　See also specific device

Endovascular diagnostics,
    significant developments
    in, 3–6
Endovascular facilities, 54–55
Endovascular graft(s)
    biomaterials considerations of,
        236–240
    intravascular ultrasound and,
        211–212
    prevention of lesion
        recurrence and, 539–549
    radial compliance of, 236
    tensile yield strength of, 238
    types of, 141–142
Endovascular intervention
    complications of, 445–454
        access-related, 446–453
        axillary-brachial access
            techniques, 453
        common, 445–446
        imaging related, 453–454
    criteria of success for, 93–94,
        105
Endovascular physicians, 54
Endovascular practice,
    components of, 128
Endovascular procedures
    anesthesia for, 59–91
    quality assurance of, 55
Endovascular service,
    establishment of, 53–58
Endovascular stent-grafts,
    375–380
Endovascular suite, operational
    plans of, 55–57
Endovascular surgery, training
    and credentialing in,
    33–39
EndoVascular Technologies
    (EVT), 367
EndoVascular Technologies
    Prosthesis, 367
Endovascular therapeutics, 3–4,
    6–10
Endovascular therapy, 3–10
    indications for, 41–52
Endovascular training, 33–39
Endovenous obliteration,
    520–523
    monopolar electrocautery, 521
    VNUS system, 521–522
Endovenous surgery, 515–529
Endovenous thrombosis, 523
Enflurane, 63, 73

Epidural analgesia, 78
Epidural hematoma, 76
Epinephrine, 147
Equipment
    for angioscopy, 177–179
    for balloon angioplasty,
        270–272
    basic, in endovascular suite,
        134–138
    for embolectomy, 293–296
    of endovascular suite, 57
    related to special procedures,
        135–139
Esters, 65–66
Etidocaine, 65
Etomidate, 62
European Wallstent Peripheral
    Artery Implant Study,
    336–338
EVT. See EndoVascular
    Technologies
EVT Prosthesis, 367
Excimer laser angioplasty,
    353–359
Expandable Access Sheath,
    303–304
External beam radiotherapy, 555
External compression devices,
    578, 586
External jugular vein
    open access to, 601–602
    percutaneous catheterization
        via, 595
Extraluminal crossover grafts,
    481–482
Extremity
    malignant tumors, 609–610, 612
    threatened, 42
    viable, 42
Eye, effect of laser light on, 127
Eyewear, lasers and, 127

False aneurysm. See
    Pseudoaneurysm
Famotidine, 60
Fasciotomy, 526–527
Fatigue ensurance limit, of metal
    used in endovascular
    implants, 231
Femoral artery
    aneurysms of, 45
    angioplasty of, 136–137,
        279–280
    antegrade puncture of, 264

    complications of access of,
        585–587
    incidence of arterial occlusion
        and, 290
    intravascular ultrasound and,
        200, 302
    management of puncture site
        and, 578
    occlusion of, operative
        procedure for, 300
    percutaneous puncture of,
        247–248
    and repair of secondary
        endoleaks, 486, 487
    retrograde puncture of, 264
    stent deployment in, 339
    stents and, 339
    Strecker stent in, 341
    superficial
        balloon sizes for, 276
        development of
            atherosclerosis and, 23
        intravascular ultrasound
            image of, 201, 203
        transluminal endarterectomy
            of, 309–314
    See also Access site
Femoral endarterectomy, 302
Femoral puncture, and
    endovascular intervention,
    446–447
Femoral vein
    percutaneous catheterization
        via, 598, 600
    and valve repair, 522
Femoropopliteal bypass, 488
Femoropopliteal percutaneous
    transluminal angioplasty,
    93
Fentanyl, 61, 72–73, 73
Fibrous cap
    erosion of, 15, 16
    formation of, 13
Film badge, radiation safety and,
    122
Film screen angiography (FSA),
    143–144
Filters
    design characteristics of,
        235–236
    Greenfield, 231, 232, 235
Fish oils, 547–548
Fixed-wire balloon catheter
    systems, 226, 227

Flexibility, of stents, 235
Flexor guiding sheath, 438, 439
Flow, oscillation of, plaque pathogenesis and, 19–20
Flow field changes, plaque pathogenesis and, 18
Flow separation and stasis, 18
Flumazenil, 60, 63, 73
Fluoroscope, invention of, 120–121
Fluoroscopic units, 35, 134–136
Fluoroscopy, 120–121, 134–136, 266
  radiation protection and, 121–122
  video, 146
Fogarty, Thomas, 6
Fogarty balloon embolectomy catheter, 293–295
Fogarty-Chin extrusion balloon, 227
Fragmin R. 402
Fretting corrosion, 228
FSA. See Film screen angiography

Galen, 3
Galvanic corrosion, 228
Gelbfish Endo-Vac System, 306, 307
General anesthesia
  for abdominal procedures, 76
  for carotid procedures, 74
  children and, 75
  induction agents for, 62–63
  for intracranial procedures, 74
  for lower extremity procedures, 76
Germ cell cancer, 604
Gianturco, Cesare, 364
Gianturco-Roehm Bird's Nest filter, 235
Gianturco coils, 231
Gianturco self-expanding stent, 338
Gianturco Zeta stent, 231, 323–324
  characteristics of, 234, 234–235
  Dacron graft attached to, 364–365
  nylon graft attached to, 364–366
  radiologic considerations and, 233–235
  use of in veins, 524
Gianturco-Roubin stent, 231, 323–324
  characteristics of, 233–235
Glioblastoma multiforme, 610
Glycopyrrolate, 60
Gold, corrosion resistance and, 228
Graduate Medical Education Directory, 33
Graft(s)
  aortofemoral, 485
  aortoiliac, 437–438
  arterial bypass, 467–471
  biomaterials considerations of, 236–240
  Corvita, 365, 374–375
  crossover, 481–482
  dialysis, 405–406
  intravascular ultrasound and, 211–212
  prosthetic versus vein, 467
  synthetic vascular, 542–544
  venous, 467
  See also Endoluminal grafts; Endovascular grafts; Intraluminal grafts
Graft stenosis, bypass, 282
Graft surveillance, 143
Graft thrombectomy catheter, 296, 298–299
Graft thrombosis, 467
Greenfield filter, 231, 232, 233, 235, 403, 406
Groshong catheter, 35
Gruntzig, Andreas, 7
Guanethidine, 68
GUIDE study, 212
Guidewire(s)
  and balloon angioplasty, 270–272
  biomaterials considerations for, 219–222
  complications of, 266
  endovascular training and, 36
  for percutaneous transluminal angioplasty, 270–272
  slippery, 219–220
  specialty, 250
  standard, 250
  steerable, 219–220, 250
  stiff, 270, 271
Guidewire-catheter mismatch, 248–249

Guiding catheters, 272
Gunter Thrombectomy Catheter, 305
Gunther filter, 405–406

H_2 receptor antagonists, 60
Hagan-Poiseuille formula, 17
Halothane, 63–64, 73
Harvey, 3
Head and neck cancer, 610–611
Healing characteristics of endovascular devices, 229–230
Heart disease, arterial occlusion and, 292
Heart rate, coronary atherosclerosis and, 20, 22
Hematoma, 585
  after balloon angioplasty, 283
  epidural, risk of, 76
  formation of, after arterial puncture, 247
  after percutaneous vascular access, 264
  spinal, risk of, 77
Hemodialysis, 606
Hemodynamic influences in atherosclerosis, 17–21
Hemodynamic monitoring
  intraoperative, 98–100
  pull-back pressures, 98
  transcranial Doppler ultrasonography, 98–99
Hemostatic introducer sheath, 266
Heparin, 546–547
  arterial occlusion and, 292
  Dispatch Catheter and, 572–573
  endarterectomy and, 313
  percutaneous access site complications and, 586
  valvulotomy and, 185–188
Hepatic artery, placement of catheters in, 607–609
High-dose isolated limb perfusion, 471–474, 475
High dose rate (HDR) afterloader, 556, 558, 559, 560
Hippocrates, 3
Hirudin, 547
Hockey-stick catheter, 251, 253, 251, 253

Index

Hodgkin's lymphoma, 604
Hoop stress, 223
Huberneedle, 603
Hydralazine, 68
Hydrogel-coated balloon
    catheter, 567, 572, 573–574
Hydrogels, 573
Hydroxyzine, 60
Hyperlipidemia, atherosclerosis
    and, 11
Hyperplasia, intimal. See Intimal
    hyperplasia
Hypertension
    abdominal aortic aneurysms
        and, 361
    anesthetic risk and, 82
    atherosclerosis and, 11, 20–21
    postoperative ischemia and,
        82
Hyperthermic regional perfusion,
    592–593
Hypertrophy, left ventricular, 82

Iliac artery(ies)
    angioplasty of, 93, 278–279,
        333–334
    balloon sizes for, 276
    common, balloon angioplasty
        of, 278–279
    computed tomography
        angiography and, 155
    dissection of, 284, 485
    incidence of arterial occlusion
        and, 290
    intravascular ultrasound, and,
        199–200, 205, 207
    operative procedure for
        occlusion of, 296, 299–300
    and Palmaz stent, 334, 336
    primary stenting of lesions of,
        338–339
    sequential approach, 489, 491,
        493
    stents and, 333–334
    Strecker stent in, 341
Iliofemoral bypass, 488
Iliofemoral deep vein
    thrombosis, 493
Iliofemoral vessels, plaque
    localization and, 21
Image production systems,
    143–159
Imager catheters, 251
Imaging systems, 143–159

two-dimensional, 137, 200–202,
    200–202
three-dimensional, 200–201,
    205–208
Impedance plethysmography, 516
In situ vein conduit preparation,
    184–187
Infection, wound, surgical
    incisions and, 266
Infectious endocarditis, 289–20
Inferior vena caval filters,
    403–410
    central lines, 407
    dialysis grafts, 405–406
    guidewire, use of, 407
    lytic treatment, 405
    pediatric patients, 407–408
    pulmonary embolectomy,
        403–404
    subclavian vein thrombosis,
        406
    thrombolysis, 405–406
Infiltration catheter, 574
Infrainguinal bypass grafting,
    angioscopy and, 184–187
Infrapopliteal angioplasty, 280
Infrared lasers, 124–125
Infrarenal flow volume, 22
Infusion port, 603
Infusion Sleeve, 568, 570–572
Innominate arteries, balloon
    angioplasty of, 281. See
    also Subclavian
    artery(ies), and PTA
Intercorunal or commissural
    space, 520
Intercostal arteries, plaque
    localization and, 21
Interface corrosion, 228
Intergranular corrosion, 229
Internal jugular vein
    open access to, 600–601
    percutaneous catheterization
        via, 595, 598
International Carotid Stent
    Survey, 440–441
International Society for
    Cardiovascular Surgery,
    104
Intimal flaps
    formation of, 264
    intravascular ultrasound and,
        204–205
Intimal hyperplasia

hemodynamic factors affecting,
    545
pharmacologic agents to
    reduce, 545
in stented arteries and
    synthetic vascular grafts,
    542–544
Intraarterial chemotherapy,
    604–611
Intraarterial digital subtraction
    angiography, 144
Intraarterial monitoring,
    intraoperatively, 137
Intracoronary stent placement,
    role of anesthesiologist in,
    75–76
Intracranial arteries, fluoroscopy
    and, 136
Intracranial procedures,
    anesthesia approach to,
    70–74
Intraluminal bypass
    abdominal aortic aneurysms
        and, 371–380
    historical perspectives of,
        361–365
    Parodi, 366–367, 371–373
    See also Grafts
Intraluminal ring grafts, 362–
    363
Intraluminal ultrasound, 96–97
Intraprocedural monitoring,
    93–102
Intravascular access, devices and
    techniques for, 259–267
Intravascular stent(s), 321–351.
    See also Stents,
    intravascular ultrasound
    and, 209–210
Intravascular ultrasound (IVUS),
    195–216
    atherosclerosis and, 204–205
    catheters used in, 195–197
    computerized image
        reconstruction and,
        200–201
    current clinical utility of, 201,
        204–213
    device design and function in,
        195–196
    diagnostic capabilities of, 201,
        204–208
    endovascular grafts and,
        211–212

Intravascular ultrasound (*cont.*)
  evaluation of atherectomy by, 210–212
  fixed versus rotational transducers in, 196–197
  future developments in, 213
  history of, 6
  image acquisition and, 197–200
  for procedural assessment, 137
  therapeutic interventions of, 208–213
  three-dimensional, 200–201, 205–207
  two-dimensional, 200–202
  vascular access and, 195–199
  versus angiography, 201, 204–205
Intravenous digital subtraction angiography, 146
Introducer sheaths, 259, 270, 271
  arteriotomy and, 266
  complications of, 267
  and femoral puncture, 449, 451, 452
  in Palmaz stent deployment, 324, 325
  placement, complications of, 266
Ionic contrast, 147
Ionic dimer, 146
Ionic monomer, 146
Iontophoresis Balloon, 567, 573–574
Iron, toxicity of, 229
Irreversible ischemia, 42
Irrigation, saline, principles of, 179–181
Irrigation pump, dedicated, 181
Ischemia
  acute limb, 457–467
  amputation and, 292
  advanced, 301–302
  chronic limb, categories of, 94
  irreversible, 42
  of lower extremity, 41–42
  noninvasive studies to assess degree of, 42–43
  postoperative, 82–83
  Rochester trial, 462–464
  segmental pressures to assess, 43–44
  STILE study of, 464–465
  TOPAS trial, 465–467
Ischemic rest pain, 41, 42

Isoflurane, 63, 73
  use of with children, 75
Isolated perfusion, 612
Isolation perfusion, 592–593, 606
IVUS. *See* Intravascular ultrasound

Jugular vein, external
  pen access to, 601–602
  percutaneous catheterization via, 595
Jugular vein, internal
  open access to, 600–601
  percutaneous catheterization via, 595, 598

Kaplan-Simpson Infusosleeve, 586
Karmody technique of aneurysm exclusion, 362
Ketamine, 68
  use of with children, 75
Ketanserin, 546
Ketorolac, 78
"Kissing balloon" technique, 278

Laparoscopic aortic surgery, 497–513
  and abdominal aortic aneurysms, 509–511
  clinical findings, 503–509
  feasibility of, 498–499
  history of, 499–500
  retroperitoneal approach, 501–503
  techniques, pneumoperitoneum versus gasless, 500–501
Laser ablation, role of anesthesiologist in, 75
Laser angioplasty
  catheters for, 354–355
  with excimer laser, 353–359
  history of, 353
  peripheral, 353–360
  success of, 93, 355–358
Laser light, characteristics of, 124–126
Laser safety, 126–128
Lasers
  advantages of, 125–126
  classes of, 127

  clinical studies, 355
  healing response to, 355–358
  physics of, 123–126
  pulsed, 354
  studies of, 355–358
  ultraviolet pulsed, 125
Left ventricular hypertrophy, 82
Lesion morphology, intravascular ultrasound and, 208
Lesion recurrence. *See* Restenosis
Leukemia, 604
  nitrogen mustard and, 591, 605
Leveen inflators with pressure gauge, 274, 275
Lidocaine, 65, 275, 276
Ligation, 592, 516–517
Limb ischemia
  acute, 457–467
  chronic, 94
Limb perfusion, isolated
  high-dose, 471–474, 475
  with thrombolytic agents, 488–489
Limb salvage
  and role of angioplasty, 423–427
    patient cohort, 423–424
    pharmacologic adjuncts, 424
    procedure, 424–425
    threatened vein grafts, 425
    results, 425–426
    techniques, alternative, 425
Linear array color transducer, 149–150
Liver tumors, 607–609, 612, 613–614
Local anesthetics, 65–66
Local drug delivery, 565–576
Local/Med InfusaSleeve, 567
Lorazepam, 60
Lovastatin, 546
Lower extremity procedures, anesthesia for, 76–78
Luminal injury, 269
Lymphoma
  Hodgkin's, 604
  nitrogen mustard and, 591, 605
Lytic agents, 455–480
Lytic therapy, systemic, 302–303

Magnetic resonance angiography (MRA)

advantages and disadvantages of, 155–157
applications of, 156–157
assessment of vascular patients with, 48–51
Magnetic resonance imaging (MRI)
advantages and disadvantages of, 155–157
applications of, 156–157
deep vein thrombosis and, 157
Metallic implants and, 233
vascular applications of, 6
of veins, 516
Malignant tumors, extremity, 609–610, 612. *See also* Tumor
Mammary artery, plaque localization and, 21
Manual pressure, to manage percutaneous puncture site, 578, 586
Maximum intensity projection, 155
Maximum permissible dose (MPD) guidelines, 121–122
May-Thurner syndrome, 525
Mechanical properties of specific metals, 231–233
Medial injury, and wall-thickening, 539–540
Medial thinning, in response to atherosclerosis, 23–24
Meperidine, 61
use of with children, BO-;
Mepivicaine, 65
Mercury strain gauge, 516
Mesenteric artery(ies)
balloon angioplasty of, 280–281
evaluation of by ultrasound, 152
occlusions of, 300
plaque localization and, 21
Metalloproteinases, 23
Methotrexate, 568
Metoclopramide, 60
Microporous balloon, 568–569
Miicroporous Infusion Catheter (MIC), 567, 568–569
Midazolam, 60, 63, 71, 73
use of with children, 75
Minoxidil, 68
Mivacurium, 65

Mobin-Uddin device, 403
Modular stent-graft contralateral leg, 394, 395
Molecular mechanisms controlling wall mass and Lumen diameter, 541
Mollring Cutter, 314–316
Mollring Cutter remote endarterectomy, 314–316
Molybdenum, 229, 231
Moniz, 3–4
Monochromaticity, of laser light, 124–125
Monopolar electrocautery, 521
Monorail balloon catheter systems, 226, 227
Morphine, 60, 61, 292
MRA. *See* Magnetic resonance angiography
MRI. *See* Magnetic resonance imaging
Muscle relaxants, 64–65
Myocardial infarction
anesthetic risk and, 82
after balloon angioplasty, 284
hypertension and, 20–21
thrombolytic agents and, 565–566
Myoglobinuria, 302
Myointimal proliferation, 310–311

Nalbuphine, 62
NeoCardia/Guidant's afterloader, 558, 560
Neostigmine, 68
Nephropathy, contrast-induced, 148
Neuromuscular blocking agents, 64–65
Nicardipine, 67
Nickel, 229, 231
Nifedipine, 67, 275, 276, 547
Nimodipine, 74
Nitinol
for endoluminal grafts, 363
mechanical and physical properties of, 231, 232–233
stents made of, 230, 323–324
toxicity of, 229
Nitrogen mustard, 591, 605
Nitroglycerin, 66, 249, 275, 276
Nitrous oxide, 64
Nonionic contrast, 147

Nonionic dimers, 146
Nonionic monomer, 146
Noninvasive studies of ischemia, 42–43
Nonreversed vein, 184
Nonsteroidal antiinflammatory drugs (NSAIDs), 77, 547
Novoste Beta-Cath System, 558, 559
NSAIDs. *See* Nonsteroidal antiinflammatory drugs
Nucletron HDR afterloader, 558, 560
Nylon
balloons made of, 224
as catheter material, 251
expandable grafts made of, 365–366

Occlusion(s)
aortic, 296, 299–300
iliac, 296, 299–300
of upper extremity, 300
See also Arterial occlusion
Occlusive arterial disease,
combined surgical and endovascular approaches for, 481–495
endarterectomy for, 488
endovascular reporting standards for, 104–105
endovascular treatment of, surveillance protocols, 105–107
stented graft revascularization for, 375–380
Oligodeoxynucleotides, antisense, 548
Open surgical incisions, to access vessel, 259, 266, 599–601
Open surgical techniques
of angioscopically directed valvulotomy, 184–186
for central venous catheter insertion, 599–601
wound infection and, 266
Operating room, requirements of with C-arm fluoroscopy unit, 135
Opioids, 61–62
Oscillating shear stress pastern, 19–20
Oscillation of flow, plaque pathogenesis and, 19–20

Osteoarthritis, compared with claudication, 41–42
Over-the-wire balloon catheter systems, 226, 227
Oximetry, transcutaneous, to evaluate limb ischemia, 44

Pain management, postoperative, 78–79
Palmaz, Julio, 8–9, 364
Palmaz stent, 230, 322–323
  characteristics of, 234, 234–235
  corrosion resistance of, 228
  complications with, 344
  covered, 371–372
  with Dacron tube, 366–367
  deployment of, 324–327, 328
  endarterectomy and, 314
  radiologic considerations and, 233–235
  in renal artery, 341–342
  in veins, 524
Pancuronium, 64, 74
Papaverine, 99
Parodi, Juan C., 9, 371–373
Parodi intraluminal grafts, 366–367, 371–373
Parodi stem-graft devices, 371–373
Particle residence time, plaque pathogenesis and, 19
Pathophysiology, of vascular disease, 11–29
Patient(s)
  assessment of, 41–52
  and distal angioplasty, 423–424
  evaluation of, preanesthetic, 83
  follow-up and monitoring, 57, 71–72
  pediatric. *See* Pediarric patients
  scheduling of, 56
  selection of, 56–57, 384, 386, 396–399
  for endovascular intervention, 51
  of endovascular suite, 56–57
  See Elderly patients
Patient-controlled analgesia, 78
PBV. *See* Percutaneous balloon valvuloplasty
Pediadtric patients
  anesthesia management and, 75

catheter selection in, 594
and inferior vena caval filters, 407–408
open saphenous vein access in, 602–603
Pelvic tumors, 611, 614
Pentobarbital, use of with children, 75
Perclose devices, 578–580, 582
  compared with conventional methods, 581–582
  complications with, 584–585
  features of, 582–585
Percutaneous access site, management of, 577–589
Percutaneous applications of angioscopy, 192–193
Percutaneous arterial puncture, 247–249
  of axillary artery, 264
  of brachial artery, 264
  of femoral artery, 247–248
  training and credentialing and, 35
Percutaneous balloon valvuloplasty (PBV), role of anesthesiologist in, 76
Percutaneous puncture site, management of, 578. *See also* Access site
Percutaneous transluminal angioplasty (PTA), 208–209, 269–287. *See also* Balloon angioplasty
  advantages of endarterectomy over, 310–311, 312
  aortoiliac, 93
  complications of, 282–284
  of femoral arteries, 279–280
  femoropopliteal, 93, 341
  guidewires for, 270–272
  history of, 269
  of iliac artery, 93, 278–279, 333–334
  indications for, 269–270
  of infrapopliteal vessels, 280
  lesions best suited for, 270
  of popliteal arteries, 279–280
  of renal artery, 280–281, 341
  restenosis after, 208, 210
  stents and, 321–351
  success of, 93
  synchronous, 488
  technique of, 275–278

versus endarterectomy, 310–311, 312
versus primary stenting, 336
Percutaneous transluminal angioplasty (PTA), 413–422
Percutaneous transluminal coronary angioplasty (PTCA)
  restenosis and, 208, 210
  role of anesthesiologist in, 75–76
Percutaneous vascular access, 259–267
  compared with surgical incisions, 266
  complications of, 264
Perforating veins, 525–527
Perforator vein interruptions, 525–527
Perfusion
  arterial, 604–611
  isolated, 612
  high-dose, 471–474, 475
  isolation, 593, 606
  regional, 593
Peripheral embolization, 485
Peripheral excimer laser angioplasty, 353–359
  follow-up, 357–358
  in-hospital complications, 357
  studies of, 355–358
  success with, 356–357
Peripheral insertion of central venous catheter (PICCl), 603–604
Peripheral laser angioplasty, 353–360
  photomechanical, 354
  photothermal, 354
Peripheral reconstruction, associated with thromboembolectomy, 301
Peripheral vascular disease
  computed tomography and, 143
  magnetic resonance imaging and, 157
  ultrasound and, 151
Personnel monitoring, radiation safety and, 122
Pharmacologic agents
  of endovascular analgesia and anesthesia, 59–68
  See also specific agent

Index

Phased array transducer, 196–197
Phenergan, 60
Phenobenzamine 73
Phenylalanine-proiine-arginine-methyl ketone, 658
Phlebography, 516
Physical properties of specific metals, 231–233
Physiologic responses to surgery and anesthesia, 69–70
PICC. See Peripheral insertion of central venous catheter
Piezoelectric pulse monitoring, intraoperative, 99–100
Piezoelectric pulse sensor, 99–100
Pigtail catheter, 251, 253
  in balloon angioplasty, 272, 273
Pipecuronium, 65, 74
Pitting corrosion, 228
Plaque
  appearance of, on intravascular ultrasound, 204
  in atherosclerosis, 11–17, 21–23
  effect of balloon angioplasty on, 269
  regression of, and aneurysm formation, 25
Platelet-derived growth factor, 541
Platinum, corrosion resistance and, 228
Plethysmography, 516
Polyester, for endovascular grafts, 236
Polyethylene
  balloons made of, 224
  as catheter material, 250–251
  terephthalate balloons, 274
Polytetrafluoroethylene grafts, 236–240
Polyurethane
  balloons made of, 224
  as catheter material, 250
Polyvinyl chloride, balloons made of, 223–224
Popliteal approach, 580–581
Popliteal artery(ies)
  aneurysms of, 474–478
  angioplasty of, 136–137, 279–280
  balloon sizes for, 276
  incidence of arterial occlusion and, 290

occlusion of, 300
  retrograde puncture of, 264
Popliteal puncture, balloon centering technique and, 258
Porosity, of vascular prosthesis, 238
Positive thrombolytic outcome, 458–462
Postintervention surveillance, 103–118
Postoperative follow-up, 103–118
Postphlebitic state, 516
Prazosin, 67, 68
Preformed angiographic catheters, 251
Pregnancy, radiation safety and, 122–123
Premedicants, 60, 78
  use of with children, 74–75
Preoperative preparation, 71
Preoperative sedation, 71–72
Priscoline, 249, 275, 276
Procaine, 65
Promethazine, 60
Propofol, 63, 72, 73, 74
  use of with children, 75
Propranolol, 66–67
Prostacyclin, 546
Prostate cancer, 611
Prosthesis, aortic, 289–290
Prosthetic materials, for endovascular grafts, 236–240
Pseudoaneurysm, 585
  in abdominal aorta, 482–484
  arterial catheterization and, 248
  as complication of balloon angioplasty, 283
  as complications of percutaneous vascular access, 266
  in internal carotid artery, 484
  at junction of supraintimal and infraintimal grafts, 484–485
  traumatic, 371–375
  treatment of, 585
PTA. See Percutaneous transluminal angioplasty
PTCA. See Percutaneous transluminal coronary angioplasty

PUCK 140–141
"Pullback," 183
Pull-back and entrapment, 305
Pull-back pressures, 98
Pulse Chek monitoring system, 99
Pulse monitoring
  device for, 106
  Piezoelectric, 99–100
Pulse volume recording (PVR), 44
  intraoperative, 99
Pulsed lasers, 354
Pushability, as catheter characteristic, 225
PVR. See Pulse volume recording

Quality assessment, of endovascular practice, 57
Quinidine therapy, 68

Rad, 121
Radial compliance, of human artery and endoascular grafts, 236
Radiation dose, absorbed, llS
Radiation exposure, 121–122
Radiation protection, 121–122
Radiation safety, 119–122
Radiation therapy. See Endoluminal radiation therapy
Radioactive liquids, 555
Radioactive stents, 555
Radiography, spot film, 144, 146
Radiologic properties of endovascular devices, 233
Radionuclide scanning, 6
Ranitidine, 60, 71
Reconstruction, thrombectomy and, 301
Recovery mechanism, of endovascular suite, 57
Recurrent stenoses. See Restenosis
Regional anesthesia, 72, 76–78
Regional chemotherapy, arterial infusion of, 592–593
Rem, 121
Remifentanil, 62
Renal artery(ies)
  balloon sizes for, 276

Renal artery(ies) (cont.)
  computed tomography and, 152
  evaluation of by ultrasound, 152
  introperative Duplex scans of, 45–46
  intravascular stents and, 341
  magnetic resonance imaging and, 48–51
  occlusion of, 300
  plaque localization and, 21
  percutaneous transluminal angioplasty of, 280–281, 341
  stenosis and, 155
  stents and, 341–344
  Strecker stent in, 343–344
  ultrasound and, 152
Renal insufficiency, 284
Renal toxicity, contrast-induced, 148
Reserpine, 68
Restenosis
  after angioplasty, 310–311, 312
  atherectomy and, 310
  biologic control of, 548
  endarterectomy and, 313–314
  local drug delivery and, 565–576
  after percutaneous transluminal angioplasty, 208, 210
  after use of Strecker stent, 341
  after peripheral excimer laser angioplasty, 356
  prevention of, 539–549
  risk of after percutaneous transluminal angioplasty, 208, 210
  stents and, 321–322
Reticular varicosities, 516
Retrograde femoral artery puncture, 264
Retrograde popliteal artery puncture, 264
Retroperitoneal hematoma, 247
Retroperitoneal hemorrhage, 283
Revascularization procedures, arterial, 93, 301, 375–380
Revascularization syndrome, 301
Reversed vein, assessment of, 184

Rhabdomyolysis, 302
Rheumatic heart disease, 289
Ring-down artifact, 196
Rochester trial, 462–464
Rocuronium, 65, 74
Roentgen, 119
Roentgen, Wilhelm, 3, 119–120
Rotating mirror devices, in intravascular ultrasound, 196
Rotating transducers, in intravascular ultrasound, 196–197

Safety monitoring, in anesthesiology service, 80–81
Saline irrigation, principles of, 179–181
Saphenofemoral junction ligation, 517, 518
Saphenous vein
  angioscopy of, 520
  in situ preparation of, 184–187
  ligation of, 517, 518
  sclerotherapy, 517, 519–520, 520
Scalenus medius, 532
Scope of service, of endovascular suite, 55–56
Scopolamine, 60
Sedation, preoperative, 71–72
Segmental pressures, to assess ischemia, 43–44
Seldinger, Sven Ivar, 5
Seldinger technique, 5, 260–261
  training and, 35
Semiclosed endarterectomy, 310, 313
Semiclosed technique, of valvulotomy, 185–187
Sequential surgical and endovascular approaches for occlusive arterial disease, 489, 491, 493
Shaded surface display, 155
Shear forces, 545
Shear stress
  oscillating pattern of, 19–20
  wall, 17–18
Sheaths, introducer, 259, 270, 271
Silastic central venous catheter, 592
Simmons catheter, 251, 253
Simpson, John B., 7–8, 309–310

Simpson atherotrac device, 305, 306
Simpson AtheroCath, 304, 309–310, 311
Single-wall arterial puncture, 261, 264
Smart needle, 586, 587
Smooth muscle cells, 539–541
Society for Vascular Surgery, 104
Society of Vascular Surgery/International Society for CardiovascularSurgery, 34
Sodium citrate, 60, 71
Sodium nitroprusside, 66
Sodium thiopental, 71
Sones, F. Mason, 5
SONOS, 137
Specific gravity, of metals used in endovascular implants, 231
Spectral analysis, stenoses and, 44–45
Spectral broadening, 150
Spectral window, loss of, 150
Spinal hernatoma, risk of, 77
Spiral computed tomography
  abdominal aorta, evaluation of scans of, 162
  and angiography, 48–49, 109, 111, 114
  and endovascular stent-grafts, 161–175
    interpretation of, 171–175
    technique for, 162–171
  scanners, current state of, 161
  See also Computed tomography
Spontaneous emission, 123–124
Spot film radiography, 144, 146
Staff requirements, of endovascular suite, 57
Stainless steel
  corrosion resistance and, 228
  mechanical and physical properties of, 231
  thromboresistance and, 229
Statistical process control, 85
Stealth single-lumen dilation catheter, 227
Steerable guidewires, 250
Stenoses
  arterial enlargement to prevent, 13–14

Index

of bypass graft, 282
computed tomography angiography and, 155
recurrent. *See* Recurrent stenosis; Restenosis
ultrasound and, 151
Stent(s), 344–346
coated, transluminal insertion of, 488–489
covered, 371–372
deployment of, 324–331
design characteristics of, 233–235
designs of, 322–324
expansion ratio of, 235
in femoral artery, 339
first, 363–364
history of, 8–9
in iliac artery, 333–334, 338–339
indications for use of, 201–210, 321–322
intracoronary placement of, 75
intravascular, 321–351
intravascular ultrasound and, 209–210
metallic, 227–230
percutaneous transluminal angioplasty and, 321–351
in renal artery, 342–344
self-expanding, 322
Tantalum-Dacron coknit, 365
thickness of, 234
in thoracic aortic aneurysm, 384, 385
results of, 387–388
types of, 233–235
in veins, 524–525
Viktor, 234
visceral artery, 344
See also specific stent
Stent-graft revascularization, 375–380
Stent-grafts
endoluminal, 371–372
endothelization of, 543–544
healing in, 541–542
history of, 8–9
insertion of, 377–380
Parodi, 371–373
See also Spiral computed tomography
Stenting
arterial injury and, 544–545
intraluminal, 93

primary, versus percutaneous transluminal angioplasty, 336–337
venous, 524–525
Steroids, 547
STILE study, 464–465
Stimulated emission, 123–124
Straight catheter, 251
Strecker stent, 139, 323–324
characteristics of, 234, 235
corrosion resistance of, 228
in femoral artery, 341
in iliac artery, 341
in renal artery, 343–344
Streptokinase, 455–456, 472, 475–476
Stroke
after balloon angioplasty, 284
hypertension and, 20–21
Subclavian artery(ies)
anatomy of, at point of entry, 264, 265
balloon angioplasty of, 281
occlusions of, 300
percutaneous puncture of, 264
thinning of media and, 230
Subclavian artery(ies), and PTA, 413–422
angioplasty, management of, 417
bypass, comparison with, 420–421
contraindications, 413–415, 416
indications, 413–415
methodology, 415–417, 418–419
results, 420
Subclavian vein
percutaneous catheterization via, 596–598
thrombosis of, 406, 493
Subfascial endoscopy, 525–527
Subintimal dissection, 283–284, 452
Sublimaze, 61
Succinylcholine, 65, 68
Sufentanil, 61, 73, 74
Suite design, endovascular intervention and, 133–142
Sulotroban, 546
Superficial femoral artery
atherosclerosis and, 22–23
balloon sizes for, 276
intravascular ultrasound and, 200, 203

transluminal endarterectomy of, 309–314
Suprarenal flow volume, 22
Surgery versus Thrombolysis for Ischemia of the Lower Extremity study. *See* STILE study
Surgery
for central venous catheter insertion, 599–601
endovenous, 515–529
physiologic responses to, 69–70
venous, 515–529
Surgical and endovascular approaches, combined, 481–495
Surgical incisions, 266
Surgical tables, 137–138
Sutureless anastomosis, 362–363
Synchronous surgical and endovascular approaches for occlusive arterial disease, 488
Synthetic vascular grafts, intimal hyperplasia in, 542–544
Systemic complications, of balloon angioplasty, 284
Systole, shear stress and, 19–20, 22

Tables, surgical, 137–138
Tantalum
corrosion resistance and, 228
mechanical and physical properties of, 231–232
thromboresistance of, 229
toxicity of, 229
Tantalum-Dacron coknit stent, 365
TEC. *See* Transluminal extraction catheter
Teflon, as catheter material, 250–251
TEGwire balloon dilation catheters, 274, 275
Telangiectasias, 516
Tennis Racquet catheter, in balloon angioplasty, 272, 273
TENS. *See* Transcutaneous electrical nerve stimulation
Tensile strength, of metal used in endovascular implants, 231

Tensile yield strength, 238
Terazosin, 68
Tetracaine, 65
Theratek Recanalization Arterial Catheter, 309–310, 312
Thiopental, 62–63, 73
Thoracic aorta, descending, 383–389
  repair, combined with open abdomenal aortic aneurysm repair, 482
Thoracic aortic aneurysms, endovascular repair of, 383–390
  device selection, 386
  imaging studies, 386
  operative approaches, 386–387
  patient selection, 384, 386
    preoperative assessment, 384, 386
  stent-graft repair, 384, 385
  results of, 387–388
  surgical repair, 384
Thoracic outlet syndrome, 531–539. See also Endoscopic transaxillary first rib resection
Thoracodorsal sympathectomy for causalgia, 538
Threatened extremity, 42
Three-dimensional computed tomography, 154–155
Three-dimensional intravascular ultrasound, 200–201, 205–207
Thrombin, smooth muscle cell growth and, 541
Thrombectomy, emerging technologies, 303–307
  aspiration, 304–305
  Expandable Access Sheath, 303–304
  Gelbfish Endo-Vac System, 306, 307
  Gunter Thrombectomy Catheter, 305
  noncirculation devices, 305, 306
    Cragg Thrombolytic Brush, 305, 306
    Simpson Atherotrac device, 305, 306
  percutaneous mechanical systems, 305–306

pull-back and entrapment, 305
recirculation techniques, 305
Simpson AthroCath, 304
Thromboembolectomy
  angioscopy and, 192–193
  balloon catheter, 457
  cardiacprocedures associated with, 302, 303
  catheter, 289–308
  evaluation of, 301
  peripheral reconstruction associated with, 301
  versus thrombolysis, 457–462
  venous, 192, 519–520
  visually assisted, 307
  See also Embolectomy
Thromboembolus, 289
Thrombolysis
  arterial applications of, 457–478
  equipment for, l 36
  and lower extremities, 405–406
  peripheral arterial applications of, 455–480
Thrombolytic agents, 455–457
  administered systemically, 565–566
  isolated limb perfusion and, 488–489
Thrombolytic therapy
  arterial bypass grafts and, 467–471
  direct intraarterial, 458
  for subclavian vein thrombosis, 493
Thromboresistance, of endovascular devices, 119
Thrombosis
  iliofemoral, 493
  See also Venous thrombosis
Thrombotic occlusion, 42, 292
Thrombotic venous disease, surgical and endovascular approaches to, 493
Thrombus, 249, 293, 295. See also Emboli; Thromboembolus
Thru-lumen embolectomy catheter, 293, 294
Tibial artery, fluoroscope and, 135
Ticlopidine, 545–546
Tissue ablation, optimal wavelength for, 354
Tissue plasminogen activator, 456–457

Tissue response to stent deployment, 229–230
Titanium
  corrosion resistance and, 228
  mechanical and physical properties of, 231, 232
  toxicity of, 229
Tolazoline, 249
TOPAS trial, 465–467
Total quality management (TQM), anesthesia and, 83–85
Toxicity, of endovascular devices, 228–229
t-PA. See Tissue plasminogen activator
TQM. See Total quality management
TRAC-WRIGHT. See Theratek Recanalization Arterial Catheter
Trackability, 225
Training, in endovascular surgery, 33–39
Tranquilizers, 60
Transaxillary surgical decompression, 531
Transcranial Doppler ultrasonography, 98–99
Transcutaneous carbon diocide tension monitoring, intraoperative, 99
Transcutaneous electrical nerve stimulation (TENS), 78
Transcutaneous oximetry, to evaluate limb ischemia 11
Transcutaneous oxygen monitoring, 99
Transcutaneous partial pressure of oxygen, 457
Transesophageal echocardiography, 154
Transesophageal ultrasound, 151
Transforming growth factor, 541
Transluminal balloon angioplasty. See Balloon angioplasty
Translulninal endarterectomy, 309–314
Transluminal Extraction Catheter (TEC), 8, 309–310, 311
Transport balloon, 569–570
Transport Catheter, 567, 570
Trapidil, 547

Traumatic aortic rupture, 155
Traumatic arteriovenous fistulas, 371–375
Traumatic pseudoaneurysms, 371–375
Triazolopyrimidine, 547
Tumor(s)
  of head, neck, and brain, 610–611
  of liver, 612, 613–614
  malignant, of extremities, 609–610, 612
  of pelvis, 613
  Wilms', 604
Tuohy-Borst adapter, 275, 276
Turbulence
  depiction of on ultrasound image, 150
  plaque pathogenesis and, 20
Two-dimensional imaging systems, 137
Two-dimensional intravascular ultrasoud, 200–202

Ultrafast computed tomography, 48
Ultrasound
  of abdominal aorta, 151
  aortic aneurysm and, 151
  aortic dissection and, 151
  of celiac axis, 152
  deep venous thrombosis and, 152
  dialysis fistulas and, 152
  Doppler, 292
  graft surveillance and, 143
  ischemia and, 44–46
  of mesenteric artery by, 152
  peripheral vascular disease and, 151
  of renal arteries by, 152
  as screening modality, 149–152
  stenosis and, 151
  transesophageal, 151
  turbulence depicted on, 150
  vascular, 150–152
  See also Duplex ultrasound
Ultraviolet pulsed lasers, 125, 354
Urokinase, 456
  acute limb ischemia and, 459
  Dispatch Catheter and, 572–573
  intraarterial use of, 472–473
  vein thrombosis and, 493

Valvular prostheses, arterial emboli and, 289–290
Valvuloplasty, 192
Valvulotomy, 185–187
Vanadium, 229
Vapiprost, 546
Varicose veins, 516
Vascular access
  devices and techniques for, 259–267
  history of, 5
  intravascular ultrasound and, 196–199
  percutaneous procedure for, 259–266
  surgery, 189–191
Vascular disease, pathophysiology of, 11–29
Vascular ultrasound, 150–152. *See also* Ultrasound
Vasodilators, 275, 276
Vecuronium, 65, 74
Vein(s)
  cephalic
    open access to, 602
    percutaneous catheterization via, 595
  contrast phlebography of, 516
  duplex examination of, 516
  external jugular
    open access to, 601–602
    percutaneous catheterization via, 595
  femoral, percutaneous catheterization via, 598–599, 600
  Gianturco Zeta stent in, 524
  internal jugular
    open access to, 600–601
    percutaneous catheterization via, 595, 598
  perforating, 525–527
  preparation of, for bypass grafting, 187
  subclavian
    thrombosis of, 493
    percutaneous catheterization via, 595, 596–598
  varicose, 516
  Wallstent used in, 524, 525
  See also Saphenous vein
Vein conduit preparation, angioscopy and, 184–187
Velocity waveform, 45

Velour Dacron grafts, 238–239
Venotomy, venous valve repair without, 192
Venous bypass
  postintervention surveillance of, 103–118
  versus endarterectomy, 314
Venous dysfunction
  compartment pressures and, 526–527
  diagnosis of, 515–516
Venous insufficiency, 516
Venous pressure recovery time, 516
Venous reflux, 516, 517, 520
Venous stenting, 523–525
Venous stripping, 517, 518
Venous surgery, 515–529
Venous thrombectomy, 519–520
  angioscopy and, 192
Venous thrombosis, 493
  and acute arterial occlusion, 301
  deep, 45, 493
  duplex ultrasonography and, 45–46
  magnetic resonance imaging and, 157
  vascular ultrasound and, 152
Venous valve repair, 192
Venous valves, types of, 519
Verapamil, 67
Vertebral artery, balloon angioplasty of, 281–282
viable extremity, 42
Video fluoroscopy, 146
Viktor stent, 234
Vincristine, 547
Visceral arteries, incidence of arterial occlusion and, 290–291
Visceral artery stents, 344
Vistaril, 60
Visualization systems, 143–159
Visually assisted thromboembolectomy, 307
Volatile anesthetic agents, 63–64
  drug interactions and, 68
Volume and flow measurements, intraoperative, 99

Wall shear stress, plaque pathogenesis and, 17–18

Wallstent, 141, 231, 323, 323
  characteristics of, 234, 234–235
  compared with balloon
    angioplasty, 340
  corrosion resistance of, 228
  deployment of, 327–331, 333
  in femoral artery, 340
  in iliac artery, 336–338
  in renal artery, 343
  in veins, 524, 525
Warfarin, 77
Wilms' tumor, 604
Wiring, in treatment of
    abdominal aortic
    aneurysms, 362
Wolinsky perforated balloon
    catheter, 567–570
Wound infection, open surgical
    incisions and, 266
Wren, Sir Christopher, 591
Wylie, Jack, 310

X-rays, history of, 119–120

Yield strength, of metal used in
    endovascular implants, 231

ISBN 0-387-98444-5